Brain Function Augmentation: Brain-Machine Interfaces

Brain Function Augmentation: Brain-Machine Interfaces

Edited by Max White

STATES
ACADEMIC PRESS
www.statesacademicpress.com

States Academic Press,
109 South 5th Street,
Brooklyn, NY 11249, USA

Visit us on the World Wide Web at:
www.statesacademicpress.com

ISBN: 978-1-63989-087-3

Cataloging-in-Publication Data

Brain function augmentation : brain-machine interfaces / edited by Max White.
p. cm.
Includes bibliographical references and index.
ISBN 978-1-63989-087-3
1. Brain-computer interfaces. 2. Cognitive neuroscience. 3. Human-computer interaction.
4. Brain--Physiology. 5. Brain--Localization of functions. 6. Neurophysiology. I. White, Max.
QP360.7 .B73 2022
612.802 85--dc23

Table of Contents

Preface

Every book is a source of knowledge and this one is no exception. The idea that led to the conceptualization of this book was the fact that the world is advancing rapidly; which makes it crucial to document the progress in every field. I am aware that a lot of data is already available, yet, there is a lot more to learn. Hence, I accepted the responsibility of editing this book and contributing my knowledge to the community.

Brain augmentation refers to the different approaches which are aimed at improving the performance of the brain. These can be aimed at people who suffer from neurological problems as well as healthy people. The three major areas which can be augmented are classified as cognitive, motor and sensory domains. The performance of the brain can also be supplemented through brain-machine interfaces (BMI). These refer to the pathways that join neuronal circuits to external assistive devices. A few of such devices are communication aids, exoskeletons and prosthesis of the limbs. Brain-machine interfaces are also useful for establishing communication in both directions, wherein artificial signals are sent to the brain while information from neural recordings is being decoded. The topics included in this book on brain augmentation are of utmost significance and bound to provide incredible insights to readers. It presents researches and studies performed by experts across the globe. Those with an interest in brain-machine interfaces would find this book helpful.

While editing this book, I had multiple visions for it. Then I finally narrowed down to make every chapter a sole standing text explaining a particular topic, so that they can be used independently. However, the umbrella subject sinews them into a common theme. This makes the book a unique platform of knowledge.

I would like to give the major credit of this book to the experts from every corner of the world, who took the time to share their expertise with us. Also, I owe the completion of this book to the never-ending support of my family, who supported me throughout the project.

Editor

1

Functional Electrical Stimulation Alters the Postural Component of Locomotor Activity in Healthy Humans

Vera Talis[1]*, *Yves Ballay*[2], *Alexander Grishin*[1] *and Thierry Pozzo*[2,3,4]

[1] *Institute for Information Transmission Problems, Moscow, Russia,* [2] *Institut National de la Santé et de la Recherche Médicale, U1093, Cognition Action Plasticité Sensorimotrice, Dijon, France,* [3] *Department of Robotics, Brain and Cognitive Sciences, Istituto Italiano di Tecnologia, Genova, Italy,* [4] *Université de Bourgogne, UFR STAPS (Sciences du Sport), Dijon, France*

Edited by:
Mikhail Lebedev,
Duke University, USA

Reviewed by:
Hari S. Sharma,
Uppsala University, Sweden
Victor Manuel Pulgar,
Wake Forest School of Medicine, USA

****Correspondence:***
Vera Talis
talis@iitp.ru

Knowledge of the effects of Functional Electrical Stimulation (FES) of different intensity on postural stability during walking in healthy subjects is necessary before these relationships in patients with postural disorders can be assessed and understood. We examined healthy subjects in Control group walking on a treadmill for 40 min and in FES group—provided with 30 min of stimulation, which intensity increased every 10 min. The main difference between Control and FES group was the progressive increase of trunk oscillations in sagittal, frontal, and horizontal planes and an increase of relative stance duration in parallel with FES intensity increase. Both Control and FES groups exhibited shank elevation angle increase as an after-effect. It is concluded, that high intensity FES significantly changes the postural component of locomotor activity, but the fatigue signs afterwards were not FES specific.

Keywords: FES, postural stability, locomotion, healthy subjects

INTRODUCTION

Human walking is characterized by the repetitive motion of limb segments aimed to propel the body forward. Joint movement is highly synchronized and muscle activity displays a typical periodical pattern (Bernstein, 1990; Perry, 1992). These rhythmic locomotor movements are produced by a brainstem-spinal central pattern generator (CPG) that is activated by descending command signals (Grillner, 1981; Grasso et al., 1998; Selionov et al., 2009). Any unpredicted disturbance during walking, such as stumbling (Eng et al., 1994; Schilling et al., 2000), could be compensated through sensory feedback. In the experimental environment, the kinematics of walking have been shown to be well preserved even under the conditions of body weight unloading (Ivanenko et al., 2002), additional loading of the legs (Smith and Martin, 2007), and during "split-belt" locomotion (Jensen et al., 1998). As an example, Ivanenko et al. (2002) has shown that dynamical change, such as an artificial decrease of foot pressure, resulted in weak changes in the coordination of segments.

A specific type of gait disturbance is the direct stimulation of muscles at the time of muscle action during the step cycle. Such a periodical stimulation could be implemented by means of electrical or vibratory intervention. Ivanenko et al. (2000) analyzed the effects of phasic leg muscle vibration on human locomotion, and have shown that the vibration of hamstring muscles produced an increase of walking speed, while the vibration of other leg muscles did not. Based on the well-known fact of position and movement illusions caused by muscle vibration in an upright standing position (Lackner and Levine, 1979; Talis and Solopova, 2000), Ivanenko and colleagues explained that hamstring vibration induced a rise in speed through the modification of kinesthetic information about joint angels consistent with the lengthening of the hamstring muscle.

In this paper, we studied the effects of electrical phasic stimulation of leg muscles (Functional Electrical Stimulation, FES) during walking. In contrast to vibratory stimulation, electrical stimulation, directly affecting the relation between motor command and force output, ensures an almost immediate muscle contraction. This increases the precision of the application of the stimulus and thus allows the stimulation of several muscles in an alternative manner through each gait cycle. The force of the muscle response to the electrical stimulation can be increased to up to 70% of maximum voluntary contraction MVC (DeVahl, 1992) [vibration elicited not more than 30% of MVC of the stimulated muscle (Matthews, 1966)]. Walking speed increase with regular use of FES in spinal cord injury (Ladouceur and Barbeau, 2000; Pomeroy et al., 2006) and stroke patients (Lindquist et al., 2007) was reported. In was shown, that this gait speed advantage lasted from weeks to a month in stroke (Bogataj et al., 1995; Alon and Ring, 2003; Daly et al., 2011) and spinal cord injury patients (Ladouceur and Barbeau, 2000; for reviews see Barbeau et al., 2002). At the same time, the origin of the retention of an increased walking speed without continued FES, meaning the long lasting effect of FES-training, called the therapeutic effect of FES-assisted walking, is unclear and even discounted (see for instance the discussion about implantable electrode technology, as a possible future of electrical stimulation in Burridge and Hughes, 2010). For instance, post-stroke gait speed increase due to FES might be because walking rate reduction was the primary reason for FES use (Taylor et al., 1999).

The rationale of the present study was to study the kinematics of healthy subjects during treadmill locomotion and compare the results of two groups, one of which was simultaneously provided with FES (FES group), and the other was not (Control group). A short account of some of the present findings was published as an abstract (Talis et al., 2011). The collected data of FES-assisted walking in healthy subjects could be implemented in the pathology of FES-assisted walking.

MATERIALS AND METHODS

Subjects

Eight healthy subjects participated in the FES group [seven males and one female, between 25 and 49 year of age, 74 ± 11 (SD) kg, 1.76 ± 0.1 m] and eight subjects in the Control group (six males and two females, between 20 and 49 year of age, 73 ± 11 kg, 1.74 ± 0.09 m, five of them from the FES group). None of the subjects had any history of neurological disease or vestibular impairment. The experiments conformed to the Declaration of Helsinki and written informed consent was obtained from all the participants according to the protocol of the Ethics Committee of the Universite de Bourgogne.

Experimental Setup and Stimulation Techniques

The subjects walked on a treadmill at individually adjusted speed of about 0.7 m/s with their shoes on. Subjects from the FES group have eight bipolar stimulation surface electrodes (5 × 5 and 5 × 10 cm) placed bilaterally on four muscles [Tibialis Anterior (TA), Gastrocnemius Medialis (GM), Quadriceps (Q), and Biceps Femoris (BF) of both legs] with the negative electrode over a motor point (DeVahl, 1992). Electrical stimulus consisted of repetitive trains of rectangular pulses with 65 mA amplitude at 65 Hz. A custom-made eight-channel stimulator delivered the desired stimulation train, triggered by the signal of the right knee goniometer in such a way, that the timing of the stimulation sequence corresponded to the timing of the activation sequence of these muscles during normal gait (Perry, 1992).

Data Recording

Body kinematics was recorded by means of the ELITE system (BTS, Italy). Nine 120-Hz TV cameras were spaced around a treadmill in a 4 × 4 × 2 m acquisition volume. Hemispherical reflective markers of 15-mm diameter attached to the skin overlying the following body landmarks for the two hemibodies: laterally on the fifth metatarsophalangeal joint (MTP), lateral malleolus (MAL), lateral tibial tables (KN), greater trochanters (GT), anterior-superior iliac spines (IS), and gleno-humeral-joints (GH).

Pain during FES-assisted walking was registered by means of a 10-cm analog pain scale, while a value close to 10 means higher pain. The pain scale was presented to the subject three times (Stim1, Stim2, and Stim3).

Experimental Protocol

Before data collection, the subject had 5–7 s to reach steady motion on the treadmill. Data collections (3 min each) were performed five times during treadmill walking: before FES (Before), three times during FES (Stim1, Stim2, and Stim3) and after FES (After). The same protocol of data collection was used in the Control group where participants walked for 40 min on the treadmill without FES.

In the FES group, the experimenter increased the intensity of stimulation every 10 min (muscle by muscle, in the range 0–250 μs of impulse duration under the verbal control of the subject—every time up to the tolerant level of pain intensity). Each increase was performed during the first minute of each 3-min interval of data collection.

Data Analysis

The spatial coordinates of each marker were recorded, the body being represented as an interconnected chain of rigid segments. Kinematics data were filtered with a low-pass zero-phase shift Butterworth filter with a 5 Hz cut-off frequency. Stride length, walking frequency and velocity were estimated using the body mid-point (average of left and right GT, IS coordinates). This resulting point provides a good estimation of the center of mass (Courtine and Schieppati, 2003).

The elevation angle of each segment in the sagittal plane corresponds to the angle between the projected segment and the vertical and were computed as:

$$\theta_{i\_sagittal} = \tan^{-1}[(X_{id} - X_{ip})/(Y_{id} - Y_{ip})],$$

where X and Y designate the coordinates of the proximal (p) and distal (d) markers for the *ith* frame of the acquisition. The elevation angle in the sagittal plane of the thigh (GT-KN), shank (KN-MAL) and foot (MAL-MTP) segments were calculated.

The elevation angle of the trunk in the sagittal, frontal, and horizontal planes corresponds to:

$$\theta_{trank\_sagittal} = \tan^{-1}\left\{\frac{\left(\frac{(X_{IS\_left}+X_{IS\_right})}{2} - \frac{(X_{GH\_left}+X_{GH\_right})}{2}\right)}{\left(\frac{(Y_{IS\_left}+Y_{IS\_right})}{2} - \frac{(Y_{GH\_left}+Y_{GH\_right})}{2}\right)}\right\}$$

and was calculated for each frame of the acquisition (Laroche et al., 2007). The trunk elevation angle in the frontal plane was computed with the same equation in the ZY plane and in the horizontal—in the XZ plane. Each trial was separated into gait cycles using the elevation angle of the lower limb axis (the line joining the MAL and GT), as described in Borghese et al. (1996). Stance phases were computed using the limb axis as described in Ivanenko et al. (2002) and was expressed in percentage of the gait cycle.

The coefficient of variation (CV) was calculated for each elevation angle to represent data variability and was calculated as the standard deviation divided by mean values across all steps of each subject during each 3 min of data collections (Bacarin et al., 2009).

Statistics

Mean and Descriptive statistics included means and the SE of the mean. Paired t-test and ANOVA were used when appropriate to compare means. In particular, to evaluate the effects of FES on the amplitude of trunk oscillations and spatio-temporal parameters, the two-way ANOVA with first factor "FES" (Before, Stim1, Stim2, Stim3 and After) and the second factor "group"(FES, Control) was used. When significant effects were found, *post-hoc* Tukey's testing was conducted to identify the loci of these effects. The level of statistical significance was set at 0.05.

RESULTS

General Gait Parameters

Figure 1 shows the mean values (over all trials and subjects) of relative stance duration, stride length, walking velocity and step frequency in the Control and FES groups. FES significantly affects stance time: in the FES group, the relative duration of a stance during Stim3 conditions was at average 65.29 ± 0.36% of the cycle; that is a larger value than that of any of the Control group. Note, that stride length was about the same in the FES and Control groups for these conditions (0.60 ± 0.02 m and 0.59 ± 0.03 m in the FES and Control groups, correspondingly). Statistical analyses revealed significant interaction between groups and conditions for relative duration of the stance [ANOVA, $F_{(4, 28)} = 6.21, p = 0.001$]. *Post-hoc* tests showed that the relative duration of the stance in the FES group was significantly larger in the Stim3 than in the Before condition. **Figure 1** also shows that control subjects exhibited the tendency of the well-known monotonic relationship of stride length and step frequency with speed increase (see Bernstein, 1935; Grillner, 1981; Winter and Scott, 1991).

Trunk Oscillations

Figure 2 shows mean individual (**Figure 2A**) and group mean data (**Figure 2B**) of trunk oscillations in sagittal (Pitch), frontal (Roll), and horizontal (Yaw) planes. Group mean data shows that before stimulation trunk oscillations were not different in Control and FES group (mean trunk oscillation in Before condition was in saggital plane 3.26 ± 0.14° and 3.45 ± 0.15°, in frontal plane 4.0 ± 0.55°, and 4.15 ± 0.55° and in horizontal plane 15.60 ± 0.57° and 13.78 ± 0.85° for FES and Control, respectively). Electrical stimulation of leg muscle significantly affects the amplitude of trunk oscillation: these amplitudes progressively increase in the FES group [ANOVA $F_{(4, 56)} = 12.28, p = 0.0002$; $F = 6.48, p = 0.0002$; $F = 5.98, p = 0.0004$ for Pitch, Roll and Yaw, correspondingly].

Limb Elevation Angels in Sagittal Plane

Figure 3 shows the profile of mean individual data (**Figure 3A**) and group mean data (**Figure 3B**) of limb elevation angels in sagittal plane. Due to stimulation, the profile of limb elevation angels didn't change, but the mean individual amplitude of foot angels decreased. Mean group data presented on **Figure 3B** also shows this tendency for distal joints, but these changes didn't approach the level of significance due to high variability of limb elevation angels due to FES. The CV of foot angle increased from 0.03 at Before up to 0.07 at Stim2 and 0.08 at Stim3 conditions (t-test, $p < 0.01$).

Perceptual Effects

All subjects in FES group reported the instability increase due to FES and the fatigue sensation afterwards. There were subjective reports during FES such as: "The locomotion is not free, my legs are out of my control, I feel my ankle joint blocked, "freezing," muscles are fatigued, I have sensation as walking in flippers." After the end of FES, several subjects sensed that the treadmill decelerated, and locomotion seemed "unusually light." Actually, some participants approached the forward part of the treadmill belt during FES. Subjective pain rating increased up to 8 cm in the Stim 3 condition (**Table 1**).

After-Effect

At the end of 40 min locomotion limb elevation angels appeared slightly increased in both groups in comparison with Before (**Figure 3B**). This increase approached the level of significance for shank angle in both groups (t-test, $p < 0.05$).

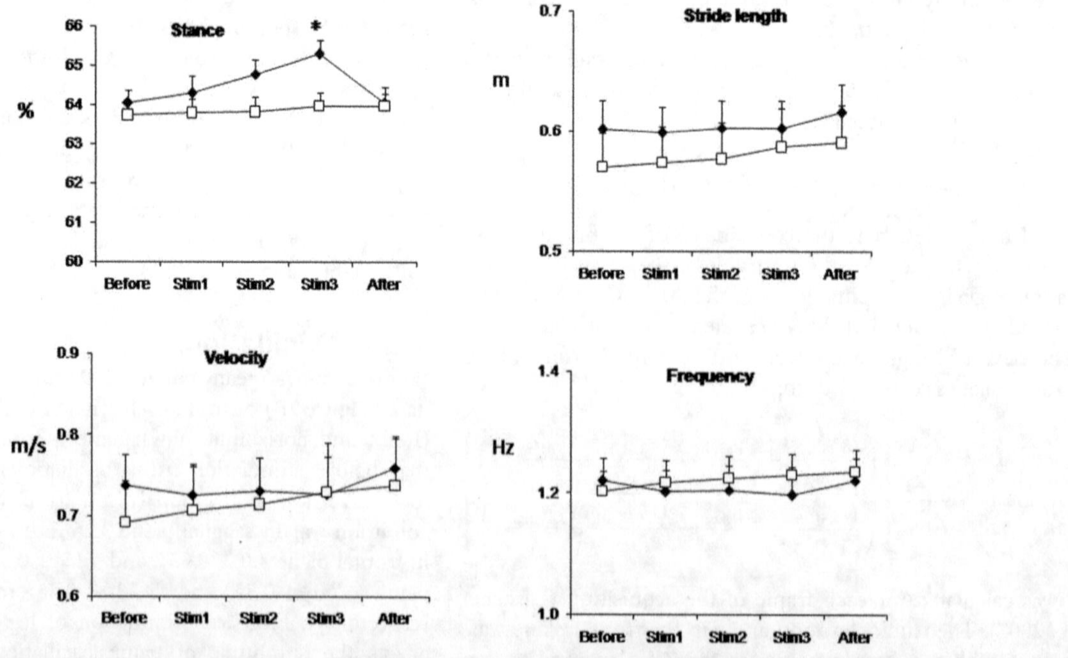

FIGURE 1 | Stance duration, stride length, velocity, and frequency of gait averaged across all trials and subjects in FES (black diamond) and Control (white square) groups. Values are mean ± SE. $^*p < 0.05$.

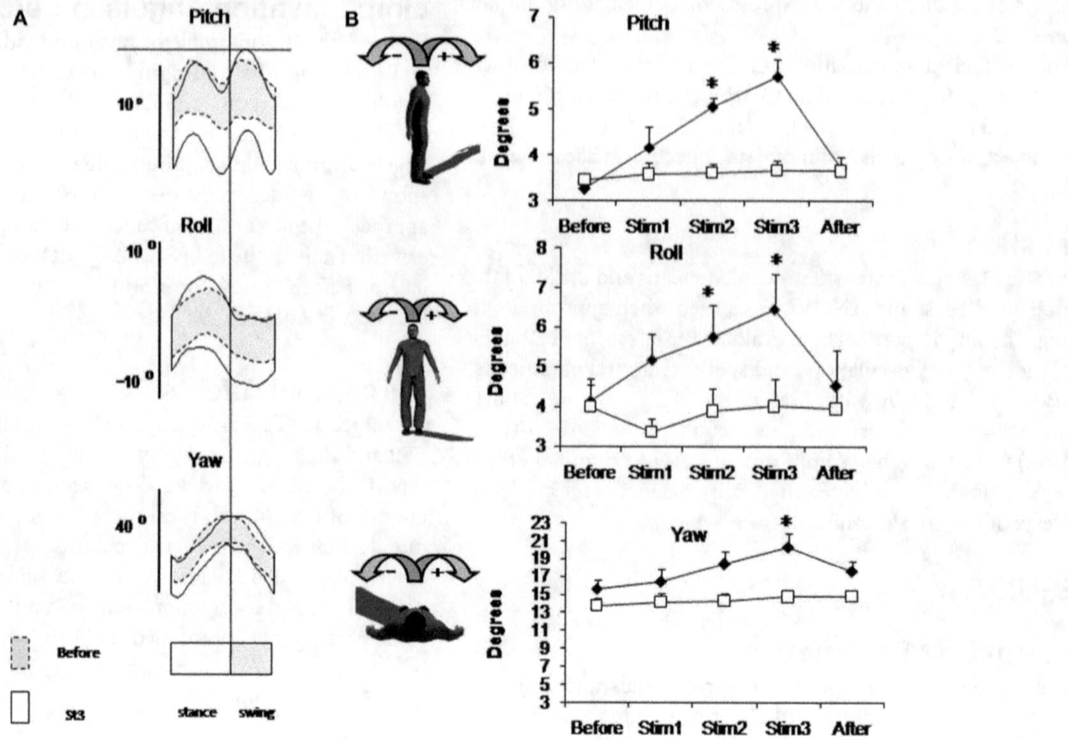

FIGURE 2 | Trunk oscillation evoked by FES. (A) Trunk motion (±SD value) in one representative subject from FES group averaged across 3-min intervals of Before (dashed lines) and Stim3 (solid lines) periods. **(B)** Peak-to-peak amplitudes of trunk oscillations averaged across FES (black diamond) and across Control (white square) groups (mean ± SE). Asterisks indicate statistical difference in Stim condition in comparison with Before condition in FES group, $^*p < 0.05$.

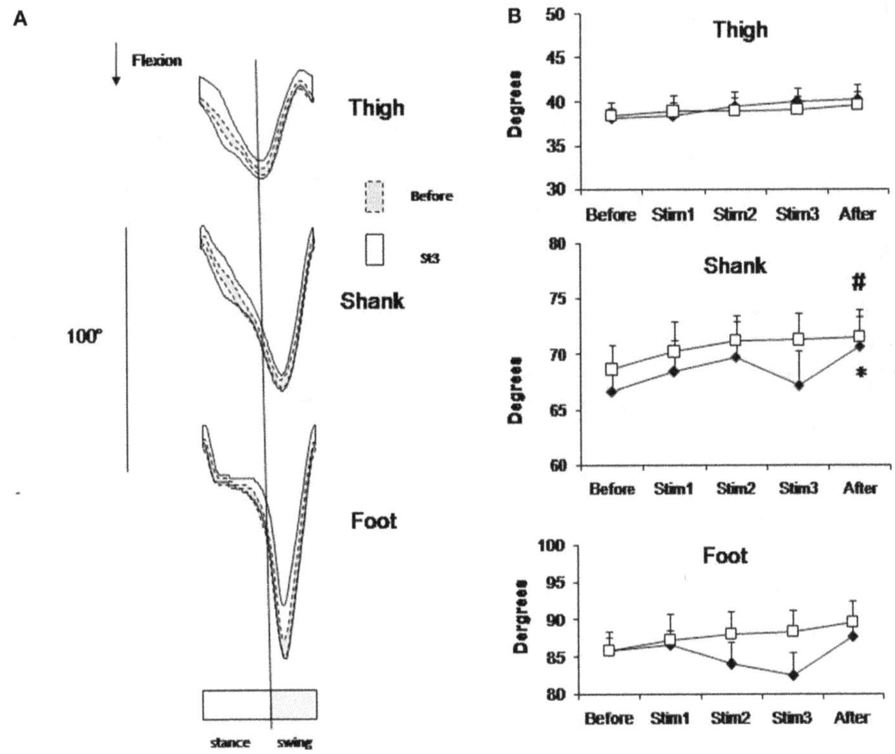

FIGURE 3 | Elevation angels in sagittal plane. (A) Segment elevation angels (±SD value) in one representative subject from FES group averaged across 3-min intervals of Before (dashed lines) Stim3 (solid lines) periods. **(B)** Peak-to-peak amplitudes of elevation angels averaged across FES (black diamond) and Control (white square) groups (mean ± SE) Asterisk (*) indicates statistical difference in the condition in comparison with Before condition in FES group; sharp (#) indicates statistical difference—in the condition in comparison with Before condition in Control group ($p < 0.05$).

TABLE 1 | Stimulation intensity (μs) of four muscles and the severity of pain for one typical subject in Stim1, Stim2 and Stim3 conditions.

Pain (cm)	Intensity of stimulation (duration of stimulation train, μs)			
	TA	GM	RF	B
5.5	60.6	82.9	92.4	92.4
7.5	143.4	162.6	162.6	130.9
8.5	226.3	239.1	258.2	334.7

DISCUSSION

In this paper, we analyzed the effects of FES on the kinematics of a healthy subjects' locomotion. The most remarkable changes caused by FES are the increase of body oscillation, accompanied by an increase in stance time duration.

Postural Instability

Although the mechanical reason of increased trunk pitch could be the excessive contraction of quadriceps muscle, the increased trunk oscillation both in sagittal, frontal and horizontal planes indicates the decrease of locomotion stability and movement disturbance caused by FES. The disruption of the normal gait by FES manifests itself as an increase in stance time, providing an increased support time—another index of instability (Bernstein, 1935; Kirtley, 2006). The fact that these parameters returned to the norm immediately after FES are in line with this explanation. Pain, especially due to strong stimulation of the tibialis muscle could also distort the sensory feedback from muscle and skin receptors and there by the descending control from the CNS.

Comparing FES-assisted and non-assisted walking of one incomplete spinal injuries patient Ladouceur and Barbeau (2000) have also found FES-induced decrease of ankle plantar flexion by 5.6°, which is similar to our data of FES-assisted walking (**Figure 3A**). The tendency of ankle and shank joints to flex less in the swing phase during intensive FES is similar to the effect of under-flexion of the knee during fatigued walking (Bernstein, 1935). However, these effects could be of a different origin: in our study the TA muscle being stimulated along the swing phase is more pain sensitive (**Table 1**). To avoid pain, the subject could aim to dorsiflex the TA muscle less than would be seen in a natural gait pattern so as to decrease the TA stimulation time and thus the amount of pain. This, in turn, resulted in excessive dorsiflexion of the ankle, which leads to a decrease of push of force.

Clinical Application

FES is a commonly used clinical tool to improve walking ability due to its simplicity, low-cost, and strong muscle response, however, muscle fatigue is a major limiting factor in FES applications (Kralj et al., 1988; Karu et al., 1995). FES is shown to have a more significant effect in comparison with physiotherapy in walking speed increase during and after FES-assisted locomotor training (see review by Taylor et al., 2013). This notion is supported by the study of Khaslavskaia et al. (2002), which has shown that the changes in healthy participants in the TA MEP during locomotion were seen over 20 min following the cessation of the stimulation of the common peroneal nerve. It is now widely accepted, that FES improves ankle dorsiflexion in the long-term perspective, increasing the corticospinal excitability and that FES-assisted training "facilitates motor relearning" in patients (Ladouceur and Barbeau, 2000; Alon and Ring, 2003; Lindquist et al., 2007; Barrett et al., 2009; Daly et al., 2011). In the present study, intensive phasic electrical stimulation was applied to both ankles and hip antagonist muscles, and similarly to leg orthosis in neurological subjects. Similarly to clinical settings, the timing of stimulation was on-line controlled trough the feedback from the current knee joint angle in each stride (this way, in clinical practice, the pathological walking is aimed to be adjusted to the typical normal walking, then the "re-education" of pathological walking is expected). Our results indicate that, in healthy subjects, the postural component of locomotor activity was changed due to strong electrical stimulation of leg muscles, while the rhythmic component remains intact. It could be speculated, that the artificial nature of muscle contractions during FES-assisted walking in healthy subjects transfers the locomotor activity from involuntary to a more voluntary controlled movement. It could be concluded, that the functional role of FES for patients is the "adaption training" rather than "re-education" of pathological walking into the typical "normal" walking.

ACKNOWLEDGMENTS

Granted by Conseil Reginal de Bourgogne, France. RFBR grant #14-04-00950.

REFERENCES

Alon, G., and Ring, H. (2003). Gait and hand function enhancement following training with a multi-segment hybrid-orthosis stimulation system in stroke patients. *J. Stroke Cerebrovasc. Dis.* 12, 209–216. doi: 10.1016/S1052-3057(03)00076-4

Bacarin, T. A., Sacco, I. C., and Hennig, E. M. (2009). Plantar pressure distribution patterns during gait in diabetic neuropathy patients with a history of foot ulcers. *Clinics (Sao Paulo)* 64, 113–120. doi: 10.1590/S1807-593220090002 00008

Barbeau, H., Ladouceur, M., Mirbagheri, M. M., and Kearney, R. E. (2002). The effect of locomotor training combined with functional electrical stimulation in chronic spinal cord injured subjects: walking and reflex studies. *Brain Res. Rev.* 40, 274–291. doi: 10.1016/S0165-0173(02)00210-2

Barrett, C. L., Mann, G. E., Taylor, P. N., and Strike, P. (2009). A randomized trial to investigate the effects of functional electrical stimulation and therapeutic exercise on walking performance for people with multiple sclerosis. *Mult. Scler.* 15, 493–504. doi: 10.1177/1352458508101320

Bernstein, N. A. (1935). *Biodynamic of Locomotion.* Moscow: VIEM.

Bernstein, N. A. (1990). *Movement Physiology and Activity. In the Series Classics of Science.* Moscow: Nauka.

Bogataj, U. L., Gros, N., Kljajic, M., Acimovic, R., and Malezic, M. (1995). The rehabilitation of gait in patients with hemiplegia: a comparison between conventional therapy and multichannel functional electrical stimulation therapy. *Phys. Ther.* 75, 490–502.

Borghese, N. A., Bianchi, L., and Lacquaniti, F. (1996). Kinematic determinants of human locomotion. *J. Physiol.* 494, 863–879. doi: 10.1113/jphysiol.1996.sp021539

Burridge, J. H., and Hughes, A. M. (2010). Potential for new technologies in clinical practice. *Curr. Opin. Neurol.* 23, 671–677. doi: 10.1097/WCO.0b013e3283402af5

Courtine, G., and Schieppati, M. (2003). Human walking along a curved path. I. Body trajectory, segment orientation and the effect of vision. *Eur. J. Neurosci.* 18, 177–190. doi: 10.1046/j.1460-9568.2003.02736.x

Daly, J. J., Zimbelman, J., Roenigk, K. L., McCabe, J. P., Rogers, J. M., Butler, K., et al. (2011). Recovery of coordinated gait: randomized controlled stroke trial of functional electrical stimulation (FES) versus no FES, with weight-supported treadmill and over-ground training. *Neurorehabil. Neural Repair* 25, 588–596. doi: 10.1177/1545968311400092

DeVahl, J. (1992). "Neuromuscular electrical stimulation (NMES) in rehabilitation," in *Electrotherapy in Rehabilitation*, ed M. R. Gersh (Philadelphia, PA: F.A. Davis Company), 227.

Eng, J. J., Winter, D. A., and Patla, A. E. (1994). Strategies for recovery from a trip in early and late swing during human walking. *Exp. Brain Res.* 102, 339–349. doi: 10.1007/BF00227520

Grasso, R., Bianchi, L., and Lacquaniti, F. (1998). Motor patterns for human gait: backward versus forward locomotion. *J. Neurophysiol.* 80, 1868–1885.

Grillner, S. (1981). "Control of locomotion in bipeds, tetra pods, and fish," in *Handbook of Physiology, Sec 1, The Nervous System II Motor Control*, ed V. B. Brooks (Bethesda: Waverly), 1179–1236.

Ivanenko, Y. P., Grasso, R., and Lacquaniti, F. (2000). Influence of leg muscle vibration on human walking. *J. Neurophysiol.* 84, 1737–1747.

Ivanenko, Y. P., Grasso, R., Macellari, V., and Lacquaniti, F. (2002). Control of foot trajectory in human locomotion: role of ground contact forces in simulated reduced gravity. *J. Neurophysiol.* 87, 3070–3089.

Jensen, L., Prokop, T., and Dietz, V. (1998). Adaptation effects during human split-belt walking: influence of afferent input. *Exp. Brain Res.* 118, 126–130. doi: 10.1007/s002210050262

Karu, Z. Z., Durfee, W. K., and Barzilai, A. M. (1995). Reducing muscle fatigue in FES applications by stimulating with N-let pulse trains. *IEEE Trans. Biomed. Eng.* 42, 809–817. doi: 10.1109/10.398642

Khaslavskaia, S., Ladouceur, M., and Sinkjaer, T. (2002). Increase in tibialis anterior motor cortex excitability following repetitive electrical stimulation on the common peroneal nerve. *Exp. Brain Res.* 145, 309–315. doi: 10.1007/s00221-002-1094-9

Kirtley, C. (2006). *Clinical Gait Analysis.* Churchill Livingstone: Elsevier.

Kralj, A., Bajd, T., and Turk, R. (1988). Enhancement of gait restoration in spinal injured patients by functional electrical stimulation. *Clin. Orthop. Relat. Res.* 233, 34–43.

Lackner, J. R., and Levine, M. S. (1979). Changes in apparent body orientation and sensory localization induced by vibration of postural muscles: vibratory myesthetic illusions. *Aviat. Space Environ. Med.* 50, 346–354.

Ladouceur, M., and Barbeau, H. (2000). Functional electrical stimulation-assisted walking for persons with incomplete spinal injuries: changes in the kinematics and physiological cost of overground walking. *Scand. J. Rehab. Med.* 32, 72–79. doi: 10.1080/003655000750045587

Laroche, D., Ornetti, P., Thomas, E., Ballay, Y., Maillefert, J. F., and Pozzo, T. (2007). Kinematic adaptation of locomotor pattern in rheumatoid arthritis patients with forefoot impairment. *Exp. Brain Res.* 176, 85–97. doi: 10.1007/s00221-006-0597-1

Lindquist, A. R., Prado, C. L., Barros, R. M., Mattioli, R., da Costa, P. H., and Salvini, T. F. (2007). Gait training combining partial body-weight support, a treadmill, and functional electrical stimulation: effects on poststroke gait. *Phys. Ther.* 87, 1144–1154. doi: 10.2522/ptj.20050384

Matthews, P. B. C. (1966). Reflex activation on the soleus muscle of the decerebrate cat by vibration. *Nature* 209, 204–205. doi: 10.1038/209204b0

Perry, J. (1992). *Gait Analysis: Normal and Pathological Function.* Thorofare, NJ: Slack.

Pomeroy, V. M., King, L., Pollock, A., Baily-Hallam, A., and Langhorne, P. (2006). Electrostimulation for promoting recovery of movement or functional ability after stroke. *Cochrane Database Syst. Rev.* 19:CD003241. doi: 10.1002/14651858.CD003241.pub2

Schillings, A. M., van Wezel, B. M., Mulder, T., and Duysens, J. (2000). Muscular responses and movement strategies during stumbling over obstacles. *J. Neurophysiol.* 83, 2093–2102.

Selionov, V. A., Ivanenko, Y. P., Solopova, I. A., and Gurfinkel, V. S. (2009). Tonic central and sensory stimuli facilitate involuntary air-stepping in humans. *J. Neurophysiol.* 101, 2847–2858. doi: 10.1152/jn.90895.2008

Smith, J. D., and Martin, P. E. (2007). Walking patterns change rapidly following asymmetrical lower extremity loading. *Hum. Mov. Sci.* 26, 412–425. doi: 10.1016/j.humov.2006.12.001

Talis, V., Ballay, Y., Grishin, A., Alexandrov, A., and Pozzo, T. (2011). "Influence of FES on healthy subject locomotion," in *Proceeding of 2nd Annual Conference of the UKRI-IFESS*, University of Dublin, Dublin, Ireland, March 10–11, 30.

Talis, V. L., and Solopova, I. A. (2000). Vibration-induced postural reaction continues after the contact with additional support. *Motor Control* 4, 407–419.

Taylor, P., Humphreys, L., and Swain, I. (2013). The long-term cost-effectiveness of the use of Functional Electrical Stimulation for the correction of dropped foot due to upper motor neuron lesion. *J. Rehabil. Med.*. 45, 154–160. doi: 10.2340/16501977-1090

Taylor, P. N., Burridge, J. H., Dunkerley, A. L., Wood, D. E., Norton, J. A., Singleton, C., et al. (1999). Clinical use of the Odstock dropped foot stimulator: its effect on the speed and effort of walking. *Arch. Phys. Med. Rehabil.* 80, 1577–1583. doi: 10.1016/S0003-9993(99)90333-7

Winter, D. A., and Scott, S. H. (1991). Technique for interpretation of electromyography for concentric and eccentric contractions in gait. *J. Electromyogr. Kinesiol.* 1, 263–269. doi: 10.1016/1050-6411(91)90013-U

2

Neurofeedback Therapy for Enhancing Visual Attention: State-of-the-Art and Challenges

Mehdi Ordikhani-Seyedlar[1]*, *Mikhail A. Lebedev*[2,3], *Helge B. D. Sorensen*[1] and *Sadasivan Puthusserypady*[1]

[1] *Division of Biomedical Engineering, Department of Electrical Engineering, Technical University of Denmark, Lyngby, Denmark,* [2] *Department of Neurobiology, Duke University, Durham, NC, USA,* [3] *Center for Neuroengineering, Duke University, Durham, NC, USA*

Edited by:
Stefano Ferraina, Sapienza University of Rome, Italy

Reviewed by:
Olivia Carter, University of Melbourne, Australia
Tomasz Maciej Rutkowski, University of Tokyo, Japan

***Correspondence:**
Mehdi Ordikhani-Seyedlar
mehdi.ordikhani@gmail.com

We have witnessed a rapid development of brain-computer interfaces (BCIs) linking the brain to external devices. BCIs can be utilized to treat neurological conditions and even to augment brain functions. BCIs offer a promising treatment for mental disorders, including disorders of attention. Here we review the current state of the art and challenges of attention-based BCIs, with a focus on visual attention. Attention-based BCIs utilize electroencephalograms (EEGs) or other recording techniques to generate neurofeedback, which patients use to improve their attention, a complex cognitive function. Although progress has been made in the studies of neural mechanisms of attention, extraction of attention-related neural signals needed for BCI operations is a difficult problem. To attain good BCI performance, it is important to select the features of neural activity that represent attentional signals. BCI decoding of attention-related activity may be hindered by the presence of different neural signals. Therefore, BCI accuracy can be improved by signal processing algorithms that dissociate signals of interest from irrelevant activities. Notwithstanding recent progress, optimal processing of attentional neural signals remains a fundamental challenge for the development of efficient therapies for disorders of attention.

Keywords: visual attention, electroencephalography, brain-computer interface, feature extraction

INTRODUCTION

The visual system in both human and non-human organisms transforms complex input information into robust neural representation of the visual world. Because the amount of information can only decrease during stochastic neural processing, it is crucial for the visual system to selectively process behaviorally relevant information (Sprague et al., 2015). For instance, when a driver approaches a busy intersection it is important to detect and respond to the relevant traffic light rather than any light source in the visual scene. Attention is the ability to block the irrelevant information to the current task and to enhance the processing of the important information. This key neural function can deteriorate due to some disorders. Patients with disorders of attention are unable to allocate their focus of attention continuously to one task or easily get distracted by irrelevant information. One of the most common disorders of attention, attention deficit hyperactivity disorder (ADHD), is a mental condition characterized by inattention, hyperactivity and impulsivity. ADHD symptoms are dominant in childhood, and extend to adulthood in 15–40%

of cases (Biederman et al., 2000; Faraone et al., 2006). ADHD impairs performance in academic, occupational and social tasks (Fleming and McMahon, 2012). According to a meta-regression analysis of 102 studies, ADHD has 5% prevalence worldwide (Polanczyk and Rohde, 2007; Skounti et al., 2007; Millichap, 2008). Treatment strategies have been mostly pharmacological, such as prescription of psychostimulants. However, long-term treatment with pharmacological agents is hindered by side-effects (Conners et al., 2001; Greenhill et al., 2001). Children develop anxiety symptoms after being treated with psychostimulants for 6 months and longer (Vance et al., 1999). There is also a considerable risk of drug misuse and abuse (Kollins, 2008; Steiner et al., 2014a). Psychological therapy, an alternative approach, relieves ADHD symptoms in 30% of cases (Zarin et al., 1998). Overall, currently available therapies for ADHD are only partially effective.

Here we review a novel strategy for enhancing the attention capability in patients with disorders of attention. This strategy is based on brain-computer interface (BCI) approach (Arns et al., 2009; Lim et al., 2010, 2012). BCIs establish uni- or bidirectional communication between the brain and external devices (Wolpaw et al., 2000; Donoghue et al., 2004; Lebedev and Nicolelis, 2006; Nicolelis and Lebedev, 2009; Lebedev, 2014; Schwarz et al., 2014). BCIs decode neural signals using mathematical algorithms. Such decoding often utilizes templates of neural patterns defined based on prior knowledge of the characteristics of different neural states. A computer algorithm then compares neural activities with the set of templates to find the best match and determine the current neural state. Additionally, the algorithm can evaluate how well the brain signals match certain requirements, and generate a feedback based on the difference. Such feedback can be used to improve neural function in patients: patients observe their own brain activity in real time, and learn to self-regulate this activity in order to bring it to normal state. This paradigm is called "*neurofeedback*" and the corresponding therapeutic approach is called "*neurofeedback therapy.*" BCIs for humans most commonly utilize electroencephalographic (EEG) recordings (Kus et al., 2013; Tonin et al., 2013; Bamdadian et al., 2014; De Vos et al., 2014; Kashihara, 2014; Yang et al., 2014). Additionally, BCIs can employ magnetoencephalography (MEG) (Mellinger et al., 2007; Bianchi et al., 2010; Ahn et al., 2013), near infrared spectroscopy (NIRS) (Coyle et al., 2004; Sitaram et al., 2007; Power et al., 2012; Waldert et al., 2012; Khan et al., 2014), functional magnetic resonance imaging (fMRI) (Logothetis, 2003; deCharms et al., 2005; Ruiz et al., 2013; Sato et al., 2013), electrocortigraphy (ECoG) (Freeman et al., 2003; Leuthardt et al., 2004, 2009; Schalk, 2010), and multi-electrode intracranial implants (Nicolelis and Ribeiro, 2002; Carmena et al., 2003; Nicolelis et al., 2003; Lebedev et al., 2005, 2011; Zacksenhouse et al., 2007; Peikon et al., 2009; Ifft et al., 2013; see **Figure 1** for comparison).

Neurofeedback therapy is applicable to a number of neurological disorders of attention (Lofthouse et al., 2012b; Hillard et al., 2013; Gevensleben et al., 2014; Steiner et al., 2014c; Zandi Mehran et al., 2014). Attention-based neurofeedback paradigms for ADHDs are usually based on visual attention (Arns et al., 2014). As to recording methods, some (EEG, NIRS, ECoG) have been already shown effective for attention control and for treatment of ADHDs, whereas the applicability of others, such as MEG and fMRI, is being researched (Ahn et al., 2013; Sulzer et al., 2013; Sokunbi et al., 2014; Stoeckel et al., 2014; Bruhl, 2015; Okazaki et al., 2015). Implementing an attention-based BCI is a challenging task because the neural representation of attention is highly complex (Ming et al., 2009; Rossini et al., 2012). A good understanding of neurophysiology of attention is required to extract attentional signals from neural recordings and dissociate them from the other ongoing activities in the brain (Sanei and Chambers, 2008). Notwithstanding these difficulties, visual-attention based BCI systems have been already developed and applied to ADHD (Christiansen et al., 2014; Heinrich et al., 2014; Holtmann et al., 2014a,b; Micoulaud-Franchi et al., 2014; Steiner et al., 2014b). In this article, we cover the current state of the art and future challenges in this research.

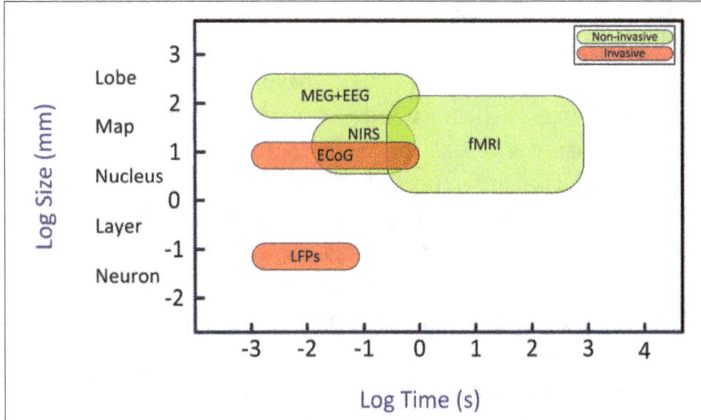

FIGURE 1 | Temporal and spatial resolution of different BCI techniques. Although EEG has a relatively poor spatial resolution, its high temporal resolution is an adequate characteristic for real-time BCIs. Abbreviations: EEG, electroencephalography; MEG, magneto-encephalogram; NIRS, near-infrared spectroscopy; fMRI, functional magnetic resonance imaging; ECoG, electro-corticogram; LFPs, local field potentials. Image is inspired from Van Gerven et al. (2009).

DECODING OF VISUAL ATTENTION FROM NEURAL SIGNALS

Neural Mechanisms of Visual Attention

In everyday life, we constantly deal with multiple sensory streams from our complex and dynamic environment. The brain starts the processing of this incoming information by filtering out irrelevant signals, which are not consciously experienced because of the filtering. Only a tiny amount of the incoming information enters the higher-order processing levels and becomes available to consciousness (Posner, 1994, 2012). Selective attention is a key function that enables the brain to effectively use its limited information processing capability when confronted with an immense number of inputs from all sensory modalities. High-level cortical areas, particularly the areas of the frontal cortex, play a key role in attentional control. It has been long known that damage to prefrontal cortex (PFC) causes mental deficits which are consistent with a loss of attentional control

(Ferrier, 1876). Neurophysiological and functional neuroimaging studies by Posner's group (Fan et al., 2005; Posner and Rothbart, 2007; Petersen and Posner, 2012) have provided a wealth of information on cortical circuitry for attentional control. The main conclusion of these studies is that attention is controlled by a network of interconnected areas that also involved in oculomotor control. These areas include the frontal eye field (FEF), parietal areas and subcortical structures, importantly superior colliculus. This attentional selection network works together with yet another, overlapping network of areas that sustains the focus of attention, called *sustained attention*. The latter system maintains the focus of attention on the selected stimulus. It is composed of the parietal cortex, right frontal cortex and locus coeruleus (Corbetta et al., 2008). Volumetric analysis in ADHD subjects showed that they have smaller frontal cortex compared to healthy subjects (He et al., 2015). This finding explains the deficits in both selective and sustained attention (Pritchard et al., 2008; Avisar and Shalev, 2011; Gomes et al., 2012; Wang et al., 2013). Notably, attention-based BCIs usually require both selecting a visual target and focusing on it (i.e., selective attention) and mental endurance training (i.e., sustained attention).

Selective attention is not a unitary process; it is driven by distinct functional sub-processes associated with different selection criteria (Brosch et al., 2011). Two major sub-processes are: stimulus-driven (exogenous) attention and observer-dependent (endogenous) attention. *Exogenous attention* is driven by intrinsic low-level features of sensory inputs (Egeth and Yantis, 1997; Wolfe and Horowitz, 2004). Low-level properties include such features as stimulus intensity, color and contrast. They all trigger involuntary responses. *Endogenous attention* refers to selection of a target based on an internal state and conscious expectation of a specific object or location (Posner et al., 1980; Desimone and Duncan, 1995). Endogenous selection is performed based on the current aim of the observer. In the classical Posner experiment that dissociated endogenous and exogenous effects, participants were instructed to press a button in response to a visual stimulus that appeared either to the left or right of a central fixation point (Posner, 1980). They were asked to keep their eyes fixed at the center of the screen throughout the task and covertly (i.e., without looking at the target) attend to the peripheral location. To guide this covert attention, a symbolic cue was presented at the center of the screen, which instructed the location to attend. This cue preceded the stimulus onset, and correctly specified the upcoming stimulus location in 80% of the trials. In the remaining 20% of trials, the target appeared at a location that disagreed with the cue. This study showed that the reaction time was significantly shorter when the stimulus was presented at the attended location than when it appeared in the opposite location and there was a misalignment between the endogenous and exogenous attention. Busse et al. investigated neurophysiological mechanisms underlying these two types of attention (Busse et al., 2008). They recorded from single neurons in macaque middle temporal area while monkeys' endogenous and/or exogenous attention was manipulated by the task events. They used a double-cueing paradigm where the first cue instructed the monkey to attend (endogenous attention) to one of three moving random dot patterns (RDPs) until a second cue. The second cue was unpredictable, and therefore captured exogenous attention. It signaled to either shift or maintain the current focus of attention. Findings of this experiment showed that the neural activity was enhanced when attention was endogenously shifted to the first cue. Then, attention was exogenously attracted to the second cue, which was manifested by a transient interruption of neural activity for approximately 70 ms, after which the endogenous attention restored neural representation of the previously relevant stimulus. These results showed that the interruption of endogenous attention by exogenous attention is not a simple refocusing to the new stimulus. Rather, there are separate ongoing processes with distinct neural correlates for endogenous and exogenous effects, as well as an interaction between these mechanisms.

Both endogenous and exogenous attention can be maintained with and without eye movements (i.e., overtly or covertly, respectively). The premotor theory of attention (Rizzolatti et al., 1987) suggests that essentially the same neural circuits in the frontal and parietal areas control the orientation of both overt and covert attention. For overt shifts of attention, eye movements are prepared and executed, whereas for covert shifts they are prepared but not executed. The premotor theory of attention is supported by the fMRI studies showing an overlap between the frontal and parietal regions activated for covert and overt attentional tasks (de Haan et al., 2008). Additionally, neurons in the intermediate layer of superior colliculus which has been long known for their involvement in saccades, are also engaged in the covert attentional shifts (Ignashchenkova et al., 2004). Golla et al. reported a clinical case of impaired overt attention in a cerebellar disorder, and suggested that the cerebellum plays a role in spatial attention (Golla et al., 2005).

Lebedev, Wise and their colleagues compared neural representation of attention with the representation of other behavioral variables, such as spatial memory, target of movement and gaze angle, which often coincide with the orientation of attention, but still can be controlled independently by the brain. In one study (Lebedev and Wise, 2001), they compared neuronal activity in monkey's dorsal premotor cortex (PMd) that reflected the orientation of selective spatial attention with neuronal activities that represented motor preparation, gaze angle, and saccades. The monkeys' attention was attracted by a robot, to which they attended in order to know when to initiate a reaching movement. The target of movement varied. It was either the location of the feeder mounted on the robot or a location of a different feeder. This study showed that approximately 20% of PMd reflected the orientation of selective spatial attention, which could be disengaged from the other spatial variables. These attention-tuned PMd neurons could account for gaze-independent (covert) attentional effects in behaviors with stimulus-response incompatibility. In another study (Lebedev et al., 2004), Lebedev et al. tested the theory that the main function of prefrontal cortex (PF) is the maintenance of working memory. To investigate alternative possibilities, activity of PF neurons was recorded while the monkeys performed an oculomotor task that required remembering one location, but attending to a different location. The largest subpopulation of

PF neurons was linked to attention, not to working memory, which indicated that PF has a major contribution to selective spatial attention. Consistent with these findings, studies in human subjects demonstrated the crucial role of frontal cortex in ADHDs (Praamstra et al., 2005; Dirlikov et al., 2015). Dirlikov et al. (2015) used brain imaging technique to explore the cortical morphology in 93 children with ADHD. They found a reduction in cortical surface of PF and premotor cortex (Dirlikov et al., 2015). Several neuroimaging studies suggested that visual attention is controlled by a network of cortical areas interconnected with the FEF. Gray matter is substantially affected in ADHD in the structures of this network, including dorsal and ventral prefrontal cortices, dorsal anterior cingulate area and inferior parietal cortex (Valera et al., 2007; Szuromi et al., 2011). Jonkman and colleagues suggested that the frontal lobe performs early selective filtering, and disorders of this function cause ADHD (Jonkman et al., 2004). A recent resting-state EEG study also suggested that frontal cortex abnormalities are a reliable marker for ADHD (Keune et al., 2015).

Neural oscillations is another neural marker of attention. Oscillations represent synchronous activity of neuronal populations of different sizes, from local to very large. They can be detected in local field potentials (LFPs) recorded with invasive electrodes, or EEGs recorded non-invasively from the scalp (Kahana, 2006). Oscillations are conventionally classified into five frequency bands: δ (1–4 Hz), θ (4–8 Hz), α (8–12 Hz), β (12–30 Hz), and γ (30–80 Hz). Attentional effects have been reported for each of these bands. For instance, attending to a spatial location and anticipating a stimulus at that location is associated with α rhythm attenuation (Rohenkohl and Nobre, 2011). α oscillations are involved in attentional gating of information flow between brain regions (Fu et al., 2001; ter Huurne et al., 2013). To investigate the relationship between brain oscillations and ADHD, ter Huurne used a motion coherence detection task where subjects were instructed to direct attention to either left or right visual field. The attended stimulus was a random dot kinematogram, a field of chaotically moving dots. Subjects were instructed to respond after the dot pattern started to move coherently in the horizontal, but not vertical dimension in the attended hemifield. Dot movements in the unattended hemifield had to be ignored. In healthy subjects, lateralized and sustained α oscillations were detected in the visual cortex during the period when the subjects prepared to respond. In patients with ADHD, oscillations started, but they were not sustained and often stopped before the stimulus onset. Furthermore, lateralization of α oscillation was highly correlated with the degree of spatial attention in the healthy group, but not in the ADHD group (ter Huurne et al., 2013). In neurofeedback training experiments, children with ADHD were able to increase α-power following 18 training sessions (Escolano et al., 2014). Overall, these studies suggest that brain oscillations can be used to monitor neural regulation of attention and improve it using neurofeedback therapy.

BCIs for Visual Attention

Early attempts to treat disorders of attention using neurofeedback date back to the mid-eighties and nineties (Elbert et al., 1980; Lutzenberger et al., 1980; Wolpaw et al., 1991). Since then, considerable progress has been made in the development of computer algorithms for the decoding of attention-related neural signals. In a typical setting, subjects endeavor to keep their visual attention while playing a video game. Attention related brain signals are extracted from the neural recordings and fed back to the subjects using visual feedback. Successful performance is rewarded. Repeated training sessions with such a BCI system engage brain plasticity mechanisms, and eventually improve attention (Dobkin, 2007; Rossini et al., 2012).

Both invasive and non-invasive recordings have been used in BCIs. Invasive BCIs utilize electrodes that penetrate the brain (LFPs and single-unit recordings) or are placed on the brain surface (ECoG). These systems require an invasive surgical procedure to implant the electrodes. Non-invasive BCIs, on the other hand, do not require any surgery and can be safely and easily implemented. Non-invasive sensors are placed on the scalp (EEG, fNIRS), or in some implementations make no contact with the head (fMRI, MEG) (see **Table 1** for details). Additionally, *hybrid* or *multimodal* BCIs employ combinations of different recording methods in order to improve performance. Fazli et al. (2012) developed a multimodal BCI consisting of the combination of EEG and NIRS that improved the signal classification accuracy in 90% of participants. That multimodal BCI had higher sensitivity and specificity and were resistant to environmental noise. Such combined EEG-NIRS neurofeedback can be used by subjects who cannot operate a BCI solely by their EEG activity (Fazli et al., 2012).

The research on BCIs that improve attention has experienced a steady growth, especially BCIs for ADHD patients. Some of these results are controversial. A number of studies reported positive outcome of neurofeedback training (Leins et al., 2007; Gevensleben et al., 2009; Steiner et al., 2011; Wangler et al., 2011), whereas others questioned these findings. In the camp of neurofeedback advocates, Arns et al. (2009) analyzed literature on neurofeedback therapy for ADHD and concluded that this treatment was "efficient and specific" (Arns et al., 2009). Lofthouse et al. (2012a) called this therapy "probably efficacious" based on their analysis of research conducted from 1994 to 2010, where the majority of studies utilized θ/β ratio (see below) (Lofthouse et al., 2012a). However, Vollebregt et al. (2014a) came to a different conclusion in their systematic review of frequency-band based BCIs for ADHD. They concluded that there was no significant effect of treatment on any neurocognitive variables affected by ADHD (Vollebregt et al., 2014a). This negative result highlights the need for further research on EEG features that would better suit attention-based BCIs. Here we review these features and the ways they could be used to improve neurofeedback therapy for ADHD.

FEATURE EXTRACTION FOR VISUAL-ATTENTION BCIs

Feature extraction is a critical part of BCI implementation and design (Shahid and Prasad, 2011). During this processing stage, a specific characteristics are extracted from brain recordings, which are then decoded and converted into control commands or neurofeedback. Depending on the recording method, different

TABLE 1 | Comparison of different signal acquisition methods used for BCI application.

BCI method (measured signal type)	Advantages	Disadvantages
LFPs (Firing rate of bundles of neurons)	High SNR; low variability during the experiment; targeting the activity in specific brain areas; higher resolution of detecting temporal and spatial features in several parallel-activated brain regions.	Intracranial surgery; very susceptible to signal-loss in long-term implantation (Shain et al., 2003; Donoghue et al., 2004); requires precise source localization in order to implant the electrodes in the right location; less common in human studies.
ECoG (Electrical activity from brain surface)	Supports accurate BCI operation with little training (Leuthardt et al., 2004); higher spatial resolution and amplitude than EEG (Freeman et al., 2000; Leuthardt et al., 2009); far less EMG and EOG artifacts (Freeman et al., 2003; Ball et al., 2009); greater long-term functionality compared to LFPs (Margalit et al., 2003); more stable SNR compared to EEG (Schalk, 2010).	Intracranial surgery; Limited long-term functional stability and signal loss (Schalk and Leuthardt, 2011); very rare research application (Sutter and Tran, 1992).
EEG (Electrical activity from the scalp)	Superior temporal resolution (suitable for real-time experiments); ease of use (non-invasive) even by inexpert individuals; inexpensive (compared to other devices); least ethical concern and medical risks compared to other methods; portable.	Susceptible to noise (EMG, EOG and environmental); Low spatial resolution (harder to localize brain activities); requires a substantial degree of user training in BCI development.
fMRI [Blood oxygenation level dependent (BOLD)]	Superior spatial resolution (deCharms et al., 2005; Lee et al., 2009); signal detection from whole brain including the subcortical structures (Logothetis, 2003; Weiskopf et al., 2004).	Signal drift due to imperfection of magnetic gradient field (Lee et al., 2009); limited to BOLD-signal-based analysis (can be done in ERP experiments but not in frequency-range analysis); less suitable for real-time BCI due to low temporal resolution; strict physical restriction of subjects inside the scanner due to motion artifacts; requires expensive devices and expertise to operate the system.
NIRS (Measure of oxygenated hemoglobin)	Robust when dealing with noise (Coyle et al., 2004; Waldert et al., 2012); superior in detection of stimulation onsets and offsets (reducing the false positive commands) (Tomita et al., 2014); precise parameter setting to extract features is not needed to detect information on the brain (Kanoh et al., 2009).	Lower temporal resolution compared to EEG (Tomita et al., 2014).
MEG (Magnetic field)	Higher spatiotemporal resolution (Mellinger et al., 2007) than EEG; less training sessions than EEG; more robust in detectability of different frequency-band compared to EEG (Mellinger et al., 2007).	Expensive (at least 10 times more expensive than EEG cost) and non-portable; lower spatial resolution compared to fMRI; poorer localization for deeper brain structures compared to fMRI.

features can be used. For example, single-unit recording are usually converted into neuronal firing rates, and EEGs are converted either into the spectral power or parameters of event related potentials. The selection of features depends on the way the user communicates with the BCI system. In the BCI design called endogenous BCI, subjects self-generate neural patterns (Nicolas-Alonso and Gomez-Gil, 2012). Alternatively, in the BCI design called exogenous BCI, neural responses are evoked by an external stimulus, and subjects modulate these responses, usually by focusing attention on relevant stimuli. **Table 2** compares these two BCI types.

Endogenous BCI

Attention-Based BCIs That Utilize Neural Oscillations

Spectral analysis of EEGs recorded at different scalp locations is commonly used to extract features for endogenous BCIs. Here, time-dependent changes in the EEG spectra for different electrodes are detected using EEG time-frequency (TF) analysis. For example, TF analysis can detect the occurrence of brain oscillations that result from transient synchronization of neuronal discharges over a millisecond time scale (Sanei and Chambers, 2008). This method can be applied to measure EEG changes associated with attention, such as synchronization of specific EEG bands associated with attention to an object. Attention-related synchronization of neural activity can be detected using a variety of recording methods, including single-unit recordings from brain neurons. Fries et al recorded from individual neurons in cortical area V4 while macaque monkeys attended to behaviorally relevant stimuli and ignored distractors (Fries et al., 2001). The neurons increased their gamma-band synchrony while decreasing low-frequency (<17 Hz) synchrony when the monkeys attended. Several studies showed attention related effects in ECoGs. Rougeul-Buser and Buser recorded ECoGs in freely moving cats and observed that 10–14 Hz oscillation over sensorimotor cortex, called μ-rhythm or "expectancy rhythm," increased when an animal actively attended

TABLE 2 | Comparison of endogenous and exogenous BCIs and their corresponding protocols.

Category	Protocol	Advantages	Drawbacks
Endogenous BCI	- Source of the brain activity - Frequency bands	- Independent of any specific task - Useful for patients with sensory deficits - Perfect for freely moving operations (since subjects are not instructed to stare at specific stimulus)	- Requires several sessions of trainings - Some patients may not be able to communicate with BCI (BCI illiterate) - Low information transfer rate - Low signal-to-noise ratio - Low spatial resolution of EEG-based BCIs (harder for source localization analysis) - Requires many EEG electrodes
Exogenous BCI	- ERP - SSVEP	- Low training session - High information transfer rate (explained in the next section) - Feasible with a few EEG channels - Higher signal-to-noise ratio	- System failure if the subject is not attending to the stimuli - Fatigue in subjects (especially in SSVEP tasks due to constant flickering objects)

to a place where a mouse was expected to appear (Rougeul-Buser and Buser, 1997). The μ-rhythm epochs were often followed by a brief 20 Hz (β-range) ECoG burst. Thorpe et al reported topographical details of these ECoG patterns. Attention was associated with μ-rhythm increases over parietal regions, whereas, β-band activity increased in motor areas (Thorpe et al., 2012). Daitch et al. suggested that these oscillatory patterns serve to increase functional connectivity between the areas that process relevant information while suppressing unwanted cross-talk within the neural network areas that could be caused by irrelevant stimuli (Daitch et al., 2013).

EEG studies have shown that high-frequency oscillations (>30 Hz) are correlated with increased attention (Kaiser and Lutzenberger, 2005; Koelewijn et al., 2013; Musch et al., 2014). Similar results were obtained using microelectrode recordings in freely behaving monkeys (Fries et al., 2001). Attention-related oscillations can have the frequency higher than the typical γ -band range (30–80 Hz) (Crone et al., 2006). Ray et al. (2008) presented human subjects with a sequence of tactile and auditory stimuli separated by pseudo-random time intervals. The tactile stimuli were delivered using a tactile stimulating cylinder, which the subjects gripped with their hands. The auditory stimuli were delivered through a headset. The subjects were instructed to attend to one of the two modalities (auditory or tactile) and respond to the attended stimulus with a button press (Ray et al., 2008). The attended stimuli enhanced high γ activity (80–150 Hz) in the cortical areas that processed the corresponding modality: attention to auditory stimuli activated auditory cortex, and attention to somatosensory stimuli activated somatosensory cortex. Additionally, these high-gamma oscillations occurred in PFC irrespective of the attended modality. This result is consistent with PFC being involved in the global attentional system (Dirlikov et al., 2015; Keune et al., 2015) regardless of the modalities of input information. Another study reported that attention in humans was associated with high frequency oscillations of approximately 350 Hz that occurred in frontal and centro-parietal regions in response to somatosensory stimuli (Ozaki et al., 2006). Several hypotheses have been proposed to explain the role of high-frequency oscillations in attention. One hypothesis states that low-amplitude, ultra-high frequency activity is a background neural noise that enhances neural processing (Benzi et al., 1982). For example, adding a small amount of noise to a neural circuit makes its component fire more synchronous (Ward et al., 2006). Here, the performance is improved due to stochastic resonance (Benzi et al., 1982), where high-frequency noise lowers detection threshold for the relevant stimulus-. The stochastic resonance driven by γ waves can play a role in high cognitive functions (Ward et al., 2006). A similar resonance can be produced by injecting noise to the brain using electrical stimulation (Medina et al., 2012).

A number of BCIs for controlling attention have been developed based on EEG spectral bands. A recent study showed that healthy subjects can quickly learn to self-modulate their γ-oscillation in superior parietal cortex by alternating between the attentive and rest states (Grosse-Wentrup and Scholkopf, 2014). This BCI system correctly decoded brain state in 70.2% of cases. Several of studies on attention-based BCIs employed the ratio of power in specific spectral bands as the signal feature to be classified. This ratio was calculated as $\beta/(\alpha+\theta)$ in many reports (Nagendra et al., 2015). The higher the ratio, the higher is the level of attention. Other studies used θ/β ratio (Clarke et al., 2013; Dupuy et al., 2013; Heinrich et al., 2014; Vollebregt et al., 2014b) that decreased with enhanced attention. These ratios reflect the fact that θ and α rhythms are stronger in drowsiness and the inattentive states; whereas, β rhythm is stronger in attentive states. For example, spectral EEG composition prior to stimulus presentation is indicative of the level of visual attention (Busch et al., 2009). Several characteristics of EEG rhythms can be also used to assess the level of attention. Instantaneous phase of EEG oscillations is one such characteristic (Busch et al., 2009). In the experiments of Busch et al. (2009), subjects were instructed to detect a brief (6 ms) light flash presented either at an attended or unattended location. Hit and miss rates were found to be correlated with the phase of EEG oscillations at the time of stimulus presentation. Additionally, stimuli preceded by strong α activity were less likely to be detected, an observation reported in the previous literature (Ergenoglu et al., 2004; Babiloni et al., 2006; Thut et al., 2006; Hanslmayr et al., 2007). In the other study on the relationship between EEG phase and detection of attended and unattended stimuli, Busch and VanRullen (Busch and VanRullen, 2010) analyzed the relationship between the pre-stimulus EEG pattern and the EEG response to the stimulus. They found that EEG responses were higher when EEG was at a certain phase the just prior to the stimulus onset and the EEG response was the lowest for the opposite EEG phase (Busch and VanRullen, 2010). The periodicity of EEG was 100–150 ms in these experiments. Several studies reported similar results (Makeig et al., 2002; Lakatos et al., 2008; Busch and VanRullen, 2010).

Exogenous BCI

Event-Related Potential (ERP) Paradigms

Event-relate potentials (ERPs) represent a compound response to a stimulus of large neuronal populations. An ERP consists of several voltage deflections that occur on a millisecond time scale. Specific ERP components have been linked to different neural origins (Cohen, 2013), including the components that are associated with attention. ERP is one of the most commonly used protocols for attention studies (Wu et al., 2009; Gherri and Eimer, 2011; Jones et al., 2013; Matheson et al., 2014; Zheng et al., 2014). ERPs recorded in primary sensory areas increase when the corresponding stimulus modality is attended to Harter et al. (1984). Selection of the appropriate ERP components and scalp locations to sample is essential to achieve good performance of an ERP-based BCI. The first ERP-based BCI was designed by Farwell and Donchin (1988). Subjects looked at a 6 × 6 matrix of alphanumeric characters. A single electrode was placed over the Pz (central-parietal) site. Subjects were instructed to attend to a specific character within the matrix while rows and columns periodically flashed. Attended stimuli evoked stronger ERPs and thus could be identified. Averaging over 30 trials was required to improve the signal-to-noise ratio and assure BCI accuracy.

For better design of ERP-based BCIs, it is important to take into consideration the detailed sequence of ERPs components. The first component is the C1-wave which is detected mostly by the posterior midline electrodes in the EEG. The onset of the C1-wave is typically 40–60 ms after the stimulus with the peak at 80–100 ms post-stimulus. C1 is generated in the primary visual cortex (Luck, 2014) and its polarity changes as a function of location of the stimulus in the visual field, i.e., whether the response comes from upper or lower bank of calcarine sulcus. This change in polarity has been identified as a unique feature for C1-wave compared to other components and has been used by many studies as a marker for V1 sources. However, later neuroimaging studies challenged this view. Ales et al. (2010) used fMRI retinotopic mapping to identify the location of V1, V2, and V3 overlaid on the high-resolution structural MRI (Ales et al., 2010). This technique allowed them to acquire a 3D shape of the upper and lower visual field projection in V1 and adjacent areas, V2 and V3. Contrary to previous studies, they found that sources in V1 do not fully conform to the sign reversal. Furthermore, V2 and V3 also showed a polarity change for upper and lower field stimuli. This suggested that the polarity inversion criterion was not a reliable method for source localization. Yet another study challenged this conclusion. Kelly et al. claimed that C1 does initiate from V1 (Kelly et al., 2013). It has been also reported that attention is not important to generate the C1 component (Martinez et al., 1999; Fu et al., 2010). According to Martinez et al., although primary visual cortex is involved in attention, it does not serve as the locus of initial sensory gain control for attended and unattended inputs. Kelly et al. (2008) disagreed with this and proposed that attentional selection occurs at the early visual processing stage reflected by C1 generation in V1 (Kelly et al., 2008). In that study, target brightness and location were adjusted for each participant in order to reduce inter-subjective variability of C1. After this correction, it became clear that C1 was enhanced due to spatial attention, which indicated that this early sensory component was adjusted before the visual information arrived in V1.

The second component is the P1-wave that starts 60–90 ms after the stimulus and peaks at 100–130 ms. It contains an early portion generated from middle occipital gyrus and a late-portion generated more ventrally, from fusiform gyrus (Di Russo et al., 2002). P1 is sensitive to the direction of spatial attention (Hillyard and Anllo-Vento, 1998). Luck and Hillyard (1995) studied attentional modulation of P1 using a stimulus display that consisted of 14 gray items and 2 colored items (Luck and Hillyard, 1995). Subjects were instructed to report presence or absence of specific colored-item (feature detection condition) or the shape of a specific colored-item (conjunction discrimination condition). Just after the onset of the search array, a task-irrelevant stimulus appeared either at the location of relevant or irrelevant items. The irrelevant stimulus evoked larger ERPs for the relevant location compared to irrelevant location. P1-wave was present in that ERP only in the discrimination condition and not in the feature detection condition, indicating that conjunction discrimination recruited additional attentional resources. In the traditional paradigm, where subjects are instructed to pay attention to one direction and ignore the other, Mangun et al. (2001) showed that the P1 magnitude is larger for the attended compared to unattended location. The study of Mangum et al. also showed that P1 response was generated not only by the contralateral hemisphere but also by the ipsilateral one, the observation that was difficult to explain in terms of redistribution of attentional resources between the hemispheres. Klimesch (2011) suggested that these results is due to inhibition effect of the P1 in two different levels. In the task-irrelevant pathways (e.g., ipsilateral hemisphere) inhibition is used to block the information processing, whereas, in the task-relevant pathways it is used to increase the SNR by enabling precisely timed activity in neurons with high level of excitation and suppressing the neurons with low-level of excitation. It seems that the inhibition increased when an attentional demand increases to make the response to the relevant stimulus sharper.

N1-wave contains an early component generated in the frontal (140 ms) and two late components between 150 and 200 ms generated parietal cortex and the lateral occipital cortex, respectively (Clark and Hillyard, 1996; Luck, 2005; Ceballos and Hernandez, 2015). The magnitude of N1-potential is highly influenced by visual spatial attention (Hillyard et al., 1998). N1 is insensitive to the physical properties of the paradigm such as light intensity and the contrast. This point was clarified in the experiment where a 6 × 6 matrix alphanumeric matrix (similar to Farwell and Donchin's paradigm) could be either high-contrast or low-contrast (Shishkin et al., 2009). Although the visual stimuli were designed in a very different contrasts, N1 characteristics between high- and low-contrast tasks remained the same. N1 is an interesting feature from two aspects: first N1 seems to be reproduce robust feature regardless of design on the paradigm which makes it suitable to compare different studies; second, there is no need to make detection paradigm hard to enhance N1 as it works well for clearly visible stimuli, and therefore, N1-based BCIs can be visually comfortable for ADHD subjects. This is important for ADHD subjects as they have higher tendency for fatigue or visual discomfort (Cao et al., 2014; Kooij and Bijlenga, 2014). It has been shown that about two-third of children with ADHD suffer from visual problems such as irritability by light (Kooij and Bijlenga, 2014). If BCIs are intended to be used on a daily basis for training and rehabilitation purposes, the rapid visual fatigue would be a great disadvantage (Sakurada et al., 2015). Therefore, presenting a paradigm with less discomfort effect should enhance the endurance of patients in long-lasting training sessions and consequently increase the chance of successful therapy.

N1 properties are influenced by repetitive training which can be a potential marker for evaluating the effect of neurofeedback therapy. For example, training to play a video game affects N1 (Latham et al., 2013). In that study, checkerboard stimuli appeared for a short time (92 ms) either in the left or right hemifield against a gray background. Subjects were instructed to respond to the flash of checkerboards by pressing a button while EEG was being recorded. Participants were divided into two groups: professional video-game players (VGP) and non-professional VGP. Expert VGPs had significantly shorter N1 latencies compared to inexperienced VGPs, and no other difference in ERP components was found between the groups.

P2-wave, that follows N1, occurs mostly for the anterior and central electrodes. P2 is larger when the stimulus occurs relatively infrequently (*oddball*). From this point of view, the anterior P2 is similar to P3-wave (see below) with the difference that P2 represents simple features (e.g., color) of the stimulus, whereas P3 is related to complex stimulus features (e.g., color and shape). For posterior electrodes, P2 component is often difficult to distinguish from the overlapping N1, N2, and P3 (Luck, 2014). P2 magnitude has been reported to differ between healthy and ADHD individuals (Banaschewski et al., 2003, 2008; Broyd et al., 2005). The P2 component is associated with automatic processing and inhibition of irrelevant information (Barry et al., 2003). Studies have shown that P2 has larger amplitude and different topographical distribution in ADHD (Banaschewski et al., 2003; Broyd et al., 2005; Barry et al., 2009; Ortega et al., 2013). Therefore, P2 amplitude could be used in BCIs as an indicator for improvement scale for ADHDs.

P3 component (also called the P300 since it peaks at 300–500 ms post-stimulus) consists of two sub-components P3a and P3b. The P3b amplitude varies between 5 and 15 μV for the parietal electrodes (Soltani and Knight, 2000). It appears following the occurrence of the oddball stimulus among a sequence of frequently repeating background stimuli. P3a, on the other hand, is distributed more in the fronto-central scalp region and peaks about 60–80 ms prior to P3b for all sensory modalities. An important characteristic of P3a component is its habituation in frontal sites within 5–10 stimulus presentations; i.e., the P3a disappears when the same type of stimulus is repeatedly presented (Lynn and Eysenck, 1966; Sokolov, 1969; Friedman et al., 2001). P3b, in many publications, is simply referred to P3 or P300. It was proposed that P3 is a possible endophenotype for ADHD (Doyle et al., 2005; Szuromi et al., 2011). Patients with ADHD have significantly lower P3 amplitude during the attention task (Szuromi et al., 2011). Szuromi et al. (2011) proposed that the P3 may be used as an ADHD marker that characterizes the deficits in the level of attentional allocation and information processing. P3 magnitude has been reported to represent the effort of attentional allocation, whereas, the latency of P3 indexes the processing speed of stimulus evaluation (Polich, 2007). Yet, P3 should be considered conservatively as a unique indicator for attention deficiency since its characteristics can be affected also by other disorders such as externalizing psychopathology (substance use, conduct disorder and antisocial behavior) (Bertoletti et al., 2014; Burwell et al., 2014).

ERP-based BCIs is one of the early developed methods in the field of BCI (Farwell and Donchin, 1988). ERP-based BCIs have a relatively low information transfer rate (ITR) or bit-rate. Bit-rate in a BCI system is an index of how much information can be communicated between the brain and the computer in the time-unit (van der Waal et al., 2012). In Farwell and Donchin's BCI, the ITR was about 12 bits min^{-1}. Zhang et al developed a visual P300-speller BCI which was able to communicate at 20 bits min^{-1}. BCI performance is substantially higher for visual ERPs compared to auditory (1.54 bit min^{-1}) and tactile (7.8 bit min^{-1}) ERPs (Furdea et al., 2009; van der Waal et al., 2012). Combination of ERP with other protocols such as steady-state visual evoked potential (SSVEP) increases the ITR up to 19.05 bit min^{-1} (Panicker et al., 2011).

ERP-based BCIs increase SNR by performing an ensemble averaging across several responses. Only the time-locked activities survive the averaging and irrelevant activities are canceled out. However, averaging is also considered as a drawback of ERP-based BCIs as the system has to obtain two or more ERP events to improve performance. Collecting data in multiple trials slows down the system speed. Thus, choosing this ERP-BCI method is a trade-off between the speed and accuracy of the system. Another limitation of ERP-based BCI is the across-trial variability in ERP amplitude and timing. The amplitude of P3 decreases if inter-trial intervals are short. To keep P3 amplitude in the standard range (10–20 μV) inter-trial interval should be around 8 s (Polich and Bondurant, 1997). This long interval limits BCI performance. In most experimental designs, intervals between oddball stimuli are random, which introduces ERP variability. Variability in the P3-characteristics makes it an unstable feature in attention experiments where the rigidity of ERP depend both on factors such as the designed paradigm and the mental states of the subjects.

Signal Characteristics in Steady-State Visual Evoked Potential (SSVEP) Paradigms

Another widely used BCI protocol is the SSVEP (Zhang et al., 2010; Palomares et al., 2012; Lesenfants et al., 2014; Wu and Su, 2014; Reuter et al., 2015). Visual evoked potential (VEP) is the brain responses to a visual stimulus such as light flash or flickering of a checker board at a specific frequency (Punsawad and Wongsawat, 2012). Presentation of a flickering visual object leads to VEPs entrained to the stimulus frequency. SSVEP-based BCIs usually detect this entrained response in the EEG of the visual and parietal cortices. These BCIs achieve high SNR over a few seconds of stimulation (Dmochowski et al., 2015). In a typical SSVEP-based BCI, several objects flicker at different frequencies while the subject attends to one the object. The subject usually looks at the attended object. SSVEP-based BCIs can be easily implemented using graphical interfaces such as video games (Leins et al., 2007; Lim et al., 2010, 2012; Bakhshayesh et al., 2011).

SSVEP-based BCIs have good accuracy and resistance to artifacts. As such, they can be used to build practical assistive systems for disabled users (Muller-Putz and Pfurtscheller, 2008). For example, Bin et al reported a SSVEP-based BCI that attained 95.3% accuracy and the ITR of 58 $\pm$ 9.6 bits min^{-1} (Bin et al., 2009). This is a substantially higher ITR compared to other BCI types, such as ERP-based BCIs. Muller and Hillyard (2000) designed a paradigm in which ERPs were embedded within a flicker sequence. They found that the magnitude of SSVEP and that of the N1 and N2 component of ERP varied together (positive correlation), whereas no significant correlation was found with other ERP components (Muller and Hillyard, 2000). SSVEP paradigms usually utilize the flickering frequency greater than 6 Hz. In a recent study (Dreyer and Herrmann, 2015), flickering frequency of up to 100 Hz was used by utilizing a novel technology. High-frequency SSVEPs are of great advantage because subjects do not perceive the flicker and are not annoyed. The flicker is not perceived for stimulus frequencies higher than 40 Hz (Lin et al., 2012). Sakurada et al. (2015) demonstrated that using BCIs with SSVEP frequency above 50–60 Hz enhanced the classification accuracy and decreased visual fatigue (Sakurada et al., 2015). Training time is also improved, particularly in ADHD subjects, as they are less irritated by light flicker (Kooij and Bijlenga, 2014).

SSVEPs can be detected not only in awake subjects, but in anesthetized subjects, as well. Several experiments employed the SSVEP technique in fully or partially anesthetized animals whose eyes were kept open in front of a visual display (Harnois et al., 1984; Xu et al., 2013). The flicker frequency was detected from the occipital electrodes.

Harmonics of the flickering frequency in some cases give a better BCI readout (Muller-Putz and Pfurtscheller, 2008; Allison et al., 2010; Ordikhani-Seyedlar et al., 2014). Müller-Putz and his colleagues reported particularly good results when they used three harmonic peaks (Muller-Putz et al., 2005). In our study (Ordikhani-Seyedlar et al., 2014) that employed a covert attention paradigm, the power of the second harmonic was higher compared to the first harmonic. This result is in agreement with Kim et al. (2011) and others Garcia et al. (2013), Zhang et al. (2015) who also reported that visual spatial attention modulates the second, but not the first harmonic of the SSVEP frequency.

PROSPECTS FOR BCIs IN RESEARCH OF ATTENTION

We are witnessing a rapid development of the BCI field. The number of peer-reviewed articles has been rapidly increasing over the past 20 years. Many of BCIs reported in the literature enable sensorimotor functions (O'Doherty et al., 2011; Ifft et al., 2013; Pais-Vieira et al., 2013; Yoo et al., 2013). While BCIs for cognitive functions are less developed, there has been a growing interest to such systems. In our opinion, the most important future challenges for attention-based BCIs include:

(1) Filtering out noise: Noise can be caused by mechanical and electrical artifacts, and it can be a neural signal that is irrelevant to the function that the BCI enables and/or augments. Noise can be reduced by proper selection of features representing a brain function of interest. Choosing the right features is especially important for therapeutic BCIs because if features are selected incorrectly, unwanted functions could be enhanced instead of the desired alleviation of an individual's disability. For instance, using the α-band to regulate attention has certain caveats. Ideally, the α-band represents suppression of irrelevant information in an attention paradigm. However, if the subject is not attending, such suppression could be confused with the drowsiness state, and the BCI would enhance drowsiness instead of working properly to enhance attention. This problem could be addressed by adding features, such as topographical information about the source of the α-oscillations.

(2) Developing of reliable criteria to quantify BCI training effects: Neurofeedback therapy is usually evaluated using a comparison of specific features before and after the training. However, enhancement in EEG features does not guarantee a behavioral improvement. For example, increase in β-band power is a popular feature indicating high attention level. If the aim is just to increase β-band oscillation, this frequency band might also be increased due to some other brain function unrelated to attention *per se*. For example, the β-band increased when motor movement had to be voluntarily suppressed in macaque monkeys (Zhang et al., 2008). Therefore, we suggest that the evaluation of neurofeedback therapy outcome should include behavioral and psychological tests to that evaluate the target function.

(3) Accounting for intra- and inter-individual variability: Sources of variability include non-stationarity of EEG signals (Vidaurre et al., 2011) as well as non-stationarities induced by the task (Iturrate et al., 2013) and different mental states of different subjects. The BCI algorithms should be able to accommodate individual characteristics of subjects, and to adapt to EEG variability during the neurofeedback therapy.

(4) Developing BCIs for individual use: current methods of NF-training require the presence of an expert to conduct the training session from the installation of scalp electrode to running the programs and maintaining the system. These

procedures impose restrictions on the usage of BCIs by patients. More user-friendly, highly automated BCIs should be developed in the future.

CONCLUSIONS

BCIs offer exciting opportunities for enhancing neural functions and developing therapies for neural disabilities, including BCIs that assist subject to regulate their neural function. Attention is a fundamental brain mechanism for selection of relevant and essential information while suppressing irrelevant signals. Disorders of this mechanism result in dysfunctions, such as ADHD. BCIs hold promise to provide effective rehabilitation strategies for individuals with impairments of attention. Several attention-based BCIs have been already developed whereas many challenges still remain. The main challenge is to combine highly technical knowledge needed to build effective BCIs with the expertise from neuroscience and psychology. Merging these multidisciplinary contributions is key to developing clinically relevant BCIs to treat attentional dysfunctions.

AUTHOR CONTRIBUTIONS

MO, ML: wrote the paper; HS, SP: edited the paper.

ACKNOWLEDGMENTS

The authors gratefully appreciate Karoline B. Doser for her valuable comments on the manuscript and Dr. Sean Bowen for editorial assistance on an earlier version of this manuscript. The original project was supported by the Department of Electrical Engineering (Biomedical Engineering) at the Technical University of Denmark (DTU), the Lundbeck Foundation and Radiometer.

REFERENCES

Ahn, M., Ahn, S., Hong, J. H., Cho, H., Kim, K., Kim, B. S., et al. (2013). Gamma band activity associated with BCI performance: simultaneous MEG/EEG study. *Front. Hum. Neurosci.* 7:848. doi: 10.3389/fnhum.2013.00848

Ales, J. M., Yates, J. L., and Norcia, A. M. (2010). V1 is not uniquely identified by polarity reversals of responses to upper and lower visual field stimuli. *Neuroimage* 52, 1401–1409. doi: 10.1016/j.neuroimage.2010.05.016

Allison, B. Z., Brunner, C., Kaiser, V., Müller-Putz, G. R., Neuper, C., and Pfurtscheller, G. (2010). Toward a hybrid brain-computer interface based on imagined movement and visual attention. *J. Neural Eng.* 7, 1–9. doi: 10.1088/1741-2560/7/2/026007

Arns, M., de Ridder, S., Strehl, U., Breteler, M., and Coenen, A. (2009). Efficacy of neurofeedback treatment in ADHD: the effects on inattention, impulsivity and hyperactivity: a meta-analysis. *Clin. EEG Neurosci.* 40, 180–189. doi: 10.1177/155005940904000311

Arns, M., Feddema, I., and Kenemans, J. L. (2014). Differential effects of theta/beta and SMR neurofeedback in ADHD on sleep onset latency. *Front. Hum. Neurosci.* 8:1019. doi: 10.3389/fnhum.2014.01019

Avisar, A., and Shalev, L. (2011). Sustained attention and behavioral characteristics associated with ADHD in adults. *Appl. Neuropsychol.* 18, 107–116. doi: 10.1080/09084282.2010.547777

Babiloni, C., Brancucci, A., Del Percio, C., Capotosto, P., Arendt-Nielsen, L., Chen, A. C., et al. (2006). Anticipatory electroencephalography alpha rhythm predicts subjective perception of pain intensity. *J. Pain* 7, 709–717. doi: 10.1016/j.jpain.2006.03.005

Bakhshayesh, A. R., Hansch, S., Wyschkon, A., Rezai, M. J., and Esser, G. (2011). Neurofeedback in ADHD: a single-blind randomized controlled trial. *Eur. Child Adolesc. Psychiatry* 20, 481–491. doi: 10.1007/s00787-011-0208-y

Ball, T., Kern, M., Mutschler, I., Aertsen, A., and Schulze-Bonhage, A. (2009). Signal quality of simultaneously recorded invasive and non-invasive EEG. *NeuroImage* 46, 708–716. doi: 10.1016/j.neuroimage.2009.02.028

Bamdadian, A., Guan, C., Ang, K. K., and Xu, J. (2014). The predictive role of pre-cue EEG rhythms on MI-based BCI classification performance. *J. Neurosci. Methods* 235, 138–144. doi: 10.1016/j.jneumeth.2014.06.011

Banaschewski, T., Brandeis, D., Heinrich, H., Albrecht, B., Brunner, E., and Rothenberger, A. (2003). Association of ADHD and conduct disorder–brain electrical evidence for the existence of a distinct subtype. *J. Child Psychol. Psychiatry* 44, 356–376. doi: 10.1111/1469-7610.00127

Banaschewski, T., Yordanova, J., Kolev, V., Heinrich, H., Albrecht, B., and Rothenberger, A. (2008). Stimulus context and motor preparation in attention-deficit/hyperactivity disorder. *Biol. Psychol.* 77, 53–62. doi: 10.1016/j.biopsycho.2007.09.003

Barry, R. J., Clarke, A. R., McCarthy, R., Selikowitz, M., Brown, C. R., and Heaven, P. C. (2009). Event-related potentials in adults with Attention-Deficit/Hyperactivity Disorder: an investigation using an inter-modal auditory/visual oddball task. *Int. J. Psychophysiol.* 71, 124–131. doi: 10.1016/j.ijpsycho.2008.09.009

Barry, R. J., Johnstone, S. J., and Clarke, A. R. (2003). A review of electrophysiology in attention-deficit/hyperactivity disorder: II. Event-related potentials. *Clin. Neurophysiol.* 114, 184–198. doi: 10.1016/S1388-2457(02)00363-2

Benzi, R., Parisi, G., Sutera, A., and Vulpiani, A. (1982). Stochastic resonance in climatic change. *Tellus* 34, 10–16. doi: 10.1111/j.2153-3490.1982.tb01787.x

Bertoletti, E., Michelini, G., Moruzzi, S., Ferrer, G., Ferini-Strambi, L., Stazi, M. A., et al. (2014). A general population twin study of conduct problems and the auditory P300 waveform. *J. Abnorm. Child Psychol.* 42, 861–869. doi: 10.1007/s10802-013-9836-7

Bianchi, L., Sami, S., Hillebrand, A., Fawcett, I. P., Quitadamo, L. R., and Seri, S. (2010). Which physiological components are more suitable for visual ERP based brain-computer interface? A preliminary MEG/EEG study. *Brain Topogr.* 23, 180–185. doi: 10.1007/s10548-010-0143-0

Biederman, J., Mick, E., and Faraone, S. V. (2000). Age-dependent decline of symptoms of attention deficit hyperactivity disorder: impact of remission definition and symptom type. *Am. J. Psychiatry* 157, 816–818. doi: 10.1176/appi.ajp.157.5.816

Bin, G., Gao, X., Wang, Y., Hong, B., and Gao, S. (2009). VEP-based brain-computer interfaces: time, frequency, and code modulations. *IEEE Comput. Intell. Mag.* 4, 22–26. doi: 10.1109/MCI.2009.934562

Brosch, T., Pourtois, G., Sander, D., and Vuilleumier, P. (2011). Additive effects of emotional, endogenous, and exogenous attention: behavioral and electrophysiological evidence. *Neuropsychologia* 49, 1779–1787. doi: 10.1016/j.neuropsychologia.2011.02.056

Broyd, S. J., Johnstone, S. J., Barry, R. J., Clarke, A. R., McCarthy, R., Selikowitz, M., et al. (2005). The effect of methylphenidate on response inhibition and the event-related potential of children with attention deficit/hyperactivity disorder. *Int. J. Psychophysiol.* 58, 47–58. doi: 10.1016/j.ijpsycho.2005.03.008

Bruhl, A. B. (2015). Making sense of real-time functional magnetic resonance imaging (rtfMRI) and rtfMRI neurofeedback. *Int. J. Neuropsychopharmacol.* 18:pyv020. doi: 10.1093/ijnp/pyv020

Burwell, S. J., Malone, S. M., Bernat, E. M., and Iacono, W. G. (2014). Does electroencephalogram phase variability account for reduced P3 brain potential in externalizing disorders? *Clin. Neurophysiol.* 125, 2007–2015. doi: 10.1016/j.clinph.2014.02.020

Busch, N. A., Dubois, J., and VanRullen, R. (2009). The phase of ongoing EEG oscillations predicts visual perception. *J. Neurosci.* 29, 7869–7876. doi: 10.1523/JNEUROSCI.0113-09.2009

Busch, N. A., and VanRullen, R. (2010). Spontaneous EEG oscillations reveal periodic sampling of visual attention. *Proc. Natl. Acad. Sci. U.S.A.* 107, 16048–16053. doi: 10.1073/pnas.1004801107

Busse, L., Katzner, S., and Treue, S. (2008). Temporal dynamics of neuronal modulation during exogenous and endogenous shifts of visual attention in macaque area MT. *Proc. Natl. Acad. Sci. U.S.A.* 105, 16380–16385. doi: 10.1073/pnas.0707369105

Cao, T., Wan, F., Wong, C. M., da Cruz, J. N., and Hu, Y. (2014). Objective evaluation of fatigue by EEG spectral analysis in steady-state visual evoked potential-based brain-computer interfaces. *Biomed. Eng. Online* 13:28. doi: 10.1186/1475-925x-13-28

Carmena, J. M., Lebedev, M. A., Crist, R. E., O'Doherty, J. E., Santucci, D. M., Dimitrov, D. F., et al. (2003). Learning to control a brain-machine interface for reaching and grasping by primates. *PLoS Biol.* 1:E42. doi: 10.1371/journal.pbio.0000042

Ceballos, G. A., and Hernandez, L. F. (2015). Non-target adjacent stimuli classification improves performance of classical ERP-based brain computer interface. *J. Neural Eng.* 12:026009. doi: 10.1088/1741-2560/12/2/026009

Christiansen, H., Reh, V., Schmidt, M. H., and Rief, W. (2014). Slow cortical potential neurofeedback and self-management training in outpatient care for children with ADHD: study protocol and first preliminary results of a randomized controlled trial. *Front. Hum. Neurosci.* 8:943. doi: 10.3389/fnhum.2014.00943

Clark, V. P., and Hillyard, S. A. (1996). Spatial selective attention affects early extrastriate but not striate components of the visual evoked potential. *J. Cogn. Neurosci.* 8, 387–402. doi: 10.1162/jocn.1996.8.5.387

Clarke, A. R., Barry, R. J., Dupuy, F. E., McCarthy, R., Selikowitz, M., and Johnstone, S. J. (2013). Excess beta activity in the EEG of children with attention-deficit/hyperactivity disorder: a disorder of arousal? *Int. J. Psychophysiol.* 89, 314–319. doi: 10.1016/j.ijpsycho.2013.04.009

Cohen, M. X. (ed.). (2013). "Overview of time-domain EEG analyses," in *Analyzing Neural Time Series Data: Theory and Practice* (London: MIT Press), 97–106.

Conners, C. K., Epstein, J. N., March, J. S., Angold, A., Wells, K. C., Klaric, J., et al. (2001). Multimodal treatment of ADHD in the MTA: an alternative outcome analysis. *J. Am. Acad. Child Adolesc. Psychiatry* 40, 159–167. doi: 10.1097/00004583-200102000-00010

Corbetta, M., Patel, G., and Shulman, G. L. (2008). The reorienting system of the human brain: from environment to theory of mind. *Neuron* 58, 306–324. doi: 10.1016/j.neuron.2008.04.017

Coyle, S., Ward, T., Markham, C., and McDarby, G. (2004). On the suitability of near-infrared (NIR) systems for next-generation brain-computer interfaces. *Physiol. Meas.* 25, 815–822. doi: 10.1088/0967-3334/25/4/003

Crone, N. E., Sinai, A., and Korzeniewska, A. (2006). High-frequency gamma oscillations and human brain mapping with electrocorticography. *Prog. Brain Res.* 159, 275–295. doi: 10.1016/S0079-6123(06)59019-3

Daitch, A. L., Sharma, M., Roland, J. L., Astafiev, S. V., Bundy, D. T., Gaona, C. M., et al. (2013). Frequency-specific mechanism links human brain networks for spatial attention. *Proc. Natl. Acad. Sci. U.S.A.* 110, 19585–19590. doi: 10.1073/pnas.1307947110

deCharms, R. C., Maeda, F., Glover, G. H., Ludlow, D., Pauly, J. M., Soneji, D., et al. (2005). Control over brain activation and pain learned by using real-time functional MRI. *Proc. Natl. Acad. Sci. U.S.A.* 102, 18626–18631. doi: 10.1073/pnas.0505210102

de Haan, B., Morgan, P. S., and Rorden, C. (2008). Covert orienting of attention and overt eye movements activate identical brain regions. *Brain Res.* 1204, 102–111. doi: 10.1016/j.brainres.2008.01.105

Desimone, R., and Duncan, J. (1995). Neural mechanisms of selective visual attention. *Annu. Rev. Neurosci.* 18, 193–222. doi: 10.1146/annurev.ne.18.030195.001205

De Vos, M., Kroesen, M., Emkes, R., and Debener, S. (2014). P300 speller BCI with a mobile EEG system: comparison to a traditional amplifier. *J. Neural Eng.* 11:036008. doi: 10.1088/1741-2560/11/3/036008

Dirlikov, B., Shiels Rosch, K., Crocetti, D., Denckla, M. B., Mahone, E. M., and Mostofsky, S. H. (2015). Distinct frontal lobe morphology in girls and boys with ADHD. *Neuroimage Clin.* 7, 222–229. doi: 10.1016/j.nicl.2014.12.010

Di Russo, F., Martinez, A., Sereno, M. I., Pitzalis, S., and Hillyard, S. A. (2002). Cortical sources of the early components of the visual evoked potential. *Hum. Brain Mapp.* 15, 95–111. doi: 10.1002/hbm.10010

Dmochowski, J. P., Greaves, A. S., and Norcia, A. M. (2015). Maximally reliable spatial filtering of steady state visual evoked potentials. *Neuroimage* 109, 63–72. doi: 10.1016/j.neuroimage.2014.12.078

Dobkin, B. H. (2007). Brain-computer interface technology as a tool to augment plasticity and outcomes for neurological rehabilitation. *J. Physiol.* 579, 637–642. doi: 10.1113/jphysiol.2006.123067

Donoghue, J. P., Nurmikko, A., Friehs, G., and Black, M. (2004). Development of neuromotor prostheses for humans. *Suppl. Clin. Neurophysiol.* 57, 592–606. doi: 10.1016/S1567-424X(09)70399-X

Doyle, A. E., Willcutt, E. G., Seidman, L. J., Biederman, J., Chouinard, V. A., Silva, J., et al. (2005). Attention-deficit/hyperactivity disorder endophenotypes. *Biol. Psychiatry* 57, 1324–1335. doi: 10.1016/j.biopsych.2005.03.015

Dreyer, A. M., and Herrmann, C. S. (2015). Frequency-modulated steady-state visual evoked potentials: a new stimulation method for brain-computer interfaces. *J. Neurosci. Methods* 241, 1–9. doi: 10.1016/j.jneumeth.2014.12.004

Dupuy, F. E., Clarke, A. R., Barry, R. J., McCarthy, R., and Selikowitz, M. (2013). EEG differences between the combined and inattentive types of attention-deficit/hyperactivity disorder in girls: a further investigation. *Clin. EEG Neurosci.* 45, 231–237. doi: 10.1177/1550059413501162

Egeth, H. E., and Yantis, S. (1997). Visual attention: control, representation, and time course. *Annu. Rev. Psychol.* 48, 269–297. doi: 10.1146/annurev.psych.48.1.269

Elbert, T., Rockstroh, B., Lutzenberger, W., and Birbaumer, N. (1980). Biofeedback of slow cortical potentials. I. *Electroencephalogr. Clin. Neurophysiol.* 48, 293–301. doi: 10.1016/0013-4694(80)90265-5

Ergenoglu, T., Demiralp, T., Bayraktaroglu, Z., Ergen, M., Beydagi, H., and Uresin, Y. (2004). Alpha rhythm of the EEG modulates visual detection performance in humans. *Brain Res. Cogn. Brain Res.* 20, 376–383. doi: 10.1016/j.cogbrainres.2004.03.009

Escolano, C., Navarro-Gil, M., Garcia-Campayo, J., Congedo, M., and Minguez, J. (2014). The effects of individual upper alpha neurofeedback in ADHD: an open-label pilot study. *Appl. Psychophysiol. Biofeedback* 39, 193–202. doi: 10.1007/s10484-014-9257-6

Fan, J., McCandliss, B. D., Fossella, J., Flombaum, J. I., and Posner, M. I. (2005). The activation of attentional networks. *Neuroimage* 26, 471–479. doi: 10.1016/j.neuroimage.2005.02.004

Faraone, S. V., Biederman, J., and Mick, E. (2006). The age-dependent decline of attention deficit hyperactivity disorder: a meta-analysis of follow-up studies. *Psychol. Med.* 36, 159–165. doi: 10.1017/S003329170500471X

Farwell, L. A., and Donchin, E. (1988). Talking off the top of your head: toward a mental prosthesis utilizing event-related brain potentials. *Electroencephalogr. Clin. Neurophysiol.* 70, 510–523. doi: 10.1016/0013-4694(88)90149-6

Fazli, S., Mehnert, J., Steinbrink, J., Curio, G., Villringer, A., Muller, K. R., et al. (2012). Enhanced performance by a hybrid NIRS-EEG brain computer interface. *Neuroimage* 59, 519–529. doi: 10.1016/j.neuroimage.2011.07.084

Ferrier, D. (1876). *The Function of the Brain.* London: Smith, Elder & Co.

Fleming, A. P., and McMahon, R. J. (2012). Developmental context and treatment principles for ADHD among college students. *Clin. Child Fam. Psychol. Rev.* 15, 303–329. doi: 10.1007/s10567-012-0121-z

Freeman, W. J., Holmes, M. D., Burke, B. C., and Vanhatalo, S. (2003). Spatial spectra of scalp EEG and EMG from awake humans. *Clin. Neurophysiol.* 114, 1053–1068. doi: 10.1016/S1388-2457(03)00045-2

Freeman, W. J., Rogers, L. J., Holmes, M. D., and Silbergeld, D. L. (2000). Spatial spectral analysis of human electrocorticograms including the alpha and gamma bands. *J. Neurosci. Methods* 95, 111–121. doi: 10.1016/S0165-0270(99)00160-0

Friedman, D., Cycowicz, Y. M., and Gaeta, H. (2001). The novelty P3: an event-related brain potential (ERP) sign of the brain's evaluation of novelty. *Neurosci. Biobehav. Rev.* 25, 355–373. doi: 10.1016/S0149-7634(01)00019-7

Fries, P., Reynolds, J. H., Rorie, A. E., and Desimone, R. (2001). Modulation of oscillatory neuronal synchronization by selective visual attention. *Science* 291, 1560–1563. doi: 10.1126/science.1055465

Fu, K. M., Foxe, J. J., Murray, M. M., Higgins, B. A., Javitt, D. C., and Schroeder, C. E. (2001). Attention-dependent suppression of distracter visual input can be cross-modally cued as indexed by anticipatory parieto-occipital alpha-band oscillations. *Brain Res. Cogn. Brain Res.* 12, 145–152. doi: 10.1016/S0926-6410(01)00034-9

Fu, S., Fedota, J. R., Greenwood, P. M., and Parasuraman, R. (2010). Dissociation of visual C1 and P1 components as a function of attentional load: an event-related potential study. *Biol. Psychol.* 85, 171–178. doi: 10.1016/j.biopsycho.2010.06.008

Furdea, A., Halder, S., Krusienski, D. J., Bross, D., Nijboer, F., Birbaumer, N., et al. (2009). An auditory oddball (P300). spelling system for brain-computer interfaces. *Psychophysiology* 46, 617–625. doi: 10.1111/j.1469-8986.2008.00783.x

Garcia, J. O., Srinivasan, R., and Serences, J. T. (2013). Near-real-time feature-selective modulations in human cortex. *Curr. Biol.* 23, 515–522. doi: 10.1016/j.cub.2013.02.013

Gevensleben, H., Holl, B., Albrecht, B., Vogel, C., Schlamp, D., Kratz, O., et al. (2009). Is neurofeedback an efficacious treatment for ADHD? A randomised controlled clinical trial. *J. Child Psychol. Psychiatry* 50, 780–789. doi: 10.1111/j.1469-7610.2008.02033.x

Gevensleben, H., Moll, G. H., Rothenberger, A., and Heinrich, H. (2014). Neurofeedback in attention-deficit/hyperactivity disorder - different models, different ways of application. *Front. Hum. Neurosci.* 8:846. doi: 10.3389/fnhum.2014.00846

Gherri, E., and Eimer, M. (2011). Active listening impairs visual perception and selectivity: an ERP study of auditory dual-task costs on visual attention. *J. Cogn. Neurosci.* 23, 832–844. doi: 10.1162/jocn.2010.21468

Golla, H., Thier, P., and Haarmeier, T. (2005). Disturbed overt but normal covert shifts of attention in adult cerebellar patients. *Brain* 128, 1525–1535. doi: 10.1093/brain/awh523

Gomes, H., Duff, M., Ramos, M., Molholm, S., Foxe, J. J., and Halperin, J. (2012). Auditory selective attention and processing in children with attention-deficit/hyperactivity disorder. *Clin. Neurophysiol.* 123, 293–302. doi: 10.1016/j.clinph.2011.07.030

Greenhill, L. L., Swanson, J. M., Vitiello, B., Davies, M., Clevenger, W., Wu, M., et al. (2001). Impairment and deportment responses to different methylphenidate doses in children with ADHD: the MTA titration trial. *J. Am. Acad. Child Adolesc. Psychiatry* 40, 180–187. doi: 10.1097/00004583-200102000-00012

Grosse-Wentrup, M., and Scholkopf, B. (2014). A brain-computer interface based on self-regulation of gamma-oscillations in the superior parietal cortex. *J. Neural Eng.* 11:056015. doi: 10.1088/1741-2560/11/5/056015

Hanslmayr, S., Aslan, A., Staudigl, T., Klimesch, W., Herrmann, C. S., and Bauml, K. H. (2007). Prestimulus oscillations predict visual perception performance between and within subjects. *Neuroimage* 37, 1465–1473. doi: 10.1016/j.neuroimage.2007.07.011

Harnois, C., Bodis-Wollner, I., and Onofrj, M. (1984). The effect of contrast and spatial frequency on the visual evoked potential of the hooded rat. *Exp. Brain Res.* 57, 1–8. doi: 10.1007/BF00231126

Harter, M. R., Aine, C., and Schroeder, C. (1984). Hemispheric differences in event-related potential measures of selective attention. *Ann. N.Y. Acad. Sci.* 425, 210–211. doi: 10.1111/j.1749-6632.1984.tb23535.x

He, N., Li, F., Li, Y., Guo, L., Chen, L., Huang, X., et al. (2015). Neuroanatomical deficits correlate with executive dysfunction in boys with attention deficit hyperactivity disorder. *Neurosci. Lett.* 600, 45–49. doi: 10.1016/j.neulet.2015.05.062

Heinrich, H., Busch, K., Studer, P., Erbe, K., Moll, G. H., and Kratz, O. (2014). EEG spectral analysis of attention in ADHD: implications for neurofeedback training? *Front. Hum. Neurosci.* 8:611. doi: 10.3389/fnhum.2014.00611

Hillard, B., El-Baz, A. S., Sears, L., Tasman, A., and Sokhadze, E. M. (2013). Neurofeedback training aimed to improve focused attention and alertness in children with ADHD: a study of relative power of EEG rhythms using custom-made software application. *Clin. EEG Neurosci.* 44, 193–202. doi: 10.1177/1550059412458262

Hillyard, S. A., and Anllo-Vento, L. (1998). Event-related brain potentials in the study of visual selective attention. *Proc. Natl. Acad. Sci. U.S.A.* 95, 781–787. doi: 10.1073/pnas.95.3.781

Hillyard, S. A., Vogel, E. K., and Luck, S. J. (1998). Sensory gain control (amplification) as a mechanism of selective attention: electrophysiological and neuroimaging evidence. *Philos. Trans. R. Soc. Lond. B. Biol. Sci.* 353, 1257–1270. doi: 10.1098/rstb.1998.0281

Holtmann, M., Pniewski, B., Wachtlin, D., Worz, S., and Strehl, U. (2014a). Neurofeedback in children with attention-deficit/hyperactivity disorder (ADHD)–a controlled multicenter study of a non-pharmacological treatment approach. *BMC Pediatr.* 14:202. doi: 10.1186/1471-2431-14-202

Holtmann, M., Sonuga-Barke, E., Cortese, S., and Brandeis, D. (2014b). Neurofeedback for ADHD: a review of current evidence. *Child Adolesc. Psychiatr. Clin. N. Am.* 23, 789–806. doi: 10.1016/j.chc.2014.05.006

Ifft, P. J., Shokur, S., Li, Z., Lebedev, M. A., and Nicolelis, M. A. (2013). A brain-machine interface enables bimanual arm movements in monkeys. *Sci. Transl. Med.* 5, 210ra154. doi: 10.1126/scitranslmed.3006159

Ignashchenkova, A., Dicke, P. W., Haarmeier, T., and Their, P. (2004). Neuron-specific contribution of the superior colliculus to overt and covert shifts of attention. *Nat. Neurosci.* 7, 56–64. doi: 10.1038/nn1169

Iturrate, I., Montesano, L., and Minguez, J. (2013). Shared-control brain-computer interface for a two dimensional reaching task using EEG error-related potentials. *Conf. Proc. IEEE Eng. Med. Biol. Soc.* 2013, 5258–5262. doi: 10.1109/embc.2013.6610735

Jones, A., Hughes, G., and Waszak, F. (2013). The interaction between attention and motor prediction. An ERP study. *Neuroimage* 83, 533–541. doi: 10.1016/j.neuroimage.2013.07.004

Jonkman, L. M., Kenemans, J. L., Kemner, C., Verbaten, M. N., and van Engeland, H. (2004). Dipole source localization of event-related brain activity indicative of an early visual selective attention deficit in ADHD children. *Clin. Neurophysiol.* 115, 1537–1549. doi: 10.1016/j.clinph.2004.01.022

Kahana, M. J. (2006). The cognitive correlates of human brain oscillations. *J. Neurosci.* 26, 1669–1672. doi: 10.1523/JNEUROSCI.3737-05c.2006

Kaiser, J., and Lutzenberger, W. (2005). Human gamma-band activity: a window to cognitive processing. *Neuroreport* 16, 207–211. doi: 10.1097/00001756-200502280-00001

Kanoh, S., Murayama, Y. M., Miyamoto, K., Yoshinobu, T., and Kawashima, R. (2009). A NIRS-based brain-computer interface system during motor imagery: system development and online feedback training. *Conf. Proc. IEEE Eng. Med. Biol. Soc.* 2009, 594–597. doi: 10.1109/IEMBS.2009.5333710

Kashihara, K. (2014). A brain-computer interface for potential non-verbal facial communication based on EEG signals related to specific emotions. *Front. Neurosci.* 8:244. doi: 10.3389/fnins.2014.00244

Kelly, S. P., Gomez-Ramirez, M., and Foxe, J. J. (2008). Spatial attention modulates initial afferent activity in human primary visual cortex. *Cereb. Cortex* 18, 2629–2636. doi: 10.1093/cercor/bhn022

Kelly, S. P., Schroeder, C. E., and Lalor, E. C. (2013). What does polarity inversion of extrastriate activity tell us about striate contributions to the early VEP? A comment on Ales et al. (2010). *Neuroimage* 76, 442–445. doi: 10.1016/j.neuroimage.2012.03.081

Keune, P. M., Wiedemann, E., Schneidt, A., and Schonenberg, M. (2015). Frontal brain asymmetry in adult attention-deficit/hyperactivity disorder (ADHD): extending the motivational dysfunction hypothesis. *Clin. Neurophysiol.* 126, 711–720. doi: 10.1016/j.clinph.2014.07.008

Khan, M. J., Hong, M. J., and Hong, K. S. (2014). Decoding of four movement directions using hybrid NIRS-EEG brain-computer interface. *Front. Hum. Neurosci.* 8:244. doi: 10.3389/fnhum.2014.00244

Kim, Y. J., Grabowecky, M., Paller, K. A., and Suzuki, S. (2011). Differential roles of frequency-following and frequency-doubling visual responses revealed by evoked neural harmonics. *J. Cogn. Neurosci.* 23, 1875–1886. doi: 10.1162/jocn.2010.21536

Klimesch, W. (2011). Evoked alpha and early access to the knowledge system: the P1 inhibition timing hypothesis. *Brain Res.* 1408, 52–71. doi: 10.1016/j.brainres.2011.06.003

Koelewijn, L., Rich, A. N., Muthukumaraswamy, S. D., and Singh, K. D. (2013). Spatial attention increases high-frequency gamma synchronisation in human medial visual cortex. *Neuroimage* 79, 295–303. doi: 10.1016/j.neuroimage.2013.04.108

Kollins, S. H. (2008). ADHD, substance use disorders, and psychostimulant treatment: current literature and treatment guidelines. *J. Atten. Disord.* 12, 115–125. doi: 10.1177/1087054707311654

Kooij, J. J., and Bijlenga, D. (2014). High prevalence of self-reported photophobia in adult ADHD. *Front. Neurol.* 5:256. doi: 10.3389/fneur.2014.00256

Kus, R., Duszyk, A., Milanowski, P., Labecki, M., Bierzynska, M., Radzikowska, Z., et al. (2013). On the quantification of SSVEP frequency responses in human EEG in realistic BCI conditions. *PLoS ONE* 8:e77536. doi: 10.1371/journal.pone.0077536

Lakatos, P., Karmos, G., Mehta, A. D., Ulbert, I., and Schroeder, C. E. (2008). Entrainment of neuronal oscillations as a mechanism of attentional selection. *Science* 320, 110–113. doi: 10.1126/science.1154735

Latham, A. J., Patston, L. L., Westermann, C., Kirk, I. J., and Tippett, L. J. (2013). Earlier visual N1 latencies in expert video-game players: a temporal basis of enhanced visuospatial performance? *PLoS ONE* 8:e75231. doi: 10.1371/journal.pone.0075231

Lebedev, M. A. (2014). How to read neuron-dropping curves? *Front. Syst. Neurosci.* 8:102. doi: 10.3389/fnsys.2014.00102

Lebedev, M. A., Carmena, J. M., O'Doherty, J. E., Zacksenhouse, M., Henriquez, C. S., Principe, J. C., et al. (2005). Cortical ensemble adaptation to represent velocity of an artificial actuator controlled by a brain-machine interface. *J. Neurosci.* 25, 4681–4693. doi: 10.1523/JNEUROSCI.4088-04.2005

Lebedev, M. A., Messinger, A., Kralik, J. D., and Wise, S. P. (2004). Representation of attended versus remembered locations in prefrontal cortex. *PLoS Biol.* 2:e365. doi: 10.1371/journal.pbio.0020365

Lebedev, M. A., and Nicolelis, M. A. (2006). Brain-machine interfaces: past, present and future. *Trends Neurosci.* 29, 536–546. doi: 10.1016/j.tins.2006.07.004

Lebedev, M. A., Tate, A. J., Hanson, T. L., Li, Z., O'Doherty, J. E., Winans, J. A., et al. (2011). Future developments in brain-machine interface research. *Clinics* 66(Suppl. 1), 25–32. doi: 10.1590/s1807-59322011001300004

Lebedev, M. A., and Wise, S. P. (2001). Tuning for the orientation of spatial attention in dorsal premotor cortex. *Eur. J. Neurosci.* 13, 1002–1008. doi: 10.1046/j.0953-816x.2001.01457.x

Lee, J. H., Ryu, J., Jolesz, F. A., Cho, Z. H., and Yoo, S. S. (2009). Brain-machine interface via real-time fMRI: preliminary study on thought-controlled robotic arm. *Neurosci. Lett.* 450, 1–6. doi: 10.1016/j.neulet.2008.11.024

Leins, U., Goth, G., Hinterberger, T., Klinger, C., Rumpf, N., and Strehl, U. (2007). Neurofeedback for children with ADHD: a comparison of SCP and Theta/Beta protocols. *Appl. Psychophysiol. Biofeedback* 32, 73–88. doi: 10.1007/s10484-007-9031-0

Lesenfants, D., Habbal, D., Lugo, Z., Lebeau, M., Horki, P., Amico, E., et al. (2014). An independent SSVEP-based brain-computer interface in locked-in syndrome. *J. Neural Eng.* 11:035002. doi: 10.1088/1741-2560/11/3/035002

Leuthardt, E. C., Freudenberg, Z., Bundy, D., and Roland, J. (2009). Microscale recording from human motor cortex: implications for minimally invasive electrocorticographic brain-computer interfaces. *Neurosurg. Focus* 27:E10. doi: 10.3171/2009.4.FOCUS0980

Leuthardt, E. C., Schalk, G., Wolpaw, J. R., Ojemann, J. G., and Moran, D. W. (2004). A brain-computer interface using electrocorticographic signals in humans. *J. Neural Eng.* 1, 63–71. doi: 10.1088/1741-2560/1/2/001

Lim, C. G., Lee, T. S., Guan, C., Fung, D. S., Zhao, Y., Teng, S. S., et al. (2012). A brain-computer interface based attention training program for treating attention deficit hyperactivity disorder. *PLoS ONE* 7:e46692. doi: 10.1371/journal.pone.0046692

Lim, C. G., Lee, T. S., Guan, C., Sheng Fung, D. S., Cheung, Y. B., Teng, S. S., et al. (2010). Effectiveness of a brain-computer interface based programme for the treatment of ADHD: a pilot study. *Psychopharmacol. Bull.* 43, 73–82.

Lin, F. C., Zao, J. K., Tu, K. C., Wang, Y., Huang, Y. P., Chuang, C. W., et al. (2012). SNR analysis of high-frequency steady-state visual evoked potentials from the foveal and extrafoveal regions of human retina. *Conf. Proc. IEEE. Eng. Med. Biol. Soc.* 2012, 1810–1814. doi: 10.1109/EMBC.2012.6346302

Lofthouse, N., Arnold, L. E., Hersch, S., Hurt, E., and DeBeus, R. (2012a). A review of neurofeedback treatment for pediatric ADHD. *J. Atten. Disord.* 16, 351–372. doi: 10.1177/1087054711427530

Lofthouse, N., Arnold, L. E., and Hurt, E. (2012b). Current status of neurofeedback for attention-deficit/hyperactivity disorder. *Curr. Psychiatry Rep.* 14, 536–542. doi: 10.1007/s11920-012-0301-z

Logothetis, N. K. (2003). MR imaging in the non-human primate: studies of function and of dynamic connectivity. *Curr. Opin. Neurobiol.* 13, 630–642. doi: 10.1016/j.conb.2003.09.017

Luck, S. J. (2005). *An Introduction to the Event-Related Potential Technique.* Cambridge, MA: MIT.

Luck, S. J. (ed.). (2014). "Overview of common ERP components" in *An Introduction to the Event-Related Potential Technique* (London: MIT Press), 71–118.

Luck, S. J., and Hillyard, S. A. (1995). The role of attention in feature detection and conjunction discrimination: an electrophysiological analysis. *Int. J. Neurosci.* 80, 281–297. doi: 10.3109/00207459508986105

Lutzenberger, W., Elbert, T., Rockstroh, B., and Birbaumer, N. (1980). Biofeedback of slow cortical potentials. II. Analysis of single event-related slow potentials by time series analysis. *Electroencephalogr. Clin. Neurophysiol.* 48, 302–311. doi: 10.1016/0013-4694(80)90266-7

Lynn, R., and Eysenck, H. J. (1966). *Attention, Arousal and the Orientation Reaction: International Series of Monographs in Experimental Psychology.* Oxford: Pergamon Press.

Makeig, S., Westerfield, M., Jung, T. P., Enghoff, S., Townsend, J., Courchesne, E., et al. (2002). Dynamic brain sources of visual evoked responses. *Science* 295, 690–694. doi: 10.1126/science.1066168

Mangun, G. R., Hinrichs, H., Scholz, M., Mueller-Gaertner, H. W., Herzog, H., Krause, B. J., et al. (2001). Integrating electrophysiology and neuroimaging of spatial selective attention to simple isolated visual stimuli. *Vision Res.* 41, 1423–1435. doi: 10.1016/S0042-6989(01)00046-3

Margalit, E., Weiland, J. D., Clatterbuck, R. E., Fujii, G. Y., Maia, M., Tameesh, M., et al. (2003). Visual and electrical evoked response recorded from subdural electrodes implanted above the visual cortex in normal dogs under two methods of anesthesia. *J. Neurosci. Methods* 123, 129–137. doi: 10.1016/S0165-0270(02)00345X

Martinez, A., Anllo-Vento, L., Sereno, M. I., Frank, L. R., Buxton, R. B., Dubowitz, D. J., et al. (1999). Involvement of striate and extrastriate visual cortical areas in spatial attention. *Nat. Neurosci.* 2, 364–369. doi: 10.1038/7274

Matheson, H., Newman, A. J., Satel, J., and McMullen, P. (2014). Handles of manipulable objects attract covert visual attention: ERP evidence. *Brain Cogn.* 86, 17–23. doi: 10.1016/j.bandc.2014.01.013

Medina, L. E., Lebedev, M. A., O'Doherty, J. E., and Nicolelis, M. A. (2012). Stochastic facilitation of artificial tactile sensation in primates. *J. Neurosci.* 32, 14271–14275. doi: 10.1523/JNEUROSCI.3115-12.2012

Mellinger, J., Schalk, G., Braun, C., Preissl, H., Rosenstiel, W., Birbaumer, N., et al. (2007). An MEG-based brain-computer interface (BCI). *Neuroimage* 36, 581–593. doi: 10.1016/j.neuroimage.2007.03.019

Micoulaud-Franchi, J. A., Geoffroy, P. A., Fond, G., Lopez, R., Bioulac, S., and Philip, P. (2014). EEG neurofeedback treatments in children with ADHD: an updated meta-analysis of randomized controlled trials. *Front. Hum. Neurosci.* 8:906. doi: 10.3389/fnhum.2014.00906

Millichap, J. G. (2008). Etiologic classification of attention-deficit/hyperactivity disorder. *Pediatrics* 121, e358–e365. doi: 10.1542/peds.2007-1332

Ming, D., Xi, Y., Zhang, M., Qi, H., Cheng, L., Wan, B., et al. (2009). Electroencephalograph (EEG) signal processing method of motor imaginary potential for attention level classification. *IEEE Eng. Med. Biol. Soc.* 2009, 4347–4351. doi: 10.1109/iembs.2009.5332743

Muller, M. M., and Hillyard, S. (2000). Concurrent recording of steady-state and transient event-related potentials as indices of visual-spatial selective attention. *Clin. Neurophysiol.* 111, 1544–1552. doi: 10.1016/S1388-2457(00)00371-0

Muller-Putz, G. R., and Pfurtscheller, G. (2008). Control of an electrical prosthesis with an SSVEP-based BCI. *IEEE Trans. Biomed. Eng.* 55, 361–364. doi: 10.1109/TBME.2007.897815

Muller-Putz, G. R., Scherer, R., Brauneis, C., and Pfurtscheller, G. (2005). Steady-state visual evoked potential (SSVEP)-based communication: impact of harmonic frequency components. *J. Neural Eng.* 2, 123–130. doi: 10.1088/1741-2560/2/4/008

Musch, K., Hamame, C. M., Perrone-Bertolotti, M., Minotti, L., Kahane, P., Engel, A. K., et al. (2014). Selective attention modulates high-frequency activity in the face-processing network. *Cortex* 60, 34–51. doi: 10.1016/j.cortex.2014.06.006

Nagendra, H., Kumar, V., and Mukherjee, S. (2015). Cognitive behavior evaluation based on physiological parameters among young healthy subjects with yoga as intervention. *Comput. Math. Methods Med.* 2015:821061. doi: 10.1155/2015/821061

Nicolas-Alonso, L. F., and Gomez-Gil, J. (2012). Brain computer interfaces, a review. *Sensors* 12, 1211–1279. doi: 10.3390/s120201211

Nicolelis, M. A., Dimitrov, D., Carmena, J. M., Crist, R., Lehew, G., Kralik, J. D., et al. (2003). Chronic, multisite, multielectrode recordings in macaque monkeys. *Proc. Natl. Acad. Sci. U.S.A.* 100, 11041–11046. doi: 10.1073/pnas.1934665100

Nicolelis, M. A., and Lebedev, M. A. (2009). Principles of neural ensemble physiology underlying the operation of brain-machine interfaces. *Nat. Rev. Neurosci.* 10, 530–540. doi: 10.1038/nrn2653

Nicolelis, M. A., and Ribeiro, S. (2002). Multielectrode recordings: the next steps. *Curr. Opin. Neurobiol.* 12, 602–606. doi: 10.1016/S0959-4388(02)00374-4

O'Doherty, J. E., Lebedev, M. A., Ifft, P. J., Zhuang, K. Z., Shokur, S., Bleuler, H., et al. (2011). Active tactile exploration using a brain-machine-brain interface. *Nature* 479, 228–231. doi: 10.1038/nature10489

Okazaki, Y. O., Horschig, J. M., Luther, L., Oostenveld, R., Murakami, I., and Jensen, O. (2015). Real-time MEG neurofeedback training of posterior alpha activity modulates subsequent visual detection performance. *Neuroimage* 107, 323–332. doi: 10.1016/j.neuroimage.2014.12.014

Ordikhani-Seyedlar, M., Sorensen, H. B., Kjaer, T. W., Siebner, H. R., and Puthusserypady, S. (2014). SSVEP-modulation by covert and overt attention: novel features for BCI in attention neuro-rehabilitation. *IEEE Eng. Med. Biol. Soc.* 2014, 5462–5465. doi: 10.1109/embc.2014.6944862

Ortega, R., Lopez, V., Carrasco, X., Anllo-Vento, L., and Aboitiz, F. (2013). Exogenous orienting of visual-spatial attention in ADHD children. *Brain Res.* 1493, 68–79. doi: 10.1016/j.brainres.2012.11.036

Ozaki, I., Yaegashi, Y., Baba, M., and Hashimoto, I. (2006). High-frequency oscillatory activities during selective attention in humans. *Suppl. Clin. Neurophysiol.* 59, 57–60. doi: 10.1016/S1567-424X(09)70012-1

Pais-Vieira, M., Lebedev, M., Kunicki, C., Wang, J., and Nicolelis, M. A. (2013). A brain-to-brain interface for real-time sharing of sensorimotor information. *Sci. Rep.* 3:1319. doi: 10.1038/srep01319

Palomares, M., Ales, J. M., Wade, A. R., Cottereau, B. R., and Norcia, A. M. (2012). Distinct effects of attention on the neural responses to form and motion processing: a SSVEP source-imaging study. *J. Vis.* 12:15. doi: 10.1167/12.10.15

Panicker, R. C., Puthusserypady, S., and Sun, Y. (2011). An asynchronous P300 BCI with SSVEP-based control state detection. *IEEE Trans. Biomed. Eng.* 58, 1781–1788. doi: 10.1109/TBME.2011.2116018

Peikon, I. D., Fitzsimmons, N. A., Lebedev, M. A., and Nicolelis, M. A. (2009). Three-dimensional, automated, real-time video system for tracking limb motion in brain-machine interface studies. *J. Neurosci. Methods* 180, 224–233. doi: 10.1016/j.jneumeth.2009.03.010

Petersen, S. E., and Posner, M. I. (2012). The attention system of the human brain: 20 years after. *Annu. Rev. Neurosci.* 35, 73–89. doi: 10.1146/annurev-neuro-062111-150525

Polanczyk, G., and Rohde, L. A. (2007). Epidemiology of attention-deficit/hyperactivity disorder across the lifespan. *Curr. Opin. Psychiatry* 20, 386–392. doi: 10.1097/YCO.0b013e3281568d7a

Sutter, E. E., and Tran, D. (1992). The field topography of ERG components in man–I. The photopic luminance response. *Vision Res.* 32, 433–446. doi: 10.1016/0042-6989(92)90235-B

Polich, J. (2007). Updating P300: an integrative theory of P3a and P3b. *Clin. Neurophysiol.* 118, 2128–2148. doi: 10.1016/j.clinph.2007.04.019

Polich, J., and Bondurant, T. (1997). P300 sequence effects, probability, and interstimulus interval. *Physiol. Behav.* 61, 843–849. doi: 10.1016/S0031-9384(96)00564-1

Posner, M. I. (1980). Orienting of attention. *Q. J. Exp. Psychol.* 32, 3–25. doi: 10.1080/00335558008248231

Posner, M. I. (1994). Attention: the mechanisms of consciousness. *Proc. Natl. Acad. Sci. U.S.A.* 91, 7398–7403. doi: 10.1073/pnas.91.16.7398

Posner, M. I. (2012). Attentional networks and consciousness. *Front. Psychol.* 3:64. doi: 10.3389/fpsyg.2012.00064

Posner, M. I., and Rothbart, M. K. (2007). Research on attention networks as a model for the integration of psychological science. *Annu. Rev. Psychol.* 58, 1–23. doi: 10.1146/annurev.psych.58.110405.085516

Posner, M. I., Snyder, C. R., and Davidson, B. J. (1980). Attention and the detection of signals. *J. Exp. Psychol.* 109, 160–174. doi: 10.1037/0096-3445.109.2.160

Power, S. D., Kushki, A., and Chau, T. (2012). Automatic single-trial discrimination of mental arithmetic, mental singing and the no-control state from prefrontal activity: toward a three-state NIRS-BCI. *BMC Res. Notes* 5:141. doi: 10.1186/1756-0500-5-141

Praamstra, P., Boutsen, L., and Humphreys, G. W. (2005). Frontoparietal control of spatial attention and motor intention in human EEG. *J. Neurophysiol.* 94, 764–774. doi: 10.1152/jn.01052.2004

Pritchard, V. E., Neumann, E., and Rucklidge, J. J. (2008). Selective attention and inhibitory deficits in ADHD: does subtype or comorbidity modulate negative priming effects? *Brain Cogn.* 67, 324–339. doi: 10.1016/j.bandc.2008.02.002

Punsawad, Y., and Wongsawat, Y. (2012). Motion visual stimulus for SSVEP-based BCI system. *IEEE Eng. Med. Biol. Soc.* 2012, 3837–3840. doi: 10.1109/embc.2012.6346804

Ray, S., Niebur, E., Hsiao, S. S., Sinai, A., and Crone, N. E. (2008). High-frequency gamma activity (80-150Hz) is increased in human cortex during selective attention. *Clin. Neurophysiol.* 119, 116–133. doi: 10.1016/j.clinph.2007.09.136

Reuter, E. M., Bednark, J., and Cunnington, R. (2015). Reliance on visual attention during visuomotor adaptation: an SSVEP study. *Exp. Brain Res.* 233, 2041–2051. doi: 10.1007/s00221-015-4275-z

Rizzolatti, G., Riggio, L., Dascola, I., and Umilta, C. (1987). Reorienting attention across the horizontal and vertical meridians: evidence in favor of a premotor theory of attention. *Neuropsychologia* 25, 31–40. doi: 10.1016/0028-3932(87)90041-8

Rohenkohl, G., and Nobre, A. C. (2011). alpha oscillations related to anticipatory attention follow temporal expectations. *J. Neurosci.* 31, 14076–14084. doi: 10.1523/JNEUROSCI.3387-11.2011

Rossini, P. M., Noris Ferilli, M. A., and Ferreri, F. (2012). Cortical plasticity and brain computer interface. *Eur. J. Phys. Rehabil. Med.* 48, 307–312.

Rougeul-Buser, A., and Buser, P. (1997). Rhythms in the alpha band in cats and their behavioural correlates. *Int. J. Psychophysiol.* 26, 191–203. doi: 10.1016/S0167-8760(97)00764-2

Ruiz, S., Birbaumer, N., and Sitaram, R. (2013). Abnormal neural connectivity in schizophrenia and fMRI-brain-computer interface as a potential therapeutic approach. *Front. Psychiatry* 4:17. doi: 10.3389/fpsyt.2013.00017

Sakurada, T., Kawase, T., Komatsu, T., and Kansaku, K. (2015). Use of high-frequency visual stimuli above the critical flicker frequency in a SSVEP-based BMI. *Clin. Neurophysiol.* 126, 1972–1978. doi: 10.1016/j.clinph.2014.12.010

Sanei, S., and Chambers, J. (2008). "Brain-computer interface," in *EEG Signal Processing*, eds S. Sanei and J. Chambers (Chichester: John Wiley & Sons), 239–261.

Sato, J. R., Basilio, R., Paiva, F. F., Garrido, G. J., Bramati, I. E., Bado, P., et al. (2013). Real-time fMRI pattern decoding and neurofeedback using FRIEND: an FSL-integrated BCI toolbox. *PLoS ONE* 8:e81658. doi: 10.1371/journal.pone.0081658

Schalk, G. (2010). Can electrocorticography (ECoG) support robust and powerful brain-computer interfaces? *Front. Neuroeng.* 3:9. doi: 10.3389/fneng.2010.00009

Schalk, G., and Leuthardt, E. C. (2011). Brain-computer interfaces using electrocorticographic signals. *IEEE Rev. Biomed. Eng.* 4, 140–154. doi: 10.1109/RBME.2011.2172408

Schwarz, D. A., Lebedev, M. A., Hanson, T. L., Dimitrov, D. F., Lehew, G., Meloy, J., et al. (2014). Chronic, wireless recordings of large-scale brain activity in freely moving rhesus monkeys. *Nat. Methods* 11, 670–676. doi: 10.1038/nmeth.2936

Shahid, S., and Prasad, G. (2011). Bispectrum-based feature extraction technique for devising a practical brain-computer interface. *J. Neural Eng.* 8:025014. doi: 10.1088/1741-2560/8/2/025014

Shain, W., Spataro, L., Dilgen, J., Haverstick, K., Retterer, S., Isaacson, M., et al. (2003). Controlling cellular reactive responses around neural prosthetic devices using peripheral and local intervention strategies. *IEEE Trans Neural. Syst. Rehabil. Eng.* 11, 186–188. doi: 10.1109/TNSRE.2003.814800

Shishkin, S. L., Ganin, I. P., Basyul, I. A., Zhigalov, A. Y., and Kaplan, A. Y. (2009). N1 wave in the P300 BCI is not sensitive to the physical characteristics of stimuli. *J. Integr. Neurosci.* 8, 471–485. doi: 10.1142/S0219635209002320

Sitaram, R., Zhang, H., Guan, C., Thulasidas, M., Hoshi, Y., Ishikawa, A., et al. (2007). Temporal classification of multichannel near-infrared spectroscopy signals of motor imagery for developing a brain-computer interface. *Neuroimage* 34, 1416–1427. doi: 10.1016/j.neuroimage.2006.11.005

Skounti, M., Philalithis, A., and Galanakis, E. (2007). Variations in prevalence of attention deficit hyperactivity disorder worldwide. *Eur. J. Pediatr.* 166, 117–123. doi: 10.1007/s00431-006-0299-5

Sokolov, E. N. (1969). *Handbook of Contemporary Soviet Psychology.* New York, NY: Basic Books.

Sokunbi, M. O., Linden, D. E., Habes, I., Johnston, S., and Ihssen, N. (2014). Real-time fMRI brain-computer interface: development of a "motivational feedback" subsystem for the regulation of visual cue reactivity. *Front. Behav. Neurosci.* 8:392. doi: 10.3389/fnbeh.2014.00392

Soltani, M., and Knight, R. T. (2000). Neural origins of the P300. *Crit. Rev. Neurobiol.* 14, 199–224. doi: 10.1615/CritRevNeurobiol.v14.i3-4.20

Sprague, T. C., Saproo, S., and Serences, J. T. (2015). Visual attention mitigates information loss in small- and large-scale neural codes. *Trends Cogn. Sci.* 19, 215–226. doi: 10.1016/j.tics.2015.02.005

Steiner, H., Warren, B. L., Van Waes, V., and Bolanos-Guzman, C. A. (2014a). Life-long consequences of juvenile exposure to psychotropic drugs on brain and behavior. *Prog. Brain Res.* 211, 13–30. doi: 10.1016/B978-0-444-63425-2.00002-7

Steiner, N. J., Frenette, E. C., Rene, K. M., Brennan, R. T., and Perrin, E. C. (2014b). In-school neurofeedback training for ADHD: sustained improvements from a randomized control trial. *Pediatrics* 133, 483–492. doi: 10.1542/peds.2013-2059

Steiner, N. J., Frenette, E. C., Rene, K. M., Brennan, R. T., and Perrin, E. C. (2014c). Neurofeedback and cognitive attention training for children with attention-deficit hyperactivity disorder in schools. *J. Dev. Behav. Pediatr.* 35, 18–27. doi: 10.1097/DBP.0000000000000009

Steiner, N. J., Sheldrick, R. C., Gotthelf, D., and Perrin, E. C. (2011). Computer-based attention training in the schools for children with attention deficit/hyperactivity disorder: a preliminary trial. *Clin. Pediatr.* 50, 615–622. doi: 10.1177/0009922810397887

Stoeckel, L. E., Garrison, K. A., Ghosh, S., Wighton, P., Hanlon, C. A., Gilman, J. M., et al. (2014). Optimizing real time fMRI neurofeedback for therapeutic discovery and development. *Neuroimage Clin.* 5, 245–255. doi: 10.1016/j.nicl.2014.07.002

Sulzer, J., Haller, S., Scharnowski, F., Weiskopf, N., Birbaumer, N., Blefari, M. L., et al. (2013). Real-time fMRI neurofeedback: progress and challenges. *Neuroimage* 76, 386–399. doi: 10.1016/j.neuroimage.2013.03.033

Szuromi, B., Czobor, P., Komlosi, S., and Bitter, I. (2011). P300 deficits in adults with attention deficit hyperactivity disorder: a meta-analysis. *Psychol. Med.* 41, 1529–1538. doi: 10.1017/S0033291710001996

ter Huurne, N., Onnink, M., Kan, C., Franke, B., Buitelaar, J., and Jensen, O. (2013). Behavioral consequences of aberrant alpha lateralization in attention-deficit/hyperactivity disorder. *Biol. Psychiatry* 74, 227–233. doi: 10.1016/j.biopsych.2013.02.001

Thorpe, S., D'Zmura, M., and Srinivasan, R. (2012). Lateralization of frequency-specific networks for covert spatial attention to auditory stimuli. *Brain Topogr.* 25, 39–54. doi: 10.1007/s10548-011-0186-x

Thut, G., Nietzel, A., Brandt, S. A., and Pascual-Leone, A. (2006). Alpha-band electroencephalographic activity over occipital cortex indexes visuospatial attention bias and predicts visual target detection. *J. Neurosci.* 26, 9494–9502. doi: 10.1523/JNEUROSCI.0875-06.2006

Tonin, L., Leeb, R., Sobolewski, A., and Millan Jdel, R. (2013). An online EEG BCI based on covert visuospatial attention in absence of exogenous stimulation. *J. Neural Eng.* 10:056007. doi: 10.1088/1741-2560/10/5/056007

Tomita, Y., Vialatte, F. B., Dreyfus, G., Mitsukura, Y., Bakardjian, H., and Cichocki, A. (2014). Bimodal BCI using simultaneously NIRS and EEG. *IEEE Trans. Biomed. Eng.* 61, 1274–1284. doi: 10.1109/TBME.2014.2300492

Valera, E. M., Faraone, S. V., Murray, K. E., and Seidman, L. J. (2007). Meta-analysis of structural imaging findings in attention-deficit/hyperactivity disorder. *Biol. Psychiatry* 61, 1361–1369. doi: 10.1016/j.biopsych.2006.06.011

Vance, A. L., Luk, E. S., Costin, J., Tonge, B. J., and Pantelis, C. (1999). Attention deficit hyperactivity disorder: anxiety phenomena in children treated with psychostimulant medication for 6 months or more. *Aust. N.Z. J. Psychiatry* 33, 399–406. doi: 10.1046/j.1440-1614.1999.00575.x

van der Waal, M., Severens, M., Geuze, J., and Desain, P. (2012). Introducing the tactile speller: an ERP-based brain-computer interface for communication. *J. Neural Eng.* 9:045002. doi: 10.1088/1741-2560/9/4/045002

Van Gerven, M., Farquhar, J., Schaefer, R., Vlek, R., Geuze, J., Nijholt, A., et al. (2009). The brain-computer interface cycle. *J. Neural Eng.* 6:041001. doi: 10.1088/1741-2560/6/4/041001

Vidaurre, C., Kawanabe, M., von Bunau, P., Blankertz, B., and Muller, K. R. (2011). Toward unsupervised adaptation of LDA for brain-computer interfaces. *IEEE Trans. Biomed. Eng.* 58, 587–597. doi: 10.1109/TBME.2010.2093133

Vollebregt, M. A., van Dongen-Boomsma, M., Buitelaar, J. K., and Slaats-Willemse, D. (2014a). Does EEG-neurofeedback improve neurocognitive functioning in children with attention-deficit/hyperactivity disorder? A systematic review and a double-blind placebo-controlled study. *J. Child Psychol. Psychiatry* 55, 460–472. doi: 10.1111/jcpp.12143

Vollebregt, M. A., van Dongen-Boomsma, M., Slaats-Willemse, D., Buitelaar, J. K., and Oostenveld, R. (2014b). How the individual alpha peak frequency helps unravel the neurophysiologic underpinnings of behavioral functioning in children with attention-deficit/hyperactivity disorder. *Clin. EEG Neurosci.* 46, 285–291. doi: 10.1177/1550059414537257

Waldert, S., Tushaus, L., Kaller, C. P., Aertsen, A., and Mehring, C. (2012). fNIRS exhibits weak tuning to hand movement direction. *PLoS ONE* 7:e49266. doi: 10.1371/journal.pone.0049266

Wang, S., Yang, Y., Xing, W., Chen, J., Liu, C., and Luo, X. (2013). Altered neural circuits related to sustained attention and executive control in children with ADHD: an event-related fMRI study. *Clin. Neurophysiol.* 124, 2181–2190. doi: 10.1016/j.clinph.2013.05.008

Wangler, S., Gevensleben, H., Albrecht, B., Studer, P., Rothenberger, A., Moll, G. H., et al. (2011). Neurofeedback in children with ADHD: specific event-related potential findings of a randomized controlled trial. *Clin. Neurophysiol.* 122, 942–950. doi: 10.1016/j.clinph.2010.06.036

Ward, L. M., Doesburg, S. M., Kitajo, K., MacLean, S. E., and Roggeveen, A. B. (2006). Neural synchrony in stochastic resonance, attention, and consciousness. *Can. J. Exp. Psychol.* 60, 319–326. doi: 10.1037/cjep2006029

Weiskopf, N., Mathiak, K., Bock, S. W., Scharnowski, F., Veit, R., Grodd, W., et al. (2004). Principles of a brain-computer interface (BCI) based on real-time functional magnetic resonance imaging (fMRI). *IEEE Trans. Biomed. Eng.* 51, 966–970. doi: 10.1109/TBME.2004.827063

Wolfe, J. M., and Horowitz, T. S. (2004). What attributes guide the deployment of visual attention and how do they do it? *Nat. Rev. Neurosci.* 5, 495–501. doi: 10.1038/nrn1411

Wolpaw, J. R., Birbaumer, N., Heetderks, W. J., McFarland, D. J., Peckham, P. H., Schalk, G., et al. (2000). Brain-computer interface technology: a review of the first international meeting. *IEEE Trans. Rehabil. Eng.* 8, 164–173. doi: 10.1109/TRE.2000.847807

Wolpaw, J. R., McFarland, D. J., Neat, G. W., and Forneris, C. A. (1991). An EEG-based brain-computer interface for cursor control. *Electroencephalogr. Clin. Neurophysiol.* 78, 252–259. doi: 10.1016/0013-4694(91)90040-B

Wu, J., Li, Q., Bai, O., and Touge, T. (2009). Multisensory interactions elicited by audiovisual stimuli presented peripherally in a visual attention task: a behavioral and event-related potential study in humans. *J. Clin. Neurophysiol.* 26, 407–413. doi: 10.1097/WNP.0b013e3181c298b1

Wu, Z., and Su, S. (2014). A dynamic selection method for reference electrode in SSVEP-based BCI. *PLoS ONE* 9:e104248. doi: 10.1371/journal.pone.0104248

Xu, P., Tian, C., Zhang, Y., Jing, W., Wang, Z., Liu, T., et al. (2013). Cortical network properties revealed by SSVEP in anesthetized rats. *Sci. Rep.* 3, 1–11. doi: 10.1038/srep02496

Yang, L., Leung, H., Peterson, D. A., Sejnowski, T. J., and Poizner, H. (2014). Toward a semi-self-paced EEG brain computer interface: decoding initiation state from non-initiation state in dedicated time slots. *PLoS ONE* 9:e88915. doi: 10.1371/journal.pone.0088915

Yoo, S. S., Kim, H., Filandrianos, E., Taghados, S. J., and Park, S. (2013). Non-invasive brain-to-brain interface (BBI): establishing functional links between two brains. *PLoS ONE* 8:e60410. doi: 10.1371/journal.pone.0060410

Zacksenhouse, M., Lebedev, M. A., Carmena, J. M., O'Doherty, J. E., Henriquez, C., and Nicolelis, M. A. (2007). Cortical modulations increase in early sessions with brain-machine interface. *PLoS ONE* 2:e619. doi: 10.1371/journal.pone.0000619

Zandi Mehran, Y., Firoozabadi, M., and Rostami, R. (2014). Improvement of neurofeedback therapy for improved attention through facilitation of brain activity using local sinusoidal extremely low frequency magnetic field exposure. *Clin. EEG Neurosci.* 46, 100–112. doi: 10.1177/1550059414524403

Zarin, D. A., Suarez, A. P., Pincus, H. A., Kupersanin, E., and Zito, J. M. (1998). Clinical and treatment characteristics of children with attention-deficit/hyperactivity disorder in psychiatric practice. *J. Am. Acad. Child Adolesc. Psychiatry* 37, 1262–1270. doi: 10.1097/00004583-199812000-00009

Zhang, D., Maye, A., Gao, X., Hong, B., Engel, A. K., and Gao, S. (2010). An independent brain-computer interface using covert non-spatial visual selective attention. *J. Neural Eng.* 7:16010. doi: 10.1088/1741-2560/7/1/016010

Zhang, Y., Chen, Y., Bressler, S. L., and Ding, M. (2008). Response preparation and inhibition: the role of the cortical sensorimotor beta rhythm. *Neuroscience* 156, 238–246. doi: 10.1016/j.neuroscience.2008.06.061

Zhang, Y., Guo, D., Cheng, K., Yao, D., and Xu, P. (2015). The graph theoretical analysis of the SSVEP harmonic response networks. *Cogn. Neurodyn.* 9, 305–315. doi: 10.1007/s11571-015-9327-3

Zheng, H. Y., Peng, G., Chen, J. Y., Zhang, C., Minett, J. W., and Wang, W. S. (2014). The influence of tone inventory on ERP without focal attention: a cross-language study. *Comput. Math. Methods Med.* 2014:961563. doi: 10.1155/2014/961563

3

Superior Memorizers Employ different Neural Networks for Encoding and Recall

Johannes Mallow[1], Johannes Bernarding[1,2], Michael Luchtmann[3], Anja Bethmann[4] and André Brechmann[4]*

[1] Institute for Biometry and Medical Informatics, Medical Faculty, Otto-von-Guericke University, Magdeburg, Germany, [2] Center for Behavioural Brain Sciences, Otto-von-Guericke University, Magdeburg, Germany, [3] University Clinic for Neurosurgery, Otto-von-Guericke University, Magdeburg, Germany, [4] Special-Lab Non-Invasive Brain Imaging, Leibniz Institute for Neurobiology, Magdeburg, Germany

Edited by:
*Mikhail Lebedev,
Duke University, USA*

Reviewed by:
*Beat Meier,
University of Bern, Switzerland
Fernand Gobet,
University of Liverpool, UK
Andres Rieznik,
CONICET, Argentina*

***Correspondence:**
*Johannes Mallow,
Institute for Biometry and Medical Informatics, Medical Faculty, Otto-von-Guericke University, Leipziger Straße 44, Magdeburg, Germany
info@johannes-mallow.de*

Superior memorizers often employ the method of loci (MoL) to memorize large amounts of information. The MoL, known since ancient times, relies on a complex process where information to be memorized is bound to landmarks along mental routes in a previously memorized environment. However, functional magnetic resonance imaging data on groups of trained superior memorizer are rare. Based on the memorizing strategy reported by superior memorizers, we developed a scheme of the processes successively employed during memorizing and recalling digits and relate these to brain activation that is specific for the encoding and recall period. In the examined superior memorizers several regions, suggested to be involved in mental navigation and digit-to-word processing, were specifically activated during encoding: bilateral early visual cortex, retrosplenial cortex, left parahippocampus, left visual cortex, and left superior parietal cortex. Although the scheme suggests that some steps during encoding and recall seem to be analog, none of the encoding areas were specifically activated during the recall. Instead, we found strong activation in left anterior superior temporal gyrus, which we relate to recalling the sequential order of the digits, and right motor cortex that may be related to reciting the digits.

Keywords: superior memorizers, method of loci, mental navigation, encoding, recall

Introduction

In the last two decades, functional magnetic resonance imaging (fMRI), with its capability to non-invasively localize activated brain areas, led to many studies investigating different aspects of memory-related processes. Although neuroimaging studies on encoding and retrieval have focused on prefrontal cortex (PFC) and the medial temporal lobe (MTL) memory system (Scoville and Milner, 1957; Squire and Zola-Morgan, 1991), several other regions have been found to play important roles as well (Kim, 2011). For one, varying paradigms were used to examine episodic memory, such as successful encoding, successful retrieval, and objective and subjective recollection. A major meta-analysis of the results, with a focus on the use of pictures, words, or faces as memoranda, was published by Spaniol et al. (2009). Furthermore, although enhancing memorization capabilities has always received attention, mind-enhancing techniques appear to be gaining increasing interest. This may be partially due to efforts to counteract a decline in memory capacities of elderly persons, especially those suffering from Alzheimer disease. However, it remains debatable whether training strategies can have a long-lasting ameliorating effect on memory capabilities. While emotional episodic memories tend to be easy to retain over long periods, abstract data such as numbers, long lists of words, or chemical formulas are usually harder to keep in mind. However, it is well known that trained memory experts ["superior memorizers" (SMs)] can achieve extraordinary results when memorizing long lists of numbers, sequences of images, or other data in a short time. In this study we wanted to compare the brain areas *specifically* activated by SMs using the method of loci (MoL) on digits during encoding with those activated during recall.

The essence of their strategy consists in visualizing simple or abstract data, such as numbers, as concrete objects and subsequently placing them on landmarks along an internal route that was previously memorized. Those landmarks can be actual objects, like a chair or a tree, but also the empty space between two buildings. The far most popular version of this is the MoL (*locus* means *place* in Latin), a technique from ancient art of mnemonics (Yates, 1966). The transformation of the digits into visual objects can be done by using a *phonetic system* (Worthen, 2010). For recall, the internal route is walked through mentally and the objects transformed back into the original data.

Up to now, only one study analyzed the brain networks employed in SMs when encoding data (Maguire et al., 2003) and one studied subjects who received short-term training in the MoL (Kondo et al., 2005). Furthermore, there are only two other studies that investigated how SMs encode and recite digits. Both studies were performed with only one subject (Hu et al., 2009; Raz et al., 2009). However, applying this method to abstract data such as digits is a very complex, poorly described process. For that reason we developed a detailed scheme of the sub-processes of memorizing and recalling digits by using introspective information from superior memorizers. We then used fMRI to identify and compare the brain areas that are selectively activated by trained memorizers when encoding and recalling a sequence of digits while applying a phonetic system and the MoL. Moreover, we present some hypotheses whether the activated regions might be connected to the presumably underlying internal processing chains, which were described in the detailed scheme.

We suggest that the memorizing of digits, while using the MoL in combination with a phonetic system, not only encompasses visuo-spatial and memory-related components, but also recruits several language-related processes such as word generation and internal speech. Thus, in addition to speech- and language-related visuo-spatial areas, auditory brain networks may be activated. We expected to replicate the findings of Maguire et al. (2003), who described brain areas that are active in SMs when encoding items (including digits). However, Maguire et al. (2003) did not analyze the brain areas that were active during the recall phase. Consequently, we did not have a specific hypothesis, except that, since successful retrieval in normal subjects is suggested to be accompanied by processes similar to those involved in encoding, one could expected at least some overlap of brain areas specifically active during recall and encoding (Rugg et al., 2008).

Scheme for Encoding and Recall

According to the first author, who is one of the best trained superior memorizer in the world and expert on the practical use of the mnemonic methods since more than 10 year, during encoding, SMs usually perform an intricate chain of nested language-related, visual-related, and spatial navigation-related processes. Before encoding, SMs choose a previously learned internal route that they are familiar with. The actual encoding process is then a repetition of the process shown in (**Figure 1**). To emphasize which intermediate steps of the process are related to previously learned information, we divided the process into two columns. The encoding process starts with mental visualization of the first landmark from the chosen route. Then, a subset of items (here two or three digits, individual to each superior memorizer) is transformed into letters using a previously learned digit–letter encoding table. Subsequently, these letters are used to generate key words according to previously learned rules. Usually the key words encode objects that can easily be visualized internally (e.g., the digit sequence "5 0 4" corresponds to "lsr" which is expanded to "laser"). A similar approach is described in (Yin et al., 2015). Finally, the imagined objects are placed on the particular landmark along the internal route. To increase efficiency, the connections between the landmarks and placed items are composed into a small story, often within an emotional context. This process is repeated until all numbers are memorized (**Figure 1**). The detailed scheme in **Figure 1** separates the sub-processes reported and confirmed by SMs when initially learning to encode digits using a phonetic system and the MoL. Note that—depending on the performance level and experience of each superior memorizer—the mental effort differs between subjects for the sub-processes involved in translating the digits into words (e.g., recall of the letter table, search for words, and silent speaking of the word). This reportedly requires less effort for experienced memorizers than for naïve subjects or when learning the mnemonic strategies.

Similar to the encoding process, recall (**Figure 2**) begins by mentally visualizing the first landmark from the used route. Now the previously created story or object pops into mind and the memorizer decodes the related key word, using the digit–letter table. After recalling this subset of digits, the memorizer moves on to the next landmark.

According to the first author, the described method seems to be used by almost everybody in the world of ranked memory championships. Anyway there may be other memory experts who uses different approaches, like shown by Richman et al. (1995).

Materials and Methods

Subjects

Eleven SMs (eight male, three female; mean age 30.8 years) and eleven control subjects (six male, five female; mean age 26.3 years) participated in the study. All of the SMs were highly trained in the MoL and have proven their abilities in public competitions of memory performance. They all had perfectly memorized at least 100 digits in 5 min and thus belong to a very exclusive group of SMs worldwide. To give an impression about the group

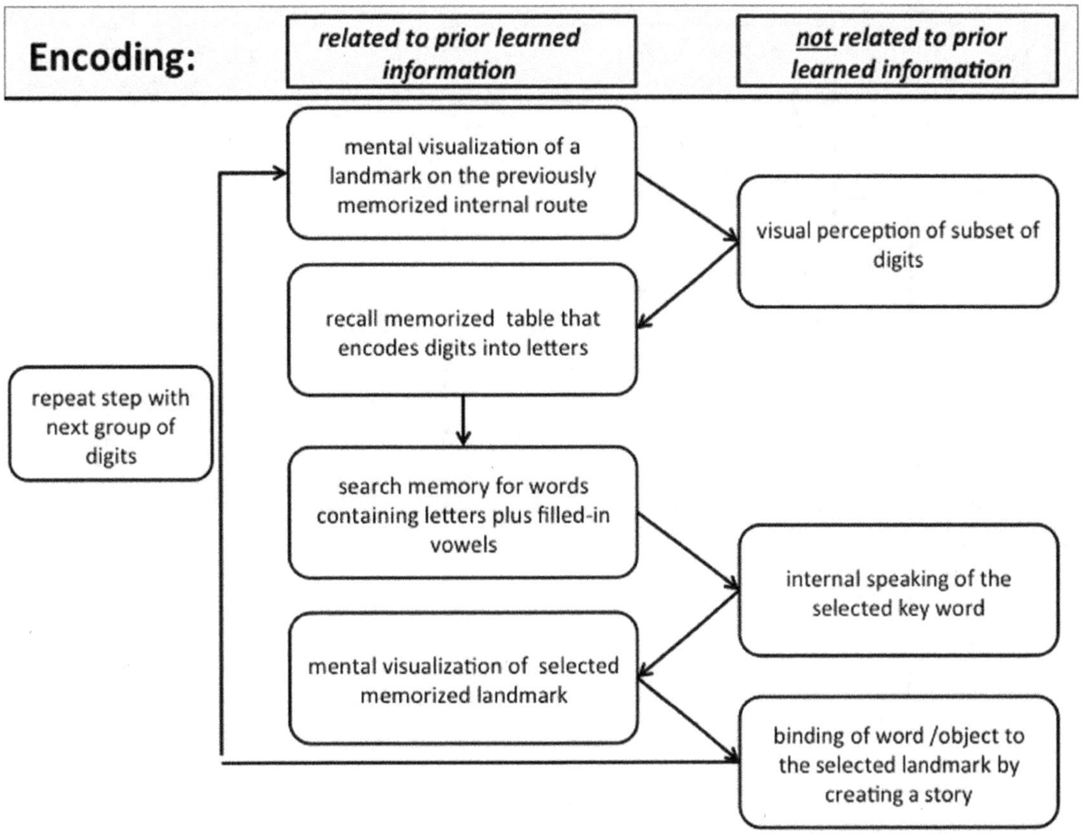

FIGURE 1 | Encoding: schematic view of a typical processing chain when encoding a sequence of digits using the method of loci (MoL). See text for further details.

size, it should be mentioned that at the time of the experiment only about 200 people worldwide had proved that capability. The performance variability for the subjects in that study was between 100 and 320 perfectly memorized digits in 5 min. All subjects confirmed to use the strategy, including the digit–letter transformation and the MoL, as shown in **Figure 1**. The reported time of experience with the methods was between 3 and 8 years. None of the control subjects reported having experience in the MoL or any other mnemonic technique and they where not provided with those strategies or any other method. The data from four SMs and four control subjects had to be excluded from the fMRI analysis due to excessive head motion (>2 mm and/or 2°). This large number of participants that has to be excluded is possibly due to the overt speech response required during the recall and rest condition. The mean age was 32.3 years for the remaining seven SMs (five male, two female, and one left-hander) and 25.1 years for the seven control subjects (four male, three female, and all right-handed). All subjects gave their written informed consent to the study, which was approved by the Local Ethics Committee of the Medical Faculty of the University of Magdeburg in compliance with national legislation and the Code of Ethical Principles for Medical Research Involving Human Subjects of the World Medical Association (Declaration of Helsinki).

Experimental Paradigm

The experiment was performed using a block design of eight blocks for the *encoding* condition (60 s duration) and eight blocks for the *attention* condition (20 s duration). During the encoding condition a complete 5 × 8 matrix of 40 digits was presented visually, and the subjects were asked to memorize as many items as possible (first row from left, then second row, etc.). This *encoding* condition was followed by a 20-s *attention* condition, where a matrix with different digits was visually presented (**Figure 3**). Here, the subjects had to indicate, by pressing one of two buttons, whether or not each digit was even and was marked by exactly two dashes when adding up the dashes below and above the digit. Zero had to be treated as an even number. The attention condition served to stop the encoding process, and thus controlled for both the visual input and attentional load.

These first two blocks were followed by a recall condition (60 s duration) in which the subjects had to recall as many digits as possible and to say the numbers aloud in the same order as they where asked to memorize them (**Figure 4**). The subjects were instructed to not move their head while talking. The sounds were recorded with a dual channel microphone (MR-Confon, Germany) that subtracted the scanner noise, which enabled the experimental supervisor in the monitor room to

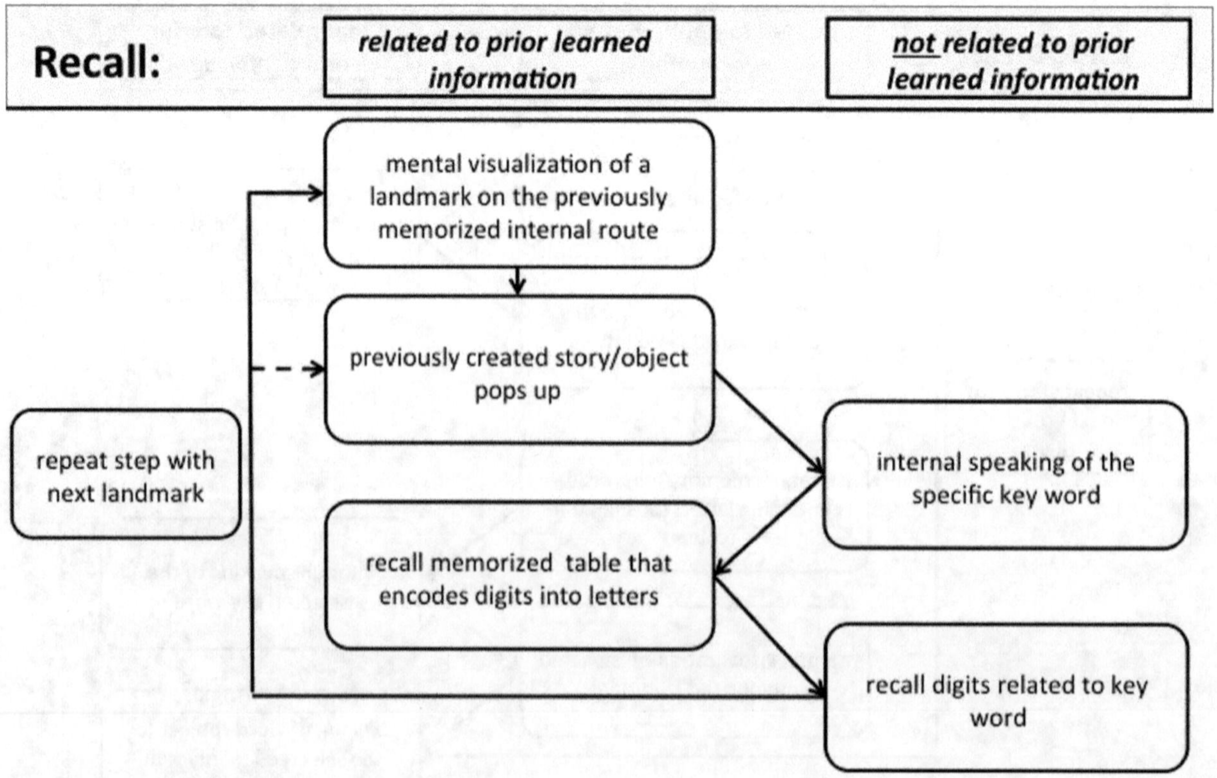

FIGURE 2 | Recall: schematic view of a typical processing chain when recalling a sequence of digits using the MoL. See text for further details.

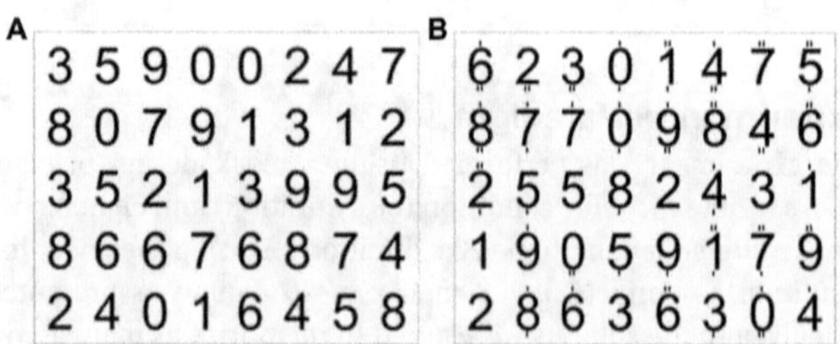

FIGURE 3 | Example of a 5 × 8 matrix of digits (A), which the subject had to encode within 60 s. (B) Digits with dashes on top or below. The subjects had to indicate by button press whether or not each digit was even (zero had to be treated as even) and marked by exactly two dashes (targets in the first row were the 2 and the 0, in the second row 0, 8, 4, 6, and in the third row 4).

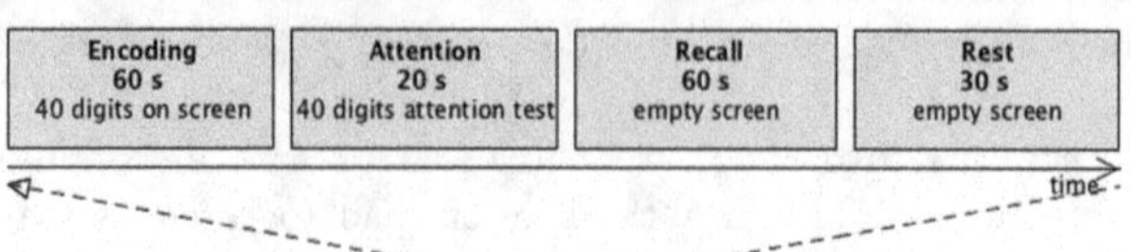

FIGURE 4 | Diagram of the trial scheme. One run consisted of a set of four blocks (encoding, attention, recall, and rest). During the recall and rest condition a fixation cross was presented. After an initial rest phase of 30 s each run was repeated eight times, resulting in 695 data sets.

easily identify the spoken numbers. The recall condition was followed by a 30-s rest condition. Here, the subjects had to recite the alphabet in silence before the next block was started. The visual stimuli were presented by a video projector onto a back-projection screen, which was viewed from inside the scanner through a mirror system. For stimulus presentation and recording of the behavioral responses, the software application *Presentation* (Neurobehavioral Systems, Albany, NY, USA) was used.

Data Acquisition and Data Analysis

Magnetic resonance imaging was carried out using a 3 T Trio MRI scanner (Siemens Medical Solutions) equipped with an eight-channel phased array coil. Anatomical data of the whole brain were acquired with high resolution using a multiplanar rapidly acquired gradient echo (MPRAGE) sequence with 1.0 mm^3 isotropic resolution. For later alignment with the anatomical data an additional inversion-recovery echo-planar imaging (IR-EPI) was acquired prior to each functional run. The IR-EPI exhibited the same geometry as the subsequent functional measurements. 695 volumes were acquired in 23 h 10 min using a gradient-recalled echo-planar imaging (EPI) pulse sequence [echo time (TE) = 30 ms; repetition time (TR) = 2000 ms; flip angle (FA) = 80°; matrix 64 × 64; field of view (FOV) = 19.2 cm; 33 slices of 3 mm, 0.3 mm gap).

The functional data were analyzed with the software system BrainVoyager^{TM}QX (Brain Innovation, Maastricht,

Netherlands). A standard chain of pre-processing steps, slice scan time correction, 3D-motion correction, linear trend removal, filtering with a high-pass of three cycles per scan, and spatial smoothing with a Gaussian filter with 4 mm full width at half maximum was applied. The functional data were projected onto the corresponding IR-EPI images, co-registered with the 3D dataset, and then transformed to Talairach space.

Due to the low number of subjects, a fixed effects analysis of the group data was performed using a conservative significance level of $p < 0.01$ (Bonferroni corrected) with a minimum cluster size of eight voxels. To determine brain regions exhibiting increased activation under specific conditions in SMs as compared to in control subjects, a conjunction analysis was performed that ensures that the resulting brain regions show a positive deflection of the BOLD response during encoding or recall vs. rest and is controlled for general attentional processes (comparison vs. attention condition). Thus, the contrast for the encoding-specific activation in SMs was: *Encode* in SMs vs. *Rest* in SMs AND *Encode* in SMs vs. *Attend* in SMs AND *Encode* in SMs vs. *Encode* in controls. The contrast for the recall-specific activation in SMs was: *Recall* in SMs vs. *Rest* in SMs AND *Recall* in SMs vs. *Attend* in SMs AND *Recall* in SMs vs. *Recall* in controls.

This analysis is rather conservative but it guarantees that the BOLD response during encoding/recall in SMs is significantly stronger. Beside the comparison between encoding in SMs and encoding in controls and the same for recall, two additional conditions must be fulfilled. Firstly, the activation of the SMs during the encoding/recall phases must be significantly stronger than during the attentional control condition of the SMs because we do not want to discuss brain areas which are strongly activated due to general attention differences between the SMs and the control group. Secondly, we only want to consider brain areas that show a positive BOLD response compared to a resting condition in which the SMs only need to recite the alphabet. This is especially important for the identification of areas involved in the recall where overt reciting of numbers is required by the memorizers. All three contrasts must be independently significant at the $p < 0.01$ level.

Results

Task Performance and fMRI Data

For the behavioral analysis we calculated the mean values and standard errors of the mean (SEM). On average, the SMs were capable to recall 34.5 of the 40 digits ($SEM = 2.37$), while the naïve subjects recalled only 10.8 digits ($SEM = 1.58$). The SMs recalled significantly more digits then the controls (t-test: $p < 0.0001$, $t = 7.6$, and effect size: $d > 4$). The mean time for recalling all numbers was 37.1 s (1.2 s/digit; $SEM = 0.15$ s) for SMs, and 24.3 s (2.5 s/digit; $SEM = 0.41$ s) for the naïve subjects. The SMs recalled the digits significantly faster (t-test: $p < 0.01$, $t = 2.86$, and effect size: $d > 1.5$). The difference in overall duration was due to fewer digits memorized by the control group, as well as to a high variation in recall speed. In some cases the number of recalled digits was too small to fill the entire recall interval. In other cases the naïve subjects recalled the numbers so slowly that the duration of the recall phase was used up completely.

Figure 5 shows the results for the conjunction analysis used to detect brain regions that were significantly more activated during the encoding process in SMs than in naïve subjects. It shows that a network of left hemisphere regions is involved in encoding, consisting of left secondary visual areas (BA 18, 19), left medial superior parietal cortex (BA 7), and left middle temporal gyrus (BA 39). The bilaterally activated retrosplenial cortex (BA 30), and posterior parahippocampal gyrus (pHi) also exhibited a very strong lateralization to the left hemisphere. The details are summarized in **Table 1**. To demonstrate the extent of the differences in brain activation between both groups, the time course of the BOLD response during the 60 s of encoding is displayed in **Figure 6** for each brain area, which was found to be significantly stronger in SMs than in naïve control subjects.

None of these regions was significantly activated in the recall condition of the SMs. **Figure 7** shows that the beta values of the recall condition were mostly negative and all significantly

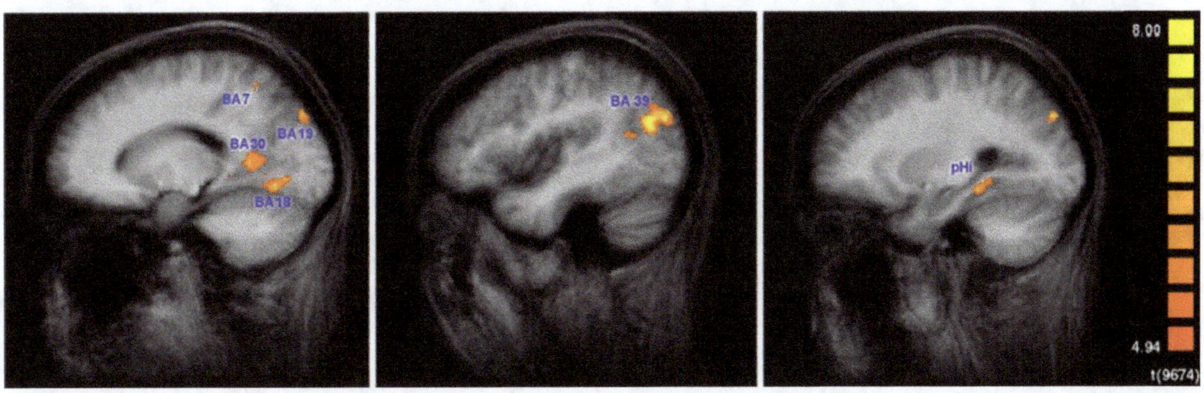

FIGURE 5 | Encoding-specific activation in superior memorizers. Contrast: *Encode* in superior memorizers vs. *Rest* in superior memorizers AND *Encode* in superior memorizers vs. *Attend* in superior memorizers AND *Encode* in superior memorizers vs. *Encode* in controls. Color-encoded activation maps overlaid on group-averaged anatomical images ($p < 0.01$, Bonferroni corrected, minimum cluster size 8 voxel) (left $x = -16$, middle $x = -42$, and right $x = -25$).

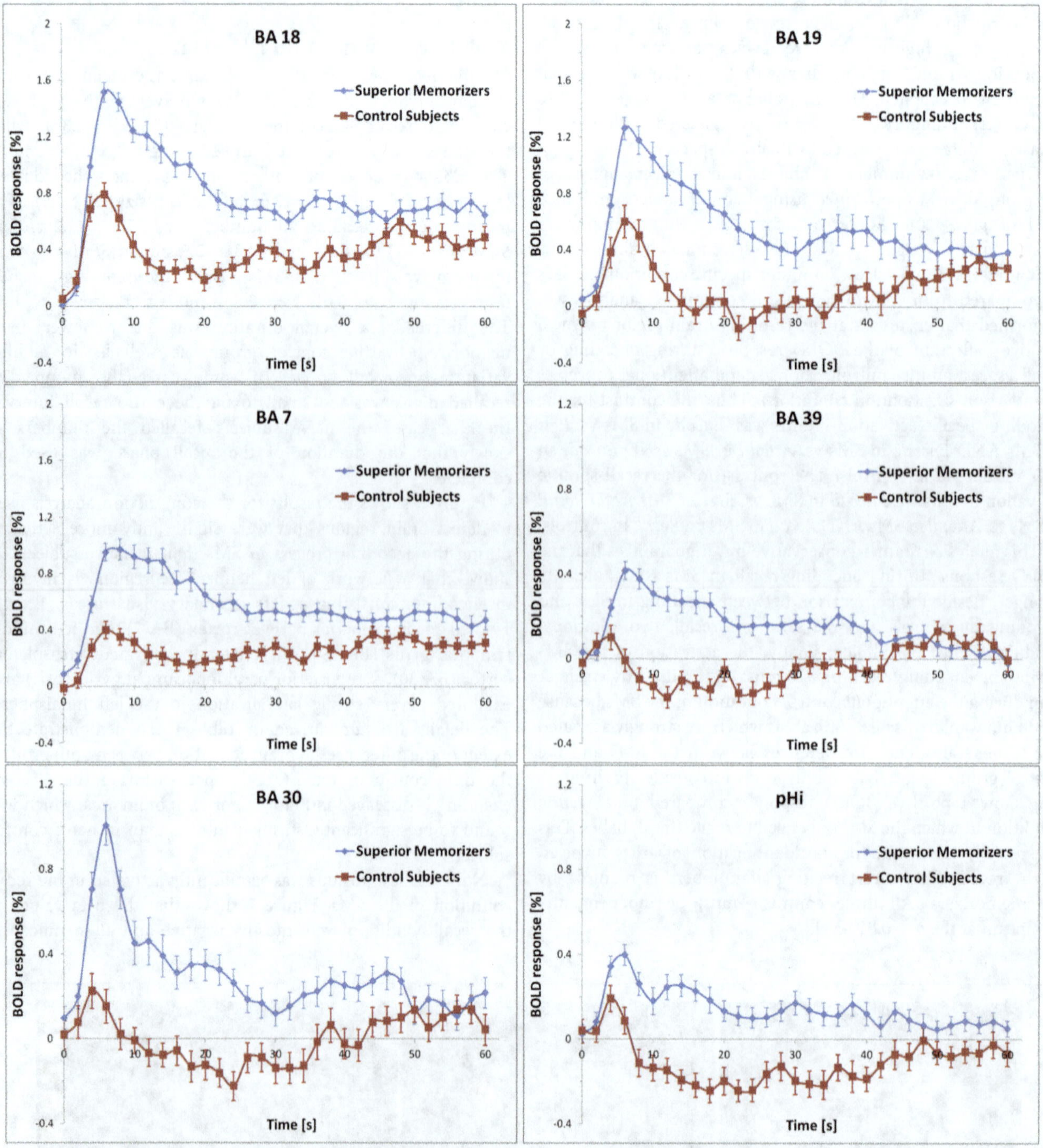

FIGURE 6 | Averaged BOLD responses of the brain areas showing encoding-specific activation in superior memorizers. Time point zero denotes the start of the encoding condition that lasted for 60 s. The baseline (0 % BOLD response) was defined as the average response within 4 s prior to the encoding condition. Note the different scaling of the ordinates. The BOLD response of control subjects is depicted for comparison.

lower than those of the encoding condition (**Figure 7**). Instead, the left anterior superior temporal gyrus (STG) and the right motor cortex were specifically activated (**Figure 8**). The BOLD response during the 60 s when recalling the digits is displayed in **Figure 9**.

Discussion

We now discuss the activated brain regions with respect to the involved processes including information transformation and binding processes of the suggested mnemonic procedure

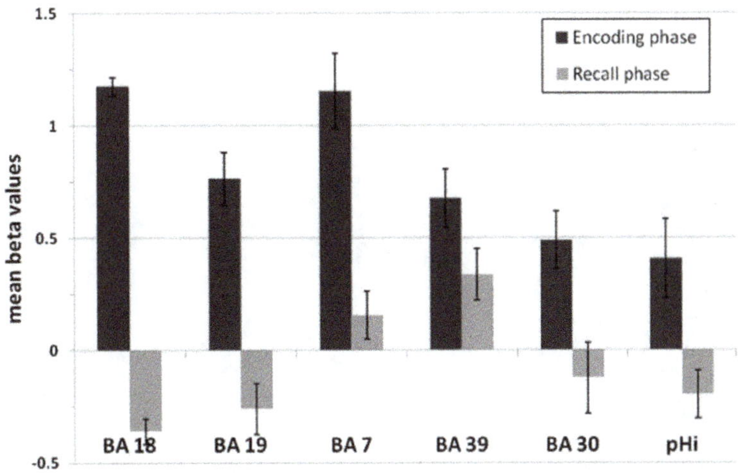

FIGURE 7 | Mean beta values of the encoding-specific areas of superior memorizers shown in Figure 5. Beta values of the encoding phase correspond to the BOLD response of the superior memorizers depicted as blue curve in **Figure 6**. The beta values of the recall phase are all significantly lower than those of the encoding phase (BA 18, BA 19, BA 7, BA 30, and pHi: $p < 0.01$; BA 39: $p < 0.05$; two sides t-test).

TABLE 1 | Regions activated to a higher degree in superior memorizers than in naïve controls ($p < 0.01$, Bonferroni corrected, minimum cluster size eight voxels).

Region	Talairach coordinates			BA	Cluster size
	x	*y*	*z*		
Encoding					
Left visual cortex	−13	−67	−3	18	1213
Right visual cortex	10	−72	−2	18	228
Left visual cortex	−20	−81	34	19	615
Left angular gyrus	−40	−65	24	39	2162
Left retrosplenial cortex	−12	−53	8	30	3914
Right retrosplenial cortex	13	−51	8	30	1047
Left superior parietal cortex	−20	−57	52	7	263
Left parahippocampus	−25	−36	−7		449
Recall					
Left anterior superior temporal gyrus	−57	−8	7	22	346
Right motor cortex	50	−8	30	4/6	676

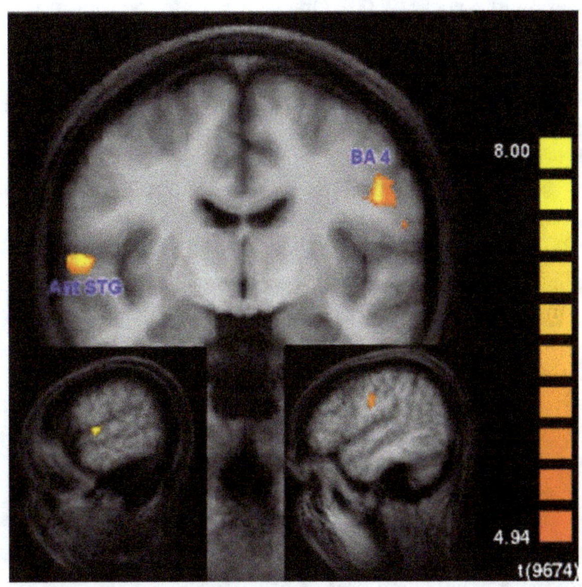

FIGURE 8 | Recall-specific activation in superior memorizers. Left anterior superior temporal gyrus (STG) and right motor cortex are the only regions that are specifically activated during the recall condition in superior memorizers. Contrast: *Recall* in superior memorizers vs. *Rest* in superior memorizers AND *Recall* in superior memorizers vs. *Attend* in superior memorizers AND *Recall* in superior memorizers vs. *Recall* in controls. ($p < 0.01$, Bonferroni corrected, minimum cluster size 8 voxel) (down left $x = -56$, down right $x = 48$, and middle $y = -8$).

(**Figure 1**). The encoding procedure includes the activation of long-term memory, which was found to be characteristic of studies when experts where involved (Guida et al., 2012). This results in mental visualization of a location on the previously memorized internal route. This explains the strong activation in visual brain regions (Johnson and Johnson, 2014). Other contributions to the activation of the visual cortex may come from several sub-processes of translating the digits into visual objects, i.e., in-depth visual perception of digits, recall of the specific letters representing these digits from the previously memorized table, and the search for a correct word containing the letters. Furthermore, several studies also suggest that BA 18 is involved in recollection processes (Spaniol et al., 2009). The fact that SMs use contextual information while applying the MoL supports these findings. Furthermore the use of long-term memory.

The left lateralized effect in BA 19 suggests the involvement of the language-related system when transforming digits into letters and subsequently into words, since a left lateralization of BA 19

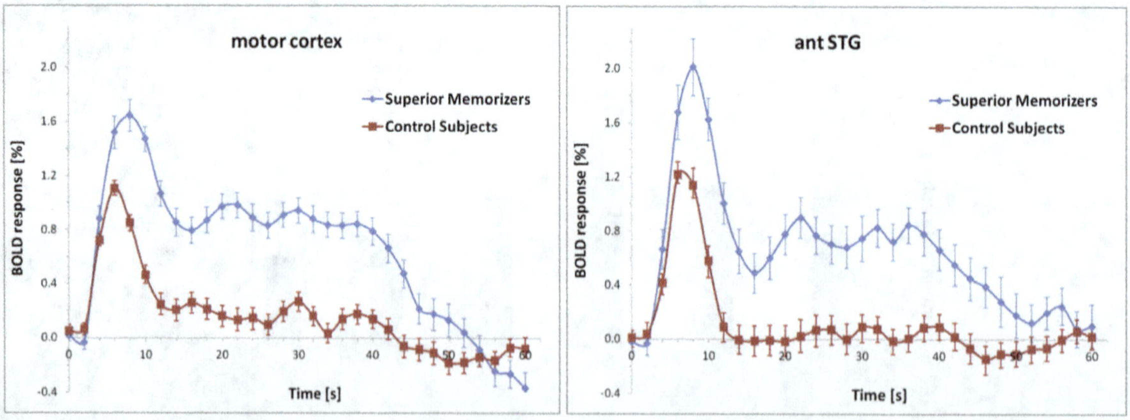

FIGURE 9 | Averaged BOLD responses of the brain areas depicted in Figure 8 showing recall-specific activation in superior memorizers. Time point zero denotes the start of the recall condition that lasted for 60 s. The baseline (0% BOLD response) was defined as the average response within four seconds prior to the recall condition. The BOLD response of control subjects is depicted for comparison.

was often found to play a role in phonological processing and forming words (Dietz et al., 2005), as well as in word recognition (Cabeza and Nyberg, 2000). One step of the proposed model in **Figure 3** involves silently speaking. However, we did not find specific activation in, e.g., Broca's area. One explanation is that the control subjects also used inner speech to encode as many digits as possible. Moreover, because the SMs in the group were highly experienced in the encoding process, some of the sub-processes involving covert speech may have required less mental effort.

When connecting the mentally visualized object to the selected landmark, the visualized object becomes navigationally relevant. This may explain why the pHi is activated (Wegman and Janzen, 2011). Moreover, the repetition of the processes depicted in (**Figure 1**) automatically results in mental navigation that is known to involve not only the pHi but also BA 7 and 30 (Ghaem et al., 1997; Maguire et al., 1998, 2003; Kondo et al., 2005; Epstein, 2008; Auger et al., 2012). With the left-hemispheric activation of BA 7 and BA 39 during encoding, we found two areas that have been also found activated by other groups during recollection (Vilberg and Rugg, 2007; Spaniol et al., 2009). Those findings imply that the encoding process of SMs is basically a mixture of encoding and retrieval, as suggested by the scheme of **Figure 1**, where it is shown that items already learned may be used to memorize other new items.

During recall none of the encoding-related areas was specifically activated and the overall number of activated voxels was much smaller than in the encoding condition. This was surprising, since a comparison of **Figures 1** and **2** leads one to expect to find at least the same areas activated for mental navigation as for encoding. This result seems to stand in some contradiction to the transfer-appropriate process theory, which proposes that successful retrieval is accompanied by neuronal processes similar to those occurring during encoding (Rugg et al., 2008). However such a conclusion must be considered very carefully since due to our conjunction analyses we only analyzed very specific activated brain regions.

During recall, the activation in the motor area may be explained by the fact that SMs had to recite significantly more digits. This is in part supported by the BOLD response (**Figure 9**) which in control subjects falls off to baseline much earlier than in SMs. The anterior temporal lobe has been shown to be involved in the retrieval of proper names (Damasio et al., 2004; Bethmann et al., 2012), which are composed of more semantic features than common objects. The left anterior temporal lobe has also been shown to be involved in syntactic processing, independent of syntactic complexity (Friederici, 2002; Dronkers et al., 2004). Hence, it has been suggested that the left anterior temporal lobe contributes to the composition of sentence meaning (Vandenberghe et al., 2002; Humphries et al., 2006). Beyond that, the anterior temporal region has been proposed to be involved in the concatenation of sentences or propositions into stories (Mar, 2004).

Taking these suggestions together, we interpret the current recall-specific activation in the anterior STG to be related to the reconstruction of the exact sequence of objects along the mental route of landmarks. Because SMs make up vivid stories of how the visual objects, which represent the encoded information, are related to the landmarks of their routes, recalling the sequence of encoded information may be interpreted as reviewing a story rather than as mental navigation along a route. Such a difference in strategy may also explain the unexpected difference in the recruitment of brain areas during the encoding compared with the recall phase. Although we think that the described process in **Figure 2** is very accurate, it has to be considered that some modifications would be appropriate. Our results show that the process of mental movement from one location to the next seems to be much less intense than during encoding. Thus it may be reasonable to link directly from the last step of the process, "recall digits related to keyword", to the step "previously created story pops up". We have shown that with the dashed arrow in **Figure 2**.

Although many aspects of memory-related processes have been investigated, little is known about persons who have trained their capabilities to memorize abstract and emotionally neutral data using the MoL (Maguire et al., 2003; Kondo et al., 2005; Konrad, 2014). The regions activated during encoding are consistent with those found by Maguire et al. (2003), except that we found activation in the pHi instead of in the hippocampus. The former was also found to be strongly activated in several other encoding studies (Spaniol et al., 2009). One explanation for the higher activation in SMs could be the fact that they encode additional information (e.g., the connection between landmark and object), since the pHi is also suggested by other studies (Epstein, 2008) to be involved in the encoding of contextual information (Davachi, 2006; Charan Ranganath, 2012) and navigationally relevant object information (Epstein, 2008; Wegman and Janzen, 2011). In another study naïve subjects were trained to use the MoL prior to the fMRI experiment (Kondo et al., 2005), which resulted in activation of the left fusiform and lingual gyrus during both encoding and recall. However, it should be noted that the subjects in this study were trained only briefly and thus were by no means SMs.

According to the hemispheric encoding/retrieval asymmetry model (HERA; Tulving et al., 1994) the left PFC should be more involved during encoding and the right PFC more involved during retrieval. We found a strong left lateralization for a few areas (**Table 1**) specifically activated by SMs during encoding but no specific activation in the PFC during encoding or during retrieval. The overall left dominance could indicate language-related and sequential processing while applying the MoL combined with a phonetic system.

In this study we aimed to interpret the fMRI data of SMs who used the MoL combined with a phonetic system to memorize long lists of digits. To understand which neuronal processes may potentially be involved, a scheme was developed of the different sub-processes that are employed when SMs fulfill this task. Although our data show some support for the proposition that language-related systems are involved in addition to the brain parts already known to play a role in encoding, this interpretation of the data is limited at the moment by the fact that the single sub-processes of the scheme cannot be separated within our experimental setup. Furthermore the overt behavior during the different conditions was different, which may cause some background noise in the data and some lack of control over all potential sub-processes. Thus there is a need for future studies focusing on partial aspects of the overall process. This could be achieved by scanning the SMs solely while they "walk" through their mental route without creating mental images or while they translate numbers into images without connecting them to specific locations.

A limitation of the fixed effects analysis is that it does not allow for inferences to the population. Nevertheless, to demonstrate the significance of the effects, we used very conservative criteria, as described in the Section "Materials and Methods". Furthermore, we show the BOLD response over time for each activated brain area that reveals how large the difference between SMs and controls is in terms of BOLD response amplitude. It also has to be stated that the potential heterogeneity of strategies of the naïve volunteers may limit the generalization of the results, which makes more specific research necessary.

In sum, we found that SMs use different networks for encoding and recall, with the latter process generating much less brain activation. This is in accordance with the everyday challenges of learning a language, playing a piece of music, or learning movement patterns. Once a pattern is learned it can be recalled and executed very quickly and with little conscious effort. However, learning strategies are seldom taught in schools or other institutions. One may speculate to which degree learning would gain efficiency when applying optimized strategies instead of trying to memorize data by endless repetition. At least our behavioral results show that the strategies of the superior memorizer are very efficient for learning digits. It would be interesting to investigate the efficiency of their strategies on general knowledge. Such a study could have an important influence on how knowledge is imparted in schools or universities.

Author Contributions

JM, ABr, and JB wrote the main manuscript text. JM also prepared **Figures 1–4**. ABr prepared **Figures 5–9**, was responsible for methods and data analysis. ABr, ABe, and ML contributed to the discussion. All authors reviewed the manuscript.

References

Auger, S. D., Mullally, S. L., and Maguire, E. A. (2012). Retrosplenial cortex codes for permanent landmarks. *PLoS ONE* 7:e43620. doi: 10.1371/journal.pone.0043620

Bethmann, A., Scheich, H., and Brechmann, A. (2012). The temporal lobes differentiate between the voices of famous and unknown people: an event-related fMRI study on speaker recognition. *PLoS ONE* 7:e47626. doi: 10.1371/journal.pone.0047626

Cabeza, R., and Nyberg, L. (2000). Imaging cognition II: an empirical review of 275 PET and fMRI studies. *J. Cogn. Neurosci.* 12, 1–47. doi: 10.1162/08989290051137585

Charan Ranganath, M. R. (2012). Two cortical systems for memory-guided behaviour. *Nat. Rev. Neurosci.* 13, 713–726. doi: 10.1038/nrn3338

Damasio, H., Tranel, D., Grabowski, T., Adolphs, R., and Damasio, A. (2004). Neural systems behind word and concept retrieval. *Cognition* 92, 179–229. doi: 10.1016/j.cognition.2002.07.001

Davachi, L. (2006). Item, context and relational episodic encoding in humans. *Curr. Opin. Neurobiol.* 16, 693–700. doi: 10.1016/j.conb.2006.10.012

Dietz, N. A. E., Jones, K. M., Gareau, L., Zeffiro, T. A., and Eden, G. F. (2005). Phonological decoding involves left posterior fusiform gyrus. 26, 81–93. doi: 10.1002/hbm.20122

Dronkers, N. F., Wilkins, D. P., Van Valin, R. D., Redfern, B. B., and Jaeger, J. J. (2004). Lesion analysis of the brain areas involved in language comprehension. *Cognition* 92, 145–177. doi: 10.1016/j.cognition.2003.11.002

Epstein, R. A. (2008). Parahippocampal and retrosplenial contributions to human spatial navigation. *Trends Cogn. Sci.* 12, 388–396. doi: 10.1016/j.tics.2008.07.004

Friederici, A. D. (2002). Towards a neural basis of auditory sentence processing. *Trends Cogn. Sci.* 6, 78–84. doi: 10.1016/S1364-6613(00)01839-8

Ghaem, O., Mellet, E., Crivello, F., Tzourio, N., Mazoyer, B., Berthoz, A., et al. (1997). Mental navigation along memorized routes activates the hippocampus, precuneus, and insula. *Neuroreport* 8, 739–744. doi: 10.1097/00001756-199702100-00032

Guida, A., Gobet, F., Tardieu, H., and Nicolas, S. (2012). How chunks, long-term working memory and templates offer a cognitive explanation for neuroimaging data on expertise acquisition: a two-stage framework. *Brain Cogn.* 79, 221–244. doi: 10.1016/j.bandc.2012.01.010

Hu, Y., Ericsson, K. A., Yang, D., and Lu, C. (2009). Superior self-paced memorization of digits in spite of a normal digit span: the structure of a memorist's skill. *J. Exp. Psychol. Learn. Mem. Cogn.* 35, 1426–1442. doi: 10.1037/a0017395

Humphries, C., Binder, J. R., Medler, D. A., and Liebenthal, E. (2006). Syntactic and semantic modulation of neural activity during auditory sentence comprehension. *J. Cogn. Neurosci.* 18, 665–679. doi: 10.1162/jocn.2006.18.4.665

Johnson, M. R., and Johnson, M. K. (2014). Decoding individual natural scene representations during perception and imagery. *Front. Hum. Neurosci.* 8:59. doi: 10.3389/fnhum.2014.00059

Kim, H. (2011). Neural activity that predicts subsequent memory and forgetting: a meta-analysis of 74 fMRI studies. *Neuroimage* 54, 2446–2461. doi: 10.1016/j.neuroimage.2010.09.045

Kondo, Y., Suzuki, M., Mugikura, S., Abe, N., Takahashi, S., Iijima, T., et al. (2005). Changes in brain activation associated with use of a memory strategy: a functional MRI study. *Neuroimage* 24, 1154–1163. doi: 10.1016/j.neuroimage.2004.10.033

Konrad, B. N. (2014). *Characteristics and Neuronal Correlates of Superior Memory Performance.* Available at: http://edoc.ub.uni-muenchen.de/16636/ [Accessed May 20, 2014]

Maguire, E. A., Burgess, N., Donnett, J. G., Frackowiak, R. S., Frith, C. D., and O'Keefe, J. (1998). Knowing where and getting there: a human navigation network. *Science* 280, 921–924. doi: 10.1126/science.280.5365.921

Maguire, E. A., Valentine, E. R., Wilding, J. M., and Kapur, N. (2003). Routes to remembering: the brains behind superior memory. *Nat. Neurosci.* 6, 90–95. doi: 10.1038/nn988

Mar, R. A. (2004). The neuropsychology of narrative: story comprehension, story production and their interrelation. *Neuropsychologia* 42, 1414–1434. doi: 10.1016/j.neuropsychologia.2003.12.016

Raz, A., Packard, M. G., Alexander, G. M., Buhle, J. T., Zhu, H., Yu, S., et al. (2009). A slice of pi: an exploratory neuroimaging study of digit encoding and retrieval in a superior memorist. *Neurocase* 15, 361–372. doi: 10.1080/13554790902776896

Richman, H. B., Staszewski, J. J., Simon, H. A., Richman, H. B., Staszewski, J. J., and Simon, H. A. (1995). Simulation of expert memory using EPAM IV. *Psychol. Rev.* 102, 305–330. doi: 10.1037/0033-295X.102.2.305

Rugg, M. D., Johnson, J. D., Park, H., and Uncapher, M. R. (2008). Encoding-retrieval overlap in human episodic memory: a functional neuroimaging perspective. *Prog. Brain Res* 169, 339–352. doi: 10.1016/S0079-6123(07)00021-0

Scoville, W. B., and Milner, B. (1957). Loss of recent memory after bilateral hippocampal lesions. *J. Neurol. Neurosurg. Psychiatry* 20, 11–21. doi: 10.1136/jnnp.20.1.11

Spaniol, J., Davidson, P. S. R., Kim, A. S. N., Han, H., Moscovitch, M., and Grady, C. L. (2009). Event-related fMRI studies of episodic encoding and retrieval: meta-analyses using activation likelihood estimation. *Neuropsychologia* 47, 1765–1779. doi: 10.1016/j.neuropsychologia.2009.02.028

Squire, L. R., and Zola-Morgan, S. (1991). The medial temporal lobe memory system. *Science* 253, 1380–1386. doi: 10.1126/science.1896849

Tulving, E., Kapur, S., Craik, F. I., Moscovitch, M., and Houle, S. (1994). Hemispheric encoding/retrieval asymmetry in episodic memory: positron emission tomography findings. *Proc. Natl. Acad. Sci. U.S.A.* 91, 2016–2020. doi: 10.1073/pnas.91.6.2016

Vandenberghe, R., Nobre, A. C., and Price, C. J. (2002). The response of left temporal cortex to sentences. *J. Cogn. Neurosci.* 14, 550–560. doi: 10.1162/08989290260045800

Vilberg, K. L., and Rugg, M. D. (2007). Dissociation of the neural correlates of recognition memory according to familiarity, recollection, and amount of recollected information. *Neuropsychologia* 45, 2216–2225. doi: 10.1016/j.neuropsychologia.2007.02.027

Wegman, J., and Janzen, G. (2011). Neural encoding of objects relevant for navigation and resting state correlations with navigational ability. *J. Cogn. Neurosci.* 23, 3841–3854. doi: 10.1162/jocn_a_00081

Worthen, J. B. (2010). *Mnemonology: Mnemonics for the 21st Century*, 1st Edn. New York, NY: Psychology Press.

Yates, F. A. (1966). *The Art of Memory.* London: University of Chicago Press.

Yin, L.-J., Lou, Y.-T., Fan, M.-X., Wang, Z.-X., and Hu, Y. (2015). Neural evidence for the use of digit-image mnemonic in a superior memorist: an fMRI study. *Front. Hum. Neurosci.* 9:109. doi: 10.3389/fnhum.2015.00109

4

Trends and Challenges in Neuroengineering: Toward "Intelligent" Neuroprostheses through Brain-"Brain Inspired Systems" Communication

Stefano Vassanelli and Mufti Mahmud*

NeuroChip Laboratory, Department of Biomedical Sciences, University of Padova, Padova, Italy

Edited by:
Mikhail Lebedev,
Duke University, USA

Reviewed by:
Dimiter Prodanov,
IMEC, Belgium
Fabian Kloosterman,
Neuroelectronics Research Flanders,
Belgium

***Correspondence:**
Stefano Vassanelli
stefano.vassanelli@unipd.it

Future technologies aiming at restoring and enhancing organs function will intimately rely on near-physiological and energy-efficient communication between living and artificial biomimetic systems. Interfacing brain-inspired devices with the real brain is at the forefront of such emerging field, with the term "neurobiohybrids" indicating all those systems where such interaction is established. We argue that achieving a "high-level" communication and functional synergy between natural and artificial neuronal networks *in vivo*, will allow the development of a heterogeneous world of neurobiohybrids, which will include "living robots" but will also embrace "intelligent" neuroprostheses for augmentation of brain function. The societal and economical impact of intelligent neuroprostheses is likely to be potentially strong, as they will offer novel therapeutic perspectives for a number of diseases, and going beyond classical pharmaceutical schemes. However, they will unavoidably raise fundamental ethical questions on the intermingling between man and machine and more specifically, on how deeply it should be allowed that brain processing is affected by implanted "intelligent" artificial systems. Following this perspective, we provide the reader with insights on ongoing developments and trends in the field of neurobiohybrids. We address the topic also from a "community building" perspective, showing through a quantitative bibliographic analysis, how scientists working on the engineering of brain-inspired devices and brain-machine interfaces are increasing their interactions. We foresee that such trend preludes to a formidable technological and scientific revolution in brain-machine communication and to the opening of new avenues for restoring or even augmenting brain function for therapeutic purposes.

Keywords: neuroengineering, biohybrid systems, neurobiohybrid systems, neuromimetic systems, brain-chip interfaces, brain machine interfaces, neurorehabilitation, artificial sensory organs

INTRODUCTION TO *NEUROBIOHYBRIDS*

An Overview on Biohybrids

The research field of biohybrid systems (or biohybrids) is capturing increasing interest across various scientific communities. The deepening of our knowledge on the physiology of living organisms –down to the cellular and molecular level– and the progress in the engineering of miniaturized interfaces between living and artificial systems, are driving research toward the creation of biohybrids where boundaries between living beings and man-made artifacts are collapsed. Classically, individual scientific communities are approaching this type of research from a different perspective. For example, within the "*robotics*" and "*biomimetics*" community, biohybrid systems are generally considered as an opportunity to exploit the unique characteristics of biological systems or their components, refined over millions of years of natural evolution, in order to solve complex or critical problems hampering artificial systems performance (Ricotti and Menciassi, 2012; Wilson et al., 2015). In this "learning from nature" endeavor, biological systems are seen as a source of inspiration for innovative solutions, toward a "soft" and "wet" robotics or "living" systems/technologies characterized by self-organization, evolvability, adaptability, and robustness (Eiben et al., 2012). Thus, biohybrid systems come here into play as workbenches where to experiment how to build "living" artificial systems.

On the other hand, biohybrids are seen by the "*life science*" community as useful tools to explore the physiology of living organisms or even as therapeutic tools. Whenever new and more advanced ways of communication with the living matter are developed, new opportunities arise to extend our capability to measure biological parameters that are relevant for understanding physiological mechanisms. Furthermore, building artificial artifacts emulating physiological operations and interacting with natural systems is a way to assess biological working hypotheses through a "reverse engineering" and reductionist approach. Biohybrids bear a huge and yet unexplored potential also for medical application, through the embodiment of natural "intelligence" and material properties in diagnostic and therapeutic tools. Neuroprostheses (Hochberg et al., 2006) and bioelectronics medicines (Birmingham et al., 2014) represent a typical example and it is easy to assume that much effort will be deployed in the future to implement artificial devices with near-physiological characteristics and communication properties for restoring function in humans. Finally, the "*materials science and engineering*" community is active in investigating fundamentals of interfacing between living matter and inorganic material. This work goes at the root of biohybrid research and has an increasing impact on other classical disciplines, including chemistry and biology. For example, thanks also to the availability of a synthetic toolbox to conjugate biomolecules and synthetic polymers in a controlled fashion, combining biomolecules, and synthetic polymers into a new class of versatile biohybrid materials following a "click" chemistry methodology has gained much interest in recent years (Dirks et al., 2007). The concept of interdisciplinary coverage of biohybrids research is sketched in **Figure 1**.

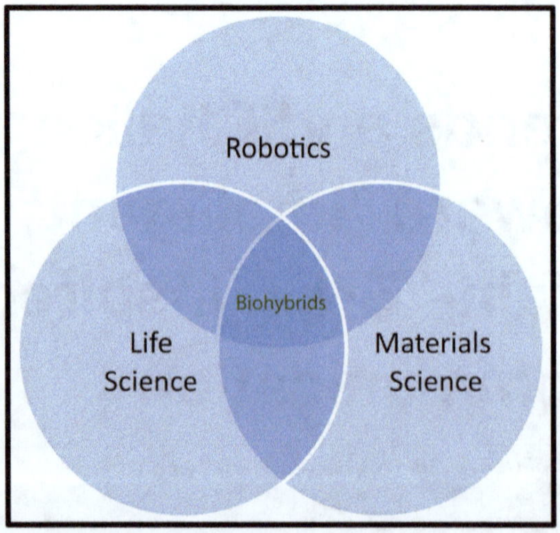

FIGURE 1 | Biohybrids as interdisciplinary research field. Within Information and Communication Technologies (ICT), Robotics, Life science, and Materials science communities are involved in biohybrids research. Scientific cooperation and interaction within the three communities is growing rapidly, although the involvement of the different actors varies by extend and typology depending on the specific research topics.

Biohybrid: A Working Definition

A common definition of biohybrid system that accepted by the scientific community is still missing. Thus, we propose a working definition to be shared with researchers interested to the field and eventually to be further refined in the future. As the term *biohybrids* encompasses a heterogeneous "melting pot" of systems spanning a range from the macro- to the nanoscale, we propose a comprehensive working definition, which highlights the importance of information exchange between living and artificial entities and its processing.

> *Biohybrid: a working definition.* A *biohybrid*, is a system formed by at least one natural and at least one artificial entity that establish close physical interactions at the molecular, cellular, or systems level, eventually leading to information flow and processing in one or both directions.

Neurobiohybrids

Within the world of biohybrids, neurobiohybrids are those where the natural component is represented by neurons. They can be present in the form of individual cells or networks, and either *in vitro* (i.e., cell culture or brain slice preparations) or *in vivo* (i.e., within the nervous system of a living animal). In general, within a neurobiohybrid, the artificial part will be composed by two functional units: (1) a device (or more devices) that have to establish the communication with neurons; (2) an interface, which mediates the physical interaction between neuron(s) and device(s), allowing the transfer of information between biological and artificial components, either in one or both directions, and its processing (**Figure 2**).

In practice, artificial devices, such as computers or bionic neuroprostheses, are communicating with neurons through energy exchange occurring in one or both directions and forming a new system acting as a whole. Whatever the approach adopted to create the neurobiohybrid system, a crucial component is represented by the interface that must include several fundamental elements to operate. First of all, in case of neuron-to-device communication, a sensor is needed, $\mathbf{S_N}$,

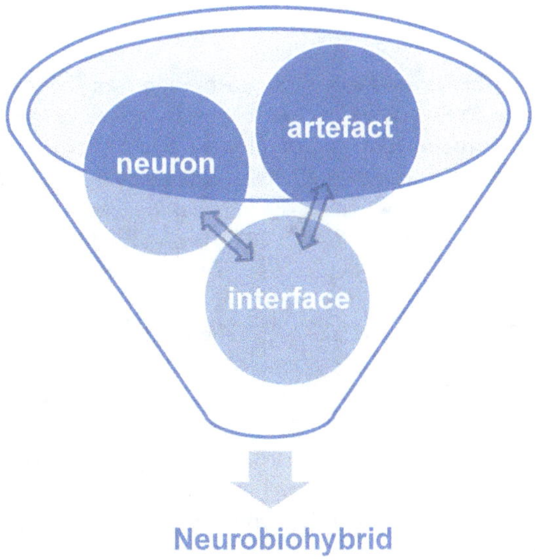

FIGURE 2 | Components of neurobiohybrid. A Neurobiohybrid is formed by three fundamental components: neuron, artifact and an interface, the latter with the function of establishing a uni- or bi-directional communication between the two.

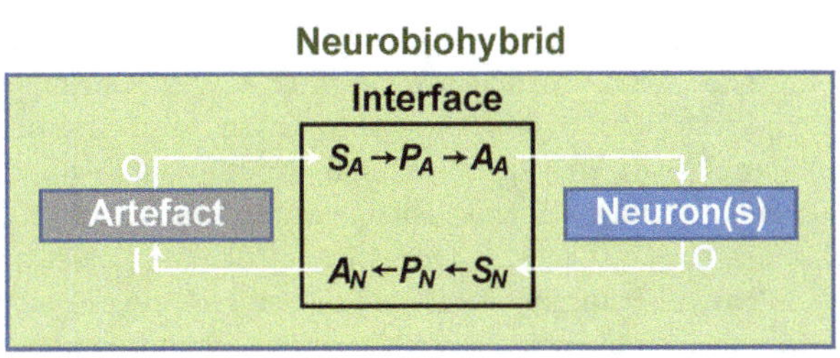

FIGURE 3 | General scheme of a neurobiohybrid. Artificial and natural components, i.e., artifact and neuron(s) respectively, communicate through a bidirectional interface. Here, signals are detected and converted by transducers, the sensor elements $\mathbf{S_A}$ and $\mathbf{S_N}$, processed by processing units, $\mathbf{P_A}$ and $\mathbf{P_N}$, and fed through actuators, $\mathbf{A_A}$ and $\mathbf{A_N}$.

transducing neuronal signals (**Figure 3**); second, a processing unit, $\mathbf{P_N}$, elaborates transduced signals; third, another transducer, the actuator $\mathbf{A_N}$, transforms the output signals from the processing unit into signals suitable to control the device. Similarly, in the opposite direction, signals from the device control the neuronal response through a chain formed by a sensor ($\mathbf{S_A}$), a processing unit ($\mathbf{P_A}$), and an actuator ($\mathbf{A_A}$) (**Figure 3**).

We must clarify how this general description of the interface is wide-ranging:

- Bidirectional communication is not an absolute requirement, as unidirectional communication is sufficient to establish a neurobiohybrid;
- Communication can occur through any type of energy conveying information (electromagnetic, chemical, mechanical). Thus, any possible mechanism allowing information exchange and processing within the neurobiohybrid is included;
- "Processing" is here intended as "operating on time-varying physical quantities." As such, the term does not solely comprise the more conventional digital or analog signal processing, but rather any type of processing that can be operated by any type of suitable processing unit, e.g., from single molecules to electronic computing architectures.

According to this introduction and the definition of biohybrid provided above, we propose a working definition of neurobiohybrid.

> *Neurobiohybrid: working definition.* A *neurobiohybrid* is a system formed by the combination of at least one neuron as natural entity and at least one device as artificial entity. To form a neurobiohybrid system, neuron(s), and device(s) establish physical interactions through an interface at the molecular, cellular, or systems level, eventually leading to information transfer and processing in one or both directions.

Noteworthy, according to such definition, all those implementations that are commonly known as brain-computer-interfaces (BCI) fall under the neurobiohybrids umbrella. Included are also those therapeutic hybrid systems working through stimulation and/or recording of the central or peripheral nervous system, and that are relying on appropriate interfacing for information transfer and processing. Typical examples based on "invasive" interfacing are deep brain stimulation (DBS, McConnell et al., 2016), neuroprosthetic limbs (e.g., Micera, 2016), cochlear implants (Roche and Hansen, 2015; Sato et al., 2016), or artificial retinas (e.g., Zeck, 2016). Interestingly, also "non-invasive" interfacing approaches such as functional electrical stimulation (FES) (for a review see Peckham and Knutson, 2005) or transcranial current stimulation (TCS, Ruffini et al., 2013) should be considered as part of the neurobiohybrids family. Given the obvious relevance of neurobiohybrids in computer science, basic neuroscience, and therapy of neurological disorders, it is no surprise that funding agencies are devoting resources to attack major challenges in the field (e.g., Miranda et al., 2015). However, we believe that, among major challenges, learning how to create functional hybrids between biological neural networks and neuromimetic architectures emulating their processing capabilities has an immense potential, particularly in the perspective of restoring or even augmenting brain function.

NEUROBIOHYBRIDS: STATE-OF-THE-ART, CURRENT TRENDS, AND CHALLENGES

In this section, a brief overview on the state-of-the-art and current trends in neurobiohybrids research is given, with particular emphasis on recent advances originating from the convergence of novel neurotechnologies and neuromimetics research. Specifically, we focus on those paving the way to "intelligent" neuroprosthetics for restoring and augmenting brain function in living animals. We identify key scientific and technological challenges as also pointed out by Thibeault (2014), and briefly discuss opportunities and threats for the development of the neurobiohybrids research community.

Neurobiohybrids: State-of-the-Art and Main Trends

We recognize in the "dynamic clamp" technique the first fundamental leap into research on neurobiohybrids. Here, although in *in vitro* conditions, artificial neuromimetic systems are physically and functionally coupled to biological neurons with mutual information exchange in a clear manner. The dynamic clamp relies on a closed-loop control over the neuronal intracellular potential and membrane conductances, the controller being an elementary analog or software-based neuronal counterpart (Sharp et al., 1993; Prinz et al., 2004). Although ground-breaking, and despite significant improvements from the time of its introduction, this method is not suited for long-term and large-scale network implementations, as it is intrinsically limited by the interfacing through intracellular electrodes.

Brain processing, instead, deeply relies on neuronal circuits. Therefore, multi-site—and minimally invasive—techniques are necessary, allowing to interface many neurons at once within the neurobiohybrid. Attempts have been made to create network-based neurobiohybrids and in the first instance, in *in vitro* systems. For example, metal multi-electrode arrays (MEA, for a historical review of MEA, see Pine, 2006) were used to interface networks of dissociated neurons to a robot actuator where the processing was taken over by software-based spike encoding/decoding algorithms (Novellino et al., 2007). In addition, parallel progress made on neural interfaces for large-scale high-resolution multi-site recording techniques and neuromimetic nanodevices and architectures, have opened up new avenues. Recording and stimulating *in vitro* with large and dense arrays of voltage transducers (Hutzler et al., 2006; Hierlemann et al., 2011; Ferrea et al., 2012; Lewandowska et al., 2016) and optical imaging techniques (Chemla and Chavane, 2010; Tian et al., 2012) allow the gathering of spiking or sub-threshold signaling events from large neuronal networks.

Studies *in vivo*, instead, have led to implant-based BCIs and brain-machine-interfaces (BMIs) taking advantage of advanced multi-site neural interfaces and real-time software-based processing for neuroprosthetic applications. Numerous examples can be found in literature, from basic research to translational medicine, and ranging from rodents (e.g., Shobe et al., 2015), to non-human primates (Zhang et al., 2016) and even to human subjects (Hochberg et al., 2006). Although constrained in terms of number of recording/stimulation sites in comparison to their *in vitro* counterpart (Csicsvari et al., 2003; Berényi et al., 2014; Vassanelli, 2014; Schroder et al., 2015), their importance for investigating neurons in an intact brain (Buzsáki et al., 2012), or as interfaces for brain-machine communication and neuroprosthetics is well recognized (Nicolelis and Lebedev, 2009; Lebedev and Nicolelis, 2011).

However, a real paradigm shift toward "intelligent" neuroprosthetics and brain augmentation can be expected from the creation of neurobiohybrids where such brain interfaces are functionally coupled to neuromimetic devices and architectures emulating brain circuits (Thibeault, 2014). In fact, in our view, similarly to what happens for cardiac pacemakers (see Miller et al., 2015; Seriwala et al., 2016) or more "classical" prostheses (e.g., orthopedic prostheses, see Goldfarb et al., 2013; Ortiz-Catalan et al., 2014; Raspopovic et al., 2014; Vujaklija et al., 2016), the challenge is to engineer artificial neuronal systems emulating as closely as possible their natural counterpart and interfacing them efficiently to the native organ to restore (or to augment) function. Recent neuromorphic architectures based on very large scale integration (VLSI) technology (Indiveri et al., 2011; Qiao et al., 2015) and the discovery of physical components with synaptic-like plasticity properties such as memristors (Strukov et al., 2008) or carbon nanotubes based circuits (Joshi et al., 2011), have set the foundations for developing such novel generation of neurobiohybrids.

Large improvements and innovations are unquestionably necessary to achieve effective communication between natural and artificial neuronal networks. Two-way (recording and stimulation), high-resolution (down to micrometers), and large-scale (hundreds to thousands of neurons) interfacing is still beyond reach. Particularly, in this context, techniques for large-scale and high-density stimulation (also known as microstimulation) are lagging behind expectations. Although optogenetic platforms may be suitable candidates (Dugue et al., 2012; Buzsáki et al., 2015; Grosenick et al., 2015; Newman et al., 2015), other means of stimulation not requiring neuronal transfection with biological agents are to be taken into account for real clinical applications (e.g., via tuneable and field-shaped electrical stimulation or localized neurotransmitters detection and release).

Scientific and Technological Challenges

Transducers (Sensing and Actuating)

As hinted above, the development of novel sensing and actuating probes is expected to play a fundamental role in the neurobiohybrids field toward application in neuroprosthetics. A wide range of probes with different materials, design, and fabrication processes, and interfacing principles have been developed and reported earlier targeting specific research needs (for reviews see Wheeler and Nam, 2011; Spira and Hai, 2013; Vassanelli, 2014; Vidu et al., 2014; Angle et al., 2015; Fekete, 2015; Giocomo, 2015; Ruther and Paul, 2015; Lee et al., 2016; Patil and Thakor, 2016; Pisanello et al., 2016; Prodanov and Delbeke, 2016). Brain-chip interfaces are among most promising strategies to support such development (Vassanelli et al., 2012) as semiconductor technology allows for integration into a single millimeter scale device of a large number (hundreds to thousands) of microtransducers for recording and stimulation of neuronal signals.

Concerning interfaces based on electrical signaling between neurons and chips (those that are most developed so far), two fundamental approaches exist depending on the nature of the transducer:

1. Neural interfaces based on metal microelectrodes were developed first, and are now available in the form of 2D or 3D arrays that can be implanted in the brain or following a different interfacing philosophy, connected to peripheral nerves (Rutten, 2002; Wise et al., 2004; Stieglitz et al., 2014). The neuroelectronic interface is established when neuron and microelectrode are "close enough," allowing signal detection (from neuron to microelectrode) or stimulation (from microelectrode to neuron). This condition can be met both *in vitro* and *in vivo*, although under different biophysical bases. In the *in vitro* case, neurons are typically cultured on the chip surface where their membrane come into close contact with microelectrodes (i.e., typically in the tens of nanometers range) by adhering to the solid chip substrate (Braun and Fromherz, 2004). Though the original brain network topology is lost, the dissociated neurons reconnect and form a more random-like network (Haider and McCormick, 2009; Kwan and Dan, 2012). Recent technological advances allowed the development of large-scale high-density metal electrode arrays (MEA) for high-resolution recording of such neuronal networks in culture (Eversmann et al., 2011; Maccione et al., 2012; Muller et al., 2015). When a MEA, instead, is implanted in the nervous system (i.e., brain or spinal cord), transducers and neurons are more separated than in *in vitro* conditions, as cell adhesion is not governing neuro-chip interaction in this context. Also, in case of chronic implants, damaged tissue first, and gliosis afterwards are commonly building a separation layer between transducers and neurons. Thus, a volume conductor of tissue surrounds the interface and ionic currents and voltage gradients developing within it are governing recording and stimulation of neurons (Mitzdorf, 1985; Gold et al., 2006; Anastassiou et al., 2010). Other types of microstructured metal electrode-based interfaces exist, as regenerating sieves (Lago et al., 2005) and cone-in-growth electrodes (Rutten, 2002). In addition, alternative to brain implantation, microfabricated cuff or intrafascicular electrodes can be used to interface peripheral nerves (Mailley et al., 2004). Whatever the site of implantation, owing to electrochemical features of the electrolyte-metal electrode interface, faradaic currents are likely to occur, particularly when relatively large potentials come into play, i.e., during stimulation (Vassanelli, 2014).
2. The second fundamental strategy for neuron-chip interfacing aims to solve this problem by using oxide-insulated semiconductor or metal-semiconductor transducers to generate a capacitive coupling with neurons (Fromherz, 2006; Eickenscheidt et al., 2012). The approach has the advantage of relying on non-faradaic currents, at least within wider voltage ranges. Basing on this approach, very high-resolution CMOS chips have been developed for electrical imaging of neurons *in vitro* (Hutzler et al., 2006) and more recently, for *in vivo* applications (Felderer and Fromherz, 2011; Schroder et al., 2015). Noteworthy, as excitatory and inhibitory neurons are expected to respond differently to appropriately selected electrical stimuli (Mahmud and Vassanelli, 2016a), it will be strategically important to achieve a high degree of control over the electrolyte-microelectrode interface to achieve a finely tuned stimulation of neurons.

Finally, it is worth to mention that electrical neural interfaces will be improved also by clever use of novel materials. For example, read-out of neuronal activity from the mammalian brain *in vivo* was achieved by means of injectable free-standing mesh electronics (Liu et al., 2015), thus potentially minimizing tissue damage and reaction and reaching and unprecedented level of intermingling between neural tissue and electronics.

With the advent of optogenetic stimulation (Dugue et al., 2012) new hybrid optoelectronic interfaces are emerging (Park et al., 2011; Armstrong et al., 2013; Wu et al., 2013; Pashaie et al., 2015). With respect to electric stimulation (Mukaino et al., 2014; Tabot et al., 2015), optogenetics offers basically two potential advantages: (i) neuronal type specificity and (ii) the possibility to inhibit and not only to excite target neurons. It is therefore easy to foresee that a considerable amount of work will be deployed to exploit these characteristics in neurobiohybrids for controlling neuronal circuit activities within a closed-loop at cellular rsolution (Packer et al., 2015).

Although invasive interfaces are the most suitable to enable a reliable and high-resolution communication with the brain, several sorts of non-invasive brain-machine interfaces are also available (Waldert, 2016). They can be indeed included within the neurobiohybrids scheme, albeit based on unidirectional communication. They include for example EEG based platforms (Friehs et al., 2004; Norton et al., 2015), but also recent developments on fMRI for real time brain-machine interfacing (Weiskopf et al., 2007; Lee et al., 2009; Ruiz et al., 2014). On the other hand, functional electrical stimulation (FES) or transcranial current (TCS) (Ali et al., 2013) or magnetic (TMS) (Camprodon, 2016) stimulation approaches are to be included as they allow for machine-to-brain communication. Although limited in spatiotemporal resolution, non-invasive interfaces offer undoubtful advantages in terms of clinical application (Ortiz-Rosario and Adeli, 2013). "Hybrid" less-invasive solutions such as high-resolution electrocorticography (ECoG), represent an interesting compromise when cortical areas are to be interfaced for recording and perhaps, stimulation (Girardi et al., 2011; Vassanelli et al., 2012; Berényi et al., 2014; Khodagholy et al., 2015) because of their limited invasiveness with respect to in-brain implants (Pei et al., 2011; Matsushita et al., 2013).

Processing Unit

Fast processing of neuronal signals is essential for real-time performance in neurobiohybrids. When dealing with one or a few neurons, this is achievable also on the basis of conventional software or analog circuits. However, when dealing with larger networks, high-performance approaches must be considered for simultaneous real-time processing of multiple neuronal signals. A detailed analysis of state-of-the art signal processing tools for brain-machine interfaces goes beyond the scope of this article and is available elsewhere (see, for example, Krusienski et al., 2011; Mahmud et al., 2012, 2014; Mahmud and Vassanelli, 2016b). However, we think that among parallel computing architectures speeding up processing times, "intelligent" neuromorphic analog processors based on artificial neuromorphic neural networks (see for example Qiao et al., 2015) will play a major role in the next generation of neurobiohybrids. As a matter of fact and similarly to other prostheses, in neuroprosthetics the ideal goal is replacing neuronal networks that have undergone injury or degeneration with artificial circuits emulating as closely as possible native functional features. Artificial neurons owning functional properties similar to their natural counterparts such as firing behavior and plasticity-based synaptic integration, will be an ideal replacement or rehabilitation support for injured or degenerating neuronal circuits in neuroprosthetics.

Dynamic Clamp

The dynamic clamp technique offers a prototypic example of such vision, where an artificial brain-inspired computing system drives the excitability of a living neuron establishing a real-time closed-loop control within a neurobiohybrid system. Beginning in the early 90s, researchers started to investigate the interaction of living nerve cells in culture with model neurons in order to understand and emulate the behavior of neural networks (Yarom, 1991; Le Masson et al., 2002). The interface connection between living and model neurons was based on intracellular electrodes, in fact obtaining a two-way artificial-natural communication within a neurobiohybrid. Due to intrinsic limitations of intracellular electrode techniques, such neurobiohybrid setup was limited to only one, or a few, biological neurons. On the other hand, having access to the intracellular potential, it had the advantage of providing high sensitivity for detecting and eliciting neuronal signals. From the neurobiohybrid perspective (see Section Neurobiohybrids), the "device" was here represented by a biomimetic artificial neuron. We may refer to this type of neurobiohybrid, where the interfaced device is a biomimetic artificial neuron, as a Neuron-Neuron Hybrid (NNH). NNH gained interest as a mean to correlate experimental and modeling studies through a sort of reverse-engineering approach, taking advantage of biological neurons to validate their emulators as well as working hypotheses on operational properties of neuronal circuits. Biomimetic neurons and their networks can be digital or analog. Elementary NNHs and their networks have been investigated through the dynamic clamp (Sharp et al., 1993; Prinz, 2004; Yang et al., 2015), which was used to monitor the membrane potential of living neurons and via numerical simulation of model neurons and synapses on a computer, to inject synaptic currents into the living neurons in real-time, as if they were "synaptically" connected to the model neurons. Alternatively, the dynamic clamp could be used to "insert" artificial membrane conductances into living neurons embedded in a network, thus exploring the role of intrinsic conductances in shaping the network's output.

From Single Neurons to Networks

In hybrid NNHs with analog model neurons and synapses, a specially designed microelectronic circuit constitutes the artificial part of the network. Such hardware model neurons and synapses can be connected to living circuits through electrodes, creating a hybrid circuit that consists of a biological network and a dedicated "neuromorphic" (or neuromimetic) silicon chip. With the development of multi-electrode approaches (Rutten, 2002), pioneering work has first succeeded to interface, through dedicated software, cultured neurons and robots, a step toward the creation of "autonomous intelligent biohybrid systems" (Novellino et al., 2007). In other examples of neurobiohybrid network applications, Nowotny et al. (2003) used a hybrid circuit with an Aplysia neuron to show that spike-timing dependent plasticity (STDP) enhances synchronization in neural networks, while Manor and Nadim (2001) demonstrated that synaptic depression in neural networks with recurrent inhibition gives rise to bistability by combining a digital model neuron with a biological pacemaker neuron. In a particular elegant study, Le Masson et al. (2002) reconstructed a thalamocortical circuit by coupling living neurons in the lateral geniculate nucleus to digital and analog model neurons. The researchers showed how feedback inhibition can functionally disconnect the cortex from sensory input in a state reminiscent of sleep, demonstrating the potential of the "Natural-Artificial-Neurohybrid" and/or hybrid NNHs approach in elucidating network function even in large circuits. Overall, when examined from a broader perspective, this sort of pioneering investigations on hybrid networks can be also interpreted as a part of a general effort in the search for novel experimental approaches to investigate neural microcircuits and to develop more efficient brain-machine interfaces for neurological therapy and rehabilitation.

Artificial Neuromorphic Neuronal Networks

Integration into a unique neurobiohybrid system of large (i.e., tens to hundreds of neurons) neuronal networks is a major challenge to be faced. To this endeavor, Very Large Scale Integrated (VLSI) devices come into play. VLSI devices comprise hybrid analog/digital circuits that implement hardware models of biological systems, using computational principles analogous to the ones used by nervous systems (Indiveri and Horiuchi, 2011; Indiveri, 2015). When implemented in VLSI technology, neuromorphic circuits use, to some extent, similar physics used in neural systems (e.g., they transport majority carriers across the channel of transistors by diffusion processes, very much like neurons transport ions inside or outside cell bodies through their ionic channels). Given the analogies at the single device level, neuromorphic circuits are ideal interfacing circuits to real neurons. Moreover, larger scale neuromorphic networks of spiking neurons share the same physical constraints of their biological counterparts (i.e., noise, temperature dependence, inhomogeneities, etc.). As a consequence, to carry out computation in a robust and reproducible manner, these architectures often have to use similar strategies for maximizing compactness, optimizing robustness to noise, minimizing power consumption, and increasing fault tolerance.

In recent years, an interesting class of neuromorphic devices implementing general-purpose computational architectures based on networks of silicon neurons and synapses emerged (Bartolozzi and Indiveri, 2007; Indiveri et al., 2011; Indiveri and Liu, 2015). Such devices range from reconfigurable arrays of basic integrate and fire neuron models to learning architectures implementing detailed models of spike-based synaptic plasticity. Spike-based plasticity circuits enable these systems to adapt to the statistics of their input signals, to learn and classify complex sequences of spatio-temporal patterns (e.g., arising from visual or auditory signals), and eventually to interact with the user and the environment. Typically, the analog circuits implemented on these devices operate in the *weak-inversion* regime, where current amplitudes are of the order of pico-Amperes and operating time-constants are of the order of milliseconds. This is a crucial characteristic that differentiates this approach with other more conventional full custom analog VLSI approaches for implementing spike-based neural networks. Conventional analog VLSI implementations of spike-based neural networks use circuits biased in the *strong-inversion* region, that produce currents of the order of micro-amperes, so the largest time-constants that can be achieved in practice are at least 1000 times smaller than biological ones. The biologically plausible time constants achieved with the neuromorphic approach are crucial, as they allow seamless interactions with real living networks. Given the types of parallel architectures that can be implemented with these silicon neurons and synapses, processing time does not increase with size, and large networks can be fabricated by (e.g., simply using more silicon real-estate) to match the numbers of recording/stimulating electrodes or real targeted neurons that one would like to interact with.

Consistent with the neuromorphic engineering approach, the strategy used to transmit signals across chip boundaries in these types of systems is inspired from the nervous system: output signals are represented by stereotyped digital pulses (spikes), and the analog nature of the signal is typically encoded in the mean frequency of the neuron's pulse sequence (spike rates). Similarly, input signals are represented by spike trains, conveyed to the chip in the form of asynchronous digital pulses, that stimulate their target synapses on the receiving chip. The circuits that generate the on-chip synaptic currents when stimulated by incoming spikes are slow low-power analog circuits. The circuits that generate and manage these streams of input/output digital pulses are fast asynchronous logic elements based on an emerging new communication standard for neuromorphic chips called the "Address-Event Representation" (AER). This representation is ideal for both implementing real-time interfaces with living networks, as well as for allowing reconfigurability of artificial network topology (e.g., via address-event source-destination lookup tables).

Memristive Plasticity

An important advancement in the field of biological networks emulation and with great potential in neuroprosthetics is the development of new nanoelectronic elements with synaptic functional properties. Carbon nanotubes (Cellot et al., 2009; Joshi et al., 2011; Fabbro et al., 2013) and particularly, memristors are emerging as a new class of devices that might serve the purpose. Resistive Random Access Memory (ReRAM) cells are nowadays classified as being memristive in nature (Chua, 2011) and have first being conceptually conceived in 1971 by Chua (1971), with the first neuromimetics applications presented at the same time. Since then, the usage of memristors in simulating artificial synapses has started to be explored (Yang et al., 2013; Kim et al., 2015; Niehrster and Thomas, 2015; Thomas et al., 2015). The functional signature of memristors is a pinched hysteresis loop in the current-voltage (i-v) domain when excited by a bipolar periodic stimulus. Such hysteresis is typically noticed for all kind of devices/materials in support of a discharge phenomenon that possess certain inertia, causing the value of a physical property to lag behind changes in the mechanism causing it, and has been common both to large scale (Prodromakis et al., 2012) as well as nanoscale dissipative devices (Strukov et al., 2008). The analogy of memristors and chemical synapses is thus made on the basis that synaptic dynamics depend upon ions flowing through the postsynaptic membrane in a similar fashion that "ionic species" can be displaced within any inorganic barrier. TiO2-based memristor models (Strukov et al., 2008; Prodromakis et al., 2011) hypothesized that solid-state devices comprise a mixture of TiO2 phases, a stoichiometric and a reduced one (TiO2-x), that can facilitate distinct resistive states via controlling the displacement of oxygen vacancies and thus the extent of the two phases. More recently however it was demonstrated that substantial resistive switching is only viable through the formation and annihilation of continuous conductive percolation channels (Shihong et al., 2012) that extend across the whole active region of a device, shorting the top (TE) and bottom (BE) electrodes; no matter what the underlying physical mechanism is.

The development of such emerging nanoscale synaptic-like computation elements may notably benefit the establishment of neuromorphic architectures and neurobiohybrids. This technology adds substantially on computation functionality, due to the rate-dependency of the underlying physical switching mechanisms. At the same time it can facilitate unprecedented complexity due to the capacity of storing and processing spiking events locally. Moreover, the minuscule dimensions and architectural simplicity of solid-state memristor implementations could be successfully exploited to substantially increase the number of cells per unit area, and effectively enhance the system's tolerance to issues stemming from device mismatch and low-yields (Gelencser et al., 2012; Gupta et al., 2016).

Toward "Intelligent" Neuroprosthetics

In perspective, neurobiohybrids, and particularly NNHs, will represent the basis for creating advanced and "intelligent" neuroprostheses. Novel generations of neuroprostheses or bioelectronic medicines (BM) acting through electrical stimulation of the central or peripheral nervous system bear a huge potential for therapy of numerous diseases, including neurological disorders, metabolic, and autonomic dysfunctions (Hyam et al., 2012; Afshar et al., 2013; Birmingham et al., 2014). In order to exploit the envisaged potential, such devices will have to be "adaptive," i.e., adjust "intelligently" and continuously their stimulation of neurons while monitoring effectiveness in real time. This is needed to counterbalance drift and intrinsic variability of the response to nerve stimulation through time, and to cope with patient-specific changes of conditions during daily life. Such a vision implies that BM must be also "precise," i.e., allow for a finely tuned control of the nervous system by means of modulating neuronal excitability. Achieving this vision and conferring such a degree of "intelligence" to a miniaturized implantable device is a tremendous challenge. As pointed out above, significant technological progress has been made in artificially emulating neurons, synapses, and neuronal networks by low-power neuromimetic microelectronics. Beyond the capability to "speak the same language" made of nerve impulses and distributed computation, such neuromimetic architectures share with biological neuronal networks other properties, as online learning and reconfigurability based upon internal plastic changes (Qiao et al., 2015). The envisioned challenge toward brain repair and augmentation is to pair neuromorphic architectures with biological neurons *in vivo*, and set it to act as "chaperon or surrogate" of neuronal circuits to intelligently restore function. The neuromorphic devices will communicate bi-directionally (i.e., both receiving and sending nerve impulses) with biological neurons in the central or peripheral nervous system through advanced neural interfaces, enabling precise, and "near-physiological" tuning of neuronal activity within an "intelligent" adaptive closed-loop. In perspective, such approach could support a variety of bioelectronic and neuroprosthetic applications, independent of the physical nature of signals measured and stimuli delivered (i.e., electrical, chemical, etc.). It will set the context and the technological grounds for a true revolution toward "intelligent" neuroprosthetics and augmentation of brain function.

Bibliometrics on Neurobiohybrids Research

The success of neurobiohybrids in neuroprosthetics will depend on community building, paralleling scientific-technological development, and directed to strenghtening of interactions, e.g., between neuroscientists, neurologists, and neurotechnologists and the communities working on brain-inspired computation and microdevices. We analyzed the development of such interactions in recent years by means of bibliometric analysis.

Bibliometrics was performed on publications related to neurobiohybrids to quantify interaction trends within the new interdisciplinary community. The details of the analysis procedure is provided in Section Methods. For the analysis, a total of 5320 journal articles and conference papers were carefully selected from three commercial scientific repositories (IEEE-Xplore, Thompson Reuters Web of Knowledge, and Elsevier's Scopus) through keyword searching for a window of 20 years (1995–2014). After careful selection, 3914 articles from 125 journals and 1406 papers from 93 conferences were taken into consideration for further analysis.

Pie-charts in **Figure 4** report the number of publications appeared in top 20 journals and top 8 conferences. It is interesting to note that the great majority of publications are mostly found in applied physics or engineering journals, with only a few appearances in multidisciplinary journals (e.g., Nature, Science and PLoS One) and even less in neuroscience journals (e.g., Neuron). From this first indications, it is tempting to conclude that the field is still very much biased toward engineering and physics communities rather than neuroscience communities. Additionally, it appears that only a few cutting edge publications have gained visibility to a wider community by publication on prestigious multidisciplinary journals. These results imply that the vast majority of researches in the neurobiohybrid field are not reaching the neuroscientific counterparts, which is a limiting factor for further development of this highly interdisciplinary field of research.

Also conference publications are dominated by engineering meetings. This can be in part explained as in neuroscience it is uncommon to publish results in conference papers, which are conversely well evaluated in the engineering environment. Again,

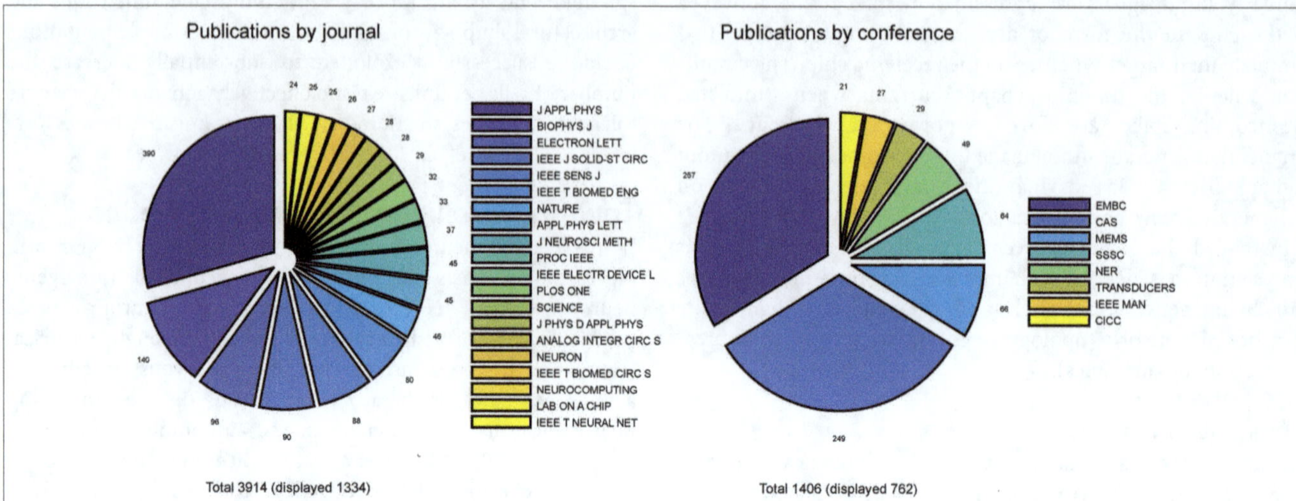

FIGURE 4 | Distribution of publications. Distribution of journal articles **(left)** and conference papers **(right)** per year are reported as slices of pies. Only journals and conferences were considered with more than 20 articles and papers in the neurobiohybrid field.

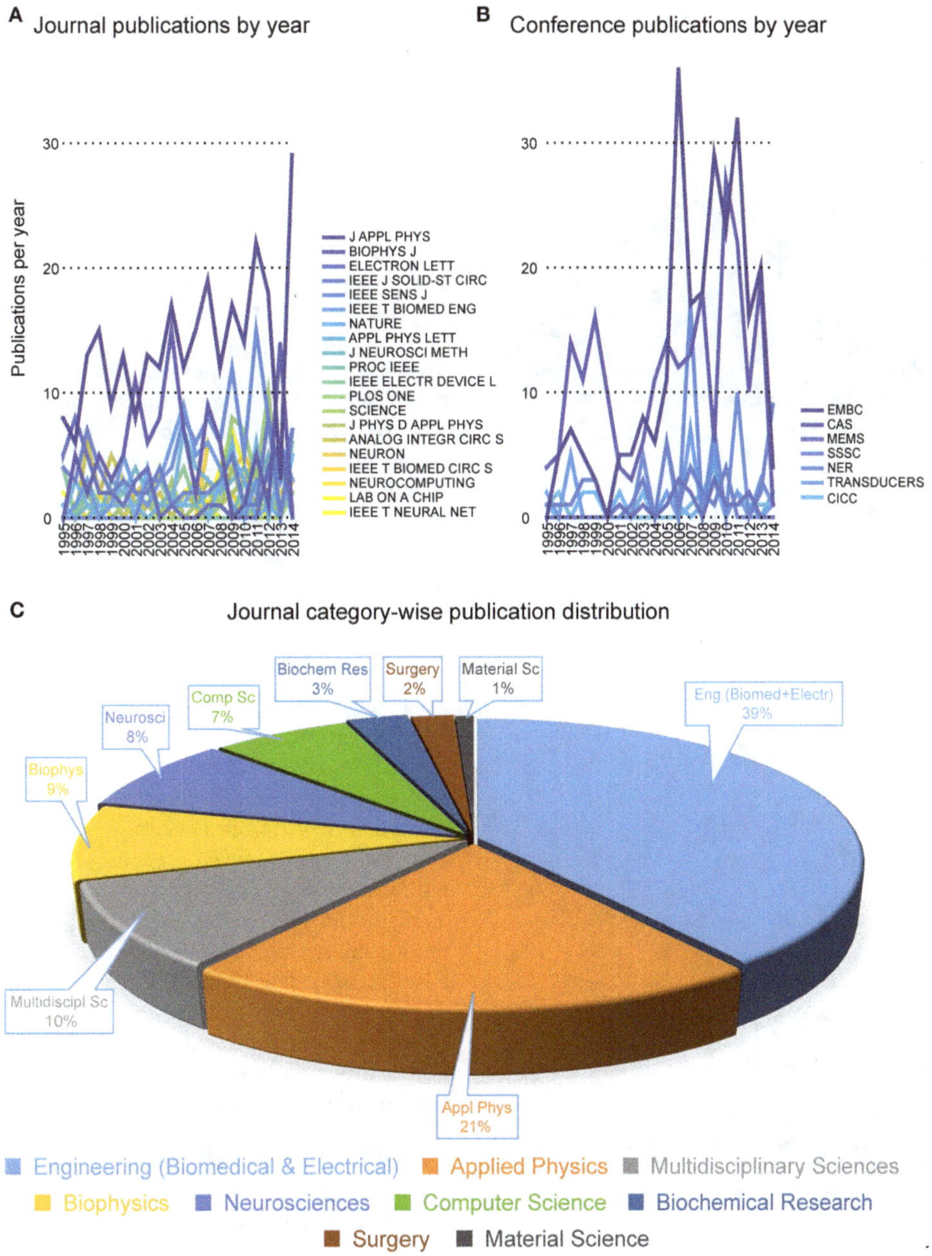

FIGURE 5 | Publication trends. Distribution of the number of publications per year in journals **(A)** and conferences **(B)**. The journal category-wise publication distribution **(C)** shows dominating appearance of publications from the Neurobiohybrid field in journals belonging to the Engineering and Physical Sciences category, in comparison to the Health and Life Sciences category.

efforts should be made to improve homogeneity of dissemination and to reach a wider audience.

Judging from the trend of the number of publications per year (**Figures 5, 6**), a reasonable growth of the field can be appreciated, although comparable with other research fields.

Most interestingly, an analysis on the impact factor (IF) distribution (**Figures 7, 8**) reveals that most publications fall within a window below impact factor 5 with a high peak at around 2. While this may be acceptable within the engineering community, it is far below average with respect to publications in the neuroscience community. This discrepancy is playing against the building of a homogeneous community with equal career opportunities for engineers or physicist, on one side, and neuroscientists on the other side. Particularly, neuroscientists working in the neurobiohybrid field seem heavily penalized in terms of IF and will struggle in the competition with colleagues of other neuroscientific disciplines. Thus, in our view, the neurobiohybrid community should invest major

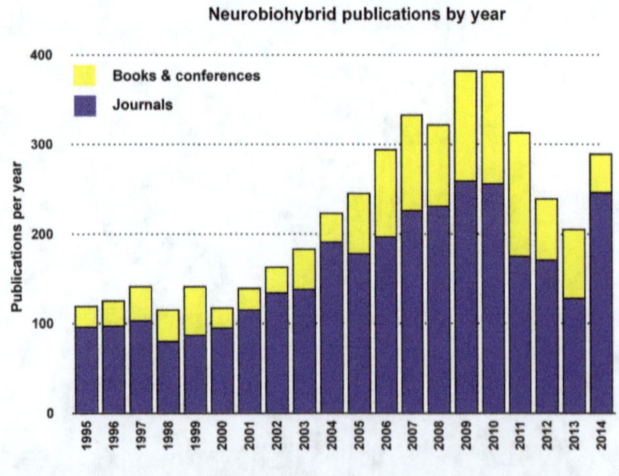

FIGURE 6 | Yearly total publications. Total number of publications appeared in journals, conference proceedings, and books per year.

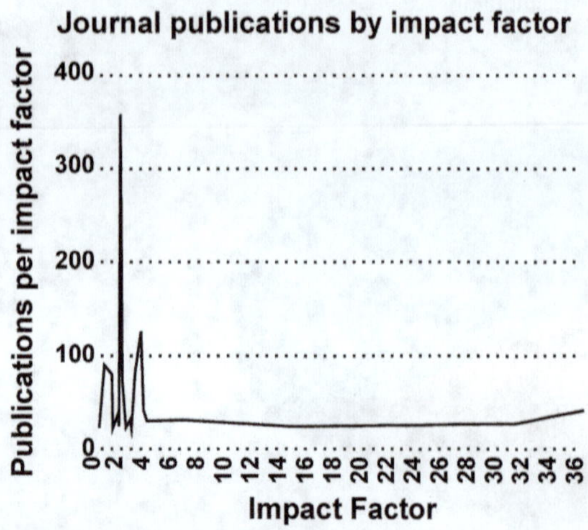

FIGURE 7 | Impact Factor distribution. Impact factor distribution of publications in the neurobiohybrid field shows that majority of the publications appeared in journals with impact factor less than 5.

efforts to improve dissemination efficacy, in particular, by increasing visibility of matured results through publications in interdisciplinary journals that can attract interest from a broader neuroscience community. In fact, as shown in **Figure 5C**, only 10% of the journal publications concerning neurobiohybrids appear in multidisciplinary journals and expanding this share will favor the communities' coalescence given the exemplary increasing interactions between the specialized subcommunities of Neuromimetics and Neuroprosthetics (**Figure 9**). Such efforts should be paralleled by organization of focused workshops and training initiatives in the neurobiohybrid field conceived in a way to attract interdisciplinary audience and to create a new generation of scientists with competences and skills spanning from neurotechnologies to neuromimetic systems and more classical neuroscience.

Word clouds of keywords used for the bibliometric analysis are reported hereafter in **Figure 10**.

DISCUSSION

Biohybrids, that is, biohybrid systems where artificial devices and living organisms establish physical interactions with information exchange, will play a pivotal role in the future development of efficient, sustainable, and powerful information and communication technologies. A clear and well known example of biohybrid application supporting such expectations is represented by cardiac pacemakers, where information needed for restoring physiological heart pacing is provided by artificial rhythm generators through implanted electrodes. Noteworthy, closed-loop bi-directional interaction between organ and artificial pacemaker is seen as an important strategy to effectively restore function through a dynamic control and prevent cardiovascular pathologies (Occhetta et al., 2003). Biohybrids will represent an essential workbench to better investigate living organisms, to assess new principles of communication between natural and artificial world, and to develop novel generations of bio-inspired devices based on non-living matter. From the application perspective, they represent an innovative strategy to improve therapy of a variety of diseases through *in vivo* implants (Nicolelis and Lebedev, 2009). Overall, from a broad perspective, biohybrid technologies may replace artificial ones, leading to higher energy efficiency and performance gain while lowering environmental impact. Among biohybrids, *neurobiohybrids* are of paramount importance. After millions of years of evolution, the nervous system of living animals, and the human brain in particular, is endowed with unique abilities to cope with information processing in an energy effective, adaptable and robust manner, outperforming artificial devices when dealing with "real world" problems. Biohybrid systems of natural and artificial neurons implanted *in vivo* will be central to explore brain operational principles and, on the clinical side, to create novel generations of "intelligent" neuroprostheses.

The Paradigm Shift

In our opinion, we are set to experience a true paradigm shift in neurobiohybrids research thanks to concomitant advances in three highly intertwined disciplines: *neurophysiology of brain microcircuits*, *neural interfaces,* and *neuromimetics* (that is, the creation of physical elements and circuits emulating living neurons and networks). For the first time, and thanks to recent development of physical elements with synaptic-like plasticity, a fascinating challenge is coming within reach: natural and hardware-based neuronal circuits could be integrated into new entities, operating *in vivo* through brain implants, and evolving together on the basis of shared plasticity and processing rules. To this endeavor, non-"von Neumann" brain-inspired architectures will have to be interfaced to their natural counterparts, the brain microcircuits. This will occur, at the physical level, through high-resolution, and bi-directional neural interfaces, and at the algorithmic level, by emulating in artificial architectures those processing rules that are key for the function of real biological brain networks. Noteworthy, however, neurobiohybrids can

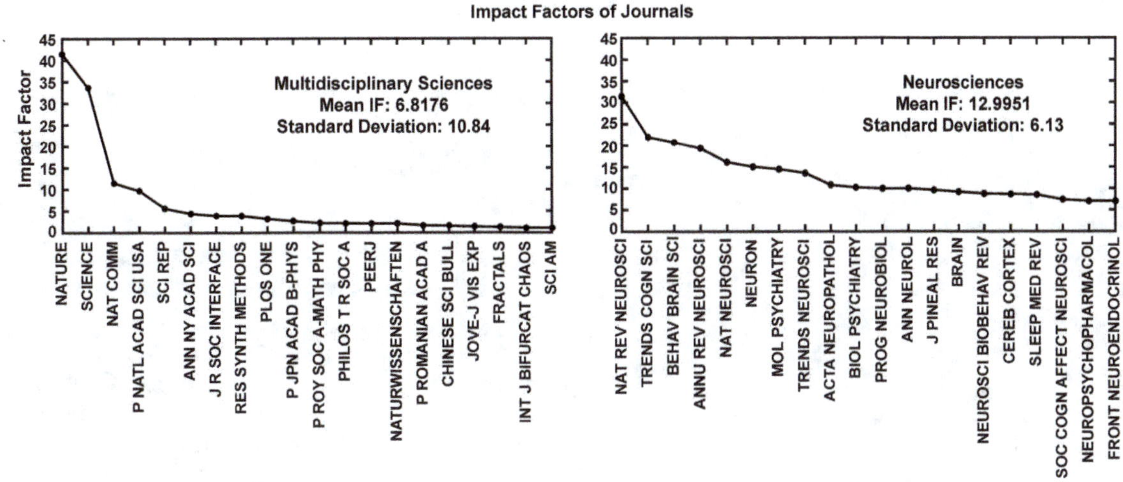

FIGURE 8 | Impact Factor comparison. Two categories of journals were compared for the impact factors (IF) during the year 2014. These journals' IFs were calculated by Thomson Reuters and reported through Journal Citation Reports (https://jcr.incites.thomsonreuters.com/). Average IFs of the journals in the multidisciplinary sciences category (left) is almost half in comparison to the neurosciences category (right). For better representation only top 20 journals from each category are shown in the figure.

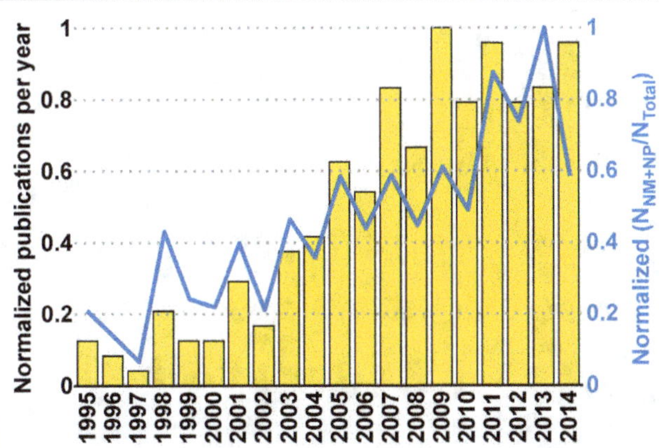

FIGURE 9 | Interaction between communities and its effect on the Neurobiohybrid publications. The bar plot (left Y-axis) shows the normalized publication frequencies calculated by extracting relevant publications through "interaction keywords"-based querying (see Section Analysis of Database) of the XML database. The increasing trend of the publication frequencies from two subcommunities ("Neuromimetics" and "Neuroprosthetics") associated to the Neurobiohybrid field demonstrates a growing interaction between them. The interaction effect on the Neurobiohybrid publications is evident in the line plot (right Y-axis) which reports the yearly normalized ratios between subsets of publications resulting from the interactions (N_{NM+NP}) and total number of journal publications in the Neurobiohybrid field (N_{Total}).

involve living networks at various levels of complexity and conditions, ranging from *in vitro* to *in vivo* systems and from "simple" nervous systems of invertebrates to the mammalian brain. Whatever the implementation strategy, the new hybrid systems will represent a technological platform with enormous potential not only for application in neuroscience and healthcare, as discussed below, but also in computer science and robotics. In fact, they will play a key role to understand operational principles of brain microcircuits and to developing new forms of brain-inspired computing devices more energy efficient and robust in dealing with real-world tasks.

From the theoretical point of view, the processing of information following the classical "von Neumann" digital computing paradigms is known to be less efficient compared to the biological counterparts, when dealing with ill-posed problems and noisy data. Though current computing technologies have reached speed and computational power figures that allows them to simulate parts of animal brains and behavior, the energy required by these systems grows exponentially with the increasing hierarchy of animal intelligence. The reason is that the biological brain is configured differently and the keys are the extremely high (~1015 synapses) connectivity between neurons in a network which offers highly parallel processing power as well as the fact that neurons are plastic and adaptive (i.e., memory dependent) signal processing and computing units. Yet, brain's most striking feature is that it is structured as an evolving system were synapses undergo "birth" and "death" as well as strengthening and weakening, reconfiguring neuronal connectivity in a self-organizing manner and allowing the networked population of neuronal processors to adapt motor and behavioral responses to the ever changing environmental inputs. Thus, by rearranging both the structural and functional topology, brain's neuronal circuits demonstrate unique evolvability, scalability, and adaptability properties that are unmatched by current computing devices. The challenge posed by neurobiohybrids research is to create networks where artificial elements overcome this deficiency by merging data storage and processing into single electronic devices, where topology can be reconfigured in a self-organizing manner, and to interface them to biological nervous systems. On-chip neuromorphic networks have recently emerged that may fulfill the purpose, and whose

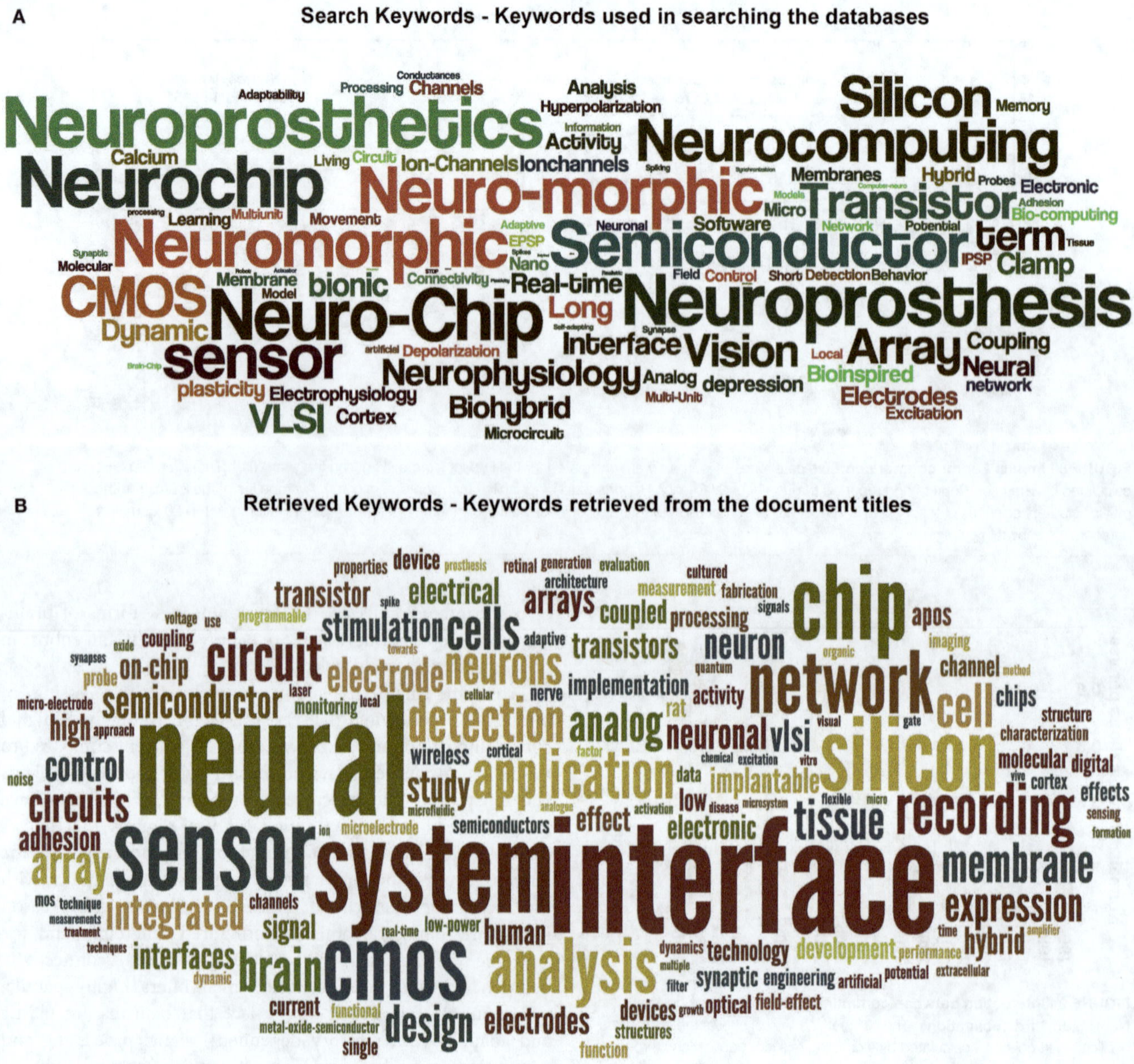

FIGURE 10 | Word cloud of keywords. Word clouds of keywords used in searching the databases **(A)** and retrieved from the publication titles **(B)**. The size of a word in **(A)** denotes the number of times it was used with other search keywords in searching for publications in the database. On the other hand, in **(B)**, the size of a word represents its number of appearances in the publication titles.

development is relying both on established microelectronic technologies (Indiveri et al., 2011; Indiveri and Liu, 2015) and novel approaches to emulate neuronal functions in single nanodevices (Indiveri et al., 2013; Gupta et al., 2016; Serb et al., 2016). Such artificial neural networks could provide the complexity, connectivity, and massive parallel information processing and thus mimic the performance of biological systems including their evolvability, self-organization, adaptability, and robustness. Following this vision, research on neurobiohybrids will on one hand enable significant progress toward novel "autonomous cognitive systems" while, on the other hand, it will promote the understanding of principles behind brain computation. The conception of brain-inspired implantable microdevices acting as "intelligent" neuroprostheses for brain rehabilitation and functional augmentation or as adaptive bioelectronic medicines will be the logical exploitation of such efforts toward clinical application.

In conclusion, we feel that we are at the beginning of a new era, where the fusion of neuromimetics and neurotechnologies for brain interfacing and creation of neurobiohybrids will lead to a new class of "smart" implantable systems with great potential for neuroscience and particularly for therapy of diseases of the nervous system. However, a process of community building is also necessary to reach the critical mass, which will have to overcome difficulties and hurdles. In particular, having a common and effective dissemination strategy, ensuring high visibility and career opportunities across all disciplines involved will be key aspect.

METHODS

The bibliometrics was performed following standard bibliometric methods as reported in Nathan et al. (2013). In short, a two-step method started with construction of an analysis database by searching and extracting information from three commercial scientific repositories using predefined search terms which was followed by analysis of the extracted publication data.

Construction of Search Terms

As part of the Convergent Science Network's (CSN) road-mapping action, we had supplied questionnaires to experts belonging to the different communities mentioned above. Mining the answers provided to the question "Relevant state-of-the-art in your field of research" we formed a "keywords pool." The unique keywords ($n = 100$) in that pool were then identified, combined and permuted to obtain the search terms ($N = 862$) which were used in querying the scientific repositories.

Construction of Analysis Database

Three commercial scientific repositories were used to gather the publication information: (i) the IEEEXplore repository (http://ieeexplore.ieee.org/), (ii) the Thomson Reuters Web of Knowledge repository (http://apps.webofknowledge.com/), and (iii) Elsevier's Scopus (http://scopus.com/) repository. Out of the three, the IEEEXplore repository was used as source of articles published in IEEE journals and conferences, and the latter two were used for other journals and conferences.

Each of these repositories were searched for priorly defined keywords (or combinations of keywords, referred as "search terms" in the subsequent text, see Section Construction of Search Terms). The search domains were restricted to science, engineering, and life sciences for the Web of knowledge and Scopus repositories. But, the IEEEXplore repository was searched only science and engineering domain articles.

These repositories were queried using their built-in search engines which compared the search terms with the stored metadata (e.g., publication title, abstract, and author-defined keywords) corresponding to each indexed article. The metadata returned by the query as a result of a match with the given search term was appended to a predefined database created in EndNote reference management software (V7.4; Thompson Reuters, Philadelphia, USA; http://endnote.com/). At the end of the querying process, the Endnote database was exported to an extensible markup language (XML, http://www.w3.org/XML/) file (referred as analysis/XML database) and an automated in-house algorithm written in MATLAB (R2015a; Mathworks Inc., Natick, USA, http://www.mathworks.com/) eliminated the redundant entries returned by overlapped queries in different repositories from the XML file. The tagged structure of XML file facilitated the application of MATLAB's standard string-manipulation functions to extract the relevant information (e.g., article title, publication year, and title, etc.) from the metadata pertaining to each publication stored in the XML database. For each unique journals, its impact factor and category were manually retrieved from the Thompson Reuters Journal Citation Reports (JCR, https://jcr.incites.thomsonreuters.com/) and appended to the database.

Analysis of Database

The pre-processed metadata belonging to publication entries in the XML database were then analyzed to extract publication titles, unique journal and conference titles, and year of publication.

The following information were then extracted from the database:

1. Yearly publication frequency in journals or conferences (as reported in **Figures 4–6**), and journal category-wise publication distribution (**Figure 5C**; top 44 journals, from a descendingly ordered list of number of appeared articles, were categorized with a total number of 1200 articles and at least 10 articles in each journal during 1994–2014).
2. Impact factor distribution of the published articles belonging to the Neurobiohybrids (as reported in **Figure 7**) field. Also, comparison of impact factors of various journals belonging to the "Multidisciplinary Sciences" and "Neurosciences" category (see **Figure 8**).

In addition, two subcategories of seven keywords each (termed as "interaction keywords") were defined by selecting popular keywords pertaining to two active subcommunities (Neuromimetics and Neuroprosthetics) in the Neurobiohybrid field. For the Neuromimetics, the selected keywords were: "neuromimetic," "neuro-morphic," "neuromorphic," "neuro-chip," "neurochip," "neurocomputing," and "sensor"; whereas for the Neuroprosthetics they were: "neuroprosthetic," "neuroprosthesis," "interface," "brain machine interface," "tissue," "slice," and "*in-vivo.*" The document titles, abstracts and author-provided keywords present in the XML database were searched for co-occurrence of at least one interaction keyword from each subcategories. The resulting publications along with their publication year were saved. The yearly publication frequency computed from the search results of the interaction keywords (see **Figure 9**) was used as a measure to determine interactions between the two subcommunities belonging to the Neurobiohybrids field.

Finally, the search terms and the retrieved keywords from the publication titles were represented as word clouds (see **Figure 10**) using a web-based free tool (wordle; http://www.wordle.net/) showing the frequencies of usage of each search keyword with another keyword (in case of search keywords cloud) and frequencies of occurrence of keywords in the publication titles (in case of retrieved keywords cloud).

AUTHOR CONTRIBUTIONS

SV and MM performed the studies reported in the article and wrote the paper. Both authors have contributed to, seen and approved the final manuscript.

FUNDING

Financial support from the 7th Framework Programme of the European Commission through "CSN II" (http://www.csnetwork.eu/, FP7-ICT-601167) and "RAMP" projects (http://www.rampproject.eu/, FP7-ICT-612058) are acknowledged.

ACKNOWLEDGMENTS

The authors are particularly thankful to the following scientists for their help and fruitful discussion: Guenther Zeck, Christian Meier, Michele Giugliano, Marco Fanciulli, Themis Prodromakis, Ralf Zeitler, Giacomo Indiveri, Peter Fromherz, Roland Thewes, Astrid Prinz, Jennifer Hasler, Andrei Zenkevich. Dr. Nathan Lepora's kind help and assistance in performing the bibliometric research is also acknowledged.

REFERENCES

Afshar, P., Khambhati, A., Stanslaski, S., Carlson, D., Jensen, R., Dani, S., et al. (2013). A translational platform for prototyping closed-loop neuromodulation systems. *Front. Neural Circuits* 6:117. doi: 10.3389/fncir.2012.00117

Ali, M. M., Sellers, K. K., and Fröhlich, F. (2013). Transcranial alternating current stimulation modulates large-scale cortical network activity by network resonance. *J. Neurosci.* 33, 11262–11275. doi: 10.1523/JNEUROSCI.5867-12.2013

Anastassiou, C. A., Montgomery, S. M., Barahona, M., Buzsáki, G., and Koch, C. (2010). The effect of spatially inhomogeneous extracellular electric fields on neurons. *J. Neurosci.* 30, 1925–1936. doi: 10.1523/JNEUROSCI.3635-09.2010

Angle, M. R., Cui, B., and Melosh, N. A. (2015). Nanotechnology and neurophysiology. *Curr. Opin. Neurobiol.* 32, 132–140. doi: 10.1016/j.conb.2015.03.014

Armstrong, C., Krook-Magnuson, E., Oijala, M., and Soltesz, I. (2013). Closed-loop optogenetic intervention in mice. *Nat. Protoc.* 8, 1475–1493. doi: 10.1038/nprot.2013.080

Bartolozzi, C., and Indiveri, G. (2007). Synaptic dynamics in analog vlsi. *Neural Comput.* 19, 2581–2603. doi: 10.1162/neco.2007.19.10.2581

Berényi, A., Somogyvári, Z., Nagy, A. J., Roux, L., Long, J. D., Fujisawa, S., et al. (2014). Large-scale, high-density (up to 512 channels) recording of local circuits in behaving animals. *J. Neurophysiol.* 111, 1132–1149. doi: 10.1152/jn.00785.2013

Birmingham, K., Gradinaru, V., Anikeeva, P., Grill, W. M., Pikov, V., McLaughlin, B., et al. (2014). Bioelectronic medicines: a research roadmap. *Nat. Rev. Drug Discov.* 13, 399–400. doi: 10.1038/nrd4351

Braun, D., and Fromherz, P. (2004). Imaging neuronal seal resistance on silicon chip using fluorescent voltage-sensitive dye. *Biophys. J.* 87, 1351–1359. doi: 10.1529/biophysj.104.039990

Buzsáki, G., Anastassiou, C. A., and Koch, C. (2012). The origin of extracellular fields and currents – eeg, ecog, lfp and spikes. *Nat. Rev. Neurosci.* 13, 407–420. doi: 10.1038/nrn3241

Buzsáki, G., Stark, E., Berényi, A., Khodagholy, D., Kipke, D. R., Yoon, E., et al. (2015). Tools for probing local circuits: high-density silicon probes combined with optogenetics. *Neuron* 86, 92–105. doi: 10.1016/j.neuron.2015.01.028

Camprodon, J. A. (2016). "Transcranial Magnetic Stimulation," in *Psychiatric Neurotherapeutics: Contemporary Surgical and Device-Based Treatments*, eds A. J. Camprodon, L. S. Rauch, D. B. Greenberg, and D. D. Dougherty (New York, NY: Springer), 165–186.

Cellot, G., Cilia, E., Cipollone, S., Rancic, V., Sucapane, A., Giordani, S., et al. (2009). Carbon nanotubes might improve neuronal performance by favouring electrical shortcuts. *Nat. Nanotech.* 4, 126–133. doi: 10.1038/nnano.2008.374

Chemla, S., and Chavane, F. (2010). Voltage-sensitive dye imaging: technique review and models. *J. Physiol. Paris* 104, 40–50. doi: 10.1016/j.jphysparis.2009.11.009

Chua, L. (1971). Memristor-the missing circuit element. *IEEE T. Circuit Theory* 18, 507–519. doi: 10.1109/TCT.1971.1083337

Chua, L. (2011). Resistance switching memories are memristors. *Appl. Phys. A* 102, 765–783. doi: 10.1007/s00339-011-6264-9

Csicsvari, J., Henze, D. A., Jamieson, B., Harris, K. D., Sirota, A., Barthó, P., et al. (2003). Massively parallel recording of unit and local field potentials with silicon-based electrodes. *J. Neurophysiol.* 90, 1314–1323. doi: 10.1152/jn.00116.2003

Dirks, A., Cornelissen, J. J. L. M., van Delft, F. L., van Hest, J. C. M., Nolte, R. J. M., Rowan, A. E., et al. (2007). From (bio)molecules to biohybrid materials with the click chemistry approach. *QSAR Comb. Sci.* 26, 1200–1210. doi: 10.1002/qsar.200740085

Dugue, G. P., Akemann, W., and Knopfel, T. (2012). A comprehensive concept of optogenetics. *Prog. Brain. Res.* 196, 1–28. doi: 10.1016/B978-0-444-59426-6.00001-X

Eiben, A. E., Kernbach, S., and Haasdijk, E. (2012). Embodied artificial evolution artificial evolutionary systems in the 21st century. *Evol. Intell.* 5, 261–272. doi: 10.1007/s12065-012-0071-x

Eickenscheidt, M., Jenkner, M., Thewes, R., Fromherz, P., and Zeck, G. (2012). Electrical stimulation of retinal neurons in epiretinal and subretinal configuration using a multicapacitor array. *J. Neurophysiol.* 107, 2742–2755. doi: 10.1152/jn.00909.2011

Eversmann, B., Lambacher, A., Gerling, T., Kunze, A., Fromherz, P., and Thewes, R. (2011). A neural tissue interfacing chip for *in-vitro* applications with 32k recording/stimulation channels on an active area of 2.6 mm2. *Proc. ESSCIRC* 211–214. doi: 10.1109/ESSCIRC.2011.6044902

Fabbro, A., Prato, M., and Ballerini, L. (2013). Carbon nanotubes in neuroregeneration and repair. *Adv. Drug Deliv. Rev.* 65, 2034–2044. doi: 10.1016/j.addr.2013.07.002

Fekete, Z. (2015). Recent advances in silicon-based neural microelectrodes and microsystems: a review. *Sens. Actuator B Chem.* 215, 300–315. doi: 10.1016/j.snb.2015.03.055

Felderer, F., and Fromherz, P. (2011). Transistor needle chip for recording in brain tissue. *Appl. Phys. A* 104, 1–6. doi: 10.1007/s00339-011-6392-2

Ferrea, E., Maccione, A., Medrihan, L., Nieus, T., Ghezzi, D., Baldelli, P., et al. (2012). Large-scale, high-resolution electrophysiological imaging of field potentials in brain slices with microelectronic multielectrode arrays. *Front. Neural Circuits* 6:80. doi: 10.3389/fncir.2012.00080

Friehs, G. M., Zerris, V. A., Ojakangas, C. L., Fellows, M. R., and Donoghue, J. P. (2004). Brain-machine and brain-computer interfaces. *Stroke* 35, 2702–2705. doi: 10.1161/01.STR.0000143235.93497.03

Fromherz, P. (2006). Three levels of neuroelectronic interfacing. *Ann. N.Y. Acad. Sci.* 1093, 143–160. doi: 10.1196/annals.1382.011

Gelencser, A., Prodromakis, T., Toumazou, C., and Roska, T. (2012). Biomimetic model of the outer plexiform layer by incorporating memristive devices. *Phys. Rev. E* 85:041918. doi: 10.1103/physreve.85.041918

Giocomo, L. M. (2015). Large scale *in vivo* recordings to study neuronal biophysics. *Curr. Opin. Neurobiol.* 32, 1–7. doi: 10.1016/j.conb.2014.09.009

Girardi, S., Maschietto, M., Zeitler, R., Mahmud, M., and Vassanelli, S. (2011). "High resolution cortical imaging using electrolyte-(metal)-oxide-semiconductor field effect transistors," in *2011 5th International*

IEEE/EMBS Conference on Neural Engineering (NER) (Cancun, QR), 269–272.

Gold, C., Henze, D. A., Koch, C., and Buzsáki, G. (2006). On the origin of the extracellular action potential waveform: a modeling study. *J. Neurophysiol.* 95, 3113–3128. doi: 10.1152/jn.00979.2005

Goldfarb, M., Lawson, B. E., and Shultz, A. H. (2013). Realizing the promise of robotic leg prostheses. *Sci. Transl. Med.* 5, 210ps15. doi: 10.1126/scitranslmed.3007312

Grosenick, L., Marshel, J. H., and Deisseroth, K. (2015). Closed-loop and activity-guided optogenetic control. *Neuron* 86, 106–139. doi: 10.1016/j.neuron.2015.03.034

Gupta, I., Serb, A., Khiat, A., Zeitler, R., Vassanelli, S., and Prodromakis, T. (2016). Real-time encoding and compression of neuronal spikes by metal-oxide memristors. *Nat. Commun.* doi: 10.5258/SOTON/400411. [Epub ahead of print].

Haider, B., and McCormick, D. A. (2009). Rapid neocortical dynamics: cellular and network mechanisms. *Neuron* 62, 171–189. doi: 10.1016/j.neuron.2009.04.008

Hierlemann, A., Frey, U., Hafizovic, S., and Heer, F. (2011). Growing cells atop microelectronic chips: interfacing electrogenic cells *in vitro* with cmos-based microelectrode arrays. *Proc. IEEE* 99, 252–284. doi: 10.1109/JPROC.2010.2066532

Hochberg, L. R., Serruya, M. D., Friehs, G. M., Mukand, J. A., Saleh, M., Caplan, A. H., et al. (2006). Neuronal ensemble control of prosthetic devices by a human with tetraplegia. *Nature* 442, 164–171. doi: 10.1038/nature04970

Hutzler, M., Lambacher, A., Eversmann, B., Jenkner, M., Thewes, R., and Fromherz, P. (2006). High- resolution multitransistor array recording of electrical field potentials in cultured brain slices. *J. Neurophysiol.* 96, 1638–1645. doi: 10.1152/jn.00347.2006

Hyam, J. A., Kringelbach, M. L., Silburn, P. A., Aziz, T. Z., and Green, A. L. (2012). The autonomic effects of deep brain stimulation-a therapeutic opportunity. *Nat. Rev. Neurol.* 8, 391–400. doi: 10.1038/nrneurol.2012.100

Indiveri, G. (2015). "Neuromorphic engineering," in *Springer Handbook of Computational Intelligence*, eds J. Kacprzyk and W. Pedrycz (Berlin: Springer), 715–725.

Indiveri, G., and Horiuchi, T. K. (2011). Frontiers in neuromorphic engineering. *Front. Neurosci.* 5:118. doi: 10.3389/fnins.2011.00118

Indiveri, G., Linares-Barranco, B., Hamilton, T. J., van Schaik, A., Etienne-Cummings, R., Delbruck, T., et al. (2011). Neuromorphic silicon neuron circuits. *Front. Neurosci.* 5:73. doi: 10.3389/fnins.2011.00073

Indiveri, G., Linares-Barranco, B., Legenstein, R., Deligeorgis, G., and Themistoklis, P. (2013). Integration of nanoscale memristor synapses in neuromorphic computing architectures. *Nanotechnology* 24:384010. doi: 10.1088/0957-4484/24/38/384010

Indiveri, G., and Liu, S. C. (2015). Memory and information processing in neuromorphic systems. *Proc. IEEE* 103, 1379–1397. doi: 10.1109/JPROC.2015.2444094

Joshi, J., Zhang, J., Wang, C., Hsu, C.-C., Parker, A., Zhou, C., et al. (2011). "A biomimetic fabricated carbon nanotube synapse for prosthetic applications," in *Life Science Systems and Applications Workshop (LiSSA) 2011 IEEE/NIH*, eds K. Peterson and E. Sanchez-Sinencio (Bethesda, MD: IEEE), 139–142.

Khodagholy, D., Gelinas, J. N., Thesen, T., Doyle, W., Devinsky, O., Malliaras, G. G., et al. (2015). NeuroGrid: recording action potentials from the surface of the brain. *Nat. Neurosci.* 18, 310–315. doi: 10.1038/nn.3905

Kim, S., Du, C., Sheridan, P., Ma, W., Choi, S., and Lu, W. D. (2015). Experimental demonstration of a second-order memristor and its ability to biorealistically implement synaptic plasticity. *Nano Lett.* 15, 2203–2211. doi: 10.1021/acs.nanolett.5b00697

Krusienski, D. J., Grosse-Wentrup, M., Galn, F., Coyle, D., Miller, K. J., Forney, E., et al. (2011). Critical issues in state-of-the-art brain-computer interface signal processing. *J. Neural Eng.* 8:025002. doi: 10.1088/1741-2560/8/2/025002

Kwan, A. C., and Dan, Y. (2012). Dissection of cortical microcircuits by single-neuron stimulation *in vivo*. *Curr. Biol.* 22, 1459–1467. doi: 10.1016/j.cub.2012.06.007

Lago, N., Ceballos, D., Rodrguez, F. J., Stieglitz, T., and Navarro, X. (2005). Long term assessment of axonal regeneration through polyimide regenerative electrodes to interface the peripheral nerve. *Biomaterials* 26, 2021–2031. doi: 10.1016/j.biomaterials.2004.06.025

Lebedev, M. A., and Nicolelis, M. A. (2011). Toward a whole-body neuroprosthetic. *Prog. Brain. Res.* 194, 47–60. doi: 10.1016/B978-0-444-53815-4.00018-2

Lee, J. H., Kim, H., Kim, J. H., and Lee, S. H. (2016). Soft implantable microelectrodes for future medicine: prosthetics, neural signal recording and neuromodulation. *Lab Chip* 16, 959–976. doi: 10.1039/C5LC00842E

Lee, J. H., Ryu, J., Jolesz, F. A., Cho, Z. H., and Yoo, S. S. (2009). Brain-machine interface via real- time fmri: preliminary study on thought-controlled robotic arm. *Neurosci. Lett.* 450, 1–6. doi: 10.1016/j.neulet.2008.11.024

Le Masson, G., Renaud-Le Masson, S., Debay, D., and Bal, T. (2002). Feedback inhibition controls spike transfer in hybrid thalamic circuits. *Nature* 417, 854–858. doi: 10.1038/nature00825

Lewandowska, M. K., Radivojević, M., Jäckel, D., Müller, J., and Hierlemann, A. R. (2016). Cortical axons, isolated in channels, display activity-dependent signal modulation as a result of targeted stimulation. *Front Neurosci.* 10:83. doi: 10.3389/fnins.2016.00083

Liu, J., Fu, T. M., Cheng, Z., Hong, G., Zhou, T., Jin, L., et al. (2015). Syringe-injectable electronics. *Nat. Nanotechnol.* 10, 629–636. doi: 10.1038/nnano.2015.115

Maccione, A., Garofalo, M., Nieus, T., Tedesco, M., Berdondini, L., and Martinoia, S. (2012). Multiscale functional connectivity estimation on low-density neuronal cultures recorded by high-density CMOS micro electrode arrays. *J. Neurosci. Methods* 207, 161–171. doi: 10.1016/j.jneumeth.2012.04.002

Mahmud, M., Bertoldo, A., Girardi, S., Maschietto, M., and Vassanelli, S. (2012). Sigmate: a matlab-based automated tool for extracellular neuronal signal processing and analysis. *J. Neurosci. Methods* 207, 97–112. doi: 10.1016/j.jneumeth.2012.03.009

Mahmud, M., Pulizzi, R., Vasilaki, E., and Giugliano, M. (2014). Qspike tools: a generic framework for parallel batch preprocessing of extracellular neuronal signals recorded by substrate microelectrode arrays. *Front. Neuroinform.* 8:26. doi: 10.3389/fninf.2014.00026

Mahmud, M., and Vassanelli, S. (2016a). Differential modulation of excitatory and inhibitory neurons during periodic stimulation. *Front. Neurosci.* 10:62. doi: 10.3389/fnins.2016.00062

Mahmud, M., and Vassanelli, S. (2016b). Processing and analysis of multichannel extracellular neuronal signals: state-of-the-art and challenges. *Front. Neurosci.* 10:248. doi: 10.3389/fnins.2016.00248

Mailley, S., Hyland, M., Mailley, P., McLaughlin, J. A., and McAdams, E. T. (2004). Thin film platinum cuff electrodes for neurostimulation: *in vitro* approach of safe neurostimulation parameters. *Bioelectrochemistry* 63, 359–364. doi: 10.1016/j.bioelechem.2003.10.033

Manor, Y., and Nadim, F. (2001). Synaptic depression mediates bistability in neuronal networks with recurrent inhibitory connectivity. *J. Neurosci.* 21, 9460–9470.

Matsushita, K., Hirata, M., Suzuki, T., Ando, H., Ota, Y., Sato, F., et al. (2013). Development of an implantable wireless ECoG 128ch recording device for clinical brain machine interface. *Conf. Proc. IEEE Eng. Med. Biol. Soc.* 2013, 1867–1870. doi: 10.1109/embc.2013.6609888

McConnell, G. C., So, R. Q., and Grill, W. M. (2016). Failure to suppress low-frequency neuronal oscillatory activity underlies the reduced effectiveness of random patterns of deep brain stimulation. *J. Neurophysiol.* 115, 2791–2802. doi: 10.1152/jn.00822.2015

Micera, S. (2016). Staying in touch: toward the restoration of sensory feedback in hand prostheses using peripheral neural stimulation. *IEEE Pulse* 7, 16–19. doi: 10.1109/MPUL.2016.2539760

Miller, M. A., Neuzil, P., Dukkipati, S. R., and Reddy, V. Y. (2015). Leadless cardiac pacemakers back to the future. *J. Am. Coll. Cardiol.* 66, 1179–1189. doi: 10.1016/j.jacc.2015.06.1081

Miranda, R. A., Casebeer, W. D., Hein, A. M., Judy, J. W., Krotkov, E. P., Laabs, T. L., et al. (2015). DARPA-funded efforts in the development of novel brain-computer interface technologies. *J. Neurosci. Methods* 244, 52–67. doi: 10.1016/j.jneumeth.2014.07.019

Mitzdorf, U. (1985). Current source-density method and application in cat cerebral cortex: investigation of evoked potentials and EEG phenomena. *Physiol. Rev.* 65, 37–100.

Mukaino, M., Ono, T., Shindo, K., Fujiwara, T., Ota, T., Kimura, A., et al. (2014). Efficacy of brain- computer interface-driven neuromuscular electrical stimulation for chronic paresis after stroke. *J. Rehabil. Med.* 46, 378–382. doi: 10.2340/16501977-1785

Muller, J., Ballini, M., Livi, P., Chen, Y., Radivojevic, M., Shadmani, A., et al. (2015). High-resolution CMOS MEA platform to study neurons at subcellular, cellular, and network levels. *Lab Chip* 15, 2767–2780. doi: 10.1039/C5LC00133A

Nathan, F., L., Paul, V., and Tony J, P. (2013). The state of the art in biomimetics. *Bioinspir. Biomim.* 8:013001. doi: 10.1088/1748-3182/8/1/013001

Newman, J. P., Fong, M., Millard, D. C., Whitmire, C. J., Stanley, G. B., and Potter, S. M. (2015). Optogenetic feedback control of neural activity. *eLife* 4:e07192. doi: 10.7554/eLife.07192

Nicolelis, M. A. L., and Lebedev, M. A. (2009). Principles of neural ensemble physiology underlying the operation of brain-machine interfaces. *Nat. Rev. Neurosci.* 10, 530–540. doi: 10.1038/nrn2653

Niehrster, S., and Thomas, A. (2015). "Preparation of Ta-O-Based tunnel junctions to obtain artificial synapses based on memristive switching," in *Methods in Molecular Biology*, Vol. 1260, ed H. Cartwright (New York, NY: Springer), 261–267.

Norton, J. J., Lee, D. S., Lee, J. W., Lee, W., Kwon, O., Won, P., et al. (2015). Soft, curved electrode systems capable of integration on the auricle as a persistent brain-computer interface. *Proc. Natl. Acad. Sci. U.S.A.* 112, 3920–3925. doi: 10.1073/pnas.1424875112

Novellino, A., D'Angelo, P., Cozzi, L., Chiappalone, M., Sanguineti, V., and Martinoia, S. (2007). Connecting neurons to a mobile robot: An *in vitro* bidirectional neural interface. *Comput. Intell. Neurosci.* 2007:12725. doi: 10.1155/2007/12725

Nowotny, T., Zhigulin, V. P., Selverston, A. I., Abarbanel, H. D., and Rabinovich, M. I. (2003). Enhance- ment of synchronization in a hybrid neural circuit by spike-timing dependent plasticity. *J. Neurosci.* 23, 9776–9785.

Occhetta, E., Bortnik, M., Vassanelli, C., and on behalf of the INVASY Italian feasibility study group (2003). The DDDR closed loop stimulation for the prevention of vasovagal syncope: results from the INVASY prospective feasibility registry. *Europace* 5, 153–162. doi: 10.1053/eupc.2002.0292

Ortiz-Catalan, M., Hakansson, B., and Branemark, R. (2014). An osseointegrated human-machine gateway for long-term sensory feedback and motor control of artificial limbs. *Sci. Transl. Med.* 6, 257re6. doi: 10.1126/scitranslmed.3008933

Ortiz-Rosario, A., and Adeli, H. (2013). Brain-computer interface technologies: from signal to action. *Rev. Neurosci.* 24, 537–552. doi: 10.1515/revneuro-2013-0032

Packer, A. M., Russell, L. E., Dalgleish, H. W. P., and Hausser, M. (2015). Simultaneous all-optical manipulation and recording of neural circuit activity with cellular resolution *in vivo*. *Nat. Meth.* 12, 140–146. doi: 10.1038/nmeth.3217

Park, H., Shin, H. J., Cho, I. J., Yoon, E. S., Suh, J. K., Im, M., et al. (2011). The first neural probe integrated with light source (blue laser diode) for optical stimulation and electrical recording. *Conf. Proc. IEEE. Eng. Med. Biol. Soc.* 2011, 2961–2964. doi: 10.1109/IEMBS.2011.6090813

Pashaie, R., Baumgartner, R., Richner, T. J., Brodnick, S. K., Azimipour, M., Eliceiri, K. W., et al. (2015). Closed-loop optogenetic brain interface. *IEEE Trans. Biomed. Eng.* 62, 2327–2337. doi: 10.1109/TBME.2015.2436817

Patil, A. C., and Thakor, N. V. (2016). Implantable neurotechnologies: a review of micro- and nanoelectrodes for neural recording. *Med. Biol. Eng. Comput.* 54, 23. doi: 10.1007/s11517-015-1430-4

Peckham, P. H., and Knutson, J. S. (2005). Functional electrical stimulation for neuromuscular applications. *Ann. Rev. Biomed. Eng.* 7, 327–360. doi: 10.1146/annurev.bioeng.6.040803.140103

Pei, X., Leuthardt, E. C., Gaona, C. M., Brunner, P., Wolpaw, J. R., and Schalk, G. (2011). Spatiotem- poral dynamics of electrocorticographic high gamma activity during overt and covert word repetition. *Neuroimage* 54, 2960–2972. doi: 10.1016/j.neuroimage.2010.10.029

Pine, J. (2006). "A history of MEA development," in *Advances in Network Electrophysiology Using Multi-Electrode Arrays*, eds M. Taketani and M. Baudry (New York, NY: Springer), 3–23.

Pisanello, F., Sileo, L., and De Vittorio, M. (2016). Micro- and nanotechnologies for optical neural interfaces. *Front. Neurosci.* 10:70. doi: 10.3389/fnins.2016.00070

Prinz, A. A. (2004). Neural networks: models and neurons show hybrid vigor in real time. *Curr. Biol.* 14, R661–R662. doi: 10.1016/j.cub.2004.08.012

Prinz, A. A., Abbott, L. F., and Marder, E. (2004). The dynamic clamp comes of age. *Trends Neurosci.* 27, 218–224. doi: 10.1016/j.tins.2004.02.004

Prodanov, D., and Delbeke, J. (2016). Mechanical and biological interactions of implants with the brain and their impact on implant design. *Front. Neurosci.* 10:11. doi: 10.3389/fnins.2016.00011

Prodromakis, T., Peh, B. P., Papavassiliou, C., and Toumazou, C. (2011). A versatile memristor model with nonlinear dopant kinetics. *IEEE T. Electron. Dev.* 58, 3099–3105. doi: 10.1109/TED.2011.2158004

Prodromakis, T., Toumazou, C., and Chua, L. (2012). Two centuries of memristors. *Nat. Mater.* 11, 478–481. doi: 10.1038/nmat3338

Qiao, N., Mostafa, H., Corradi, F., Osswald, M., Stefanini, F., Sumislawska, D., et al. (2015). A reconfigurable on-line learning spiking neuromorphic processor comprising 256 neurons and 128K synapses. *Front. Neurosci.* 9:141. doi: 10.3389/fnins.2015.00141

Raspopovic, S., Capogrosso, M., Petrini, F. M., Bonizzato, M., Rigosa, J., Pino, G. D., et al. (2014). Restoring natural sensory feedback in real-time bidirectional hand prostheses. *Sci. Transl. Med.* 6, 222ra19. doi: 10.1126/scitranslmed.3006820

Ricotti, L., and Menciassi, A. (2012). Bio-hybrid muscle cell-based actuators. *Biomed. Microdevices* 14, 987–998. doi: 10.1007/s10544-012-9697-9

Roche, J. P., and Hansen, M. R. (2015). On the horizon: cochlear implant technology. *Otolaryngol. Clin. North Am.* 48, 1097–1116. doi: 10.1016/j.otc.2015.07.009

Ruffini, G., Wendling, F., Merlet, I., Molaee-Ardekani, B., Mekonnen, A., Salvador, R., et al. (2013). Transcranial Current Brain Stimulation (tCS): models and technologies. *IEEE Trans. Neural Syst. Rehabil. Eng.* 21, 333–345. doi: 10.1109/TNSRE.2012.2200046

Ruiz, S., Buyukturkoglu, K., Rana, M., Birbaumer, N., and Sitaram, R. (2014). Real-time fmri brain computer interfaces: self-regulation of single brain regions to networks. *Biol. Psychol.* 95, 4–20. doi: 10.1016/j.biopsycho.2013.04.010

Ruther, P., and Paul, O. (2015). New approaches for CMOS-based devices for large-scale neural recording. *Curr. Opin. Neurobiol.* 32, 31–37. doi: 10.1016/j.conb.2014.10.007

Rutten, W. L. C. (2002). Selective electrical interfaces with the nervous system. *Annu. Rev. Biomed. Eng.* 4, 407–452. doi: 10.1146/annurev.bioeng.4.020702.153427

Sato, M., Baumhoff, P., and Kral, A. (2016). Cochlear implant stimulation of a hearing ear generates separate electrophonic and electroneural responses. *J. Neurosci.* 36, 54–64. doi: 10.1523/JNEUROSCI.2968-15.2016

Schroder, S., Cecchetto, C., Keil, S., Mahmud, M., Brose, E., Dogan, O., et al. (2015). "Cmos-compatible purely capacitive interfaces for high-density *in-vivo* recording from neural tissue," in *2015 IEEE Biomedical Circuits and Systems Conference (BioCAS)* (Atlanta, GA), 1–4.

Serb, A., Johannes, B., Khiat, A., Berdan, R., Legenstein, R., and Prodromakis, T. (2016). Unsupervised learning in probabilistic neural networks with multi-state metal-oxide memristive synapses. *Nat. Commun.* [Epub ahead of print].

Seriwala, H. M., Khan, M. S., Munir, M. B., Riaz, I. B., Riaz, H., Saba, S., et al. (2016). Leadless pacemakers: a new era in cardiac pacing. *J. Cardiol.* 67, 1–5. doi: 10.1016/j.jjcc.2015.09.006

Sharp, A. A., O'Neil, M. B., Abbott, L. F., and Marder, E. (1993). Dynamic clamp: computer-generated conductances in real neurons. *J. Neurophysiol.* 69, 992–995.

Shihong, M. W., Prodromakis, T., Salaoru, I., and Toumazou, C. (2012). Modelling of current percolation channels in emerging resistive switching elements. *ArXiv e-prints*.

Shobe, J. L., Claar, L. D., Parhami, S., Bakhurin, K. I., and Masmanidis, S. C. (2015). Brain activity mapping at multiple scales with silicon microprobes containing 1,024 electrodes. *J. Neurophysiol.* 114, 2043–2052. doi: 10.1152/jn.00464.2015

Spira, M. E., and Hai, A. (2013). Multi-electrode array technologies for neuroscience and cardiology. *Nat. Nano.* 8, 83–94. doi: 10.1038/nnano.2012.265

Stieglitz, T., Neves, H., and Ruther, P. (2014). Neural probes–microsystems to interface with the brain. *Biomed. Tech. (Berl.)* 59, 269–271. doi: 10.1515/bmt-2012-0094

Strukov, D. B., Snider, G. S., Stewart, D. R., and Williams, R. S. (2008). The missing memristor found. *Nature* 453, 80–83. doi: 10.1038/nature06932

Tabot, G. A., Kim, S. S., Winberry, J. E., and Bensmaia, S. J. (2015). Restoring tactile and proprioceptive sensation through a brain interface. *Neurobiol. Dis.* 83, 191–198. doi: 10.1016/j.nbd.2014.08.029

Thibeault, C. M. (2014). A role for neuromorphic processors in therapeutic nervous system stimulation. *Front. Syst. Neurosci.* 8:187. doi: 10.3389/fnsys.2014.00187

Thomas, A., Niehorster, S., Fabretti, S., Shepheard, N., Kuschel, O., Kupper, K., et al. (2015). Tunnel junction based memristors as artificial synapses. *Front. Neurosci.* 9:241. doi: 10.3389/fnins.2015.00241

Tian, L., Hires, S. A., and Looger, L. L. (2012). Imaging neuronal activity with genetically encoded calcium indicators. *Cold Spring Harb. Protoc.* 2012, 647–656. doi: 10.1101/pdb.top069609

Vassanelli, S. (2014). "Multielectrode and multitransistor arrays for *in vivo* recording," in *Nanotechnology and Neuroscience: Nano-Electronic, Photonic and Mechanical Neuronal Interfacing*, eds M. De Vittorio, L. Martiradonna, and J. Assad (New York, NY: Springer), 239–267.

Vassanelli, S., Mahmud, M., Girardi, S., and Maschietto, M. (2012). On the way to large-scale and high-resolution brain-chip interfacing. *Cogn. Comput.* 4, 71–81. doi: 10.1007/s12559-011-9121-4

Vidu, R., Rahman, M., Mahmoudi, M., Enachescu, M., Poteca, T. D., and Opris, I. (2014). Nanostructures: a platform for brain repair and augmentation. *Front. Syst. Neurosci.* 8:91. doi: 10.3389/fnsys.2014.00091

Vujaklija, I., Farina, D., and Aszmann, O. (2016). New developments in prosthetic arm systems. *Orthop. Res. Rev.* 8, 31–39. doi: 10.2147/ORR.S71468

Waldert, S. (2016). Invasive vs. Non-invasive neuronal signals for brain-machine interfaces: will one prevail? *Front. Neurosci.* 10:295. doi: 10.3389/fnins.2016.00295

Weiskopf, N., Sitaram, R., Josephs, O., Veit, R., Scharnowski, F., Goebel, R., et al. (2007). Real-time functional magnetic resonance imaging: methods and applications. *Magn. Reson. Imaging* 25, 989–1003. doi: 10.1016/j.mri.2007.02.007

Wheeler, B. C., and Nam, Y. (2011). *In vitro* microelectrode array technology and neural recordings. *Crit. Rev. Biomed. Eng.* 39, 45–61. doi: 10.1615/CritRevBiomedEng.v39.i1.40

Wilson, S. P., Verschure, P. F. M. J., Mura, A., and Prescott, T. J. (eds.). (2015). *Biomimetic and Biohybrid Systems.* Cham: Springer International Publishing.

Wise, K. D., Anderson, D. J., Hetke, J. F., Kipke, D. R., and Najafi, K. (2004). Wireless implantable microsystems: high-density electronic interfaces to the nervous system. *Proc. IEEE* 92, 76–97. doi: 10.1109/JPROC.2003.820544

Wu, F., Stark, E., Im, M., Cho, I. J., Yoon, E. S., Buzsaki, G., et al. (2013). An implantable neural probe with monolithically integrated dielectric waveguide and recording electrodes for optogenetics applications. *J. Neural Eng.* 10:056012. doi: 10.1088/1741-2560/10/5/056012

Yang, J. J., Strukov, D. B., and Stewart, D. R. (2013). Memristive devices for computing. *Nat. Nano.* 8, 13–24. doi: 10.1038/nnano.2012.240

Yang, Y., Adowski, T., Ramamurthy, B., Neef, A., and Xu-Friedman, M. A. (2015). High-speed dynamic-clamp interface. *J. Neurophysiol.* 113, 2713–2720. doi: 10.1152/jn.00543.2014

Yarom, Y. (1991). Rhythmogenesis in a hybrid system - interconnecting an olivary neuron to an analog network of coupled oscillators. *Neuroscience* 44, 263–275. doi: 10.1016/0306-4522(91)90053-Q

Zeck, G. (2016). Aberrant activity in degenerated retinas revealed by electrical imaging. *Front. Cell. Neurosci.* 10:25. doi: 10.3389/fncel.2016.00025

Zhang, S., Song, Y., Wang, M., Zhang, Z., Fan, X., Song, X., et al. (2016). A silicon based implantable microelectrode array for electrophysiological and dopamine recording from cortex to striatum in the non-human primate brain. *Biosens. Bioelectron.* 85, 53–61. doi: 10.1016/j.bios.2016.04.087

5

Evaluating the Effect of Repetitive Transcranial Magnetic Stimulation on Disorders of Consciousness by Using TMS-EEG

Yang Bai[1†], Xiaoyu Xia[2,3†], Jiannan Kang[4], Xiaoxiao Yin[2], Yi Yang[2], Jianghong He[2] and Xiaoli Li[5,6*]*

[1] Department of Automation, Institute of Electrical Engineering, Yanshan University, Qinhuangdao, China, [2] Department of Neurosurgery, PLA Army General Hospital, Beijing, China, [3] Department of Biomedical Engineering, Medical School, Tsinghua University, Beijing, China, [4] Department of Biomedical Engineering, Institute of Electronic Information Engineering, Hebei University, Baoding, China, [5] State Key Laboratory of Cognitive Neuroscience and Learning & IDG/McGovern Institute for Brain Research, Beijing Normal University, Beijing, China, [6] Center for Collaboration and Innovation in Brain and Learning Sciences, Beijing Normal University, Beijing, China

Edited by:
Ioan Opris,
University of Miami, USA

Reviewed by:
Fengyu Cong,
Dalian University of Technology, China
Cristian Donos,
University of Bucharest, Romania

Correspondence:
Jianghong He
he_jianghong@sina.cn
Xiaoli Li
xiaoli@bnu.edu.cn

[†] These authors have contributed equally to this work.

Background: The modulation efficacy of Transcranial magnetic stimulation (TMS) on consciousness improvement of patient with disorder of consciousness (DOC) has not been definitely confirmed.

Objective: This study proposes TMS-EEG to assess effects of repetitive TMS (rTMS) on brain modulation of DOC.

Methods: Twenty sessions of 10 Hz rTMS were applied over the dorsolateral prefrontal cortex for a patient with DOC. Measures of Coma Recovery Scale-Revised (CRS-R) score, TMS-evoked potential (TEP), perturbation complexity index (PCI), and global mean field power (GMFP) were used to evaluate the consciousness level of the patient at three intervals: before the rTMS protocol (T0), immediately after one session rTMS (T1), and immediately after 20 sessions (T2).

Results: It was found that the patient was diagnosed of a minimally conscious state minus (MCS-) by means of CRS-R at the interval of T0, however the TEP and PCI indicated the patient was vegetative state (VS). At the interval of T1, there was not any clinical behavioral improvement in CRS-R, but we could find significant changes in TEP, PCI, and GMFP. At the interval of T2 there was a significant increase of consciousness level according by CRS-R score, PCI value, TEP, and GMFP after 20 sessions of 10 Hz rTMS on the patient with DOC.

Conclusions: We demonstrated that TMS-EEG might be an efficient assessment tool for evaluating rTMS protocol therapeutic efficiency in DOC.

Keywords: TMS-EEG, disorder of consciousness, rTMS, perturbation complexity index, EEG

INTRODUCTION

Although, some studies have attempted to demonstrate some pharmacologic or nonpharmacologic effects, until now there were no evidence-based guidelines regarding the treatment of patients with DOC (Bernat et al., 2006). Recently, few case reports have addressed the application of rTMS on consciousness improve in patients of vegetative state (VS) or minimally consciousness state (MCS) (Lefaucheur et al., 2014). Effects of high frequency rTMS on MCS have been reported in several patients. A recent case report demonstrated that a patient in MCS has meaningful behaviors increase after received three sessions 20 Hz rTMS on the primary motor cortex (M1), it suggested that the rTMS might improve consciousness of MCS patient (Piccione et al., 2011). In a previous study (Manganotti et al., 2013), six patients in VS and MCS received one session of 20 Hz rTMS on M1 region, and one MCS patient has significant clinical and EEG modification. In a study (Naro et al., 2015), by using a protocol of 10 Hz rTMS over dorsolateral prefrontal cortex (DLPFC), three of ten patients with MCS have significant clinical improvement. Also, it was found that there was a significant improvement for VS patients after rTMS modulation. Until now, a case study was only reported that, when TMS deliver to DLPFC, a 30 sessions rTMS protocol could improve neurobehavioral change of VS patient (Louise-Bender Pape et al., 2009). Basically, rTMS modulation for DOC patient might be available.

How to evaluate the modulation of rTMS on the DOC patient is a critical issue. The current gold standard for assessing consciousness state is based on the standard behavioral assessment (Monti and Sannita, 2016). However, possible confounding factors and mechanisms underlying impaired brain function may not be fully considered. The absence of behavioral evidence of command following was not necessarily indicative of the true absence of consciousness (Owen et al., 2006). It was reported that the behavioral abilities could fluctuate across time which would cause mis-diagnostic (Monti and Sannita, 2016). Recently, several "stimulate-response" methods, such as short-latency evoked potentials (Cavinato et al., 2009; Ragazzoni et al., 2013), event-related potentials (Kotchoubey et al., 2005; Rohaut et al., 2015), and motor evoked amplitude (Naro et al., 2015) have been used as more objective assessment methods for the consciousness level of patient with DOC. However, the proposed methods did not consider the integrity of sensory or peripheral nerve pathways of DOC. Thus, it is necessary to develop a new and reliable method to accurately assess the clinical variety in DOC treatment.

Recently TMS-EEG was proposed to evaluate the consciousness state in severely brain-injured and disable of communication patients (Rosanova et al., 2012), and it could invariably trigger complex activations that sequentially involved distant cortical areas ipsi- and contralateral to the site of stimulation in MCS which was different from VS. TMS-EEG technique could directly detect the relationship between non-invasive stimulation and cortical response, and it should not depend on the condition of participant.

Although, TMS-EEG has been demonstrated helpful in differentiating MCS from VS, there were rarely studies using this technology to assess the efficiency of present therapy in DOC. The primary aim of this study was to explore TMS-EEG evidence in consciousness recovery during a therapy of rTMS protocol. The second aim was to support an example of using TMS-EEG to assess the therapy efficiency in DOC.

BACKGROUND

The patient is a woman age 47 with brain injury induced by hypertensive cerebral hemorrhage of right basal ganglia region. Post-injury, the patient remained behaviorally unresponsive for a period of 2 months based on available records and appeared unstable source location of pain after 8 weeks of injury. At about 10 weeks post-injury, the patient was transferred to a comprehensive inpatient brain injury rehabilitation program where physical, occupational, speech, and related therapies were performed for the next 7 months. But no distinct behaviorally improvement during this period. It was 9 months after-injury when she began to accept rTMS therapy, she was diagnosed as MCS- by CRS-R. She could open her eyes spontaneously, and blink when received big sound stimulation like clap but can't locate the sound source, noxious stimulation withdrawing the respective limb from the pain source. She can't sound and had no any commands following response, her mouth had reflex movement. Her caregivers reports that, she had relative stable sleeping time in afternoon and after midnight.

MATERIALS AND METHODS

Subjects

Written informed consent to participate in the study was obtained from the patient's caregivers. In order to indicate the difference of TMS-evoked potential (TEP) between the patient with DOC and controls, five age matched female healthy subjects age 43–50 participated to this study to obtain the mean control TEP. Written informed consent to subjects in the study was obtained. The present study was approved by ethics committee of Beijing Army General Hospital.

Stimulation Protocol

The process of the intervention and evaluation could be found in **Figure 1**. The patient received active 10 Hz rTMS over left DLPFC. Different from similar study (Naro et al., 2015), our protocol lasted 20 consecutive days. Daily sessions of intervention consisted of 1000 pulses (10 Hz) at an intensity of 90% RMT. The stimulation of one session included 10 trains, each train lasted 10 s with a 60 s inter-train pause. The rise time of the magnetic monophasic stimulus was about 100 μs and time to zero was about 800 μs. TMS pulses were delivered using a Magstim R^2 stimulator with a 70 mm figure-of-eight coil (Magstim Company Limited, Whitland, UK). Stimulation intensity varied across this experiment was determined relative to the resting motor threshold (RMT), defined as the lowest TMS intensity which could evoke at least 5 out of 10 EMG with an amplitude >50 μV peak-to-peak in the relaxed first dorsal interosseous muscle of the right hand. To avoid

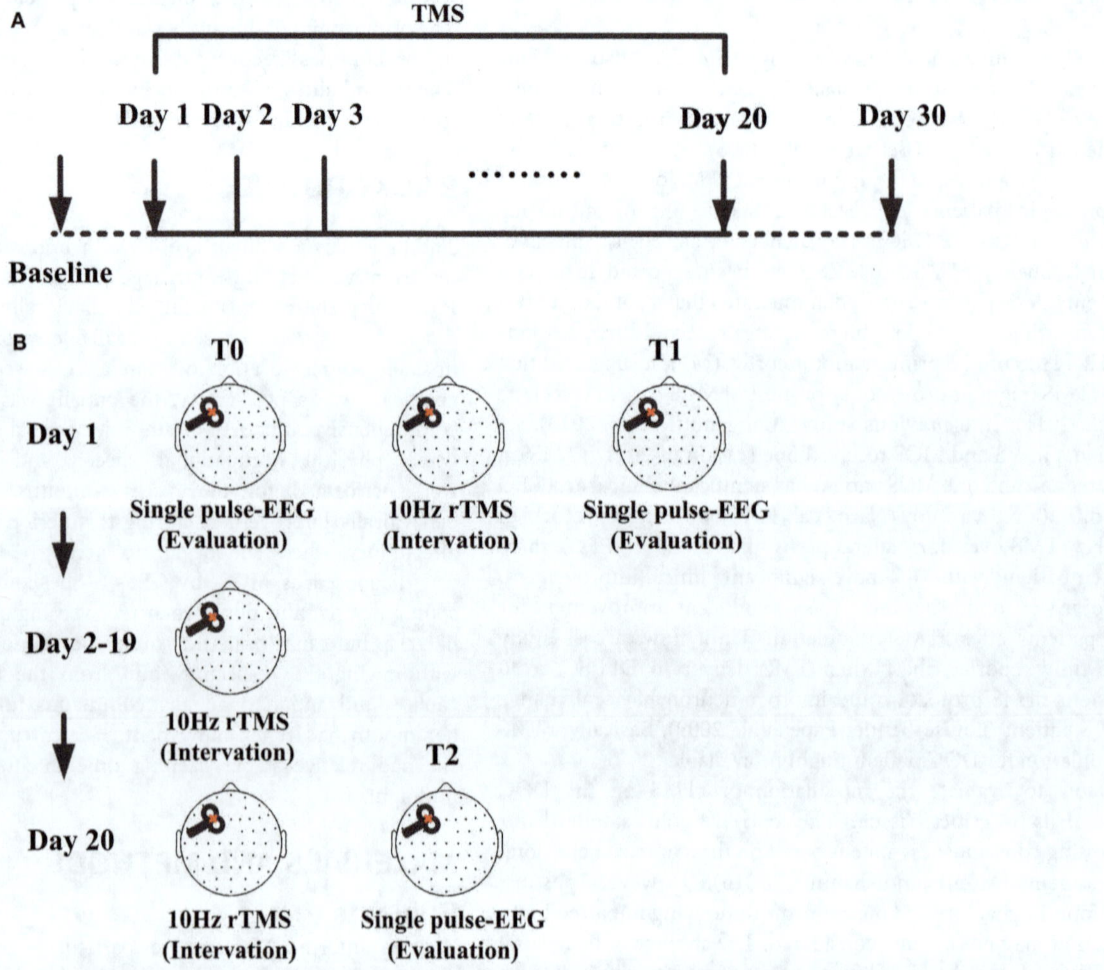

FIGURE 1 | TMS protocol for the patient. (A) Time points of the protocol, TMS were delivered at left-DLPFC lasting for 20 consecutive days. CRS-R score was assessed each day from the baseline to day 30. **(B)** Single pulse TMS evoked EEG recording before the protocol were used as baseline (T0) and that immediately after one session were used as the one session assessment (T1). From day 2 to day 19, there were no TMS and EEG evaluation. Single pulse TMS evoked EEG recorded immediately after the 20 sessions were used as assessment of the whole protocol (T2).

contamination of TMS-evoked potential by auditory potentials evoked by the click associated with the TMS discharge, patient was wearing inserted earplugs continuously playing a masking noise.

CSR-R

The CRS-R is a tool to characterize the level of consciousness and to monitor neuro-behavioral recovery in patients with DOC (Giacino et al., 2004). Scoring is based on the presence or absence of specific behavioral responses to sensory stimuli administered in a standardized manner, with low item represents reflexive activity and high items represent cognitively mediated behaviors. In this study, CRS-R was assessed daily from 1 day before rTMS protocol to30 days after this protocol.

TMS-EEG Recordings

In the experiment, we used TMS-compatible EEG recorder (BrainAmp 64 MRplus, BrainProducts), EEG was continuously acquired from 62 channels with positions of the international 10–10 system. The equipment used TMS-compatible sintered Ag/AgCl-pin electrodes. We set a band-pass filtered at DC to 1000 Hz in the recorder, and the EEG signal was digitized at a sampling rate of 2.5 kHz. During the experiment, the skin/electrode impedance was maintained below 5 kΩ. EEG was recorded in day 1 and day 20. As shown in **Figure 1B**, at T0, 200 single pulses were delivered before the protocol as baseline assessment and TMS evoked EEG immediately recorded after 10 Hz rTMS to evaluate the efficacy of one session rTMS. At T2, 200 single pulses were delivered immediately after rTMS to assess the performance of whole protocol. EEG recordings were carried out while patients were behaviorally awake (eyes open, EO) during the modulation and assessment. If the patient showed signs of sleepiness (prolonged eye closure, EC), the CRS-R arousal facilitation protocol was applied, or the experiment was suspended.

EEG Analysis

Evoked Potential by TMS

Off-line analysis was performed with EEGLAB 12.0.2.5b, running in a MATLAB environment (Version 2013b, MathWorks Inc., Natick, USA). The continuous EEG signal was segmented into epochs starting the TMS pulse onset and ending 300 ms (Massimini et al., 2005; Ferrarelli et al., 2010; Ferreri et al., 2011) after it. After this, data 20 ms after TMS pulse were removed from each trial to exclude the TMS artifact through the cubic interpolation function of MATLAB (Thut et al., 2011). Independent component analysis (ICA) function was used to identify the TMS unrelated artifacts (such as eye movement and muscle artifacts). Then each component was visually inspected in terms of scalp distribution, frequency, timing, and amplitude. The components deemed as artifact were removed with ICA (Casula et al., 2014). The 50 Hz artifact was removed from remaining trials using a notch filter. Then, EEG data were average referenced; down-sampled to 500 Hz, band pass filtered (1–80 Hz), and baseline corrected over 300 ms pre-stimulus. Single trails were carefully inspected to ensure absence of residual TMS artifacts. Each TMS-evoked response was obtained by averaging 150–200 artifact-free trials.

Perturbation Complexity Index

An index of consciousness, called the perturbation complexity index (PCI), was applied to evaluate the consciousness level of the patient. The PCI was proposed before (Casali et al., 2013), the calculation mainly includes three steps. Firstly, TMS evoked cortical perturbation (300 ms after TMS pulse) which was recorded by high-density EEG (62 channels in this study). Then source modeling was performed and nonparametric statistics extracted a binary matrix $[SS(x, t)]$ which describes the spatiotemporal pattern of activation caused by the TMS perturbation. At last, the Lempel-Ziv complexity index was used to compress the matrix. The PCI index was calculated as the normalized Lempel-Ziv complexity. The PCI is expected to be low if there is reduced interaction among cortical areas and will be high if interaction of the cortical areas increased. As suggested (Casali et al., 2013), the PCI values in VS were range of 0.19–0.31 and in MCS were range of 0.32–0.49.

Global Mean Field Power

In order to obtain the overall amount of electrical activity induced by TMS, the global mean field power (GMFP) was calculated with the multichannel average signals as follows (Lehmann and Skrandies, 1980):

$$\text{GMFP (t)} = \sqrt{\frac{\sum_i^k (V_i(t) - V_{mean}(t))^2}{k}} \quad (1)$$

where k means the number of channels, V_i means the amplitude of channel I, and V_{mean} is the mean value of the amplitude across all channels.

RESULTS

CRS-R

CRS-R were used to assess the consciousness level of the patient (**Table 1**). CRS-R score of 8 was marked at baseline. With the rTMS protocol starting, the score remained unchanged for the first 8 days. Although the patient care claimed that the patient showed more excitation, more sensitive to stimulation and less sleeping time, there were no significant clinical behavioral improvement expressed in CRS-R. In the day 9, some simple finger movements were found, and the CRS-R score increased to 10. From the day 15 to 20, the patient represented stable simply movement following the command with score of 13, and her eyes could track movement of objects like mobile phone with video. In the last week of this protocol, there was one score increased for her concentration on something for a time. The shadow area in the **Table 1** shows the CRS-R values in 20 days with 10 Hz rTMS. In the shadow area, the consciousness level of the patient arose from MCS− to MCS+ with score from 8 to 13.

TMS-EEG

TEP

Single pulse evoked potential over DLPFC was calculated at T0, T1, and T2, could be seen in **Figure 2A**. Black line shows the TEP over DLPFC calculating of mean of healthy subjects. We could see that the TEP of T0 shows simple positive-negative EEG response with positive peak at about 35 ms and negative peak at about 60 ms. The TEP of the T1 shows more channels' response activity than T0 while the TEP of the T2 shows more complex than the T1 with bigger amplitude of the fluctuation. Comparing with the TEP of the healthy subjects, the TEP of T2 appears similar fluctuation: positive peak at about 180 ms, which never occurred before.

Figures 2B–D show the butterfly plots of the TEP at three time point, respectively. There have nearly same temporal distribution of the peaks for T0 and T1, but very different from T2. Then PCI was calculated for quantifying the TEP. The first row under the butterfly plot shows the source modeling of corresponding TEP peaks. And then nonparametric statistics was performed to obtain a significant activation distribution (last row of each figure), where the black regions in the cortical represent significant cortical activation induced by the stimulation. The

TABLE 1 | Data of the CRS-R score in this protocol.

Time	CRS-R							CS
(day)	Auditory	Visual	Motor	Oro-motor	Comm	Arousal	Total	
Baseline	1	1	3	1	0	2	8	MCS−
1–8	1	1	3	1	0	2	8	MCS−
9–14	3	1	3	1	0	2	10	MCS+
15–20	4	3	3	1	0	2	13	MCS+
20–22	4	3	3	1	0	2	13	MCS+
23–30	4	3	3	1	0	3	14	MCS+

Shadow area shows the score during rTMS sessions. Comm, communication; CS, consciousness state.

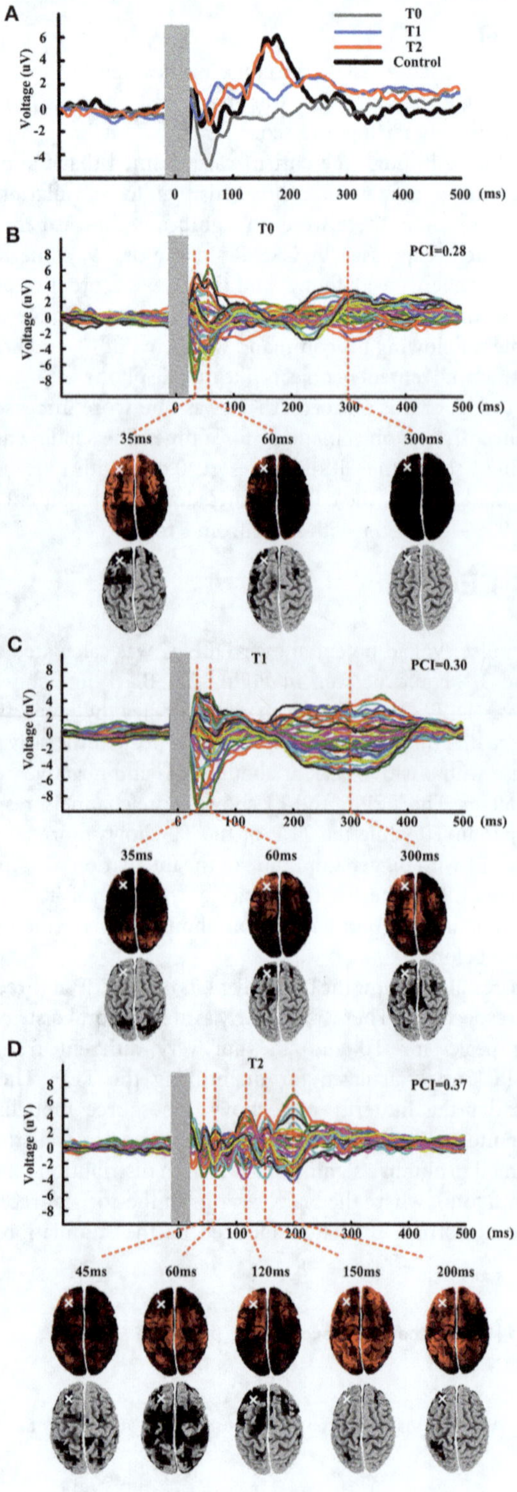

FIGURE 2 | TMS evoked potential and butterfly plots at three time points: T0, T1, and T2. (A) TMS evoked potentials of mean of healthy subjects and patient at three time points. Shadow area means 10 ms before to 20 ms after the TMS onset. **(B–D)** Butterfly plots of patient at three time points. Source modeling corresponding to each TEP peaks is given under the butterfly plots. Last row of each figure gives the significant activation distribution. White cross shows the stimulation site.

activation distribution of T0-T1-T2 indicate a trend of from local to global and from ipsilateral to contralateral. After compressing the binary matrix, the PCI was obtained. At T0, the PCI value was 0.28 and after one session rTMS, the PCI value raised to 0.30. After all the protocol, the PCI value raised to 0.37.

GMFP

The GMFP is depicted in **Figure 3**. The black line shows the mean GMFP of the healthy subjects and the red lines show the GMFP of the patient at three different time. The correlation coefficient (Matlab code: corrcoef.m) were calculated of the GMFP after stimulation between the patient and the healthy subjects. At T0, the correlation is 0.2 and T1 the correlation arose to 0.22. Different from the mean value of healthy subjects, the activation power of the global brain for the T0 and T1 mainly distributed within 100 ms after stimulation. And during the time window from 250 to 400 ms, the global brain power were activated at T0 and T1 while the healthy subject didn't show any activation. After all the rTMS protocol, the GMFP pattern of the patient was similar with the mean GMFP of healthy subjects with correlation 0.86. Meanwhile, the time window of main activation power of the patient was well-matched with the healthy subjects, and main power occurred within 300 ms after stimulation.

DISCUSSION

TEP

Measuring the EEG responses to TMS to differentiate different consciousness states had been proposed (Rosanova et al., 2012). Similar with that observed in unconscious sleeping or anesthetized subjects (Massimini et al., 2005; Ferrarelli et al., 2010), in awake VS patients, TMS triggered a simple, local slow response that indicated a breakdown in effective connectivity. While TMS triggered complex activations that sequentially involved distant cortical areas ipsilateral and contralateral stimulation site in MCS patients. The baseline TEP of the patient in this study showed a relative simple and slow curve similar with VS introduced by Rosanova et al. (2012). It did exactly matched the clinical behavioral result which was diagnosed as MCS- with CRS-R score of 8. The possible reason is due to the fluctuations in behavioral abilities across time. After one session rTMS, TMS triggered more channels' activity. After all the rTMS protocol, the TEP represented a more complex curve, which combined with the theory linking integration and differentiation to consciousness indicated a positive modulation effects of rTMS on this patient.

PCI

The PCI is a measurement to quantify the complexity of TEP and it measures the amount of information integration and differentiation within the brain's response to perturbation. The PCI value of the patient in this study arose from 0.28 to 0.37. As described by Casali et al. (2013) the PCI ranged from 0.19 to 0.31 for a stable clinical diagnosis of VS, and ranged from 0.32 to 0.49 for MCS patients. Therefore, according to the PCI values, the patient was diagnosed as a VS before rolling in this TMS

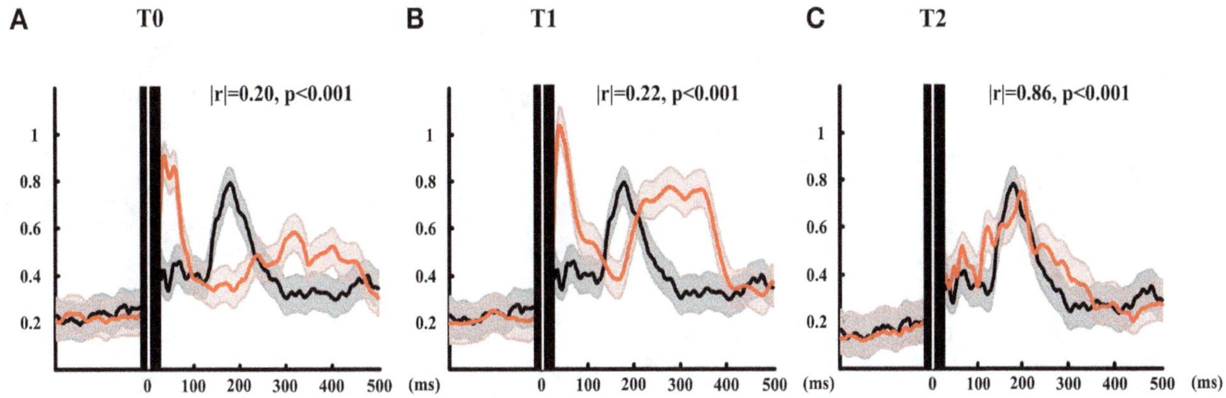

FIGURE 3 | GMFP calculated of patient at three time points and the mean of healthy subjects. Red lines show the GMFP curves of the patient at T0 **(A)**, T1 **(B)**, and T2 **(C)**. Black lines show the mean GMFP curves of healthy subjects. The gray and red shadow means standard deviation of patient and healthy subjects, respectively. Black area with white line show 10 ms before and 20 ms after TMS onset.

protocol, and it was still staying in VS after one rTMS session despite an increase of PCI value. After all the protocol rTMS, the PCI indicated that the patient was staying in MCS+. The TEP results and CRS-R score were consistent with the variation tendency of PCI and both indexes indicated an improvement of consciousness state. But the PCI values showed VS state of the patient at baseline which was not agreement with the CRS-R score. Consistent with the TEP results, the PCI values also showed that patient was still in vegetate state, although appeared much fast oscillation in TEP after one session rTMS, it indicated the patient didn't emerge from vegetate state. Indeed, the boundary of PCI used to differentiate VS from MCS was not perfectly accurate as the study just enrolled few patients for calculating, six for VS and six for MCS. But the PCI values might be useful as a significant potential diagnostic tool for consciousness evaluation.

GMFP

The GMFP results of this study showed that, at a global level, one session rTMS over the left DLPFC increased cortical excitability in temporal windows of 30–100 and 200–400 ms after stimulation. Interestingly, when comparing with healthy subjects, there was a global activation after 300 ms of stimulation for baseline and one session TEP, which nearly impossibly occurred in healthy subjects even in consciousness reduced states such as anesthesia (Ferrarelli et al., 2010) and sleep state (Massimini et al., 2005). The possible reason is that the "overtime" activation may be induced by abnormally electrical transmission evoked by damaged brain region. Then after 20 sessions rTMS, the brain activation pattern (amplitude and time) was tend to well-matched with the healthy brain. Hence, combined with the clinical behavioral assessment in CRS-R scores, we suggested that GMFP might be also a significant marker for consciousness recovery of DOC.

Overall, although there had some diversity in evaluating the base line and one session, all the assessment methods proposed in this case study consistently indicated that the consciousness state was improved after all the rTMS protocol. This divergence of the baseline assessment might be induced by fluctuation of state of the patient and the sensitivity of assessment method should be tested in quantity application. On the other hand, as demonstrated in Naro et al. (2015), we suggest that one session rTMS indeed has transiently improvement but it may difficult leading to permanent clinical behavioral change. Thereby, in this study, we used 20 sessions to use the accumulation efficacy of the rTMS modulation. The incubation time was 8 days in this study but 10 days was reported in a patient in Louise-Bender Pape et al. (2009), we think that this modification efficiency may be variable in individual level and depend on the time and intensity of rTMS.

CONCLUDING REMARKS

This was first study on reporting TMS-EEG based characteristic of consciousness recovery during rTMS protocol. The results indicated that the TMS-EEG might lead to more objectively evaluation of consciousness and might be an efficient assessment tool for rTMS protocol therapeutic efficiency evaluation. Our study was an example of using TMS-EEG method to assess an therapy efficiency in DOC. And we suggest that methods of TMS-EEG supported in this study may facilitate therapy improvement in DOC.

AUTHOR CONTRIBUTIONS

All authors listed, have made substantial, direct and intellectual contribution to the work, and approved it for publication. YB had full access to all the data in the study and takes responsibility for the integrity of the data and the accuracy of the data analysis. Study concept and design, acquisition, analysis, or interpretation of data: YB and XX. Administrative, technical, or material support: XX, JK, XY, and YY. Study supervision and obtained funding: JH and XL.

REFERENCES

Bernat, J. L., D'Alessandro, A. M., Port, F. K., Bleck, T. P., Heard, S. O., Medina, J., et al. (2006). Report of a National Conference on Donation after cardiac death. *Am. J. Transplant.* 6, 281–291. doi: 10.1111/j.1600-6143.2005.01194.x

Casali, A. G., Gosseries, O., Rosanova, M., Boly, M., Sarasso, S., Casali, K. R., et al. (2013). A theoretically based index of consciousness independent of sensory processing and behavior. *Sci. Transl. Med.* 5, 198ra105. doi: 10.1126/scitranslmed.3006294

Casula, E. P., Tarantino, V., Basso, D., Arcara, G., Marino, G., Toffolo, G. M., et al. (2014). Low-frequency rTMS inhibitory effects in the primary motor cortex: insights from TMS-evoked potentials. *Neuroimage* 98, 225–232. doi: 10.1016/j.neuroimage.2014.04.065

Cavinato, M., Freo, U., Ori, C., Zorzi, M., Tonin, P., Piccione, F., et al. (2009). Post-acute P300 predicts recovery of consciousness from traumatic vegetative state. *Brain Inj.* 23, 973–980. doi: 10.3109/02699050903373493

Ferrarelli, F., Massimini, M., Sarasso, S., Casali, A., Riedner, B. A., Angelini, G., et al. (2010). Breakdown in cortical effective connectivity during midazolam-induced loss of consciousness. *Proc. Natl. Acad. Sci. U.S.A.* 107, 2681–2686. doi: 10.1073/pnas.0913008107

Ferreri, F., Pasqualetti, P., Määttä, S., Ponzo, D., Ferrarelli, F., Tononi, G., et al. (2011). Human brain connectivity during single and paired pulse transcranial magnetic stimulation. *Neuroimage* 54, 90–102. doi: 10.1016/j.neuroimage.2010.07.056

Giacino, J. T., Kalmar, K., and Whyte, J. (2004). The JFK coma recovery scale-revised: measurement characteristics and diagnostic utility. *Arch. Phys. Med. Rehabil.* 85, 2020–2029. doi: 10.1016/j.apmr.2004.02.033

Kotchoubey, B., Lang, S., Mezger, G., Schmalohr, D., Schneck, M., Semmler, A., et al. (2005). Information processing in severe disorders of consciousness: vegetative state and minimally conscious state. *Clin. Neurophysiol.* 116, 2441–2453. doi: 10.1016/j.clinph.2005.03.028

Lefaucheur, J.-P., André-Obadia, N., Antal, A., Ayache, S. S., Baeken, C., Benninger, D. H., et al. (2014). Evidence-based guidelines on the therapeutic use of repetitive transcranial magnetic stimulation (rTMS). *Clin. Neurophysiol.* 125, 2150–2206. doi: 10.1016/j.clinph.2014.05.021

Lehmann, D., and Skrandies, W. (1980). Reference-free identification of components of checkerboard-evoked multichannel potential fields. *Electroencephalogr. Clin. Neurophysiol.* 48, 609–621. doi: 10.1016/0013-4694(80)90419-8

Louise-Bender Pape, T., Rosenow, J., Lewis, G., Ahmed, G., Walker, M., Guernon, A., et al. (2009). Repetitive transcranial magnetic stimulation-associated neurobehavioral gains during coma recovery. *Brain Stimul.* 2, 22–35. doi: 10.1016/j.brs.2008.09.004

Manganotti, P., Formaggio, E., Storti, S. F., Fiaschi, A., Battistin, L., Tonin, P., et al. (2013). Effect of high-frequency repetitive transcranial magnetic stimulation on brain excitability in severely brain-injured patients in minimally conscious or vegetative state. *Brain Stimul.* 6, 913–921. doi: 10.1016/j.brs.2013.06.006

Massimini, M., Ferrarelli, F., Huber, R., Esser, S. K., Singh, H., and Tononi, G. (2005). Breakdown of cortical effective connectivity during sleep. *Science* 309, 2228–2232. doi: 10.1126/science.1117256

Monti, M. M., and Sannita, W. G. (2016). *Brain Function and Responsiveness in Disorders of Consciousness.* Chem: Springer International Publishing.

Naro, A., Russo, M., Leo, A., Bramanti, P., Quartarone, A., and Calabrò, R. S. (2015). A single session of repetitive transcranial magnetic stimulation over the dorsolateral prefrontal cortex in patients with unresponsive wakefulness syndrome: preliminary results. *Neurorehabil. Neural Repair* 29, 603–613. doi: 10.1177/1545968314562114

Owen, A. M., Coleman, M. R., Boly, M., Davis, M. H., Laureys, S., and Pickard, J. D. (2006). Detecting awareness in the vegetative state. *Science* 313, 1402. doi: 10.1126/science.1130197

Piccione, F., Cavinato, M., Manganotti, P., Formaggio, E., Storti, S. F., Battistin, L., et al. (2011). Behavioral and neurophysiological effects of repetitive transcranial magnetic stimulation on the minimally conscious state: a case study. *Neurorehabil. Neural Repair* 25, 98–102. doi: 10.1177/1545968310369802

Ragazzoni, A., Pirulli, C., Veniero, D., Feurra, M., Cincotta, M., Giovannelli, F., et al. (2013). Vegetative versus minimally conscious states: a study using TMS-EEG, sensory and event-related potentials. *PLoS ONE* 8:e57069. doi: 10.1371/journal.pone.0057069

Rohaut, B., Faugeras, F., Chausson, N., King, J. R., Karoui, I. E., Cohen, L., et al. (2015). Probing ERP correlates of verbal semantic processing in patients with impaired consciousness. *Neuropsychologia* 66, 279–292. doi: 10.1016/j.neuropsychologia.2014.10.014

Rosanova, M., Gosseries, O., Casarotto, S., Boly, M., Casali, A. G., Bruno, M. A., et al. (2012). Recovery of cortical effective connectivity and recovery of consciousness in vegetative patients. *Brain* 135(Pt 4), 1308–1320. doi: 10.1093/brain/awr340

Thut, G., Veniero, D., Romei, V., Miniussi, C., Schyns, P., and Gross, J. (2011). Rhythmic TMS causes local entrainment of natural oscillatory signatures. *Curr. Biol.* 21, 1176–1185. doi: 10.1016/j.cub.2011.05.049

6

Invasive vs. Non-Invasive Neuronal Signals for Brain-Machine Interfaces: Will One Prevail?

Stephan Waldert *

Sobell Department of Motor Neuroscience and Movement Disorders, University College London Institute of Neurology, University College London, London, UK

Edited by:
Mikhail Lebedev, Duke University, USA

Reviewed by:
Thomas G. Brochier, Centre National de la Recherche Scientifique France, France

***Correspondence:**
Stephan Waldert
s.waldert@ucl.ac.uk

Keywords: Brain computer interface (BCI), intracortical, action potentials, LFP, EEG, neuroprosthetics, microstimulation, Ethics

Brain-machine interfaces (BMI) translate neuronal activity of the brain into signals driving an external effector or affecting internal body parts and functions. Initially, their applications were seen in the field of rehabilitation and medical care for patients to restore social interaction or movement capabilities. Inspired by their success we can already witness the advent of bidirectional and commercial BMIs.

Contemporary BMIs allow for real-time control of prostheses (Gilja et al., 2015), communication (Chen et al., 2015) and "sensation" (O'doherty et al., 2011), notably, the cochlea implant could be considered as the most successful BMI. These applications exemplify that performance can be high but is far from natural interaction with the environment and success depends on manifold factors.

This Opinion is not about algorithms and paradigms but about possibilities and limitations of invasive vs. non-invasive means to *electrically* interface the brain, argued in the realm of BMIs for direct and intuitive motor control.

Current techniques allow to interface electric neuronal activity *in vivo* ranging from intracellular potentials over extracellular action potentials (APs) up to local field potentials (LFPs). These neurophysiological processes are inherently coupled: neurons can interact ephaptically and via electric synapses, spikes change LFPs via synaptic input which in turn influences spiking activity, electric fields of APs can influence LFPs directly without involvement of synaptic currents. Although the LFP is difficult to interpret (Einevoll et al., 2013), correlations between APs and LFPs vary (Buzsaki et al., 2012) and the information they convey can be independent (Belitski et al., 2008), this coupling may have given rise to discussions I have come across and which have triggered this Opinion: the misconception that, to a certain extent, information conveyed by invasive (APs/LFPs) vs. non-invasive (EEG) signals are similar enough for non-invasive signals, and thus non-invasive BMIs, not to be subject to intrinsic impediments.

Such speculations may have been nourished by studies showing similar performance for intracortical BMIs based on APs vs. LFPs (Mehring et al., 2003) as the latter are detectable by EEG techniques. Similar performance might be evident for multi-unit APs vs. high-frequency LFPs ($>\approx$200 Hz), which contain extracellular fields of APs. However, also low/band-pass filtered LFPs below 8 Hz, generally free of such direct AP influences (Waldert et al., 2013), can show similar BMI performance as APs and are suitable for online BMIs (Stavisky et al., 2015). Importantly, this LFP component also carries information about movement parameters if recorded non-invasively (MEG, EEG; Waldert et al., 2008).

Non-invasive EEG yields lower performance than APs or LFPs (Waldert et al., 2009) but with the findings mentioned above and novel approaches: Could non-invasive BMIs catch up?

The source of neuronal signals extracted from EEG after thorough removal of noise, muscle, eye, and movement artifacts, are post-synaptic extracellular currents; in fact, the same currents that contribute to spike-free LFPs. Despite this common source, there are several differences, most of which well-documented, between invasive and non-invasive signals.

First, number and type of neurons: As electric fields produced by neurons decay exponentially with distance, the number of neurons that have to be simultaneously active in a confined area for the fields to superimpose and produce a detectable signal, is magnitudes smaller for LFP than EEG. Hence, the activity of small neuronal clusters is undetectable or recorded at a lower SNR with EEG. In addition, EEG signals are dominated by fields of pyramidal neurons as only their morphology (long, parallel dendrites) and high number in the cortex allow fields to add up and reach the scalp. In contrast, LFPs reflect a superposition of a variety of electrophysiological processes, those underlying EEG plus interneurons, APs, etc.

Second, signal composition: Tissue acts as a low-pass filter generally attenuating high-frequency signals to the extent that buries them in background noise. Hence, with the exception of AP bursts in neuronal populations (Waterstraat et al., 2015), non-invasive signals mainly allow analysis of low-frequency neuronal activity ($<\approx 90$ Hz, lower for dry EEG electrodes). Invasive signals convey information up to several kHz. Moreover, frequency-dependent phase shifts might be stronger when signals spread across larger distances (EEG) and might disintegrate temporal consistency across signal components.

Third, spatial distortion: The extracellular space is composed of media with different electrophysiological properties, which influence how fields spread before being detected as LFPs. On top of this, fields spread in the cerebrospinal fluid, skull, and scalp, causing further spatial distortion before reaching EEG electrodes. Sophisticated head models and algorithms in combination with high-density EEG montages mitigate distortion (Michel and Murray, 2012) for signals above a certain noise level. To be similar to invasive signals, such models might need to be obtained *in vivo* for each user individually, rely on stable sensor positions, necessitate finite-element analysis and run near real-time (BMI performance depends on small delays, Cunningham et al., 2011).

These limitations are intrinsic to EEG and cannot be practicably (or theoretically) overcome. However, EEG offers the paramount advantage to monitor large-scale neuronal activity of the entire brain adjacent to the neurocranium at a low cost and risk-free. Invasive recordings can be deeper but cannot cover the whole neocortex and are initially more laborious due to surgical interventions.

Invasive electrodes come in many forms: single electrodes, electrodes with multiple contacts at the tip or along the shaft, multi-electrode arrays (MEA), or combinations of these in different designs. Electrodes can have arbitrary lengths up to several cm or, for example, up to 1.5 mm (Utah, Blackrock Microsystems) or 10 mm (FMA, MicroProbes) in a MEA. Intracortical electrodes typically yield LFPs and detectable APs of 0–5 identifiable neurons per intact contact. Electrodes can be specifically targeted at arbitrary cerebral areas although accuracy decreases with implantation depth (unless aided by MRI and/or CT).

Nevertheless, for several reasons high implantation accuracy seems not to be crucial for invasive motor BMIs as long as contacts remain in gray matter. The general aim is to record APs and LFPs. In motor cortex, LFPs are recorded at different depths and convey information about movement parameters; recorded APs are faint at layer 1 and usually increase in amplitude with electrode depth up to layer 5 because the size of pyramidal cell somas tends to increase from layer 3 to 5, possibly to support the longer dendrites necessary to project to superficial (input) layers, and because layer 5 is the place of large corticospinal neurons, a main cortical output to control motor functions. This region may therefore often be targeted in invasive motor BMIs for high performance. Importantly, even MEAs with relatively short electrodes (Utah) should have access to this activity because: layer 4 is very thin in motor cortex (Rockel et al., 1980), floating MEAs sink into cortical tissue and APs of large pyramidal neurons can be recorded at several 100 μm distance (experimental and analytical experiences here in the Sobell Department, UCL). For deeper regions, like the anterior wall of the central sulcus, MEAs with longer electrodes can be used to follow layers into the sulcus.

Overall and in contrast to non-invasive signals, invasive signals reflect input to, local processing and output of cortical areas. They may even allow to deduce on intracellular states of neurons (Henze et al., 2000).

Hence, a main advantage of intracortical over non-invasive approaches are inherently possible higher information transfer rates. This and two further advantages are decisive for the future of motor BMIs: tuning and sensation.

BMI performance is still far from natural. After BMI initiation this is partly due to an undersampling of the neuronal network required for natural motor control. Performance then increases during BMI usage as the neurons' tuning "improves" (Carmena et al., 2003), i.e., plasticity enables the brain to learn to control the BMI (closed-loop). This works with arbitrary neurons (Fetz, 1969) and is facilitated by using already tuned neuronal activity (Ganguly and Carmena, 2009) accompanied by a transition from externally assisted to full brain control (Collinger et al., 2013). LFPs seem to be more stable (Flint et al., 2013; Perge et al., 2014), i.e., less easy to tune; probably as in contrast to spiking activity of some neurons, activity of a neuronal cluster needs to change coherently. Although possible (Okazaki et al., 2015), this holds even more so for EEG.

Feedback in closed-loop BMIs has been mainly visual or acoustic. Such inadequate feedback also accounts for low BMI performance as the absence of direct forms of feedback (touch and proprioception) impoverishes information contained in brain signals (Galan et al., 2014) and can disturb the generation of appropriate motor commands (Galan and Baker, 2015). Researchers have begun to employ intracortical microstimulation to establish a direct BMI input channel (Klaes et al., 2014) with possible long-term stability (Callier et al., 2015). This should eventually improve performance as feedback may be delivered specifically to task-relevant cortical areas, which closes the output-feedback loop adequately. As electrodes may be used for stimulation and recording; stimulation could be adapted to ongoing brain activity to improve efficacy.

In contrast to non-invasive BMIs, the great opportunity offered by invasive BMIs thus lies in accurate control, a prerequisite for user acceptance, combined with restoration of somatosensation: Prostheses will be controlled using high-dimensional BMI output signals (Wodlinger et al., 2015) while at the same time BMI input signals, obtained from skin prostheses (Kim et al., 2014) during interaction with the environment, will be transmitted to cortical sensory areas. Providing such information may remain far off evoking natural percepts but the brain will learn to make use of such artificial input channels.

User acceptance is lower for invasive than non-invasive BMIs (Blabe et al., 2015). Invasive BMIs will for many years remain to be used in patients, either for research or if no other remedy is available. Present commercial BMIs are all non-invasive.

This lower acceptance mainly arises from medical concerns related to neurosurgery and the implant. Such risks are clearly not negligible but seem to be partly overrated. For example, validation of DBS showed that complications are rare and, with appropriate procedures, are reduced to 0.9% transient and no permanent deficits (Zrinzo et al., 2012). Even if multiple subpial transection, a series of long cuts in gray matter used to treat epilepsy, is performed in the primary motor cortex, patients are left with no permanent motor deficits (Blount et al., 2004). Implanting electrode arrays for invasive motor BMIs should appear innocuous against this procedure. They have been used in many laboratories for years now and also here in the Sobell Department, UCL, we have not experienced any motor deficits after array implantations. Medical concerns might subside with better awareness of such evidence.

It is now crucial to overcome current challenges of invasive BMIs: better understanding of the "neuronal code," implant miniaturization, wireless signal transmission (Borton et al., 2013), implants charged from outside (Ho et al., 2014) or by harvesting energy from the body (Hannan et al., 2014). BMIs need to be asynchronous for unrestricted control, adaptable to unstable signals and require better sensory-motor prostheses. A major challenge of intracortical implants is biocompatibility, time-dependent degradation of recording quality, and eventually implant failure due to tissue damage during implantation, array micromotion, and a breach of the blood-brain-barrier triggering glial scarring, neurodegeneration, and neuronal death. Only few APs are still recorded years after implantation (Hochberg et al., 2012). LFPs also deteriorate but might show better long-term stability (Flint et al., 2013; Perge et al., 2014). To increase longevity and yield, electrodes need to be reduced in size, coated with neurointegrative, anti-inflammatory factors (Gunasekera et al., 2015), and/or redesigned (e.g., carbon nanotubes, Vitale et al., 2015; Lopez et al., 2016).

As an invasive but extracortical technique, miniaturized ECoG causes lesser cortical tissue damage/irritation and allows for epicortical recordings of LFPs at high spatial resolution and, as recently shown, also of spiking activity (Khodagholy et al., 2015). Benefits derivable from such advances, especially regarding increased information transfer rates, biocompatibility, and long-term signal stability (Chao et al., 2010) over years, are being investigated and might be decisive for the development of future BMIs.

Once invasive BMIs are fully body-embeddable and their benefits outweigh concerns, they might become acceptable to the majority (of patients). However, other, non-medical concerns have to be addressed as well. As invasive BMIs allow access to the brain, i.e., the individual as such, it is necessary to discuss (and regulate) socio-ethical issues: privacy, "mind reading," remote control, brain enhancement, which accuracy legitimates control of potentially hazardous devices, liability, and eventually self-perception and perception through others.

This Opinion is not a polemic against EEG. EEG is a prime tool for many applications, e.g., medical, rehabilitation, current BMIs for communication.

The conclusion of this Opinion is that once technical, socio-ethical, and neuroscientific challenges are resolved, user concerns might subside, and invasive BMIs (using primarily intracortical and potentially epicortical recordings) will prevail in most applications; certainly those for restoration of motor functions and perhaps even in applications not medically indicated.

AUTHOR CONTRIBUTIONS

SW conceived and wrote the paper.

FUNDING

This work was supported by the Wellcome Trust (WT102849MA).

REFERENCES

Belitski, A., Gretton, A., Magri, C., Murayama, Y., Montemurro, M. A., Logothetis, N. K., et al. (2008). Low-frequency local field potentials and spikes in primary visual cortex convey independent visual information. *J. Neurosci.* 28, 5696–5709. doi: 10.1523/JNEUROSCI.0009-08.2008

Blabe, C. H., Gilja, V., Chestek, C. A., Shenoy, K. V., Anderson, K. D., and Henderson, J. M. (2015). Assessment of brain-machine interfaces from the perspective of people with paralysis. *J. Neural Eng.* 12:043002. doi: 10.1088/1741-2560/12/4/043002

Blount, J. P., Langburt, W., Otsubo, H., Chitoku, S., Ochi, A., Weiss, S., et al. (2004). Multiple subpial transections in the treatment of pediatric epilepsy. *J. Neurosurg.* 100, 118–124. doi: 10.3171/ped.2004.100.2.0118

Borton, D. A., Yin, M., Aceros, J., and Nurmikko, A. (2013). An implantable wireless neural interface for recording cortical circuit dynamics in moving primates. *J. Neural Eng.* 10:026010. doi: 10.1088/1741-2560/10/2/026010

Buzsaki, G., Anastassiou, C. A., and Koch, C. (2012). The origin of extracellular fields and currents–EEG, ECoG, LFP and spikes. *Nat. Rev. Neurosci.* 13, 407–420. doi: 10.1038/nrn3241

Callier, T., Schluter, E. W., Tabot, G. A., Miller, L. E., Tenore, F. V., and Bensmaia, S. J. (2015). Long-term stability of sensitivity to intracortical microstimulation of somatosensory cortex. *J. Neural Eng.* 12:056010. doi: 10.1088/1741-2560/12/5/056010

Carmena, J. M., Lebedev, M. A., Crist, R. E., O'doherty, J. E., Santucci, D. M., Dimitrov, D. F., et al. (2003). Learning to control a brain-machine interface for reaching and grasping by primates. *PLoS Biol.* 1:e42. doi: 10.1371/journal.pbio.0000042

Chao, Z. C., Nagasaka, Y., and Fujii, N. (2010). Long-term asynchronous decoding of arm motion using electrocorticographic signals in monkeys. *Front. Neuroeng.* 3:3. doi: 10.3389/fneng.2010.00003

Chen, X., Wang, Y., Gao, S., Jung, T. P., and Gao, X. (2015). Filter bank canonical correlation analysis for implementing a high-speed SSVEP-based brain-computer interface. *J. Neural Eng.* 12:046008. doi: 10.1088/1741-2560/12/4/046008

Collinger, J. L., Wodlinger, B., Downey, J. E., Wang, W., Tyler-Kabara, E. C., Weber, D. J., et al. (2013). High-performance neuroprosthetic control by an individual with tetraplegia. *Lancet* 381, 557–564. doi: 10.1016/S0140-6736(12)61816-9

Cunningham, J. P., Nuyujukian, P., Gilja, V., Chestek, C. A., Ryu, S. I., and Shenoy, K. V. (2011). A closed-loop human simulator for investigating the role of feedback control in brain-machine interfaces. *J. Neurophysiol.* 105, 1932–1949. doi: 10.1152/jn.00503.2010

Einevoll, G. T., Kayser, C., Logothetis, N. K., and Panzeri, S. (2013). Modelling and analysis of local field potentials for studying the function of cortical circuits. *Nat. Rev. Neurosci.* 14, 770–785. doi: 10.1038/nrn3599

Fetz, E. E. (1969). Operant conditioning of cortical unit activity. *Science* 163, 955–958. doi: 10.1126/science.163.3870.955

Flint, R. D., Wright, Z. A., Scheid, M. R., and Slutzky, M. W. (2013). Long term, stable brain machine interface performance using local field potentials and multiunit spikes. *J. Neural Eng.* 10:056005. doi: 10.1088/1741-2560/10/5/056005

Galan, F., Baker, M. R., Alter, K., and Baker, S. N. (2014). Degraded EEG decoding of wrist movements in absence of kinaesthetic feedback. *Hum. Brain Mapp.* 36, 643–654. doi: 10.1002/hbm.22653

Galan, F., and Baker, S. N. (2015). Deafferented controllers: a fundamental failure mechanism in cortical neuroprosthetic systems. *Front. Behav. Neurosci.* 9:186. doi: 10.3389/fnbeh.2015.00186

Ganguly, K., and Carmena, J. M. (2009). Emergence of a stable cortical map for neuroprosthetic control. *PLoS Biol.* 7:e1000153. doi: 10.1371/journal.pbio.1000153

Gilja, V., Pandarinath, C., Blabe, C. H., Nuyujukian, P., Simeral, J. D., Sarma, A. A., et al. (2015). Clinical translation of a high-performance neural prosthesis. *Nat. Med.* 21, 1142–1145. doi: 10.1038/nm.3953

Gunasekera, B., Saxena, T., Bellamkonda, R., and Karumbaiah, L. (2015). Intracortical recording interfaces: current challenges to chronic recording function. *ACS Chem. Neurosci.* 6, 68–83. doi: 10.1021/cn5002864

Hannan, M. A., Mutashar, S., Samad, S. A., and Hussain, A. (2014). Energy harvesting for the implantable biomedical devices: issues and challenges. *Biomed. Eng.* 13:79. doi: 10.1186/1475-925X-13-79

Henze, D. A., Borhegyi, Z., Csicsvari, J., Mamiya, A., Harris, K. D., and Buzsaki, G. (2000). Intracellular features predicted by extracellular recordings in the hippocampus *in vivo*. *J. Neurophysiol.* 84, 390–400.

Ho, J. S., Yeh, A. J., Neofytou, E., Kim, S., Tanabe, Y., Patlolla, B., et al. (2014). Wireless power transfer to deep-tissue microimplants. *Proc. Natl. Acad. Sci. U.S.A.* 111, 7974–7979. doi: 10.1073/pnas.1403002111

Hochberg, L. R., Bacher, D., Jarosiewicz, B., Masse, N. Y., Simeral, J. D., Vogel, J., et al. (2012). Reach and grasp by people with tetraplegia using a neurally controlled robotic arm. *Nature* 485, 372–375. doi: 10.1038/nature11076

Khodagholy, D., Gelinas, J. N., Thesen, T., Doyle, W., Devinsky, O., Malliaras, G. G., et al. (2015). NeuroGrid: recording action potentials from the surface of the brain. *Nat. Neurosci.* 18, 310–315. doi: 10.1038/nn.3905

Kim, J., Lee, M., Shim, H. J., Ghaffari, R., Cho, H. R., Son, D., et al. (2014). Stretchable silicon nanoribbon electronics for skin prosthesis. *Nat. Commun.* 5, 5747. doi: 10.1038/ncomms6747

Klaes, C., Shi, Y., Kellis, S., Minxha, J., Revechkis, B., and Andersen, R. A. (2014). A cognitive neuroprosthetic that uses cortical stimulation for somatosensory feedback. *J. Neural Eng.* 11:056024. doi: 10.1088/1741-2560/11/5/056024

Lopez, C. M., Mitra, S., Putzeys, J., Raducanu, B., Ballini, M., Andrei, A., et al. (2016). "A 966-electrode neural probe with 384 configurable channels in 0.13μm SOI CMOS," in *IEEE International Solid-State Circuits Conference (ISSCC)* (San Fransisco, CA), 392–393. doi: 10.1109/ISSCC.2016.7418072

Mehring, C., Rickert, J., Vaadia, E., Cardoso De Oliveira, S., Aertsen, A., and Rotter, S. (2003). Inference of hand movements from local field potentials in monkey motor cortex. *Nat. Neurosci.* 6, 1253–1254. doi: 10.1038/nn1158

Michel, C. M., and Murray, M. M. (2012). Towards the utilization of EEG as a brain imaging tool. *Neuroimage* 61, 371–385. doi: 10.1016/j.neuroimage.2011.12.039

O'doherty, J. E., Lebedev, M. A., Ifft, P. J., Zhuang, K. Z., Shokur, S., Bleuler, H., et al. (2011). Active tactile exploration using a brain-machine-brain interface. *Nature* 479, 228–231. doi: 10.1038/nature10489

Okazaki, Y. O., Horschig, J. M., Luther, L., Oostenveld, R., Murakami, I., and Jensen, O. (2015). Real-time MEG neurofeedback training of posterior alpha activity modulates subsequent visual detection performance. *Neuroimage* 107, 323–332. doi: 10.1016/j.neuroimage.2014.12.014

Perge, J. A., Zhang, S., Malik, W. Q., Homer, M. L., Cash, S., Friehs, G., et al. (2014). Reliability of directional information in unsorted spikes and local field potentials recorded in human motor cortex. *J. Neural Eng.* 11:046007. doi: 10.1088/1741-2560/11/4/046007

Rockel, A. J., Hiorns, R. W., and Powell, T. P. (1980). The basic uniformity in structure of the neocortex. *Brain* 103, 221–244. doi: 10.1093/brain/103.2.221

Stavisky, S. D., Kao, J. C., Nuyujukian, P., Ryu, S. I., and Shenoy, K. V. (2015). A high performing brain-machine interface driven by low-frequency local field potentials alone and together with spikes. *J. Neural Eng.* 12, 036009. doi: 10.1088/1741-2560/12/3/036009

Vitale, F., Summerson, S. R., Aazhang, B., Kemere, C., and Pasquali, M. (2015). Neural stimulation and recording with bidirectional, soft carbon nanotube fiber microelectrodes. *ACS Nano* 9, 4465–4474. doi: 10.1021/acsnano.5b01060

Waldert, S., Lemon, R. N., and Kraskov, A. (2013). Influence of spiking activity on cortical local field potentials. *J. Physiol.* 591, 5291–5303. doi: 10.1113/jphysiol.2013.258228

Waldert, S., Pistohl, T., Braun, C., Ball, T., Aertsen, A., and Mehring, C. (2009). A review on directional information in neural signals for brain-machine interfaces. *J. Physiol. Paris* 103, 244–254. doi: 10.1016/j.jphysparis.2009.08.007

Waldert, S., Preissl, H., Demandt, E., Braun, C., Birbaumer, N., Aertsen, A., et al. (2008). Hand movement direction decoded from MEG and EEG. *J. Neurosci.* 28, 1000–1008. doi: 10.1523/JNEUROSCI.5171-07.2008

Waterstraat, G., Burghoff, M., Fedele, T., Nikulin, V., Scheer, H. J., and Curio, G. (2015). Non-invasive single-trial EEG detection of evoked human neocortical population spikes. *Neuroimage* 105, 13–20. doi: 10.1016/j.neuroimage.2014.10.024

Wodlinger, B., Downey, J. E., Tyler-Kabara, E. C., Schwartz, A. B., Boninger, M. L., and Collinger, J. L. (2015). Ten-dimensional anthropomorphic arm control in a human brain-machine interface: difficulties, solutions, and limitations. *J. Neural. Eng.* 12, 016011. doi: 10.1088/1741-2560/12/1/016011

Zrinzo, L., Foltynie, T., Limousin, P., and Hariz, M. I. (2012). Reducing hemorrhagic complications in functional neurosurgery: a large case series and systematic literature review. *J. Neurosurg.* 116, 84–94. doi: 10.3171/2011.8.JNS101407

7

Brain Enhancement through Cognitive Training: A New Insight from Brain Connectome

Fumihiko Taya*[1], *Yu Sun*[1], *Fabio Babiloni*[2], *Nitish Thakor*[1,3,4] and *Anastasios Bezerianos*[1]

[1] Centre for Life Sciences, Singapore Institute for Neurotechnology (SINAPSE), National University of Singapore, Singapore, Singapore, [2] Department of Molecular Medicine, University "Sapienza" of Rome, Rome, Italy, [3] Department of Electrical and Computer Engineering, National University of Singapore, Singapore, Singapore, [4] Department of Biomedical Engineering, Johns Hopkins University, Baltimore, MD, USA

Edited by:
Mikhail Lebedev, Duke University, USA

Reviewed by:
Yong He, Beijing Normal University, China
Joydeep Bhattacharya, Goldsmiths, University of London, UK
Tal Dotan Ben-Soussan, Research Institute for Neuroscience, Italy

****Correspondence:***
Anastasios Bezerianos, Centre for Life Sciences, Singapore Institute for Neurotechnology (SINAPSE), National University of Singapore, 28 Medical Drive, #05-Cor, 117456 Singapore, Singapore
tassos.bezerianos@nus.edu.sg

Owing to the recent advances in neurotechnology and the progress in understanding of brain cognitive functions, improvements of cognitive performance or acceleration of learning process with brain enhancement systems is not out of our reach anymore, on the contrary, it is a tangible target of contemporary research. Although a variety of approaches have been proposed, we will mainly focus on cognitive training interventions, in which learners repeatedly perform cognitive tasks to improve their cognitive abilities. In this review article, we propose that the learning process during the cognitive training can be facilitated by an assistive system monitoring cognitive workloads using electroencephalography (EEG) biomarkers, and the brain connectome approach can provide additional valuable biomarkers for facilitating leaners' learning processes. For the purpose, we will introduce studies on the cognitive training interventions, EEG biomarkers for cognitive workload, and human brain connectome. As cognitive overload and mental fatigue would reduce or even eliminate gains of cognitive training interventions, a real-time monitoring of cognitive workload can facilitate the learning process by flexibly adjusting difficulty levels of the training task. Moreover, cognitive training interventions should have effects on brain sub-networks, not on a single brain region, and graph theoretical network metrics quantifying topological architecture of the brain network can differentiate with respect to individual cognitive states as well as to different individuals' cognitive abilities, suggesting that the connectome is a valuable approach for tracking the learning progress. Although only a few studies have exploited the connectome approach for studying alterations of the brain network induced by cognitive training interventions so far, we believe that it would be a useful technique for capturing improvements of cognitive functions.

Keywords: cognitive training, brain connectome, electroencephalography (EEG), functional magnetic resonance imaging (fMRI), biomarkers

Introduction

Recent developments in neuroimaging techniques and related mathematical tools have extended our understanding of neural mechanisms underlying brain cognitive functions. As such, enhancement of cognitive performance or speeding-up learning process through a brain enhancement system is a tangible target of contemporary research. Thus, the enhancement of brain functions has been studied for a wide range of cognitive functions using a variety of techniques (Clark and Parasuraman, 2014).

Such a system for brain enhancement would be beneficial for a wide variety of people and can be based on several techniques. Firstly, patients with neurological disorders (e.g., Alzheimer's disease, dementia, stroke) or psychiatric disorder (e.g., schizophrenia, major depression, bipolar disorder) would be greatly benefitted if undesirable symptoms can be diminished or rehabilitation can be speeded up by the system (Farah et al., 2004). So far, two enhancement approaches, psychopharmacology and the brain stimulation, have a long history of researches and medical applications. Secondly, healthy elderly people with declined cognitive functions due to aging can be benefited from such a system, as the quality of their daily life would be improved. It is known that aging has detrimental effects on several cognitive functions such as processing speed, working memory (WM) function, executive function, reasoning, and long-term memory (LTM; Park et al., 2002) although some other cognitive functions such as vocabulary (Schaie, 1994) and implicit memory (Fleischman et al., 2004) remain relatively stable or even get improved. Also, substantial evidences have emerged to show that brain can be modified or reorganized throughout the lifespan (Gutchess, 2014). Thirdly, people who are working under extreme circumstances, such as traffic controllers, military personnel, and surveillance system operators, will have a great profit from the brain enhancement system as they need to engage in operations for a long duration with high workloads and pressure, and even a small error in the operations could result in fatal accidents (Pop et al., 2012). Fourthly, struggling students could be benefited from a system that accelerates their learning performance when they are cramming for their examinations, and thus improving their chances for a good job status and salary, which are often dependent on their educational backgrounds (Deary et al., 2007). In fact, it is known that a psychostimulant called methylphenidate (MPH), also known as Ritalin, is sometimes misused by students for boosting cognitive abilities (Talbot, 2009). Finally, even ordinary people can be benefitted from the advantages of such a system, since their quality of life, their reputation in public community, or their performance at workplace could be improved along with the enhancement of the memory function, the attention levels, or emotional states. For the purpose, a variety of interventions such as cognitive training (Klingberg, 2010), neurofeedback (Sulzer et al., 2013), or more directly by brain stimulations, e.g., TMS, tDCS (Hamilton et al., 2011), or psychopharmacological drugs, e.g., MPH, modafini (Repantis et al., 2010) have extensively been studied.

In this review article, we will mainly focus on the brain enhancement through the cognitive training interventions, in which people perform specific cognitive tasks for improving their cognitive functions (Klingberg, 2010). We will propose that electroencephalography (EEG) biomarkers of cognitive workload can be used for a brain enhancement system to improve the outcome of cognitive training interventions, and the connectome approach can provide further valuable metrics for the assessment of effectiveness of the interventions. For this purpose, three general topics will be covered: cognitive training interventions, EEG biomarkers for cognitive workload, and the brain connectome approach (**Figure 1**). The purpose of this review article is to bridge between these three different topics. A similar attempt has been made for the combination of brain stimulation and connectome, which will not be covered here (Luft et al., 2014).

Firstly, we will introduce studies on cognitive training interventions, and their effects on the brain activities (Klingberg, 2010). Generally, the cognitive training interventions without any physical or pharmacological interventions would be more desirable for most people because of its relatively low-costs and lower potential risks—undesirable side effects (e.g., headache, dizziness, nervousness, sleep disturbances) can be avoided. Neurofeedback, in which individuals are presented with a feedback signal derived from brain activity that indicates their learning goals, is another technique for brain enhancement which requires no physical interventions and has several common characteristics with the cognitive training. However a significant difference might be the fact that while cognitive training goals include improvements of behavioral performance and accompanying modifications in brain activations, neurofeedback is targeting directly in improving brain activations and consequently increasing cognitive performance.

Secondly, we will introduce EEG biomarkers for cognitive workload, and propose that an adaptive training system using EEG biomarkers based on real-time monitoring of cognitive workload can improve gains of the cognitive training interventions as cognitive overload or mental fatigue during the course of training would reduce or even eliminate the gains of cognitive training (Baldwin and Penaranda, 2012). Owing to recent developments and spreads of neuroimaging techniques such as EEG and MRI, tremendous amounts of studies have been done for investigating associations between mental states and brain activities. Meanwhile, a lot of researchers have developed mathematical methods for revealing biomarkers of brain functions mainly based on advances in signal processing and machine learning techniques (Kothe and Makeig, 2011). The combination of extended knowledge of the mechanism underlying brain cognitive functions and the advanced mathematical techniques would provide more elaborated ways for boosting learning processes during cognitive training.

Finally, we will propose that the brain connectome approach, mainly based on graph theory (Sporns, 2014), would provide further valuable biomarkers for monitoring mental states to accelerate learning process by optimizing cognitive workload during the performance of training tasks. The brain connectome is a relatively new approach for investigating topological architecture of the brain network. Because the brain is a complex network consisting of a number of brain areas dedicated to different functions, it has been suggested that cognitive functions emerged from the dynamic interactions of the distributed areas in large-scale network (Bressler and Menon, 2010). Therefore, brain network analysis would provide further

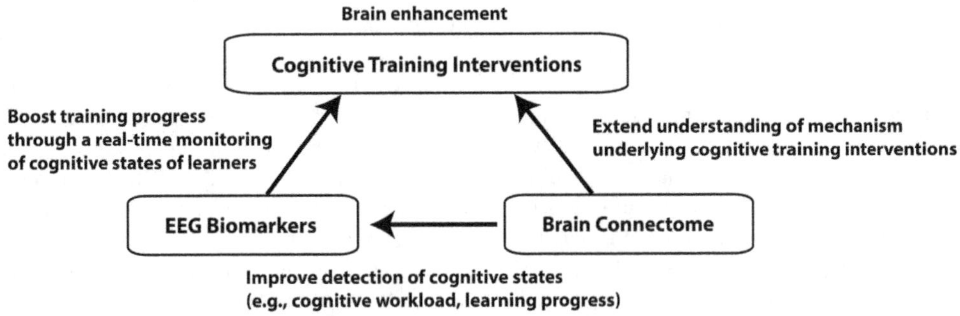

FIGURE 1 | A schematic diagram depicting connections between the three different topics. Improvement of cognitive functions through cognitive training interventions is the ultimate goal of the brain enhancement system we propose. EEG biomarkers can facilitate learners' learning process through a real-time monitoring of cognitive states while brain connectome approach can improve detection of cognitive states as well as understanding of neural mechanism underlying cognitive training.

insights into the mechanism underlying the cognitive training, and the graph theoretical network metrics would be useful for discriminating different brain states during the training. We will first provide a general introduction of the network science, and then introduce studies applying the connectome approach to the brain connectivity. Next, we will present our attempts to employ the connectome approach for discriminating different cognitive states as well as relevant studies that demonstrated cognitive state dependent differences in brain networks or changes in brain network evoked by prior experience or cognitive training. Although so far only one study directly examined the changes in network metrics induced by cognitive training interventions (Langer et al., 2013), the studies showing changes of brain connectivity and differences in graph theoretical network metrics would suggest a potential use of the network metrics for the brain enhancement system assisting learners' learning processes.

Cognitive Training

Cognitive Training Interventions

Cognitive training has emerged as a promising alternative to improve cognitive abilities (Lustig et al., 2009; Karbach and Schubert, 2013; Moreau and Conway, 2013). Several studies have been performed to explore the effectiveness of the cognitive training and its effects on neural activities (Klingberg, 2010; Jolles and Crone, 2012). It has also been suggested that even just playing video games could improve perceptual or cognitive abilities (Green and Bavelier, 2003). Because of its ease of use and the numerous potential applications, the cognitive training has attracted substantial public attention, and a lot of computer software for "brain training" are available on web, PCs or smartphones, e.g., Lumosity,[1] CogniFit,[2] Cogmed.[3]

In this section, we will introduce neuroimaging studies on cognitive training, which demonstrated changes of brain activations or morphological changes in the brain induced by the cognitive training interventions. Understanding the neural process underlying the cognitive training interventions is of great importance in order to develop the brain enhancement system facilitating learners' learning processes. The theoretical framework capturing the neural plasticity behind cognitive training is introduced by Hebb, known as Hebbian learning theory (Hebb, 1949). According to this theory, any two neurons or group of neurons that are repeatedly active at the same time they will tend to form stronger associations, and consequently, activity in one will be facilitating activity in the other. Briefly, when neurons fire together, the connection between them is strengthened. This means that when executing a cognitive task repeatedly, the brain areas associated with the cognitive functions engaged in the task will form stronger associations. Hence, we could improve our cognitive abilities through modifications of the brain activations induced by cognitive training interventions.

Major criticism on the cognitive training is about the transferability of training-related performance gain (Lustig et al., 2009). It is likely that performance of the trained task would be improved by the training, but its effects could be limited to the particular trained task (Jaeggi et al., 2008). What most of the people expect of the cognitive training is an improvement of their general cognitive abilities useful in everyday life, not just a better performance specific to the trained task. Therefore, it is of great importance to succeed in reproducing the improved performance gained from training in one task, on another, different task with no prior training on the second (Karbach and Schubert, 2013). Improved performance on untrained, but directly related tasks to the trained task is called "near transfer", while improvements on untrained tasks which are related, but not directly related to the cognitive abilities is called "far transfer". In fact, several studies have shown the possibility of such far transfer of practice effect beyond task-specific performance (Klingberg et al., 2002), although its generality remains controversial (Colom et al., 2010). The basic theory behind the transfer is also simple. If a brain sub-network that is engaged in a trained task overlaps with

[1] www.lumosity.com
[2] www.cognifit.com
[3] www.cogmed.com

networks related to untrained tasks, these networks will be also strengthened following the Hebbian learning rule, and consequently result in improved cognitive performance on the untrained tasks.

In search of training schemes that can induce transfer effects, WM training has been studied intensively. It is believed that the WM is essential for a variety of higher cognitive functions such as reasoning, problem solving, and decision making (Klingberg, 2010), and moreover, it is considered to be the basis for the general intelligence (Conway et al., 2003). Additionally, WM capacity is crucial for knowledge and skill acquisition, and is closely related to academic achievements and educational success, engaging intense interest from a broad range of people. For this reason, many programs for cognitive training including commercial products such as Cogmed WM Training[4] or Jungle Memory Program[5] (Shipstead et al., 2012), are designed to target on the WM capacity. Some studies have demonstrated that the gain of WM oriented cognitive training can be transferred to cognitive control mechanisms (Klingberg et al., 2002), the WM updating process (Dahlin et al., 2008), reading comprehension (Chein and Morrison, 2010), and even to measures of fluid intelligence, a cognitive ability of abstract thinking and adaptation to novel problems (Jaeggi et al., 2008). The fluid intelligence is known to be closely related to professional and educational success (Neisser et al., 1996). Although it is believed that the fluid intelligence is unsusceptible to influences of education, Halford et al. proposed a hypothesis that the WM and reasoning share a common mechanism, providing a framework for improvements of the general intelligence through WM oriented cognitive training (Halford et al., 2007). To verify the hypothesis, Jaeggi et al. trained subjects for 8–19 days with an adaptive dual *n*-back task, in which subjects were required to update the information about spatial locations of visual stimuli and auditory information concurrently, and found the improvements of the fluid intelligence measured by Raven's Advanced Progressive Matrices test and the Bochumer Matrizen-Test (Jaeggi et al., 2008). Stephenson et al. also found improved scores in two out of four tests for the fluid intelligence by the dual *n*-back task training (Stephenson and Halpern, 2013). Despite a number of successful observations of transfer effects of WM training gain, neural mechanism underlying the WM training interventions remains elusive. Some studies have suggested that the improvements of fluid intelligence could be achieved through cognitive training other than WM training. Colom et al. found similar improvements in two out of four scores measuring fluid intelligence induced by simple speed tasks (Colom et al., 2010). Also the improvement of fluid intelligence was observed only for participants who underwent cognitive training with visuospatial components, and even a visuospatial short-term memory (STM) training improved the fluid intelligence (Stephenson and Halpern, 2013). One promising account for the effects of WM training is that participants' short-term storage capacity, which is a common factor among STM, WM, executive function, attention, and general fluid intelligence, is expanded through intensive performance of the cognitive training (Colom et al., 2013).

Effects of Cognitive Training on Brain Activations

In order to develop the brain enhancement system which facilitates cognitive training processes, it is also of great importance to investigate the effects of cognitive training on the brain and to understand what is actually accomplished by the cognitive training. Modulation of brain activation has been demonstrated with a variety of cognitive training interventions, such as the WM training (Hempel et al., 2004; Olesen et al., 2004; Jolles et al., 2010), an attentional training (Mozolic et al., 2010), dual tasks (Erickson et al., 2007), video games training (Maclin et al., 2011), and even meditation training (Tang and Posner, 2014).

A number of studies using functional magnetic resonance imaging (fMRI) have shown that besides improving behavioral performance, intense cognitive training resulted also in changes of the brain activations that were related to the cognitive functions implicated in the tasks used as cognitive interventions were changed by intense cognitive training, accompanying with improvements of behavioral performance (Hempel et al., 2004). Olesen et al. found an increase of brain activity in the areas related to the WM induced by 5 weeks practice of WM tasks (Olesen et al., 2004) while Hempel et al. showed increased activations after 2 weeks of training on a WM task and decreased activations after 4 weeks, suggesting two distinct mechanisms mediating the training effects: an enhancement mechanism for WM and a suppressive mechanism related to automation of processing (Hempel et al., 2004). Furthermore, a training of multi-task processing revealed training-induced reductions in activity of brain areas responsible for stimulus-response associations, attentional control, and response selection process as well as an increase of activity in a region related to executive control (Erickson et al., 2007). Such reductions in brain activity induced by training may reflect increased task selectivity within the areas (Dux et al., 2009). Even thirty hours of training on a video game can induce reduction of activation in attentional control areas, suggesting a reduction of attentional demands after the training (Lee et al., 2012). Interestingly, a WM training has also induced less deactivation in "default-mode network", which is usually deactivated during cognitive tasks, suggesting more automatic processing after practice (Jolles et al., 2010).

In addition to the changes of activation at brain regions specific to trained tasks, several neuroimaging studies demonstrated transfer effects of cognitive interventions (Dahlin et al., 2008). Dahlin et al. examined whether transfer effect was induced by training on a task that involved "updating", which is a basic executive function relating to intelligence, WM, and manipulation of information (Dahlin et al., 2008). After 5 weeks of training on a letter memory task, young subjects showed improved performance on 3-back task, but no improvement in the Stroop task. A comparison between pre- and post-changes in the fMRI data that were collected during the training task showed increased activity in the left striatum and decreased activity in fronto-parietal network. As

[4]www.cogmed.com/program
[5]junglememory.com/

far as the transfer task is concerned, training-induced increases in brain activations were found in the left striatum and the frontal cortex for the 3-back task, but no significant changes were detected for the Stroop task. Additionally, a conjunction analysis revealed that overlap region exclusive to letter memory and 3-back was the left striatum, which is associated with updating, suggesting that the activation of the overlapping brain region during the training induced the transfer to the untrained 3-back task. No transfer was observed in older adults who showed no significant activation in the striatum during the letter memory task. Transfer effect was also examined for affective cognitive control (Schweizer et al., 2013). They found that twenty days of a dual *n*-back task with emotional stimuli (eWM task) induced improved emotional regulation and increased activations in the fronto-parietal demand network, including the dorsal and subgenual anterior cingulate (sgACC), on another task that required emotional regulation. Furthermore, several studies have examined cross-modal transfer effects of WM training (Schneiders et al., 2011, 2012; Buschkuehl et al., 2014). Buschkuel et al. have examined cross-modal transfer effects of 7 days of training of a visuospatial *n*-back task to an auditory *n*-back task, and investigated longitudinal changes of brain activities using perfusion (arterial spin labeling; ASL) (Buschkuehl et al., 2014). They found a transfer effects across modalities, and observed increased perfusion in right superior frontal gyrus, which is thought to be involved in executive control and WM processing. On the contrary, Schneiders et al. failed to observe cross-modal transfer effects for a visual and an auditory WM tasks (Schneiders et al., 2011, 2012). They found a modality-specific training effect for the visual WM training in the right middle frontal gyrus, which is to some extent specific to the maintenance of visual objects in WM, (Schneiders et al., 2011), and that for the auditory WM training in the right inferior frontal gyrus responsible for maintaining auditory information (Schneiders et al., 2012). However, no across-modal transfer effects were detected. One possible account for this discrepancy is that WM training would once increase brain activations in areas associated with executive control, which is shared between WM tasks with different modalities, but further training would decrease the brain activation along with a decrease in cognitive efforts necessary for the performance of the WM tasks (Chein and Schneider, 2005).

Furthermore, such modifications of brain activations induced by cognitive training can also be captured by EEG as well (Maclin et al., 2011). Changes in activtions related to attentional processes triggered by complex game learning were detected in P3 ERP component as well as in δ and α EEG spectral power (Maclin et al., 2011). Moreover, frontal EEG α power during early phase of the game training predicted subsequent learning rates (Mathewson et al., 2012). An improvement of the fluid intelligence induced by WM training and increases in θ and α synchronization have suggested that the WM training has improved not only WM maintenance functions, but also central executive and attentional control (Jaušovec and Jaušovec, 2012). A first-person shooter (FPS) video game enhanced neural processes that support spatial selective attention, as it was shown by increased amplitudes of the later visual ERPs in high-performing FPS players (Wu et al., 2012). Improvements of visual attention allocation, executive attention, and updating function in WM representation has been indicated by increases in ERP components (N160, P200 and P300) after training on a WM task that engaged updating function (Zhao et al., 2013). Modifications of EEG signals induced by training on a game involving dual tasks or a WM task along with behavioral improvements were also observed for elderly adults (Anguera et al., 2013) and dysphoric participants (Owens et al., 2013). Moreover, a meditation training such as integrative body-mind training (IBMT) improved attention, mood, and stress regulation, while it increased frontal midline θ power, where the anterior cingulate cortex (ACC) is suggested to be the generator of the activity (Tang et al., 2009). Thus, several cognitive training programs have shown alterations in brain activities as well as their effectiveness in improvements of cognitive performance. In **Table 1**, we provide a summary of existing neuroimaging studies showing changes in brain activations induced by cognitive training interventions.

Structural Brain Changes Induced by Cognitive Training Interventions

In addition to the training-induced changes in brain activity, morphological changes can be induced by cognitive practice in the adult brain despite a belief that changes in brain structure are limited to the critical period of development (Draganski and May, 2008). Repeated practice of skills during professional career can induce long-lasting changes in structure of the brain: i.e., London taxi drivers who have substantial experiences to use spatial knowledge for navigation in the complex city were found to have larger gray matter volumes in hippocampus (Maguire et al., 2006), professional typists devoted to the prolonged practice of typing show increased gray matter volume in brain regions related to programming of motor tasks such as supplementary motor area, prefrontal cortex and cerebellum (Cannonieri et al., 2007), violinists and other string players who use the second to the fifth digits of the left hand for fingering the string have larger cortical representation of the digits of the left hand in the primary somatosensory cortex (Elbert et al., 1995).

More directly, several studies have examined the effects of training on the structure of the brain. Modulations of neural structures and functions of the brain can occur for a relatively short period of time as demonstrated by MR-based morphology in conjunction with longitudinal design. Three months of training on juggling task induced a transient expansion of gray matter in the brain areas associated with the processing and storage of complex visual motion for both young and older participants (Draganski et al., 2004; Boyke et al., 2008). Even seven days of the juggling training induced a change in gray matter (Driemeyer et al., 2008) and 6 weeks of the training induced changes in white matter measured with diffusion tensor imaging (DTI) as well as in gray matter density (Scholz et al., 2009). Additionally, real-life intervention such as an intensive preparation for the medical examination, which requires acquisition of substantial amount of new information,

TABLE 1 | Studies showing changes in brain activations induced by cognitive interventions.

Study	Modality	Training task	Control group	Population	Training period
McKendrick et al. (2014)	NIRS	a dual verbal and spatial WM task	a yoked condition group	YA	5 days
Heinzel et al. (2014)	fMRI	an adaptive *n*-back task	-	OA and YA	4 weeks
Buschkuehl et al. (2014)	ASL	adaptive visuaospatial *n*-back	vocabulary and general knowledge questions	YA	7 days
Zhao et al. (2013)	EEG	Three memory tasks	no training	YA	21–23 days
Schweizer et al. (2013)	fMRI	adaptive emotional dual *n*-back	a feature match training	YA	20 days
Owens et al. (2013)	EEG	an online dual *n*-back task	a nonadaptive dual 1-back task	YA (dysphoric)	2 weeks
Anguera et al. (2013)	EEG	NeuroRacer (a dual task)	single task and no-contact control	OA	4 weeks
Wu et al. (2012)	EEG	a FPS video game	nonaction game control group	YA	10 h
Schneiders et al. (2012)	fMRI	adaptive auditory *n*-back	-	YA	2 weeks
Prakash et al. (2012)	fMRI	Space Fortress vidoegame	only limited game experience	YA	30 h
Mathewson et al. (2012)	EEG	Space Fortress vidoegame	-	YA	20 h
Lee et al. (2012)	fMRI	Space Fortress videogame	only limited game experience	YA	30 h
Jaušovec and Jaušovec (2012)	EEG, NIRS	Five different WM tasks	communication and social skills	YA	30 h
Schneiders et al. (2011)	fMRI	adaptive visual or auditory *n*-back	no training	YA	2 weeks
Maclin et al. (2011)	EEG	Space Fortress vidoegame	-	YA	20 h
Jolles et al. (2010)	fMRI	a verbal WM task	no training	YA	6 weeks
Dux et al. (2009)	fMRI	sensory-motor task (single or dual task trials)	-	YA	2 weeks
Tang et al. (2009)	EEG	a meditation training	a relaxation training	YA	5 days
Dahlin et al. (2008)	fMRI	a letter memory task	no training	OA and YA	5 weeks
Erickson et al. (2007)	fMRI	a dual tasks and a single task	no training	YA	2–3 weeks
Olesen et al. (2004)	fMRI	WM tasks	-	YA	5 weeks
Hempel et al. (2004)	fMRI	*n*-back	-	YA	4 weeks

Note: EEG: electroencephalography, fMRI: functional magnetic resonance imaging, NIRS: near-infrared spectroscopy, ASL: arterial spin labeling, YA: young adults, OA: old adults.

could also induce the increment of gray matter in the brain areas known to be involved in memory processes (Draganski et al., 2006). Furthermore, a variety of training tasks other than the juggling training have induced alterations in brain structures. A Morse code training, a sort of language learning, induced a gray matter increase in the left occipitotemporal cortex, which projects to the area involved in language perception (Schmidt-Wilcke et al., 2010). A complex motor skill learning task induced an increase in gray matter volume in the prefrontal cortex, which was positively correlated with performance improvements over time, and a decrease in white matter volume in the prefrontal cortex (Taubert et al., 2010). A memory training induced cortical thickness changes in the right fusiform and lateral orbitofrontal cortex correlated with improvements in memory performance (Engvig et al., 2010). A WM training increased myelination measured by fractional anisotropy (FA) of fiber tracts in the white matter regions adjacent to the intraparietal sulcus and the anterior part of the body of the corpus callosum, both of which are considered to be critical in WM (Takeuchi et al., 2010). A mental calculation training that required WM function induced a decrease in regional gray matter volume in the WM-related regions, which could be attributed to the usage-dependent selective elimination of synapses (Takeuchi et al., 2011). A meditation training increased white matter efficiency in areas surrounding the ACC that is implicated in cognitive control (Tang et al., 2012). Furthermore, a logical reasoning training gain to fluid intelligence was associated with an increase in structural integrity in corpus and genu of the corpus callosum, which connect between homologous cortical areas of the two hemispheres and are considered to be involved in executive functions and WM (Wolf et al., 2014). Taken together, structural brain changes in response to cognitive training interventions were observed for a variety of training schemes, and such changes were mainly found in the brain areas that were supposed to be involved in the training tasks. These observed structural plasticity can be a basis of improvements in cognitive functions through the interventions, suggesting a potential effectiveness of the cognitive training. We provide a brief summary of structural changes in the brain induced by training intervention in **Table 2**.

Summary of Effects of Cognitive Training

In summary, cognitive training can modify activations or the structure of the brain regions directly related to the training tasks along with improvements in behavioral performance of the tasks. As different training tasks can induce changes of brain activations at different brain areas, the selection of training tasks is also an important issue. Although the brain areas engaged by the training tasks can be different dependent on sensory modality, the cognitive tasks recruiting

TABLE 2 | Studies showing structural brain changes induced by training interventions.

Study	Modality	Training task	Control group	Population	Training period
Wolf et al. (2014)	DTI	logical reasoning training	-	OA	4 weeks
Tang et al. (2012)	DTI	a meditation training	a relaxation training	YA	4 weeks
Takeuchi et al. (2011)	gray matter volume	mental calculation	placebo, no training	YA	5 days
Takeuchi et al. (2010)	DTI	WM program	-	YA	2 months
Engvig et al. (2010)	cortical thickness	memory training	no training	OA	8 weeks
Taubert et al. (2010)	DTI, gray matter volume	a complex motor skill learning	-	YA	6 weeks
Schmidt-Wilcke et al. (2010)	gray matter density	a Morse code learning	no training	YA	2.5–8 months
Scholz et al. (2009)	DTI, gray matter	juggling	no training	YA	6 weeks
Driemeyer et al. (2008)	gray matter density	juggling	-	YA	7 days
Boyke et al. (2008)	gray matter density	juggling	-	OA	3 months
Draganski et al. (2006)	gray matter density	studying for medical exam	-	YA (medical students)	3 months
Draganski et al. (2004)	gray matter density	juggling	jugglers vs. non-jugglers	YA	3 months

Notes: DTI: diffusion tensor imaging, YA: young adults, OA: old adults.

higher cognitive functions, such as WM training or attentional training, are likely to show some transfer effects. Most of the demanding tasks usually recruit higher cognitive functions such as executive function, cognitive control, and attentional control (Buschkuehl et al., 2014). For example, WM training is supposed to induce changes in brain activity in frontal and parietal cortex, both of which are associated with WM capacity (Klingberg, 2010), a WM task that demands emotional regulation evoked increased activation in a part of the ACC, which has been shown to be involved in cognitive control and emotional regulation (Schweizer et al., 2013), an attention training program altered a part of the attentional control system in the prefrontal cortex (Mozolic et al., 2010), sensory motor tasks such as a juggling and a videogame modified cortical regions involved in spatial attention (Prakash et al., 2012) or visual areas specific to motion processing (Draganski and May, 2008), and meditation training program changed brain activities associated with attention, mood, and stress regulation (Tang and Posner, 2014). These results suggest that higher cognitive functions can be improved by cognitive training interventions regardless of sensory modality involved, and the changes in brain activations after cognitive training can be captured by a variety of neuroimaging techniques including fMRI, EEG, fNIRS and structural MRI. Although it is difficult to utilize functional or structural MRI for real-time tracking of training-induced changes of the brain due to their costs and portability, some of the neuroimaging techniques such as EEG can be useful for monitoring alterations in brain activity during the course of cognitive training.

EEG Biomarkers for Cognitve Workload

In the previous section, we introduced studies showing functional and structural changes of the brain induced by cognitive training interventions. These studies have shown that human cognitive functions could be improved through cognitive interventions if the brain regions implicated in trained tasks overlap between trained and untrained target tasks. In the cognitive training, subjects are required to repeatedly perform behavioral tasks such as WM tasks or video games. As a result of intense involvements of the brain regions during the course of the training, connections among the regions would be enhanced, leading to improved cognitive performance. To engage the brain regions effectively, individualized adaptive training platforms can be useful tools. Also, the neuroimaging techniques including EEG can capture changes in cognitive performance which could be potentially used as biomarkers for the brain enhancement system and facilitate learners' learning process through tracking learning progress or monitoring mental states.

For example, cognitive overload would induce a reduction of learner's motivation and mental fatigue, both of which hamper the effectiveness of cognitive training interventions. Thus, the cognitive training can be facilitated using passive Brain-Computer Interface (BCI) system, which utilizes biomarkers derived from the brain signal and adapts to the user's performance without the purpose of voluntary control of the system (Zander and Kothe, 2011). Through a real-time monitoring of cognitive workload of learners, the system can flexibly be adjusted to avoid overloading learners' cognitive resources and to keep the learners' engagement and motivation, speeding up the learning progress (Baldwin and Penaranda, 2012). Additionally, individual differences in learners' learning rate can be predicted by EEG biomarker (Mathewson et al., 2012), suggesting that combinations with other cognitive training or neurofeedback training which improve the EEG biomarker could optimize training of targeted cognitive functions. In this section, we will first provide a general introduction of EEG biomarkers, which have been studied mainly for BCI and Neurofeedback, and discuss a potential use of biomarkers for increasing effectiveness of cognitive training interventions. As it is practically difficult to use fMRI or structural MRI to monitor learners' learning process in real-time due to its costs and portability, we will focus on EEG biomarkers here. Then, examples of neurophysiological biomarkers for cognitive workload will be introduced, which can be used for optimizing cognitive workload of a training task to keep learners' concentration and motivation.

EEG Biomarkers: BCI and Neurofeedback

The biomarkers based on EEG have been studied extensively for the BCI, which enables users to control computers or devices through the neurophysiological signals, mainly because of ease of use and low cost (Graimann et al., 2010). Mathematical techniques developed for the BCI system can also be employed for the assistive system of cognitive training interventions. In general, the detection of mental states consists of three stages: pre-processing, feature extraction and selection, and classification. The pre-processing can include artifact removals, spatial filtering, and temporal filtering. After the pre-processing, specific properties of the signal will be extracted over window, useful features will be selected for dimensional reduction, and the selected features will be subjected to classification, which accounts for difference in mental states. Classification enables the system to adapt to individual difference in learners, but the selection of feature space to be extracted is critical for detection of cognitive states, and requires understanding of mechanism behind the cognitive states.

In the BCI systems, various types of EEG signals such as modulations of sensorimotor rhythms (SMR) during motor imagery (Pfurtscheller et al., 1997), event-related potentials (Farwell and Donchin, 1988) or slow cortical potentials (SCPs; Birbaumer et al., 1999) are utilized for discriminating mental states. In any case, it is well known that users often have to be trained to control the BCI system properly, suggesting a need of adjustments to individual difference in signals (Neuper and Pfurtscheller, 2010). In the course of the training for the control of BCI, the user is repeatedly presented with feedbacks indicating performance of the system, and needs to learn voluntarily generating specific patterns of brain signal, which is detectable by the BCI system. Thus, a kind of neurofeedback training for the BCI control is necessary. Actually, the only difference between typical BCI systems and neurofeedback training is how to use biomarkers. For the BCI system, detected mental states would be used for controlling devices and the training would be done through improvements of behavioral performance in the control while the neurofeedback training would be achieved through direct modulations of brain signal.

EEG-neurofeedback has been examined with various types of EEG biomarkers, e.g., up- or down-training of the SMR, the β1 ratio, the θ/α ratio, γ, etc., and improved cognitive functions including sustained attention, orienting, executive functions, spatial rotation, procedural memory, recognition memory have been repeatedly reported through the EEG-neurofeedback training (Gruzelier, 2014). The successful outcomes of the neurofeedback training suggest that the mental state revealed by the EEG biomarkers could provide quantitative metrics for guiding learners to obtain certain mental state suitable for efficient learning or performing specific tasks. In the neurofeedback training, the desired brain state would be achieved through associative learning, in which the association between the desired state and reinforcing feedback stimulus revealing the brain activity is learned (Sulzer et al., 2013). For the adaptive system for effective training, such neurofeedback techniques could be used to optimize learners' mental state to facilitate their learning progress.

Neurophysiological Biomarkers for Cognitive Workload

The assessment of cognitive workload based on neurophysiological biomarkers, particularly EEG biomarker has been of great interest and been extensively studied (Kothe and Makeig, 2011), and the spectral analysis of the EEG waveforms is a powerful tool for the assessment of the mental states during performance of cognitive tasks (Kohlmorgen et al., 2007).

To search for features of EEG signals associated with task demands, an increase of the EEG power-spectrum in the θ bands (4–7 Hz) at frontal sites and a decrease in the α bands (8–12 Hz) over parietal sites have been investigated (Borghini et al., 2014). The increase of frontal θ activity has been observed for high cognitive demand or high mental effort (Berka et al., 2007), and is considered to reflect attentional process to allocate cognitive resources (Gomarus et al., 2006) while the decrease of α power may reflect semantic LTM processing (Klimesch, 1999).

These kinds of neurophysiological biomarkers can be used for on-line monitoring of mental states. Aricò et al. developed a framework for classification of multiple levels of mental workload during a simulated flight based on EEG and ECG signals (Aricò et al., 2014). In this study, subjects performed the Multi Attribute Task Battery (MATB; Comstock and Arnegard, 1992), which includes a variety of simulated tasks involved in a flight scene, over three different difficulty levels (cruise flight phase, flight level maintaining, and emergencies) during recordings of EEG and ECG signals. The classifiers were trained offline for discriminating cognitive workload, and then tested with the other data where difficulty levels were changed dynamically. The stability of the classifier parameters was tested as well. The workload was assessed based on fusion workload index: a combination of EEG and ECG based workload indices. For the EEG-based workload index, the power spectral density (PSD) was evaluated, and the stepwise linear discrimination analysis (SWLDA) was used to select the most relevant spectral features to discriminate workload levels. For the ECG-based workload index, the PSD was estimated for R-peaks extracted from the ECG signal, and the relevant features were selected using the SWLDA. The derived workload indices were subjected to the SWLDA to calculate the best estimation of coefficients of a linear combination of the EEG and ECG-based workload indices for discriminating the workload levels. The authors demonstrated that the proposed system was able to evaluate multiple levels of mental workload, and the classification parameters were stable within a week.

The frontal θ and parietal α power can be changed along with a change of cognitive efforts induced by training of a task. In the study by Borghini et al., subjects trained on the MATB for 5 days while EEG signals were recorded at first (T1), third (T3) and fifth (T5) day of the training (Borghini et al., 2015). The frontal θ power increased from T1 to T3, and then decreased at T5 and the parietal α power showed an opposite pattern while performances of the MATB task continued to improve during the training. This result seems to reflect changes in attentional demands in the course of the training. We may be able to monitor the progress of cognitive training through such biomarkers associated with allocation of attentional resources.

In summary, there exist several evidences showing that neurophysiological biomarkers can discriminate between different levels of cognitive workload. Although further developments would be necessary for applications based on integration of such biomarkers into an adaptive training system, classification of cognitive workload can be a useful measure for assisting cognitive training and increase its effectiveness by controlling the difficulty levels of the training task. Actually, as mentioned above, some studies have shown changes in frontal θ power after WM training (Jaušovec and Jaušovec, 2012) or training that uses a complex video game (Anguera et al., 2013), suggesting that these EEG biomarkers can be useful for tracking the progress of cognitive training.

Brain Connectome Approach

The brain connectome is a useful approach not only for understanding brain cognitive functions, but also for extracting biomarkers that could discriminate between different brain states. By using network metrics to represent a feature space for classification, detection of mental states of learners could be enhanced. In this section, we will introduce the network science and its application to brain networks. Firstly, a general introduction of the network science will be provided. Secondly, prior studies using brain connectome approach will be introduced. Then, we will discuss why the connectome approach is beneficial to the brain enhancement system and how it can boost the learning progress. Finally, we will introduce prior studies showing differences or modifications of the brain connectivity patterns, which suggest potential use of brain connectome approach for the brain enhancement system.

Network Science

It is widely known that brain is a complex network consisting of brain regions dedicated to different kinds of cognitive functions. Furthermore, accumulating evidences support that cognitive functions emerge from the dynamic interactions of distributed brain areas in large-scale networks (Bressler and Menon, 2010). Thus, in order to understand the neural mechanism behind the cognitive training interventions, it would also be important to study alterations in the brain network. The network science, largely based on graph theory, is a useful methodology for investigating an architecture of a complex network and has been employed for studying the brain network (Bullmore and Sporns, 2009; Sporns, 2014). Graph theory is a field of mathematics, aiming at studying topological architecture of networks, and has a long history, dating back to 1736 when a pioneering Swiss mathematician, Leonhard Euler, published the paper on the famous "Seven Bridges of Königsberg" problem. More recently, Watts and Strogatz employed graph theoretical approach to show "small-world" structure of complex networks derived from empirical data (Watts and Strogatz, 1998), leading to the rise of network science as a mathematical tool for studying structure and functions of a wide variety of complex systems from neuroscience, social science, physics, biology, computer science, etc.

In graph theory, networks are represented as "graphs" that consist of objects ("nodes" or "vertices") and connections or relationships between them ("edges"). The topological properties of complex network are quantified by a wide variety of measures, such as small-worldness, modularity, hierarchy, centrality, and the distribution of network hubs (Bullmore and Sporns, 2009). For example, the degree of a node is the number of connections linking to the other nodes, and the probability distribution of the node degree over the whole network is called the degree distribution: a useful measure for investigating a global architecture of a network. Clustering coefficients quantify the degree of mutual connections between the nearest neighbors of a node. High clustering leads to high efficiency of local interactions and robustness. Shortest path length is the minimum number of edges necessary for a node to reach to another. The inverse of the path length can be used to quantify global efficiency of information transfer of the network. Connection density is a proportion of actual connections to the total possible connections. High connection density indicates high physical cost of a network. The centrality of a node represents its importance in communication, and several measures for node centrality has been proposed, such as degree centrality, eigenvector centrality, closeness centrality, betweennes centrality, and so on. For example, the degree centrality is the simplest centrality measure: the degree of a node, while Betweenness centrality is measured by counting the number of paths between the other nodes passing through the node for taking the shortest route. Nodes with high centrality are called hubs, and can be used for assessing robustness of the network by deleting them. Complex networks often consist of a number of modules composed of locally interconnected nodes with few connections to those in different modules. Hubs can have different roles in this complex network architecture. Provincial hubs are connected mainly to nodes inside their own modules while connector hubs have connections with nodes in other modules. Further details about the formulation of these network metrics and their interpretation can be found in recent reviews of this topic (e.g., Rubinov and Sporns, 2010).

Graph theoretical network analysis allows us to quantitatively study topology of networks. A number of studies utilizing graph theoretical measures have revealed that most real world networks including brain network had non-trivial topological features. Watts and Storogatz have shown that a variety of networks have "small-world" properties, based on empirical examples including social network of film actors, power grid, and the neural network of the worm Caenorhabditis elegans (C. elegans) (Watts and Strogatz, 1998). The "small-world" network, by analogy with the small-world phenomenon (popularly known as six degrees in separation), has topological properties somewhere between two extreme cases, i.e., regular and random networks. The small-world network can be characterized by two independent graph theoretical measures introduced above, namely the clustering coefficients and average shortest path length. Regular network is highly clustered, but has a large path length: it is robust, yet inefficient in information transfer. Random network, on the other hand, has a small path length along with a small clustering coefficient, indicating that it is efficient, but is not robust. Small-world network is the intermediate between the regular and the random network, and consists of a number of clusters or modules, interlinking with each other via hubs. Such modular architecture of the small-world network enables global efficiency of information transfer and robustness to perturbations at the same time. It is believed that the small-world architecture is a fundamental principle of a diversity of complex networks, e.g., social, economical, biological, and neurological networks.

Scale-free network, whose degree distribution follows a power law, is also an important concept in the network science (Barabási, 2013). The scale-free property of the network means that some "hub" nodes have a large number of connections while a majority of nodes have only a few connections, which is considered to enable rapid information transfer, minimal wiring costs, and balancing between local and global communications. Such scale-free property has also been found in a variety of networks in the natural world.

Brain Connectome Approach to Large-Scale Human Brain Network

A number of studies have attempted to employ graph theoretical approaches for the brain network analysis (Sporns, 2014). For large-scale human brain networks, the nodes are usually considered to be brain regions or sensors (e.g., voxels for fMRI and electrodes for EEG/magnetoencephalography (MEG)) while the edges can be derived from different, but relevant forms of connectivity, i.e., anatomical connectivity (AC), functional connectivity (FC), or effective connectivity (EC). AC, also called structural connectivity, is the axonal-fibers (white matter) pathways usually acquired by DTI or diffusion spectrum imaging (DSI). FC is defined as temporal dependency between activities of distributed and often spatially distant brain regions without explicit reference to causal effects, normally monitored via fMRI. EC represents causal interactions between brain regions, defined as an influence of one system on another. The causality can be inferred through network perturbations, or the temporal ordering of events. As estimations of EC usually require high temporal resolution, signals from EEG, electrocorticogram (ECoG) or MEG are used. The distinction between FC and EC in neuroimaging studies is important when considering several aspects of functional organization (Friston, 1994). Once the connectivity pattern is provided, regardless of which modality is employed for deriving the network, graph theoretical approaches can be applied for investigating its network architecture. The functional and EC derived from functional data can dynamically change even at rest and do not necessarily match with the AC and should not be interpreted as it is (Honey et al., 2009; Hermundstad et al., 2013).

To obtain connectivity patterns of the large-scale network from brain activity, a variety of techniques have been proposed. For FC, correlation analysis can be used regardless of the modality of signals while several techniques have been proposed for EC, depending on modality of signals. To derive EC from electrophysiological signals such as EEG and ECoG, the Granger causality analysis based on multivariate autoregressive model (MVAR) can be used to determine the directional interaction among electrophysiological signals (Astolfi et al., 2007). The directed transfer function (DTF; Kamiński and Blinowska, 1991) and the partial directed coherence (PDC; Baccalá and Sameshima, 2001) have been used to estimate such causal relationships. To derive EC from fMRI data, Granger Causality Modeling (GCM) and Dynamic Causal Modeling (DCM) have been proposed (Valdes-Sosa et al., 2011). Approximately, GCM is data-driven while DCM is hypothesis-driven. Once connectivity maps are obtained regardless of techniques used for deriving connectivity patterns, graph theoretical approaches can be employed to investigate the network properties.

Graph theoretical network metrics demonstrate topological architecture of the brain network, such as global or local efficiency of information transfer, small-worldness, and a modular structure of the network. Studies employing graph theoretical metrics on human large-scale structural brain network have exhibited robust small-world properties, i.e., high clustering coefficients with relatively small mean path length, for structural brain networks derived from diffusion MRI (Hagmann et al., 2007) as well as those from cortical thickness (He et al., 2007). Similarly, the small-world properties have also been shown for human brain functional networks based on neurophysiological data, such as a task fMRI (Eguíluz et al., 2005; Kinnison et al., 2012; Breckel et al., 2013), resting-state fMRI (Salvador et al., 2005; Achard et al., 2006; Achard and Bullmore, 2007; van den Heuvel et al., 2008), EEG (Micheloyannis et al., 2006, 2009; Stam et al., 2007; Smit et al., 2008; Boersma et al., 2011; Langer et al., 2012; Sun et al., 2014a), and MEG (Stam, 2004; Deuker et al., 2009). Also, the scale-free organization has been reported for the functional network derived from fMRI (Eguíluz et al., 2005; Achard et al., 2006; van den Heuvel et al., 2008) and EEG (Lee et al., 2010). These findings consistent among structural and functional brain network reveal that the small-world and scale-free property are fundamental principles of the brain networks, suggesting that the brain networks have evolved to achieve high efficiency of information transfer between nodes at low connection cost with robustness to perturbations.

Furthermore, several studies have shown that the human brain network has some "hub" regions that work as core regions linking between brain regions (van den Heuvel and Sporns, 2013b). The hub regions were identified for both structural brain networks (He et al., 2007; Hagmann et al., 2008; Iturria-Medina et al., 2008; Gong et al., 2009; van den Heuvel and Sporns, 2011, 2013a; Nijhuis et al., 2013) and functional brain networks (Achard et al., 2006; Cole et al., 2010b; Tomasi and Volkow, 2011a,b; Zuo et al., 2012). The identified hub areas were relatively consistent among the studies regardless of the modality used for obtaining the brain networks, and mostly included parietal and prefrontal regions, such as precuneus, anterior and posterior cingulate gyrus, and the superior frontal gyrus (Bullmore and Sporns, 2009; van den Heuvel and Sporns, 2013b). These hub regions are believed to be responsible for multimodal or integrative function. In fact, the precuneus is a part of the default mode network, and has been suggested to be involved in visuospatial imagery, episodic memory retrieval, self-processing, and consciousness (Cavanna and Trimble, 2006), while the superior frontal gyrus contributes to various cognitive functions, such as WM and attention (Petrides, 2005). The damage to these regions could result in drastic changes of stability and efficiency of the network (Sporns and Zwi, 2004). Such hub regions, in particular the fronto-parietal brain network (FPN), may work as a flexible hub, which implement cognitive control by biasing information flow across sub-networks depending on task demands (Cole et al., 2013).

As revealed by the graph theoretical approach, the brain has a modular architecture with small-world network attributes. Each module, probably corresponding to anatomically or functionally defined brain regions, has dense connections within the module for local processing of information, and is implicated in a particular function, exhibiting functional segregation of local areas. On the other hand, the modules are interconnected with each other through short- or long-range connections through hubs, implying functional integration of globally distributed brain areas. In fact, human brain structural network derived from co-variation of regional gray matter volumes measured using MRI and DSI exhibited hierarchical modular architecture with 2–3 levels (Bassett et al., 2010). It is likely that such hierarchical small-world network architecture enables the coexistence of functional segregation and functional integration within a single brain network. Also, these findings are consistent with those for the resting-state FC, which have shown the existence of a number of sub-networks consisting of functionally linked brain regions (Cole et al., 2010a). Therefore, the brain has an inhomogeneous architecture, and each brain region has different functions with different degree of importance. As such, brain regions dedicated to the relevant cognitive functions are engaged depending on cognitive demands, and work together as a network to communicate and influence one-another to produce coherent experiences and behavior. Such sub-networks could be divided into "intrinsic" and "evoked" functional network architecture, where the intrinsic network serves as a standard state of the brain and relatively small changes of the task-evoked networks support task-specific demands (Cole et al., 2014).

In summary, functional and structural connectivity patterns of the human large-scale brain network can be obtained by means of a variety of neuroimaging and mathematical techniques. A number of studies have been conducted to investigate the topological architecture of the brain network using graph theoretical network metrics, and have shown that the human brain network had small-world network characteristics, scale-free organization, and a modular structure, suggesting applicability of network analysis for elucidating neural underpinnings of human cognitive functions.

For the brain enhancement through cognitive training, elucidation of the brain network architecture is of great importance for several reasons. Firstly, cognitive training can affect sub-network consisting of spatially distributed, but functionally relevant brain regions even when improvement of activation in a single brain region is targeted. Secondly, a degree of impact of cognitive intervention can differ among brain regions, depending on its topological property of the brain network. To be specific, hub regions that link with other sub-network can have greater influence compared to other brain areas. Thirdly, the graph theoretical network metrics can simply be additional biomarkers for monitoring mental states of learners during the training, enabling the adaptive learning system depending on the learner's mental state to facilitate the learning progress. Finally, although reduced activation in brain regions responsible for attentional control and mental efforts has been observed after the cognitive training and is considered to indicate relative automaticity of behavior induced by the training (Prakash et al., 2012), it cannot be accounted for in terms of the improved "efficiency" of neural function (Poldrack, 2015). The connectome approach can provide another perspective for the effects of the cognitive training in terms of changes in cost of information transfer within the network. Additionally, FC strength was spatially correlated with regional cerebral blood flow (rCBF), particularly in the default mode network and executive control network, and the coupling between blood supply and FC in the lateral-parietal lobe was modulated with task demands (Liang et al., 2013), suggesting that FC analysis would provide effective tools for measuring changes of energy consumption induced by cognitive training interventions. Therefore, it is getting more important to consider about modulations of the brain network architecture induced by the cognitive training in order to develop the assistance system for the cognitive training.

We have introduced graph theory as a tool for investigating the topological architecture of complex networks, and its applications to the human large-scale brain network. In the studies introduced above, the graph theoretical network metrics have been used to show prevailing attributes of the brain network, such as small-world architecture, scale-free organization, or hub brain regions. In the next section, we will discuss its applicability for demonstrating difference in the brain functional network architecture, which could discriminate cognitive states.

Difference in the Brain Functional Network

The FC patterns of the brain network can be different depending on cognitive states or states of mind, suggesting that functional brain network can be used as biomarkers for detecting mental states. For example, the functional interaction between cell assemblies revealed by the human EEG coherence, which is the correlation coefficient in the frequency domain, was higher during memory encoding phase for subsequently recalled words compared to forgotten words (Weiss and Rappelsberger, 2000). In one study, Astolfi et al. showed different cortical connectivity pattern during observations of TV commercials between subsequently remembered and forgotten ones (Astolfi et al., 2008). They also demonstrated that the parietal areas received a larger amount of the incoming flow of information during the observation of TV commercials that were remembered than that of forgotten ones. Even more precise differences in cognitive states can be predicted by connectivity patterns of the brain network. Through calculating

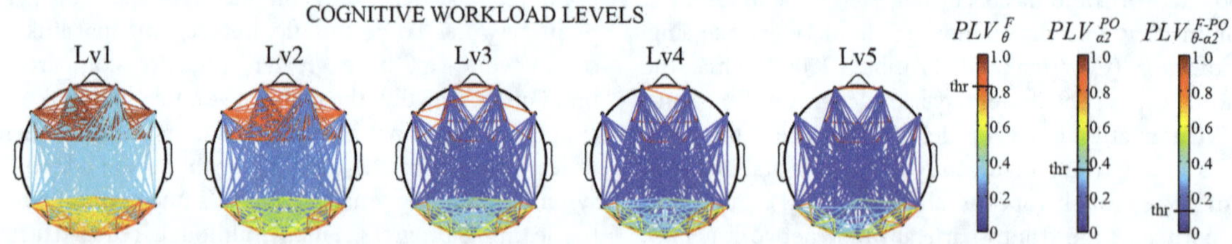

FIGURE 2 | Cross-frequency causal interactions revealed by Phase Locking Values (PLV) for multiple cognitive workload levels during a mental arithmetic task. Three different thresholds have been applied to each type of coupling (F/θ, POα2, CFC) (Adapted from Dimitriadis et al., 2014). a permission will be obtained from the publisher after acceptance, the image will be replaced with high-resolution version.

the cross-frequency causal interactions (Canolty and Knight, 2010) between frontal and parieto-occipital sites, Dimitriadis et al. estimated effective networks derived from EEG signals during a mental arithmetic task with different cognitive workload levels (Dimitriadis et al., 2014). The tensor subspace analysis (TSA) based learning was then used to extract features that can discriminate different cognitive workload levels based on FC patterns. These features achieved a remarkable high correct-recognition-rate (96%) for classification of the task difficulties, suggesting that the FC patterns based on cross-frequency couplings between subregions can become powerful biomarkers for measuring cognitive workload levels (**Figure 2**). Also, multivariate pattern analysis (MVPA) on EEG FC patterns demonstrated successful classification of mental fatigue states from vigilant state at an accuracy of 81.5% (Sun et al., 2014b). These results have suggested that a combination of FC patterns and advanced mathematical tools could provide powerful biomarkers of cognitive states.

In addition to the FC pattern itself, differences in the topological architecture of the brain functional network can be quantified in terms of graph theoretical network metrics. Kitzbichler et al. have found that the brain functional network derived from human MEG data became more globally efficient, less clustered, and less modular network configuration as cognitive efforts got greater during a WM task (Kitzbichler et al., 2011). Furthermore, Sun et al. employed the graph theoretical metrics on FC patterns derived from lower α band (8–10 Hz) of EEG data to investigate small-world network properties due to a decline in vigilance caused by performing an attention demanding task (Psychomotor Vigilance Test; PVT; Sun et al., 2014a). They found a decrease in efficiency of global information transfer revealed by increased weighted characteristic path length, and an asymmetrical pattern of connectivity (right > left) in fronto-parietal regions due to mental fatigue (**Figure 3**). Such difference in graph theoretical network metrics was found between rest and a task performance for the functional network derived from MEG (Bassett et al., 2006) and fMRI (Cao et al., 2014; Taya et al., 2014). Also, the graph theoretical metrics on fMRI functional network could discriminate between resting-state and sensory stimulation (Moussa et al., 2011), different cognitive load during a WM task (Ginestet and Simmons, 2011), different cognitive states in an emotional and a motivational task (Kinnison et al., 2012), and between an intentional and an incidental learning of words during neuropsychological tests (Kuhnert et al., 2013). The small-worldness of EEG functional network was different between during rest and mathematical thinking (Micheloyannis et al., 2009) and some network metrics of a combined EEG and MEG functional network was different between low- and high-memory load during a visual WM retention period (Palva et al., 2010). Furthermore, graph theoretical network metrics or network modularity of fMRI functional network were different depending on sleep levels or conscious levels (Ferri et al., 2007; Spoormaker et al., 2010; Tagliazucchi et al., 2013; Uehara et al., 2014).

The graph theoretical network metrics can be effective in discriminating individual differences in mental or cognitive abilities as well. Van den Heuvel et al. have demonstrated a strong negative association between the normalized characteristic path length of the intrinsic brain network derived from resting-state fMRI data and intelligence quotient (IQ), suggesting that human intellectual performance is related to how efficiently the brain integrates information between brain regions (van den Heuvel et al., 2009). Moreover Langer et al. have shown that clustering coefficient and path length of the functional network derived from resting EEG were strongly related to general intelligence evaluated by Ravens advanced progressive matrices: higher small-worldness for higher general intelligence (Langer et al., 2012). Although the network metrics can also be useful biomarkers for diagnosis of mental disorders (Bassett and Bullmore, 2009), we will not discuss about this case here.

In summary, the brain functional network can show different connectivity patterns depending on cognitive states such as cognitive workloads or sleep stages, and such difference can be extracted and be classified using advanced mathematical techniques. Furthermore, the graph theoretical metrics that quantify topological architecture of complex networks can also discriminate between cognitive states and individual differences in intelligence. These results have suggested that graph theoretical network metrics on functional network can be useful biomarkers for monitoring and optimizing cognitive states of learners during cognitive training.

Modulations of the Brain Network Induced by Cognitive Training Interventions

We have introduced a number of examples showing that the brain FC patterns could be different depending on cognitive

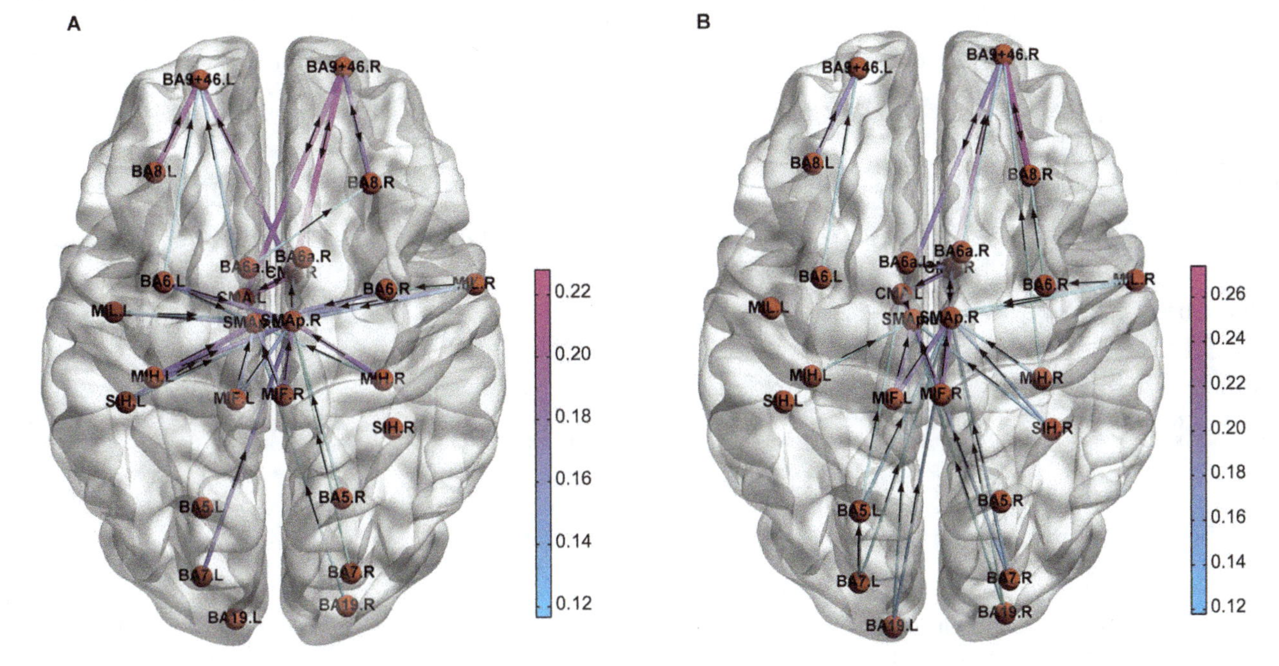

FIGURE 3 | Functional connectivity patterns in the low alpha (8–10 Hz) frequency band obtained for (A) 1st and (B) 4th quartile during the PVT task performance. The cortical connections are weaker at left prefrontal cortex compared to right one in the 4th quartile (Adapted from Sun et al., 2014a).

states or even individual cognitive abilities. For assisting the cognitive training, it is important to know whether the brain functional network could be changed through cognitive interventions. Although only one study has directly examined the effect of cognitive training interventions on topological architecture of the brain functional network so far (Langer et al., 2013), a number of studies have examined the effect of cognitive interventions on the brain network in different time scales, and found the modulation of the brain network induced by prior experiences including the cognitive training, as introduced below.

There are a number of studies showing modifications of the brain FC induced by cognitive or perceptual task performance. Albert et al. (2009) have shown that a motor learning could modulate subsequent neural activity during rest and the changes in resting activity were not limited to immediately after the learning, but persisted after 4 min of unrelated task. Stevens et al. (2010) have examined the effects of preceding exposure of visual stimuli from distinct categories (i.e., faces or scenes) on FC between frontal networks and category-preferential visual regions during rest. They found that increased couplings between a frontal brain region (rIFG) and category-preferential visual regions after each task, and subsequent memory performance was predicted by the degree of modulation of the couplings. These findings have indicated that resting-state FC could be modulated by perceptual or cognitive tasks at least in a short-term (minutes).

Such modulations of resting-state connectivity induced by prior experience can last for longer duration (days or weeks). Lewis et al. (2009) have investigated the effects of intense training (2–9 days) on a visual perceptual task on resting-state FC, and found that the FC between trained visual cortex and dorsal attention regions became more negatively correlated while that between untrained visual cortex and several default regions became less negatively correlated after learning. Changes of resting-state FC were found for WM training as well. Six weeks of a verbal WM training induced modifications in resting-state FC and the change of frontoparietal connectivity was positively related to performance improvement while that of default network connectivity was negatively correlated (Jolles et al., 2013). Also, 27 days of the WM training program increased FC between mPFC and precuneus and that between mPFC and right posterior parietal cortex and right lPFC (Takeuchi et al., 2013). Even some weeks of training of video games changed FC during game playing (Voss et al., 2012) and rest (Strenziok et al., 2014).

The changes in brain network induced by cognitive training interventions can be observed in structural connectivity as well. Takeuchi et al. have demonstrated that 2 months of WM training increased FA in the white matter regions, possibly attributable to increased myelination after training (Takeuchi et al., 2010). Additionally, Wolf et al. investigated the transfer capability of general fluid intelligence related cognitive training in elderly subjects (Wolf et al., 2014). They examined structural integrity measured by DTI immediately after a 4-week training and a 3-month follow-up period. Although only 22% of subjects showed successful long-term transfer effects, transfer of training gains was associated with a higher degree of structural integrity.

In addition to the individual connectivity between brain regions, the graph theoretical approaches can be employed to

TABLE 3 | Neuroimaging studies showing changes in brain FC induced by cognitive interventions.

Study	Modality	Training task	Control group	Population	Training period
Strenziok et al. (2014)	fMRI, DTI	Rise of Nations, Brain Fitness, Space Fortress	-	OA	6 weeks
Jolles et al. (2013)	fMRI	a verbal WM task	-	YA and CH	6 weeks
Takeuchi et al. (2013)	fMRI, ASL	WMT program	no training	YA	27 days
Langer et al. (2013)	EEG	Tatool (adaptive WM training)	tasks with low WM demand	YA	4 weeks
Heitger et al. (2012)	fMRI	a motor learning task	-	YA	4 days
Voss et al. (2012)	fMRI	Space Fortress	-	YA	20 h
Bassett et al. (2011)	fMRI	a motor learning task	-	YA (musical instruments)	5 days
Stevens et al. (2010)	fMRI	visual semantic classification tasks	-	YA	15 min
Albert et al. (2009)	fMRI	a motor learning task	a motor performance task	YA	11 min
Lewis et al. (2009)	fMRI	a shape-identification task	-	YA	2–9 days

YA: young adults, OA: old adults, CH: children.

examine changes in global characteristics of the brain network. Bassett et al. investigated reconfiguration of modular structure of the FC induced by 3 days of a motor learning task (Bassett et al., 2011). They found that some of the brain regions showed consistent community allegiance (low-flexibility nodes) while other regions constantly shift allegiance (high-flexibility nodes). Additionally, the network flexibility first increased and then decreased during the learning process. The authors have also examined changes of modular structure over thirty-day of a motor skill training, and demonstrated that the separation between core and periphery nodes decreased over the course of training, and good learners tend to have greater separation than poor learners (Bassett et al., 2013). Even 4 days of learning of complex hand coordination pattern induced changes in topological architecture of the fMRI functional network (Heitger et al., 2012). Additionally, Breckel et al. have demonstrated prolonged changes in the global architecture of the resting-state brain network during a series of task performance (Breckel et al., 2013). They compared topological properties of the functional brain network derived from fMRI data before a sustained attentional task performance and those after the task, and showed that the post-task functional network had more clustering, less global efficiency, and less long-distance connections, suggesting a reduction in network integration due to the task performance. These changes in network architecture were still observed after 6 min of resting state. Interestingly, such changes in information transfer efficiency of the brain functional network were induced by a cognitive training intervention (Langer et al., 2013). Langer et al. investigated effects of intensive WM training on the EEG functional network. They first confirmed that WM performance was correlated with power in the θ frequency band, and the WM training increased the θ power. Then, they found the global efficiency of the functional network in the θ band was correlated with higher WM performance before training, and WM training induced increase of small-world topology revealed by an increase of the clustering coefficient and a decrease of the path length in the majority of the subjects.

Taken together, prior sensory or cognitive experience and cognitive training interventions can have even prolonged effects on the brain structural and FC. In addition, motor training and WM training induced changes in topological architecture of the brain network. Although only one study has directly examined the effect of cognitive training interventions using brain connectome approach so far (Langer et al., 2013), alterations in the brain connectivity patterns can also be captured by graph theoretical network metrics such as clustering coefficients or path length. Such changes in topological architecture and information transfer efficiency of the brain functional network can be attributed to improvements in cognitive processing related to the trained tasks, enhancements of general intelligence, changes in attentional levels, difference in cognitive workload, or reconfiguration of brain sub-networks involved. These results have suggested that the network metrics can be useful biomarkers, not only for monitoring cognitive states, but also for tracking effects of the cognitive training interventions. A summary for existing studies showing changes in functional brain connectivity induced by cognitive training interventions is given in **Table 3**.

Conclusion

In this review article, we proposed that biomarkers based on brain connectome approach could be useful for a brain enhancement system by optimizing effectiveness of cognitive training interventions on learners' learning process. For this purpose, we first introduced studies on cognitive training interventions. A number of studies have shown that the brain cognitive functions could be improved through cognitive training interventions such as WM training or video game training, and brain activities were modulated as a result of the training (Klingberg, 2010). Although such cognitive interventions are effective, their effectiveness can be different among individuals and they may even vary depending on mental state at the moment of the training. If the task that the learner is performing is too difficult or too demanding, it would be difficult for them to keep the motivation and concentration on the facing task and some of them can be exhausted from the excess of cognitive workload, resulting in a poor or a lack of improvement in cognitive functions. An adaptive assistance system for cognitive training through monitoring the learners' mental states such as cognitive workload using objective biomarkers is a useful approach to facilitation and optimization of the learning progress. As introduced above, a number of biomarkers have been proposed for monitoring mental states including cognitive workloads. Most of the biomarkers are based on spectral properties of EEG signals or ERPs, and the extracted features are often subjected to cutting-edge mathematical tools based on machine learning theory to discriminate mental states (Kothe and Makeig, 2011). Additionally, some biomarkers can be used to predict individuals' intelligence or learners' subsequent learning rate (Langer et al., 2012). If optimal mental states for ongoing training can be replicated in the brain through the adjustment of the cognitive workload, neurofeedback, or other cognitive training scheme, we could optimize the effectiveness of the training process.

Furthermore, we have introduced the functional connectome approach, which is mainly based on the graph theory (Sporns, 2014). The brain is a complex network consisting of spatially distributed regions dedicated to different functions, and it is proposed that cognitive functions emerge from dynamic interactions of several brain areas, not a result of an activation of a single brain region (Bressler and Menon, 2010). As such, the number of publications regarding brain network is drastically increasing (Friston, 2011). We have proposed here that the brain connectome can be a useful approach not only for elucidating mechanisms underlying brain cognitive functions, but also for detection of mental states. The graph theoretical network metrics can be biomarkers of cognitive states, as shown in previous studies on cognitive workload (Ginestet and Simmons, 2011; Kitzbichler et al., 2011) or mental fatigue (Breckel et al., 2013; Sun et al., 2014a). Several studies have shown that the brain functional and structural network connectivity can be altered through cognitive interventions, and the graph theoretical network metrics have shown the reorganization of topological architecture of the brain functional network over multiple temporal scales (i.e., minutes, days, weeks). These results suggest that the functional connectome approach as well as conventional biomarkers would be effective methods for boosting learning progress of learners during the course of cognitive training.

Acknowledgments

The authors appreciate the National University of Singapore for supporting the Cognitive Engineering Group at the Singapore Institute for Neurotechnology (SINAPSE) under WBS Number R-719-001-102-232 and Ministry of Education of Singapore for funding support under the grant number MOE2014-T2-1-115.

References

Achard, S., and Bullmore, E. (2007). Efficiency and cost of economical brain functional networks. *PLoS Comput. Biol.* 3:e17. doi: 10.1371/journal.pcbi.0030017

Achard, S., Salvador, R., Whitcher, B., Suckling, J., and Bullmore, E. (2006). A resilient, low-frequency, small-world human brain functional network with highly connected association cortical hubs. *J. Neurosci.* 26, 63–72. doi: 10.1523/jneurosci.3874-05.2006

Albert, N. B., Robertson, E. M., and Miall, R. C. (2009). The resting human brain and motor learning. *Curr. Biol.* 19, 1023–1027. doi: 10.1016/j.cub.2009.04.028

Anguera, J. A., Boccanfuso, J., Rintoul, J. L., Al-Hashimi, O., Faraji, F., Janowich, J., et al. (2013). Video game training enhances cognitive control in older adults. *Nature* 501, 97–101. doi: 10.1038/nature12486

Aricò, P., Borghini, G., Graziani, I., Taya, F., Sun, Y., Bezerianos, A., et al. (2014). Towards a multimodal bioelectrical framework for the online mental workload evaluation. *Conf. Proc. IEEE Eng. Med. Biol. Soc.* 2014, 3001–3004. doi: 10.1109/EMBC.2014.6944254

Astolfi, L., Cincotti, F., Mattia, D., Marciani, M. G., Baccala, L. A., de Vico Fallani, F., et al. (2007). Comparison of different cortical connectivity estimators for high-resolution EEG recordings. *Hum. Brain Mapp.* 28, 143–157. doi: 10.1002/hbm.20263

Astolfi, L., De Vico Fallani, F., Cincotti, F., Mattia, D., Bianchi, L., Marciani, M. G., et al. (2008). Neural basis for brain responses to TV commercials: a high-resolution EEG study. *IEEE Trans. Neural Syst. Rehabil. Eng.* 16, 522–531. doi: 10.1109/TNSRE.2008.2009784

Baccalá, L. A., and Sameshima, K. (2001). Partial directed coherence: a new concept in neural structure determination. *Biol. Cybern.* 84, 463–474. doi: 10.1007/pl00007990

Baldwin, C. L., and Penaranda, B. N. (2012). Adaptive training using an artificial neural network and EEG metrics for within- and cross-task workload classification. *Neuroimage* 59, 48–56. doi: 10.1016/j.neuroimage.2011.07.047

Barabási, A. L. (2013). Network science. *Philos. Trans. A Math. Phys. Eng. Sci.* 371:20120375. doi: 10.1098/rsta.2012.0375

Bassett, D. S., and Bullmore, E. T. (2009). Human brain networks in health and disease. *Curr. Opin. Neurol.* 22, 340–347. doi: 10.1097/WCO.0b013e32832d93dd

Bassett, D. S., Greenfield, D. L., Meyer-Lindenberg, A., Weinberger, D. R., Moore, S. W., and Bullmore, E. T. (2010). Efficient physical embedding of topologically complex information processing networks in brains and computer circuits. *PLoS Comput. Biol.* 6:e1000748. doi: 10.1371/journal.pcbi.1000748

Bassett, D. S., Meyer-Lindenberg, A., Achard, S., Duke, T., and Bullmore, E. (2006). Adaptive reconfiguration of fractal small-world human brain functional networks. *Proc. Natl. Acad. Sci. U S A* 103, 19518–19523. doi: 10.1073/pnas.0606005103

Bassett, D. S., Wymbs, N. F., Porter, M. A., Mucha, P. J., Carlson, J. M., and Grafton, S. T. (2011). Dynamic reconfiguration of human brain networks during learning. *Proc. Natl. Acad. Sci. U S A* 108, 7641–7646. doi: 10.1073/pnas.1018985108

Bassett, D. S., Wymbs, N. F., Rombach, M. P., Porter, M. A., Mucha, P. J., and Grafton, S. T. (2013). Task-based core-periphery organization of human brain dynamics. *PLoS Comput. Biol.* 9:e1003171. doi: 10.1371/journal.pcbi.1003171

Berka, C., Levendowski, D. J., Lumicao, M. N., Yau, A., Davis, G., Zivkovic, V. T., et al. (2007). EEG correlates of task engagement and mental workload in vigilance, learning and memory tasks. *Aviat. Space Environ. Med.* 78, B231–B244.

Birbaumer, N., Ghanayim, N., Hinterberger, T., Iversen, I., Kotchoubey, B., Kübler, A., et al. (1999). A spelling device for the paralysed. *Nature* 398, 297–298. doi: 10.1038/18581

Boersma, M., Smit, D. J. A., de Bie, H. M. A., Van Baal, G. C. M., Boomsma, D. I., de Geus, E. J. C., et al. (2011). Network analysis of resting state EEG in the developing young brain: structure comes with maturation. *Hum. Brain Mapp.* 32, 413–425. doi: 10.1002/hbm.21030

Borghini, G., Aricò, P., Graziani, I., Salinari, S., Sun, Y., Taya, F., et al. (2015). Quantitative assessment of the training improvement in a motor-cognitive task by using EEG, ECG and EOG signals. *Brain Topogr.* doi: 10.1007/s10548-015-0425-7. [Epub ahead of print].

Borghini, G., Astolfi, L., Vecchiato, G., Mattia, D., and Babiloni, F. (2014). Measuring neurophysiological signals in aircraft pilots and car drivers for the assessment of mental workload, fatigue and drowsiness. *Neurosci. Biobehav. Rev.* 44, 58–75. doi: 10.1016/j.neubiorev.2012.10.003

Boyke, J., Driemeyer, J., Gaser, C., Büchel, C., and May, A. (2008). Training-induced brain structure changes in the elderly. *J. Neurosci.* 28, 7031–7035. doi: 10.1523/JNEUROSCI.0742-08.2008

Breckel, T. P. K., Thiel, C. M., Bullmore, E. T., Zalesky, A., Patel, A. X., and Giessing, C. (2013). Long-term effects of attentional performance on functional brain network topology. *PLoS One* 8:e74125. doi: 10.1371/journal.pone.0074125

Bressler, S. L., and Menon, V. (2010). Large-scale brain networks in cognition: emerging methods and principles. *Trends Cogn. Sci.* 14, 277–290. doi: 10.1016/j.tics.2010.04.004

Bullmore, E., and Sporns, O. (2009). Complex brain networks: graph theoretical analysis of structural and functional systems. *Nat. Rev. Neurosci.* 10, 186–198. doi: 10.1038/nrn2575

Buschkuehl, M., Hernandez-Garcia, L., Jaeggi, S. M., Bernard, J. A., and Jonides, J. (2014). Neural effects of short-term training on working memory. *Cogn. Affect. Behav. Neurosci.* 14, 147–160. doi: 10.3758/s13415-013-0244-9

Cannonieri, G. C., Bonilha, L., Fernandes, P. T., Cendes, F., and Li, L. M. (2007). Practice and perfect: length of training and structural brain changes in experienced typists. *Neuroreport* 18, 1063–1066. doi: 10.1097/wnr.0b013e3281a030e5

Canolty, R. T., and Knight, R. T. (2010). The functional role of cross-frequency coupling. *Trends Cogn. Sci.* 14, 506–515. doi: 10.1016/j.tics.2010.09.001

Cao, H., Plichta, M. M., Schäfer, A., Haddad, L., Grimm, O., Schneider, M., et al. (2014). Test-retest reliability of fMRI-based graph theoretical properties during working memory, emotion processing and resting state. *Neuroimage* 84, 888–900. doi: 10.1016/j.neuroimage.2013.09.013

Cavanna, A. E., and Trimble, M. R. (2006). The precuneus: a review of its functional anatomy and behavioural correlates. *Brain* 129, 564–583. doi: 10.1093/brain/awl004

Chein, J. M., and Morrison, A. B. (2010). Expanding the mind's workspace: training and transfer effects with a complex working memory span task. *Psychon. Bull. Rev.* 17, 193–199. doi: 10.3758/PBR.17.2.193

Chein, J. M., and Schneider, W. (2005). Neuroimaging studies of practice-related change: fMRI and meta-analytic evidence of a domain-general control network for learning. *Brain Res. Cogn. Brain Res.* 25, 607–623. doi: 10.1016/j.cogbrainres.2005.08.013

Clark, V. P., and Parasuraman, R. (2014). Neuroenhancement: enhancing brain and mind in health and in disease. *Neuroimage* 85(Pt. 3), 889–894. doi: 10.1016/j.neuroimage.2013.08.071

Cole, M. W., Bassett, D. S., Power, J. D., Braver, T. S., and Petersen, S. E. (2014). Intrinsic and task-evoked network architectures of the human brain. *Neuron* 83, 238–251. doi: 10.1016/j.neuron.2014.05.014

Cole, M. W., Pathak, S., and Schneider, W. (2010b). Identifying the brain's most globally connected regions. *Neuroimage* 49, 3132–3148. doi: 10.1016/j.neuroimage.2009.11.001

Cole, M. W., Reynolds, J. R., Power, J. D., Repovs, G., Anticevic, A., and Braver, T. S. (2013). Multi-task connectivity reveals flexible hubs for adaptive task control. *Nat. Neurosci.* 16, 1348–1355. doi: 10.1038/nn.3470

Cole, D. M., Smith, S. M., and Beckmann, C. F. (2010a). Advances and pitfalls in the analysis and interpretation of resting-state FMRI data. *Front. Syst. Neurosci.* 4:8. doi: 10.3389/fnsys.2010.00008

Colom, R., Quiroga, M. Á., Shih, P. C., Martínez, K., Burgaleta, M., Martínez-Molina, A., et al. (2010). Improvement in working memory is not related to increased intelligence scores. *Intelligence* 38, 497–505. doi: 10.1016/j.intell.2010.06.008

Colom, R., Román, F. J., Abad, F. J., Shih, P. C., Privado, J., Froufe, M., et al. (2013). Adaptive n-back training does not improve fluid intelligence at the construct level: gains on individual tests suggest that training may enhance visuospatial processing. *Intelligence* 41, 712–727. doi: 10.1016/j.intell.2013.09.002

Comstock, J. R., and Arnegard, R. J. (1992). *The Multi-Attribute Task Battery for Human Operator Workload and Strategic Behavior Research.* Hampton, VA: National Aeronautics and Space Administration, Langley Research Center.

Conway, A. R., Kane, M. J., and Engle, R. W. (2003). Working memory capacity and its relation to general intelligence. *Trends Cogn. Sci.* 7, 547–552. doi: 10.1016/j.tics.2003.10.005

Dahlin, E., Neely, A. S., Larsson, A., Bäckman, L., and Nyberg, L. (2008). Transfer of learning after updating training mediated by the striatum. *Science* 320, 1510–1512. doi: 10.1126/science.1155466

Deary, I. J., Strand, S., Smith, P., and Fernandes, C. (2007). Intelligence and educational achievement. *Intelligence* 35, 13–21. doi: 10.1016/j.intell.2006.02.001

Deuker, L., Bullmore, E. T., Smith, M., Christensen, S., Nathan, P. J., Rockstroh, B., et al. (2009). Reproducibility of graph metrics of human brain functional networks. *Neuroimage* 47, 1460–1468. doi: 10.1016/j.neuroimage.2009.05.035

Dimitriadis, S. I., Sun, Y., Kwok, K., Laskaris, N. A., Thakor, N., and Bezerianos, A. (2014). Cognitive workload assessment based on the tensorial treatment of EEG estimates of cross-frequency phase interactions. *Ann. Biomed. Eng.* doi: 10.1007/s10439-014-1143-0. [Epub ahead of print].

Draganski, B., Gaser, C., Busch, V., Schuierer, G., Bogdahn, U., and May, A. (2004). Neuroplasticity: changes in grey matter induced by training. *Nature* 427, 311–312. doi: 10.1038/427311a

Draganski, B., Gaser, C., Kempermann, G., Kuhn, H. G., Winkler, J., Büchel, C., et al. (2006). Temporal and spatial dynamics of brain structure changes during extensive learning. *J. Neurosci.* 26, 6314–6317. doi: 10.1523/jneurosci.4628-05.2006

Draganski, B., and May, A. (2008). Training-induced structural changes in the adult human brain. *Behav. Brain Res.* 192, 137–142. doi: 10.1016/j.bbr.2008.02.015

Driemeyer, J., Boyke, J., Gaser, C., Büchel, C., and May, A. (2008). Changes in gray matter induced by learning–revisited. *PLoS One* 3:e2669. doi: 10.1371/journal.pone.0002669

Dux, P. E., Tombu, M. N., Harrison, S., Rogers, B. P., Tong, F., and Marois, R. (2009). Training improves multitasking performance by increasing the speed of information processing in human prefrontal cortex. *Neuron* 63, 127–138. doi: 10.1016/j.neuron.2009.06.005

Eguíluz, V. M., Chialvo, D. R., Cecchi, G. A., Baliki, M., and Apkarian, A. V. (2005). Scale-free brain functional networks. *Phys. Rev. Lett.* 94:018102. doi: 10.1103/physrevlett.94.018102

Elbert, T., Pantev, C., Wienbruch, C., Rockstroh, B., and Taub, E. (1995). Increased cortical representation of the fingers of the left hand in string players. *Science* 270, 305–307. doi: 10.1126/science.270.5234.305

Engvig, A., Fjell, A. M., Westlye, L. T., Moberget, T., Sundseth, Ø., Larsen, V. A., et al. (2010). Effects of memory training on cortical thickness in the elderly. *Neuroimage* 52, 1667–1676. doi: 10.1016/j.neuroimage.2010.05.041

Erickson, K. I., Colcombe, S. J., Wadhwa, R., Bherer, L., Peterson, M. S., Scalf, P. E., et al. (2007). Training-induced functional activation changes in dual-task processing: an FMRI study. *Cereb. Cortex* 17, 192–204. doi: 10.1093/cercor/bhj137

Farah, M. J., Illes, J., Cook-Deegan, R., Gardner, H., Kandel, E., King, P., et al. (2004). Neurocognitive enhancement: what can we do and what should we do? *Nat. Rev. Neurosci.* 5, 421–425. doi: 10.1038/nrn1390

Farwell, L. A., and Donchin, E. (1988). Talking off the top of your head: toward a mental prosthesis utilizing event-related brain potentials. *Electroencephalogr. Clin. Neurophysiol.* 70, 510–523. doi: 10.1016/0013-4694(88)90149-6

Ferri, R., Rundo, F., Bruni, O., Terzano, M. G., and Stam, C. J. (2007). Small-world network organization of functional connectivity of EEG slow-wave activity during sleep. *Clin. Neurophysiol.* 118, 449–456. doi: 10.1016/j.clinph.2006.10.021

Fleischman, D. A., Wilson, R. S., Gabrieli, J. D., Bienias, J. L., and Bennett, D. A. (2004). A longitudinal study of implicit and explicit memory in old persons. *Psychol. Aging* 19, 617–625. doi: 10.1037/0882-7974.19.4.617

Friston, K. J. (1994). Functional and effective connectivity in neuroimaging: a synthesis. *Hum. Brain Mapp.* 2, 56–78. doi: 10.1002/hbm.460020107

Friston, K. J. (2011). Functional and effective connectivity: a review. *Brain Connect.* 1, 13–36. doi: 10.1089/brain.2011.0008

Ginestet, C. E., and Simmons, A. (2011). Statistical parametric network analysis of functional connectivity dynamics during a working memory task. *Neuroimage* 55, 688–704. doi: 10.1016/j.neuroimage.2010.11.030

Gomarus, H. K., Althaus, M., Wijers, A. A., and Minderaa, R. B. (2006). The effects of memory load and stimulus relevance on the EEG during a visual selective memory search task: an ERP and ERD/ERS study. *Clin. Neurophysiol.* 117, 871–884. doi: 10.1016/j.clinph.2005.12.008

Gong, G., He, Y., Concha, L., Lebel, C., Gross, D. W., Evans, A. C., et al. (2009). Mapping anatomical connectivity patterns of human cerebral cortex using *in vivo* diffusion tensor imaging tractography. *Cereb. Cortex* 19, 524–536. doi: 10.1093/cercor/bhn102

Graimann, B., Pfurtscheller, G., and Allison, B. Z. (2010). *Brain-Computer Interfaces: Revolutionizing Human-Computer Interaction.* Heidelberg, Berlin: Springer.

Green, C. S., and Bavelier, D. (2003). Action video game modifies visual selective attention. *Nature* 423, 534–537. doi: 10.1038/nature01647

Gruzelier, J. H. (2014). EEG-neurofeedback for optimising performance. I: a review of cognitive and affective outcome in healthy participants. *Neurosci. Biobehav. Rev.* 44, 124–141. doi: 10.1016/j.neubiorev.2013.09.015

Gutchess, A. (2014). Plasticity of the aging brain: new directions in cognitive neuroscience. *Science* 346, 579–582. doi: 10.1126/science.1254604

Hagmann, P., Cammoun, L., Gigandet, X., Meuli, R., Honey, C. J., Wedeen, V. J., et al. (2008). Mapping the structural core of human cerebral cortex. *PLoS Biol.* 6:e159. doi: 10.1371/journal.pbio.0060159

Hagmann, P., Kurant, M., Gigandet, X., Thiran, P., Wedeen, V. J., Meuli, R., et al. (2007). Mapping human whole-brain structural networks with diffusion MRI. *PLoS One* 2:e597. doi: 10.1371/journal.pone.0000597

Halford, G. S., Cowan, N., and Andrews, G. (2007). Separating cognitive capacity from knowledge: a new hypothesis. *Trends Cogn. Sci.* 11, 236–242. doi: 10.1016/j.tics.2007.04.001

Hamilton, R., Messing, S., and Chatterjee, A. (2011). Rethinking the thinking cap: ethics of neural enhancement using noninvasive brain stimulation. *Neurology* 76, 187–193. doi: 10.1212/WNL.0b013e318205d50d

He, Y., Chen, Z. J., and Evans, A. C. (2007). Small-world anatomical networks in the human brain revealed by cortical thickness from MRI. *Cereb. Cortex* 17, 2407–2419. doi: 10.1093/cercor/bhl149

Hebb, D. (1949). *The Organization of Behavior: A Neuropsychological Theory.* New York: John Wiley and Sons.

Heinzel, S., Lorenz, R. C., Brockhaus, W. R., Wustenberg, T., Kathmann, N., Heinz, A., et al. (2014). Working memory load-dependent brain response predicts behavioral training gains in older adults. *J. Neurosci.* 34, 1224–1233. doi: 10.1523/JNEUROSCI.2463-13.2014

Heitger, M. H., Ronsse, R., Dhollander, T., Dupont, P., Caeyenberghs, K., and Swinnen, S. P. (2012). Motor learning-induced changes in functional brain connectivity as revealed by means of graph-theoretical network analysis. *Neuroimage* 61, 633–650. doi: 10.1016/j.neuroimage.2012.03.067

Hempel, A., Giesel, F. L., Garcia Caraballo, N. M., Amann, M., Meyer, H., Wüstenberg, T., et al. (2004). Plasticity of cortical activation related to working memory during training. *Am. J. Psychiatry* 161, 745–747. doi: 10.1176/appi.ajp.161.4.745

Hermundstad, A. M., Bassett, D. S., Brown, K. S., Aminoff, E. M., Clewett, D., Freeman, S., et al. (2013). Structural foundations of resting-state and task-based functional connectivity in the human brain. *Proc. Natl. Acad. Sci. U S A* 110, 6169–6174. doi: 10.1073/pnas.1219562110

Honey, C. J., Sporns, O., Cammoun, L., Gigandet, X., Thiran, J. P., Meuli, R., et al. (2009). Predicting human resting-state functional connectivity from structural connectivity. *Proc. Natl. Acad. Sci. U S A* 106, 2035–2040. doi: 10.1073/pnas.0811168106

Iturria-Medina, Y., Sotero, R. C., Canales-Rodríguez, E. J., Alemán-Gómez, Y., and Melie-García, L. (2008). Studying the human brain anatomical network via diffusion-weighted MRI and graph theory. *Neuroimage* 40, 1064–1076. doi: 10.1016/j.neuroimage.2007.10.060

Jaeggi, S. M., Buschkuehl, M., Jonides, J., and Perrig, W. J. (2008). Improving fluid intelligence with training on working memory. *Proc. Natl. Acad. Sci. U S A* 105, 6829–6833. doi: 10.1073/pnas.0801268105

Jaušovec, N., and Jaušovec, K. (2012). Working memory training: improving intelligence–changing brain activity. *Brain Cogn.* 79, 96–106. doi: 10.1016/j.bandc.2012.02.007

Jolles, D. D., and Crone, E. A. (2012). Training the developing brain: a neurocognitive perspective. *Front. Hum. Neurosci.* 6:76. doi: 10.3389/fnhum.2012.00076

Jolles, D. D., Grol, M. J., Van Buchem, M. A., Rombouts, S. A. R. B., and Crone, E. A. (2010). Practice effects in the brain: changes in cerebral activation after working memory practice depend on task demands. *Neuroimage* 52, 658–668. doi: 10.1016/j.neuroimage.2010.04.028

Jolles, D. D., van Buchem, M. A., Crone, E. A., and Rombouts, S. A. (2013). Functional brain connectivity at rest changes after working memory training. *Hum. Brain Mapp.* 34, 396–406. doi: 10.1002/hbm.21444

Kamiński, M. J., and Blinowska, K. J. (1991). A new method of the description of the information flow in the brain structures. *Biol. Cybern.* 65, 203–210. doi: 10.1007/bf00198091

Karbach, J., and Schubert, T. (2013). Training-induced cognitive and neural plasticity. *Front. Hum. Neurosci.* 7:48. doi: 10.3389/fnhum.2013.00048

Kinnison, J., Padmala, S., Choi, J. M., and Pessoa, L. (2012). Network analysis reveals increased integration during emotional and motivational processing. *J. Neurosci.* 32, 8361–8372. doi: 10.1523/JNEUROSCI.0821-12.2012

Kitzbichler, M. G., Henson, R. N., Smith, M. L., Nathan, P. J., and Bullmore, E. T. (2011). Cognitive effort drives workspace configuration of human brain functional networks. *J. Neurosci.* 31, 8259–8270. doi: 10.1523/JNEUROSCI.0440-11.2011

Klimesch, W. (1999). EEG alpha and theta oscillations reflect cognitive and memory performance: a review and analysis. *Brain Res. Brain Res. Rev.* 29, 169–195. doi: 10.1016/s0165-0173(98)00056-3

Klingberg, T. (2010). Training and plasticity of working memory. *Trends Cogn. Sci.* 14, 317–324. doi: 10.1016/j.tics.2010.05.002

Klingberg, T., Forssberg, H., and Westerberg, H. (2002). Training of working memory in children with ADHD. *J. Clin. Exp. Neuropsychol.* 24, 781–791. doi: 10.1076/jcen.24.6.781.8395

Kohlmorgen, J., Dornhege, G., Braun, M., Blankertz, B., Müller, K.-R., Curio, G., et al. (2007). "Improving human performance in a real operating environment through real-time mental workload detection," in *Toward Brain-Computer Interfacing*, eds G. Dornhege, J. D. R. Millán, T. Hinterberger, D. J. Mcfarland and K.-R. Müller (Cambridge, MA: MIT Press), 409–422.

Kothe, C. A., and Makeig, S. (2011). Estimation of task workload from EEG data: new and current tools and perspectives. *Conf. Proc. IEEE Eng. Med. Biol. Soc.* 2011, 6547–6551. doi: 10.1109/IEMBS.2011.6091615

Kuhnert, M.-T., Bialonski, S., Noennig, N., Mai, H., Hinrichs, H., Helmstaedter, C., et al. (2013). Incidental and intentional learning of verbal episodic material differentially modifies functional brain networks. *PLoS One* 8:e80273. doi: 10.1371/journal.pone.0080273

Langer, N., Pedroni, A., Gianotti, L. R., Hänggi, J., Knoch, D., and Jäncke, L. (2012). Functional brain network efficiency predicts intelligence. *Hum. Brain Mapp.* 33, 1393–1406. doi: 10.1002/hbm.21297

Langer, N., von Bastian, C. C., Wirz, H., Oberauer, K., and Jäncke, L. (2013). The effects of working memory training on functional brain network efficiency. *Cortex* 49, 2424–2438. doi: 10.1016/j.cortex.2013.01.008

Lee, U., Oh, G., Kim, S., Noh, G., Choi, B., and Mashour, G. A. (2010). Brain networks maintain a scale-free organization across consciousness, anesthesia and recovery: evidence for adaptive reconfiguration. *Anesthesiology* 113, 1081–1091. doi: 10.1097/ALN.0b013e3181f229b5

Lee, H., Voss, M. W., Prakash, R. S., Boot, W. R., Vo, L. T., Basak, C., et al. (2012). Videogame training strategy-induced change in brain function during a complex visuomotor task. *Behav. Brain Res.* 232, 348–357. doi: 10.1016/j.bbr.2012.03.043

Lewis, C. M., Baldassarre, A., Committeri, G., Romani, G. L., and Corbetta, M. (2009). Learning sculpts the spontaneous activity of the resting human brain. *Proc. Natl. Acad. Sci. U S A* 106, 17558–17563. doi: 10.1073/pnas.0902455106

Liang, X., Zou, Q., He, Y., and Yang, Y. (2013). Coupling of functional connectivity and regional cerebral blood flow reveals a physiological basis for network hubs of the human brain. *Proc. Natl. Acad. Sci. U S A* 110, 1929–1934. doi: 10.1073/pnas.1214900110

Luft, C. D., Pereda, E., Banissy, M. J., and Bhattacharya, J. (2014). Best of both worlds: promise of combining brain stimulation and brain connectome. *Front. Syst. Neurosci.* 8:132. doi: 10.3389/fnsys.2014.00132

Lustig, C., Shah, P., Seidler, R., and Reuter-Lorenz, P. A. (2009). Aging, training and the brain: a review and future directions. *Neuropsychol. Rev.* 19, 504–522. doi: 10.1007/s11065-009-9119-9

Maclin, E. L., Mathewson, K. E., Low, K. A., Boot, W. R., Kramer, A. F., Fabiani, M., et al. (2011). Learning to multitask: effects of video game practice on electrophysiological indices of attention and resource allocation. *Psychophysiology* 48, 1173–1183. doi: 10.1111/j.1469-8986.2011.01189.x

Maguire, E. A., Woollett, K., and Spiers, H. J. (2006). London taxi drivers and bus drivers: a structural MRI and neuropsychological analysis. *Hippocampus* 16, 1091–1101. doi: 10.1002/hipo.20233

Mathewson, K. E., Basak, C., Maclin, E. L., Low, K. A., Boot, W. R., Kramer, A. F., et al. (2012). Different slopes for different folks: alpha and delta EEG power predict subsequent video game learning rate and improvements in cognitive control tasks. *Psychophysiology* 49, 1558–1570. doi: 10.1111/j.1469-8986.2012.01474.x

McKendrick, R., Ayaz, H., Olmstead, R., and Parasuraman, R. (2014). Enhancing dual-task performance with verbal and spatial working memory training: continuous monitoring of cerebral hemodynamics with NIRS. *Neuroimage* 85(Pt. 3), 1014–1026. doi: 10.1016/j.neuroimage.2013.05.103

Micheloyannis, S., Pachou, E., Stam, C. J., Vourkas, M., Erimaki, S., and Tsirka, V. (2006). Using graph theoretical analysis of multi channel EEG to evaluate the neural efficiency hypothesis. *Neurosci. Lett.* 402, 273–277. doi: 10.1016/j.neulet.2006.04.006

Micheloyannis, S., Vourkas, M., Tsirka, V., Karakonstantaki, E., Kanatsouli, K., and Stam, C. J. (2009). The influence of ageing on complex brain networks: a graph theoretical analysis. *Hum. Brain Mapp.* 30, 200–208. doi: 10.1002/hbm.20492

Moreau, D., and Conway, A. R. (2013). Cognitive enhancement: a comparative review of computerized and athletic training programs. *Int. Rev. Sport Exerc. Psychol.* 6, 155–183. doi: 10.1080/1750984x.2012.758763

Moussa, M. N., Vechlekar, C. D., Burdette, J. H., Steen, M. R., Hugenschmidt, C. E., and Laurienti, P. J. (2011). Changes in cognitive state alter human functional brain networks. *Front. Hum. Neurosci.* 5:83. doi: 10.3389/fnhum.2011.00083

Mozolic, J. L., Hayasaka, S., and Laurienti, P. J. (2010). A cognitive training intervention increases resting cerebral blood flow in healthy older adults. *Front. Hum. Neurosci.* 4:16. doi: 10.3389/neuro.09.016.2010

Neisser, U., Boodoo, G., Bouchard, T. J. Jr., Boykin, A. W., Brody, N., Ceci, S. J., et al. (1996). Intelligence: knowns and unknowns. *Am. Psychol.* 51, 77–101. doi: 10.1037/0003-066X.51.2.77

Neuper, C., and Pfurtscheller, G. (2010). "Neurofeedback training for BCI control," in *Brain-Computer Interfaces*, eds B. Graimann, G. Pfurtscheller, and B. Allison (London: Springer), 65–78.

Nijhuis, E. H., van Cappellen van Walsum, A. M., and Norris, D. G. (2013). Topographic hub maps of the human structural neocortical network. *PLoS One* 8:e65511. doi: 10.1371/journal.pone.0065511

Olesen, P. J., Westerberg, H., and Klingberg, T. (2004). Increased prefrontal and parietal activity after training of working memory. *Nat. Neurosci.* 7, 75–79. doi: 10.1038/nn1165

Owens, M., Koster, E. H., and Derakshan, N. (2013). Improving attention control in dysphoria through cognitive training: transfer effects on working memory capacity and filtering efficiency. *Psychophysiology* 50, 297–307. doi: 10.1111/psyp.12010

Palva, S., Monto, S., and Palva, J. M. (2010). Graph properties of synchronized cortical networks during visual working memory maintenance. *Neuroimage* 49, 3257–3268. doi: 10.1016/j.neuroimage.2009.11.031

Park, D. C., Lautenschlager, G., Hedden, T., Davidson, N. S., Smith, A. D., and Smith, P. K. (2002). Models of visuospatial and verbal memory across the adult life span. *Psychol. Aging* 17, 299–320. doi: 10.1037//0882-7974.17.2.299

Petrides, M. (2005). Lateral prefrontal cortex: architectonic and functional organization. *Philos. Trans. R. Soc. Lond. B Biol. Sci.* 360, 781–795. doi: 10.1098/rstb.2005.1631

Pfurtscheller, G., Neuper, C., Flotzinger, D., and Pregenzer, M. (1997). EEG-based discrimination between imagination of right and left hand movement. *Electroencephalogr. Clin. Neurophysiol.* 103, 642–651. doi: 10.1016/s0013-4694(97)00080-1

Poldrack, R. A. (2015). Is "efficiency" a useful concept in cognitive neuroscience? *Dev. Cogn. Neurosci.* 11, 12–17. doi: 10.1016/j.dcn.2014.06.001

Pop, V. L., Stearman, E. J., Kazi, S., and Durso, F. T. (2012). Using engagement to negate vigilance decrements in the nextgen environment. *Int. J. Hum. Comput. Interact.* 28, 99–106. doi: 10.1080/10447318.2012.634759

Prakash, R. S., De Leon, A. A., Mourany, L., Lee, H., Voss, M. W., Boot, W. R., et al. (2012). Examining neural correlates of skill acquisition in a complex videogame training program. *Front. Hum. Neurosci.* 6:115. doi: 10.3389/fnhum.2012.00115

Repantis, D., Schlattmann, P., Laisney, O., and Heuser, I. (2010). Modafinil and methylphenidate for neuroenhancement in healthy individuals: a systematic review. *Pharmacol. Res.* 62, 187–206. doi: 10.1016/j.phrs.2010.04.002

Rubinov, M., and Sporns, O. (2010). Complex network measures of brain connectivity: uses and interpretations. *Neuroimage* 52, 1059–1069. doi: 10.1016/j.neuroimage.2009.10.003

Salvador, R., Suckling, J., Coleman, M. R., Pickard, J. D., Menon, D., and Bullmore, E. (2005). Neurophysiological architecture of functional magnetic resonance images of human brain. *Cereb. Cortex* 15, 1332–1342. doi: 10.1093/cercor/bhi016

Schaie, K. W. (1994). The course of adult intellectual development. *Am. Psychol.* 49, 304–313. doi: 10.1037//0003-066x.49.4.304

Schmidt-Wilcke, T., Rosengarth, K., Luerding, R., Bogdahn, U., and Greenlee, M. W. (2010). Distinct patterns of functional and structural neuroplasticity associated with learning Morse code. *Neuroimage* 51, 1234–1241. doi: 10.1016/j.neuroimage.2010.03.042

Schneiders, J. A., Opitz, B., Krick, C. M., and Mecklinger, A. (2011). Separating intra-modal and across-modal training effects in visual working memory: an fMRI investigation. *Cereb. Cortex* 21, 2555–2564. doi: 10.1093/cercor/bhr037

Schneiders, J. A., Opitz, B., Tang, H., Deng, Y., Xie, C., Li, H., et al. (2012). The impact of auditory working memory training on the fronto-parietal working memory network. *Front. Hum. Neurosci.* 6:173. doi: 10.3389/fnhum.2012.00173

Scholz, J., Klein, M. C., Behrens, T. E., and Johansen-Berg, H. (2009). Training induces changes in white-matter architecture. *Nat. Neurosci.* 12, 1370–1371. doi: 10.1038/nn.2412

Schweizer, S., Grahn, J., Hampshire, A., Mobbs, D., and Dalgleish, T. (2013). Training the emotional brain: improving affective control through emotional working memory training. *J. Neurosci.* 33, 5301–5311. doi: 10.1523/JNEUROSCI.2593-12.2013

Shipstead, Z., Redick, T. S., and Engle, R. W. (2012). Is working memory training effective? *Psychol. Bull.* 138, 628–654. doi: 10.1037/a0027473

Smit, D. J. A., Stam, C. J., Posthuma, D., Boomsma, D. I., and de Geus, E. J. C. (2008). Heritability of "small-world" networks in the brain: a graph theoretical analysis of resting-state EEG functional connectivity. *Hum. Brain Mapp.* 29, 1368–1378. doi: 10.1002/hbm.20468

Spoormaker, V. I., Schröter, M. S., Gleiser, P. M., Andrade, K. C., Dresler, M., Wehrle, R., et al. (2010). Development of a large-scale functional brain network during human non-rapid eye movement sleep. *J. Neurosci.* 30, 11379–11387. doi: 10.1523/JNEUROSCI.2015-10.2010

Sporns, O. (2014). Contributions and challenges for network models in cognitive neuroscience. *Nat. Neurosci.* 17, 652–660. doi: 10.1038/nn.3690

Sporns, O., and Zwi, J. D. (2004). The small world of the cerebral cortex. *Neuroinformatics* 2, 145–162. doi: 10.1385/ni:2:2:145

Stam, C. J. (2004). Functional connectivity patterns of human magnetoencephalographic recordings: a 'small-world' network? *Neurosci. Lett.* 355, 25–28. doi: 10.1016/j.neulet.2003.10.063

Stam, C. J., Jones, B. F., Nolte, G., Breakspear, M., and Scheltens, P. (2007). Small-world networks and functional connectivity in Alzheimer's disease. *Cereb. Cortex* 17, 92–99. doi: 10.1093/cercor/bhj127

Stephenson, C. L., and Halpern, D. F. (2013). Improved matrix reasoning is limited to training on tasks with a visuospatial component. *Intelligence* 41, 341–357. doi: 10.1016/j.intell.2013.05.006

Stevens, W. D., Buckner, R. L., and Schacter, D. L. (2010). Correlated low-frequency BOLD fluctuations in the resting human brain are modulated by recent experience in category-preferential visual regions. *Cereb. Cortex* 20, 1997–2006. doi: 10.1093/cercor/bhp270

Strenziok, M., Parasuraman, R., Clarke, E., Cisler, D. S., Thompson, J. C., and Greenwood, P. M. (2014). Neurocognitive enhancement in older adults: comparison of three cognitive training tasks to test a hypothesis of training transfer in brain connectivity. *Neuroimage* 85(Pt. 3), 1027–1039. doi: 10.1016/j.neuroimage.2013.07.069

Sulzer, J., Haller, S., Scharnowski, F., Weiskopf, N., Birbaumer, N., Blefari, M. L., et al. (2013). Real-time fMRI neurofeedback: progress and challenges. *Neuroimage* 76, 386–399. doi: 10.1016/j.neuroimage.2013.03.033

Sun, Y., Lim, J., Kwok, K., and Bezerianos, A. (2014a). Functional cortical connectivity analysis of mental fatigue unmasks hemispheric asymmetry and changes in small-world networks. *Brain Cogn.* 85, 220–230. doi: 10.1016/j.bandc.2013.12.011

Sun, Y., Lim, J., Meng, J., Kwok, K., Thakor, N., and Bezerianos, A. (2014b). Discriminative analysis of brain functional connectivity patterns for mental fatigue classification. *Ann. Biomed. Eng.* 42, 2084–2094. doi: 10.1007/s10439-014-1059-8

Tagliazucchi, E., von Wegner, F., Morzelewski, A., Brodbeck, V., Borisov, S., Jahnke, K., et al. (2013). Large-scale brain functional modularity is reflected in slow electroencephalographic rhythms across the human non-rapid eye movement sleep cycle. *Neuroimage* 70, 327–339. doi: 10.1016/j.neuroimage.2012.12.073

Takeuchi, H., Sekiguchi, A., Taki, Y., Yokoyama, S., Yomogida, Y., Komuro, N., et al. (2010). Training of working memory impacts structural connectivity. *J. Neurosci.* 30, 3297–3303. doi: 10.1523/JNEUROSCI.4611-09.2010

Takeuchi, H., Taki, Y., Nouchi, R., Hashizume, H., Sekiguchi, A., Kotozaki, Y., et al. (2013). Effects of working memory training on functional connectivity and cerebral blood flow during rest. *Cortex* 49, 2106–2125. doi: 10.1016/j.cortex.2012.09.007

Takeuchi, H., Taki, Y., Sassa, Y., Hashizume, H., Sekiguchi, A., Fukushima, A., et al. (2011). Working memory training using mental calculation impacts regional gray matter of the frontal and parietal regions. *PLoS One* 6:e23175. doi: 10.1371/journal.pone.0023175

Talbot, M. (2009). Brain gain: the underground world of neuroenhancing drugs. *New Yorker* 27, 32–43.

Tang, Y. Y., Lu, Q., Fan, M., Yang, Y., and Posner, M. I. (2012). Mechanisms of white matter changes induced by meditation. *Proc. Natl. Acad. Sci. U S A* 109, 10570–10574. doi: 10.1073/pnas.1207817109

Tang, Y. Y., Ma, Y., Fan, Y., Feng, H., Wang, J., Feng, S., et al. (2009). Central and autonomic nervous system interaction is altered by short-term meditation. *Proc. Natl. Acad. Sci. U S A* 106, 8865–8870. doi: 10.1073/pnas.0904031106

Tang, Y.-Y., and Posner, M. I. (2014). Training brain networks and states. *Trends Cogn. Sci.* 18, 345–350. doi: 10.1016/j.tics.2014.04.002

Taubert, M., Draganski, B., Anwander, A., Müller, K., Horstmann, A., Villringer, A., et al. (2010). Dynamic properties of human brain structure: learning-related changes in cortical areas and associated fiber connections. *J. Neurosci.* 30, 11670–11677. doi: 10.1523/JNEUROSCI.2567-10.2010

Taya, F., Sun, Y., Thakor, N., and Bezerianos, A. (2014). "Information transfer efficiency during rest and task a functional connectome approach," in *IEEE Biomedical Circuits and Systems Conference* (Lausanne).

Tomasi, D., and Volkow, N. D. (2011a). Association between functional connectivity hubs and brain networks. *Cereb. Cortex* 21, 2003–2013. doi: 10.1093/cercor/bhq268

Tomasi, D., and Volkow, N. D. (2011b). Functional connectivity hubs in the human brain. *Neuroimage* 57, 908–917. doi: 10.1016/j.neuroimage.2011.05.024

Uehara, T., Yamasaki, T., Okamoto, T., Koike, T., Kan, S., Miyauchi, S., et al. (2014). Efficiency of a "small-world" brain network depends on consciousness level: a resting-state FMRI study. *Cereb. Cortex* 24, 1529–1539. doi: 10.1093/cercor/bht004

Valdes-Sosa, P. A., Roebroeck, A., Daunizeau, J., and Friston, K. (2011). Effective connectivity: influence, causality and biophysical modeling. *Neuroimage* 58, 339–361. doi: 10.1016/j.neuroimage.2011.03.058

van den Heuvel, M. P., and Sporns, O. (2011). Rich-club organization of the human connectome. *J. Neurosci.* 31, 15775–15786. doi: 10.1523/JNEUROSCI.3539-11.2011

van den Heuvel, M. P., and Sporns, O. (2013a). An anatomical substrate for integration among functional networks in human cortex. *J. Neurosci.* 33, 14489–14500. doi: 10.1523/JNEUROSCI.2128-13.2013

van den Heuvel, M. P., and Sporns, O. (2013b). Network hubs in the human brain. *Trends Cogn. Sci.* 17, 683–696. doi: 10.1016/j.tics.2013.09.012

van den Heuvel, M. P., Stam, C. J., Boersma, M., and Hulshoff Pol, H. E. (2008). Small-world and scale-free organization of voxel-based resting-state functional connectivity in the human brain. *Neuroimage* 43, 528–539. doi: 10.1016/j.neuroimage.2008.08.010

van den Heuvel, M. P., Stam, C. J., Kahn, R. S., and Hulshoff Pol, H. E. (2009). Efficiency of functional brain networks and intellectual performance. *J. Neurosci.* 29, 7619–7624. doi: 10.1523/JNEUROSCI.1443-09.2009

Voss, M. W., Prakash, R. S., Erickson, K. I., Boot, W. R., Basak, C., Neider, M. B., et al. (2012). Effects of training strategies implemented in a complex videogame on functional connectivity of attentional networks. *Neuroimage* 59, 138–148. doi: 10.1016/j.neuroimage.2011.03.052

Watts, D. J., and Strogatz, S. H. (1998). Collective dynamics of 'small-world' networks. *Nature* 393, 440–442. doi: 10.1038/30918

Weiss, S., and Rappelsberger, P. (2000). Long-range EEG synchronization during word encoding correlates with successful memory performance. *Brain Res. Cogn. Brain Res.* 9, 299–312. doi: 10.1016/s0926-6410(00)00011-2

Wolf, D., Fischer, F. U., Fesenbeckh, J., Yakushev, I., Lelieveld, I. M., Scheurich, A., et al. (2014). Structural integrity of the corpus callosum predicts long-term transfer of fluid intelligence-related training gains in normal aging. *Hum. Brain Mapp.* 35, 309–318. doi: 10.1002/hbm.22177

Wu, S., Cheng, C. K., Feng, J., D'Angelo, L., Alain, C., and Spence, I. (2012). Playing a first-person shooter video game induces neuroplastic change. *J. Cogn. Neurosci.* 24, 1286–1293. doi: 10.1162/jocn_a_00192

Zander, T. O., and Kothe, C. (2011). Towards passive brain-computer interfaces: applying brain-computer interface technology to human-machine systems in general. *J. Neural Eng.* 8:025005. doi: 10.1088/1741-2560/8/2/025005

Zhao, X., Zhou, R., and Fu, L. (2013). Working memory updating function training influenced brain activity. *PLoS One* 8:e71063. doi: 10.1371/journal.pone.0071063

Zuo, X. N., Ehmke, R., Mennes, M., Imperati, D., Castellanos, F. X., Sporns, O., et al. (2012). Network centrality in the human functional connectome. *Cereb. Cortex* 22, 1862–1875. doi: 10.1093/cercor/bhr269

8

Prospects for Optogenetic Augmentation of Brain Function

*Sarah Jarvis and Simon R. Schultz**

Centre for Neurotechnology and Department of Bioengineering, Imperial College London, London, UK

Edited by:
Mikhail Lebedev,
Duke University, USA

Reviewed by:
Elena Rusconi,
University College London, UK
Leonardo Sacconi,
University of Florence, Italy
Marco Canepari,
Institut National de la Santé et de la Recherche Médicale, France

***Correspondence:**
Simon R. Schultz
s.schultz@imperial.ac.uk

The ability to optically control neural activity opens up possibilities for the restoration of normal function following neurological disorders. The temporal precision, spatial resolution, and neuronal specificity that optogenetics offers is unequalled by other available methods, so will it be suitable for not only restoring but also extending brain function? As the first demonstrations of optically "implanted" novel memories emerge, we examine the suitability of optogenetics as a technique for extending neural function. While optogenetics is an effective tool for altering neural activity, the largest impediment for optogenetics in neural augmentation is our systems level understanding of brain function. Furthermore, a number of clinical limitations currently remain as substantial hurdles for the applications proposed. While neurotechnologies for treating brain disorders and interfacing with prosthetics have advanced rapidly in the past few years, partially addressing some of these critical problems, optogenetics is not yet suitable for use in humans. Instead we conclude that for the immediate future, optogenetics is the neurological equivalent of the 3D printer: its flexibility providing an ideal tool for testing and prototyping solutions for treating brain disorders and augmenting brain function.

Keywords: optogenetics, neural augmentation, neural coding and decoding, neural engineering, neural modulation, neural prosthetics, BMI (brain machine interface)

1. INTRODUCTION

Combining genetic targeting with optical excitation, optogenetics offers the ability to not only record the activity of large populations of neurons but also manipulate the activity of individual cells. Recording neural activity is achieved by selective expression of activity sensitive fluorophores (such as those from the GCaMP and VSFP protein families, reviewed by Knöpfel, 2012) into neurons, whose activity can then be read out by optical imaging. Manipulation of neural activity can be achieved via the insertion of light-sensitive proteins (opsins) that act as ion channels or pumps into a neuron's membrane and are preferentially controlled by photons of different wavelengths, providing temporal control on the order of milliseconds. Together, this cell type specificity and temporal control results in a tool that can perturb neural circuits with high precision. Since its first application to neural populations in 2005 (Boyden et al., 2005), it has already had substantial impact as a popular technique within the neuroscientific toolkit.

In addition to its use as a research tool, optogenetic stimulation has been suggested as a new approach for neuroprosthetics and treatment of brain disorders. While therapies in these domains have traditionally used electrical or pharmacological techniques, optogenetics has one particular advantage over electrical stimulation in being able to target specific cell classes through gene expression. As a result, specific neuronal populations can in principle be controlled without potential brain-wide, side effects. Likewise, the extremely fine temporal precision it offers on the scale of milliseconds, due to its optical activation, has the advantage over pharmacology of not only acting immediately but also having no washout time. Together, these characteristics have led to optogenetics to be proposed as a viable approach for improved deep brain stimulation (Kravitz et al., 2010), reinstatement of functionality following spinal cord injury (Alilain et al., 2008) and retinal prostheses (Degenaar et al., 2009; Busskamp et al., 2012), amongst other potential clinical applications in humans, following studies using mice, rats and non-human primates as animal models.

The blurred boundary between restoring function and functional enhancement is present for any biomedical intervention. From improving existing function to the incorporation of new streams of information, augmentation of the central nervous system raises specific challenges, from technical issues that are shared with the development of neural therapies, to the more fundamental difficulty of identifying where and how to best modify existing activity to move to the new neural trajectory. In addition, the ethics of the benefits and unintended consequences of intervening in the brain are substantial, as discussed in a recent report by the Nuffield Council on Bioethics 2013.

Does the usefulness of optogenetics as a tool for probing neural circuits automatically translate to its use for neuroaugmentation? Or instead, is it at best limited to the rapid prototyping of novel approaches for enhancing neural processing, much like 3D printers have accelerated for the development of biomedical devices such as prosthetics (including ears, prosthetics and sockets), with the benefit of allowing easy customization? In this article, we examine how well suited is it as a tool for improving, and not merely probing, neural function. By identifying the advantages optogenetics offers over traditional tools for treatment of dysfunction, as well as the hurdles facing neuroaugmentation, we evaluate the use of optogenetics as a practical tool for neural enhancement.

2. OPTOGENETIC TREATMENT AND NEUROPROSTHETICS

A long-held goal of neuroscience has been to identify the specific roles that various neuronal populations play in neural information processing, in order to develop novel therapeutic approaches for brain disorders. The development of light sensitive tools, including opsins and optically activated G protein–coupled receptors (GPCRs), has provided an exceptional tool with which to dissect out the roles of neuronal populations. Critically, their specificity to target neurons by neuronal class and location is a unique advantage, and the ability to test without inducing irreversible changes allows confirmation without long-term damage. In rodent models, optogenetics has been used for investigating disorders such as Parkinson's Disease (Gradinaru et al., 2010), drug addiction (Witten et al., 2010), epilepsy (Bernstein and Boyden, 2011; Tye and Deisseroth, 2012), post-traumatic stress disorder (Sparta et al., 2013) and obesity (Krashes and Kravitz, 2014), among others. Subsequently, refining our understanding of neuronal processing has led to improving treatments by either refining the stimulation protocol or identifying a different target population.

The potential of optogenetics as a more finely targeted alternative to traditional neuromodulatory treatments, such as deep brain stimulation (DBS), has led to the development of optical DBS in rodent models (Aravanis et al., 2007) and proposals for its use in primates (Han and Boyden, 2007; Han, 2012). More recently, combining optical DBS with online monitoring of state has been possible: By integrating optogenetics with fMRI (Lee et al., 2010; Kahn et al., 2013), thus providing the critical link for evaluating the efficacy of the intervention. Specifically, this has been utilized to evaluate the use of optogenetics for the effective control of epileptic seizures, thus allowing the development of less disruptive interventions for temporal lobe epilepsy than are currently clinically available (Armstrong et al., 2013; Krook-Magnuson et al., 2013).

The ability to either increase or decrease activity is an essential aspect of making defined manipulations of targeted elements of the cortical circuit. However, identifying the optimal opsin for a given effect and target neuronal population is challenging. This is illustrated by the recent history of the development of optogenetic retinal prostheses. Originally, channelrhodopsin-2, an excitatory opsin, was proposed to be used to replace function in the retinal ganglion cells layers in conditions such as Retinitis Pigmentosa (RP) and Macular Degeneration (MD). Despite initially promising reports (reviewed in Busskamp et al., 2012), a later study concluded that channelrhodopsin-2 (ChR2) lacks the necessary sensitivity to make its use in a retinal prosthesis viable (Lagali et al., 2008). Soon after, halorhodopsin, an inhibitory opsin, was instead targeted to the photoreceptors. By changing the targeted circuit element, and sign of the perturbation applied, it was possible to significantly improve performance (Busskamp et al., 2010). Given that the retinal circuit has been mapped and extensively studied, this highlights the difficulty in identifying the optimal population to be targeted for even relatively simple networks.

The prospect of viable optically targeted treatments has been further advanced by the development of opsins that have effects beyond their immediate photoactivation, such as step-function opsins (SFO; Berndt et al., 2009) and stabilized step-function opsins (SSFO; Yizhar et al., 2011) that are able to sustain a photocurrent for longer durations (on the order of 30 min) before deactivation via illumination at another wavelength. These opsins thus offer the potential to alter the balance between excitation and inhibition over long-time scales. By doing so over large cortical areas, they offer the possibility to modulate activity which make them suited for treating conditions that are characterized gain dysfunction, such as depression, anxiety, autism, schizophrenia and attention deficit disorders (Yizhar et al., 2011), while minimizing the need for sustained activation. Independently of other clinical hurdles, the reality of this approach hinges on the stability of SFO and SSFOs to sustain a photocurrent over far longer durations, which drastically limits its potential as a therapy in itself. However, a substantial advantage of these opsins is that the strength of their modulation is dependent on the irradiance, which could provide a effective method by which to evaluate the magnitude of the shift required to restore healthy neural functioning, thus indirectly assisting in the development of alternative therapies.

A further use of optogenetics exploits its ability for altering neural activity with high temporal precision. By using short, well-timed pulses, it is possible to not only induce short-term plasticity but also induce long-term potentiation and/or depression (Zhang and Oertner, 2006). This suggests the possibility of reprogramming circuits by either strengthening or weakening connections (Gu and Yakel, 2011; Larsen et al., 2014). The same technique has also been applied to promote regrowth following peripheral nerve injury (Li et al., 2011).

Together, these studies demonstrate that optogenetic technology has many useful properties, including specificity for targeting neuronal populations, activation flexibility due to the range of opsins available, and excellent spatiotemporal control. Given this, we now examine how well suited optogenetics is for augmenting brain function.

3. EXTENDING NEURAL FLOW OF INFORMATION THROUGH OPTICAL CONTROL

Neural augmentation technologies aim to enhance the cognitive capacity or sensorimotor function of the brain. The underlying principles here are conceptually similar to those of neuroprosthetics, in that they both involve altering neural activity or neural circuits in order to redefine input-output relationships. However, there is a fundamental difference. Replacing functionality requires only a crude approximation of absent activity, while enhancement can involve either refining existing activity whilst preserving the brain's ability to process existing signals, or alternatively incorporating new streams of information, thus allowing a neuron to sample input from additional stimuli. The difficulty in interfacing with the CNS whilst preserving natural activity can be observed even at the single cell level. In optogenetics, using high levels of illumination lead to optical initiation of an action potential that effectively overrides the neuron's behavior, so that it produces a spike irregardless of its inputs. A subtler approach to integrating additional signals into the nervous system might instead superimpose such signals onto the existing inputs to the neuron, thus allowing the addition of new information streams into neural circuits without necessarily disrupting the processing of existing streams.

The obstacle of effectively blending information in the brain is well-illustrated in the history of the visual prosthesis. Following earlier observations that applying electrical current to the occipital lobe resulted in the perception of phosphenes (Foerster, 1929), the first visual prosthesis was implanted into the cortex (Brindley and Lewin, 1968), preceding the first retinal prosthesis by nearly a decade (Dawson and Radtke, 1977). Despite improvements to electrode design in the decades since, such as increasing the density of cortical electrodes, as well as an ever-increasing understanding of the visual system, cortical visual prostheses have not yet matched the clinical success of retinal prostheses (Eiber et al., 2013), highlighting the difficulties of artificially altering neural activity within the brain. This is despite the presence of organizational features of the visual cortical areas, such as the retinotopic map, providing a topography for mapping information onto the surface of the cortex which could be coopted for brain-machine interfacing purposes. As one progresses synaptically further from the retina, visual information is organized along more complex—and generally less well understood—dimensions. Consequently, the lack of a well-understood topographic map makes neural interfacing with association areas more difficult. This is even more true of higher cortical areas, such as the prefrontal cortex, which receive information from multiple areas. Thus, although information relating to our interaction with the world may be mapped in some kind of ordered fashion onto its surface, our understanding of that map is incomplete and we are therefore currently unable to exploit it for brain augmentation.

However, there is evidence demonstrating that optogenetic manipulation for augmenting simple stimuli is possible. In a recent study, mice were trained to discriminate the location of a bar during whisking (O'Connor et al., 2013). After identifying the coding scheme used within the barrel cortex to encode the location of the bar stimulus, optogenetic perturbations were then applied that would encode, if successful, for the other potential position. The mice reported the bar in the incorrect (virtual) location. While this study was important for the insight it provided into the mechanisms of whisker stimulus encoding, it also provides us with a glimpse into the possibilities provided by illusionary or virtual stimuli. If it is possible to optically signal a false bar position during whisking, then it also hints at the potential of refining sensory inputs based upon additional, non-biological sensors—or potentially even of integrating entirely new sensory inputs into conscious awareness. For instance, it may be possible to augment conscious perception with input from non-visible parts of the electromagnetic spectrum, in order to provide additional sensory capability for working in dangerous environments (**Figure 1A**).

Augmenting sensory function supplies additional input to the relevant sensory cortex and require a detailed topological map of the neural organization. Similarly, motor outputs can be remapped onto robotic manipulators, allowing augmented motor functionality for external actuators. Neuroprostheses for augmenting motor functionality might use open-loop systems, requiring only the reading of signals from motor cortex. However, closed loop neural interfaces have proved to be important for making BMI a completely integrated replacement for motor function (Donoghue, 2002). In the context of optogenetic brain augmentation, this might involve a fully optical system (e.g., reading out signals from motor cortex using optical imaging of a genetically encodable calcium indicator, together with writing feedback signals into, for instance, somatosensory cortex using optical stimulation of opsins). This potentially also opens up the opportunity to improve learning by augmenting the trajectory error, which provides vital feedback during normal motor learning tasks (**Figure 1B**). Studies have shown that for gross movements, both error amplification and offsetting improve the amount and speed of adaptation during motor learning, using protocols normally targeted at

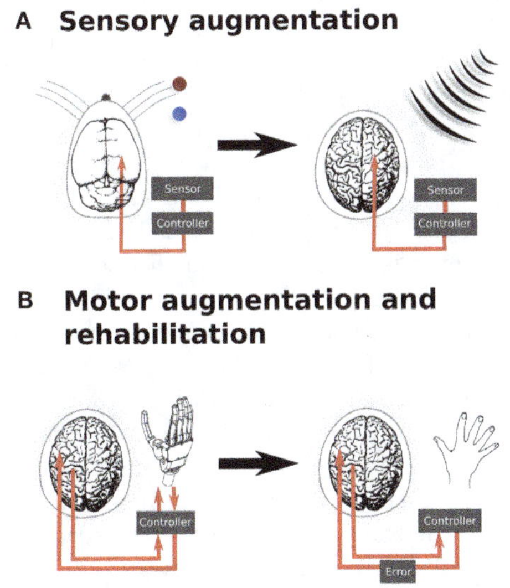

FIGURE 1 | Translation from experimental and existing therapeutics to clinical applications of neural augmentation using optogenetics. (A) Manipulation of somatosensory codes has been achieved in mouse barrel cortex, whereby optogenetically perturbing the sensory code caused the mouse to incorrectly report the location of the real bar as being in the blue position when the correct location was the red position (O'Connor et al., 2013). In a similar manner, directly interfacing into human somatosensory when an external sensor detects signals that are imperceptible for humans, such as electromagnetic radiation, may allow for additional sensory capabilities. **(B)** Currently, BMI applications only offer the possibility of open-loop applications, by reading neural activity to drive interfaces. Optogenetics could potentially extend BMI to provide currently sensory feedback from the prosthetic back, thus closing the feedback loop (left). This could be extended to refine motor control (right), by supplying an additional sensory error which has been proposed to improve motor rehabilitation following stroke (Wei et al., 2005; Celik et al., 2009). Together, these applications highlight the potential to develop applications from both animal models as well as existing applications, such as BMI. Images: prosthetic hand taken from Patent US Patent App. 10/488,008. Human brain (Wikimedia Commons); Mouse brain (Green, 1966).

motor rehabilitation following stroke (Wei et al., 2005; Celik et al., 2009). While these studies have been limited to error augmentation to gross movements, the spatial specificity of optogenetics when applied to topological maps presents the possibility for artificially inducing errors in either a motor-related cortices, to induce a trajectory bias (Wei et al., 2005), or with more difficulty, to generate errors related to subject's knowledge of the current state (Celik et al., 2009).

One requirement for a closed-loop system is the need for optimizing information transfer rates. Motivated by the need for more efficient methods for patients with neuromuscular disorders, much effort has been dedicated to developing classification schemas to optimize information transfer rates (Wolpaw et al., 2002; McFarland et al., 2003). Many BMIs currently use EEG, which is slower and population based, or implanted cortical electrodes, which improve on temporal and spatial resolution for decoding neural activity but lack encoding specificity, particularly for neural stimulation. By replacing this with optogenetics, it becomes possible to record signals with higher temporal and spatial resolution, thereby increasing accuracy, as well as stimulating defined cell types and patterns. This offers the potential of precise decoding of the activity of neural ensembles, which has implications beyond clinical BMI applications. In principle, the provision of a high bit-rate bidirectional interface between the brain and a computer would enable additional computational operations to be outsourced to a computer. This includes, for instance, possibilities ranging from decoding encrypted content using visualized passcodes, through to the external storage of memories (Berger et al., 2011). However, the development of such applications requires human subjects, and is thus unlikely to achieve ethical approval for these applications alone. Yet, as with electrode-based interfaces, such applications of optogenetic brain-machine interfaces may emerge as a by-product of clinical research.

In addition to memory, there is already some evidence that optogenetics can successfully alter cognitive and behavioral processing. In a recent study, it was possible to induce a negative behavior similar to obsessive-compulsive disorder (OCD) by targeting cortico-striatal projections, thus inducing behavior directly (Ahmari et al., 2013). The aim of the study was to test whether hyperstimulation of this pathway in mice would result in OCD-like behavior, which is unable to be tested clinically, but their success demonstrates that optogenetic intervention can change behavioral characteristics—with changes lasting up to weeks after the experiment ended. Similarly, another recent report investigated the role of serotonergic neurons within the dorsal raphe nucleus, which were already known to be involved in signalling reward. Using optogenetics, Miyazaki et al. (2014) established that mice extended their waiting time with a probability that inversely correlated with the delay before serotonergic neurons were optogenetically activated, leading them to conclude that precisely timed stimulation of serotonin neuron correlates with the willingness to wait—a quality they referred to as "patience."

From sensory and motor augmentation, through to modification of cognitive and behavioral traits, optogenetics uniquely has the specificity and precision to affect the neural correlates of these processes and to improve them. Yet for all the promise, this is still hampered by a common limitation: a deep understanding of the topographic mapping of information onto the relevant cortical areas and of the fine-grained neural coding of cognitive signals. Considerable progress in optogenetic augmentation of cognitive capacity will therefore have to wait for a more detailed understanding of "the cognitive neural code" before augmented neural function becomes an achievable reality.

4. CLINICAL CHALLENGES FOR OPTOGENETIC AUGMENTATION

Despite the very clear advantages that optogenetics offers for controlling neural activity, there are also four technical hurdles that exist before its translation to applied clinical use. These are opsin delivery, opsin choice, illumination strategies and optical actuators. Additionally, the ethical and regulatory hurdles raised by augmentation using optogenetics are manifold.

To date, the majority of optogenetic studies use mice, due to the large number of transgenic murine strains available for cellular targeting (e.g., using Cre recombinase, Madisen et al., 2012, and now intersectional genetic targeting approaches, Madisen et al., 2015). Cre recombinase targeting is however inapplicable in humans, thus an alternative method must be used. The most likely remaining candidate for opsin delivery is viral transfection, which uses viruses as carriers, such as adeno-associated viruses (AAV) or lentiviruses. Recent studies have confirmed that opsin delivery via AAV can be performed in species other than mice, including rats (Bass et al., 2010; Witten et al., 2010; Stefanik et al., 2013) and primates (Han, 2012). Furthermore, AAVs have been approved by the FDA for use in clinical trials (1995 for the first application; 2005 for the first application within the brain; Carter, 2005), thus removing a key hurdle for the use of optogenetics in clinical trials. An alternative strategy uses transplantable cells deliver opsins to marked sites (Weick et al., 2010); although this approach can suffer from extended opsin expression time, it raises the intriguing prospect of incorporating optogenetic addressability into new tissue formed by stem cell approaches to brain repair.

Different opsin variants have been shown to modify neuronal firing patterns in different ways. The insertion of CatCh, an excitatory opsin, prevented spikes following an initial volley spiking in fast-spiking cells, while the same cell class demonstrated sustained spiking when another actuating opsin, channelrhodopsin fast receiver (FR), was used instead (Mattis et al., 2012). The improvement of opsin design is ongoing, aiming for faster kinetics, preferred excitation wavelength, increased sensitivity and faster recovery (Lin, 2011). Among the newer generation of opsins are Chronos, a improved channelrhodopsin (Klapoetke et al., 2014), and JAWS, a red-shifted light-driven chloride pump (Chuong et al., 2014). As exhaustively testing all combinations of opsins and neuronal populations is impossible, this issue highlights the importance of good opsin characterization and models for determining suitable opsin-neuron combinations within any given neural circuit. In this, the development of accurate computational models of neurons, circuits (Potjans and Diesmann, 2014) and opsins (Nikolic et al., 2009; Grossman et al., 2013; Nikolic et al., 2013) will be vital for refining the matching of opsin to neuronal population and illumination protocols (Lin, 2011; Mattis et al., 2012; Jarvis et al., 2014).

A more practical concern is the light source, which can either be externally located or implantable. Similarly to the limitations that have troubled other biomedical devices, such as electrical DBS or retinal implants, both external and implantable devices have limitations: respectively, these are the need to open a pathway through the skin, and the need to provide power, either by an implanted battery or by transcutaneous transmission (O'Handley et al., 2008). Further practical limitations apply due to the need to deliver light to structures that can be located deep within the brain. Light penetration through tissue is limited by scattering. This is already limiting in mice (although new redshifted opsins such as ReaChR Lin et al., 2013 and JAWS Chuong et al., 2014, are increasing the achievable penetration depth). This factor becomes a major hurdle upon scaling up to human subjects. One approach to the solution of this problem is to target deep brain structures using penetrating optrodes, analogous to the use of penetrating electrodes in DBS. An additional issue that may arise in larger animals is to ensure the uniform spread of light over a wide area of tissue, i.e., ensuring that the falloff rate for illumination is sufficiently low such that the entirety of targeted areas are illuminated, whilst avoiding tissue damage due to overheating (Han, 2012).

Additionally, it is currently unclear that actuating an entire population of cells will be sufficient to provide useful input to the brain. While population firing rate codes have been demonstrated in some cortical areas (Georgopoulos et al., 1986), even firing rate codes may be "labeled line" codes in which cell identity matters (Montani et al., 2007; Schultz et al., 2009). Processing in some brain circuits has been proposed to occur through precise phase latencies within oscillatory activity (Engel et al., 2001), and the mechanisms underlying coding of cognitive information within the brain are still far from clear. For these latter schemes, whole field illumination of neurons in even a class-specific manner will clearly not be effective. Instead, only a specific subset of cells, such as an orientation column, should be targeted which is currently impossible using whole-field illumination.

This leads directly on to the last significant technical hurdle for clinical optogenetics: how can a large number of neurons within a population be driven with precise spatial, and defined temporal, resolution? The majority of optogenetic experiments to date have employed single photon excitation of opsins, typically supplied by a light emitting diode or fibre-coupled laser. The disadvantage with such approaches is that optogenetic activation is then not spatially limited, and consequently all opsin-expressing cells within an area of tissue are affected (**Figure 2A**). For some optogenetic applications, this may not be sufficient. Instead, it is critical to target subpopulations of neurons, then alternatives are available, such as the use of techniques such as multi-site light emitting diode arrays (Grossman et al., 2010). However, such approaches are in practice limited to the retina or *in vitro* preparations, as they provide negligible to no confinement within the axial plane (**Figure 2B**).

Two further possibilities exist that exploit optical technology to provide precise spatiotemporal patterning. The first is multiphoton excitation (Rickgauer and Tank, 2009), typically 2-photon (2P), which is spatially confined enough to allow the optical activation of individual cells. By using the interaction of two photons of longer wavelengths, which have less scatter, a small point spread function (PSF) is created that is constrained in the axial as well as lateral dimension (**Figure 2C**) and can be relocated in space, thus activating individual neurons throughout the tissue volume. However, as the PSF is typically smaller than the soma, 2P excitation is insufficient to initiate an action potential without scanning within the cell—which in turn reduces the temporal resolution of the technique (Rickgauer and Tank, 2009). Another recent approach uses wavefront shaping methods, such as digital holography or generalized phase contrast (**Figure 2D**), and by manipulating the phase of light with a spatial light modulator, create a defined spatial pattern of light that can similarly scan multiple neurons in a volume of tissue (Papagiakoumou et al., 2010; Oron et al., 2012). Both

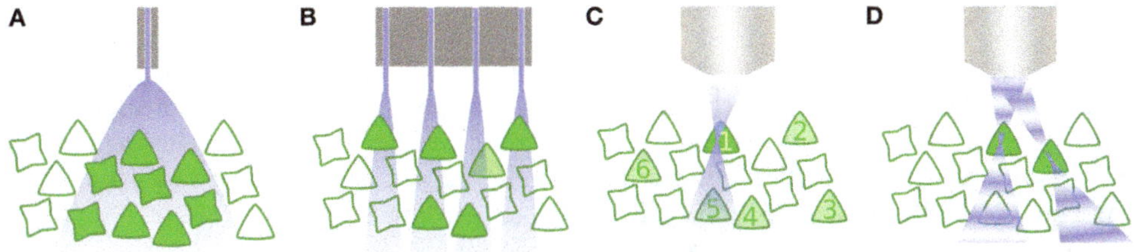

FIGURE 2 | Activating neurons to drive activity. (A) Whole field illumination via diode, either located at the cortical surface or inserted within the tissue. In both instances, all neurons within the illuminated area are activated. **(B)** An array of photodiodes illuminates subpopulations in the lateral plane, illustrated here in combination with opsin specificity for only one class of neuron. However, targeting is not constrained in the axial dimension and likewise drives multiple neurons within a column corresponding to each individual diode. **(C)** Multiphoton excitation results in a spatially constrained point spread function (PSF) in lateral and axial planes. Here, the 2P beam is targeted for the first neuron, whose soma is significantly larger than the PSF thus requiring scanning the neuron and increasing the dwell time. Driving other selected neurons within the population (2–6) is performed sequentially. **(D)** Digital holography utilizes wavefront shaping, in which a spatial light modulator alters the phase of beams in order to create multiple PSFs, allowing multiple neurons to be simultaneously but independently driven.

multiphoton excitation and wavefront shaping are limited at a rate proportional to the population size of the neurons to be targeted. Furthermore, despite being tested *in vivo* as well as *in vitro*, they only exist for head-fixed subjects, thus currently preventing its application for experiments including freely behaving subjects. Yet, as precise spatiotemporal patterning is likely to be necessary to take advantage of the full capabilities of optogenetic manipulation of brain circuitry, particularly where synaptic plasticity mechanisms are involved, this area of technological development is one to watch closely.

In addition to technical hurdles, the regulatory requirements for bringing optogenetics to clinical reality are also substantial. As discussed, the FDA has already cleared the use of AAV-delivered, providing an option for opsin delivery (Carter, 2005). However, opsin expression application in human, in which light-sensitive proteins are inserted into cellular membrane via genetic manipulation, has not been cleared and would likely require similar clearance to other gene therapies. This is compounded with the difficulty in determining the correct levels of opsin expression, as overexpression has been demonstrated to have cytotoxic effects. The FDA has recently cleared an application for optogenetic gene therapy for the treatment of RP, which will allow clinical trials in humans to commence (Francis et al., 2013; RetroSense, 2015). The treatment aims to restore photosensitivity of photoreceptors, bypassing the need for a separate light activation source. This is in contrast to cortical optogenetic application which would additionally require implanted optrodes, placing them in the highest band for both the FDA and EU regulatory approval. In addition to the usual considerations associated with implantable device, implanted optical devices have an additional constraint of minimization of energy via heat lost to prevent tissue damage. Determining the distribution of energy by optical delivery devices has been modeled (Ozden et al., 2013), however althought the FDA have determined power limits for MRI that allow temperature changes of 1°C, there are, as yet, no limits for power limits for chronically implanted optrodes (Ozden et al., 2013). For chronic usage, this may require significantly lower limits for power, thus restricting the range of illumination.

Finally, the ethical considerations that surround neuroenhancement are substantial and have been discussed elsewhere, including in this issue (Clark, 2014; Shook et al., 2014). Many of the same arguments for enhancement of cognitive abilities via pharamacological (Hyman, 2011), transcranial or electrical means are similarly applicable here for optogenetics: the development of a cognitive "arms race"; the question of who is in control of the augmenting device; and safety, both due to unintended consequences of manipulating neural activity as well as from the treament itself. The latter is particularly pertinent for the application of optogenetics, as it is highly invasive, requiring both manipulation of genetic material as well as the subcranial placement of devices to provide optical activation. This raises the ethical cost of optogenetics, such that its capacity for neuroenhancement must be substantially higher in comparison to other treatments to warrant its use preferentially. However, this provides an ethical impasse: how should these critera be tested and developed for optogenetics, while the risk and invasiveness of clinical optogenetics remains high? It may well be that such clinical trials may emerge as a by-product of optogenetic therapies for treatment of existing dysfunction or BMIs, rather than augmentation; or instead that it will ultimately require the use of similar but separate therapies, such as targeted nanoparticles (Carvalho-de Souza et al., 2015) which have the same advantages as optogenetics, but with diminished risks, to make neuroenhancement not only ethically more attractive but also clinically attainable.

5. CONCLUSION

Optogenetics has opened up a variety of new experimental paradigms in neuroscience. Its key advantage lies in the ability to target neuronal populations with precise spatiotemporal activation with immediate and reversible effect, which has been advantageous for untangling the contribution of neuronal populations in neural processing in both anatomical and behavioral studies (Tye and Deisseroth, 2012). These advantages also place optogenetics as a well-suited tool to assist in the *development* of neurological therapies and, correspondingly, neural enhancements.

The application of optogenetics as a tool for *direct use* in neural modulation itself is less certain. The technological development of optogenetics is still in progress, with opsin molecular engineering, opsin delivery and optical stimulation techniques advancing rapidly, which will undoubtedly increase the precision of optogenetics and with it, our ability to manipulate neural circuits. However, the translation of optogenetics from research tool to clinical application has additional stipulations, particularly for its use in humans. From the challenges of opsin delivery to the difficulties in optically driving neurons with implantable devices, applying optogenetics outside of research remains a remote possibility in the foreseeable future. Yet in themselves, these elements are not the most significant constraint on the application of optogenetics for neural augmentation, which is instead our understanding of the neural codes that we are attempting to adapt. In the meantime, optogenetics offers a viable possibility for the development of novel neural therapies, by providing a robust capability to technically refine stimulation protocols and evaluate the effect of modulating activity levels of different neuronal populations.

ACKNOWLEDGMENTS

The authors would like to thank Konstantin Nikolic and Stephen Brickley for useful discussions on the uses and limitations of optogenetics, and the EU seventh framework programme (award PIEF-GA-2013-628086) and the BBSRC (awards BB/L018268/1and BB/K001817/1) for financial support.

REFERENCES

Ahmari, S. E., Spellman, T., Douglass, N. L., Kheirbek, M. A., Simpson, H. B., Deisseroth, K., et al. (2013). Repeated cortico-striatal stimulation generates persistent OCD-like behavior. *Science* 340, 1234–1239. doi: 10.1126/science.1234733

Alilain, W. J., Li, X., Horn, K. P., Dhingra, R., Dick, T. E., Herlitze, S., et al. (2008). Light-induced rescue of breathing after spinal cord injury. *J. Neurosci.* 28, 11862–11870. doi: 10.1523/JNEUROSCI.3378-08.2008

Aravanis, A. M., Wang, L.-P., Zhang, F., Meltzer, L. A., Mogri, M. Z., Schneider, M. B., et al. (2007). An optical neural interface: *in vivo* control of rodent motor cortex with integrated fiberoptic and optogenetic technology. *J. Neural Eng.* 4, S143–S156. doi: 10.1088/1741-2560/4/3/s02

Armstrong, C., Krook-Magnuson, E., Oijala, M., and Soltesz, I. (2013). Closed-loop optogenetic intervention in mice. *Nat. Protocols* 8, 1475–1493. doi: 10.1038/nprot.2013.080

Bass, C. E., Grinevich, V. P., Vance, Z. B., Sullivan, R. P., Bonin, K. D., and Budygin, E. A. (2010). Optogenetic control of striatal dopamine release in rats. *J. Neurochem.* 114, 1344–1352. doi: 10.1111/j.1471-4159.2010.06850.x

Berger, T. W., Hampson, R. E., Song, D., Goonawardena, A., Marmarelis, V. Z., and Deadwyler, S. A. (2011). A cortical neural prosthesis for restoring and enhancing memory. *J. Neural Eng.* 8:046017. doi: 10.1088/1741-2560/8/4/046017

Berndt, A., Yizhar, O., Gunaydin, L. a., Hegemann, P., and Deisseroth, K. (2009). Bi-stable neural state switches. *Nat. Neurosci.* 12, 229–234. doi: 10.1038/nn.2247

Bernstein, J. G. and Boyden, E. S. (2011). Optogenetic tools for analyzing the neural circuits of behavior. *Trends Cogn. Sci.* 15, 592–600. doi: 10.1016/j.tics.2011.10.003

Boyden, E. S., Zhang, F., Bamberg, E., Nagel, G., and Deisseroth, K. (2005). Millisecond-timescale, genetically targeted optical control of neural activity. *Nat. Neurosci.* 8, 1263–1268. doi: 10.1038/nn1525

Brindley, G. S. and Lewin, W. S. (1968). The sensations produced by electrical stimulation of the visual cortex. *J. Physiol.* 196, 479–493. doi: 10.1113/jphysiol.1968.sp008519

Busskamp, V., Duebel, J., Balya, D., Fradot, M., Viney, T. J., Siegert, S., et al. (2010). Genetic reactivation of cone photoreceptors restores visual responses in retinitis pigmentosa. *Science* 329, 413–417. doi: 10.1126/science.1190897

Busskamp, V., Picaud, S., Sahel, J. A., and Roska, B. (2012). Optogenetic therapy for retinitis pigmentosa. *Gene Ther.* 19, 169–175. doi: 10.1038/gt.2011.155

Carter, B. J. (2005). Adeno-associated virus vectors in clinical trials. *Hum. Gene Ther.* 16, 541–550. doi: 10.1089/hum.2005.16.541

Carvalho-de Souza, J. L., Treger, J. S., Dang, B., Kent, S. B., Pepperberg, D. R., and Bezanilla, F. (2015). Photosensitivity of neurons enabled by cell-targeted gold nanoparticles. *Neuron* 86 207–217. doi: 10.1016/j.neuron.2015.02.033

Celik, O., Powell, D., and Malley, M. K. (2009). "Impact of visual error augmentation methods on task performance and motor adaptation," in *Rehabilitation Robotics, 2009. ICORR 2009. IEEE International Conference on* (Kyoto: IEEE). 793–798.

Chuong, A. S., Miri, M. L., Busskamp, V., Matthews, G. A. C., Acker, L. C., Sø rensen, A. T., et al. (2014). Noninvasive optical inhibition with a red-shifted microbial rhodopsin. *Nat. Neurosci.* 17, 1123–1129. doi: 10.1038/nn.3752

Clark, V. P. (2014). The ethical, moral, and pragmatic rationale for brain augmentation. *Front. Syst. Neurosci.* 8:130. doi: 10.3389/fnsys.2014.00130

Dawson, W. W. and Radtke, N. D. (1977). The electrical stimulation of the retina by indwelling electrodes. *Invest. Ophthalmol. Vis. Sci.* 16, 249–252.

Degenaar, P., Grossman, N., Memon, M. A., Burrone, J., Dawson, M., Drakakis, E., et al. (2009). Optobionic vision–a new genetically enhanced light on retinal prosthesis. *J. Neural Eng.* 6:035007. doi: 10.1088/1741-2560/6/3/035007

Donoghue, J. P. (2002). Connecting cortex to machines: recent advances in brain interfaces. *Nat. Neurosci.* 5(Suppl.), 1085–1088. doi: 10.1038/nn947

Eiber, C. D., Lovell, N. H., and Suaning, G. J. (2013). Attaining higher resolution visual prosthetics: a review of the factors and limitations. *J. Neural Eng.* 10:011002. doi: 10.1088/1741-2560/10/1/011002

Engel, A. K., Fries, P., and Singer, W. (2001). Dynamic predictions: oscillations and synchrony in top-down processing. *Nat. Rev. Neurosci.* 2, 704–716. doi: 10.1038/35094565

Foerster, O. (1929). Beiträge zur Pathophysiologie der Sehbahn und der Sehsphäre. *J. Psychol. Neurol. (Leipzig)* 39, 463–485.

Francis, P. J., Mansfield, B., and Rose, S. (2013). Proceedings of the first international optogenetic therapies for vision symposium. *Transl. Vis. Sci. Technol.* 2:4. doi: 10.1167/tvst.2.7.4

Georgopoulos, A. P., Schwartz, A. B., and Kettner, R. E. (1986). Neuronal population coding of movement direction. *Science* 233, 1416–1419.

Gradinaru, V., Zhang, F., Ramakrishnan, C., Mattis, J., Prakash, R., Diester, I., et al. (2010). Molecular and cellular approaches for diversifying and extending optogenetics. *Cell* 141, 154–165. doi: 10.1016/j.cell.2010.02.037

Green, E. L. (ed.). (1966). *Biology of the Laboratory Mouse.* New York, NY: McGraw-Hill Book Co.

Grossman, N., Poher, V., Grubb, M. S., Kennedy, G. T., Nikolic, K., McGovern, B., et al. (2010). Multi-site optical excitation using ChR2 and micro-LED array. *J. Neural Eng.* 7:16004. doi: 10.1088/1741-2560/7/1/016004

Grossman, N., Simiaki, V., Martinet, C., Toumazou, C., Schultz, S. R., and Nikolic, K. (2013). The spatial pattern of light determines the kinetics and modulates backpropagation of optogenetic action potentials. *J. Comput. Neurosci.* 34, 477–488. doi: 10.1007/s10827-012-0431-7

Gu, Z. and Yakel, J. L. (2011). Timing-dependent septal cholinergic induction of dynamic hippocampal synaptic plasticity. *Neuron* 71, 155–165. doi: 10.1016/j.neuron.2011.04.026

Han, X. (2012). Optogenetics in the nonhuman primate. *Prog. Brain Res.* 196, 215–233. doi: 10.1016/B978-0-444-59426-6.00011-2

Han, X. and Boyden, E. S. (2007). Multiple-color optical activation, silencing, and desynchronization of neural activity, with single-spike temporal resolution. *PLoS ONE* 2:e299. doi: 10.1016/b978-0-444-59426-6.00011-2

Hyman, S. E. (2011). Cognitive enhancement: promises and perils. *Neuron* 69, 595–598.

Jarvis, S. J., Nikolic, K., and Schultz, S. R. (2014). Optical coactivation in cortical cells: reprogramming the excitation-inhibition balancing act to control neuronal gain in abstract and detailed models. *BMC Neurosci.* 15(Suppl. 1):F1. doi: 10.1186/1471-2202-15-S1-F1

Kahn, I., Knoblich, U., Desai, M., Bernstein, J., Graybiel, A. M., Boyden, E. S., et al. (2013). Optogenetic drive of neocortical pyramidal neurons generates fMRI signals that are correlated with spiking activity. *Brain Research* 1511, 33–45. doi: 10.1016/j.brainres.2013.03.011

Klapoetke, N. C., Murata, Y., Kim, S. S., Pulver, S. R., Birdsey-Benson, A., Cho, Y. K., et al. (2014). Independent optical excitation of distinct neural populations. *Nat. Methods* 11, 338–346. doi: 10.1038/nmeth.2836

Knöpfel, T. (2012). Genetically encoded optical indicators for the analysis of neuronal circuits. *Nat. Rev. Neurosci.* 13, 687–700. doi: 10.1038/nrn3293

Krashes, M. J. and Kravitz, A. V. (2014). Optogenetic and chemogenetic insights into the food addiction hypothesis. *Front. Behav. Neurosci.* 8:57. doi: 10.3389/fnbeh.2014.00057

Kravitz, A. V., Freeze, B. S., Parker, P. R. L., Kay, K., Thwin, M. T., Deisseroth, K., et al. (2010). Regulation of parkinsonian motor behaviours by optogenetic control of basal ganglia circuitry. *Nature* 466, 622–626. doi: 10.1038/nature09159

Krook-Magnuson, E., Armstrong, C., Oijala, M., and Soltesz, I. (2013). On-demand optogenetic control of spontaneous seizures in temporal lobe epilepsy. *Nat. Commun.* 4, 1376. doi: 10.1038/ncomms2376

Lagali, P. S., Balya, D., Awatramani, G. B., Münch, T. A., Kim, D. S., Busskamp, V., et al. (2008). Light-activated channels targeted to ON bipolar cells restore visual function in retinal degeneration. *Nat. Neurosci.* 11, 667–675. doi: 10.1038/nn.2117

Larsen, R. S., Smith, I. T., Miriyala, J., Han, J. E., Corlew, R. J., Smith, S. L., et al. (2014). Synapse-specific control of experience-dependent plasticity by presynaptic NMDA receptors. *Neuron* 83, 879–893. doi: 10.1016/j.neuron.2014.07.039

Lee, J. H., Durand, R., Gradinaru, V., Zhang, F., Goshen, I., Kim, D.-S., et al. (2010). Global and local fMRI signals driven by neurons defined optogenetically by type and wiring. *Nature* 465, 788–792. doi: 10.1038/nature09108

Li, N., Downey, J. E., Bar-Shir, A., Gilad, A. A., Walczak, P., Kim, H., et al. (2011). Optogenetic-guided cortical plasticity after nerve injury. *Proc. Natl. Acad. Sci. U.S.A.* 108, 8838–8843. doi: 10.1073/pnas.1100815108

Lin, J. Y. (2011). A user's guide to channelrhodopsin variants: features, limitations and future developments. *Exp. Physiol.* 96, 19–25. doi: 10.1113/expphysiol.2009.051961

Lin, J. Y., Knutsen, P. M., Muller, A., Kleinfeld, D., and Tsien, R. Y. (2013). ReaChR: a red-shifted variant of channelrhodopsin enables deep transcranial optogenetic excitation. *Nat. Neurosci.* 16, 1499–1508. doi: 10.1038/nn.3502

Madisen, L., Garner, A. R., Shimaoka, D., Chuong, A. S., Klapoetke, N. C., Li, L., et al. (2015). Transgenic mice for intersectional targeting of neural sensors and effectors with high specificity and performance. *Neuron* 85, 942–958. doi: 10.1016/j.neuron.2015.02.022

Madisen, L., Mao, T., Koch, H., Zhuo, J.-m., Berenyi, A., Fujisawa, S., et al. (2012). A toolbox of Cre-dependent optogenetic transgenic mice for light-induced activation and silencing. *Nat. Neurosci.* 15, 793–802. doi: 10.1038/nn.3078

Mattis, J., Tye, K., and Ferenczi, E. (2012). Principles for applying optogenetic tools derived from direct comparative analysis of microbial opsins. *Nat. Methods* 9, 159–172. doi: 10.1038/nmeth.1808

McFarland, D. J., Sarnacki, W. A., and Wolpaw, J. R. (2003). Brain-computer interface (BCI) operation: optimizing information transfer rates. *Biol. Psychol.* 63, 237–251. doi: 10.1016/S0301-0511(03)00073-5

Miyazaki, K., Miyazaki, K., Tanaka, K., Yamanaka, A., Takahashi, A., Tabuchi, S., et al. (2014). Optogenetic activation of dorsal raphe serotonin neurons enhances patience for future rewards. *Curr. Biol.* 24, 2033–2040. doi: 10.1016/j.cub.2014.07.041

Montani, F., Kohn, A., Smith, M. A., and Schultz, S. R. (2007). The role of correlations in direction and contrast coding in the primary visual cortex. *J. Neurosci.* 27, 2338–2348. doi: 10.1523/JNEUROSCI.3417-06.2007

Nikolic, K., Grossman, N., Grubb, M. S., Burrone, J., Toumazou, C., and Degenaar, P. (2009). Photocycles of channelrhodopsin-2. *Photochem. Photobiol.* 85, 400–411. doi: 10.1111/j.1751-1097.2008.00460.x

Nikolic, K., Jarvis, S., Grossman, N., and Schultz, S. (2013). Computational models of optogenetic tools for controlling neural circuits with light. *IEEE Eng. Med. Biol. Soc.* 5, 2–5. doi: 10.1109/embc.2013.6610903

Nuffield Council on Bioethics (2013). *Novel Neurotechnologies: Intervening in the Brain.* London: Nuffield Council on Bioethics.

O'Connor, D. H., Hires, S. A., Guo, Z. V., Li, N., Yu, J., Sun, Q.-Q., et al. (2013). Neural coding during active somatosensation revealed using illusory touch. *Nat. Neurosci.* 16, 958–965. doi: 10.1038/nn.3419

O'Handley, R. C., Huang, J. K., Bono, D, C., and Simon, J. (2008). Improved wireless, transcutaneous power transmission for *in vivo* applications. *Sens. J. IEEE* 8, 57–62.

Oron, D., Papagiakoumou, E., Anselmi, F., and Emiliani, V. (2012). Two-photon optogenetics. *Prog. Brain Res.* 196, 119–143. doi: 10.1016/B978-0-444-59426-6.00007-0

Ozden, I., Wang, J., Lu, Y., May, T., Lee, J., Goo, W., et al. (2013). A coaxial optrode as multifunction write-read probe for optogenetic studies in non-human primates. *J. Neurosci. Methods* 219, 142–154. doi: 10.1016/j.jneumeth.2013.06.011

Papagiakoumou, E., Anselmi, F., Bègue, A., de Sars, V., Glückstad, J., Isacoff, E. Y., et al. (2010). Scanless two-photon excitation of channelrhodopsin-2. *Nat. Methods* 7, 848–854. doi: 10.1038/nmeth.1505

Potjans, T. C. and Diesmann, M. (2014). The cell-type specific cortical microcircuit: relating structure and activity in a full-scale spiking network model. *Cereb. Cortex* 24, 785–806. doi: 10.1093/cercor/bhs358

RetroSense (2015). *Retrosense Therapeutics Lead Gene Therapy Candidate Gets Fda Clearance to Proceed to First-in-human Clinical Trials.* Available online at: http://www.businesswire.com/news/home/20150824005576/en/RetroSense-Therapeutics (Accessed on Augest 24, 2015)

Rickgauer, J. P. and Tank, D. W. (2009). Two-photon excitation of channelrhodopsin-2 at saturation. *Proc. Natl. Acad. Sci. U.S.A.* 106, 15025–15030. doi: 10.1073/pnas.0907084106

Schultz, S. R., Kitamura, K., Post-Uiterweer, A., Krupic, J., and Häusser, M. (2009). Spatial pattern coding of sensory information by climbing fiber-evoked calcium signals in networks of neighboring cerebellar Purkinje cells. *J. Neurosci.* 29, 8005–8015. doi: 10.1523/JNEUROSCI.4919-08.2009

Shook, J. R., Galvagni, L., and Giordano, J. (2014). Cognitive enhancement kept within contexts: neuroethics and informed public policy. *Front. Syst. Neurosci.* 8:228. doi: 10.3389/fnsys.2014.00228

Sparta, D. R., Jennings, J. H., Ung, R. L., and Stuber, G. D. (2013). Optogenetic strategies to investigate neural circuitry engaged by stress. *Behav. Brain Res.* 255, 19–25. doi: 10.1016/j.bbr.2013.05.007

Stefanik, M. T., Moussawi, K., Kupchik, Y. M., Smith, K. C., Miller, R. L., Huff, M. L., et al. (2013). Optogenetic inhibition of cocaine seeking in rats. *Addict. Biol.* 18, 50–53. doi: 10.1111/j.1369-1600.2012.00479.x

Tye, K. M. and Deisseroth, K. (2012). Optogenetic investigation of neural circuits underlying brain disease in animal models. *Nat. Rev. Neurosci.* 13, 251–266. doi: 10.1038/nrn3171

Wei, Y., Bajaj, P., Scheidt, R., and Patton, J. (2005). "Visual error augmentation for enhancing motor learning and rehabilitative relearning, " in *Rehabilitation Robotics, 2005. ICORR 2005. 9th International Conference on* (Chicago, IL: IEEE), 505–510.

Weick, J. P., Johnson, M. A., Skroch, S. P., Williams, J. C., Deisseroth, K., and Zhang, S.-C. (2010). Functional control of transplantable human ESC-derived neurons via optogenetic targeting. *Stem cells* 28, 2008–2016. doi: 10.1002/stem.514

Witten, I. B., Lin, S.-C., Brodsky, M., Prakash, R., Diester, I., Anikeeva, P., et al. (2010). Cholinergic interneurons control local circuit activity and cocaine conditioning. *Science* 330, 1677–1681. doi: 10.1126/science.1193771

9

Neostriatal Neuronal Activity Correlates Better with Movement Kinematics under Certain Rewards

Ioan Opris[1], Mikhail A. Lebedev[2] and Randall J. Nelson[3]*

[1] Miami Project, University of Florida, Miami, FL, USA, [2] Department of Neurobiology, Duke University, Durham, NC, USA, [3] Department of Anatomy and Neurobiology, The University of Tennessee Health Science Center, Memphis, TN, USA

Edited by:
Yoshio Sakurai,
Doshisha University, Japan

Reviewed by:
Vassiliy Tsytsarev,
University of Maryland School of Medicine, USA
Christian K. E. Moll,
University Medical Center Hamburg-Eppendorf, Germany

***Correspondence:**
Ioan Opris
ioanopris.phd@gmail.com;
ixo82@med.miami.edu

This study investigated how the activity of neostriatal neurons is related to the kinematics of movement when monkeys performed visually and vibratory cued wrist extensions and flexions. Single-unit recordings of 142/236 neostriatal neurons showed pre-movement activity (PMA) in a reaction time task with unpredictable reward. Monkeys were pseudo-randomly (75%) rewarded for correct performance. A regression model was used to determine whether the correlation between neostriatal neuronal activity and the kinematic variables (position, velocity, and acceleration) of wrist movement changes as a function of reward contingency, sensory cues, and movement direction. The coefficients of determination (CoD) representing the proportion of the variance in neuronal activity explained by the regression model on a trial by trial basis, together with their temporal occurrences (time of best regression/correlation, ToC) were compared across sensory modality, movement direction, and reward contingency. The best relationship (correlation) between neuronal activity and movement kinematic variables, given by the average coefficient of determination (CoD), was: (a) greater during trials in which rewards were certain, called "A" trials, as compared with those in which reward was uncertain called ("R") trials, (b) greater during flexion (Flex) trials as compared with extension (Ext) trials, and (c) greater during visual (VIS) cued trials than during vibratory (VIB) cued trials, for the same type of trial and the same movement direction. These results are consistent with the hypothesis that predictability of reward for correct performance is accompanied by faster linkage between neostriatal PMA and the vigor of wrist movement kinematics. Furthermore, the results provide valuable insights for building an upper-limb neuroprosthesis.

Keywords: basal ganglia, neostriatum, neuronal activity, movement preparation, hand movement, multilinear regression, reward uncertainty, motivation

INTRODUCTION

A significant proportion of neurons from neostriatum (NS) modulate their firing rate in response to environmental stimuli and/or fire before movement initiation and/or execution (Aldridge et al., 1980; Liles, 1985; Schultz and Romo, 1988; Alexander and Crutcher, 1990; Kimura, 1990; Romo and Schultz, 1990; Gardiner and Nelson, 1992; Lebedev and Nelson, 1999; Opris et al., 2011a). Several studies indicate that NS neurons may also participate in associating task stimuli with rewards (Schultz and Romo, 1990; Apicella et al., 1991; Robbins and Everitt, 1996; Opris et al., 2009; Schultz, 2010) or in modulating movement vigor (Opris et al., 2011a).

This connection between reinforcement and behavior may be mediated by the dopaminergic system at either sub-cortical or cortical levels (Robbins and Everitt, 1996; Schultz et al., 1997). After behaviors are learned, a state of expectation about the time of occurrence of reward delivery relative to requested behaviors is created (Apicella et al., 1991, 1992; Schultz et al., 1992, 1993).

It has also been suggested that during goal-oriented behavior NS neurons exhibit context-dependent behavioral responses that may vary depending on changes in the predictability of the linkage between stimuli and rewards (Schultz and Romo, 1990; Apicella et al., 1992; Schultz et al., 1992; Mirenowicz and Schultz, 1994). Moreover, several lines of evidence indicate that the NS neuronal activity may become better related to movements and sensory cues when behavioral conditions are novel (Mirenowicz and Schultz, 1994; Nelson et al., 1996; Berns et al., 1997). Sensitivity to novelty seems to be a property of neurons in the substantia nigra, the ventral striatum, and the prefrontal cortex (Apicella et al., 1991; Schultz et al., 1992, 1993; Watanabe, 1996; Berns et al., 1997; Schultz, 2010). Surmeier and Kitai (1997) indicated that the dopaminergic inputs to neostriatum may "shape" the activity of NS neurons involved in motor behavior. Therefore, the substantia nigra, ventral striatum and prefrontal cortex may influence segments of the so-called "motor loop" (which includes the dorsal striatum) where pre-movement activity (PMA) often occurs (Alexander et al., 1986; Hoover and Strick, 1993; Graybiel et al., 1994; Watanabe, 1996; Berns et al., 1997).

We hypothesize that primate dorsal striatum (Putamen and Caudate Nucleus) is part of a system that modulates the behavioral parameters (i.e., movement kinematics: position, speed, and acceleration), depending on the probability of the expected reward (Fu et al., 1995; Fiorillo et al., 2003; Lee and Assad, 2003; Stark et al., 2007; Pekny et al., 2015; Reppert et al., 2015). Dorsal striatum may be responsible for enhancing movement vigor when rewards are certain and decreasing the vigor when rewards become uncertain (Turner and Desmurget, 2010; Opris et al., 2011a). This hypothesis is supported by the finding that changes in dorsal striatal activity occur shortly after go cues and clearly earlier than the movements (100–200 ms before movements). Therefore, *certain rewards* may mediate a stronger correlation (Opris et al., 2011a) between neostriatal PMA and the kinematics of wrist movements.

Below, we describe the changes in NS neuronal activity in relation to movement kinematics by using a multilinear regression analysis (Ashe and Georgopoulos, 1994). Furthermore, we believe that striatal modulations can provide a good motor signal for neuroprosthetics (Lebedev and Nicolelis, 2006; Nicolelis and Lebedev, 2009). The goals of this study was to: (a) determine if the correlation between NS firing rates and the movement kinematics varies as a function of go-cue modality, movement directions, behavioral contexts; and (b) quantify the occurrence and timing of best relationship/correlation between NS neuronal activity and hand movement kinematics. Moreover, since changes in movement related NS activity often occur 100–200 ms before movements, it is possible that unpredictable behavioral conditions modify NS activity that is involved in movement preparation and initiation. The results are relevant for the decoding of wrist kinematics for building an upper-limb neuroprosthesis (Lebedev et al., 2005; Aggarwal et al., 2009).

MATERIALS AND METHODS

Experimental Apparatus and Behavioral Paradigm

Two adult male rhesus monkeys (*Macaca mulatta*: E, N) were trained to make wrist flexion and extension movements in response to vibratory or visual stimuli (Lebedev and Nelson, 1995; Liu et al., 2005; Opris et al., 2011a). The monkeys were cared for in accordance with the National Research Council Guide for the Care and Use of Laboratory Animals. Experimental protocols were approved by the Animal Care and Use Committee of The University of Tennessee Health Science Center, Memphis. Detailed descriptions of the experimental apparatus have been provided elsewhere (Gardiner and Nelson, 1992; Lebedev and Nelson, 1995; Liu et al., 2005, 2008). A brief description is provided below.

Each monkey sat in an acrylic monkey chair, with its right palm on a movable plate (**Figure 1A**). One end of the plate was attached to the axle of a brushless D.C. torque motor (Colburn and Evarts, 1978). A load of 0.07 Nm was applied to the plate. The load assisted wrist extensions and opposed wrist flexions. Feedback of current wrist position was provided by a visual display consisting of 31 light-emitting diodes (LEDs), located 35 cm in front of the animal. The middle, red LED corresponded to a centered wrist position. Yellow LEDs (above and below the middle LED) indicated successive angular deviations of 1°. Two instructional LEDs were located in the upper left corner of the visual display. When the first red LED was illuminated at the start of a trial, it indicated that extension movements should be made; otherwise flexions were required. When the second, green LED was illuminated, it informed the monkey that the go-cue for that trial would be a palmar vibration; otherwise, the go-cue was the illumination of one of two LEDs which were each 5° from the center. Vibratory go-cues of 27, 57, and 127 Hz were routinely used. In this paper we consider only records of neuronal activity triggered by vibratory cues at 57 Hz and/or visual go-cues.

The behavioral paradigm is illustrated schematically in **Figure 1B** and the partition of reaction time (RT) interval in **Figure 1C**. Each trial began when the monkey centered the plate. At this time a movement direction request was given by the instructional LED as described above. The monkey was required to hold the plate in the centered position for 0.5, 1.0, 1.5, 2.0 s (pseudo-randomized) without moving, until a go cue (visual or vibrotactile) was presented. If the animal moved prior to the completion of the hold period, the trial was canceled. If the monkey made the requested movement of 5° or greater, he received a fruit juice reward. The reward delivery for blocks of 10 trials per direction was pseudorandom with correct performance being rewarded on average 75% of the time. Two unrewarded trials were never imposed sequentially. The type of trials under this pseudorandom reward schedule included: (i) rewarded trials, for which the current and the immediately

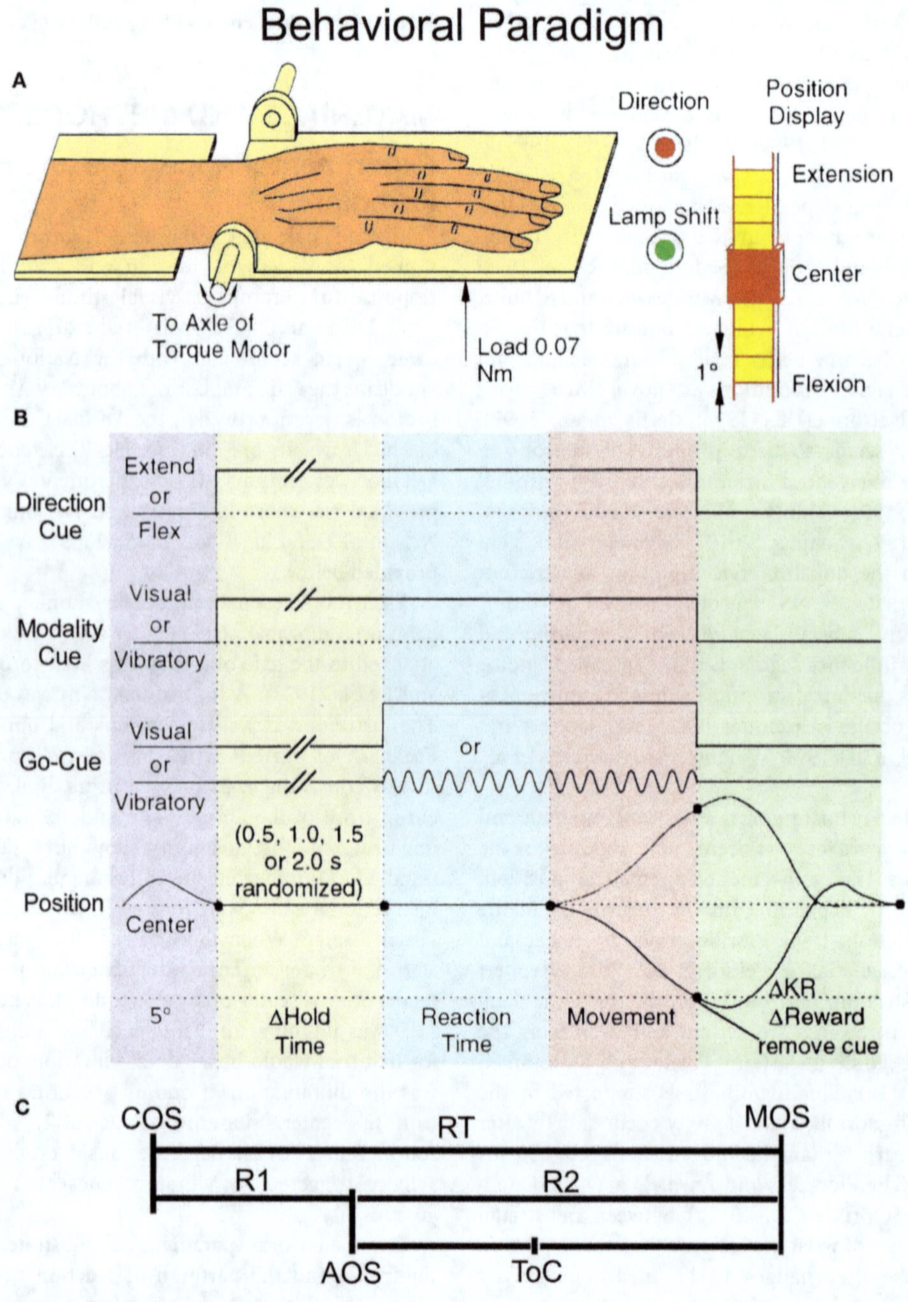

FIGURE 1 | Behavioral paradigm. (A) The experimental setup showing monkey's hand on the handle together with the instruction LEDs. **(B)** Schematic diagram of the unpredictable task. The direction cue was given by a red LED that was illuminated during extension trials, but not during flexion trials. The modality cue was a green LED that was illuminated during vibratory cued trials but not during visually cued trials. The onset of these instructional cues was coincident with the onset of the hold period. They remained lit until the end of the trial, coincident with reward delivery. Go-cues that signaled the monkeys could initiate wrist movements were presented after a variable time delay of 0.5, 1.0, 1.5, or 2.0 s (pseudo-randomized). **(C)** Divisions of the Reaction Time (RT) interval. RT has been split into two intervals: R1, the latency from cue onset (COS) to premovement activity onset (AOS), and R2, the time from AOS until movement onset (MOS). ToC represents the time of best correlation (time at best CoD).

preceding trial were rewarded, called regular ("R") trials, (ii) unrewarded trials, and (iii) trials immediately following withheld rewards, called after ("A") trials or *certain reward* trials (while reward in all other trials was *uncertain*). In some instances there were trials in which the animal failed to perform properly (i.e., made a movement in the wrong direction). For analyses we required that each neuron must have at least 4 valid trials per condition. If any single group of records had fewer than 4 trials, the data from that group were not included in the analyses.

Electrophysiological Recordings and Histology

Once an animal reached a stable daily performance level (~2000 rewarded trials per experimental session), it was prepared for recording. A stainless steel recording chamber was surgically implanted over the skull to allow for extracellular recordings of the activity of basal ganglia neurons by using platinum-iridium microelectrodes with impedances of 1–2 MOhms (see Nelson et al., 1991; Gardiner and Nelson, 1992). Transdural penetrations began no sooner than 1 week after the chamber implantation. In each recording session, a microelectrode was lowered into the striatum and the activity of single units was amplified, discriminated, and stored in a computer by conventional means (Lebedev and Nelson, 1995; Liu et al., 2005). Neuronal receptive fields (RFs) were examined by lightly touching punctuate skin surfaces, manipulating joints, and palpating muscles. On occasion, the electromyographic (EMG) activity patterns of forearm muscles acting across the wrist were recorded using intramuscular EMG wires (see Nelson, 1987). EMG activity was converted into pulse data (Nelson, 1987; Vaadia et al., 1988). On the last recording day, electrolytic lesions were made to mark some recording locations by passing 10 μA of current for 10–20 s. These lesions provided references for the histological reconstruction of the recording sites. The animal was then deeply anesthetized with sodium pentobarbital and transcardially perfused with 10% buffered formol-saline. The brain was removed from the skull, and cut on a freezing microtome into 50 μm thick coronal sections. Histological sections of the basal ganglia (**Figure 2**) were stained for Nissl substance. Recording sites were reconstructed based on the depth of each electrode penetration and its location with respect to the marking lesions (Nelson, 1988; Nelson et al., 1991).

Data Analysis

Neuronal activity data, recorded on-line (Lebedev and Nelson, 1995, 1996; Liu et al., 2005; Opris et al., 2011a), were processed by off-line analysis programs and displayed as rasters, peri-event time histogram (PETH), fractional interspike interval (ISI) histogram (FISIH; Ashe and Georgopoulos, 1994), and traces of position, velocity, and acceleration, aligned on important events in the animal's behavior. A multilinear regression analysis (Ashe and Georgopoulos, 1994) has been used to regress low-pass filtered single trial spike functions coming from a FISIH, against position, velocity, and acceleration traces.

Multilinear Regression Analysis

An important step in our implementation of the regression analysis is the formulation of a FISIH from single trial neuronal activity records. We followed almost precisely the published methods (Ashe and Georgopoulos, 1994; Taira et al., 1996). This type of histogram is a filtered version of a binned PETH, in which the fraction of each ISI that is distributed across a given bin is calculated. The whole ISI is equal to unity, whereas each bin receives fractional contributions relative to the interval of that bin. We have employed single trial FISIHs, as well as, composite FISIH representing up to 40 trials. Each spike train was binned in 5 ms bins and the time-varying frequency of cell discharge, d(t), was computed from FISIHs. The resulting spike function, f(t), was smoothed using a 5-point low-pass filter, then the squared root of each point comprising the function was taken (Cox and Lewis, 1966; Ashe and Georgopoulos, 1994) and the resultant was divided by the binwidth (bw; in seconds), to convert this function to units proportional to the instantaneous firing rate:

$$f(t) = \mathrm{sqrt}(d(t))/bw \tag{1}$$

The position trace was smoothed using a single 5-point low-pass filter while the velocity and acceleration were obtained from the smoothed position trace as single or double discrete time derivatives.

A multilinear regression algorithm (Sokal and Rohlf, 1981) was applied to epochs of single trials so that portion of the single trial FISIH was expressed as a function of the animal's hand position, velocity, and acceleration during the initial phase of the movement. The regression analysis compares, on a trial-by-trial basis (**Figure 3A**), the frequency of cell discharge, f, at time $t_0 + \tau$, where τ is the variable time shift of a "sliding window" (**Figure 3B**), relative to movement onset, and the duration of t_0 is equal to the movement time. The window was advanced in time steps of 5 ms over the behaviorally important epoch T (the number of steps being T/bw). The variable T is defined as the interval that begins 50 ms after the cue onset, and ends at the time at which the movement reached amplitude of 5° from center. The square root of the discharge frequency, f, at time $t_0 + \tau$, was expressed as a function of the position (°), velocity (°/sec), and acceleration (°/sec^2) of monkey's hand at time t_1, where t_1 always began at movement onset (MOS). The regression equation is:

$$\begin{aligned} f(t_0 + t) &= \mathrm{const} + c1\varphi1(t1) + c2\varphi2(t1) + c3\varphi3(t1) \\ &+ \varepsilon,\ t_0 + \tau < T\ \mathrm{and} |t_0| = |t1| \end{aligned} \tag{2}$$

where c1, c2, and c3 are the regression coefficients of position, velocity, and acceleration. The terms $\varphi1(t1)$, $\varphi2(t1)$ and $\varphi3(t1)$ are the time-dependent variables of position, velocity, and acceleration, and ε is an error term. The coefficient of determination (CoD) is defined as the proportion of variance accounted for by the neuronal activity-to-movement correlation. Average CoDs were calculated only for valid trials having significant activity changes within the period of consideration.

The output of the regression analysis program provided averaged values of the CoD together with the time shift representing the time of best correlation (ToC) at which the best CoD occurred, as well as the partial regression coefficients at that point. The values of CoD ranged from 0 (the absence of correlation) to 1, where a full correlation of spike function and movement variables occurs. The analysis has been performed on single trial basis, but the results are displayed in normalized composite histograms for convenience and clarity (**Figures 3A,C**).

The changes in neuronal activity and their relationship to movement initiation and/or execution can be easily appreciated by visually estimating the outline of the composite histogram. FISIH patterns depict the activity of a cell, as indicated by the shape of the composite histogram and the site ToC relative to the shape of the composite histogram.

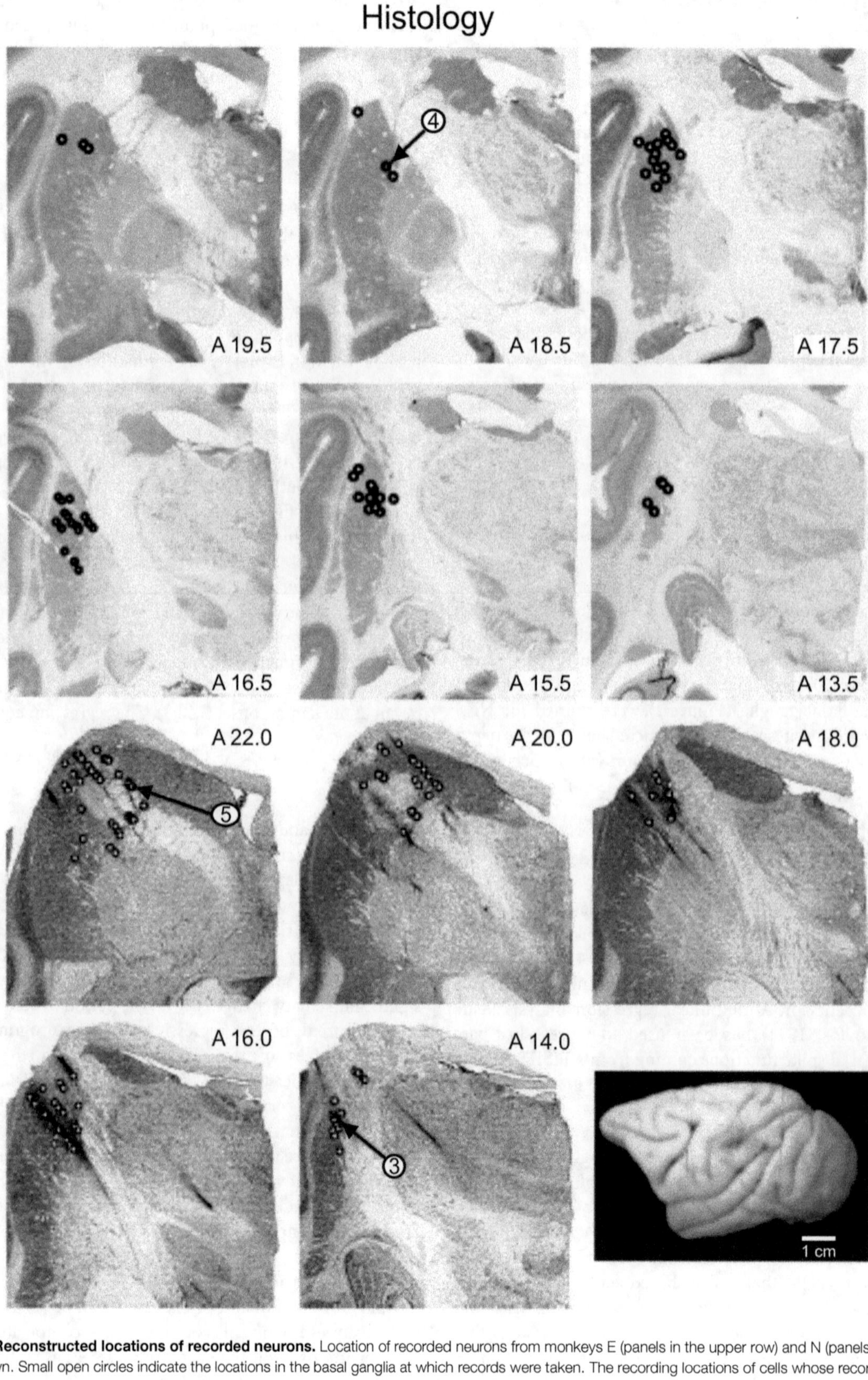

FIGURE 2 | Reconstructed locations of recorded neurons. Location of recorded neurons from monkeys E (panels in the upper row) and N (panels in the lower row) are shown. Small open circles indicate the locations in the basal ganglia at which records were taken. The recording locations of cells whose records have been illustrated are indicated by the arrows. A drawing of the dorsolateral surface of monkey E is shown in the lower right panel.

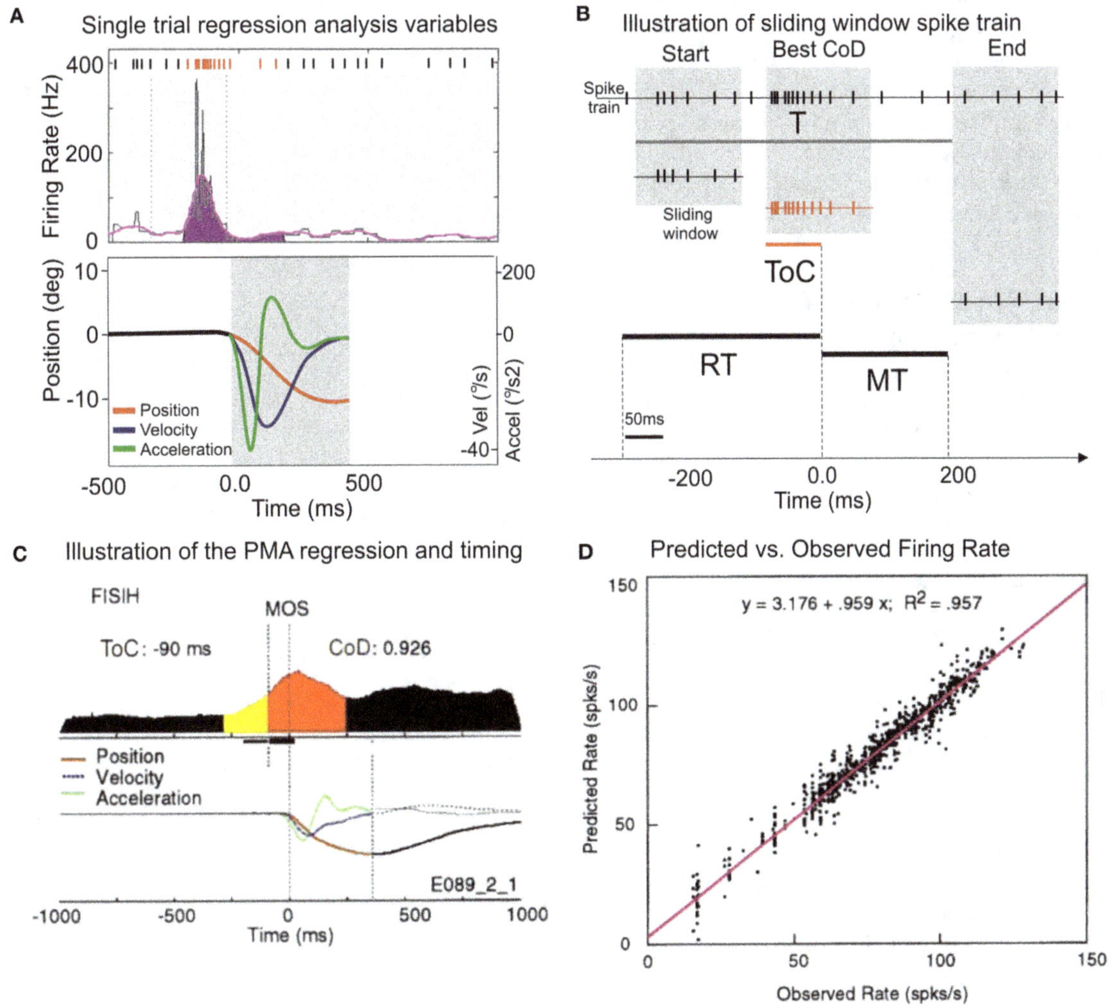

FIGURE 3 | Illustration of the application of multilinear regression analysis. (A) A single trial histogram of the neuronal activity expressed as mean firing rate (in spikes/s), together with the kinematic variables of position, velocity, and accelaration. **(B)** Illustration of the sliding window regression analysis. RT, reaction time; MT, movement time; ToC is the time of best correlation (at best CoD). **(C)** A typical putamen neuron with increased premovement activity during vibratory cued trials is shown. The display of the average kinematics for uncertain reward flexion trials R, are centered on MOS, on both panels. **(D)** The scatter diagram of the predicted discharge rate plotted against the observed rate. Regression equation of predicted vs. observed mean firing rates and the regression coefficient in the upper part of the panel.

Analysis of Changes in Neuronal Activity

The changes of neuronal activity associated with wrist movement were analyzed using multilinear regression in single trial (**Figure 3A**). Data from a putamen neuron, recorded during vibratory cued "R" trials, is presented in **Figure 3C**. The baseline activity (Bkg) of each recorded neuron was calculated as its mean firing rate during the 250 ms prior to the presentation of go-cues, while the animal held his wrist in a centered position. The first change in the cumulative sum of more than three standard deviations (SDs), lasting for at least 40 ms, was designated as the activity onset (Onset or AOS). The total number of spikes occurring from AOS until movement onset (**Figure 3C** the yellow segment) divided by the interval divided by the number of trials was designated as the cell's pre-movement firing response (Resp). Mean firing rates of Bkg and Resp (4.9 and 24.7 spikes/s) together with the AOS (−147 ms) are further compared across cells and conditions (see **Figure 6B**). The period between AOS and MOS (R2) is defined in **Figure 1C**.

The regression analysis describes the covariant relationship between changes in NS activity and movement variables. The best covariance between activity and kinematics (cT) occurred ~90 ms before MOS. The average CoD of this cell was 0.926 and indicates that the neuronal activity has 92.6% of the variance explained by the multilinear regression analysis. This implies that the correlation between neuronal activity and the subsequent movement occurred at a time that proceeds the average onset time of electromyographic activity in this task (Gardiner and Nelson, 1992; Lebedev and Nelson, 1995). The time course of position, velocity, and acceleration are displayed beneath the FISIH; the regression analysis is described by Equation (2). To compare the actual firing properties with those predicted by the regression model, **Figure 3D** shows a scatter-gram of the predicted discharge rate plotted against the observed rate. Each column of dots is a trial, and each window shift is a dot. The plot indicates a consistent linear relationship between the predicted firing rate as calculated by the regression model and the rate recorded during experiments. This relationship suggests that the methods are reliable and compatible with those used by other investigators (Ashe and Georgopoulos, 1994; Taira et al., 1996).

Quantitative Criteria for PMA Directionality

To determine the directionality of PMA, we calculated the difference between the Resp and the Bkg, and dubbed this difference the activity change (Act). In the cases in which Act was <1 spike/s, Act was recorded as 0 spike/s. If the sign of Act for a neuron differed as a function of movement direction, then that neuron was classified as "reciprocal" (encoding both flexions and extensions). In addition, we compared Act for flexion and extension movements and calculated their difference and sum. The ratio between difference and sum yields a scalar that should theoretically range between −1 and +1. Cases in which the ratio was −1 or +1, corresponded to those in which there was no change in activity for one direction of movement. These were coded as "directional." Cases in which the scalar was > +1 or < −1 were instances in which PMA had the opposite sign as a function of movement direction, and were thus "reciprocal." For those cases with scalars between −1 and +1, we took the standard score of the mean value, (about zero) and then defined cases that were between ±2 SDs from the mean and the extremes as being "directional." Cases with values falling within the ±2 SD limits were classified as non-directional. The distribution of PMA directionality of NS neurons by location is shown in **Table 1**.

TABLE 1 | The distribution of recorded neurons by location.

Category	Putamen		Caudate		Bridge		Total	
Recorded cells	104	73%	20	14%	18	13%	142	100%
RFs tested	81	78%	16	80%	16	89%	113	80%
Cutaneous	7	9%	1	6%	2	13%	10	7%
Deep	27	33%	3	19%	4	25%	34	24%
No Clear RF	47	58%	12	75%	10	62%	69	49%
PMA								
Cue	11	11%	2	10%	1	6%	14	10%
Movement	85	82%	17	85%	17	94%	119	84%
Intermediate	8	8%	1	5%	0	0%	9	6%
PMA DIR R Trials								
Reciprocal	36	35%	6	30%	5	28%	47	13%
Directional	4	4%	0	0%	0	0%	4	3%
Non-Directional	64	62%	14	70%	13	72%	91	64%
PMA DIR A Trials								
Reciprocal	35	34%	5	25%	3	17%	43	30%
Directional	2	2%	1	5%	0	0%	3	2%
Non-Directional	67	67%	14	70%	15	83%	96	68%

RF type and RF location. PMA relationship to cue and movement. PMA changes during certain/uncertain "A" and "R" trials.

Statistical Analysis

Analyses of the characteristics of activity-to-movement relationships for different NS neurons were examined for statistical significance using repeated measures ANOVA, including Scheffe's *post hoc* test and *t*-test. The observations were also checked using the nonparametric Mann Whitney *U*-test and Kruskal–Wallis tests to determine the significance levels of the differences in CoDs and ToCs, for groups separated by trial type (regular or after), go-cue (visual or vibratory), and movement direction (flexion or extension).

RESULTS

Database

A total of 236 recorded neurons, 142 (~60%) were selected, because each neuron: (i) had activity changes (PMA) following the vibratory or visual go-cue onset and prior to MOS, (ii) had a PMA firing rate that was at least 3 SDs different from the Bkg activity firing rate, and (iii) was held long enough to record at least 25 trials for each movement direction. Of these, 102/142 (~72%) also had a complete set of recordings during visually cued trials. Of the selected NS neurons, 104/142 (~73%) neurons were located in putamen, 20/142 (~14%) in the caudate nucleus, and 18/142 (~13%) in the cellular bridges in between these structures. We eliminated 3/142 neurons from consideration because their activity was completely suppressed during the PMA interval. Also, the activity of 3/142 neurons during flexion movements and of 7/142 neurons during extension movements had CoDs outside the range that included ±4 SDs from the distribution of the main population and were thus excluded as outliers. This left for statistical consideration the records of 136/142 (96%) cells for flexion movements and 130/142 (92%) cells for extensions. Receptive fields (RF) were found for 44/142 (~31%) NS neurons; 69/136 (~49%) had no clear RFs and 29/142 (~20%) were not tested. Of the cells exhibiting RFs, 10/44 had cutaneous RFs and 34/44 had deep RFs. **Table 1** shows the distribution of NS neurons by location and RF type.

The activity patterns of the striatal neurons could not be defined as a homogeneous group. Separation was required because these neurons had significant differences in their activity-to-movement relationship as a function of trial type, cue, movement direction, and location revealed by factorial ANOVA and Scheffe's *post hoc* comparisons. Therefore, our data were grouped by these variables.

PMA and Movement Initiation

Significant changes in neuronal activity, defined as a deviation of at least ±3 SDs from the baseline that lasted more than 40 ms (see Nelson and Douglas, 1989; Gardiner and Nelson, 1992) were commonly related either to the go-cue or to the movement. Neuronal firing changes were considered to be cue-related if they occurred in a consistent temporal relationship with the cue and followed its presentation after a relatively short latency (<100 ms). Of the total number, 14/142 (~10%) had cue-related activity, while 9/142 (~6%) had very early PMA which we termed "intermediate" responses. Each of these also had movement related activity as did the 119/142 (~84%) which show activity changes only in relationship to movement onset (see **Table 1** for their distribution by location). Significant changes in firing rate that were time locked with MOS, but that preceded MOS, were considered to be PMA (Gardiner and Nelson, 1992; Lebedev et al., 1994; Lebedev and Nelson, 1995; Opris et al., 2011a). Changes in neuronal firing rates that occurred during the execution of wrist movement (i.e., from MOS until potential reward delivery) were classified as "movement-associated activity." Movement related cells exhibiting PMA may be involved in either movement initiation or execution, depending on the time of occurrence of their activity changes.

Neural Activity to Movement Kinematics Relationship

Consistent with the motor role of dorsal striatum, the firing rate of a subpopulation of neurons in putamen reflect the encoding of hand kinematics (position, velocity, and acceleration).

Examples of Differential Firing during Encoding of Hand Position

Figure 4A shows the PMA of a putamen neuron classified as "reciprocal" that exhibits a strong suppression during flexion trials while during extension trials this cell's firing is substantially increased. This differential mean firing rate during flexion and extension movements likely reflects the encoding of hand position in the two opposite movement directions (flexions and extensions). At the population level, the encoding of position occurred in 47/142 (33%) VIB cued neurons during uncertain reward "R" trials and 43/142 (30%) during certain reward "A" trials, and in 32/102 VIS cued neurons during uncertain reward "R" trials and of 38/102 NS neurons during certain reward "A" trials. Only 4 NS neurons were "directional" during "R" trials and three cells were "directional" during "A" trials. A minority of the population changed the type of direction-related activity between "R" and "A" trials.

The non-directional NS cell subpopulation which included the vast majority of the studied neurons (*vibration cues*: 91/142 neurons during "R" trials and 96/142 neurons during "A" trials; *visual cues*: 66/102 neurons during "R" trials and 60/102 neurons during "A" trials) had characteristics consistent with the encoding of the magnitude of the position (distance from the center) shown for the population, as a whole, in **Tables 1, 2**. This type of non-directional modulation was noticed in most of the cells, regardless of go-cue modality. That is, the sign of the activity changes of these neurons was the same regardless of the direction of the movements that followed the onset of this activity (Gardiner and Nelson, 1992).

Examples of Differential Firing with Hand Velocity and Acceleration Encoding

In **Figure 4B** is shown the PMA of a putamen neuron, cued by vibratory stimuli ("A" trials) with firing rate mimicking the velocity profile (on the left). On the other hand, **Figure 4C** shows a sharper PMA modulation of a putamen neuron, cued by visual stimuli ("A" trials) with firing rate mimicking the acceleration profile (on the right). It is noticeable a sharper firing peak encoding acceleration that is accompanied by a deeper inhibition trough than in the case of cell encoding velocity. Bkg and Resp firing rates (**Figures 4B,C**) were again slightly higher during "A" trials (not shown) than in "R" trials.

Neural Activity-to-Movement Kinematics Analysis

The regression analysis described above was used to investigate changes in NS activity associated with movement initiation under two conditions. Comparisons were made between trials with uncertain rewards ("R" trials) and trials with certain rewards ("A" trials). We illustrate the activity patterns of a representative putamen neuron recorded during vibratory go-cue trials, in **Figure 5A**, and the pattern of the same neuron recorded during visual go-cue trials, in **Figure 5B**. The records of "R" trials (left panel, **Figure 5A**) and "A" trials (right panel, **Figure 5A**) are illustrated for flexion movements. This cell exhibited an increased discharge, before MOS (**Figure 5A**), and thus PMA preceding wrist flexion (position traces displayed for both "R" and "A" conditions). The neuron was more active in the blocks of vibratory cued "A" trials than during R trials (left panel, **Figure 5A**). Bkg and Resp were also higher when rewards were certain. In addition to PMA changes associated with unpredictable reward conditions, this putamen neuron's activity became better correlated with animal's movement. This is accompanied by changes in the average CoDs, which were greater during "A" trials than during "R" trials (0.941 vs. 0.920). The time occurrence of the best correlation (ToC) was ~117 ms before MOS during "A" trials and ~99 ms, during regular reward.

This same putamen neuron, whose visually cued trial records are shown in **Figure 5B** exhibited a higher firing rate during the "A" trials for flexion movement under this cueing condition, as well. The Bkg and Resp are higher during "A" trials (26.8 and 52.2 spks/s) than during regularly "R" rewarded ones (21.3 and 49.3 spks/s). The PMA changes occur quite early, before MOS. The increase in CoDs in "A" trials, as compared with "R" trials, indicates that PMA becomes better correlated with the movement after withheld rewards (0.954 vs. 0.942). Comparing the neuronal activity during visual go-cue trials with vibratory go-cue trials, one can note an average increase (of 10 spks/s) in the mean firing rate of PMA that occurred during the former. However, average CoDs during visually cued A trials were greater than during cued trials (0.954 vs. 0.941).

At the population level, NS firing was significantly higher in the Resp vs. Bkg conditions for the majority of cells ($p < 0001$, *post hoc*). However, when comparing mean firing rate across trial type, go-cue type or movement direction the effects varied (see **Table 2**). Bkg and Resp firing rates were slightly higher during "A" vs. "R" trials (**Figure 5C**) and during VIS vs. VIB trials ($P < 0.001$, *post hoc*; $n = 91$ vs. 66).

Additional information about the timing of this relationship can be derived from the examination of the time of occurrence of best CoDs i.e., (ToCs), which indicate the time of best CoDs at either MOS or AOS, respectively (see **Table 2**). A comparison of PMA onsets and ToCs for vibratory cued trials

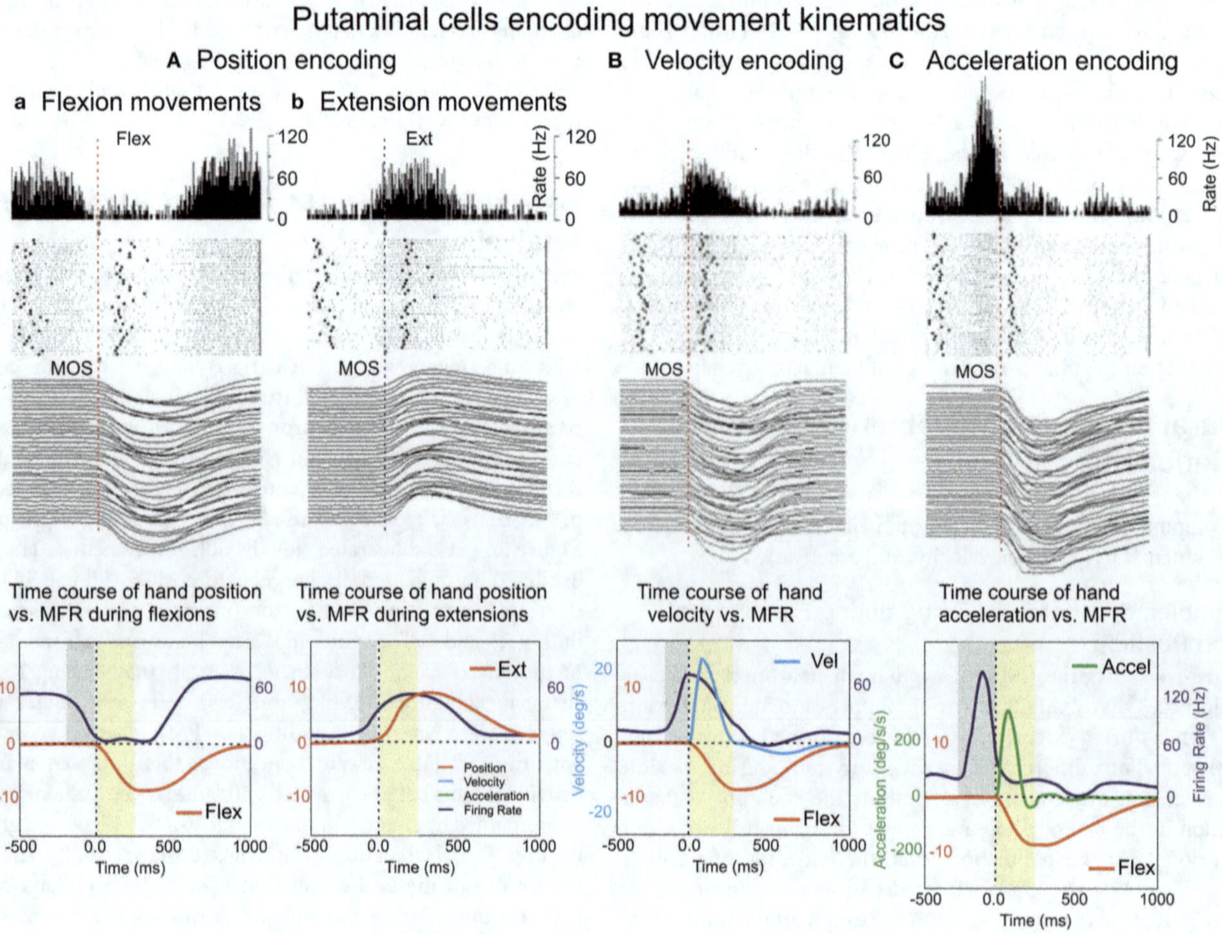

FIGURE 4 | Examples of encoding the variables of movement kinematics. Putamen neurons show encoding of hand position (**Aa**, flexions and **b**, for extensions) movement velocity **(B)** and acceleration **(C)**. Peri-event histograms (PEHs), rasters, and movement trajectories were plotted for R flexions and extensions **(Aa,b)**, velocity **(B)**, and acceleration **(C)**. The PEHs of the neuronal activity expressed as mean firing rate (in spikes/s), with a bin size equal to 5 ms and a raster display. In the raster display, rows represent individual trials, dots represent single spikes, while the left and right bold dots represent vibratory cue onset and reward delivery, respectively.

TABLE 2 | The means and standard deviations for Bkg and Resp neural activity, premovement onset R2s, time of best regression/correlation ToC, and the coefficients of determination CoD for flexions and extensions trials, under certain vs. uncertain rewards.

Go Cue	Vibratory				Visual			
Direction	**Flexions**		**Extensions**		**Flexions**		**Extensions**	
Trial Type	**R Trials**	**A Trials**	**R Trials**	**A Trials**	**R Trials**	**A Trials**	**R Trials**	**A Trials**
Bkg (Hz)	21 ± 14	21 ± 14	20 ± 14	21 ± 13	19 ± 13	20 ± 14	20 ± 14	20 ± 13
Resp (Hz)	25 ± 16	26 ± 16	24 ± 14	25 ± 14	24 ± 15	24 ± 16	24 ± 14	24 ± 14
R2 (ms)	187 ± 74	160 ± 54	173 ± 52	158 ± 49	228 ± 70	215 ± 60	185 ± 42	185 ± 50
ToC (ms)	88 ± 70	84 ± 60	73 ± 62	68 ± 58	154 ± 59	161 ± 52	121 ± 51	121 ± 46
CoD	0.871 ± 0.054	0.888 ± 0.056	0.861 ± 0.054	0.867 ± 0.054	0.902 ± 0.04	0.908 ± 0.033	0.903 ± 0.039	0.908 ± 0.033

Comparison between values for certain vs. uncertain rewards, in respectively, "A" and "R" trials. Statistical significance was determined using repeated measures ANOVA, including Scheffe's post hoc test and t-test (See Text for abbreviations).

is shown in **Figure 5D**. The ToCs during visually cued trials occur much earlier than during vibratory cue trials. The ToCs in "A" vs. "R" trials for flexion movements were significantly different only with visual go-cues (see **Table 2**). There was also a statistical significance in the ToCs for flexions and extensions triggered by visual cues (not shown). Although we were unable to distinguish between direction and load effects (since monkeys always performed the movements against a load which assisted

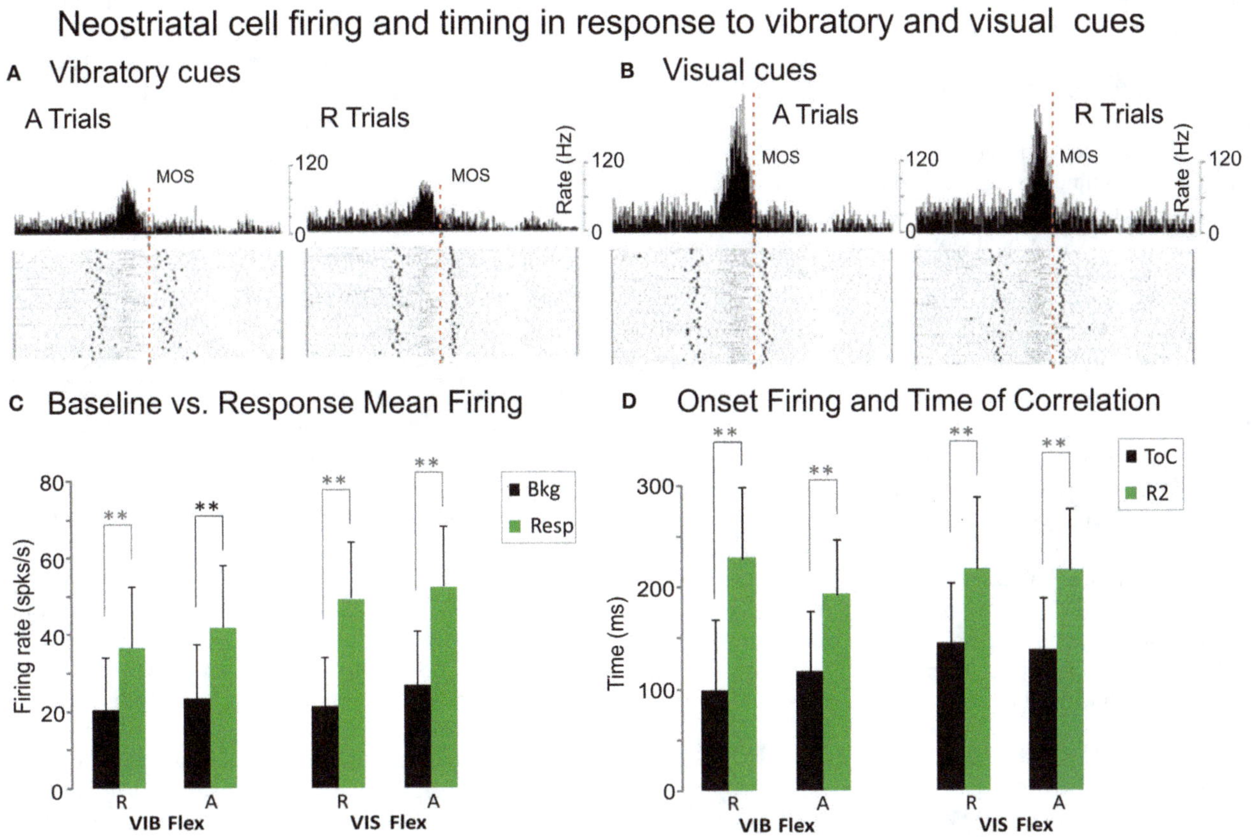

FIGURE 5 | Premovement firing and timing. (A,B) Example of putaminal cell that exhibited PMA under vibratory **(A)** and visual **(B)** stimuli. Each histogram illustrates neuronal activity expressed as mean firing rate together with raster displays aligned on MOS. The left panels display the NS activity during "A" flexion trials and the right panels represent the activity during "R" flexion trials. Wrist position traces for each trial are presented at the bottom of each panel. Coefficients of Determination (CoDs) which quantify the best relationship, are: 0.920 ± 0.044 during R trials and 0.941 ± 0.024 during "A" trials (**Figure 4A**). CoDs for R and A trials are: 0.942 ± 0.021 and 0.954 ± 0.021, (**Figure 4B**) respectively. This cell exhibited increased discharge during flexion movements that occurred well before MOS. Baseline firing BKG and RESP are higher during trials following withheld rewards than during R trials. PMA onsets together with ToCs suggest that the cell may have been involved in movement initiation. **(C)** Comparison of premovement mean firing rates of NS cells during baseline BKG and response RESP for flexions and extensions under vibratory and visual cues. **(D)** Comparison of the premovement activity timing for response onsets and of best correlation time ToC for flexions and extensions under vibratory and visual cues. Statistical significance was determined using repeated measures. $^{**}p < 0.001$ ANOVA, including Scheffe's *post hoc* test and *t*-test.

wrist extensions and opposed flexions), the effects of direction and load were evident through the fact that interfered with each other.

PMA onsets for single trials were measured relative to two events: go-cue onsets (COS) and movement onsets (MOS; see **Figure 1**). R1s, measured from COS, during vibrotactile stimulation, for both flexion and extension movements were significantly shorter in the A trials (see **Table 2**). R2s, measured from MOS, were calculated by subtracting the R1 from the RT (**Figure 1**). Flexion movements had R2s that were significantly shorter during "A" trials regardless of go-cue modality. Thus, PMA during vibratory cued trials started ~27 ms closer to MOS in the "A" trials when compared with "R" trials. During visually cued flexion trials, it started closer to MOS by ~13 ms. R2s were significantly different during visually cued flexion and extension movements, but not different during vibratory cued trials.

Statistical analyses of the activity-movement kinematics relation under unpredictable reward conditions are presented in **Table 2**. We have considered the trial type as a repeated measure and split each of the PMA-related variables by the go cue type and movement direction. Significant differences in the variables between conditions ("R" and "A" trials) were obtained by repeated measures ANOVA.

Coefficients of Determination

A measure of the correlation's strength in "R" and "A" trials is provided by the average CoDs. In general, the average CoDs showed a tight relationship between NS neuronal activity and monkey's kinematics (see **Table 2**). Flexion movement CoDs were significantly greater during "A" trials than during "R" trials ($p < 0.01$; ANOVA) regardless of the modality of go cues (see **Table 2**). The occurrence of enhanced activity-to-movement correlation in trials following withheld rewards is illustrated in

Figure 6. Cumulative sum plots of CoDs for "R" and "A" trials show a consistent shift to the right for the "A" trials ($p < 0.001$ for vibratory flexions; $p < 0.01$ for vibratory extensions; $p < 0.01$ for visual flexions; $p \sim$ ns for visual extensions; ANOVA), independent of go-cue modality.

There was also a directional effect, in that CoDs after withheld rewards were significantly greater during flexion trials than during extension trials ($p < 0.001$ for flexions; $p < 0.01$, for extensions, ANOVA), for both vibratory cued trials and visually cued trials (**Table 2**). In general, there was a better correlation of NS neuronal activity with kinematics in visual go-cue trials compared with that in vibratory go-cue trials ($p < 0.001$ for flexions). The average CoDs for visually cued flexions during "A" trials were greater during vibratory go-cued flexion "A" trials.

Given the existence of the activity-to-movement relationship (measured by the CoD) during trials following withheld rewards, we noticed three distinct effects: first, an effect of unpredictable reward which results in a better activity-to-movement correlation for certain rewarded "A" trials than for "R" trials; second, a directional effect which results in a better correlation for flexion than for extension movements for both cues, and third, a modality effect as indicated by better relationship for visually cued as compared with vibratory cued movements.

Electromyographic Activity

We compared average onsets of electromyographic (EMG) activity between flexion (**Figure 7A**) and extension (**Figure 7B**) movements for both "Regular" and "After" trials. With few exceptions, for most muscles the EMG activity starts earlier in the "After" trials than in "Regular" trials. Brachioradialis has the opposite trend in the "After" vs. "Regular" trials for both flexions and extensions. All together the EMG and behavioral measures seem to have a consistent agreement with NS pre-movement neural activity supporting the hypothesis that under certain rewards NS neuronal activity becomes better correlated to movement kinematics.

DISCUSSION

In the present study we recorded the activity of neostriatal neurons in two rhesus monkeys performing wrist movements in a pseudo-random reward task. We examined the relationship between PMA and kinematic variables (position, velocity, and acceleration) under three conditions: (a) reward contingency, (b) vibratory vs. visual go-cues, and (c) flexions vs. extensions movements (Opris et al., 2011a).

The results of this study indicate that NS neurons have PMA which is functionally correlated with movement kinematics. This correlation varies as a function of reward contingency (unpredictable vs. predictable delivery of reward for correct performance). Our goal was to determine whether there is a relationship between NS PMA and movement kinematics and to quantify this relationship in terms of coefficients of determination (CoDs) and relationship occurrence times (ToCs). These parameters varied significantly not only as a function of rewarding conditions, but also with variations in the modality of sensory triggering stimuli and with the direction of movement. In addition, we found that reaction times RTs and PMA onsets are also significantly different as a function of reward schedule and go-cue modality. These results suggest that it is likely that the NS is involved in sensorimotor-related activity that is combined with attentional, decision, and motivational influences (Schultz, 1997, 2010; Schultz et al., 1997; Opris and Bruce, 2005; Samejima et al., 2005).

Neural Firing to Movement Correlation Under Unpredictable Task

The statistically significant differences in CoDs for "R" and "A" trials may be related to attention and motivational factors associated with reward (Watanabe, 1996; Ueda and Kimura, 2003). Changes in the predictability of reward delivery, assumed to occur after withheld rewards, are accompanied by increases in CoDs and decreases in reaction times. Furthermore, changes in the predictability of reward delivery are accompanied by increases in CoDs, suggesting that the changes in CoDs are related to an animal's increased attention.

Differences in CoDs as a function of go-cue modality may be related to the gating of somatosensory inputs that often accompanies sensory-triggered movements. Our results indicate that the CoDs associated with NS neural activity during vibratory cued trials have significantly lower values as compared with those occurring during visual go-cued trials. Vibratory stimuli are one type of peripheral input to SI neurons that may be gated before active movements (Lebedev and Nelson, 1995). Because somatosensory cortex projects extensively to the neostriatum (see Parent and Hazrati, 1995 for review), it seems reasonable to suggest that gating in the cortex could ultimately result in modulation of NS activity. Changes in CoDs as a function of go-cue modality may be a reflection of alterations in cortical inputs to NS, as well as modulatory effects by dopaminergic systems (Lebedev and Nelson, 1995; Kiyatkin and Rebec, 1996). It has been suggested that changes in behavioral motivation may be mediated by dopaminergic neurons (Apicella et al., 1991; Schultz et al., 1992, 1993). Therefore, the dopaminergic pathways arising from the pars compacta of substantia nigra (SNc) and projecting to dorsal striatum (Lynd-Balta and Haber, 1994; Parent and Hazrati, 1995) may be involved in the motivational process underlying the learning and maintenance of goal driven behavior (Mirenowicz and Schultz, 1994; Schultz et al., 1997).

Statistically significant differences in CoDs between trials involving flexion and extension movements may be due to the fact that the movements were performed against a load which assisted wrist extensions and opposed flexions. Flexion trials had CoDs that were significantly higher than those during extension movements. The presence of the load may add a small contribution to the relationship during flexion movements or subtract that contribution when moving with the load (Liles, 1985; Alexander and Crutcher, 1990; Gardiner and Nelson, 1992). Sensorimotor territories of NS may also show differential firing as a result of cortical load effects, since it has been suggested that there are several parallel pathways of somatotopic input to NS (Alexander et al., 1986; Graybiel et al., 1994). Therefore, the difference in CoDs as a function of movement direction may be influenced by load, the movement direction itself, or both.

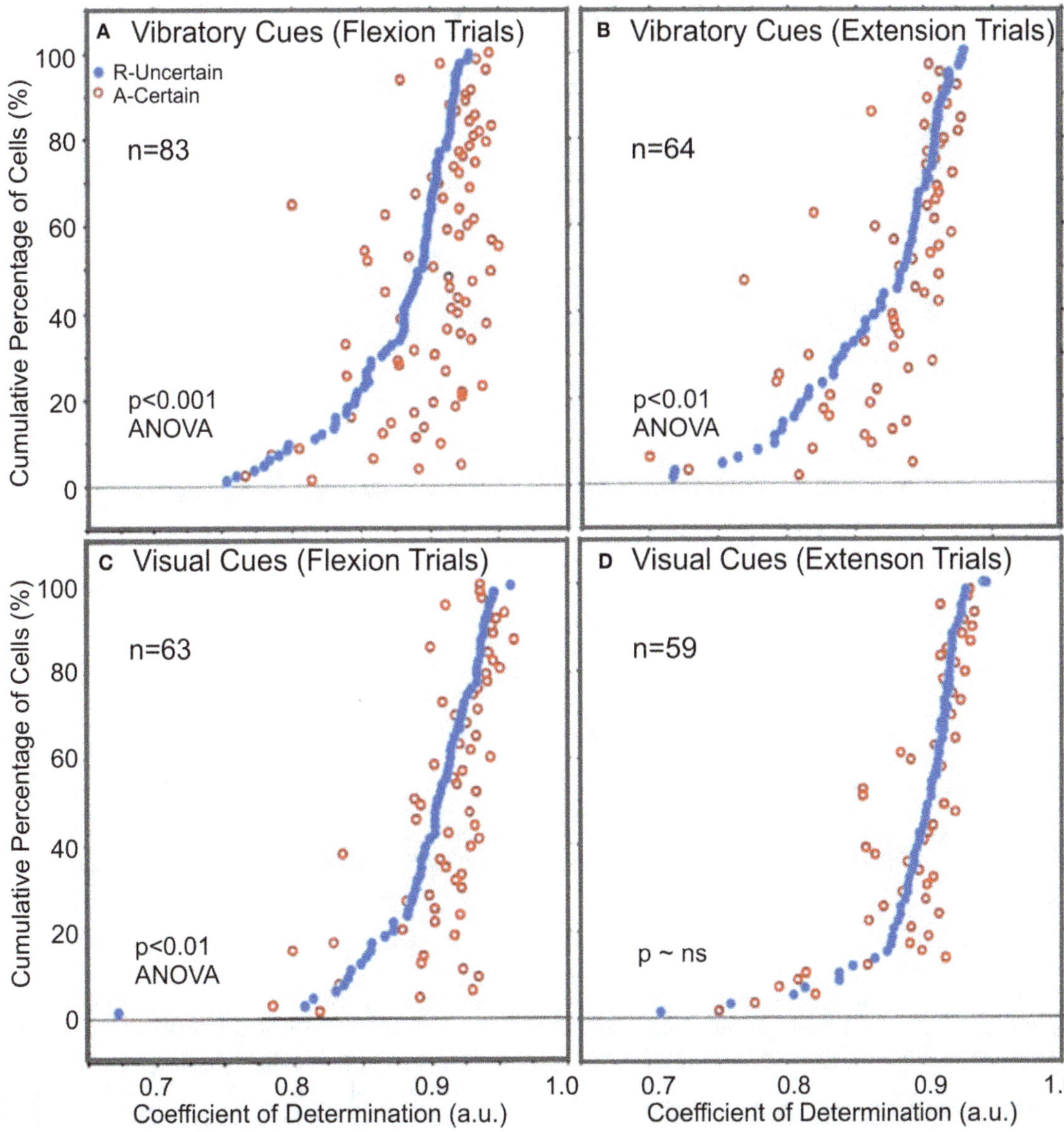

FIGURE 6 | The comparison of regression coefficients. Paired coefficients of determination, CoDs, for both vibratory and visually cued trials: **(A,B)** Certain "A" and uncertain "R" rewarded trials for vibratory cued trials and **(C,D)** for visually cued trials. In both instances, CoDs of the uncertain R trials (black dots) were arranged in ascending order from left to right. The certain trial CoDs corresponding to each uncertain trial CoDs were plotted at the appropriate height. Open dots to the right of the black dots indicate instances where the neuronal activity was better related (CoDs were greater) for movements made in the certain reward A trials.

Pre-movement Activity and Regression Times as a Function of Reward Schedule

In general, PMA activity was well correlated with wrist movement variables. The average CoD of the whole NS neuronal population was >0.85 for each modality, movement direction, recording location, and rewarding schedule. During vibratory cued trials which follow withheld rewards, there is a shift in PMA onset toward MOS despite the fact that reaction times become shorter. Schultz and co-workers have demonstrated that leftward shifts in the onset of activity occur in the firing patterns of dopaminergic neurons when tasks become more predictable (Schultz et al., 1992, 1993). The corollary of this would be that if the process was reversed and task requirements become more unpredictable, rightward shifts in activity onsets might be observed as was indeed observed in this study. Similar shifts in PMA were seen by Kimura (1990) when the amount of prior task information about behavioral requirements was varied. In our task, shifts in reaction times and PMA onsets, as shown in **Figure 6A**, occur after withheld rewards (Kimura et al., 2003; Churchland et al., 2006; Hori et al., 2009). Despite these shifts, the onsets of PMA and ToCs are early enough to suggest that the activity of NS neurons may be associated with the initiation

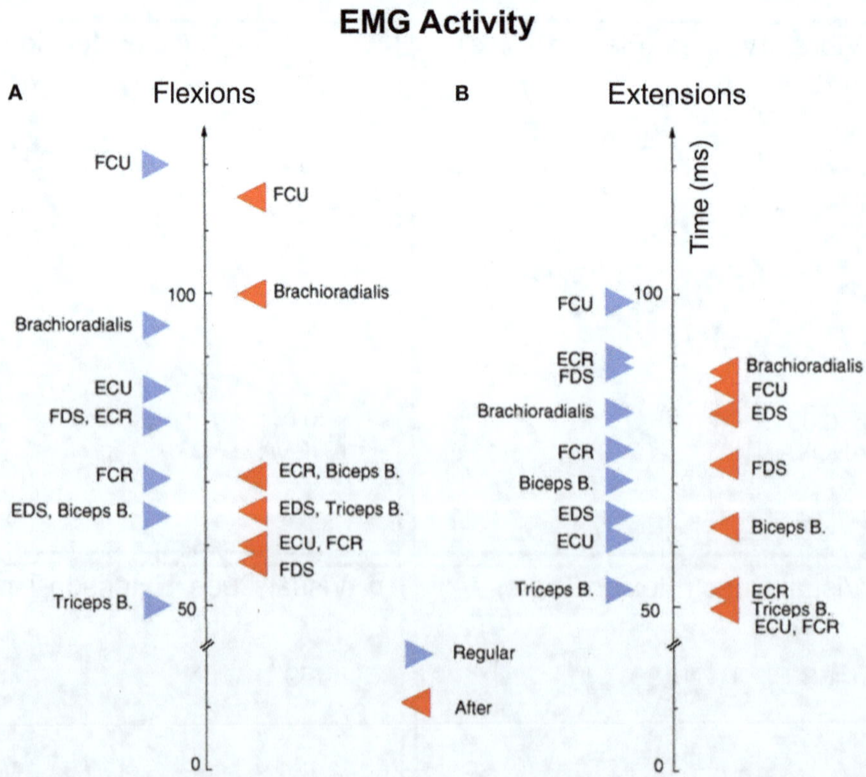

FIGURE 7 | Average onsets of electromyographic (EMG) activity. EMG activity between flexion **(A)** and extension **(B)** movements for both certain and uncertain reward trials. Each triangle (red for certain and blue for uncertain reward trials) represents the average EMG onset for at least 40 trials recorded consecutively. Biceps B, biceps brachii; BR, brachioradialis; ECR, extensor carpi radialis; ECU, extensor carpi ulnaris; EDS, extensor digitorum superficialis; FCR, flexorcarpi radialis; FDS, flexor digitorum superficialis; FCU, flexor carpi ulnaris; FDS, flexor digitorium superficialis; Triceps B, triceps brachii.

of wrist movements, as well as its execution (Graybiel, 1990; Romo et al., 1992; Nelson et al., 1996). The onset of PMA in NS occurred earlier than did PMA onset for somatosensory cortical neurons when monkeys performed the same task (unpublished observations).

Functional Consequences of Unpredictable Reward

The mechanisms contributing to sensorimotor integration in the NS, as perhaps indicated by PMA, are not completely understood. However, part of a mechanism necessary for the shaping of NS activity during the initiation and execution of motor behavior has been suggested to involve the dopaminergic (DA) modulation (Surmeier and Kitai, 1997). There are several relevant features of DA modulation. DA modulation is a dynamic process that, depending on the level of membrane depolarization, causes an increase in the NS neuron firing rate if the membrane is in an "up" state or a decrease in firing rate if the membrane is in the "down" state (Hernández-López et al., 1997).

According to Berns et al. (1997) the withholding of rewards may be considered to be a context violation which may be thought of as a breach in expectation. These authors suggest that ventral striatum becomes activated when contexts are violated by stimuli that appear unexpectedly. It is reasonable to assume that the absence of reward, when it is expected, is itself, an unexpected stimulus. Dopamine neurons become activated during unpredictable behavioral conditions, thereby providing contrast to previously fully predicted stimuli (Mirenowicz and Schultz, 1994). As a working hypothesis, we suggest that the dopamine system, through its projections to NS, may influence neuronal activity (Schultz and Romo, 1988; Pasquereau et al., 2007), resulting in an increase of covariant relationship between PMA neuronal activity and movement variables (Nelson et al., 1996). Moreover, learning theories suggest that the learning process is driven by the unpredictability of reward, and that little or no further learning takes place when reward is entirely predicted (see Schultz et al., 1997 for review). Dealing with unpredictable aspects of behavior seems to involve a higher order processing of information in basal ganglia and require multiple processing channels (Hoover and Strick, 1993).

The results presented in this work are consistent with the view that NS may provide an "interface" between sensorimotor, limbic and association subcortical territories and cortical areas involved in higher brain functions such as motivation, attention, and memory (Evarts and Wise, 1984; Schultz et al., 1997; Opris et al., 2011a,b, 2013; Santos et al., 2014). The complete understanding of these functions requires more experimental and theoretical work. However, it is likely that cerebral cortex and basal ganglia structures utilize different modular subsets at any given time during highly dynamic processing involved in sensorimotor integration (Evarts et al., 1984).

SUMMARY

When monkeys are rewarded pseudo-randomly (75% of the correct trials) in a task requiring either vibratory or visually-cued wrist movements, neostriatal PMA is tightly correlated with movement kinematics. There are two different modes of this activity-to-movement correlation. The correlation between neuronal activity and movement, during flexion trials but not extension trials, was higher in trials with certain rewards as compared to the trials with uncertain rewards. The improvement in the activity-to-movement correlation was accompanied by shifts in PMA onsets so that they occurred closer to movement onset and by shorter reaction times (Opris et al., 2011a). Thus, the changes in the predictability of behavioral requirements are reflected in the correlation between neostriatal PMA and the kinematics of wrist movements. These observations are consistent with the hypothesized modulation of neostriatal activity by the dopaminergic systems during certain vs. uncertain behavioral situations.

AUTHOR CONTRIBUTIONS

IO performed the data analyses and wrote the manuscript. ML collected the data. RN supervised all aspects of the research.

ACKNOWLEDGMENTS

The authors wish to thank John M. Denton who assisted during the gathering of data that was presented in this manuscript and Ben Bennet, D. James Surmeier, and Charles J. Wilson for detailed comments on versions of this manuscript. This work was supported by NIH Program Project Grant NS26473.

REFERENCES

Aggarwal, V., Tenore, F., Acharya, S., Schieber, M. H., and Thakor, N. V. (2009). Cortical decoding of individual finger and wrist kinematics for an upper-limb neuroprosthesis. *Conf. Proc. IEEE Eng. Med. Biol. Soc.* 2009, 4535–4538. doi: 10.1109/iembs.2009.5334129

Aldridge, J. W., Anderson, R. J., and Murphy, J. T. (1980). The role of basal ganglia in controlling a movement initiated by a visually presented cue. *Brain Res.* 192, 3–16. doi: 10.1016/0006-8993(80)91003-3

Alexander, G. E., and Crutcher, M. D. (1990). Preparation for movement: neural representations of intended direction in three motor areas of the monkey. *J. Neurophysiol.* 64, 133–150.

Alexander, G. E., DeLong, M. E., and Strick, P. L. (1986). Parallel organization of functionally segregated circuits linking basal ganglia and cortex. *Ann. Rev. Neurosci.* 9, 357–381. doi: 10.1146/annurev.ne.09.030186.002041

Apicella, P., Ljungberg, T., Scarnati, E., and Schultz, W. (1992). Neuronal activity in the monkey striatum related to the expectation of predictable environmental events. *J. Neurophysiol.* 68, 945–960.

Apicella, P., Scarnati, E., and Schultz, W. (1991). Tonically discharging neurons of monkey striatum respond to preparatory and rewarding stimuli. *Exp. Brain Res.* 84, 672–675. doi: 10.1007/BF00230981

Ashe, J., and Georgopoulos, A. P. (1994). Movement parameters and neural activity in motor cortex and area 5. *Cereb. Cortex* 6, 590–600. doi: 10.1093/cercor/4.6.590

Berns, G. S., Cohen, J. D., and Mintun, M. A. (1997). Brain regions responsive to novelty in the absence of awareness. *Science* 276, 1272–1275.

Churchland, M. M., Santhanam, G., and Shenoy, K. V. (2006). Preparatory activity in premotor and motor cortex reflects the speed of the upcoming reach. *J. Neurophysiol.* 96, 3130–3146. doi: 10.1152/jn.00307.2006

Colburn, T. R., and Evarts, E. V. (1978). "Long-loop adjustments during intended movements: use of brushless DC. torque motors in studies of neuromuscular function," in *Progress in Clinical Neurophysiology*, Vol. 4, ed J. E. Desmedt (New York, NY: Karger), 153–166.

Cox, D. R., and Lewis, P. A. W. (1966). *The Statistical Analysis of Series of Events.* London: Chapman and Hall.

Evarts, E. V., Kimura, M., Wurtz, R. H., and Hikosaka, O. (1984). Behavioral correlates of activity in basal ganglia neurons. *Trends Neurosci.* 7, 447–453. doi: 10.1016/S0166-2236(84)80151-4

Evarts, E. V., and Wise, S. P. (1984). Basal ganglia outputs and motor control. *Ciba Found. Symp.* 107, 83–102. doi: 10.1002/9780470720882.ch6

Fiorillo, C. D., Tobler, P. N., and Schultz, W. (2003). Discrete coding of reward probability and uncertainty by dopamine neurons. *Science* 299, 1898–1902. doi: 10.1126/science.1077349

Fu, Q. G., Flament, D., Coltz, J. D., and Ebner, T. J. (1995). Temporal encoding of movement kinematics in the discharge of primate primary motor and premotor neurons. *J. Neurophysiol.* 73, 836–854.

Gardiner, T. W., and Nelson, R. J. (1992). Striatal neuronal activity during the initiation of hand movements made in response to visual and vibratory cues. *Exp. Brain Res.* 92, 15–26. doi: 10.1007/BF00230379

Graybiel, A. M. (1990).The basal ganglia and the initiation of movement. *Rev. Neurol. (Paris)* 146, 570–574.

Graybiel, A. M., Aosaki, T., Flaherty, A. W., and Kimura, M. (1994). The basal ganglia and adaptive motor control. *Science* 265, 1826–1831. doi: 10.1126/science.8091209

Hernández-López, S., Bargas, J., Surmeier, D. J., Reyes, A., and Galarraga, E. (1997). D1 receptor activation enhances evoked discharge in neostriatal medium spiny neurons by modulating an L-type Ca2+ conductance. *J. Neurosci.* 17, 3334–3342.

Hoover, J. E., and Strick, P. L. (1993). Multiple output channels in the basal ganglia. *Science* 259, 819–821. doi: 10.1126/science.7679223

Hori, Y., Minamimoto, T., and Kimura, M. (2009). Neuronal encoding of reward value and direction of actions in the primate putamen. *J. Neurophysiol.* 102, 3530–3543. doi: 10.1152/jn.00104.2009

Kimura, M. (1990). Behaviorally contingent property of movement-related activity of the primate putamen. *J. Neurophysiol.* 63, 1277–1296.

Kimura, M., Yamada, H., and Matsumoto, N. (2003). Tonically active neurons in the striatum encode motivational contexts of action. *Brain Dev.* 25(Suppl. 1), S20–S23. doi: 10.1016/S0387-7604(03)90003-9

Kiyatkin, E. A., and Rebec, G. V. (1996). Dopaminergic modulation of glutamate-induced excitations of neurons in the neostriatum and nucleus accumbens of awake unrestrained rats. *J. Neurophysiol.* 75, 142–152.

Lebedev, M. A., Carmena, J. M., O'Doherty, J. E., Zacksenhouse, M., Henriquez, C. S., Principe, J. C., et al. (2005). Cortical ensemble adaptation to represent velocity of an artificial actuator controlled by a brain-machine interface. *J. Neurosci.* 25, 4681–4693. doi: 10.1523/JNEUROSCI.4088-04.2005

Lebedev, M. A., Denton, J. M., and Nelson, R. J. (1994). Vibration-entrained and premovement activity in monkey primary somatosensory cortex. *J. Neurophysiol.* 72, 1654–1673.

Lebedev, M. A., and Nelson, R. J. (1995). Rhythmically firing, 20-50 Hz neurons in monkey primary somatosensory cortex: activity patterns during initiation of vibratory-cued hand movements. *J. Comp. Neurosci.* 2, 313–334. doi: 10.1007/BF00961443

Lebedev, M. A., and Nelson, R. J. (1996). High-frequency vibratory neurons in monkey primary somatosensory cortex: entrained and nonintrained responses to vibration during the performance of vibratory-cued hand movements. *Exp. Brain Res.* 111, 313–325. doi: 10.1007/BF00228721

Lebedev, M. A., and Nelson, R. J. (1999). Rhythmically firing neostriatal neurons in monkey: activity patterns during reaction-time hand movements. *J. Neurophysiol.* 82, 1832–1842.

Lebedev, M. A., and Nicolelis, M. A. (2006). Brain-machine interfaces: past, present and future. *Trends Neurosci.* 29, 536–546. doi: 10.1016/j.tins.2006.07.004

Lee, H., and Assad, J. (2003). Putaminal activity for simple reactions or self-timed movements. *J. Neurophysiol.* 89, 2528–2537. doi: 10.1152/jn.01055.2002

Liles, S. L. (1985). Activity of neurons in putamen during active and passive movements of the wrist. *J. Neurophysiol.* 53, 217–235.

Liu, Y., Denton, J. M., and Nelson, R. J. (2005). Neuronal activity in primary motor cortex differs when monkeys perform somatosensory and visually guided wrist movements. *Exp. Brain Res.* 167, 571–586. doi: 10.1007/s00221-005-0052-8

Liu, Y., Denton, J. M., and Nelson, R. J. (2008). Monkey primary somatosensory cortical activity during the early reaction time period differs with cues that guide movements. *Exp. Brain Res.* 187, 349–358. doi: 10.1007/s00221-008-1307-y

Lynd-Balta, E., and Haber, S. N. (1994). The organization of midbrain projections to the ventral striatum in the primate: a comparison of the sensorimotor-related striatum and the ventral striatum. *J. Comp. Neurol.* 345, 562–578. doi: 10.1002/cne.903450407

Mirenowicz, J., and Schultz, W. (1994). Importance of unpredictability for reward responses in primate dopamine neurons. *J. Neurophysiol.* 72, 1024–1027.

Nelson, R. J. (1987). Activity of monkey primary somatosensory cortical neurons changes prior to active moment. *Brain Res.* 406, 402–407. doi: 10.1016/0006-8993(87)90815-8

Nelson, R. J. (1988). Set related and premovement related activity of primate somatosensory cortical neurons depends upon stimulus modality and subsequent movement. *Brain Res. Bull.* 21, 411–424. doi: 10.1016/0361-9230(88)90153-0

Nelson, R. J., and Douglas, V. D. (1989). Changes in premovement activity in primary somatosensory cortex differ when monkey make hand movements in response to visual vs. vibratory cues. *Brain Res.* 484, 43–56. doi: 10.1016/0006-8993(89)90346-6

Nelson, R. J., Lebedev, M. A., Opris, I., and Denton, J. M. (1996). Neostriatal neuronal activity becomes better related to movements when conditions become unpredictable. *Soc. Neurosci. Abstr.* 22, 1085.

Nelson, R. J., Smith, B. N., and Douglas, V. D. (1991). Relationship between sensory responsiveness and premovement activity of quickly adapting neurons in areas 3b and 1 of monkey primary somatosensory cortex. *Exp. Brain Res.* 71, 431–436. doi: 10.1007/bf00231763

Nicolelis, M. A., and Lebedev, M. A. (2009). Principles of neural ensemble physiology underlying the operation of brain-machine interfaces. *Nat. Rev. Neurosci.* 10, 530–540. doi: 10.1038/nrn2653

Opris, I., and Bruce, C. J. (2005). Neural circuitry of judgment and decision mechanisms. *Brain Res. Rev.* 48, 509–528. doi: 10.1016/j.brainresrev.2004.11.001

Opris, I., Hampson, R. E., and Deadwyler, S. A. (2009). The encoding of cocaine vs. natural rewards in the striatum of nonhuman primates: categories with different activations. *Neuroscience* 163, 40–54. doi: 10.1016/j.neuroscience.2009.06.002

Opris, I., Hampson, R. E., Stanford, T. R., Gerhardt, G. A., and Deadwyler, S. A. (2011b). Neural activity of frontal cortical layers: evidence for columnar sensorimotor processing. *J. Cogn. Neurosci.* 23, 1507–1521 doi: 10.1162/jocn.2010.21534

Opris, I., Santos, L., Gerhardt, G. A., Song, D., Berger, T. W., Hampson, R. E., et al. (2013). Prefrontal cortical microcircuits bind perception to executive control. *Sci. Rep.* 3:2285. doi: 10.1038/srep02285

Opris, I., Lebedev, M., and Nelson, R. J. (2011a). Motor planning under unpredictable reward: Modulations of movement vigor and primate striatum activity. *Front. Neurosci.* 5:61. doi: 10.3389/fnins.2011.00061

Parent, A., and Hazrati, L.-N. (1995). Functional anatomy of the basal ganglia. I. The cortico-basal ganglia-thalamo-cortical loop. *Brain Res. Rev.* 20, 91–127. doi: 10.1016/0165-0173(94)00007-C

Pasquereau, B., Nadjar, A., Arkadir, D., Bezard, E., Goillandeau, M., Bioulac, B., et al. (2007). Shaping of motor responses by incentive values through the basal ganglia. *J. Neurosci.* 27, 1176–1183. doi: 10.1523/JNEUROSCI.3745-06.2007

Pekny, S. E., Izawa, J., and Shadmehr, R. (2015). Reward-dependent modulation of movement variability. *J. Neurosci.* 35, 4015–4024. doi: 10.1523/JNEUROSCI.3244-14.2015

Reppert, T. R., Lempert, K. M., Glimcher, P. W., and Shadmehr, R. (2015). Modulation of Saccade Vigor during Value-Based Decision Making. *J. Neurosci.* 35, 15369–15378. doi: 10.1523/JNEUROSCI.2621-15.2015

Robbins, T. W., and Everitt, B. J. (1996). Neurobehavioral mechanisms of reward and motivation. *Curr. Opin. Neurobiol.* 6, 228–236. doi: 10.1016/S0959-4388(96)80077-8

Romo, R., Scarnati, E., and Schultz, W. (1992). Role of primate basal ganglia and frontal cortex in the internal generation of movements. *Exp. Brain Res.* 91, 385–395. doi: 10.1007/BF00227835

Romo, R., and Schultz, W. (1990). Dopamine neurons of the monkey midbrain: Contingencies of responses to active touch during self-initiated arm movements. *J. Neurophysiol.* 63, 592–606.

Samejima, K. Ueda, Y., Doya, K., and Kimura, M. (2005). Representation of action-specific reward values in the striatum. *Science* 310, 1337–1340. doi: 10.1126/science.1115270

Santos, L. M., Opris, I., Hampson, R. E., Godwin, D. W., Gerhardt, G. A., and Deadwyler, S. A. (2014). Functional dynamics of primate cortico-striatal networks during volitional movements. *Front. Syst. Neurosci.* 8:27. doi: 10.3389/fnsys.2014.00027

Schultz, W. (1997). Dopamine neurons and their role in reward mechanisms. *Curr. Opin. Neurobiol.* 7, 191–197. doi: 10.1016/S0959-4388(97)80007-4

Schultz, W. (2010). Dopamine signals for reward value and risk: basic and recent data. *Behav. Brain Funct.* 6:24. doi: 10.1186/1744-9081-6-24

Schultz, W., Apicella, P., and Ljungberg, T. (1993). Response of monkey dopamine neurons to reward and conditioned stimuli during successive steps of learning a delayed response task. *J. Neurosci.* 13, 900–913.

Schultz, W., Apicella, P., Scarnati, E., and Ljungberg, T. (1992). Neuronal activity in monkey ventral striatum related to the expectation of reward. *J. Neurosci.* 12, 4595–4610.

Schultz, W., Dayan, P., and Read-Montague, P. (1997). A neural substrate of prediction and reward. *Science* 275, 1593–1599. doi: 10.1126/science.275.5306.1593

Schultz, W., and Romo, R. (1988). Neuronal activity in the monkey striatum during the initiation of movements. *Exp. Brain Res.* 71, 431–436. doi: 10.1007/BF00247503

Schultz, W., and Romo, R. (1990). Dopamine neurons of the monkey midbrain: contingencies of responses to active touch during self-initiated arm movements. *J. Neurophysiol.* 63, 607–624.

Sokal, R. R., and Rohlf, F. J. (eds.). (1981). *Biometry: The Principles and Practice of Statistics in Biological Research.* San Francisco, CA: W. H. Freeman. Available online at: https://books.google.com/books/about/Biometry.html?id=C-OTQgAACAAJ

Stark, E., Drori, R., Asher, I., Ben-Shaul, Y., and Abeles, M. (2007). Distinct movement parameters are represented by different neurons in the motor cortex. *Eur. J. Neurosci.* 2007, 1055–1066. doi: 10.1111/j.1460-9568.2007.05711.x

Surmeier, D. J., and Kitai, S. T. (1997). State-dependent regulation of neuronal excitability by dopamine. *Jpn. J. Psychopharmacol.* 17, 105–110.

Taira, M., Boline, J., Smyrnis, N., Georgopoulos, A. P., and Ashe, J. (1996). On the relations between single cell activity in the motor cortex and the direction and magnitude of three-dimensional static force. *Exp. Brain Res.* 109, 367–376. doi: 10.1007/BF00229620

Turner, R. S., and Desmurget, M. (2010). Basal ganglia contributions to motor control: a vigorous tutor. *Curr. Opin. Neurobiol.* 20, 704–716. doi: 10.1016/j.conb.2010.08.022

Ueda, Y., and Kimura, M. (2003). Encoding of direction and combination of movements by primate putamen neurons. *Eur. J. Neurosci.* 18, 980–994. doi: 10.1046/j.1460-9568.2003.02814.x

Vaadia, E., Kurata, K., and Wise, S. P. (1988). Neuronal activity preceding directional and nondirectional cues in the premotor cortex of rhesus monkeys. *Somatosens. Motor Res.* 6, 207–230. doi: 10.3109/08990228809144674

Watanabe, M. (1996). Reward expectancy in primate prefrontal neurons. *Nature* 382, 629–632. doi: 10.1038/382629a0

10

Remotely-Supervised Transcranial Direct Current Stimulation (tDCS) for Clinical Trials: Guidelines for Technology and Protocols

Leigh E. Charvet[1], Margaret Kasschau[1], Abhishek Datta[2], Helena Knotkova[3], Michael C. Stevens[4], Angelo Alonzo[5], Colleen Loo[5], Kevin R. Krull[6] and Marom Bikson[7]*

[1] Department of Neurology, Stony Brook Medicine, Stony Brook, NY, USA, [2] Soterix Medical Inc., NY, USA, [3] MJHS Institute for Innovation in Palliative Care, NY, USA, [4] Olin Neuropsychiatry Research Center, Yale University School of Medicine, New Haven, CT, USA, [5] School of Psychiatry, University of New South Wales, Black Dog Institute, Randwick, Australia, [6] Department of Epidemiology and Cancer Control, St. Jude Children's Research Hospital, Memphis, Tennessee, USA, [7] Department of Biomedical Engineering, The City College of New York of CUNY, NY, USA

Edited by:
Mikhail Lebedev,
Duke University, USA

Reviewed by:
Andre R. Brunoni,
Universidade de São Paulo, Brazil
Thiago Leiros Costa,
Universidade de São Paulo, Brazil
Zaghloul Ahmed,
The College of Staten Island, USA

***Correspondence:**
Leigh E. Charvet,
Department of Neurology,
Stony Brook Medicine, HSC T12,
Stony Brook NY 11794-8121, USA
leigh.charvet@stonybrookmedicine.edu

The effect of transcranial direct current stimulation (tDCS) is cumulative. Treatment protocols typically require multiple consecutive sessions spanning weeks or months. However, traveling to clinic for a tDCS session can present an obstacle to subjects and their caregivers. With modified devices and headgear, tDCS treatment can be administered remotely under clinical supervision, potentially enhancing recruitment, throughput, and convenience. Here we propose standards and protocols for clinical trials utilizing remotely-supervised tDCS with the goal of providing safe, reproducible and well-tolerated stimulation therapy outside of the clinic. The recommendations include: (1) training of staff in tDCS treatment and supervision; (2) assessment of the user's capability to participate in tDCS remotely; (3) ongoing training procedures and materials including assessments of the user and/or caregiver; (4) simple and fail-safe electrode preparation techniques and tDCS headgear; (5) strict dose control for each session; (6) ongoing monitoring to quantify compliance (device preparation, electrode saturation/placement, stimulation protocol), with corresponding corrective steps as required; (7) monitoring for treatment-emergent adverse effects; (8) guidelines for discontinuation of a session and/or study participation including emergency failsafe procedures tailored to the treatment population's level of need. These guidelines are intended to provide a minimal level of methodological rigor for clinical trials seeking to apply tDCS outside a specialized treatment center. We outline indication-specific applications (Attention Deficit Hyperactivity Disorder, Depression, Multiple Sclerosis, Palliative Care) following these recommendations that support a standardized framework for evaluating the tolerability and reproducibility of remote-supervised tDCS that, once established, will allow for translation of tDCS clinical trials to a greater size and range of patient populations.

Keywords: tDCS, clinical trials, attention deficit hyperactivity disorder, depression, multiple sclerosis, palliative care

Introduction

Transcranial direct current stimulation (tDCS) is a noninvasive brain stimulation (NIBS) technique that utilizes low amplitude direct currents (typically less than 2.5 mA current and 0.08 mA/cm^2 average electrode current density) to induce changes in cortical excitability. Advantages of tDCS compared to other methods of NIBS, such as transcranial magnetic stimulation (TMS), include ease-of-use, low cost, and tolerability (Vanneste et al., 2010). Using clinical grade equipment and following strict protocols with trained operators, tDCS has been tested in hundreds of clinical trials and is considered to be both safe and well-tolerated for study in a wide range of subjects (Nitsche et al., 2008; Brunoni et al., 2012b; Kalu et al., 2012).

tDCS can influence sensory, motor, cognitive and psychiatric processes that could be applied directly to the treatment of common yet refractory symptoms that represent major areas of unmet treatment need, such as depressed mood, pain, fatigue, sensory and motor recovery, and cognitive impairment (Ball et al., 2002; Fregni et al., 2006; Mori et al., 2010, 2013; Andrews et al., 2011; Acler et al., 2013; Brunoni et al., 2013b; Cuypers et al., 2013; Bennabi et al., 2014), typically occurring in the context of a neurologic or psychiatric condition.

Remote Delivery Will Expand tDCS Clinical Study

Neurophysiologic and clinical trials with tDCS increasingly reinforce that efficacy increases with multiple sessions (Mori et al., 2010, 2013; Acler et al., 2013; Ferrucci et al., 2014; Meesen et al., 2014; Tecchio et al., 2014), with effects thought to be cumulative. Many clinical investigators apply tDCS in conjunction with a behaviorally-based treatment approach to improve outcome (Demirtas-Tatlidede et al., 2013; Martin et al., 2013b; Brunoni and Vanderhasselt, 2014; Brunoni et al., 2014; Flöel, 2014), which must be repeated alongside tDCS. The clinical utility of tDCS must be established through trials that are sufficiently-powered, with adequate dose (Peterchev et al., 2012) and session number, and with precise protocol control. However, multiple sessions require subjects to repeatedly travel to the clinic for each treatment, placing significant and often insurmountable burden to patients and their caregivers, at the same time associated with significant provider time and cost, especially as the sample size increases (Brunoni et al., 2012a; Holland and Crinion, 2012; Ferrucci et al., 2014; Meesen et al., 2014; Shiozawa et al., 2014; Vaseghi et al., 2014). For example, in a sample of 64 subjects treated for depression, Loo et al. administered 30 sessions across 6 weeks (Loo et al., 2012), followed by up to 20 maintenance treatment sessions spaced over 6 months (Martin et al., 2013a). Similarly, during the 6 month follow up of a depression trial, Valiengo and colleagues showed a dropout rate of 17 of 42 subjects—with almost all dropouts citing the burden of regular visits to the clinic (Valiengo et al., 2013).

A remedy to this feasibility problem is controlled remote tDCS application, with a common protocol that ensures safe, well-tolerated and reproducible remotely-supervised tDCS. Combining this remote approach with behaviorally-based treatments (e.g., cognitive or physical rehabilitation exercises completed at home, or behavioral therapy delivered through remote, web-based platforms) will allow investigators to reach subjects either through satellite clinic locations or directly from their home or care facility.

While there has not yet been a clinical trial involving remotely-supervised tDCS, the home use of tDCS over a 3 year period has been reported as both safe and effective in the case of a patient with schizophrenia through 20 minute daily sessions administered by a medically licensed caregiver (Andrade, 2013).We propose here a protocol for remotely-supervised delivery of tDCS for clinical trials, with the expectation of maintaining the same level of uniformity and compliance that would be seen with tDCS sessions administered in the clinic. This step represents an extension of currently-accepted tDCS methodology to allow for trials to include more subjects and to remove any logistical limits on the number of sessions studied.

The approach proposed for remotely-supervised tDCS can be applied to double-blind trials. tDCS clinical trial devices have been developed which deliver active or sham stimulation depending on the individual subject code keyed in, leaving both device operator and subject blinded to treatment assignment. There is no reason why blinding should be any less available when the subject (or proxy) operates the device under remote supervision.

The Potential and Limitations of tDCS Away From Clinic

Below, we outline a set of what we consider to be essential features for this next step of remotely-supervised tDCS delivery. While the tDCS may be self- or proxy-administered, an important distinction is the difference with this controlled and remotely-supervised extension as compared to direct home use. One recent report described the challenges of prescribing tDCS directly for self-administered home use, without remote supervision. Using a crossover design to treat pain in patients with trigeminal neuralgia, investigators (Hagenacker et al., 2014), instructed subjects and one other adult to apply tDCS at home using a device pre-programmed to alternate active and sham stimulation across 14 sessions over 2 weeks, recording any adverse effects in a diary. All subjects tolerated the stimulation well with no adverse events reported; active treatment was found to be effective in reducing pain. However, many subjects reported difficulty with the tDCS application with an associated high dropout rate (41%). The authors concluded that a more specific and detailed education and training protocol could improve delivery. Of further concern, there was minimal guidance or structure during the course of sessions, possibly leading to variability of method across subjects and no explicit safety monitoring.

It is clear that a structured protocol is needed to identify subjects who are appropriate candidates for remote study, and to ensure that they—or a proxy who will administer the tDCS for them (e.g., caregiver)—are adequately trained. This training and certification, must be gauged against the usability of the (specially-designed) device and headgear, the likelihood that the subject may fluctuate in ability to operate the equipment (e.g., due to fluctuations in physical or mental state), the risks associated with the specific trial, and other relevant study factors such as the nature of ongoing monitoring.

As a qualifier, specialized equipment designed for this remote study purpose is a minimum requirement. State-of-the-art clinical tDCS equipment and accessories have been developed and validated in controlled clinical trials, with trained operators. It is not safe or prudent to simply provide subjects with specialized clinical equipment, including devices and headgear, not designed for home use. Doing so without accounting for variability in skill, training, and environment puts subjects at risk and compromises reproducibility (e.g., dose control). The distinction between medical equipment designed for professional operators vs. subjects and their caregivers is evident across physical medicine, and is no less important for tDCS. It is misguided to conflate the inherent simplicity and tolerability of clinical tDCS with the assumption that devices not designed for subject use applied by untrained operators pose no risk (Bikson et al., 2013) and allow for reproducible protocols (Peterchev et al., 2012).

Our guidelines are built around ongoing supervision in real-time, even with subjects who have completed training and demonstrated competency to self-administer. While the level of supervision may vary across patient group or risk level at the subject level, we believe that consistency is essential for every tDCS session to ensure safety and tolerability, as well as to maintain the standards of administration set by tDCS sessions in the clinic.

Subject take-home tDCS checklist

Subject: ______________________ Date: __________

Assessor: ______________________

The following abilities should be demonstrated:

Head and Electrode Preparation	**Satisfactory / Comments**
Parting hair to expose stimulation area (if applicable) and gently swabbing the skin with alcohol	
Check the skin for signs of redness, cuts, grazes, pimples, etc.	
Check the electrodes for signs of wear and tear	
Prepare sponges with the correct amount of saline (approx. 6 mL for each side of the sponge)	
Correctly insert electrodes into the sponges (check for right surface facing up and orientation of sponge)	
Correctly attach the sponge electrodes onto the headband	
Correctly place and secure the band on the head with the electrodes in the right position	
Adjust band placement as needed	
Machine Preparation and Stimulation	
Correctly connect the leads to the stimulator (red wire must be inserted into the red slot and black wire into the black slot; red = ANODE, black = CATHODE)	
Correctly connect the leads to the electrodes on the head (anode = left, cathode = right) and place leads over the head crosswise	
Understanding the electrode contact quality read-outs and adjusting the electrode and headband accordingly, adding saline if necessary	
Correctly entering the activation code to initiate stimulation	
During Stimulation	
Remain seated, relaxed and unoccupied during the stimulation	
Monitor contact quality and add saline at designated intervals	
After Stimulation	
Removing the electrodes, disposing of sponges and cleaning of electrodes	
Recharge/replace batteries when required	

☐ The subject was assessed to be competent at delivering tDCS

☐ The subject is not competent at delivering tDCS and needs to be reassessed

Signed by:

Name: ______________________ Date: ____________

FIGURE 1 | Example of subject checklist.

Requirements for Remotely-Supervised tDCS: Essential Features

The recommendations listed here are governed by the principle that remote tDCS administration must be safe, structured and reproducible across study sites. Items are generally categorized by training of staff and subjects/caregivers, design of headgear and stimulators, and ongoing monitoring. These items are interrelated and are itemized here for emphasis of key points—in clinical trial design they will be implemented holistically.

Training of the tDCS Research Staff

Study research staff will first be trained in tDCS treatment technique and in administering tDCS to others. Staff will be trained using standard-operating-procedures (SOP) specifying all subject interactions as well as device usage. In terms of subject interaction, study research staff will be trained to monitor for study-specific "stop" criteria following a decision-tree-based flowchart that allows for evaluation of eligibility to continue at each progressive step. At baseline visits (in clinic) tDCS research staff will complete a checklist to screen subjects for at home tDCS (see **Figure 1** for an example).

Following training on screening procedures, study research staff will be briefed on the usage of the device and the location of headset placement. In addition, selected research staff will be trained with and have access to a guide that details (e.g., the device manual), in a step-by-step fashion, the procedures that are required to configure and program devices prior to release to subjects, for example programming device unlock codes for one-time use to be provided prior to each session. Prior to releasing a device to a subject, selected research staff must program the intensity, duration, and condition (active or sham) of each planned session, along with code that limits the number and frequency of sessions. In the case of code-based session release, research staff will be instructed to withhold any one-time use codes until subject device placement and setup are deemed appropriate.

Research staff will be trained in the preparation and testing of any devices and accessories (e.g., kits) release to subjects, as documentation of material release. Through the duration of the study, technicians will be trained to monitor subjects for any unexpected adverse events (e.g., atypical discomfort) or misuse of the device. At the end of the study, technicians will be instructed on how to evaluate retrieved physical device materials (e.g., headgear/stimulator condition, expendables) and download any data stored on the device (e.g., completion codes for each subject's study sessions, stimulation history of each code issued) as relevant to confirm compliance (**Figure 2**).

In addition to training specific to the implementation of remotely-supervised tDCS as describe above, the clinical research

Training of Research Staff and Subjects/Caregivers

- Training of research staff
  - Manual of standard operating procedures
  - Completion of standardized training
    - Experience administering tDCS to others
    - Knowledge of study equipment and its operation for material release
  - Subject screening and clearance procedures to issue tDCS dose delivery
  - Evaluation of equipment and session results at study end
- Training of subjects/caregivers
  - Screening for eligibility and suitability for remotely-supervised delivery
    - Ability for subject or proxy/caregiver to correctly place headset and operate equipment
    - Testing for tolerability of tDCS session
  - If to be self-administered, at least two in-person training sessions with a study staff member, with built in contingencies to identify and provide for those who require additional training
  - Agreement for remote participation
    - Loan of study equipment
    - Connection with study staff on schedule
    - Cooperation with all study procedures
- Detailed user manual and materials (e.g., training video) for subject reference
- Study-specific subject binder to record self-reported data

FIGURE 2 | Guidelines for training.

team needs to be skilled in other aspects of clinical trial methodology, including screening of subjects, monitoring of subject progress and evaluation of outcomes.

Initial and Ongoing Assessment of the User's Capability to Participate in tDCS Remotely

A precisely defined protocol (decision-tree-based flowchart) will be closely followed through the duration of the study for each subject. Study "stop" criteria (**Figure 3**) will be reviewed at each stage of the trial: screening, baseline, study sessions, and follow-up. If stop criteria are met at any time throughout the study, the session and/or trial participation will be terminated as specified in the protocol. Following an initial screening, at least one baseline visit will confirm the subject's tDCS aptitude and tolerability. Before any subject is sent home with a device, it will be determined whether the subject-or designated proxy- can properly follow the steps to ensure correct electrode preparation and placement, low impedance and safe removal of the device, and whether the subject can tolerate the stimulation period.

Throughout the study, general compliance will be maintained through stop criteria that exclude subjects who continually fail to set up a device properly or fail to attend regularly scheduled sessions. In addition, if any subject reports an unexpected level of discomfort, pain, or desire to withdraw, the session and/or ongoing study participation may be terminated. At the end of the study, the record of completed and uncompleted sessions, recorded by the device itself, will be reviewed for all subjects who successfully met study criteria. This will be used to determine both individual subject and overall trial compliance based on pre-determined criteria.

Supportive Training Procedures and Materials (Including Assessments of the User and/or Caregiver)

The protocol will be supported by a manual of operating procedures for study staff. For designs with remote supervision of self- or proxy-administered tDCS, that there be at least two in-person training sessions with study staff, including training and practice for the real-time remote supervision procedures (e.g., a training session with a study staff member that includes connection to another remotely-located study staff member via secure internet-based video conference).

For subjects who meet criteria for study continuation, subsequent sessions will be completed with the remote technician alone, with the nature and length of ongoing monitoring to be specific to the subject or trial. For instance, some subjects may require remote monitoring indefinitely, while other trials may use remote monitoring for a training period only.

The protocol will include sequential safety, tolerability and compliance "stops" administered by the supervising study staff throughout the course of the treatment sessions to ensure appropriate use. For instance, potential concerns include failure to place the headset and electrodes correctly, selecting incorrect electrode polarity, inadequate electrode saturation, lack of compliance, and loss of precision in electrode placement.

Each subject will be provided with supportive and readily-accessible training materials (**Figure 2**). These should include an instruction manual (potentially supported with an instructional video) and a method to self-report (electronic or binder). These materials are designed as a resource to the subject to reference or confirm study details. In addition, they serve the purpose of remotely training subjects or caregivers who look to clarify

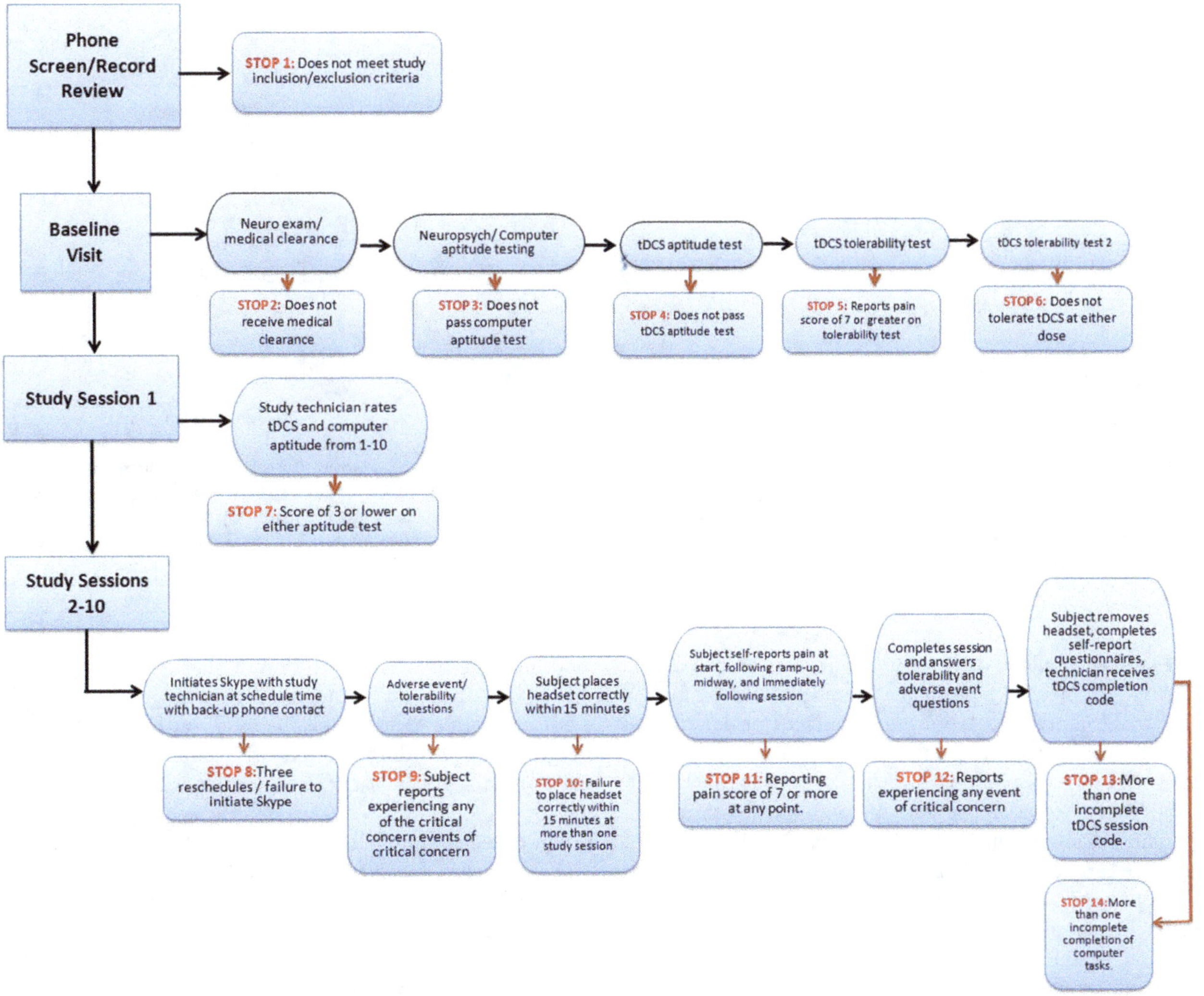

FIGURE 3 | Example of study flowchart with stop criteria.

items of set-up or device usage. The self-report binder will provide the subject with forms that measure adverse events, assess tolerance, along with study-specific measures (e.g., mood). While the manual and video (if used) will serve as ongoing training procedures, the self-report forms will enable the subject and caregiver to assess the experience throughout the study. Any remotely-delivered adjunctive behavioral therapy (e.g., cognitive or physical training) will be trial-specific with a supplemental protocol and procedures.

Simple and Fail-Safe Electrode Preparation and Positioning

The essential aspects of reproducible tDCS dose (defined in Peterchev et al., 2012) are electrode preparation and montage (addressed in this section) and waveform (addressed in the next). Remotely-supervised tDCS administration would reduce barriers to reliably apply tDCS away from the treatment center.

The headgear should be designed to allow simple and consistent placement of electrode at desired locations on the scalp (**Figures 4, 5**)—for example headband snaps for the sponges to be placed on the headband to ensure consistent correct placement.

Subjects will be screened for aptitude with the specific headgear as part of inclusion/enrollment. Participation is contingent on the ability to properly apply the headset and correctly operate the device. The headgear may be marked in a way that facilitates reliable setup, for example the headset will be labeled "RED" and "BLACK" to confirm that color coded cables are properly placed, ensuring anode (RED) and cathode (BLACK) placement (white can be substituted for red if color blindness is a concern). The headset should be designed to fit reliably on the head, for example designed with a market to align with the bridge of the nose at midline. Headsets may come in multiple sizes and/or allow adjustment by research staff. The device includes an impedance meter and will not allow access until headgear and electrodes are accurately and correctly placed.

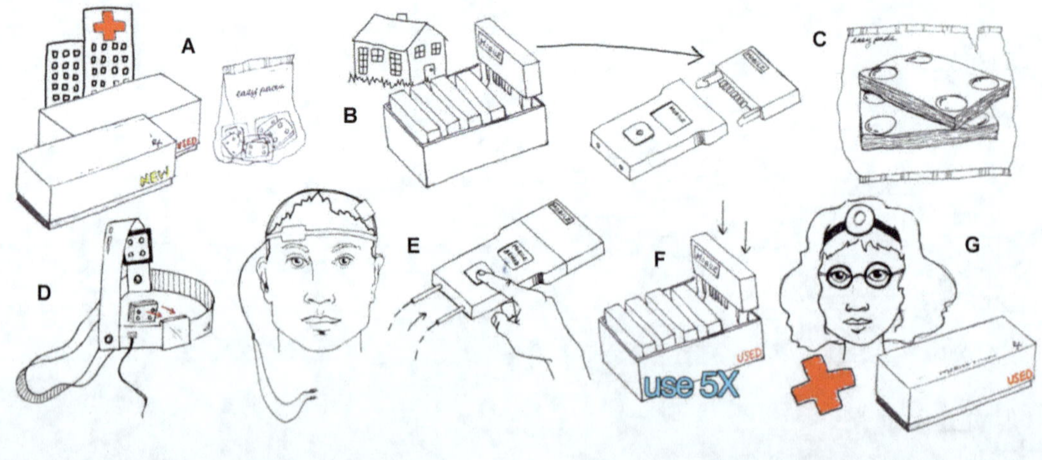

FIGURE 4 | Example of hardware-based waveform control. Users are provided with an individual device and accessories such as the 5x-Session Home Kit **(A)**The subject checks in with the supervisor before and after each session **(B)**. The supervisor unlocks operation before each session by providing a code **(B)**. The subject enters only the code provided with no access to device programming or stimulation settings. The subject uses custom fit headgear to position electrodes **(C,D)**. The device automatically collects compliance data and may also prompt the user for information **(E)**. Details of implementation will be customized to each clinical trial while maintaining the principles of supervised neuromodulation **(F,G)**. *(Image courtesy of Soterix Medical Inc.)*

The headset should be designed to minimize error in electrode placement, ideally allowing just the montage designed for the specific trial (**Figure 6**), e.g., bifrontal montage (for dorsolateral prefrontal cortex target application) or M1-SO montage (for motor cortex target applications).

Subjects/proxies should be provided with kits which include all of the necessary supplies for the entire study or until expendable can be replenished (by either a visit to the clinic or visit by study personnel to the subjects' home or care-facility). Components should be labeled properly in order to simplify application, minimize confusion, and prevent error (e.g., mark each pair of sponges by session number). The subject manual should clearly explain the contents of the kit and the correct use of each component.

Also of note, re-use of sponges across subjects is not hygienic. Re-use of the sponge across sessions, even when cleaned, is not recommended for supervised home use- single-use sponges increase tolerability, cleanliness, and reproducibility. Medical grade sponges are required to comply with biocompatibility requirements, and labeling for re-use would require testing under the intended conditions of use—which are complex and variable in the case of home-application. Reliable control of cleanliness, much less contamination, would prove difficult in home use (would not for example be reliably detected by impedance check or remote observation).In addition, attempt to remediate these sponge re-use concerns would increase the operator and patient burden for monitoring and preparation (e.g., concerns about storage, residue from skin/hair product).

Strict Dose Control for Each Session

Control of stimulation parameters is the second essential aspect after electrode placement. For tDCS essential parameters are the intensity, duration (along with any ramp), and condition (active or sham) of stimulation. For multiple sessions, the number and interval of sessions is critical. For remotely-supervised tDCS, limitations on the number and timing of sessions, along with control of each session intensity and duration is pivotal (**Figure 6**). Providing subjects with clinical stimulators that do not limit either is not safe or supportive of reproducible protocols.

Two general approaches to control stimulation parameters under remotely supervised-tDCS can be considered. In the first case, "hardware" based limitation (**Figure 4**) provides subjects with equipment that is pre-programmed to provide a limited number of sessions with limited interval. For example, the stimulator will provide only 10 sessions, with pre-set intensity, duration, and condition, with a maximum of one session every 23 h. Once 10 sessions have exhausted, the device no longer provides output until the entire hardware or a component (storage disk) is replaced. With "hardware" limitations, it is not necessarily possible to remotely stop use before the 10 sessions are activated. The Soterix Medical/Neuroconn Mobile transcranial Direct Current Stimulator (Mobile) and Magstim/Neuronica HDC-Kit are example of "hardware" based limitation. Subjects or caregivers are required to return to the clinic to replenish expended hardware—supervisors may be provide a "pack" containing multiple dose-control hardware units (e.g., 10 storage disks with 10 sessions each for 100 sessions) but this effectively extends the window where control of dose is limited.

In the second case, "software" based limitation (**Figure 5**) subjects are provided with a device which is deactivated until a code is provided by the research staff. The code typically unlocks a single session which a pre-set duration and intensity. After a single discharge, the device is inert until a new code is provided. This allows the remote supervisor to tightly control compliance, for example not providing a code until proper electrode set-up is confirmed by video,

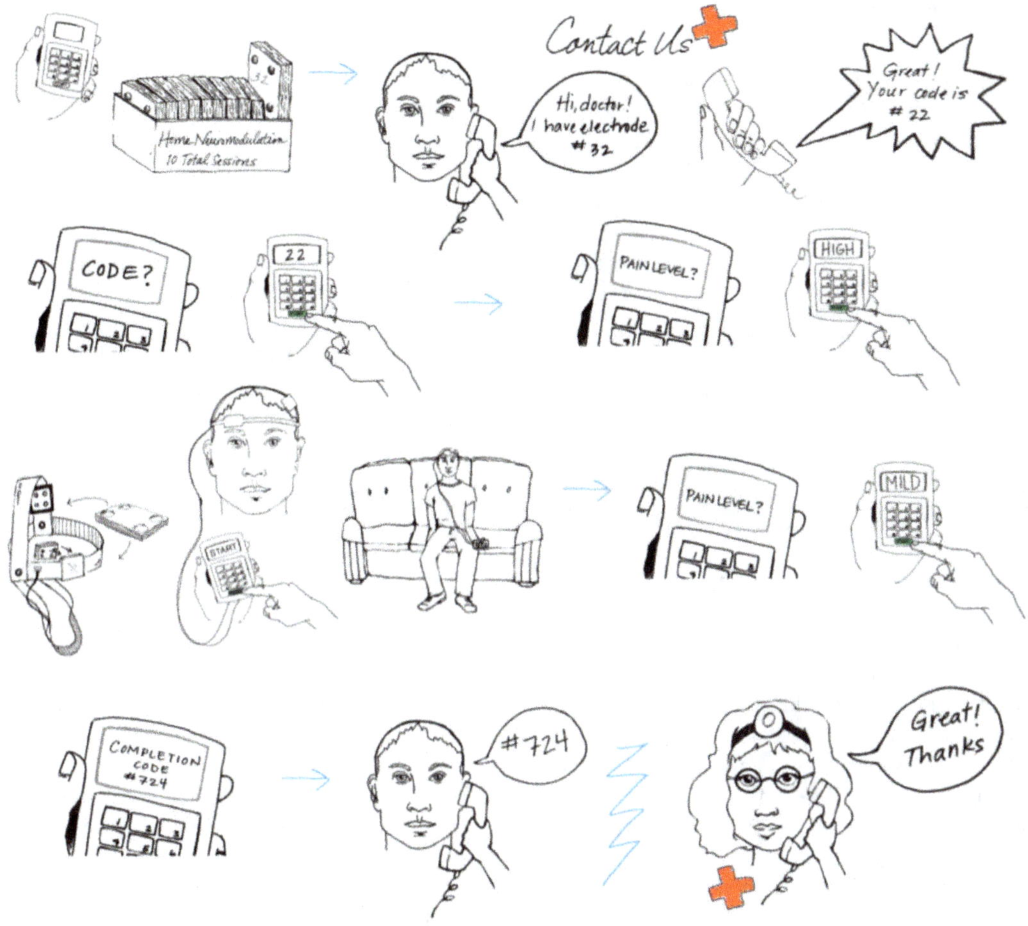

FIGURE 5 | Example of software-based waveform control. Users are provided with an individual stimulator, a discharge key, and accessories such as the 5x-Session Home Kit. The supervisor limits stimulation by programming the discharge key. The subject plugs the discharge key into the device and presses a single button to activate stimulation. The subject uses custom fit headgear to position electrodes. The device automatically collects compliance data which is stored in the discharge key. Details of device implementation will be customized to each clinical trial while maintaining the principles of supervised neuromodulation. *(Image courtesy of Soterix Medical Inc.)*

provides an opportunity for supervisor to directly interact with subject and gather feedback and data for each trial. In this situation, the remote supervisor may vary the provided code based on subject experience. Soterix Medical transcranial Direct Current Stimulator mini-Clinical Trials system (Mini-CT) is one example of "software" based limitation. Given stimulators can be programmed with excess of codes (e.g., thousands), there is no need for subjects to return to the clinic to replenish hardware.

In both "hardware" and "software" based governing for remote supervision, the subject or caregiver does not program session intensity of duration which enhances safety and reproducibility. In case of blinded treatment, the subject may not know which device/code is real or sham treatment. Double blinding may also be implemented by blinding the remote supervisor.

The user manual should clearly explain the hardware contents of the kit and the correct set-up of the device, such as entering a code or reading the display.

Ongoing Monitoring for Compliance

While in-person monitoring will be completed during the initial sessions, subjects may be monitored and/or contacted to confirm compliance throughout the remaining sessions. Subject interaction will be maintained (e.g., through secure video) to quantify compliance (device preparation, electrode saturation/placement, stimulation protocol) with corresponding corrective steps. As an example, secure video will be scheduled and maintained with each subject daily. Visual confirmation will ensure proper set up, appropriate home environment, and acceptable impedance. Following these checks during monitoring, subjects will be given their one time use code for that session (**Figure 7**).

Ongoing Monitoring for Treatment-Emergent Adverse Effects

Before starting a session, study staff will ask the subject about any adverse events since the last session, with clearly defined stop criteria if anything is reported that is of clinical concern

Design of Headgear and Stimulators Strict Dose Control

- Electrode Preparation and Placement
  - Subjects and/or their proxy will be screened for ability to operate and place headgear
    - Headgear designed to allow simple and consistent electrode placement
      - Markers for reliable setup
      - Allowing only one trial-specific montage
  - Study kit for organization and maintenance of clearly-labelled materials
  - Disposal of sponges after each use
- Strict Dose Control
  - Remote devices must include dosing limits and controls
    - Hardware-based limitations (e.g., "pack" of dose-control hardware units)
    - Software-based limitations (e.g., dose unlock code provided by study staff)

FIGURE 6 | Guidelines for study equipment.

related to safety or tolerability. In addition, subjects will be asked to report pain and/or discomfort level at set points during the stimulation. If pain crosses a given threshold, there will be an immediate stop in place in order to prevent any risk of skin burn (Loo et al., 2011) and the supervising staff will assess whether this has occurred due to suboptimal treatment technique. If tDCS causes pain above the given threshold despite adequate treatment technique, subjects will be withdrawn from the study. After the session, subjects will be again assessed by study staff for any adverse events. Subjects will also record their experience in the study-specific materials.

Guidance to Identify and Implement Discontinuation of a Session and/or Study Participation (Including Emergency Failsafe Procedures) Tailored to the Treatment Population's Level of Need

Finally, during training and in reference materials, subjects will be instructed to abort the session if they need to immediately discontinue stimulation by allowing ramp down and then removing their headset. These instructions will be used if any subject reports significant discomfort or other adverse event, otherwise needs to discontinue a session, or if study staff determines that the session should be discontinued.

Examples of Clinical Trial Applications and Population-specific Adaptations

The authors' interest in remote (non-clinic) tDCS for clinical trials has facilitated effort to develop study protocols for specific patient populations. Below, we provide examples of population-specific considerations that may navigate tailoring the guidelines described above to specific populations with differing limitations and needs. These summaries are not intended to be exhaustive but rather illustrate salient features of applying the above eight principles to specific applications. Once population specific protocols have been implemented, and the feasibility of these methods has been confirmed within the target groups, more expansive clinical trials can apply them to study the effectiveness of the treatment.

Attention Deficit Hyperactivity Disorder (ADHD)

The immediate facilitatory effects of tDCS on cognitive abilities often seen impaired in ADHD has prompted interest in whether or not the technique might have a therapeutic effect. For instance, a recent study of ADHD-diagnosed children in another experiment showed that 0.75 Hz oscillating tDCS increased EEG-recorded slow wave oscillation during sleep, and subsequent memory recall the next day (Prehn-Kristensen et al., 2014). One brief tDCS trial in non-ADHD subjects showed better response inhibition task performance after 5 consecutive days of training with concurrent 1.5 mA anodal tDCS stimulation than training alone (Ditye et al., 2012). The latter suggests that tDCS paired with cognitive training/rehabilitation techniques might have the highest potential for efficacy in minimizing ADHD-related behavioral dysfunction. However, previous trials that combine these therapeutic approaches typically last 1–3 weeks, making clinic visits impractical for a typical family that contends with school demands and extra-curricular activities, worsened when there is more than one school-aged child in the home. Any clinic-based tDCS trial for ADHD not only would be plagued by poor compliance and high dropout, but it is also likely that only the most motivated of families and subjects would complete treatment, complicating generalizability and efficacy inferences.

Remotely-supervised tDCS performed is an obvious approach to circumvent the main obstacles, but the age and behavioral characteristics of the patient population introduce unique issues to any home-based tDCS clinical trial. ADHD is a behavioral disorder whose hallmarks are distractibility, restlessness, and motivational issues--all of which must be managed effectively within a standardized tDCS delivery protocol. Although self-administered tDCS for adults diagnosed with ADHD

Ongoing Assessment of the User to Proceed

- Method for real-time subject connection, such as the use internet-enabled secured video connection
  - For continued training by study staff
  - For evaluation of study continuation criteria (e.g., to confirm correct headgear placement or to issue an unlock code)
- Study stop criteria implemented by study staff using a decision-tree-based flowchart, with determinations for safety, tolerability and compliance
  - Adverse events assessed before after each session, with a study stop if any event of concern is reported (e.g., severe headache)
  - Tolerability assessed before, during and after each session, with a study stop if deemed clinically significant
  - Compliance includes connecting with study staff at appointment times, following study staff instructions and all study procedures
- Clearly-defined and demonstrated procedures to safely abort a session and remove headgear

FIGURE 7 | Guidelines for ongoing assessment.

certainly is feasible, it is more likely that trials will consider tDCS with older children or adolescents, as tDCS has been shown to be safe with these age groups. However, most institutional review boards will not likely approve trial protocols where youth are asked to set up and administer tDCS themselves, suggesting effective trials must plan to overcome and troubleshoot issues arising from parent training to administer tDCS properly. Such issues include effective parent screening/training, attention to how dyadic interactions influence motivation, and special care in assessing compliance and outcome. To accommodate these special considerations, we recommend a trial design that at minimum includes: (1) a clinic visit for consent, clinical assessment, and training with particular attention paid to educating families that treatment must be a "whole family" cooperative effort, (2) an "at home" visit prior to treatment so that research staff can assess and advise tDCS equipment set up and other technical issues, (3) careful consideration of whether every tDCS session should be remotely-supervised (e.g., via video teleconferencing) to ensure optimal protocol adherence; and (4) formal consideration in trial design of how ADHD-related behavior interacts with both treatment delivery, motivation, or outcome.

Some specific recommendations for ADHD protocols include:

- *Parent preparedness, training, and motivational issues*: Informed consent for a remotely-supervised tDCS trial should emphasize the multiple types of training required for parents who will administer tDCS. At minimum, parental tDCS technical proficiency should be demonstrated as suggested above, with at least 1 clinic visit and 1 remotely-supervised session, if not at each daily session. If computer-administered cognitive training techniques will accompany tDCS stimulation, separate training should be provided in how to start, stop, and evaluate the successful implementation of such techniques. In addition, parent training should be provided in how to properly motivate their ADHD-diagnosed child. Obviously, an important goal is to avoid punitiveness or coercion that might occur if parents are more motivated than their children, but it is equally as important is to standardize and measure motivation across the trial. For example, simple behavioral contingency management techniques should be considered as standard, especially for younger age groups. Protocol-specific guidelines on how and when to provide positive reinforcements should be made explicit; their use should be quantified by trial staff weekly.
- *Dyadic interaction impact*: It is not yet known what interaction styles or personality factors might make some parents more effective in operating and supervising tDCS at home than others. Until such study has been done, we recommend that each trial should make effort to formally assess the nature of parent-child dyadic interactions or familial relationships styles to see if they moderate treatment compliance or outcome.
- *Preparation for tDCS delivery and Monitoring of Potential Treatment Barriers*: Homes with children are different than those without. For tDCS with a child or teenager, tDCS should be set up in a specially-designated quiet room and performed without distraction or interruption, preferably with the cooperation of the whole family during treatment delivery to reduce distractions. Protocols should set clear guidelines for whether or not breaks are permitted during training and set guidelines for them. A standardized compliance checklist should be used for each session, which emphasizes whether ADHD-related behaviors that could have interfered with treatment occurred and how they were managed. Any concurrently-done computer-administered cognitive training ideally will be internet-enabled. This will allow research staff to remotely verify that any exercises were set up and run correctly, as well as offers the potential for any behavioral performance data to be uploaded for secure storage at the clinic site after each treatment session.

- *Careful Choice of Outcome Measures*: Although it is likely that the primary outcome measures of any tDCS trial would be performance on tests of a specific cognitive domain, (either because it is specifically targeted by concurrent cognitive training or merely because it is one of several domains often impaired in ADHD), secondary outcome measures should include ADHD symptom severity checklists or ADHD "problem behavior" inventories (e.g., Brown ADD Scales). Because of the subjective nature of the latter types of assessments, it is important to use multiple respondents (e.g., parent and teacher). Similarly, the most effective trials will include appropriate placebo conditions in order to mitigate expectancy effects.

Depression

There is a long history of the use of "brain polarization", essentially an earlier form of tDCS often given at lower stimulus intensities, to treat depression (Arul-Anandam and Loo, 2009). Over the last decade, in the context of the emergence of brain stimulation treatments for depression (e.g., transcranial magnetic stimulation) and developments in tDCS equipment, methodology and scientific understanding, interest has rapidly emerged in tDCS as a treatment for depression. tDCS has been applied both to treatment resistant depression (i.e., in subjects who have failed to improve after treatment with antidepressant medication) and to non pharmacotherapy resistant depression, as some patients may prefer a non medication form of treatment. From 2006, evidence from several placebo-controlled, randomized clinical trials has indicated significant antidepressant effects for tDCS (Loo et al., 2012; Brunoni et al., 2013a; Shiozawa et al., 2014). A key barrier to the widespread use of tDCS for this common disorder is the requirement to travel to a treatment center for multiple sessions as repeated treatment sessions, typically given on consecutive weekdays over several weeks, are often required to optimize clinical response. For example, the Loo et al. (2012) study suggested that extension of the treatment period from three to 6 weeks resulted in greater clinical improvement. After the acute treatment course, ongoing "maintenance" tDCS, given weekly to fortnightly, has also been reported to be useful in maintaining improvement gained in the acute phase and preventing relapse of depression (Martin et al., 2013a).

Several specific issues need to be considered when applying tDCS in depression trials:

- An important precaution in this patient group is suicide risk, which may fluctuate from day to day and should be closely monitored. It is unknown if tDCS may lead to increased suicide risk early in the treatment course (as has been proposed with antidepressant medications), either due to improved motivation, or specific treatment-related effects.
- Dose-control, i.e., control of access and restriction of stimulation to pre-programmed stimulation is important as a safeguard so that the device cannot be used for deliberate self-harm.
- The research team should closely monitor fluctuations in mental state, which may impinge on the subject's ability to adequately perform the tDCS procedure at home, for example, due to changes in motivation or concentration. Thus, it is possible that a subject initially assessed as capable of performing remotely supervised tDCS at home, later becomes unable to adequately continue treatment at home—contingencies should be made for this event. Conversely, given findings that tDCS improves information processing speed in depressed patients (Loo et al., 2012) it is also possible that subjects initially assessed as not capable of performing remotely supervised tDCS at home, who may need to commence acute treatment at the treatment center, may later be able to continue the acute treatment course and ongoing maintenance treatments at home under supervision.
- As part of the initial assessment of suitability for home-based, remotely supervised tDCS, a thorough psychiatric assessment by an experienced clinician is required, evaluating not only mood, but also personality style, current stressors and social and family support. All of these factors should be considered in evaluating a person's ability to comply with tDCS procedures, likely fluctuations in mental state and risk.
- The majority of depressed patients presenting for treatment are likely to be on a combination of psychotropic medications, including antidepressants, atypical antipsychotics, anxiolytics, lithium and anticonvulsant mood stabilizers. Further, alterations in concurrent medication treatment may occur frequently common in order to manage side effects, achieve better antidepressant response or provide symptomatic relief (e.g., sleep, anxiety). As there is evidence that anticonvulsant and benzodiazepine medications may affect the efficacy of tDCS, these medications are best avoided if possible. The tDCS team should maintain close liaison with the subject's treating doctor(s) throughout the tDCS treatment course, to optimize concurrent medications and to establish procedures for clear and prompt communication about any alterations in medications.

Multiple Sclerosis (MS)

For those living with MS, treatments using tDCS have the potential to directly alleviate common yet refractory symptoms including pain, fatigue, depression, and sensory and motor dysfunction (Palm et al., 2014). An important first step is to establish the procedures for feasible at home use, with consideration of potential motor and cognitive impairments.

For this patient population, the emphasis is on extensive and ongoing screening procedures, as well as streamlined and simplified equipment design and set up. To ensure compliance, safety, and assist with training, a secure, daily video monitoring protocol should be implemented.

Further recommendations for MS protocols include the following:

- Screening is an important first step as remotely-supervised tDCS will not be appropriate for all MS patients. A treating neurologist should ensure that the subject has potential suitability for operating the headgear and device. This would include cutoffs for minimal neurological (motor) and cognitive function. For instance, severe motor impairment can be screened for using the Expanded Disability Status Scale (EDSS) score (Kurtzke, 1983), excluding those with scores of 6.5 or greater. In addition, subjects should be excluded from a remotely-supervised protocol if any visual, auditory, or motor deficits prevent the ability to understand the study instructions or operate the device or laptop computer (**Figures 1, 3**). Minimal cognitive ability for participation could also be defined, for example by establishing cutoffs using the Brief International Cognitive Assessment in MS (BICAMS; Benedict et al., 2012) to exclude those with severe cognitive deficits.

- The study device should be simple to operate and engineered to unlock single tDCS sessions through a one-time use passcode. Headgear should also be simplified for use. For example, headgear should be modified with a hat-like design to ensure minimal motor requirements. In addition, device kits should be prepared and organized to ensure maximal ease in terms of sponge pocket set-up and daily materials.
- Clinical and research staff should be trained through a study technician manual on the device setup (programming sessions, retrieving session codes), headgear placement, and subject interactions (requirements for a successful session, items that qualify as "stop" criteria, and troubleshooting). In addition, research staff should be trained on how to safely abort a subject session and on procedures to reestablish video connection if lost.
- Subject training should occur during an initial in-person training session where each subject will view an instructional video, practice the technique in full and ultimately complete their first tDCS session. Beyond training, these initial visits will ensure inclusion and exclusion criteria are met. Subjects must have a suitable home environment (e.g., distraction free location and space to complete the sessions) access to internet, and the ability to commit to tDCS sessions.
- An instructional video should support training and implementation, be accessible to the subject throughout the study, and cover all details necessary to complete a session. The video should contain information on general materials, a step by step guide to set up the device, how to abort a session in case of emergency, and the means of properly ending a session and disposing of materials.
- Stop criteria (assessed at baseline, during sessions, and at follow-up) should be used as a gateway for the subject to proceed at each step (**Figure 3**). The protocol should be designed with a series of checkpoints to be met to address compliance (attendance, ability to complete the procedures as instructed, following study guidelines) and tolerability (at any time if any predefined events are reported or if pain crosses a threshold).

Palliative Care

Palliative care is an interdisciplinary model of care for patients with serious or life-threatening illnesses. The goal of palliative care is to manage symptoms of the disease and to mitigate illness burden for the patient and family from the time of diagnosis until the end of life. In the U.S., palliative care is available through both hospital-based and community-based palliative care programs (Hauser and Kramer, 2004; Defilippi and Cameron, 2010; Connell et al., 2013; Kamal et al., 2013). An overall goal of community-based palliative care is to provide adequate support in symptom management, and psychological and spiritual support to the patient and family so that the patient can remain at home, even during the terminal phase of the disease. Therefore, the development of novel home-based approaches for symptom control is highly relevant for this patient population.

Although outcomes targeted in existing tDCS studies, such as pain, mood, sleep, cognitive performance, or overall quality of life, are highly relevant for palliative care patients, there are numerous barriers of an access of palliative care patients to the tDCS studies. The burden of repeated visits to the research facility in order to receive the tDCS application has been among the major obstacles. Therefore, the development of the mini-CT tDCS enabling home-application provides an opportunity for the palliative care patients to be included in tDCS studies. However, designing study protocols of remotely-supervised tDCS for palliative care patients requires specific considerations, such as the following:

- *Involvement of family caregiver:* Palliative care subjects frequently rely on an assistance of family caregivers. Therefore, it is likely that the home-based tDCS application will be delivered by the family caregiver rather than self-performed by the subject. Thus, both the subject and the family caregiver may need to be included in the study.
- *Minimizing burden to the subject and the family caregiver:* It has to be kept in mind that both the subject and the caregiver bear the burden of the illness, and the level of their overall distress may be high. Therefore, study procedures pertaining to the tDCS procedure and data collection have to be user friendly, easy and not time-demanding. Further, time planning of study procedures should leave reasonable margins acceptable for both the dyad of subject-caregiver and the study personnel, for example when scheduling the real-time video monitoring of the procedure. Further, it needs to be taken to the account that the tDCS stimulation usually takes 15–20 min during which the subject has to remain seated or in the bed, without walking around. Therefore, subjects who for variety of reasons, such as restlessness, are not comfortably able to comply with that requirement are not good candidates for the tDCS procedure. Another aspect to consider in this category is data collection, especially in study population involving palliative care subjects at advanced stage of the illness. While data collection in healthy populations may include extensive questionnaire sets and testing, data collection in palliative care subjects should very carefully reflect the specifics of the involved population.
- *Polypharmacy*: Symptom management in palliative care frequently relies on pharmacological treatments, often including multiple medications. There is growing evidence indicating that certain agents (such as NMDA antagonists or amphetamine) may alter (inhibit or enhance) tDCS effects. This requires careful consideration when planning the tDCS protocol, because it is unlikely that medication wash-out prior

the study participation would be feasible in palliative care patients.

- *Feasibility*: Overall, the feasibility of the home-delivered remotely-monitored tDCS in palliative care patient population is multifaceted, including (but not limited to) the following elements:
- The patient's and family caregiver's understanding of the procedure, their willingness and ability to participate in the study.
- Caregiver's ability to perform tDCS specific procedures [after training]: Establishing videoconference connection; Assembling the electrodes and the head set; Positioning the headset on the subject's head; Turning on-off the tDCS unit; and the procedure has to be regarded by the involved caregiver as acceptable for him/her and the subject;
- Subject's acceptability and tolerability of the procedure: Able to remain seated or in bed for the 20-min stimulation [does not interrupt the stimulation session by walking around]; Able to provide a brief feedback or numerical rating when asked; Regards the procedure as acceptable; Tolerates the tDCS procedure (in the means of adverse events);
- Home environment: the Internet connectivity sufficient for the videoconference connection; sufficient space to accommodate the tDCS and videoconferencing devices.

Conclusion

Remotely-supervised tDCS can serve as an extension of in-clinic administered tDCS sessions. Proper frameworks around clinical staff training, user capability, training and monitoring guides are intended to maintain the same level of safety and tolerability experienced within the clinic setting. Careful consideration of each of these criteria is essential to a remotely-supervised trial. Future expansion toward a more robust training method for clinical staff on the technique will further optimize its application. In addition, following the completion of each clinical trial, population-specific modifications will be considered within the training, design, and monitoring of such patient populations. For some subjects or populations, prescription for direct home use may ultimately be the resulting clinical application, while others may be eligible only for continued remotely-supervised use. Validation of the compliance experienced in remotely-supervised tDCS trials will serve as a means of comparison to the level of compliance observed within in-clinic trials. Expanding the patient populations able to comply with a tDCS trial through remote supervision can ultimately broaden the reach of clinical trials, helping to deepen the current understanding of tDCS. With these principles in place, tDCS clinical trials will expand with results to ultimately guide appropriate and effective clinical use.

References

Acler, M., Bocci, T., Valenti, D., Turri, M., Priori, A., and Bertolasi, L. (2013). Transcranial direct current stimulation (tDCS) for sleep disturbances and fatigue in patients with post-polio syndrome. *Restor. Neurol. Neurosci.* 31, 661–668. doi: 10.3233/RNN-130321

Andrade, C. (2013). Once- to twice-daily, 3-year domiciliary maintenance transcranial direct current stimulation for severe, disabling, clozapine-refractory continuous auditory hallucinations in schizophrenia. *J. ECT* 29, 239–242. doi: 10.1097/YCT.0b013e3182843866

Andrews, S. C., Hoy, K. E., Enticott, P. G., Daskalakis, Z. J., and Fitzgerald, P. B. (2011). Improving working memory: the effect of combining cognitive activity and anodal transcranial direct current stimulation to the left dorsolateral prefrontal cortex. *Brain Stimul.* 4, 84–89. doi: 10.1016/j.brs.2010.06.004

Arul-Anandam, A. P., and Loo, C. (2009). Transcranial direct current stimulation: a new tool for the treatment of depression? *J. Affect. Disord.* 117, 137–145. doi: 10.1016/j.jad.2009.01.016

Ball, K., Berch, D. B., Helmers, K. F., Jobe, J. B., Leveck, M. D., Marsiske, M., et al. (2002). Effects of cognitive training interventions with older adults: a randomized controlled trial. *JAMA* 288, 2271–2281. doi: 10.1001/jama.288.18.2271

Benedict, R. H., Amato, M. P., Boringa, J., Brochet, B., Foley, F., Fredrikson, S., et al. (2012). Brief International Cognitive Assessment for MS (BICAMS): international standards for validation. *BMC Neurol.* 12:55. doi: 10.1186/1471-2377-12-55

Bennabi, D., Pedron, S., Haffen, E., Monnin, J., Peterschmitt, Y., and Van Waes, V. (2014). Transcranial direct current stimulation for memory enhancement: from clinical research to animal models. *Front. Syst. Neurosci.* 8:159. doi: 10.3389/fnsys.2014.00159

Bikson, M., Bestmann, S., and Edwards, D. (2013). Neuroscience: transcranial devices are not playthings. *Nature* 501:167. doi: 10.1038/501167b

Brunoni, A. R., Boggio, P. S., De Raedt, R., Benseñor, I. M., Lotufo, P. A., Namur, V., et al. (2014). Cognitive control therapy and transcranial direct current stimulation for depression: a randomized, double-blinded, controlled trial. *J. Affect. Disord.* 162, 43–49. doi: 10.1016/j.jad.2014.03.026

Brunoni, A. R., Ferrucci, R., Fregni, F., Boggio, P. S., and Priori, A. (2012a). Transcranial direct current stimulation for the treatment of major depressive disorder: a summary of preclinical, clinical and translational findings. *Prog. Neuropsychopharmacol. Biol. Psychiatry* 39, 9–16. doi: 10.1016/j.pnpbp.2012.05.016

Brunoni, A. R., Nitsche, M. A., Bolognini, N., Bikson, M., Wagner, T., Merabet, L., et al. (2012b). Clinical research with transcranial direct current stimulation (tDCS): challenges and future directions. *Brain Stimul.* 5, 175–195. doi: 10.1016/j.brs.2011.03.002

Brunoni, A. R., Valiengo, L., Baccaro, A., Zanão, T. A., de Oliveira, J. F., Goulart, A., et al. (2013a). The sertraline vs. electrical current therapy for treating depression clinical study: results from a factorial, randomized, controlled trial. *JAMA Psychiatry* 70, 383–391. doi: 10.1001/2013.jamapsychiatry.32

Brunoni, A. R., and Vanderhasselt, M. A. (2014). Working memory improvement with non-invasive brain stimulation of the dorsolateral prefrontal cortex: a systematic review and meta-analysis. *Brain Cogn.* 86, 1–9. doi: 10.1016/j.bandc.2014.01.008

Brunoni, A. R., Zanao, T. A., Ferrucci, R., Priori, A., Valiengo, L., de Oliveira, J. F., et al. (2013b). Bifrontal tDCS prevents implicit learning acquisition in antidepressant-free patients with major depressive disorder. *Prog. Neuropsychopharmacol. Biol. Psychiatry* 43, 146–150. doi: 10.1016/j.pnpbp.2012.12.019

Connell, T., Fernandez, R. S., Tran, D., Griffiths, R., Harlum, J., and Agar, M. (2013). Quality of life of community-based palliative care clients and their caregivers. *Palliat. Support. Care* 11, 323–330. doi: 10.1017/s1478951512000260

Cuypers, K., Leenus, D. J., Van Wijmeersch, B., Thijs, H., Levin, O., Swinnen, S. P., et al. (2013). Anodal tDCS increases corticospinal output and projection strength in multiple sclerosis. *Neurosci. Lett.* 554, 151–155. doi: 10.1016/j.neulet.2013.09.004

Defilippi, K. M., and Cameron, S. (2010). Expanding the reach of palliative care to community-based home care programs. *J. Pain Symptom Manage.* 40, 3–5. doi: 10.1016/j.jpainsymman.2010.04.004

Demirtas-Tatlidede, A., Vahabzadeh-Hagh, A. M., and Pascual-Leone, A. (2013). Can noninvasive brain stimulation enhance cognition in neuropsychiatric disorders? *Neuropharmacology* 64, 566–578. doi: 10.1016/j.neuropharm.2012.06.020

Ditye, T., Jacobson, L., Walsh, V., and Lavidor, M. (2012). Modulating behavioral inhibition by tDCS combined with cognitive training. *Exp. Brain Res.* 219, 363–368. doi: 10.1007/s00221-012-3098-4

Ferrucci, R., Vergari, M., Cogiamanian, F., Bocci, T., Ciocca, M., Tomasini, E., et al. (2014). Transcranial direct current stimulation (tDCS) for fatigue in multiple sclerosis. *NeuroRehabilitation* 34, 121–127. doi: 10.3233/NRE-131019

Flöel, A. (2014). tDCS-enhanced motor and cognitive function in neurological diseases. *Neuroimage* 85(Pt. 3), 934–947. doi: 10.1016/j.neuroimage.2013.05.098

Fregni, F., Boggio, P. S., Lima, M. C., Ferreira, M. J., Wagner, T., Rigonatti, S. P., et al. (2006). A sham-controlled, phase II trial of transcranial direct current stimulation for the treatment of central pain in traumatic spinal cord injury. *Pain* 122, 197–209. doi: 10.1016/j.pain.2006.02.023

Hagenacker, T., Bude, V., Naegel, S., Holle, D., Katsarava, Z., Diener, H. C., et al. (2014). Patient-conducted anodal transcranial direct current stimulation of the motor cortex alleviates pain in trigeminal neuralgia. *J. Headache Pain* 15:78. doi: 10.1186/1129-2377-15-78

Hauser, J. M., and Kramer, B. J. (2004). Family caregivers in palliative care. *Clin. Geriatr. Med.* 20, 671–688, vi. doi: 10.1016/j.cger.2004.07.003

Holland, R., and Crinion, J. (2012). Can tDCS enhance treatment of aphasia after stroke? *Aphasiology* 26, 1169–1191. doi: 10.1080/02687038.2011.616925

Kalu, U. G., Sexton, C. E., Loo, C. K., and Ebmeier, K. P. (2012). Transcranial direct current stimulation in the treatment of major depression: a meta-analysis. *Psychol. Med.* 42, 1791–1800. doi: 10.1017/s0033291711003059

Kamal, A. H., Currow, D. C., Ritchie, C. S., Bull, J., and Abernethy, A. P. (2013). Community-based palliative care: the natural evolution for palliative care delivery in the U.S. *J. Pain Symptom Manage.* 46, 254–264. doi: 10.1016/j.jpainsymman.2012.07.018

Kurtzke, J. F. (1983). Rating neurologic impairment in multiple sclerosis: an expanded disability status scale (EDSS). *Neurology* 33, 1444–1452. doi: 10.1212/WNL.33.11.1444

Loo, C. K., Alonzo, A., Martin, D., Mitchell, P. B., Galvez, V., and Sachdev, P. (2012). Transcranial direct current stimulation for depression: 3-week, randomised, sham-controlled trial. *Br. J. Psychiatry* 200, 52–59. doi: 10.1192/bjp.bp.111.097634

Loo, C. K., Martin, D. M., Alonzo, A., Gandevia, S., Mitchell, P. B., and Sachdev, P. (2011). Avoiding skin burns with transcranial direct current stimulation: preliminary considerations. *Int. J. Neuropsychopharmacol.* 14, 425–426. doi: 10.1017/s1461145710001197

Martin, D. M., Alonzo, A., Ho, K. A., Player, M., Mitchell, P. B., Sachdev, P., et al. (2013a). Continuation transcranial direct current stimulation for the prevention of relapse in major depression. *J. Affect. Disord.* 144, 274–278. doi: 10.1016/j.jad.2012.10.012

Martin, D. M., Liu, R., Alonzo, A., Green, M., Player, M., Sachdev, P., et al. (2013b). Can transcranial direct current stimulation enhance outcomes from cognitive training? A randomized controlled trial in healthy participants. *Int. J. Neuropsychopharmacol.* 16, 1927–1936. doi: 10.1017/S1461145713000539

Meesen, R. L., Thijs, H., Leenus, D. J., and Cuypers, K. (2014). A single session of 1 mA anodal tDCS-supported motor training does not improve motor performance in patients with multiple sclerosis. *Restor. Neurol. Neurosci.* 32, 293–300. doi: 10.3233/RNN-130348

Mori, F., Codecà, C., Kusayanagi, H., Monteleone, F., Buttari, F., Fiore, S., et al. (2010). Effects of anodal transcranial direct current stimulation on chronic neuropathic pain in patients with multiple sclerosis. *J. Pain* 11, 436–442. doi: 10.1016/j.jpain.2009.08.011

Mori, F., Nicoletti, C. G., Kusayanagi, H., Foti, C., Restivo, D. A., Marciani, M. G., et al. (2013). Transcranial direct current stimulation ameliorates tactile sensory deficit in multiple sclerosis. *Brain Stimul.* 6, 654–659. doi: 10.1016/j.brs.2012.10.003

Nitsche, M. A., Cohen, L. G., Wassermann, E. M., Priori, A., Lang, N., Antal, A., et al. (2008). Transcranial direct current stimulation: state of the art 2008. *Brain Stimul.* 1, 206–223. doi: 10.1016/j.brs.2008.06.004

Palm, U., Ayache, S. S., Padberg, F., and Lefaucheur, J. P. (2014). Non-invasive brain stimulation therapy in multiple sclerosis: a review of tDCS, rTMS and ECT results. *Brain Stimul.* 7, 849–854. doi: 10.1016/j.brs.2014.09.014

Peterchev, A. V., Wagner, T. A., Miranda, P. C., Nitsche, M. A., Paulus, W., Lisanby, S. H., et al. (2012). Fundamentals of transcranial electric and magnetic stimulation dose: definition, selection and reporting practices. *Brain Stimul.* 5, 435–453. doi: 10.1016/j.brs.2011.10.001

Prehn-Kristensen, A., Munz, M., Göder, R., Wilhelm, I., Korr, K., Vahl, W., et al. (2014). Transcranial oscillatory direct current stimulation during sleep improves declarative memory consolidation in children with attention-deficit/hyperactivity disorder to a level comparable to healthy controls. *Brain Stimul.* 7, 793–799. doi: 10.1016/j.brs.2014.07.036

Shiozawa, P., Fregni, F., Benseñor, I. M., Lotufo, P. A., Berlim, M. T., Daskalakis, J. Z., et al. (2014). Transcranial direct current stimulation for major depression: an updated systematic review and meta-analysis. *Int. J. Neuropsychopharmacol.* 17, 1443–1452. doi: 10.1017/S1461145714000418

Tecchio, F., Cancelli, A., Cottone, C., Zito, G., Pasqualetti, P., Ghazaryan, A., et al. (2014). Multiple sclerosis fatigue relief by bilateral somatosensory cortex neuromodulation. *J. Neurol.* 261, 1552–1558. doi: 10.1007/s00415-014-7377-9

Valiengo, L., Benseñor, I. M., Goulart, A. C., de Oliveira, J. F., Zanao, T. A., Boggio, P. S., et al. (2013). The sertraline versus electrical current therapy for treating depression clinical study (select-TDCS): results of the crossover and follow-up phases. *Depress. Anxiety* 30, 646–653. doi: 10.1002/da.22079

Vanneste, S., Plazier, M., Ost, J., van der Loo, E., van de Heyning, P., and De Ridder, D. (2010). Bilateral dorsolateral prefrontal cortex modulation for tinnitus by transcranial direct current stimulation: a preliminary clinical study. *Exp. Brain Res.* 202, 779–785. doi: 10.1007/s00221-010-2183-9

Vaseghi, B., Zoghi, M., and Jaberzadeh, S. (2014). Does anodal transcranial direct current stimulation modulate sensory perception and pain? A meta-analysis study. *Clin. Neurophysiol.* 125, 1847–1858. doi: 10.1016/j.clinph.2014.01.020

11

Augmenting brain function with Meditation: can Detachment coincide with Empathy?

*Shirley Telles *, Nilkamal Singh and Acharya Balkrishna*

Patanjali Research Foundation, Haridwar, India

Keywords: meditation, detachment, empathy, dmPFC, vmPFC

Edited by:
Mikhail Lebedev,
Duke University, USA

Reviewed by:
Maria V. Sanchez-Vives,
ICREA-Institut d'Investigacions Biomèdiques August Pi i Sunyer, Spain
Mikhail Lebedev,
Duke University, USA
Jooseph John Loizzo,
Weill Cornell Medical College, USA
Michael Stephen Ball,
Northumbria University, UK

****Correspondence:***
Shirley Telles
shirleytelles@gmail.com

Background and Aim

Meditation practices aim at modifying the emotions by reducing reactivity to both pleasant and unpleasant emotions (Sperduti et al., 2012; Reva et al., 2014). Meditation also regulates the attention by reducing distractibility and directing focused attention to the object of meditation (Sperduti et al., 2012). In many meditation techniques attention is directed to ongoing experiences without the intention to analyze, judge, get involved, or expect anything which can lead to detachment (Tei et al., 2009). Detachment here was taken to mean reducing or removing the need to control, possess, and be influenced by the actions of people or circumstances. Detachment or remaining dispassionate is ideally combined with empathy. The aim of the present article is to discuss the neurophysiological basis by which detachment and empathy may co-exist in meditation.

Review of Relevant Articles

Tei et al. (2009) found differences between Qigong meditators and controls in the resting state using standardized low resolution electromagnetic tomography (sLORETA; *t*-tests for unpaired data, Tei et al., 2009). The Qigong meditation includes practices for self-regulation of the body and mind (Pan et al., 1994). In the study by Tei et al. (2009) differences between groups were seen in the delta EEG band. In meditators brain areas involved in detecting and integrating internal and external sensory information were activated, whereas appraisal systems were inhibited. In non-meditators film generated emotion which is emotion in response to external stimuli was associated with activity in the occipitotemporoparietal cortex, lateral cerebellum, hypothalamus, and regions involving the anterior temporal cortex, amygdala, and hippocampal formation; whereas recall generated emotion, associated with the response to interoceptive sensory stimuli was associated with activation in the anterior insular cortex (Reiman et al., 1997).

A quantitative meta-analysis of 10 neuroimaging studies with 91 meditators, tested the hypothesis that a common neural network exists for different meditations since all meditations aim at inducing relaxation, regulating attention, and developing detachment from one's thoughts (Sperduti et al., 2012). An activation likelihood estimation (ALE) of the 10 fMRI studies showed activation during meditation in the left caudate nucleus (body of the caudate), entorhinal cortex and medial prefrontal cortex. This suggests that a common neural network may exist for meditation techniques which have comparable regulation of attention and goals. Changes in activity in the medial prefrontal cortex (MPFC) can be associated with mental activity during introspection (Gusnard et al., 2001). The ventral MPFC shows task-induced decreases in activity even when the task consists, for example, of lying quietly (Shulman et al., 1997). Hence, the ventral MPFC is believed to be engaged in actively maintaining a default state, which gets attenuated even by passive activities (e.g., lying quietly with eyes closed or passively viewing a stimulus; Raichle et al., 2001). In addition as detailed below the ventral MPFC, along with the temporo-parietal junction and medial temporal lobe are involved in cognitive aspects of empathy (Shamay-Tsoory, 2011). In contrast to the ventral MPFC, changes in the dorsal MPFC include both increases and decreases in activity (Pardo et al., 1993; Shulman et al., 1997). Increased activity was found in BA 8, 9, and 10 and the adjacent paracingulate sulcus of the dorsal MPFC (Castelli et al., 2000). Gusnard and others showed increased activity in the dorsal MPFC during mental activity associated with introspection (Gusnard et al., 2001).

Mental activity associated with introspection is possibly part of a continuum in the mental state induced by meditation which could lead to detachment (Atchley, 1997).

This is supported by a sLORETA study of experienced meditators practicing five types of techniques, viz., Tibetan-Buddhist, Qigong, Sahaja-Yoga, Ananda Marga Yoga, and Zen (Lehmann et al., 2012). Eight EEG frequency bands (delta through gamma) were computed for 171 functional connectivities between regions (t-tests for unpaired data), and showed "lagged coherence." All significant differences between meditation and before/after states showed lower coherence during meditation for the five meditations and eight EEG bands. This suggested that functional interdependence between brain regions was globally reduced. The reduced functional interdependence was considered to be related to minimized interaction and constraints on the self process (which includes self-awareness and embodiment), leading to non-involvement and detachment (Lehmann et al., 2012). Detachment can help an individual to get mental peace (Sonnetag et al., 2010). However, in order to contribute usefully to society empathy and compassion are essential. Empathy and compassion are seemingly similar social emotions, however they alter brain activation in distinct, non-overlapping neural networks, and change affective responses with opposite valence (Klimecki et al., 2014).

Empathy is the ability to understand other's feelings (Bird et al., 2010). However, when faced with the suffering of others, intense sharing of the pain experiences by others can cause empathic distress, and reduce helping behavior (Batson et al., 1987; Eisenberg et al., 1989). It was speculated by Klimecki et al. (2014) that compassion could be a potential remedy. Compassion has been defined as a feeling of concern for the suffering of others, associated with the motivation to help (Keltner and Goetz, 2007). Klimecki et al. (2014) demonstrated that after empathy training viewing videos depicting suffering resulted in negative affect and brain activation in regions previously associated with empathy for pain. The areas were the anterior insula, and anterior mid cingulate cortex (Fan et al., 2011; Lamm et al., 2011). When the same individuals (Klimecki et al., 2014) were subsequently given training in compassion and asked to view videos depicting comparable suffering, the negative affect was reversed and brain activations occurred in non-overlapping areas including the ventral striatum, pregenual anterior cingulate cortex, and medial orbito frontal cortex. Klimecki et al. (2014) concluded that compassion training could actually reduce empathic distress and increase emotional resilience. Compassion is an inherent part of a meditation technique called compassion-meditation (CM), which is closely related to two other widely studied meditation techniques, that is, mindfulness-based meditation (MM) and Loving-Kindness meditation (LKM; Hofmann et al., 2011).

There is evidence which supports two separate systems for cognitive and for emotional aspects of empathy apart from the areas involved in empathy training described earlier (Klimecki et al., 2014). The areas involved in cognitive empathy, are particularly relevant to this article. They are the ventral MPFC, temporo-parietal junction, and medial temporal lobe (Shamay-Tsoory, 2011). As discussed above the dorsal MPFC is associated with detachment (Gusnard et al., 2001). Hence, the MPFC in addition to other functions, is concerned with both empathy (the ventral MPFC) and with detachment (the dorsal MPFC).

Brain activity using fMRI was assessed while novice and experienced meditators practiced loving-kindness-compassion meditation (LKCM; Lutz et al., 2008). Affective reactivity was probed by presenting emotional and neutral sounds during meditation and control periods. When emotional sounds were presented there was activation in the insula and cingulate cortices during meditation compared to rest (ANOVA; paired t-tests). Also, during meditation (compared to rest), in response to emotional and neutral sounds, there was increased activation in the amygdala, right temporo-parietal junction, and right posterior superior temporal sulcus. The results support the speculation that LKCM activates brain circuits related to empathy in response to emotional stimuli.

The studies cited above suggest that LKM causes functional changes in specific areas and in inter-connections between areas, to generate social consciousness and empathy. However, as the names suggest, LKM and CM emphasize loving kindness and compassion, respectively, in addition to empathy.

A study was designed to examine the effects of focused-attention meditation (FAM) and loving-kindness meditation (LKM) during the performance of cognitive and affective tasks (Lee et al., 2012). There were 22 practitioners of FAM (11 experts and 11 novices) and similarly for LKM, 11 experts and 11 novices. Comparisons were between states (meditation vs. baseline) and expertise (experts vs. novices; paired and unpaired t-tests). A conjunction approach was used to reveal regions common to the expert meditation state. Both FAM and LKM appeared to influence the neural responses to affective pictures.

The difference between FAM and LKM was apparent when participants were given emotion-processing tasks, involving viewing affective pictures. When viewing sad faces the FAM practitioners showed activation in areas related to attention whereas in the LKM practitioners changes occurred in areas associated with compassion and emotional regulation.

Summary

These findings showed that different meditations are associated with distinct neural activity during sustained attention and processing emotions. Hence, meditation causes changes in parts of the brain and modifies brain activity, in distinct ways based on the meditation technique.

To our knowledge no study has checked whether detachment and empathy can co-exist as a result of meditation; and the pathway has not been determined. The dorsal MPFC showed increased activation associated with mental activity during introspection (Gusnard et al., 2001), which is believed to lead to detachment (Raichle et al., 2001). The ventral MPFC has been associated with cognitive empathy (Shamay-Tsoory, 2011). The ventral and dorsal MPFC are functionally connected via the amygdala (Kim et al., 2011). It is speculated that this neural circuit, involving the dorsal and ventral MPFC and the amygdala, a circuit which could be the basis for simultaneous detachment and empathy. It hence appears that detachment and empathy are associated with activation in closely connected areas of the brain.

Recommendations for Future Studies

The above discussion suggests that detachment and empathy can be experienced simultaneously through meditation. A study of the effects of meditation would be interesting to test whether detachment and empathy can indeed co-exist. It would also be of interest to understand whether following the necessary training empathy could lead to compassion. The present speculation suggests that through meditation an individual can reach a mental state which is disengaged and detached, but retains the choice to engage with specific situations based on empathy.

References

Atchley, R. C. (1997). Everyday mysticism: spiritual development in later adulthood. *J. Adult Dev.* 4, 123–134.

Batson, C. D., Fultz, J., and Schoenrade, P. A. (1987). Distress and empathy: two qualitatively distinct vicarious emotions with different motivational consequences. *J. Pers.* 55, 19–39.

Bird, G., Silani, G., Brindley, R., White, S., Frith, U., and Singer, T. (2010). Empathic brain responses in insula are modulated by levels of alexithymia but not autism. *Brain* 133, 1515–1525. doi: 10.1093/brain/awq060

Castelli, F., Happé, F., Frith, U., and Frith, C. (2000). Movement and mind: a functional imaging study of perception and interpretation of complex intentional movement patterns. *Neuroimage* 12, 314–325. doi: 10.1006/nimg.2000.0612

Eisenberg, N., Fabes, R. A., Miller, P. A., Fultz, J., Shell, R., Mathy, R. M., et al. (1989). Relation of sympathy and personal distress to prosocial behavior: a multimethod study. *J. Pers. Soc. Psychol.* 57, 55–66.

Fan, Y., Duncan, N. W., de Greck, M., and Northoff, G. (2011). Is there a core neural network in empathy? an fMRI based quantitative meta-analysis. *Neurosci. Biobehav. Rev.* 35, 903–911. doi: 10.1016/j.neubiorev.2010.10.009

Gusnard, D. A., Akbudak, E., Shulman, G. L., and Raichle, M. E. (2001). Medial prefrontal cortex and self-referential mental activity: relation to a default mode of brain function. *Proc. Natl. Acad. Sci. U.S.A.* 98, 4259–4264. doi: 10.1073/pnas.071043098

Hofmann, S. G., Grossman, P., and Hinton, D. E. (2011). Loving-kindness and compassion meditation: potential for psychological interventions. *Clin. Psychol. Rev.* 31, 1126–1132. doi: 10.1016/j.cpr.2011.07.003

Keltner, D., and Goetz, J. L. (2007). "Compassion," in *Encyclopedia of Social Psychology*, eds R. F. Baumeister and K. D. Vohs (Thousand Oaks, CA: Sage Publications), 159–161.

Kim, M. J., Gee, D. G., Loucks, R. A., Davis, F. C., and Whalen, P. J. (2011). Anxiety dissociates dorsal and ventral medial prefrontal cortex functional connectivity with the amygdale at rest. *Cereb. Cortex*21, 1667–1673. doi: 10.1093/cercor/bhq237

Klimecki, O. M., Leiberg, S., Ricard, M., and Singer, T. (2014). Differential pattern of functional brain plasticity after compassion and empathy training. *Soc. Cogn. Affect. Neurosci.* 9, 873–879. doi: 10.1093/scan/nst060

Lamm, C., Decety, J., and Singer, T. (2011). Meta-analytic evidence for common and distinct neural networks associated with directly experienced pain and empathy for pain. *Neuroimage* 54, 2492–2502. doi: 10.1016/j.neuroimage.2010.10.014

Lee, T. M, Leung, M. K., Hou, W. K., Tang, J. C., Yin, J., So, K. F., et al. (2012). Distinct neural activity associated with focused-attention meditation and loving-kindness meditation. *PLoS ONE*7:e40054. doi: 10.1371/journal.pone.0040054

Lehmann, D., Faber, P. L., Tei, S., Pascual-Marqui, R. D., Milz, P., Kochi, K., et al. (2012). Reduced functional connectivity between cortical sources in five meditation traditions detected with lagged coherence using EEG tomography. *Neuroimage* 60, 1574–1586. doi: 10.1016/j.neuroimage.2012.01.042

Lutz, A., Brefczynski-Lewis, J., Johnstone, T., and Davidson, R. J. (2008). Regulation of the neural circuitry of emotion by compassion meditation: effects of meditative expertise. *PLoS ONE*3:e1897. doi: 10.1371/journal.pone.0001897

Pan, W., Zhang, L., and Xia, Y. (1994). The difference in EEG theta waves between concentrative and non-concentrative Qi-Gong states – a power spectrum and topographic mapping study. *J. Tradit. Chin. Med.* 14, 212–218.

Pardo, J. V., Pardo, P. J., and Raichle, M. E. (1993). Neural correlates of self-induced dysphoria. *Am. J. Psychiatry* 150, 713–719.

Raichle, M. E., MacLeod, A. M., Snyder, A. Z., Powers, W. J., Gusnard, D. A., and Shulman, G. L. (2001). A default mode of brain function. *Proc. Natl. Acad. Sci. U.S.A.* 98, 676–682. doi: 10.1073/pnas.98.2.676

Reiman, E. M., Lane, R. D., Ahern, G. L., Schwartz, G. E., Davidson, R. J., Friston, K. J., et al. (1997). Neuroanatomical correlates of externally and internally generated human emotion. *Am. J. Psychiatry* 154, 918–925.

Reva, N. V., Pavlov, S. V., Loktev, K. V., Korenyok, V. V., and Aftanas, L. I. (2014). Influence of long-term Sahaja Yoga meditation practice on emotional processing in the brain: an ERP study. *Neuroscience* 281, 195–201. doi: 10.1016/j.neuroscience.2014.09.053

Shamay-Tsoory, S. G. (2011). The neural bases for empathy. *Neuroscientist* 17, 18–24. doi: 10.1177/1073858410379268

Shulman, G. L., Fiez, J. A., Corbetta, M., Buckner, R. L., Miezin, F. M., Raichle, M. E., et al. (1997). Common blood flow changes across visual tasks: II. decreases in cerebral cortex. *J. Cogn. Neurosci.* 9, 648–663.

Sonnetag, S., Kuttler, I., and Fritz, C. (2010). Job stressor, emotional exhaustion, and need for recovery: a multi-source study on the benefits of psychological detachment. *J. Vocat. Behav.* 76, 355–365. doi: 10.1016/j.jvb.2009.06.005

Sperduti, M., Martinelli, P., and Piolino, P. (2012). A neurocognitive model of meditation based on activation likelihood estimation (ALE) meta-analysis. *Conscious. Cogn.* 21, 269–276. doi: 10.1016/j.concog.2011.09.019

Tei, S., Faber, P. L., Lehmann, D., Tsujiuchi, T., Kumano, H., Pascual-Marqui, R. D., et al. (2009). Meditators and non-meditators: EEG source imaging during resting. *Brain Topogr.* 22, 158–165. doi: 10.1007/s10548-009-0107-4

12

Bidirectional Interactions between Neuronal and Hemodynamic Responses to Transcranial Direct Current Stimulation (tDCS): Challenges for Brain-State Dependent tDCS

Anirban Dutta[1,2]*

[1] *INRIA (Sophia Antipolis) – CNRS: UMR5506 – Université Montpellier, Montpellier, France,* [2] *Laboratoire d'Informatique de Robotique et de Microélectronique de Montpellier (LIRMM), CNRS: UMR5506 – Université Montpellier, Montpellier, France*

Edited by:
Mikhail Lebedev,
Duke University, USA

Reviewed by:
Victor Manuel Pulgar,
Wake Forest School of Medicine, USA
Armando López-Cuevas,
Center for Research and Advanced Studies, Mexico

***Correspondence:**
Anirban Dutta,
INRIA (Sophia Antipolis) – CNRS: UMR5506 – Université Montpellier, Batiment 5 - 860 Rue de Saint Priest, Montpellier 34095, France
adutta@ieee.org

Transcranial direct current stimulation (tDCS) has been shown to modulate cortical neural activity. During neural activity, the electric currents from excitable membranes of brain tissue superimpose in the extracellular medium and generate a potential at scalp, which is referred as the electroencephalogram (EEG). Respective neural activity (energy demand) has been shown to be closely related, spatially and temporally, to cerebral blood flow (CBF) that supplies glucose (energy supply) via neurovascular coupling. The hemodynamic response can be captured by near-infrared spectroscopy (NIRS), which enables continuous monitoring of cerebral oxygenation and blood volume. This neurovascular coupling phenomenon led to the concept of neurovascular unit (NVU) that consists of the endothelium, glia, neurons, pericytes, and the basal lamina. Here, recent works suggest NVU as an integrated system working in concert using feedback mechanisms to enable proper brain homeostasis and function where the challenge remains in capturing these mostly nonlinear spatiotemporal interactions within NVU for brain-state dependent tDCS. In principal accordance, we propose EEG-NIRS-based whole-head monitoring of tDCS-induced neuronal and hemodynamic alterations during tDCS.

Keywords: transcranial direct current stimulation, electroencephalogram, near-infrared spectroscopy, hemo-neural hypothesis, neurovascular coupling

Challenges in Clinical Translation of Transcranial Brain Stimulation—An Introduction

Transcranial direct current stimulation (tDCS)—an electrically based intervention directed at the central nervous system level—is a promising tool to alter cortical excitability and facilitate neuroplasticity (Nitsche and Paulus, 2011). However, inter-subject variability and intra-subject reliability currently limits clinical translation (Horvath et al., 2014). Indeed, a recent meta-analysis showed that the treatment effects of transcranial brain stimulation in patients with stroke are rather inconsistent across studies and the evidence for therapeutic efficacy is still uncertain (Raffin and Siebner, 2014). Here, it may be possible to reduce inter-subject variability and improve intra-subject reliability using simultaneous neuroimaging that can objectively quantify the individual brain-state before and during tDCS. Non-invasive neuroimaging techniques that have previously been combined with tDCS include electrophysiological, e.g., electroencephalogram (EEG; Schestatsky et al., 2013) and hemodynamic, e.g., functional magnetic resonance imaging (fMRI; Meinzer et al., 2014) and near-infrared spectroscopy (NIRS; McKendrick et al., 2015) approaches. Here, NIRS presents several advantages relative to fMRI, such as measurement of concentration changes in both oxygenated (HbO_2) and deoxygenated (HHb) hemoglobin, finer temporal resolution, ease of administration and relative insensitivity to movement artifacts. Although fMRI has become the benchmark for *in vivo* imaging of the human brain, in practice, NIRS and EEG are more convenient and less expensive technology than fMRI for simultaneous neuroimaging for brain-state dependent tDCS. However, the challenge remains in modeling whole-head spatiotemporal coupling of neuronal and hemodynamic alterations induced by tDCS where such brain-state dependent tDCS need not only to consider the brain as a dynamical system but also need to consider that its parameters will be inter-individually heterogeneous, dependent on brain injury (and maladaptive plasticity, e.g., reactive gliosis, Buffo et al., 2008), task characteristics (e.g., attention issues) and other factors (Raffin and Siebner, 2014).

Biophysical Models for Capturing Hemodynamic Alterations Induced by tDCS

Neural activity has been shown to be closely related, spatially and temporally, to cerebral blood flow (CBF) that supplies glucose via neurovascular coupling (Girouard and Iadecola, 2006). The hemodynamic response to neural activity can be captured by NIRS, which enables continuous monitoring of cerebral oxygenation and blood volume (Siesler et al., 2008). The regulation of CBF and its spatiotemporal dynamics may be probed with short-duration anodal tDCS which challenges the system with a vasoactive stimulus in order to observe the system response. Based on prior works (Nitsche and Paulus, 2000; Dutta et al., 2015), such short-duration (<1 min) anodal tDCS is postulated to cause no aftereffects and may be used to probe neurovascular coupling (and neurovascular unit, NVU; Jindal et al., 2015b). Here, CBF is increased in brain regions with enhanced neural activity via metabolic coupling mechanisms (Attwell et al., 2010) while cerebral autoregulation mechanisms ensure that the blood flow is maintained during changes of perfusion pressure (Lucas et al., 2010). During such a short-duration anodal tDCS experiment, cerebrovascular reactivity (CVR) can be measured as the change in CBF per unit change in relation to anodal tDCS intensity. Moreover, the rate of change of hemodynamic responses to same tDCS intensity may explain inter-individual differences in tDCS after-effects (Han et al., 2014). Also, phenomological model for metabolic coupling mechanisms (Attwell et al., 2010) can be used to capture CVR that represents the capacity of blood vessels to dilate during anodal tDCS due to neuronal activity-related increased demands of oxygen (Dutta et al., 2013). Here, CVR reflects the capacity of blood vessels to dilate, and is an important marker for brain vascular reserve (Markus and Cullinane, 2001). Indeed pressure–perfusion–cognition relationships may be monitored with the brain vascular reserve (Novak, 2012) where the CVR distributes CBF toward the brain areas in need of increased perfusion due to enhanced neural activity.

Prior work has shown a significant correlation between tDCS current strength and increase in regional CBF in the on-period relative to the pre-stimulation baseline (Zheng et al., 2011). We investigated regional CVR during anodal tDCS by adapting an arteriolar compliance model of the CBF response to a neural stimulus (Behzadi and Liu, 2005). Regional CVR was defined as the coupling between changes in CBF and cerebral metabolic rate of oxygen ($CMRO_2$) during anodal tDCS-induced local brain activation (Leontiev and Buxton, 2007). The complex path from the tDCS-induced change of the synaptic transmembrane current, $u(t)$ (only excitatory effects considered; Molaee-Ardekani et al., 2013) to a change in the concentration of multiple vasoactive agents (such as NO, potassium ions, adenosine), represented by a single vascular flow-inducing vasoactive signal, s, was captured by a first-order Friston's model (Friston et al., 2000). Chander and Chakravarthy (2012) presented a computational model that studied the effect of metabolic feedback on neuronal activity to bridge the gap between measured hemodynamic response and ongoing neural activity. Here, the NVU (see **Figure 1**) consists of the endothelium, glia, neurons, pericytes, and the basal lamina that has been proposed to maintain the homeostasis of the brain microenvironment (Iadecola, 2004). In this connection, the role of lactate as a signaling molecule was described recently (Yang et al., 2014), which supports a (delayed) "reverse" influence in the NVU from the vessel back to neuron via lactate (Chander and Chakravarthy, 2012). Recently, a detailed biophysical model of the brain's metabolic interactions was presented by Jolivet et al. (2015). This not only supported the astrocyte-neuron lactate shuttle (ANLS) hypothesis that the lactate produced in astrocytes (a type of glial cell) can also fuel neuronal activity but it also provided a quantitative mathematical description of the metabolic activation in neurons and glial cells, as well as of the macroscopic measurements obtained during brain imaging. Indeed, this model captured the pattern of neurovascular responses observed in rodents in response to sustained sensory stimulation where CBF only starts to increase above its baseline ~0.5–1 s after the onset of stimulation (Jolivet et al., 2015). We also found such onset effects (called "initial dip") of anodal tDCS in stroke patients (Dutta et al., 2015). Moreover, Jolivet et al. (2015) highlighted the neuron-astrocyte cross-talk during oscillations linked to blood oxygenation levels (DiNuzzo et al., 2011) where such oscillations also occurred after anodal tDCS-based perturbation of the neuroglial networks in our EEG-NIRS stroke study (Dutta et al., 2015). We therefore postulate that short-duration anodal tDCS can be used to perturb neuroglial networks in health and disease to probe the

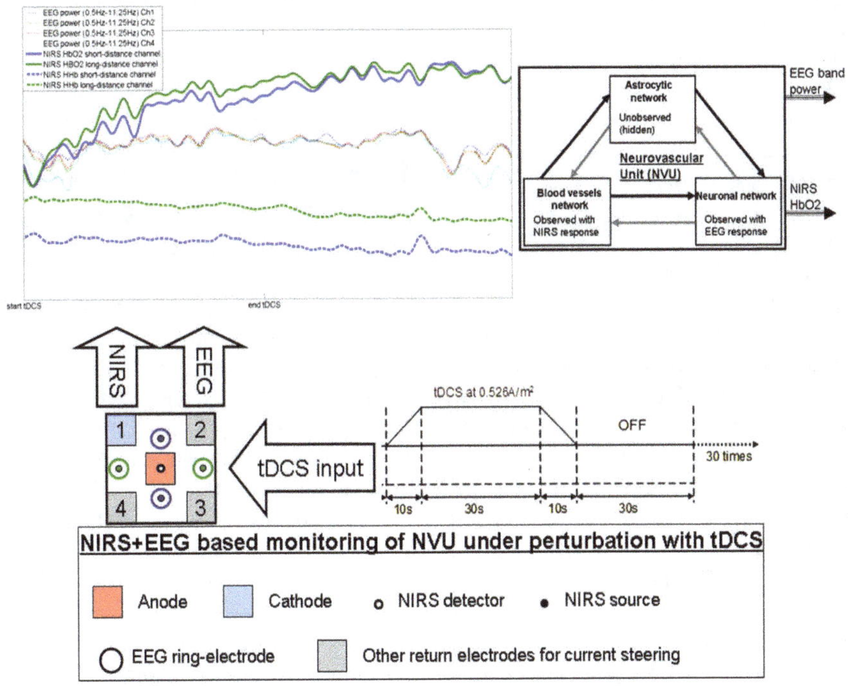

FIGURE 1 | Illustration of the effects of transcranial direct current stimulation (tDCS) from simultaneous recording of electroencephalogram (EEG) and near infra red spectroscopy (NIRS). The colors on the plot corresponds to the sensors. Here, only one anode and one cathode is highlighted for tDCS, however, local current steering based on NIRS-EEG feedback is possible to optimally orient the electric field with multiple return electrodes (Khadka et al., 2015). Here, neurovascular unit (NVU) consists of the endothelium, glia, neurons, pericytes, and the basal lamina in which neurons, astrocytes, and vessels are semi-independent networks operating in tandem. Neuronal network activity drives functional hyperemia via direct effects on the blood vessels network as well as indirect effects via the astrocytic network. Also, the hemodynamics changes can impact neuronal network activity via direct (diffusible messengers, electromechanical and thermal interactions) and indirect (via astrocytic network) pathways.

spatiotemporal dynamics of the NVU based on simultaneous EEG-NIRS neuroimaging (Dutta, 2014; Dutta et al., 2015) and biophysical model (Jolivet et al., 2015) based analysis.

Neural Mass or Field Models for Capturing Neuronal Alterations Induced by tDCS

During neural activity, the electric currents from excitable membranes of brain tissue superimpose at a given location in the extracellular medium and generate a potential, which is referred to as the EEG (Nunez and Srinivasan, 2006). Here, neural mass models (NMM) can provide insights into the neuromodulatory mechanisms underlying alterations of cortical activity induced via tDCS (Molaee-Ardekani et al., 2013). Specifically, the origin of tDCS-induced alterations in the EEG power spectrum was captured using a thalamocortical NMM (Dutta and Nitsche, 2013). The NMM for a single cortical source comprises of four neuronal subpopulations, excitatory pyramidal neurons (ePN), excitatory interneurons (eIN), slow inhibitory interneurons (siIN), and fast inhibitory interneurons (fiIN; Zavaglia et al., 2006). The NMM for the cortical source was coupled with another representing the thalamus (Sotero et al., 2007), which comprises of two neuronal subpopulations—an excitatory thalamocortical (eTCN) and an inhibitory reticular-thalamic (iRT). The basis of our cortical NMM is the Friston model (Moran et al., 2007) that emulates the activity of a cortical area using three neuronal subpopulations, ePN, eIN, and siIN. A population of ePN (output) cells receives inputs from inhibitory and excitatory populations of interneurons via intrinsic connections (intrinsic connections are confined to the cortical sheet). An extrinsic thalamo-cortico-thalamic loop consists of eTCN and iRT in the thalamic NMM (Ursino et al., 2010). Our lumped thalamo-cortico-thalamic network model can be used to simulate the subject-specific EEG power spectral density changes during/following tDCS (Dutta and Nitsche, 2013) by modifying the model parameters (e.g., average gain of synapses, their time constants; Zavaglia et al., 2006). We found that anodal tDCS enhances activity and excitability of the excitatory pyramidal neuron at a population level in a non-specific manner and mu-rhythm desynchronization is generated (Dutta and Nitsche, 2013). The tDCS effects on the population kinetics depend on the direction of cortical current flow determining the relative influence of acute tDCS on the cellular targets responsible for modulation of synaptic efficacy, which are primarily somata and axon terminals (Rahman et al., 2013). Basal and apical dendrites can be concomitantly polarized in opposite directions, and Layer V pyramidal neurons exhibit the highest measured somatic sensitivities to subthreshold fields (Rahman et al., 2013). Therefore, not all neural tissue will be equally affected by a given stimulation protocol which may distinctly affect neuronal populations/neuronal compartments. Indeed, a recent computational modeling study suggested that tDCS may induce opposing effects on different types of interneurons (Molaee-Ardekani et al., 2013). Here, the excitation vs. inhibition effects (Krause et al., 2013) of tDCS on the population kinetics can produce a whole spectrum of EEG signals within the oscillatory regime of a neural mass model (David and Friston, 2003).

There are several prior works that have shown both "online" effects of tDCS on EEG with EEG performed during tDCS as well as "offline" effects with EEG performed after tDCS. Here, it is important to separate studies where tDCS is applied during a rest state (Ardolino et al., 2005; Zaehle et al., 2011; Spitoni et al., 2013) or an active task state (Matsumoto et al., 2010; Mangia et al., 2014). We computationally found (Dutta and Nitsche, 2013) in concordance with the experimental results of Matsumoto et al. (2010) that tDCS effects on mu-rhythm desynchronization depend on the direction of cortical current flow determining the relative influence of acute tDCS on the cellular targets. Matsumoto et al. (2010) found that tDCS applied over the left primary motor area for 10 min at 1 mA with a 35 cm^2 electrode influenced event-related desynchronization (ERD) during right hand grasping where the mu ERD increased after anodal tDCS and decreased after cathodal tDCS. Here, not only the "local" effects but the "distant" effects of tDCS are also relevant where Polanía et al. (2012) reported that the functional connectivity patterns significantly increased after anodal tDCS (i.e., "offline" effects) over the primary motor cortex where tDCS modulated functional connectivity of cortico-striatal and thalamo-cortical circuits. Notturno et al. (2014) showed spatial diffusion of anodal tDCS (during a motor task) effects where an increment of low alpha band power over the course of pre- and post-stimulation recording sessions was found during motor task that was localized in the sensorimotor and parieto-occipital regions. Indeed, not only the "offline" effects, but changes in functional connectivity patterns may start evolving during tDCS (i.e., "online" effects) as shown by our modeling study (Dutta and Nitsche, 2013). tDCS/EEG co-registration studies have shown that anodal tDCS mostly modulate spontaneous cortical activity in the alpha band where alpha-rhythm states have a significant effect on perceptual learning (Sigala et al., 2014). In fact, more than 60% of the observed inter-subject variability in perceptual learning can be ascribed to ongoing alpha activity where Sigala et al. (2014) highlighted the need for multidisciplinary approaches combining assessment of behavior and multi-scale neuronal activity, active modulation of ongoing brain states and computational modeling to reveal the mathematical principles of the complex neuronal interactions. We therefore postulate that concurrent EEG-NIRS-based neuroimaging of the short-duration tDCS-induced modulation can be analyzed by combining a biophysical model (Jolivet et al., 2015) of the NVU with the computational model (neural mass or field model) of multi-scale neuronal activity of the whole brain (Sigala et al., 2014) to capture the spatiotemporal dynamics of the interactions between the neuronal and hemodynamic responses in health and disease. Here, the challenges remain in ensuring the observability of the NVU with intelligent placement of EEG-NIRS sensors since presence of symmetry in the nonlinear network of NVU (see **Figure 1**) may decrease observability (although networks containing only rotational symmetries remain observable; Whalen et al., 2015).

Bidirectional Interactions Between Neuronal and Hemodynamic Responses to tDCS—A Discussion

In our prior work (Dutta et al., 2015), we found an initial dip in the oxy-hemoglobin concentration and concomitant increase in the mean power spectral density within lower (<12 Hz) EEG frequency band. It was postulated that the immediate need to fuel neuronal energy recovery was via the lactate shuttle (Pellerin and Magistretti, 1994) where blood glucose supply has a longer delay (Gruetter et al., 1996). A detailed biophysical model of the brain's metabolic interactions by Jolivet et al. (2015) also supported the ANLS hypothesis. Moreover, recent works showed that lactate can modulate the activity of primary cortical neurons through a receptor-mediated pathway (Bozzo et al., 2013) and vasomotion rhythms can influence neural firing patterns (Nikulin et al., 2014). Also, lactate promotes plasticity gene expression by potentiating NMDA signaling in neurons, and the action of lactate is mediated by the modulation of NMDA receptor activity (Yang et al., 2014). These dynamic ANLS interactions leave us to question its role in tDCS facilitated neuroplasticity and learning (Suzuki et al., 2011). Also, the spatiotemporal dynamics of the millisecond-to-second-range direct (diffusible messengers, electromechanical and thermal interactions) and seconds-to-tens-of-seconds-range indirect interaction in the NVU following tDCS, i.e., the hemo-neural hypothesis (Moore and Cao, 2008), may at least partially explain the time course of the induction of homeostatic plasticity generated by repeated tDCS of the human motor cortex (Fricke et al., 2011). Fricke et al. (2011) hypothesized a role of L-type voltage-gated Ca^{2+} channels (L-VGCC) in short-term homeostatic plasticity, since tDCS has been shown to induce a long-lasting disturbance of Ca^{2+} homeostasis (Islam et al., 1995) and induce calcium-dependent plasticity (Nitsche et al., 2003). Here, the glial network may have an important role (i.e., spatial buffering) in regulating neural activity by distributing ions (Halnes et al., 2013) in seconds-to-tens-of-seconds-range where an influence of long-lasting disturbance of Ca^{2+} homeostasis via tDCS on the myogenic and the metabolic control of cerebral circulation cannot be excluded. In fact, astrocytes, a sub-type of glia in the central nervous system, can integrate a large number of synapses and can respond to neuronal activity via neurotransmitter-evoked activation of astrocytic receptors (Araque et al., 2001). Indeed, neuronal activity can mobilize internal calcium in astrocytes and the calcium wave in different spatial–temporal dimensions can result in a higher level of brain integration (Volterra et al., 2014) where the evidence for tDCS-induced large scale changes in brain synchronization and topological functional organization has been shown after acute stimulation (Polanía et al., 2011).

Based on these prior works, we recently proposed EEG-NIRS-based monitoring of neurovascular coupling functionality under perturbation with tDCS (Jindal et al., 2015b). Here, neuronal and hemodynamic responses measured with EEG-NIRS neuroimaging can be represented abstractly as the system response of the NVU to tDCS perturbation (see **Figure 1**) where presence of symmetry in the nonlinear network of NVU (see **Figure 1**) may decrease observability (Whalen et al., 2015). Since no real-world network has exact symmetries so with intelligent placement of EEG-NIRS sensors (e.g., to avoid systemic interference; Sood et al., 2015) along with system identification and parameter estimation techniques, it may be possible to track the spatiotemporal change of the states of the NVU. This observer model can then be used to drive multi-electrode tDCS (Dmochowski et al., 2011) for active spatiotemporal modulation of the brain states (e.g., posterior alpha-rhythm). Here, we base our discussions on the recent advances in Kalman filtering approaches to spatiotemporal nonlinear systems (Schiff and Sauer, 2008) and an understanding from group representation theory in controller or observer design by obtaining a modal decomposition into decoupled controllable and uncontrollable (observable and unobservable) subspaces (Whalen et al., 2015). Specifically, Schiff and Sauer (2008) showed the feasibility of unscented Kalman filter (UKF) for recursive estimation of system state for nonlinear systems, including unobserved variables and parameter tracking, in a spatiotemporal model of cortex where such a nonlinear system is controllable using an adaptive feedback electrical field. Here, discretization of the whole-brain detailed biophysical model of NVU (Jolivet et al., 2015), for example with Galerkin methods that are used quite robustly in fluid dynamics, will be necessary where each discrete element corresponds to a volume of tissue imaged as well as stimulated with the EEG-NIRS/tDCS unit (see **Figure 1**). As an alternative to a fundamental NVU model (Jolivet et al., 2015) for the volume of tissue imaged and stimulated with EEG-NIRS/tDCS unit, we tried (Dutta et al., 2015) to find an empirical model where we performed empirical mode decomposition (EMD) and the Hilbert spectrum (Huang et al., 1998) to model the system dynamics and found a negative cross-correlation between one of the intrinsic mode function (IMF) of the HbO_2 time-series and log-transformed mean-power time-course of EEG primarily within 0.5–11.25 Hz frequency band (i.e., one of the EEG IMFs). In principal accordance, for whole-head monitoring, we propose independent component analysis (ICA) to transform multi-channel EEG-NIRS/tDCS unit imaging data to a spatially transformed "virtual channel" (i.e., a spatial filter; Jung et al., 2001). Then, the "virtual channel" activity (e.g., posterior alpha band activity) can be subjected to EMD (i.e., a temporal filter) to reduce the dimension of the observable dynamics (i.e., further observer model reduction) before developing the Kalman filter observer (Schiff and Sauer, 2008) using the IMFs. For EEG-NIRS-based monitoring of NVU under perturbation with tDCS, as shown in the **Figure 2**, the NVU dynamics is captured by the function F and the IMF observations by the function W. The UKF approach should match the nonlinear IMF dynamics up to the second order statistics where

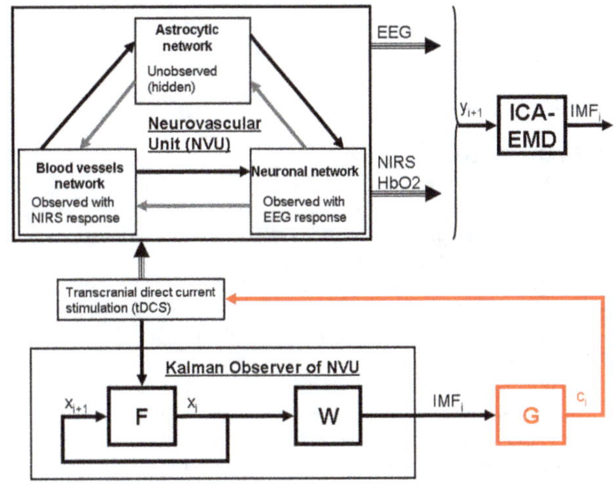

FIGURE 2 | State modulation of the NVU with (tDCS) to facilitate a brain state, e.g., spatiotemporal alpha-rhythm state. F is the function to capture NVU system, W is the function to capture observations, ICA is independent component (IC) analysis is a linear decomposition method to transform EEG—NIRS data collected at single scalp channels to a spatially transformed "virtual channel" (i.e., a spatial filter on multi-channel EEG-NIRS data), empirical mode decomposition (EMD) is empirical model decomposition of the "virtual channel" observations that provide intrinsic mode functions (IMF) for proportional control (gain is G) of individual "virtual channel" activity or IC (e.g., posterior alpha band activity) with tDCS.

the feasibility remains to be tested experimentally in future studies. Furthermore, it may be possible to use the Kalman observer to calculate proportional control (see **Figure 2**) of the brain-state (e.g., cortical excitability; Jindal et al., 2015a) with tDCS. Here, intelligent placement of EEG-NIRS sensors and tDCS effectors is necessary to ensure observability and controllability (Whalen et al., 2015) where Whalen et al. (2015) suggested in general that more direct incoming connections into an observed node lead to higher observability and more direct outgoing connections from a controlled node lead to higher controllability. Furthermore, controllability may be enhanced with multi-modal non-invasive brain stimulation (NIBS), e.g., with direct electrical stimulation (Pulgar, 2015) and photobiostimulation (Gonzalez-Lima and Barrett, 2014), which needs to be investigated.

Towards such brain-state dependent tDCS, the challenges include the nature of observability and controllability in whole-brain complex NVU networks as well as the subtleties of the tDCS interaction with the whole-brain NVU (e.g., based on heterogeneous geometrical characteristics, Molaee-Ardekani et al., 2013) that can also have multi-timescale cross-talk and resulting complex non-linear dynamics (Jolivet et al., 2015) where the spatiotemporal observability and controllability remains to be verified in future studies.

Acknowledgments

Research was conducted within the context of the regional NUMEV funding, Franco-German PHC-PROCOPE 2014 funding, and Franco-Indian INRIA-DST funding. The help and advice received from the German collaborator (Dr. med. Michael A. Nitsche), Indian collaborators (Dr. med. Abhijit Das, Dr. Shubhajit Roy Chowdhury, and Dr. Dipanjan Roy), and the French collaborators (Dr. Mitsuhiro Hayashibe, Dr. Stephane Perrey and Dr. Mark Muthalib) are gratefully acknowledged.

References

Araque, A., Carmignoto, G., and Haydon, P. G. (2001). Dynamic signaling between astrocytes and neurons. *Annu. Rev. Physiol.* 63, 795–813. doi: 10.1146/annurev.physiol.63.1.795

Ardolino, G., Bossi, B., Barbieri, S., and Priori, A. (2005). Non-synaptic mechanisms underlie the after-effects of cathodal transcutaneous direct current stimulation of the human brain. *J. Physiol. Lond.* 568, 653–663. doi: 10.1113/jphysiol.2005.088310

Attwell, D., Buchan, A. M., Charpak, S., Lauritzen, M., Macvicar, B. A., and Newman, E. A. (2010). Glial and neuronal control of brain blood flow. *Nature* 468, 232–243. doi: 10.1038/nature09613

Behzadi, Y., and Liu, T. T. (2005). An arteriolar compliance model of the cerebral blood flow response to neural stimulus. *Neuroimage* 25, 1100–1111. doi: 10.1016/j.neuroimage.2004.12.057

Bozzo, L., Puyal, J., and Chatton, J.-Y. (2013). Lactate Modulates the Activity of Primary Cortical Neurons through a Receptor-Mediated Pathway. *PLoS One* 8:e71721. doi: 10.1371/journal.pone.0071721

Buffo, A., Rite, I., Tripathi, P., Lepier, A., Colak, D., Horn, A.-P., et al. (2008). Origin and progeny of reactive gliosis: A source of multipotent cells in the injured brain. *Proc. Natl. Acad. Sci. U S A* 105, 3581–3586. doi: 10.1073/pnas.0709002105

Chander, B. S., and Chakravarthy, V. S. (2012). A Computational Model of Neuro-Glio-Vascular Loop Interactions. *PLoS One* 7:e48802. doi: 10.1371/journal.pone.0048802

David, O., and Friston, K. J. (2003). A neural mass model for MEG/EEG: coupling and neuronal dynamics. *Neuroimage* 20, 1743–1755. doi: 10.1016/j.neuroimage.2003.07.015

DiNuzzo, M., Gili, T., Maraviglia, B., and Giove, F. (2011). Modeling the contribution of neuron-astrocyte cross talk to slow blood oxygenation level-dependent signal oscillations. *J. Neurophysiol.* 106, 3010–3018. doi: 10.1152/jn.00416.2011

Dmochowski, J. P., Datta, A., Bikson, M., Su, Y., and Parra, L. C. (2011). Optimized multi-electrode stimulation increases focality and intensity at target. *J. Neural Eng.* 8:046011. doi: 10.1088/1741-2560/8/4/046011

Dutta, A. (2014). "EEG-NIRS based low-cost screening and monitoring of cerebral microvessels functionality," in *International Stroke Conference 2014, At San Diego, Volume: Junior Investigator Session II: Invited Symposium*, San Diego, CA.

Dutta, A., Chowdhury, S. R., Dutta, A., Sylaja, P. N., Guiraud, D., and Nitsche, M. (2013). "A phenomological model for capturing cerebrovascular reactivity to anodal transcranial direct current stimulation," in *6th International IEEE/EMBS Conference on Neural Engineering (NER)*, (San Diego, CA), 827–830.

Dutta, A., Jacob, A., Chowdhury, S. R., Das, A., and Nitsche, M. A. (2015). EEG-NIRS Based Assessment of Neurovascular Coupling During Anodal Transcranial Direct Current Stimulation - a Stroke Case Series. *J. Med. Syst.* 39:205. doi: 10.1007/s10916-015-0205-7

Dutta, A., and Nitsche, M. (2013). "Neural mass model analysis of online modulation of electroencephalogram with transcranial direct current stimulation," in *6th International IEEE/EMBS Conference on Neural Engineering (NER)*, (San Diego, CA), 206–210.

Fricke, K., Seeber, A. A., Thirugnanasambandam, N., Paulus, W., Nitsche, M. A., and Rothwell, J. C. (2011). Time course of the induction of homeostatic plasticity generated by repeated transcranial direct current stimulation of the human motor cortex. *J. Neurophysiol.* 105, 1141–1149. doi: 10.1152/jn.00608.2009

Friston, K. J., Mechelli, A., Turner, R., and Price, C. J. (2000). Nonlinear responses in fMRI: the Balloon model, Volterra kernels and other hemodynamics. *NeuroImage* 12, 466–477. doi: 10.1006/nimg.2000.0630

Girouard, H., and Iadecola, C. (2006). Neurovascular coupling in the normal brain and in hypertension, stroke and Alzheimer disease. *J. Appl. Physiol. (1985)* 100, 328–335. doi: 10.1152/japplphysiol.00966.2005

Gonzalez-Lima, F., and Barrett, D. W. (2014). Augmentation of cognitive brain functions with transcranial lasers. *Front. Syst. Neurosci.* 8:36. doi: 10.3389/fnsys.2014.00036

Gruetter, R., Novotny, E. J., Boulware, S. D., Rothman, D. L., and Shulman, R. G. (1996). 1H NMR Studies of Glucose Transport in the Human Brain. *J. Cereb. Blood Flow Metab.* 16, 427–438. doi: 10.1097/00004647-199605000-00009

Halnes, G., Ostby, I., Pettersen, K. H., Omholt, S. W., and Einevoll, G. T. (2013). Electrodiffusive model for astrocytic and neuronal ion concentration dynamics. *PLoS Comput. Biol.* 9:e1003386. doi: 10.1371/journal.pcbi.1003386

Han, C.-H., Song, H., Kang, Y.-G., Kim, B.-M., and Im, C.-H. (2014). Hemodynamic responses in rat brain during transcranial direct current stimulation: a functional near-infrared spectroscopy study. *Biomed. Opt. Express* 5, 1812–1821. doi: 10.1364/BOE.5.001812

Horvath, J. C., Carter, O., and Forte, J. D. (2014). Transcranial direct current stimulation: five important issues we aren't discussing (but probably should be). *Front. Syst. Neurosci.* 8:2. doi: 10.3389/fnsys.2014.00002

Huang, N. E., Shen, Z., Long, S. R., Wu, M. C., Shih, H. H., Zheng, Q., et al. (1998). The empirical mode decomposition and the Hilbert spectrum for nonlinear and non-stationary time series analysis. *Proc. R. Soc. Lond. Ser. Math. Phys. Eng. Sci.* 454, 903–995. doi: 10.1098/rspa.1998.0193

Iadecola, C. (2004). Neurovascular regulation in the normal brain and in alzheimer's disease. *Nat. Rev. Neurosci.* 5, 347–360. doi: 10.1038/nrn1387

Islam, N., Aftabuddin, M., Moriwaki, A., Hattori, Y., and Hori, Y. (1995). Increase in the calcium level following anodal polarization in the rat brain. *Brain Res.* 684, 206–208. doi: 10.1016/0006-8993(95)00434-r

Jindal, U., Sood, M., Chowdhury, S. R., Das, A., Kondziella, D., and Dutta, A. (2015a). "Corticospinal excitability changes to anodal tDCS elucidated with NIRS-EEG joint-imaging: an ischemic stroke study," in *Conference Proceedings IEEE Engineering in Medicine and Biology Society*, Milan, Italy.

Jindal, U., Sood, M., Dutta, A., and Chowdhury, S. R. (2015b). Development of point of care testing device for neurovascular coupling from simultaneous recording of EEG and NIRS during anodal transcranial direct current stimulation. *IEEE J. Transl. Eng. Health Med.* 3, 1–12. doi: 10.1109/jtehm.2015.2389230

Jolivet, R., Coggan, J. S., Allaman, I., and Magistretti, P. J. (2015). Multi-timescale modeling of activity-dependent metabolic coupling in the neuron-glia-vasculature ensemble. *PLoS Comput. Biol.* 11:e1004036. doi: 10.1371/journal.pcbi.1004036

Jung, T.-P., Makeig, S., McKeown, M. J., Bell, A. J., Lee, T.-W., and Sejnowski, T. J. (2001). Imaging brain dynamics using independent component analysis. *Proc. IEEE Inst. Electr. Electron. Eng.* 89, 1107–1122. doi: 10.1109/5.939827

Khadka, N., Truong, D. Q., and Bikson, M. (2015). Principles of within electrode current steering1. *J. Med. Devices* 9:020947. doi: 10.1115/1.4030126

Krause, B., Márquez-Ruiz, J., and Cohen Kadosh, R. (2013). The effect of transcranial direct current stimulation: a role for cortical excitation/inhibition balance? *Front. Hum. Neurosci.* 7:602. doi: 10.3389/fnhum.2013.00602

Leontiev, O., and Buxton, R. B. (2007). Reproducibility of BOLD, perfusion and CMRO2 measurements with calibrated-BOLD fMRI. *NeuroImage* 35, 175–184. doi: 10.1016/j.neuroimage.2006.10.044

Lucas, S. J. E., Tzeng, Y. C., Galvin, S. D., Thomas, K. N., Ogoh, S., and Ainslie, P. N. (2010). Influence of Changes in Blood Pressure on Cerebral Perfusion and Oxygenation. *Hypertension* 55, 698–705. doi: 10.1161/HYPERTENSIONAHA.109.146290

Mangia, A. L., Pirini, M., and Cappello, A. (2014). Transcranial direct current stimulation and power spectral parameters: a tDCS/EEG co-registration study. *Front. Hum. Neurosci.* 8:601. doi: 10.3389/fnhum.2014.00601

Markus, H., and Cullinane, M. (2001). Severely impaired cerebrovascular reactivity predicts stroke and TIA risk in patients with carotid artery stenosis and occlusion. *Brain* 124, 457–467. doi: 10.1093/brain/124.3.457

Matsumoto, J., Fujiwara, T., Takahashi, O., Liu, M., Kimura, A., and Ushiba, J. (2010). Modulation of mu rhythm desynchronization during motor imagery by transcranial direct current stimulation. *J. Neuroeng. Rehabil.* 7:27. doi: 10.1186/1743-0003-7-27

McKendrick, R., Parasuraman, R., and Ayaz, H. (2015). Wearable functional near infrared spectroscopy (fNIRS) and transcranial direct current stimulation (tDCS): expanding vistas for neurocognitive augmentation. *Front. Syst. Neurosci.* 9:27. doi: 10.3389/fnsys.2015.00027

Meinzer, M., Lindenberg, R., Darkow, R., Ulm, L., Copland, D., and Flöel, A. (2014). Transcranial direct current stimulation and simultaneous functional magnetic resonance imaging. *J. Vis. Exp.* e51730. doi: 10.3791/51730

Molaee-Ardekani, B., Márquez-Ruiz, J., Merlet, I., Leal-Campanario, R., Gruart, A., Sánchez-Campusano, R., et al. (2013). Effects of transcranial Direct Current Stimulation (tDCS) on cortical activity: a computational modeling study. *Brain Stimul.* 6, 25–39. doi: 10.1016/j.brs.2011.12.006

Moore, C. I., and Cao, R. (2008). The hemo-neural hypothesis: on the role of blood flow in information processing. *J. Neurophysiol.* 99, 2035–2047. doi: 10.1152/jn.01366.2006

Moran, R. J., Kiebel, S. J., Stephan, K. E., Reilly, R. B., Daunizeau, J., and Friston, K. J. (2007). A neural mass model of spectral responses in electrophysiology. *Neuroimage* 37, 706–720. doi: 10.1016/j.neuroimage.2007.05.032

Nikulin, V. V., Fedele, T., Mehnert, J., Lipp, A., Noack, C., Steinbrink, J., et al. (2014). Monochromatic ultra-slow (~0.1 Hz) oscillations in the human electroencephalogram and their relation to hemodynamics. *NeuroImage* 97, 71–80. doi: 10.1016/j.neuroimage.2014.04.008

Nitsche, M. A., Fricke, K., Henschke, U., Schlitterlau, A., Liebetanz, D., Lang, N., et al. (2003). Pharmacological modulation of cortical excitability shifts induced by transcranial direct current stimulation in humans. *J. Physiol.* 553, 293–301. doi: 10.1113/jphysiol.2003.049916

Nitsche, M. A., and Paulus, W. (2000). Excitability changes induced in the human motor cortex by weak transcranial direct current stimulation. *J. Physiol.* 527, 633–639. doi: 10.1111/j.1469-7793.2000.t01-1-00633.x

Nitsche, M. A., and Paulus, W. (2011). Transcranial direct current stimulation – update 2011. *Restor. Neurol. Neurosci.* 29, 463–492. doi: 10.3233/RNN-2011-0618

Notturno, F., Marzetti, L., Pizzella, V., Uncini, A., and Zappasodi, F. (2014). Local and remote effects of transcranial direct current stimulation on the electrical activity of the motor cortical network. *Hum. Brain Mapp.* 35, 2220–2232. doi: 10.1002/hbm.22322

Novak, V. (2012). Cognition and Hemodynamics. *Curr. Cardiovasc. Risk Rep.* 6, 380–396. doi: 10.1007/s12170-012-0260-2

Nunez, P. L., and Srinivasan, R. (2006). *Electric Fields of the Brain: The Neurophysics of EEG,* 2nd Edn. Oxford: Oxford University Press.

Pellerin, L., and Magistretti, P. J. (1994). Glutamate uptake into astrocytes stimulates aerobic glycolysis: a mechanism coupling neuronal activity to glucose utilization. *Proc. Natl. Acad. Sci. U S A* 91, 10625–10629. doi: 10.1073/pnas.91.22.10625

Polanía, R., Nitsche, M. A., and Paulus, W. (2011). Modulating functional connectivity patterns and topological functional organization of the human brain with transcranial direct current stimulation. *Hum. Brain Mapp.* 32, 1236–1249. doi: 10.1002/hbm.21104

Polanía, R., Paulus, W., and Nitsche, M. A. (2012). Modulating cortico-striatal and thalamo-cortical functional connectivity with transcranial direct current stimulation. *Hum. Brain Mapp.* 33, 2499–2508. doi: 10.1002/hbm.21380

Pulgar, V. M. (2015). Direct electric stimulation to increase cerebrovascular function. *Front. Syst. Neurosci.* 9:54. doi: 10.3389/fnsys.2015.00054

Raffin, E., and Siebner, H. R. (2014). Transcranial brain stimulation to promote functional recovery after stroke. *Curr. Opin. Neurol.* 27, 54–60. doi: 10.1097/wco.0000000000000059

Rahman, A., Reato, D., Arlotti, M., Gasca, F., Datta, A., Parra, L. C., et al. (2013). Cellular effects of acute direct current stimulation: somatic and synaptic terminal effects. *J. Physiol. Lond.* 591, 2563–2578. doi: 10.1113/jphysiol.2012.247171

Schestatsky, P., Morales-Quezada, L., and Fregni, F. (2013). Simultaneous EEG monitoring during transcranial direct current stimulation. *J. Vis. Exp.* e50426. doi: 10.3791/50426

Schiff, S. J., and Sauer, T. (2008). Kalman filter control of a model of spatiotemporal cortical dynamics. *J. Neural Eng.* 5, 1–8. doi: 10.1088/1741-2560/5/1/001

Siesler, H. W., Ozaki, Y., Kawata, S., and Heise, H. M. (2008). *Near-Infrared Spectroscopy: Principles, Instruments, Applications,* 1st Edn. Weinheim: Wiley-VCH.

Sigala, R., Haufe, S., Roy, D., Dinse, H. R., and Ritter, P. (2014). The role of alpha-rhythm states in perceptual learning: insights from experiments and computational models. *Front. Comput. Neurosci.* 8:36. doi: 10.3389/fncom.2014.00036

Sood, M., Jindal, U., Chowdhury, S. R., Das, A., Kondziella, D., and Dutta, A. (2015). "Anterior temporal artery tap to identify systemic interference using short-separation NIRS measurements: a NIRS/EEG-tDCS study," in *Conference Proceedings IEEE Engineering in Medicine and Biology Society,* Milan, Italy.

Sotero, R. C., Trujillo-Barreto, N. J., Iturria-Medina, Y., Carbonell, F., and Jimenez, J. C. (2007). Realistically coupled neural mass models can generate EEG rhythms. *Neural Comput.* 19, 478–512. doi: 10.1162/neco.2007.19.2.478

Spitoni, G. F., Cimmino, R. L., Bozzacchi, C., Pizzamiglio, L., and Di Russo, F. (2013). Modulation of spontaneous alpha brain rhythms using low-intensity transcranial direct-current stimulation. *Front. Hum. Neurosci.* 7:529. doi: 10.3389/fnhum.2013.00529

Suzuki, A., Stern, S. A., Bozdagi, O., Huntley, G. W., Walker, R. H., Magistretti, P. J., et al. (2011). Astrocyte-neuron lactate transport is required for long-term memory formation. *Cell* 144, 810–823. doi: 10.1016/j.cell.2011.02.018

Ursino, M., Cona, F., and Zavaglia, M. (2010). The generation of rhythms within a cortical region: analysis of a neural mass model. *NeuroImage* 52, 1080–1094. doi: 10.1016/j.neuroimage.2009.12.084

Volterra, A., Liaudet, N., and Savtchouk, I. (2014). Astrocyte Ca 2+ signalling: an unexpected complexity. *Nat. Rev. Neurosci.* 15, 327–335. doi: 10.1038/nrn3725

Whalen, A. J., Brennan, S. N., Sauer, T. D., and Schiff, S. J. (2015). Observability and controllability of nonlinear networks: the role of symmetry. *Phys. Rev. X* 5:011005. doi: 10.1103/physrevx.5.011005

Yang, J., Ruchti, E., Petit, J.-M., Jourdain, P., Grenningloh, G., Allaman, I., et al. (2014). Lactate promotes plasticity gene expression by potentiating NMDA signaling in neurons. *Proc. Natl. Acad. Sci. U S A* 111, 12228–12233. doi: 10.1073/pnas.1322912111

Zaehle, T., Sandmann, P., Thorne, J. D., Jäncke, L., and Herrmann, C. S. (2011). Transcranial direct current stimulation of the prefrontal cortex modulates working memory performance: combined behavioural and electrophysiological evidence. *BMC Neurosci.* 12:2. doi: 10.1186/1471-2202-12-2

Zavaglia, M., Astolfi, L., Babiloni, F., and Ursino, M. (2006). A neural mass model for the simulation of cortical activity estimated from high resolution EEG during cognitive or motor tasks. *J. Neurosci. Methods* 157, 317–329. doi: 10.1016/j.jneumeth.2006.04.022

Zheng, X., Alsop, D. C., and Schlaug, G. (2011). Effects of transcranial direct current stimulation (tDCS) on human regional cerebral blood flow. *Neuroimage* 58, 26–33. doi: 10.1016/j.neuroimage.2011.06.018

13

The Temple University Hospital EEG Data Corpus

*Iyad Obeid * and Joseph Picone*

Electrical and Computer Engineering, Temple University, Philadelphia, PA, USA

Keywords: EEG, database, machine learning, clinical trials as topic, big data

Edited by:
Mikhail Lebedev, Duke University, USA

Reviewed by:
Duygu Kuzum, University of California, San Diego, USA
Ervin Sejdic, University of Pittsburgh, USA
Ivan Selesnick, New York University, USA
Xiaomu Song, Widener University, USA
Zhanpeng Jin, Binghamton University, USA

****Correspondence:***
Iyad Obeid
iobeid@temple.edu

INTRODUCTION

The electroencephalogram (EEG) is an excellent tool for probing neural function, both in clinical and research environments, due to its low cost, non-invasive nature, and pervasiveness. In the clinic, the EEG is the standard test for diagnosing and characterizing epilepsy and stroke, as well as a host of other trauma and pathology related conditions (Tatum et al., 2007; Yamada and Meng, 2009). In research laboratories, EEG is used to study neural responses to external stimuli, motor planning and execution, and brain-computer interfaces (Lebedev and Nicolelis, 2006; Wang et al., 2013). While human interpretation is still the gold standard for EEG analysis in the clinic, a host of software tools exist to facilitate the process or to make predictive analyses such as seizure prediction.

Recently, a confluence of events has underscored the need for robust EEG tools. First, there has been a renewed push via the White House BRAIN initiative to understand neural function and disease (Weiss, 2013). Secondly, there is an increased awareness on brain injury owing to both the influx of injured warfighters and numerous high-profile athletes found to have chronic brain damage (McKee et al., 2009; Stern et al., 2011). And thirdly, a wave of consumer grade scalp sensors has entered the market, allowing end users to monitor sleep, arousal, and mood (Liao et al., 2012).

In all these applications, there is a need for robust signal processing tools to analyze the EEG data. Historically, EEG signal processing tools have been devised using either ad hoc heuristic methods, or by training pattern recognition engines on small data sets (Gotman, 1982). These methods have yielded limited results, owing mostly to the fact that brain signals (and EEG in particular) are characterized by great variability, which can only be properly interpreted by building statistical models using massive amounts of data (Alotaiby et al., 2014; Ramgopal et al., 2014). Unfortunately, despite EEG being perhaps the most pervasive modality for acquiring brain signals, there is a severe lack of data in the public domain. For example, the "EEG Motor Movement/Imagery Dataset" (http://www.physionet.org/pn4/eegmmidb/) contains ~1500 recordings of 1 or 2 min duration apiece from 109 subjects (Goldberger et al., 2000; Schalk et al., 2004). The CHB-MIT database contains data from 22 subjects, mostly pediatric (Shoeb, 2009). A database from Karunya University contains 175 16-channel EEGs of duration 10 s (Selvaraj et al., 2014). One of the most extensive databases for supporting epilepsy research is the European Epilepsy Database (http://epilepsy-database.eu/), which contains 250 datasets from 30 unique patients, but sells for €3000. Other databases, such as ieee.org, contain a wealth of data from more invasive modalities such as electrocorticogram, but little or no EEG.

This lack of publically available data is ironic considering that hundreds of thousands of EEGs are administered annually in clinical settings around the world. Relatively little of this data is publicly available to the research community in a form that is useful to machine learning research. Massive amounts of EEG data would allow the use of state-of-the-art machine learning algorithms to discover new diagnostics and validate clinical practice. Furthermore, it is desirable that such data be collected in clinical settings, as opposed to tightly controlled research environments, since "clinical-grade" data is inherently more variable with respect to parameters such as electrode location, clinical environment, equipment, and noise. Capturing this variability is critical to the development of robust, high performance technology that has real-world impact.

In this work, we describe a new corpus, the TUH-EEG Corpus, which is an ongoing data collection effort that has recently released 14 years of clinical EEG data collected at Temple University Hospital. The records have been curated, organized, and paired with textual clinician reports that describe the patients and scans. The corpus is publicly available from the Neural Engineering Data Consortium (www.nedcdata.org) (Picone and Obeid, 2016).

METHODS

Clinical EEG data were collected from archival records at Temple University Hospital (TUH). All work was performed in accordance with the Declaration of Helsinki and with the full approval of the Temple University IRB. All personnel in contact with privileged patient information were fully trained on patient privacy and were certified by the Temple IRB.

Archival EEG signal data were recovered from CD-ROMs. Files were converted from their native proprietary file format (Nicolet's NicVue) to an open format EDF standard. Data was then rigorously de-identified to conform to the HIPAA Privacy Rule by eliminating 18 potential identifiers including patient names and dates of birth. Patient medical record numbers were replaced with randomized database identifiers, with a key to that mapping being saved to a secure off-line location. Importantly, our process captured instances in which the same patient received multiple EEGs over time and assigned database IDs accordingly. Data de-identification was performed by combining automated custom-designed software tools with manual editing and proofreading. All storage and manipulation of source files was conducted on dedicated non-network connected computers that were physically located within the TUH Department of Neurology.

We also manually paired each retrieved EEG with its corresponding clinician report. These reports are generated by the neurologist after analyzing the EEG scan and are the official hospital summary of the clinical impression. These reports are comprised of unstructured text that describes the patient, relevant history, medications, and clinical impression. Reports were mined from the hospital's central electronic medical records archives and typically consisted of image scans of printed reports. Various levels of image processing were employed to improve the image quality before applying optical character recognition (OCR) to convert the images into text. A combination of software and manual editing was used to scrub protected health information (PHI) from the reports and to correct errors in OCR transcription. Only sessions with both an EEG and a corresponding clinician report were included in the final corpus.

The corpus was defined with a hierarchical Unix-style filetree structure. The top folder, `edf`, contains 109 numbered folders, each of which contain numbered folders for up to 100 patients. Each of these patient folders contains sub-folders that correspond to individual recording sessions. Those folder names reflect the session number and date of recording. Finally, each session folder includes one or more EEG (`.edf`) data files as well as the clinician report in `.txt` format. **Figure 1** summarizes the corpus file structure and gives examples of text and signal data.

RESULTS

The completed corpus comprises 16,986 sessions from 10,874 unique subjects. Each of these sessions contains at least one EDF file (more in the case of long term monitoring sessions that were broken into multiple files) and one physician report. Corpus metrics are summarized in **Figure 2**. Subjects were 51% female and ranged in age from less than 1 year to over 90 (average 51.6, stdev 55.9; see **Figure 2** bottom left). The average number of sessions per patient was 1.56, although as many as 37 EEGs were

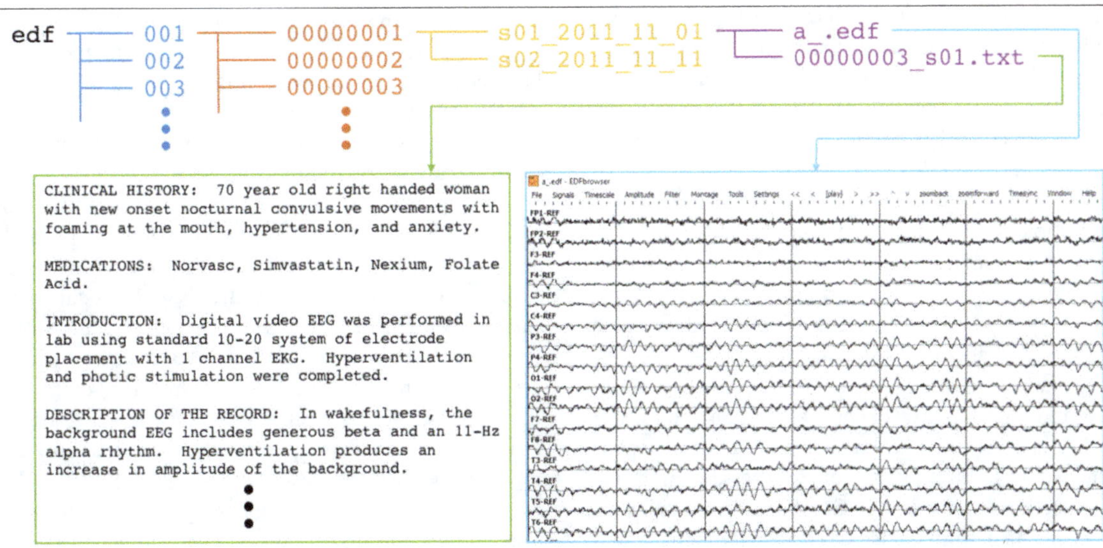

FIGURE 1 | Directory and file structure of the TUH-EEG database. Data is organized by patient (orange) and then by session (yellow). Each session contains one or more signal (edf) and physician report (txt) files. To accommodate file system management issues, patients are grouped into sets of about 100 (blue).

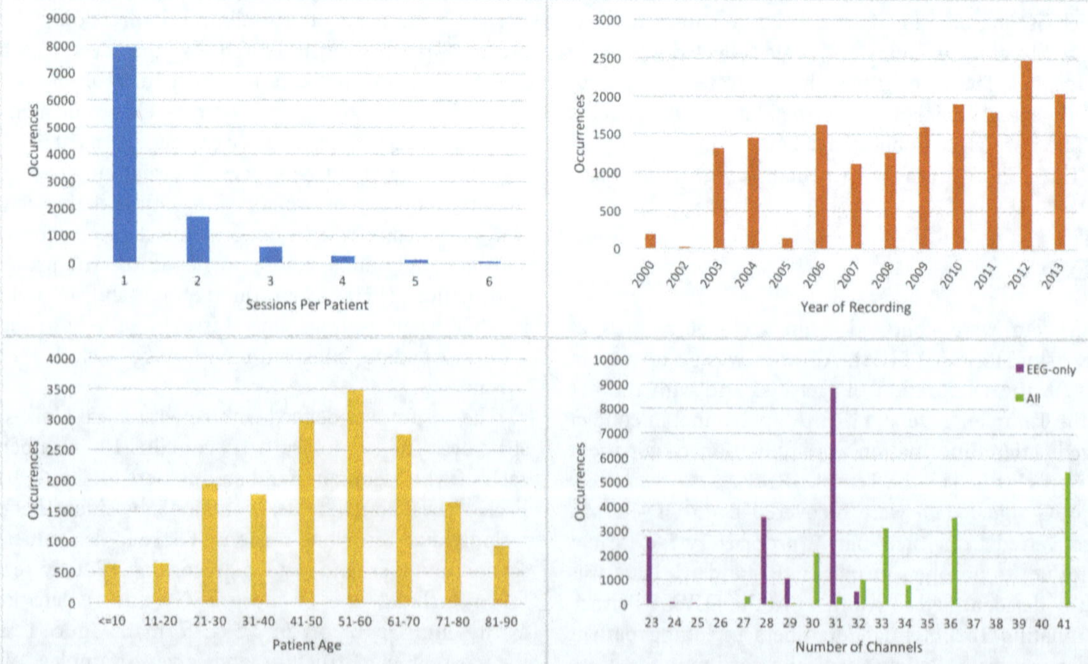

FIGURE 2 | Metrics describing the TUH-EEG corpus. [**Top left**] histogram showing number of sessions per patient; [**top right**] histogram showing number of sessions recorded per calendar year; [**bottom left**] histogram of patient ages; [**bottom right**] histogram showing number of EEG-only channels (purple); and total channels (green).

recorded for a single patient over an 8-month period (**Figure 2** top left). The number of sessions per year varies from ~1000 to 2500 (with the exception of years 2000–2002, and 2005, in which limited numbers of complete reports were found in the various electronic medical record archives; see **Figure 2** top right).

There was a substantial degree of variability with respect to the number of channels included in the corpus (see **Figure 2** bottom right). EDF files typically contained both EEG-specific channels as well as supplementary channels such as detected bursts, EKG, EMG, and photic stimuli. The most common number of EEG-only channels per EDF file was 31, although there were cases with as few as 20. A majority of the EEG data was sampled at 250 Hz (87%) with the remaining data being sampled at 256 Hz (8.3%), 400 Hz (3.8%), and 512 Hz (1%).

An initial analysis of the physician reports reveals a wide range of medications and medical conditions. Unsurprisingly, the most common listed medications were anti-convulsants such as Keppra and Dilantin, as well as blood thinners such as Lovenox and heparin. Approximately 87% of the reports included the text string "`epilep`," and about 12% included "`stroke`." Only 48 total reports included the string "`concus`."

The TUH-EEG corpus v0.6.0 has been released and is freely available online at www.nedcdata.org. Users must register with a valid email address. The uncompressed EDF files and reports together comprise 572 GB. For convenience, the website stores all data from each patient as individual `gzip` files with a median filesize of 4.1 MB; all 10,874 `gzips` together comprise 330GB. Users wanting to access the entire database are encouraged to physically mail a USB hard drive to the authors in order to avoid the downloading process.

DISCUSSION

This work presents the world's largest publically available corpus of clinical EEG data, representing a grand total of 29.1 years (total duration summed over all EEG channels) of EEG data. In addition to its size, this corpus features a wide variation of patient ages, diagnoses, medications, channel counts, and sampling rates. Furthermore, the corpus continues to be expanded at a rate of ~2500 new sessions per year.

Biomedicine is entering a new age of data-driven discovery driven by ubiquitous computing power, inexpensive data storage, the machine learning revolution, and high speed internet connections. Access to massive quantities of properly curated data is now the critical bottleneck to advancement in many areas of biomedical research. Ironically, doctors and clinicians generate enormous quantities of data every day, but that information is almost exclusively sequestered in secure archives where it cannot be used for research by the biomedical research community. The quantity, quality, and variability of such data represent a significant unrealized potential, which is doubly unfortunate considering that the cost of generating that data has already been borne. Although, there has been some advancement with respect to publishing databases of patient metadata, curated *signal* databases are much less commonly available, especially in quantities that would be sufficient to train most contemporary machine learning engines.

In this work, we have endeavored to achieve two goals. The first is to create a corpus of clinical EEG signals and their corresponding physician reports. The second is to establish best practices for the curation and publication of clinical signal data, which is an inherently different entity than discrete metadata. The EEG corpus we present here is the first of its kind, both in terms of volume and heterogeneity, both of which are critical factors for training machine learning engines. Typically, "research-grade" data is created by tightly controlling as many external factors as possible. In contrast, "clinical-grade" data is inherently heterogeneous with respect to those same external factors. Whereas certain classes of research questions can only be answered using well-controlled data, others benefit from variability. For example, an epilepsy detection algorithm that is trained using 31 specific EEG channels may not be effective if one or more of those channels are not connected, or if the electrodes are improperly located or affixed to the scalp. Algorithms that must be sufficiently robust to function under a plurality of conditions must be trained with data that is sufficiently heterogeneous.

Our work has shown that, although clinical signal data is ubiquitous and inherently valuable to the research community, it requires substantial manipulation before it can be released as an adequately curated data corpus. This effort is non-trivial, both in terms of time and cost. Our team's activities ranged from the mundane (e.g., manually copying archival hospital data from over 1500 CD-ROMs) to more technical challenges (e.g., developing software for detecting data entry errors in the clinical records). Physician reports had to be located through one of five different EMR portals, often manually. A battery of tests was created to validate that each record was complete, unique, error-free, and completely free of privileged patient information. A rigorous accounting system was created to track and organize the tens of thousands of files and their status.

The cost to develop the TUH EEG Corpus has been relatively low, totaling less than $100 K in direct charges. As medical record technology improves, the cost of this collection can be reduced even further. On the balance, these types of large-scale collections are a worthwhile investment, since costs are minor relative to the cost of acquiring the data or conducting research on the data. In general, the authors expect that a dedicated community-wide data facility would be best suited to curate data of the magnitude and complexity described here because there are significant on-going costs associated with such an activity.

An example of these on-going costs is annotation of the data—a critical issue for machine learning research. In most semi-supervised machine learning applications, one of the first steps is to annotate the data, a process in which important elements of the signal are marked as such. This can be performed either manually by a human domain expert, or automatically with a bootstrap-style algorithm. In addition to the EEG data itself, we are releasing a collection of annotations which may be downloaded separately if they are of interest to the user. The annotations contain the start and stop time and an event label and are specific to each channel. Six classes of events are included: (1) spike and/or sharp waves (SPSW), (2) periodic lateralized epileptiform discharges (PLED), and (3) generalized periodic epileptiform discharges (GPED). SPSW events are epileptiform transients that are typically observed in patients with epilepsy. PLED events are indicative of EEG abnormalities and often manifest themselves with repetitive spike or sharp wave discharges that can be focal or lateralized over one hemisphere. These signals display quasi-periodic behavior. GPED events are similar to PLEDs, and manifest themselves as periodic short-interval diffuse discharges, periodic long-interval diffuse discharges and suppression-burst patterns according to the interval between the discharges. Triphasic waves, which manifest themselves as diffuse and bilaterally synchronous spikes with bifrontal predominance, typically at a rate of 1–2 Hz, are also included in this class.

Three events are used to model background noise: (1) artifacts (ARTF) are recorded electrical activity that is not of cerebral origin, such as those due to the equipment, patient behavior or the environment; (2) eye movement (EYEM) are common events that can often be confused with a spike; (3) background (BCKG) is used for all other signals.

These six classes (three signal classes and three noise classes) were arrived at through several iterations of a study conducted with Temple University Hospital neurologists. Automatic labeling of these events allows a neurologist to rapidly search long-term EEG recordings for anomalous behavior. However, there are many more annotations that need to be developed for this data. For example, we are currently developing technology to automatically annotate seizures. There are many other events of interest that need annotation (e.g., sleep states). We expect to be continually enhancing the value of the TUH EEG Corpus.

AUTHOR CONTRIBUTIONS

JP led the database creation effort and co-wrote the manuscript. IO contributed to the database creation effort, performed data metrics, and co-wrote the manuscript.

FUNDING

This work has been supported by DARPA award D13AP00065, NSF awards 1305190 and 1458411, and by the Research Office and Dean of Engineering at Temple University.

REFERENCES

Alotaiby, T. N., Alshebeili, S. A., Alshawi, T., Ahmad, I., and Abd El-Samie, F. E. (2014). EEG seizure detection and prediction algorithms: a survey. *EURASIP J. Adv. Signal Process.* 2014:183. doi: 10.1186/1687-6180-2014-183

Goldberger, A. L., Amaral, L. A., Glass, L., Hausdorff, J. M., Ivanov, P. C., Mark, R. G., et al. (2000). Physiobank, physiotoolkit, and physionet components of a new research resource for complex physiologic signals. *Circulation* 101, e215–e220. doi: 10.1161/01.CIR.101.23.e215

Gotman, J. (1982). Automatic recognition of epileptic seizures in the EEG. *Electroencephalogr. Clin. Neurophysiol.* 54, 530–540. doi: 10.1016/0013-4694(82)90038-4

Lebedev, M., and Nicolelis, M. (2006). Brain–machine interfaces: past, present and future. *Trends Neurosci.* 29, 536–546. doi: 10.1016/j.tins.2006.07.004

Liao, L. D., Lin, C. T., McDowell, K., Wickenden, A. E., Gramann, K., Jung, T. P., et al. (2012). Biosensor technologies for augmented brain – computer interfaces in the next decades. *Proceed. IEEE* 100, 1553–1566. doi: 10.1109/JPROC.2012.2184829

McKee, A. C., Cantu, R. C., Nowinski, C. J., Hedley-Whyte, E. T., Gavett, B. E., Budson, A. E., et al. (2009). Chronic traumatic encephalopathy in athletes: progressive tauopathy after repetitive head injury. *J. Neuropathol. Exp. Neurol.* 68, 709–35. doi: 10.1097/NEN.0b013e3181a9d503

Picone, J., and Obeid, I. (2016). *Temple University Hospital EEG Corpus, Neural Engineering Data Consortium, v0.6.3.* Available online at: www.nedcdata.org

Ramgopal, S., Thome-Souza, S., Jackson, M., Kadish, N. E., Sánchez Fernández, I., Klehm, J., et al. (2014). Seizure detection, seizure prediction, and closed-loop warning systems in Epilepsy. *Epilepsy Behav.* 37, 291–307. doi: 10.1016/j.yebeh.2014.06.023

Schalk, G., McFarland, D. J., Hinterberger, T., Birbaumer, N., and Wolpaw, J. R. (2004). BCI2000: a general-purpose Brain-Computer Interface (BCI) system. *IEEE Trans. Bio Med. Eng.* 51, 1034–1043. doi: 10.1109/TBME.2004.827072

Selvaraj, T. G., Ramasamy, B., Jeyaraj, S. J., and Suviseshamuthu, E. S. (2014). EEG database of seizure disorders for experts and application developers. *Clin. EEG Neurosci.* 45, 304–309. doi: 10.1177/1550059413500960

Shoeb, A. (2009). *Application of Machine Learning to Epileptic Seizure Onset Detection and Treatment.* Cambridge, MA: MIT.

Stern, R. A., Riley, D. O., Daneshvar, D. H., Nowinski, C. J., Cantu, R. C., and McKee, A. C. (2011). Long-term consequences of repetitive brain trauma: chronic traumatic encephalopathy. *PM R* (10 Suppl. 2), S460–S467. doi: 10.1016/j.pmrj.2011.08.008

Tatum, W., Husain, A., Benbadis, S., and Kaplan, P. (2007). *Handbook of EEG Interpretation.* New York, NY: Demos Medical Publishing.

Wang, W., Collinger, J. L., Degenhart, A. D., Tyler-Kabara, E. C., Schwartz, A. B., Moran, D. W., et al. (2013). An electrocorticographic brain interface in an individual with tetraplegia. *PLoS ONE* 8:e55344. doi: 10.1371/journal.pone.0055344

Weiss, P. S. (2013). President obama announces the BRAIN initiative. *ACS Nano* 7, 2873–2874. doi: 10.1021/nn401796f

Yamada, T., and Meng, E. (2009). *Practical Guide for Clinical Neurophysiologic Testing: EEG.* Philadelphia, PA: Lippincott Williams & Wilkins.

14

A Novel Wireless Recording and Stimulating Multichannel Epicortical Grid for Supplementing or Enhancing the Sensory-Motor Functions in Monkey (*Macaca fascicularis*)

Antonio G. Zippo[1], *Pantaleo Romanelli*[2]*, *Napoleon R. Torres Martinez*[3], *Gian C. Caramenti*[4], *Alim L. Benabid*[3] *and Gabriele E. M. Biella*[1]*

[1] *Institute of Molecular Bioimaging and Physiology, National Research Council, Segrate, Italy,* [2] *Ab Medica, Lainate, Italy,* [3] *Commissariat à l'Energie Atomique et aux Energies Alternatives, Laboratoire d' Électronique des Technologies de l'Information, CLINATEC, Grenoble, France,* [4] *Institute of Biomedical Technology, Segrate, Italy*

Edited by:
Mikhail Lebedev, Duke University, USA

Reviewed by:
Yoshio Sakurai, Kyoto University, Japan
Kazutaka Takahashi, University of Chicago, USA
Ioan Opris, Wake Forest University School of Medicine, USA

***Correspondence:**
Pantaleo Romanelli, Via Nerviano 31, 20020 Lainate, Milan, Italy
radiosurgery2000@yahoo.com
Gabriele E. M. Biella, Via Nerviano 31, Lainate, Milan, Italy
gembiella@gmail.com

Artificial brain-machine interfaces (BMIs) represent a prospective step forward supporting or replacing faulty brain functions. So far, several obstacles, such as the energy supply, the portability and the biocompatibility, have been limiting their effective translation in advanced experimental or clinical applications. In this work, a novel 16 channel chronically implantable epicortical grid has been proposed. It provides wireless transmission of cortical recordings and stimulations, with induction current recharge. The grid has been chronically implanted in a non-human primate (*Macaca fascicularis*) and placed over the somato-motor cortex such that 13 electrodes recorded or stimulated the primary motor cortex and three the primary somatosensory cortex, in the deeply anaesthetized animal. Cortical sensory and motor recordings and stimulations have been performed within 3 months from the implant. In detail, by delivering motor cortex epicortical single spot stimulations (1–8 V, 1–10 Hz, 500 ms, biphasic waves), we analyzed the motor topographic precision, evidenced by tunable finger or arm movements of the anesthetized animal. The responses to light mechanical peripheral sensory stimuli (blocks of 100 stimuli, each single stimulus being <1 ms and interblock intervals of 1.5–4 s) have been analyzed. We found 150–250 ms delayed cortical responses from fast finger touches, often spread to nearby motor stations. We also evaluated the grid electrical stimulus interference with somatotopic natural tactile sensory processing showing no suppressing interference with sensory stimulus detection. In conclusion, we propose a chronically implantable epicortical grid which can accommodate most of current technological restrictions, representing an acceptable candidate for BMI experimental and clinical uses.

Keywords: brain-machine interface, sensory-motor recordings, sensory-motor stimulation, *Macaca fascicularis*, epicortical grid, chronic implantation

Introduction

It is now almost 50 years that brain-machine interfaces (BMI) are used both in research and in the clinics (Lebedev and Nicolelis, 2006; Graimann et al., 2010; Borton et al., 2013; Wenger et al., 2014) with an expanding range of applications and a growing complexity of exploited tasks. BMIs have been originally devoted to create implantable devices or external frames able to substitute failing brain functions by invasive surgery with e.g., stimulating electrodes (Hochberg et al., 2006; George et al., 2007; Schulze-Bonhage, 2009; Géléoc and Holt, 2014) or by peripheral auxiliary tutors such as cochlear or motor prostheses (Esquenazi and Packel, 2012; Jackson and Zimmermann, 2012). A further issue is represented by the signal quality: the higher the signal to noise ratio, the better the signal representation and the better the output will be presented. Novel applications are also gradually introduced with the aim to enhance brain functions (Deca and Koene, 2014). BMIs are, however, progressively refining on emergent knowledge of brain dynamics and in particular on the assessment that neuronal populations better tune outputs than the activity modulation of single neurons (Nicolelis and Lebedev, 2009). A cooperative, not merely additive, model of brain operation modes turns to be a greater hurdle in completing integrative devices upscaling in complexity, a matter still far from a rigorous understanding (Baranauskas, 2014) though promising preliminary results (Ifft et al., 2012). Along with these functional requirements, a compliant neural interface has also to meet constraints of biological tolerability in order to reduce or block adverse responses from hosting tissues (Groothuis et al., 2014). These prerequisites appear crucial for lifelong neuromorpho implants. In summary, a sort of BMI "ecology" to interlace to local structures and activities appears necessary (Freire et al., 2011; Andersen et al., 2014; Orsborn et al., 2014). Indeed, promising solutions have been since successively proposed in these years (Lebedev and Nicolelis, 2006). From then now, a further new research path has grown related to exploring possible enhancements of brain functions (Deca and Koene, 2014), virtually enabling expanded aptitudes (in strength, fatigue resistance, sensory perspicuity a.s.o.) or working in special or hostile environments (Lebedev et al., 2011). As from the above description, planning a new brain stimulating device settles as a strongly demanding topic, with a large front of vital requirements. In an earlier work on another monkey a prototype grid had been previously implanted with no additional feature for stimulating and recording (Piangerelli et al., 2014). In this paper we tried to focus, beyond the experimental application of stimulation and recording we further checked two of those themes mentioned above, namely the noiseless data transmission accompanied to high biological compatibility and the biological tolerance during long term experiments. We show here the electrophysiological results obtained by the epicortical grid in the monkey. The grid has a matrix of 16 recording and stimulating channels mounted over a thinnest (15 μm) plastic support and connected with a subcutaneously implantable wireless and power supply. The final goal of this device is meant to sense and counteract anomalous excitation in epilepsy with easier localization of epileptic foci or to balance activity disorders in chronic pain. Two experimental series, with recording and stimulating sessions, have been performed, while checking long term performance of the grid within 3 months from the device placement analysing the single channel resistance. In the first experimental series an analysis of the fine grained stimulation of single fingers by the epicortical probes has been evaluated. In the second series the recording properties from the sensory cortical potentials elicited by peripheral electrical and natural stimuli, as well as the electrical interference on the naturally evoked stimuli have been estimated.

Methods

Surgical Procedure and Implanted Device

The grid was implanted by one of the authors (Pantaleo Romanelli) in a non-human primate (*Macaca fascicularis*) over the sensorimotor cortex to record somatosensory potentials, to check the grid efficiency in eliciting fine finger or gross arm movements through remotely-driven cortical stimulation. Briefly, a male macaque monkey, weighting 7.07 kg, was used in this study. The experimental protocol was approved by the regional committee (Cometh Grenoble) and registered to the national committee under the number 12/136 Clinatec-NTM-01 and complied with the EU directive 22nd September 2010 (2010/63/EU) on the care and use of laboratory animals (for an extensive description of the surgical preparation used in former experiments on a prototype of this grid see Piangerelli et al., 2014 on a different monkey). The new grid was equipped with the technical facilities for wireless recording and stimulating to and to from each of its channels. This enabled us to program experimental sessions with diverse protocols. The protocols aimed, to map the cortical responsiveness to light sensory stimuli delivered onto somatotopically competent peripheral areas, and explored the interference of stimuli delivered by the grid electrodes on the epicortical foci with the peripheral stimuli. Briefly, the animal was anesthetized using Xylazine (5 mg/kg), and Ketamine hydrochloride (20 mg/kg), intramuscular (IM), and then a maintenance dose of 1.25 mg/kg, 5 mg/kg Xylazine/Ketamine. All the vital parameters (Heart rate, ECG, respiration, oxygenation, and body temperature) were constantly monitored by the veterinary staff (monitor Infinity® Delta XL; DRAGER, Luebeck, Germany). Surgical procedures took place in standard aseptic conditions. In deep anesthesia with the animal secured to a stereotaxic frame, a craniotomy was performed over the left motor cortex (M1) in Brodmann area 4 and, posteriorly, gyrus of the corresponding primary somatosensory cortex (SS1) removing a rectangular (3 × 2.5 cm) bone tile. After bone removal, the epidural site was tested using ISIS IOM Neuromonitoring© cortical stimulator (INOMED Medizintechnik; Emmendingen, GERMANY) which delivered biphasic train pulses between poles, to identify the hand area. The *dura mater* was then opened by a Y-shaped cut, exposing the surface of M1 and the anterior margin of the corresponding primary somatosensory cortex (SS1). The location of the grid electrodes was determined by identifying topic anatomical landmarks (the central, the intraparietal, and the arcuate sulci). Retesting was conducted and hand area identification was refined with the same INOMED stimulator directly in contact to the cortex and EMG of the right hand (Cortical stimulation parameters were 100 μs, 5 mA, 7 Hz). The device was positioned orthogonally and the grid was centered above the hand knob of the left motor cortex. The grid Channels 1, 2, and 3 were placed over the sensory cortex in correspondence of cortical stations responsive to light peripheral stimuli on contralateral thumb, index and middle fingers. Channels 4 to 16 covered the motor cortex able to generate fine movements in the contralateral upper limb. The electrode impedance has been measured during the months of the experiment, allowing for comparisons among the experimental recording or stimulating procedures in time. The signals were recorded using commercial software for Epicortical Grid (EcoG) recording provided by Micromed, Treviso, Italy. The technical characteristics of this new grid, different from those shown in the previous work by Piangerelli et al., are summarized in **Table 1**. In detail, the grid was made by a thin (15 μm) foil of flexible polyimide with printed platinum (Pt) small plaquettes (16 plaques in a 4 × 4 matrix, 200 nm thick, interplaque distance of slightly less than 3 mm). Two reference Pt electrodes were printed posteriorly to the plan of application of the grid. The grid was built with direct connection with a battery (Li ions, rechargeable) case (Peek polymer, 800 μm thick) including the electronic components for wireless transmission. The recording features were realized with a detection range of ±780 μV in a bandwidth of 0–500 Hz at gain 12. The available variable gains were (1, 2, 3, 4, 6, 8, 10, 12). The programmable waveforms were between ±3 V at impedance of 10Ω (**Figure 2E**).

The Cortical Recordings and Stimulations

Recordings and stereoselective somatic stimulations (13 electrodes placed over the primary motor cortex and 3 on the primary somatosensory cortex) were performed within 3 months from the implant. A sampling rate of 512 Hz (@16 bit) was used for the grid recordings. Electrical stimulations were delivered on the spontaneous activity background either *per se*, to evaluate the magnitude of the elicited motor responses or concurrently to peripheral light threshold stimuli to check the spatiotemporal electrical interference of artificial inputs over the sensory responses. In **Figure 1** the elements of the grid and of the wireless transmitting and recharging device are shown. **Figure 1A**: the constructive elements of the grid and of the power supply are reported. **Figure 1B**: a view in detail of the grid circuitry is shown. The recording and stimulating plaquettes and their schematized circuitry along with the analytic spatial measures of its architecture are also shown. **Figure 1C**: the grid to be implanted is shown. **Figure 1D**: the apparatuses for wireless recording and stimulus delivery with the anesthetized monkey are shown. During the experiments the monkey was covered with a blanket to avoid loss of temperature of the animal. In **Figure 1E**, the recording device alone is shown. The grid was recharged by induction into a dedicated cage (not shown here). Thirteen electrodes (4–16) were placed over the motor fields. Electrodes 1–3 face the sensory cortical surface. In **Figure 2** the technical details of the grid stimulating output and the Arduino driven sensory stimuli device are shown. In detail, in **Figures 2A,B** the electrical scheme and the controller with optic insulator for the electrical grid stimulus control are respectively displayed. In **Figure 2C** the home-made device able to release point-like (1 mm^2) sub-millisecond random stimuli (see Zippo et al., 2014) are shown. **Figure 2D**: The overall 16 channel impedance profiles during the implantation period. **Figure 2E**: The peripheral signal as delivered by the microcontroller. As evident from the reported trace, sensory inputs are elicited in random sequence.

The Peripheral Stimulator

The peripheral stimulation device is composed by an Arduino® electronic card able to deliver 1 kHz outputs in random sequences (See **Figures 2C,D**). The output device is composed by a woofer with a pipette tip mounted vertically over the cusp of the woofer dust cap. The stimuli had to be as fast and spatially selective as possible in order to reduce the "background noise" and sharpen the signals of interest. To this purpose, we used the stimulation device together with a novel stimulus delivery protocol and a predictive computational framework. The protocol of randomizing stimuli offered the advantage of paired pulses and reduced the possibility of spurious locking between stimuli and spontaneous periodical bursts of neuronal activity and sensory habituation with waning responses to equal subsequent stimuli (Zippo et al., 2013, 2014).

The Grid Stimulation

Bipolar stimulations were delivered by rectangular 0.5 ms pulses and anodal monophasic current. This stimulation technique consists of a train of five pulses delivered at 1 Hz with an interstimulus interval of 100 ms. The stimulus intensity was regulated between 1 and 3 mA at constant voltage of 3.3 V.

In **Tables 1, 2**, the technical data of the EcoG pads and of the Grid (Cyberbrain, AB Medica) electronic properties are reported.

We followed three experimental protocols to analyze, respectively, the stability of the spontaneous activity with the cortical responses to peripheral light threshold stimuli, the spontaneous activity with the responses to grid driven electrical stimuli, and, finally, the interference induced by the grid electrical stimuli on the sensory patterns elicited by the sensory peripheral stimuli.

Protocols

(1) Protocol 1

   (a) 15 min (three sessions of 5 min each) of spontaneous activity recording have been performed from all the available channels
   (b) Natural Peripheral Stimulations: Short, non-nociceptive, point-like sensory stimuli have been delivered on the finger tips by the pipette tip mounted over a woofer dust-cap driven by an Arduino electronically controlled output (Zippo et al., 2014). Each finger-tip was stimulated by trains of light touches (100 stimuli randomised in order to avoid habituation). Each 100 stimulus train lasted 90 s. An trigger to the recording

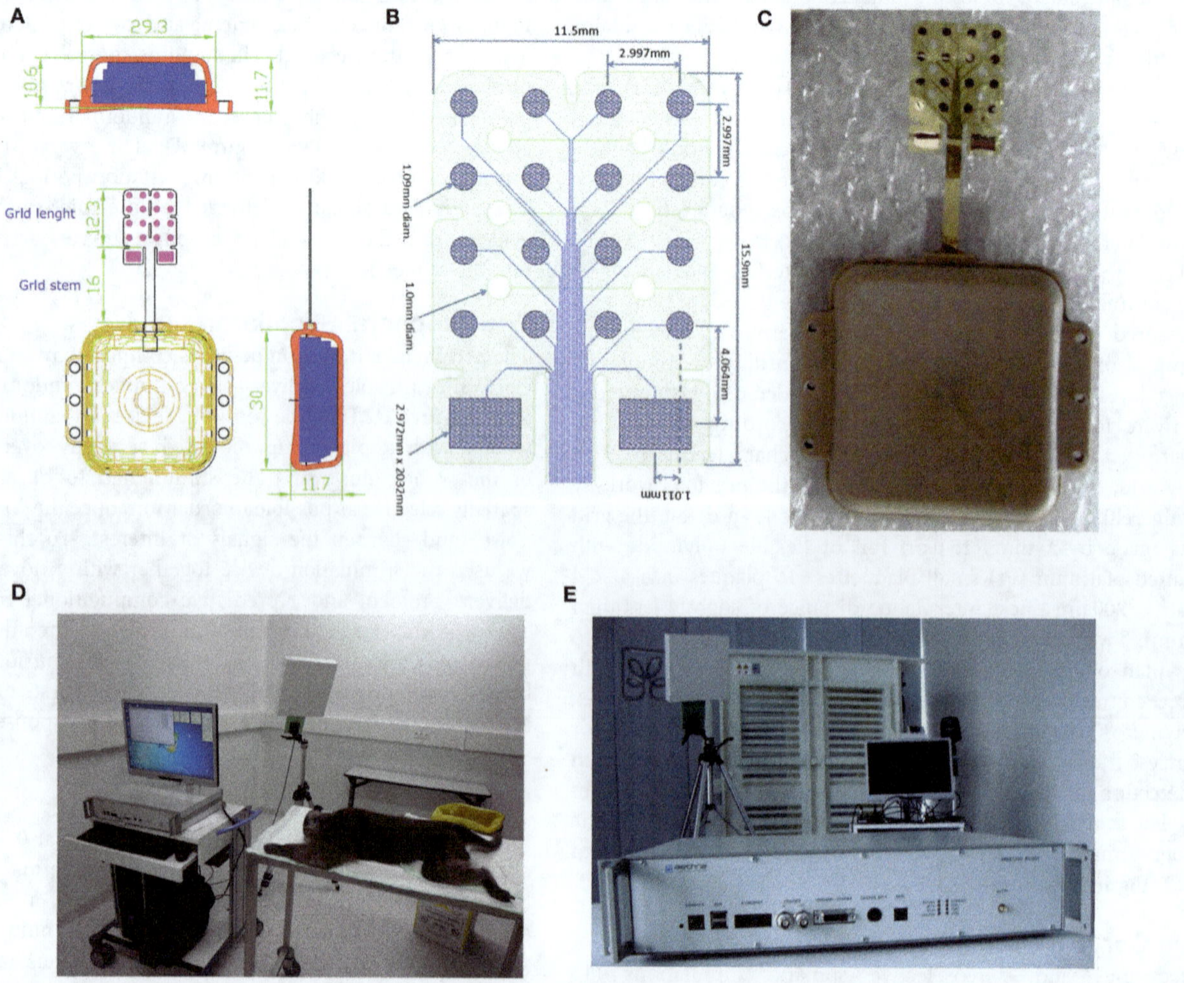

FIGURE 1 | Characteristics of the epicortical grid. (A,B) Shape and measures of the grid. **(C)** Picture of the grid. **(D)** Experimental configuration with wireless data transmission device. **(E)** Wireless data transmission device in detail.

device from the Arduino card was provided in order to synchronize the stimulus signals with the recorded electrocorticographic activities.

(2) Protocol 2

  (a) 15 min (three sessions of 5 min each) of spontaneous activity recording from all the available channels
  (b) Grid Stimulations: Stimuli have been delivered by the ECoG device. Stimuli will be separately delivered at each electrode placed over the sensory cortex. 2 min of 1, 7, and 30 Hz of 100 to 500 μs stimulation cycles have been recorded from the other two sensory electrodes. Some 5 min of resting activity recordings among the stimulation trains was left.

(3) Protocol 3

  (a) Concurrent Grid and peripheral stimulations: The peripheral stimuli were delivered with comparable scheme (see above) to the responsive fingers after 1 min of Grid electrical stimuli. Plaquette current sources were chosen with the criterion of proximity to those showing maximal sensory responses. These observations have been done in order to evaluate the effects of central electrical stimuli on the peripheral natural stimuli cortical estimates.

Analysis of Epicortical Evoked Potentials

The effects of the different stimulation protocols were evaluated by averaging the recorded potentials among all trials (100) and all experimental sessions (2). Each recording session was split into 100 time windows taking into account 125 ms before the onset of the stimulus (both tactile peripheral and electrical) and 1 s after the onset of the stimulus. Therefore we had 1125 ms windows in all stimulation protocols. To evaluate the null hypothesis, that the observed potentials were not due to our stimulation protocols (SHAM), we randomized the time occurrences of the stimuli and we repeated the same averaging technique used in the previous description.

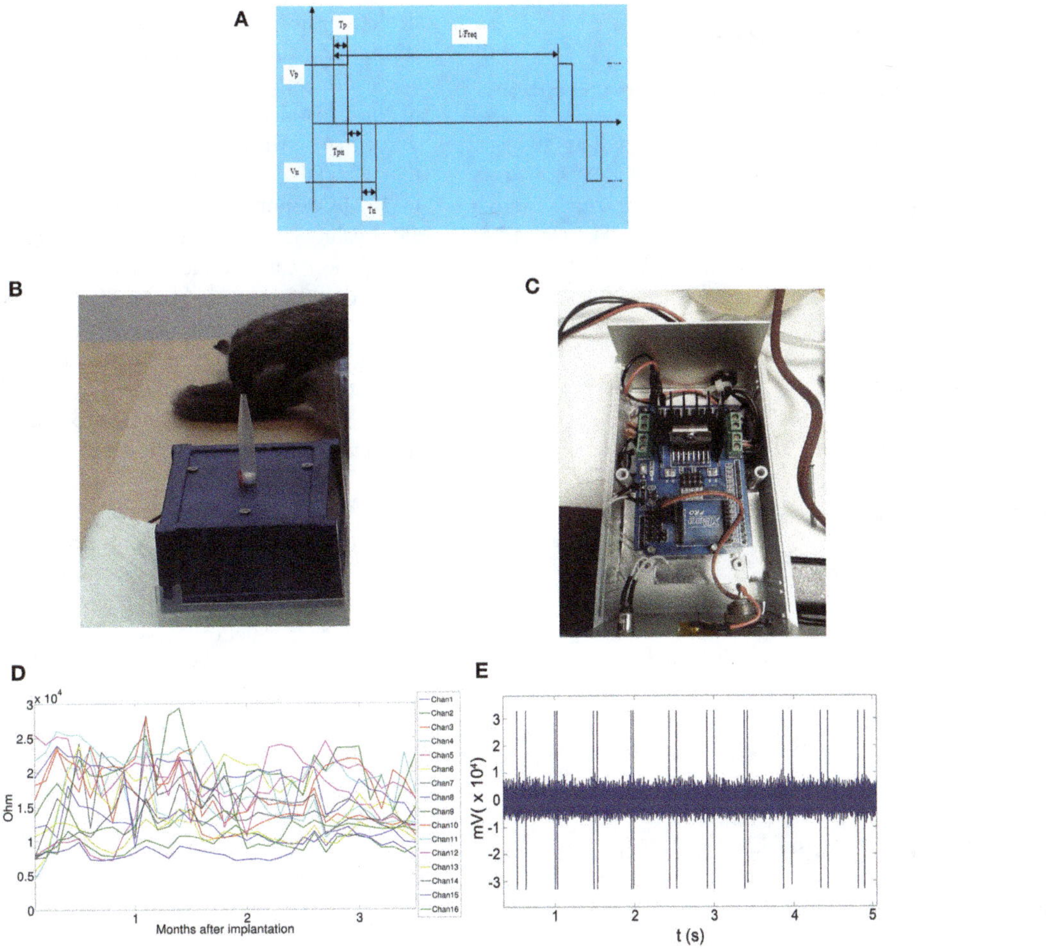

FIGURE 2 | Features of the electrical and tactile stimulation setups. **(A)** Wave-front of the Arduino delivered stimuli. **(B)** The stimulus delivery device. The pipette base is sealed on a midrange loudspeaker dust-cap moved at 1 kHz. The tip was placed just on hand fingertips, *thenar* or *hypothenar* eminences or on foot fingertips. **(C)** The electronic card Arduino driving the woofer dustcap. **(D)** Impedences of the grid during the period of the experimental sensory-motor measurements. **(E)** Stimulus artifacts over the magnified trace of the stimulus recording channel.

Statistical Tests

To assess statistical differences between evoked potential patterns we used an *ad hoc* hypothesis test. Given the evoked potentials by N trials of all the 16 electrodes in two sites, $A = A_{1,\dots,}A_N$ and $B = B_{1,\dots,}B_N$, we computed the correlation coefficient (R) between A_i and B_j, $\forall i, j \in \{1, \dots, N\}$.

Subsequently we arbitrarily set a threshold of 0.5 for the correlation coefficient: A_i and B_j are considered different matrices if R was below the threshold, similar otherwise. An exploratory analysis revealed that R values (99.87%) were clustered into two groups: those in the range [0, 0.23] and those in the range [0.7, 1]. Therefore the arbitrary choice of the used threshold (0.5) did not produce effects on results. Finally, to estimate the p-value we computed the ratio of comparisons with a R value above the threshold among the set of all comparisons between the trials of two stimulation sites.

To establish the statistical significance of the impedance measures (16 electrodes per day of sampling) over time, we used the Kruskal-Wallis test avoiding the assumption of normality of the data.

Results

We performed repeated the same experimental protocol (see Methods Section) in two dates: the first, approximately 1 month after (D34) the day of surgical implantation and the second after 3 months (D92). In each session we applied the same experimental protocol divided into parts: in the first we produced tactile stimulations through the Arduino microntroller in five different sites, namely the thumb, the index, the middle and the anular fingers of the right forelimb, and the big toe finger of the right hindlimb. In the second part we combined the tactile stimulations with trains of direct current stimulations delivered by the epicortical grid.

Prior to analyze the electrical potentials evoked by stimulation protocols we wondered whether the electrode impedance

TABLE 1 | Physical features of the epicortical grid.

EcoG 16 PADS MATERIALS		
Components	**Materials**	**Characteristics**
Grid	Flexible polymide	15 μm thickness
Electrodes	Platinum	200 nm thickness
Case	Peek (invibio)	0.8 mm thickness
Adhesives	Fast-cure silicone adhesives (Nusil)	MED1-4213, MED2-4213, MED3-4213
	Solicon primer (Nasil)	MED-163
	Epoxy resin (Epoxy Technology)	EPO-TEK 301-2
EMC	Alumina thick film	0.5 mm thickness
Battery	Rechargeable lithium ion polymer cell	
Electronic circuits	Electronics components	

TABLE 2 | Technical features of the grid.

ANALOG FRONT END	
Numer of channels	16
Variable Gain	1, 2, 3, 4, 6, 8, 12
Detection range	± 780 μV (@ Gain 12)
Bandwidth	0–500 Hz (@ 2 Ksps)
Resolution	16 bit Σ/Δ
Input noise	1 μVrms (G = 12 @ 500 Hz BW)
Sampling frequency	250 Hz to 2 KHz
Lead off detection	DC and 250 Hz @ 24 nA
MICROCONTROLLER AND PERIPHERAL	
Microcontroller	Kinetic MK40N512K 100 MHz Freescale
External SRAM	16 Mbits (2 M × 8 bit)
Sensors	3 Axis g, Temperature, Charge current
STIMULUS	
Waveform	Programmable waveforms
Amplitude	± 3V and ± 1.65 V (between Ref and Pad)
Impedance	10 Ω
INDUCTIVE WIRELESS POWER	
Inductive local coil frequency	145 KHz (Charge current 20 mA @ 3.7 V
Magnetic cage	145 KHz (Charge current 20 mA @ 3.7 V)
BATTERY	
Li Ion rechargeable	3.6 V 140 mA/h
	Battery Life ~3h @38 mA
	Recharging Period >12 h (Cage)
POWER CONSUMPTION	
16CH @ 500SPS + TX_RF	38 mA
16CH @ 500SPS	33 mA

(measured once a day) changed along the 3 months (104 days). We found that no significant modifications of the electrode impedance emerged during these months ($P = 0.591$, $N = 1664$, Kruskal-Wallis test). Furthermore, no conspicuous immune response or evident grid rejection signs were noticed neither at the interface with the cortical surface nor by the removed *dura mater* during the period of electrophysiological observation.

From the electrophysiological point of view the grid efficiently detected the fine-grain tactile information from peripheral stimuli and the central electrically evoked potentials. By using a specific statistical hypothesis test we evaluated the stability of the evoked potentials in a stimulation site or the statistical difference between the responses of two different sites. We found that evoked potentials of each of the five sites corresponded to stable response patterns (see the diagonal of the **Table 3**, all *P*-values are close to 1). In addition we wondered if each stimulation site produced a specific response pattern and we found that this was the case. Indeed, each site evoked a particular and an unequivocal potential along the recording electrodes that fully identified the stimulus location (non-diagonal values of **Table 3** that are all smaller than 0.1). Here below are reported the results of the three experimental conditions we tested the grid. In **Figure 3** are reported the recorded somatosensory responses to the peripheral point-like stimuli delivered by the Arduino driven device. Stimuli were delivered on four fingertips of the right arm (**Figures 3B–D**), contralateral to the stimulated cortex as well to the homologous big toe (**Figure 3A**). Clear patterns of responses are reported in color-code raster images (Blue to Brick Red representing a scale from no to "strong" cortical response, normalized on these maxima). It is interesting to note that the four stimulated fingers produced four different patterns of response. Namely, index and thumb showed precocious responses within 125 ms while the responses to the big toe and the hand middle finger had delayed response onset latency around 250 ms.

Eventually, we investigated the potential effects of epicortical current stimulations (whose effects are shown in **Video 1**) on the somatosensory processing caused by tactile stimulations. This has been planned in order to examine the effects of repeated electrical stimulations over the timing and patterning of the natural peripheral stimuli. For this reason we applied the same statistical framework to verify whether the responses from a given site were statistically similar or different. Taking into consideration the large variability of the responses to peripheral stimuli, no significant influence after the discontinuation of the grid electrical stimuli was noticed in the response profile of sensory peripheral stimuli. As expected by a first visual inspection, electrical stimulation did not interfere with the normal somatosensory processing (see *P*-values in the last column of **Table 3**, all close to 1).

In **Figure 4** are reported the results from the concurrent electrical vs. natural peripheral stimuli. Left column—Above: the picture shows an example of cortical responses to low-threshold peripheral stimuli delivered to a finger. Bottom: the peripheral stimuli have been delivered after a cycle of grid driven electrical stimuli on the same recording plaquettes. Where the fine grain of the responses was slightly interfered, there was no gross suppression or distortion of sensory signaling after the electrical stimuli delivery.

Discussion

In this paper we propose a novel ultrathin 16 channel grid apparatus to record/stimulate the cerebral cortex in

TABLE 3 | Statistical comparisons among the tactile stimulation sites.

Site	Thumb (Forelimb)	Index (Forelimb)	Middle (Forelimb)	Anular (Forelimb)	Big Toe (Forelimb)	DCS
Thumb (Forelimb)	$P = 0.872$, $N = 200$	$P = 0.012$, $N = 40{,}000$	$P = 0.015$, $N = 40{,}000$	$P = 0.013$, $N = 40{,}000$	$P = 0.058$, $N = 40{,}000$	$P = 0.992$, $N = 200$
INdex (Forelimb)	$P = 0.013$, $N = 40{,}000$	$P = 0.939$, $N = 200$	$P = 0.017$, $N = 40{,}000$	$P = 0.015$, $N = 40{,}000$	$P = 0.017$, $N = 40{,}000$	$P = 0.988$, $N = 200$
Middle (Forelimb)	$P = 0.079$, $N = 40{,}000$	$P = 0.125$, $N = 40{,}000$	$P = 0.973$, $N = 200$	$P = 0.127$, $N = 40{,}000$	$P = 0.013$, $N = 40{,}000$	$P = 0.975$, $N = 200$
Anular (Forelimb)	$P = 0.014$, $N = 40{,}000$	$P = 0.099$, $N = 40{,}000$	$P = 0.124$, $N = 40{,}000$	$P = 0.994$, $N = 200$	$P = 0.014$, $N = 40{,}000$	$P = 0.966$, $N = 200$
Big Toe (Hindlimb)	$P = 0.015$, $N = 40{,}000$	$P = 0.018$, $N = 40{,}000$	$P = 0.010$, $N = 40{,}000$	$P = 0.016$, $N = 40{,}000$	$P = 0.894$, $N = 200$	$P = 0.981$, $N = 200$

We exerted each stimulation site of the right forelimb and hindlimb 200 times: 100 times in the first experimental session after 1 month and 100 in the second experimental session after 3 months of the grid surgical implantation. P-values toward 1 on the table diagonal ensured that the response patterns were stable both within each experimental session and between the experimental sessions. Instead, small p-values indicated that each stimulation site produces an unequivocal activation pattern detected by the epicortical grid that characterized the somatosensory response. The similarity between responses was asserted by computing the correlation coefficient between the resulting matrices (see Methods section).

diverse clinical conditions such as epilepsy or chronic pain. Brain Machine Interfaces (BMIs) are multipurpose devices instrumental in a number of brain pathological conditions from replacement of injured brain circuits to sustenance of weakened functions or of circuitry intermittent failures or again to their supervision (Nicolelis, 2012; Rao, 2013).

The BMI Puzzle

More recently the concept of brain function augmentation has also been set forth with the aim of supporting particularly demanding performances as for instance actions in adverse environments (e.g., in outer space missions or in memory challenging assignments) (Hampson et al., 2012; Deca and Koene, 2014). Most of these applications come from practice on "normal" experimental animals and prospected to find application in pathology (as for instance to vascular, degenerative or traumatic pathologies). Hence, it is advisable to point-out that resident "functional engrams" simply activated in "normal conditions" don't overlap pathological conditions where exogenous "neural programs" are to be re-assigned *ab-externo* (Birbaumer et al., 2006; Andersen et al., 2014; Grahn et al., 2014; Hu et al., 2014; Lebedev, 2014). The grid presented in this paper has been planned to evolve in a frame apt to intercept anomalous insurgence of seizure signals, to localize them on the cortical thread and ultimately generate interfering or blocking hyper-synchronization codes of epileptic waves. Eventually, it has been, as well, designed to balance the electrical anomalies steadily present in chronic pain. Along a theoretic approach stemmed in our labs, chronic pain relates to a collapse of information transmission within supraspinal sensory networks (Zippo et al., 2011). As prediction, an admittance of coherent information to the involved networks is critical to reestablish natural conditions abating stereotyped signal recursions. Cortically applied magnetic fields or electrical currents have been indeed shown to control chronic pain symptoms (Passard et al., 2007; Fricová et al., 2013; Lefaucheur et al., 2014; Moreno-Duarte et al., 2014). Instead, diversely from these settings, the disruption of epileptic hyper-synchronizations meets less "refined" problems, the goal being to stop abruptly diffuse and "sudden" excitatory wave fronts. Currently, there are no clear indications on "prospective" electrodynamical solutions to balance or cancel these anomalies but thinking of electrical interferences halting the anomalous signal regeneration with different DBS or peripheral stimulation approaches (Goodman, 2004; Boon et al., 2009; Fisher and Velasco, 2014). On a theoretic ground, these devices should subserve fast "interpretations" of degeneracy codes and deliver tuned outputs or re-drive networks within normal ranges. The "interference" over epileptic backgrounds, presents, thus, distinct aims from the "ecological coherences" needed by BMIs in other contexts (e.g., trial and error routines to drive external prostheses; Dromerick et al., 2008; Bongers et al., 2011). A provisional measure counteracting the epileptic surge is expected to either provide rough "antagonistic" currents or to generate "seizure contextual" outputs, a very remote goal because of the poor decoding of epileptic waves achieved until now, but for snapshots of non-deterministic analyses of ictal and interictal epochs (Knowlton et al., 2004a,b; Dwyer et al., 2010).

Function Restorations

A different planning would be obviously to be provided for substitutive tasks, such as in motor and motor-like functions, requiring to re-allocating lost abilities within a (slow) trial-and-error learning context. Surprisingly, in these experiments carried on normal experimental animals, it has been shown that the number of involved neurons seemingly sufficient in prosthesis motion appears notably small with consistent conservation of the collective neuronal frequency (with multiple single unit and unit ensemble tuning; Nicolelis and Lebedev, 2009). These features may hypostatize future synthetic bases enriched with multiple network activation loci where the recruitment of a limited number of neurons for each locus may facilitate textured activations. However these assumptions may be biased by the mismatch between experimental trials on healthy circuits and those providing restitutive implants for lost functions. Namely, in the former conditions, long

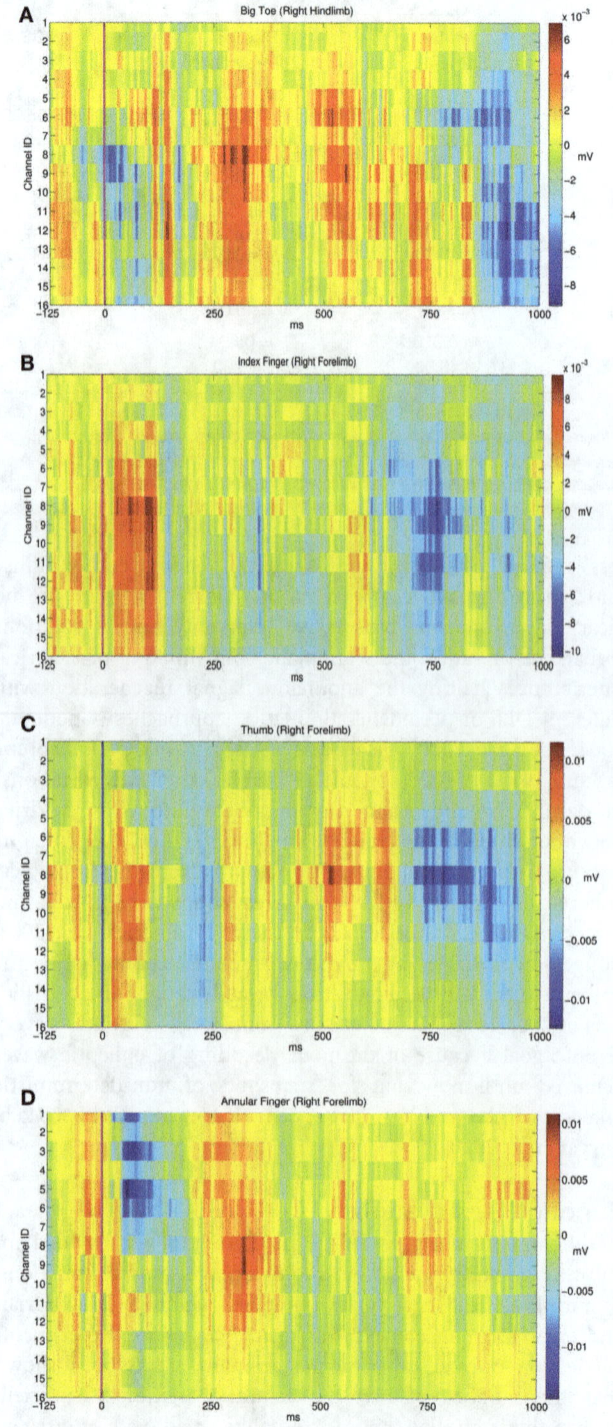

FIGURE 3 | Average evoked potentials of the cortical recorded responses to the peripheral sensory stimuli (Arduino driven fingertip stimuli) on four regions. Responses from respectively **(A)** the right big toe. **(B)** The right index fingertip. **(C)** The right index fingertip. **(D)** The right ring (or annular) fingertip.

processes of environmental adaptation and learning may have reduced the network dimensionality by gradual pruning of prototypal neuronal ensembles in conjunction to budding memories and plasticity processes (Koralek et al., 2012; Di Pino et al., 2014) to realize complex outputs with parsimonious expenditures and scaled modulations (Ganguly et al., 2011; Marblestone et al., 2013). In case of brain damages, machines have to be merged within erratic environment connectivity, hardly an achievable context by current devices (Mandonnet and Duffau, 2014). Cutting edge technologies, now, prompt to deep functional refinements such as interventions on cortical minicolumn coherence or stabilization of engrams generated by the prosthetic devices or again able to spot not only surface but also intrasulcal electrocorticographic signals (Ganguly and Carmena, 2009; Matsuo et al., 2011; Opris and Casanova, 2014) or again on intrinsic oscillatory circuit properties to coordinate dispersed neuronal populations (Canolty et al., 2010). These issues don't change even in functional disorders accompanied by cortical microstructural misalignments, such as chronic pain. It has been shown that exogenous transcranial magnetic or epicortical inputs significantly reduce chronic pain symptoms and these results go along with our theory on chronic pain as the result of collapsed information and the assumed symptom conversion by reinstatement of information. This strengthens the idea to adopt implantable brain machine devices injecting opportune or comparable currents to durably control chronic pain.

Advancement of Interface Material

All the above hints highlight the technical novelties to be imported onto future devices. Technical novelties grow significantly and allow for a wide range of applications with constructive (as for instance in sensory-motor supply), modulatory (as in chronic pain control) or disruptive (to counteract epileptic foci dynamic anomalies) scopes. Basic requirements are, obviously, features like adjustable intensity of output and functional coherence with the extant tissue. Examples have been realized recently for extreme flexibility of newly conceived devices (Yin et al., 2011) as well as for even neuroprosthetic device learning reactivation (Gulati et al., 2014). A further step has, been recently done by an organic material-based, biocompatible neural interface array apt to record both local field potentials (LFPs) and action potentials from superficial cortical neurons without penetrating the brain surface, a crucial leap forward in the technique of cortical grids when enabled to be mounted on human patients (Khodagholy et al., 2015). The grid we present here delivers strength enough to provoke sudden gross arm displacements as well as tunings able to elicit fine movements of single fingers. This suggests that, in the first mode, a "stop" sequence might be generated strong enough to halt even a generalized seizure (where a mere quantitative criterion could be held). On the other side the grid, selectively arousing smooth and independent finger movements, prospectively adapts to generate finest motor plans in suitable contexts. The subject becomes even more delicate with future BMIs applied on sensory compartments. Aside from the delivery of conventional stimulus sequences to elicit raw sensory information, BMIs would be loaded by semantics apt to encode the environment information features and keep into account corollary problems such as the forward effects of sensory

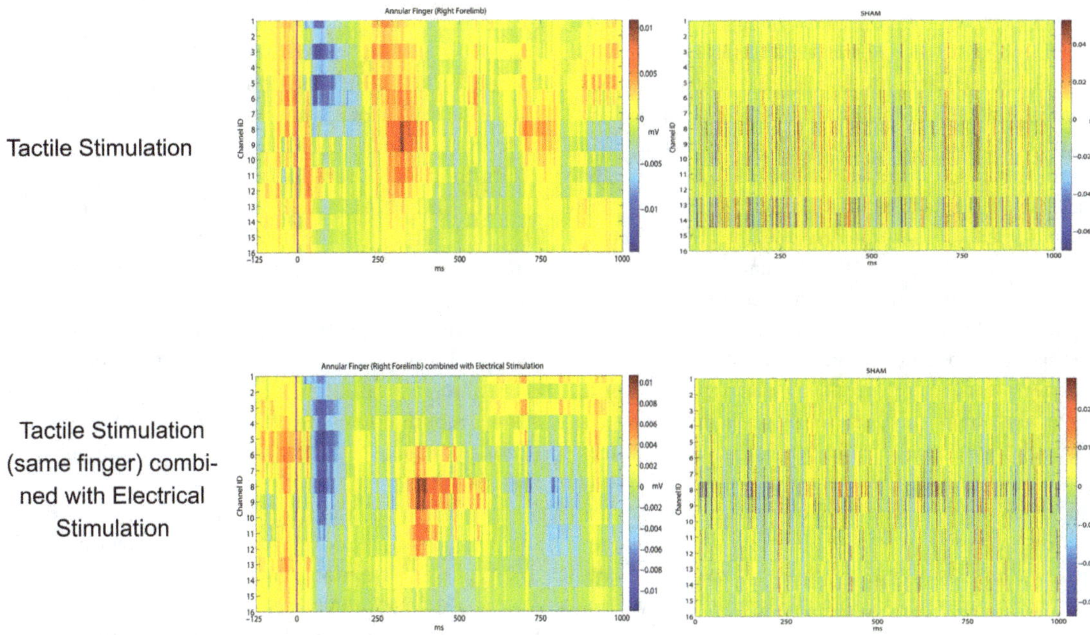

FIGURE 4 | Average evoked potentials from the ring (annular) finger. Row above: peripheral Arduino driven sensory stimuli (left). With no peripheral stimuli (right). Bottom row: peripheral Arduino driven sensory stimuli just after the central grid driven electrical stimuli on the most responding channels (left). Recording just after the central grid driven electrical stimuli with no peripheral Arduino driven sensory stimuli (right).

generated motor activations (O'Doherty et al., 2011; Opris et al., 2013), or input induced sensory learning (Koralek et al., 2012; Tabot et al., 2014). In fact, in experiments on rats, repetitive sensory or prefrontal cortical stimuli have shown coherent motor learning enhancements (Opris et al., 2013).

The Sensorimotor Pathway

Along these lines, we then explored the effect of epicortical stimulus patterns and their potential spreading to nearby grid plaquettes and, in conjunction, we analyzed the interferences of epicortical stimuli with concurrent peripheral sensory stimuli, in keeping with the core idea that local synthetic activations could drift natural stimuli. Indeed, in experiments on rats, mismatches between active and passive activations of the sensory cortex have been reported (Krupa et al., 2004). In our experiments, epicortical stimuli, although disturbing parallel natural sensory stimuli, once discontinued, did not show any extra interference with the responses to those stimuli. The natural stimuli were very light threshold sensory touches, repeatedly presented on single fingertips by a device delivering less than one millisecond-long inputs over some 1 mm^2 (Zippo et al., 2014). They were apt to elicit extremely evident responses on a significant cluster of recording electrodes with evident stereotactical distribution. On the other side, artificial grid stimuli were of low or mean intensity (see **Table 2**) and suitably delivered in turn from one single of the 16 plaquette. As noted above, the four stimulated fingers produced four different patterns of response. Namely, index and thumb showed precocious responses within 125 ms while the responses to the big toe and the hand middle finger had delayed response onset latency around 250 ms. These discrepancies may be explained by potential somatotopic coherence of the stimulated regions with the responding electrode. If the epicortical plaquette was place over the correct somatotopic projection area of the stimulated finger, the response could be clearly and quickly identified. If a mismatch between the projection field and the finger was relevant, it is conceivable to hypothesize that intra-cortical ("horizontal") paths could transport delayed activations from sources in the focus of inputs but far from the plaquettes. An alternative explanation could hold and namely that the stimulus competent (but non-recorded) cortex could recruit the thalamus (backward recruitment within local recurrent thalamic-cortico-thalamic loops). The thalamus could, in turn, forwardly recruit non-competent (but recorded) cortical areas. The mechanism could simply generate there a "warning sensory condition" in non-somatotopic areas declining in case of stimulus cessation. A balance between specific and non-specific (or core and matrix) thalamic activations could also be prospected. Whatever the origin, a delayed response was well detectable. Handiness and precision thus provide a path for future complex input constructs, meeting at least a number of requirements.

Limitations and Conclusions

As further note, the BMI driven function enhancement deserves some additional reflection. Supplementary feature integrations within natural networks urge questioning on the essence of the envisioned functional increment and, in greater detail, on how and what to achieve it. The increments themselves appear planned imbalances within however "normal" circuitries, well far from the conventional BMI roles in circuit degeneracies

(Hu et al., 2014), devoted to achievements in shorter time or with higher efficiency, time endurance or, again, by helping fatigued brain circuitries in defiant conditions. All in all, in a "connectome" perspective, both subsidiary and vicarious devices must recognize spatio-temporal alignments in hosting tissue to avoid anomalous avalanches and signal propagation within the biological environment (Deca, 2012). Finally, biologically-oriented manufacture and dedicated architectures are required to circumvent or strongly reduce immuno-rejection or inflammatory foci hampering the implanted devices by responses such as partial or complete connective encapsulation (McConnell et al., 2009). For instance, gelatine (Lind et al., 2010) or other treatments provided interesting experimental results to counter these effects and, more recently special probe shaping showed improvements in tissue tolerance by reducing the effects of sustained trauma (Sohal et al., 2014). No particular treatment has been operated over the grid, yet obtaining satisfying results during period of the electrophysiological study, due to the particularly suited polymer material surrounding the plaquettes (no apparent reaction observed during the period of the electrophysiological observations). Interesting results have also been obtained with other materials, however only in laboratory experiments and not in surgical epicortical implants (Chou et al., 2013). As a rule, however, the epicortical devices are usually placed for short or very short periods for diagnostic aims and then quickly removed. A long-term placement with negligible or no cortical damage could overcome the conventional diagnostic limits to switch them to long term application. The grid has been in-site showing no generalized rejection signs from an electrophysiological point of view and no blinding of the local electrical cortical contacts. The subtlety of the plastic contact carrier appears, then, contributing to its good tolerance. A prospective suitably engineered grid conformation could extend its application range, by encompassing more than one single cortical region and allow for the accurate studies of intra-cortical stimuli conduction and the careful activations of collection or single mini-electrodes exploring selected subsets of cortical regions.

In conclusion, the grid used in these experiments enabled the fine detail recordings and the conveyance of long-term fine-grain information from and to cortical surfaces. These features will potentially help for future therapeutic applications in sensorimotor and neurodegenerative diseases.

References

Andersen, R. A., Kellis, S., Klaes, C., and Aflalo, T. (2014). Toward more versatile and intuitive cortical brain-machine interfaces. *Curr. Biol.* 24, R885–R897. doi: 10.1016/j.cub.2014.07.068

Baranauskas, G. (2014). What limits the performance of current invasive brain machine interfaces? *Front. Syst. Neurosci.* 8:68. doi: 10.3389/fnsys.2014.00068

Birbaumer, N., Weber, C., Neuper, C., Buch, E., Haagen, K., and Cohen, L. (2006). "Physiological regulation of thinking: brain-computer interface (BCI) research, Chap. 24," in *Progress in Brain Research,* Vol. 159, eds Neuper and Klimesch, 369–391. doi: 10.1016/S0079-6123(06)59024-7

Bongers, R. M., Bouwsema, H., and van der Sluis, C. K. (2011). "Motor control processes when learning to use a prosthetic device. MEC 11 raising the standard," in *Proceedings of the 2011 MyoElectric Controls/Powered Prosthetics Symposium Fredericton August 14-19, 2011* (New Brunswick, NJ: Copyright University of New Brunswick).

Boon, P., Raedt, R., de Herdt, V., Wyckhuys, T., and Vonck, K. (2009). Electrical stimulation for the treatment of epilepsy. *Neurotherapeutics* 6, 218–227. doi: 10.1016/j.nurt.2008.12.003

Borton, D. A., Yin, M., Juan, A., and Nurmikko, A. (2013). An implantable wireless neural interface for recording cortical circuit dynamics in moving primates. *J. Neural Eng.* 10:026010. doi: 10.1088/1741-2560/10/2/026010

Canolty, R., Ganguly, K., Kennerley, S., Cadieu, C., Koepsell, K., Wallis, J., et al. (2010). Oscillatory phase coupling coordinates anatomically-dispersed functional cell assemblies. *Proc. Natl. Acad. Sci. U.S.A.* 107, 17356–17361. doi: 10.1073/pnas.1008306107

Chou, N., Yoo, S., and Sohee Kim, S. (2013). A largely deformable surface type neural electrode array based on PDMS. *IEEE Trans. Neural. Syst. Rehabil. Eng.* 21, 544–553. doi: 10.1109/TNSRE.2012.2210560

Deca, D. (2012). The Connectome, WBE and AGI. *Artif. Gen. Intell. Lect. Notes Comp. Sci.* 7716, 41–49. doi: 10.1007/978-3-642-35506-6_5

Deca, D., and Koene, R. A. (2014). Experimental enhancement of neurphysiological function. *Front. Syst. Neurosci.* 8:189. doi: 10.3389/fnsys.2014.00189

Di Pino, G., Maravita, A., Zollo, L., Guglielmelli, E., and Di Lazzaro, V. (2014). Augmentation-related brain plasticity. *Front. Syst. Neurosci.* 8:109. doi: 10.3389/fnsys.2014.00109

Dromerick, A. W., Schabowsky, C. N., Holley, R. J., Monroe, B., Markotic, A., and Lum, P. S. (2008). Effect of training on upper-extremity prosthetic performance and motor learning: a single-case study. *Arch. Phys. Med. Rehabil.* 89, 1199–1204. doi: 10.1016/j.apmr.2007.09.058

Dwyer, J., Lee, H., Martell, A., Stevens, R., Hereld, M., and van Drongelen, W. (2010). Oscillation in a network model of neocortex. *Neurocomputing* 73, 1051–1056. doi: 10.1016/j.neucom.2009.12.021

Esquenazi, A., and Packel, A. (2012). Robotic-assisted gait training and restoration. *Am. J. Phys. Med. Rehabil.* 91(11 Suppl. 3), S217–S227. doi: 10.1097/PHM.0b013e31826bce18

Fisher, R. S., and Velasco, A. L. (2014). Electrical brain stimulation for epilepsy. *Nat. Rev. Neurol.* 10, 261–270. doi: 10.1038/nrneurol.2014.59

Freire, M. A., Morya, E., Faber, J., Santos, J. R., Guimaraes, J. S., Lemos, N. A., et al. (2011). Comprehensive analysis of tissue preservation and recording quality from chronic multielectrode implants. *PLoS ONE* 6:e27554. doi: 10.1371/journal.pone.0027554

Fricová, J., Klírová, M., Masopust, V., Novák, T., Vérebová, K., and Rokyta, R. (2013). Repetitive transcranial magnetic stimulation in the treatment of chronic orofacial pain. *Physiol Res.* 62(Suppl. 1), S125–S134.

Ganguly, K., and Carmena, J. M. (2009). Emergence of a stable cortical map for neuroprosthetic control. *PLoS Biol.* 7:e1000153. doi: 10.1371/journal.pbio.1000153

Ganguly, K., Dimitrov, D. F., Wallis, J. D., and Carmena, J. M. (2011). Reversible large-scale modification of cortical networks during neuroprosthetic control. *Nat. Neurosci.* 14, 662–667. doi: 10.1038/nn.2797

Géléoc, G. S., and Holt, J. R. (2014). Sound strategies for hearing restoration. *Science* 344:1241062. doi: 10.1126/science.1241062

George, M. S., Nahas, Z., Borckardt, J. J., Anderson, B., Burns, C., Kose, S., et al. (2007). Vagus nerve stimulation for the treatment of depression and other neuropsychiatric disorders. *Expert Rev. Neurother.* 7, 63–74. doi: 10.1586/14737175.7.1.63

Goodman, J. H. (2004). Brain stimulation as a therapy for epilepsy. *Adv. Exp. Med. Biol.* 548, 239–247. doi: 10.1007/978-1-4757-6376-8_17

Grahn, P. J., Mallory, G. W., Berry, B. M., Hachmann, J. T., Lobel, D. A., and Lujan, J. L. (2014). Restoration of motor function following spinal cord injury via optimal control of intraspinal microstimulation: toward a next generation closed-loop neural prosthesis. *Front. Neurosci.* 8:296. doi: 10.3389/fnins.2014.00296

Graimann, B., Allison, B., and Pfurtscheller, G. (2010). Brain–computer interfaces: a gentle introduction. *Brain Comput. Interfaces* 1–27. doi: 10.1007/978-3-642-02091-9_1

Groothuis, J., Ramsey, N. F., Ramakers, G. M., and van der Plasse, G. (2014). Physiological challenges for intracortical electrodes. *Brain Stimul.* 7, 1–6. doi: 10.1016/j.brs.2013.07.001

Gulati, T., Ramanathan, D. S., Wong, C. C., and Ganguly, K. (2014). *Nat. Neurosci.* 17, 1107–1113. doi: 10.1038/nn.3759

Hampson, R. E., Gerhardt, G. A., Marmarelis, V., Song, D., Opris, I., Santos, L., et al. (2012). Facilitation and restoration of cognitive function in primate prefrontal cortex by a neuroprosthesis that utilizes minicolumn-specific neural firing. *J. Neural. Eng.* 9:056012. doi: 10.1088/1741-2560/9/5/056012

Hochberg, L. R., Serruya, M. D., Friehs, G. M., Mukand, J. A., Saleh, M., Caplan, A. H., et al. (2006). Neuronal ensemble control of prosthetic devices by a human with tetraplegia. *Nature* 442, 164–171. doi: 10.1038/nature04970

Hu, X., Wang, Y., Zhao, T., and Gunduz, A. (2014). Neural coding for effective rehabilitation. *Biomed Res. Int.* 2014:286505. doi: 10.1155/2014/286505

Ifft, P. J., Lebedev, M. A., and Nicolelis, M. A. L. (2012). Reprogramming movements: extraction of motor intentions from cortical ensemble activity when movement goals change. *Front. Neuroeng.* 5:16. doi: 10.3389/fneng.2012.00016

Jackson, A., and Zimmermann, J. B. (2012). Neural interfaces for the brain and spinal cord–restoring motor function. *Nat. Rev. Neurol.* 8, 690–699. doi: 10.1038/nrneurol.2012.219

Khodagholy, D., Gelinas, J. N., Thesen, T., Doyle, W., Devinsky, O., Malliaras, G. et al. (2015). NeuroGrid: recording action potentials from the surface of the brain. *Nat. Neurosci.* 18, 310–315. doi: 10.1038/nn.3905

Knowlton, R. C., Lawn, N. D., Mountz, J. M., Buddhiwardhan, O., Miller, S., Burneo, J. G., et al. (2004b). Ictal single-photon emission computed tomography imaging in extra temporal lobe epilepsy using statistical parametric mapping. *J. Neuroimaging* 14, 324–330. doi: 10.1177/1051228404268570

Knowlton, R. C., Lawn, N. D., Mountz, J. M., and Kuzniecky, R. I. (2004a). Ictal SPECT analysis in epilepsy: subtraction and statistical parametric mapping techniques. *Neurology* 63, 10–15. doi: 10.1212/01.WNL.0000132885.83350.45

Koralek, A., Jin, X., Long, J., Costa, R., and Carmena, J. M. (2012). Corticostriatal plasticity is necessary for learning intentional neuroprosthetic skills. *Nature* 483, 331–335. doi: 10.1038/nature10845

Krupa, D. J., Wiest, M. C., Shuler, M. G., Laubach, M., and Nicolelis, M. A. (2004). Layer-specific somatosensory cortical activation during active tactile discrimination. *Science* 304, 1989–1992. doi: 10.1126/science.1093318

Lebedev, M. (2014). Brain-machine interfaces: an overview. *Transl. Neurosci.* 5, 99–110. doi: 10.2478/s13380-014-0212-z

Lebedev, M. A., and Nicolelis, M. A. (2006). Brain-machine interfaces: past, present and future. *Trends Neurosci.* 29, 536–46. doi: 10.1016/j.tins.2006.07.004

Lebedev, M. A., Tate, A. J., Hanson, T. L., Li, Z., O'Doherty, J. E., Winans, J. A., et al. (2011). Future developments in brain-machine interface research. *Clinics* 66, 25–32. doi: 10.1590/S1807-59322011001300004

Lefaucheur, J. P., André-Obadia, N., Antal, A., Ayache, S. S., Baeken, C., Benninger, D. H., et al. (2014). Evidence-based guidelines on the therapeutic use of repetitive transcranial magnetic stimulation (rTMS). *Clin. Neurophysiol.* 125, 2150–2206. doi: 10.1016/j.clinph.2014.05.021

Lind, G., Eriksson Linsmeier, C., Thelin, J., and Schouenborg, J. (2010). Gelatine-embedded electrodes—a novel biocompatible vehicle allowing implantation of highly flexible microelectrodes. *J. Neural Eng.* 7:046005. doi: 10.1088/1741-2560/7/4/046005

Mandonnet, E., and Duffau, H. (2014). Understanding entangled cerebral networks: a prerequisite for restoring brain function with brain-computer interfaces. *Front. Syst. Neurosci.* 8:82. doi: 10.3389/fnsys.2014.00082

Marblestone, A. H., Zamft, B. M., Maguire, Y. G., Shapiro, M. G., Cybulski, T. R., Glaser, J. I., et al. (2013). Physical principles for scalable neural recording. *Front. Comput. Neurosci.* 7:137. doi: 10.3389/fncom.2013.00137

Matsuo, T., Kawasaki, K., Osada, T., Sawahata, H., Suzuki, T., Shibata, M., et al. (2011). Intrasulcal electrocorticography in macaque monkeys with minimally invasive neurosurgical protocols. *Front. Syst. Neurosci.* 5:34. doi: 10.3389/fnsys.2011.00034

McConnell, G. C., Rees, H. D., Levey, A. I., Gutekunst, C. A., Gross, R. E., and Bellamkonda, R. V. (2009). Implanted neural electrodes cause chronic, local inflammation that is correlated with local neurodegeneration. *J. Neural Eng.* 6:056003. doi: 10.1088/1741-2560/6/5/056003

Moreno-Duarte, I., Morse, L. R., Alam, M., Bikson, M., Zafonte, R., and Fregni, F. (2014). Targeted therapies using electrical and magnetic neural stimulation for the treatment of chronic pain in spinal cord injury. *Neuroimage* 85(Pt 3), 1003–113. doi: 10.1016/j.neuroimage.2013.05.097

Nicolelis, M. A. L. (2012). *Beyond Boundaries: The New Neuroscience of Connecting Brains with Machines and How It Will Change Our Lives.* New York, NY: Times Books; Henry Holt and Company.

Nicolelis, M. A., and Lebedev, M. A. (2009). Principles of neural ensemble physiology underlying the operation of brain-machine interfaces. *Nat. Rev.* 10, 530–540. doi: 10.1038/nrn2653

O'Doherty, J. E., Lebedev, M. A., Ifft, P. J., Zhuang, K. Z., Shokur, S., Bleuler, H., et al. (2011). Active tactile exploration enabled by a brain-machine-brain interface. *Nature* 479, 228–231. doi: 10.1038/nature10489

Opris, I., and Casanova, M. F. (2014). Prefrontal cortical minicolumn: from executive control to disrupted cognitive processing. *Brain* 137(Pt 7), 1863–1875. doi: 10.1093/brain/awt359

Opris, I., Santos, L. M., Song, D., Gerhardt, G. A., Berger, T. W., Hampson, R. E., et al. (2013). Prefrontal cortical microcircuits bind perception to executive control. *Sci. Rep.* 3:2285. doi: 10.1038/srep02285

Orsborn, A., Moorman, H., Overduin, S., Shanechi, M., Dimitrov, D., and Carmena, J. M. (2014). Closed-loop decoder adaptation shapes neural plasticity for skillful neuroprosthetic control. *Neuron* 82, 1–14. doi: 10.1016/j.neuron.2014.04.048

Passard, A., Attal, N., Benadhira, R., Brasseur, L., Saba, G., Sichere, P., et al. (2007). Effects of unilateral repetitive transcranial magnetic stimulation of the motor cortex on chronic widespread pain in fibromyalgia. *Brain* 130(Pt 10), 2661–2670. doi: 10.1093/brain/awm189

Piangerelli, M., Ciavarro, M., Paris, A., Marchetti, S., Cristiani, P., Puttilli, C., et al. (2014). A fully integrated wireless system for intracranial direct cortical stimulation, real-time electrocorticography data transmission, and smart cage for wireless battery recharge. *Front. Neurol.* 5:156. doi: 10.3389/fneur.2014.00156

Rao, R. P. N. (2013). *Brain-Computer Interfacing: An Introduction.* New York, NY: Cambridge University Press

Schulze-Bonhage, A. (2009). Deep brain stimulation: a new approach to the treatment of epilepsy. *Dtsch Arztebl Int.* 106, 407–412. doi: 10.3238/arztebl.2009.0407

Sohal, H. S., Jackson, A., Jackson, R., Clowry, G. J., Vassilevski, K., O'Neill, A., et al. (2014). The sinusoidal probe: a new approach to improve electrode longevity. *Front. Neuroeng.* 7:10. doi: 10.3389/fneng.2014.00010

Tabot, G. A., Kim, S. S., Winberry, J. E., and Bensmaia, S. J. (2014). Restoring tactile and proprioceptive sensation through a brain interface. *Neurobiol. Dis.* 260–265. doi: 10.1016/j.nbd.2014.08.029

Wenger, N., Moraud, E. M., Raspopovic, S., Bonizzato, M., DiGiovanna, J., Musienko, P., et al. (2014). Closed-loop neuromodulation of spinal sensorimotor circuits controls refined locomotion after complete spinal cord injury. *Sci. Transl. Med.* 6, 255. doi: 10.1126/scitranslmed.3008325

Yin, M., Borton, D. A., Komar, J., Agha, N., Lu, Y., Li, H., et al. (2011). Wireless Neurosensor for Full-Spectrum Electrophysiology Recordings during Free Behavior. *Neuron* 84, 1170–1182. doi: 10.1016/j.neuron.2014.11.010

Zippo, A. G., Nencini, S., Caramenti, G. C., Valente, M., Storchi, R., and Biella, G. E. M. (2014). A simple stimulatory device for evoking point-like tactile stimuli: a searchlight for LFP to spike transitions. *J. Vis. Exp. 25, 85* doi: 10.3791/50941

Zippo, A. G., Storchi, R., Nencini, S., Caramenti, G. C., Valente, M., and Biella, G. E. M. (2013). Neuronal functional connection graphs among multiple areas of the rat somatosensory system during spontaneous and evoked activities. *PLoS Comput. Biol.* 9:e1003104. doi: 10.1371/journal.pcbi.1003104

Zippo, A. G., Storchi, R., Valente, M., Caramenti, G. C., and Biella, G. E. M. (2011). Neural substrates of chronic pain in the thalamocortical circuit. *Nat. Preceed.*

15

A Framework for Combining rTMS with Behavioral Therapy

*K. Zoe Tsagaris[1], Douglas R. Labar[1,2] and Dylan J. Edwards[1,2]**

[1] Non-Invasive Brain Stimulation and Human Motor Control Laboratory, Burke Medical Research Institute, White Plains, NY, USA, [2] Department of Neurology, New York Presbyterian, Weill Cornell Medicine, New York, NY, USA

Edited by:
Mikhail Lebedev,
Duke University, USA

Reviewed by:
Patrizia Silvia Bisiacchi,
University of Padua, Italy
Rachel M. Sherrard,
Pierre-and-Marie-Curie University, France

***Correspondence:**
Dylan J. Edwards
dje2002@med.cornell.edu

Upon its inception, repetitive transcranial magnetic stimulation (rTMS) was delivered at rest, without regard to the potential impact of activity occurring during or around the time of stimulation. rTMS was considered an experimental intervention imposed on the brain; therefore, the myriad features that might suppress or enhance its desired effects had not yet been explored. The field of rTMS has since grown substantially and therapeutic benefits have been reported, albeit with modest and inconsistent improvements. Work in this field accelerated following approval of a psychiatric application (depression), and it is now expanding to other applications and disciplines. In the last decade, experimental enquiry has sought new ways to improve the therapeutic benefits of rTMS, intended to enhance underlying brain reorganization and functional recovery by combining it with behavioral therapy. This concept is appealing, but poorly defined and requires clarity. We provide an overview of how combined rTMS and behavioral therapy has been delineated in the literature, highlighting the diversity of approaches. We outline a framework for study design and reporting such that the effects of this emerging method can be better understood.

Keywords: repetitive transcranial magnetic stimulation (rTMS), non-invasive brain stimulation, neurological rehabilitation, behavioral interventions, therapy

INTRODUCTION

The brain is never at rest; the *default-mode network* comprised of coherent and connected brain networks (cingulate cortices, inferior parietal, and medial prefrontal regions), operative at times of behavioral rest, has been examined through the use of blood oxygenation level-dependent (BOLD) signals. Functional MRI testing has shown the default-mode network is active at rest and in the presence of volitional behavior (e.g., repetitive task practice), decreases in activation. This deactivation may allow for associated activity-dependent plasticity in other parts of the motor system. Because of the default-mode network's activation/deactivation patterns, it appears the motor cortex does not work in isolation during volitional behavior, motor learning, recovery and reorganization (Sanes and Donoghue, 2000; Gusnard and Raichle, 2001; Damoiseaux et al., 2006). Instead, the motor cortex injury-response functional reorganization appears to occur through use-dependent alteration of outputs, which result from behavioral experiences, such as repetitive task practice (Nudo et al., 2001). Interventions promoting recovery should attend to this complex dynamic process, and likely utilize a multi-faceted approach for optimal outcome.

Background

The initial application of spatially targeted non-invasive brain stimulation (NIBS) as treatment to improve function was not temporally linked to meaningful voluntary brain activity; instead was delivered in isolation of standard therapy practice techniques (Amassian and Maccabee, 2006). Such applications would seem to tap into only a fraction of the complex multi-faceted systems changes involved in learning and memory. Influencing brain areas remote from, but functionally connected to, a primary target, and influencing brain activity at critical time periods relative to practice and therapy timing, may be important additional considerations in this domain.

Hardwired existing pathways (e.g., skilled movement, speech, or executive function) may have lower threshold for activation by transcranial magnetic stimulation (TMS), and therefore be preferentially predisposed to modulation by NIBS. For example, in the motor system, Rothwell et al. (1987) studied a healthy population at rest and found the largest electromyographic (EMG) responses in distal muscles (which have the finest movements associated with them) versus lower EMG responses in proximal muscles. Furthermore, upon simultaneous voluntary contraction, the EMG response latency to brain TMS shortens, becomes larger, and the threshold is lower. Therefore, if voluntary activation is absent or decreased, such as in a diseased brain state, the modulation possible with NIBS may be altered. Conversely, TMS may affect a patient's ability to produce a voluntary motor activation. Thus the quality and duration of responses seem likely to be influenced by the interactions of interdependent complex systems. The efficacy of stand-alone NIBS is influenced by its stimulation variables, which include: frequency, intensity, coil positioning, stimulation site, and number of sessions delivered (Nollet et al., 2003; Goetz et al., 2016). Therefore, TMS protocols may be adapted to modulate the motor response through excitatory or depressive methods dependent on stimulation parameters, providing opportunity for custom programs based on the population, person, and pathology.

rTMS and Behavioral Intervention: Current Focus

One contemporary approach is to link NIBS with behavioral techniques, in hopes of producing more robust and durable outcomes. The logic for doing so stems from the idea that effects of repetitive TMS (rTMS) and behavioral therapy will sum or that rTMS will enhance, or consolidate, the effects of therapy. For instance, Mills and Schubert (1995) suggest TMS during sustained voluntary, tonic activity may increase synchronicity of common input fibers and motor neurons. This improved synchrony may promote increased motor cortex plasticity, compared to one intervention alone. Finding the optimal pairing of intensity, duration, frequency, and site, for both rTMS and therapy, would be important for the strongest enhancement, but also to avoid maladaptive plasticity.

Thus one can learn from analyzing the variety of approaches that have been employed previously and assess outcome. In the present paper we aimed to: (a) outline what is meant by *combined therapy* in the context of historical literature [this is examining how traditional therapies (occupational, speech, physical, cognitive-behavioral, or task practice) are combined with rTMS either on or off-line]; (b) provide a snapshot of the literature showing the diverse range of approaches, and outcomes; and (c) propose a framework for how combined therapy should be reported in the literature moving forward.

Most *combined therapy* studies have been on stroke survivors to date and have been intuitively and practically based (Supplementary Table S1). For example, time considerations such as equipment practicality, busy clinical setting, staffing, training, and availability, may affect feasibility of temporally combined therapies. Additionally, the participant's cognitive or physical state during rTMS delivery is rarely reported in the literature but may influence intervention efficacy (e.g., patient engaged in conversation, use of mobile device, listening to music). Despite increasing application of TMS in the field of psychiatry and FDA approval for refractory depression, very little has been done in examining the combination of rTMS with behavioral interventions, such as cognitive behavioral therapy (Micoulaud-Franchi et al., 2013; *note French language*). Instead, most commonly, papers describe using rTMS in isolation for patients with medication-resistant depression (Lam et al., 2008; Slotema et al., 2010). It would be of considerable interest for systematic research on *combined therapy* to expand beyond the motor function domain, and study brain processes such as depression or learning in the future. Hopefully this would lead to a better understanding of broader principles concerning the effects of rTMS as an adjunct to older, traditional, well-accepted therapy approaches.

Cumulative Effect

Research to determine the cumulative effect and duration of results of NIBS intervention is ongoing. This cumulative effect was examined in a healthy population by Baumer et al. (2003) who found repeated sessions of rTMS (two trains of inhibitory, sub-motor threshold rTMS over the pre-motor cortex) delivered within 24 h, or no greater than 7 days later (consecutive days), induced plastic changes of intrinsic motor cortex excitability. Khedr et al. (2006) and Lomarev et al. (2006) found a cumulative effect of rTMS in individuals with Parkinson's Disease (eight sessions of 25 Hz rTMS over 4 weeks) which lasted 1 month or more. It appears that multiple sessions of rTMS will lead to a cumulative effect, identified as regions of sustained membrane polarization (Pell et al., 2011). With this effect it may be possible to build on neuromodulatory changes in subsequent sessions to promote recovery or slow disease progression. Similarly, in behavioral therapy, efficacy of treatment may be affected by factors including: duration, intensity, type of intervention, and modality used. These therapeutic variables, specifically intensity and duration of therapy, may carry varying levels of importance dependent on individual functional status, though there is still much debate regarding this (Winstein et al., 2016). Thus there are striking similarities between NIBS and traditional therapy variables, in that frequency, intensity, site or system, and duration of the intervention affect outcome.

LITERATURE SEARCH

The intent of this search was to identify and summarize published studies combining rTMS with behavioral intervention for clinical benefit. Therefore, we have limited the search to a neurological patient population. All articles were found through the PubMed database and excluded: non-English, case studies, drug studies, transcranial direct current stimulation (tDCS) or other non-invasive stimulation methods, and/or healthy subjects. The acronym *rTMS* was used in combination with the following search terms (relevant/hits): physical therapy (23/267), occupational therapy (8/35), speech therapy (10/54), behavioral intervention (0/95), task training (2/23), motor practice (3/42), motor training (3/50), rehabilitation (8/232), cognition (0/144), cognitive rehabilitation (0/24), cognitive behavioral therapy (2/144), CBT (0/7), cognitive training (0/19). A summary of hits for tDCS in combination with the above search terms is located in Supplementary Figure S1, however, will not be further reviewed in this paper.

LITERATURE ANALYSIS

The majority of rTMS papers report application of the full stimulation protocol at rest, i.e., not during associated therapy (37/50). A smaller proportion of experimental studies used an interleaved approach of combined therapy, performing the therapeutic task during inter-train intervals (5/50). Less than twenty percent of studies fell into the following categories; unspecified timing (2/50), used high or low frequency dependent on experimental group (3/50), delivered rTMS and therapy simultaneously (2/50) or completed rTMS and therapy on different days (1/50).Within these experimental studies, there was great diversity in the stimulation and therapy variables used for each diagnosis within the neurological population (**Figure 1**). Despite differences, the majority of papers show improvement in clinical outcomes. However, vague and inconsistent reporting of the combined intervention, as well as diverse approaches, impede advancement of understanding toward optimizing intervention and maximizing clinical efficacy. Elements of rTMS application that varied most commonly between studies include; rTMS timing relative to therapy, and either inhibitory (low-frequency), or excitatory (high-frequency) rTMS (Supplementary Table S1). Detailed reporting and standardization for both rTMS and therapy characteristics is a strategy for taking into consideration variations between clinicians, locations, resources, and type of intervention.

Stimulation Targeting

Of studies investigating chronic motor impairment following stroke (24/50), all but one targeted the primary motor cortex, the exception targeted the somatosensory cortex (Supplementary Table S1, Study #18). The majority of these studies targeted the unaffected hemisphere (17/24). The remaining studies stimulated the affected hemisphere (5/24; Supplementary Table S1, Study #5, 16, 18, 20, 23), or stimulated bilaterally (3/24; Supplementary Table S1, Study #6, 9, 13). With regards to pulse frequency in this population, 14/24 stimulated with low, 7/24 with high (Supplementary Table S1, Study # 5, 14, 16, 18, 20, 23, 26), and 3/24 alternated between high-frequency stimulation (affected hemisphere) and low-frequency (unaffected hemisphere).

All papers (6/50) addressing motor impairment in a sub-acute stroke population targeted the primary motor cortex. Three studies stimulated the unaffected hemisphere at low-frequency (Supplementary Table S1, Study #33, 34, 35), 1 stimulated the affected hemisphere at high-frequency (Supplementary Table S1, Study #32), and 1 stimulated both hemispheres (unaffected at low-frequency, affected at high-frequency) dependent on treatment group (Supplementary Table S1, Study #31). Cha and Kim (2016) stimulated the cortical representation of the first right dorsal interosseous muscle at a low-frequency in their study examining unilateral neglect and motor control.

Additional studies in the stroke population were completed in acute stroke [>1 month post onset (Emara et al., 2010)] or in sub-acute and chronic patients [3+ months post onset (Chang et al., 2012)]. In the acute population patients were stimulated at high-frequency (affected motor cortex) or low-frequency (unaffected). Chang et al. (2012) stimulated the affected primary motor cortex at high-frequency. Other motor impairment studies were completed in patients with congenital hemiparesis (children), Parkinson's disease, and hand dystonia (Supplementary Table S1, Study # 1, 2, 3, respectively). Gillick et al. (2014) stimulated the unaffected primary motor cortex with priming rTMS (high then low-frequency) for children with congenital hemiparesis. Yang et al. (2013) stimulated the contralateral primary motor cortex at high-frequency to "more affected side" in patients with Parkinson's disease. Kimberley et al. (2015) stimulated the unaffected pre-motor cortex at low-frequency in patients with hand dystonia. One study (Lim et al., 2010) studied hemispatial neglect and stimulated the left parietal area (P5; affected side for all participants) at low-frequency.

Studies examining speech impairments following stroke ($n = 11$) were completed in sub-acute (<6 months post-onset; 6/11) and chronic populations (>6 months post-onset; 5/11). Within the speech domain, Momosaki et al. (2014) studied oral motor control and stimulated two times daily (low then high-frequency) to the pharyngeal muscles representation. Of studies examining aphasia ($n = 10$), four stimulated Broca's Area (i.e., pars triangularis); 3/4 delivered a low-frequency (Supplementary Table S1, Study #40, 42, 46), while 1/4 stimulated with priming rTMS [high then low-frequency (Khedr et al., 2014)]. Abo et al. (2012) differentially defined the stimulation target based on aphasia-type, as determined by fMRI activation (inferior frontal gyrus in non-fluent aphasia and superior temporal gyrus in fluent aphasia) and stimulated at low-frequency.

Studies targeting cognitive impairment were completed in Alzheimer's (2/3), and chronic stroke populations (1/3). In the Alzheimer's studies, high-frequency stimulation was delivered to cortical targets including: Broca's Area, Wernicke's Area, right dorsolateral prefrontal cortex, and left parietal somatosensory association cortex (two targets stimulated one day, third target on another) (Supplementary Table S1, Study #49, 50). Park and Yoon (2015) targeted the left prefrontal cortex in stroke, the affected hemisphere for all participants, at high-frequency.

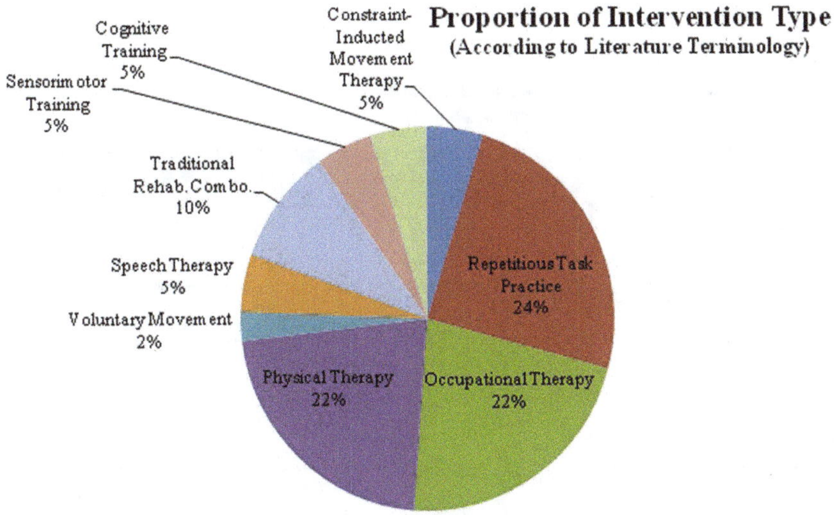

FIGURE 1 | The majority of research in repetitive transcranial magnetic stimulation (rTMS) and behavioral intervention has been completed with rTMS in conjunction with motor training. rTMS paired with speech therapy, cognitive training, and sensorimotor training account for only 30%. rTMS in conjunction with cognitive therapies has not been widely studied, despite FDA approval for use in refractory depression. This graph shows the distribution of behavioral interventions used in conjunction with rTMS. Despite there being a fairly wide variety of interventions utilized there are great differences in protocol design and stimulation parameters, which makes comparing protocols or drawing firm conclusions difficult.

Thus no clearly superior targeting strategy has emerged. Stimulation of a primary lesion area, stimulation of other areas with significant network connections to a primary lesion area, and stimulation of a focal area in the presence of a widespread brain disease process, all seem effective.

Outcomes with Respect to Timing

The relative timing of combined therapy has not been well explored, and is one of the most poorly reported variables in rTMS studies; however, none of the papers examined in this review reported a negative response, regardless of timing. In papers examining rTMS prior to behavioral intervention, 86.5% (32/37) cited a positive response, while 5/37 (Supplementary Table S1, Study #3, 20, 28, 35, 42) report a neutral response. The second most frequent approach (5/50) involved alternating protocols (behavioral intervention during the inter-train interval), all of which indicate a positive result in outcome (Supplementary Table S1, Study #5, 23, 30, 31, 32). Out of the remaining 20% of identified studies, 7/8 reported a positive response (Supplementary Table S1, Study #1, 10, 16, 26, 46, 49, 50), while 1/10 reported a neutral response (Supplementary Table S1, Study #48). Thus, as in the case of stimulation targeting, discussed above, no clearly superior strategy for temporal pairing of rTMS and behavioral therapy has emerged. However, firm conclusions cannot be drawn due to small sample sizes and need for additional randomized, controlled clinical trials.

For future research and reporting, we propose the temporal relationship of rTMS application with behavioral intervention be defined as: *concurrent* (rTMS being applied at the same time as the behavior is expressed); *sequential* (one intervention follows the other), *interleaved* (rTMS trains are alternating with behavioral expression/repetition) (**Figure 2**).

One could consider an ongoing pharmacological intervention paired with rTMS a concurrent application of combined therapy, and studies are underway of this nature. Sequential stimulation can occur at numerous time points prior to or following therapy (e.g., volitional activity), ranging from seconds to days. For instance, pulses can be delivered in an event-triggered manner, perhaps with an electroencephalogram (EEG) defined trigger; where important EEG changes known within the neural systems are presently under investigation. Therapeutic rTMS could plausibly be delivered seconds before a task through a clinician prompted visual or verbal cue to promote cognitive effort or movement. Indeed, a single case with positive outcome was reported in the literature for depression where rTMS was combined with a form of cognitive behavioral therapy; here, the cognitive effort was performed in between trains of rTMS – so in this case, combined, but alternating (Vedeniapin et al., 2010). Behavioral intervention can be initiated within minutes following stimulation through use of a defined time window to ensure consistency [i.e., therapy starts 5–10 min after rTMS completion, as in clinical trial NCT02089464 (Nexstim Ltd, 2015)]. Stimulation can be delivered within hours or days of therapeutic intervention (i.e., rTMS in morning, therapy in the afternoon or next day). Optimal timing may vary depending on diagnosis and behavioral intervention type, and further research is needed in this area, as 74% of papers delivered rTMS before behavioral intervention (37/50).

While the physiologic effects of rTMS and behavioral therapy are likely different; a key commonality in both is that after-effects have been linked to adaptive behavioral response, and attributed to lasting modification of synaptic strength in cortical networks subserving the behavior (Butefisch et al., 1995; Silasi and Murphy, 2014), which can be local (e.g., primary motor cortex), or distant

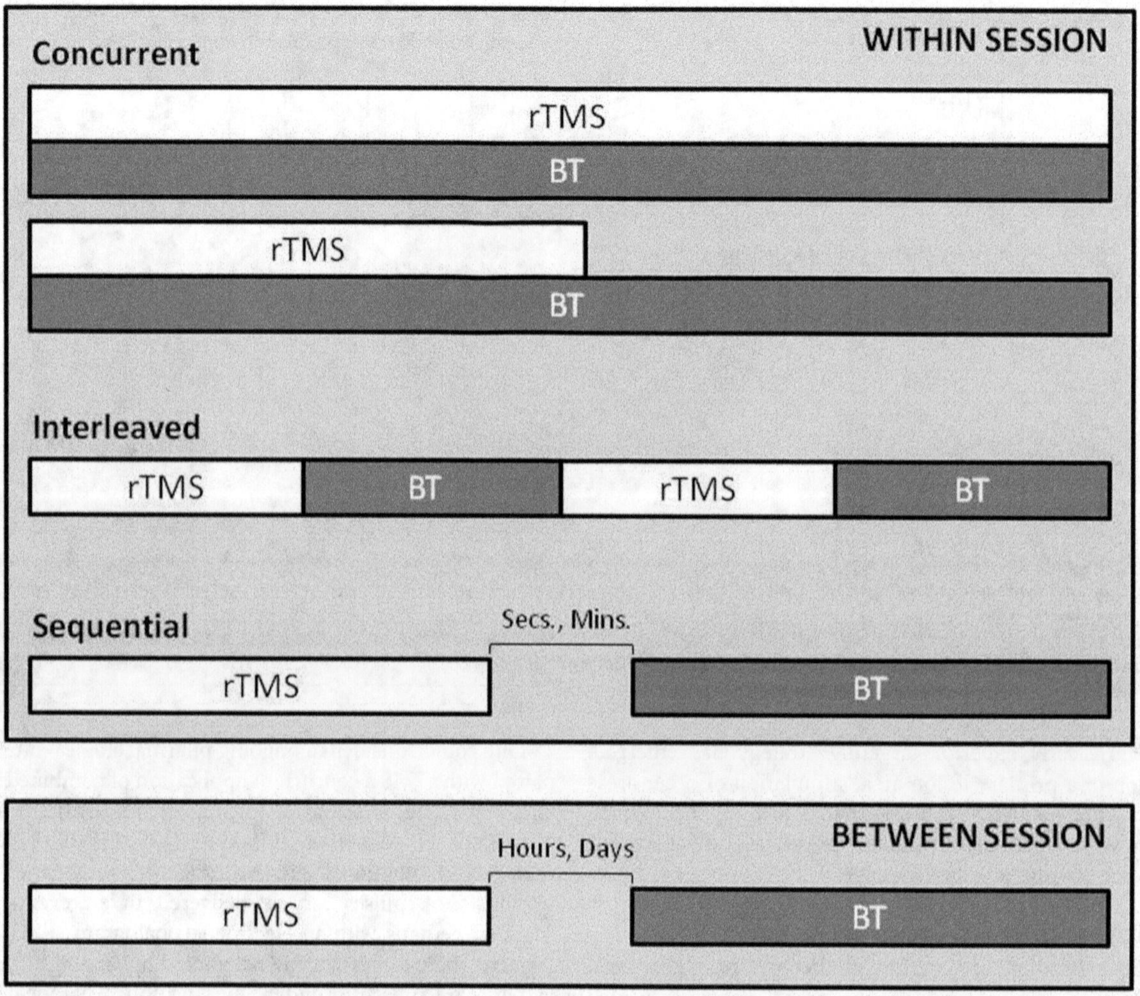

FIGURE 2 | A conceptual guide for timing of rTMS and behavioral therapy. The within session and between session temporal relationship, influences *during* and *after-effect* interactions, depending on the time-course of combination. The relationship can be defined as; 1. *concurrent*, rTMS is applied at the same time as the behavior is expressed (reporting should include if one intervention outlasts the other), 2. *interleaved*, rTMS trains are alternating with behavioral expression/repetition, 3. *sequential*, one intervention follows the other. Note: Separation of the two techniques by hours or days may not harness the interactions of short term after effects of each.

through functionally connected networks. The physiological interaction of brain stimulation and discrete voluntary behaviors has been well reported experimentally in healthy subjects (Iyer et al., 2003; Daskalakis et al., 2006; Buch et al., 2011), with striking interactive effects, including augmentation, cancelation, and reversal of effect, depending on the circumstances of the interaction. In the context of the present review, the data suggest a more uniform positive response to intervention, which may be troubling. The authors suggest a framework for reporting research methods in studies examining paired rTMS and behavioral interventions (Supplementary Table S2).

rTMS and Behavioral Therapy in Other Functional Domains and Adverse Events

Currently there is a lack of research on combined applications studying functional domains outside of motor and speech. In the future, rTMS may be a promising approach for increasing the efficacy of currently accepted, traditional behavioral interventions. There were no serious adverse events reported in our reviewed studies, and only mild headaches were reported in a few papers.

CONCLUSION

Combined therapy of rTMS paired with behavioral intervention has gained traction in the scientific field. Historically, rTMS was delivered in isolation, yet with positive results. Researchers are now examining how rTMS may be used as an adjuvant to more traditional therapies (e.g., physical, occupational, speech, or cognitive therapies) to maximize the benefit of both interventions. To date, the majority of research has been completed in the motor-domain of a stroke population and has examined delivering rTMS prior to the behavioral intervention. Of the studies reviewed, combined therapy appears to be safe, since only minor adverse effects (primarily mild headache) were reported in a few papers. Further research is needed to examine the optimal pairing of rTMS and behavioral intervention. Focused attention to all rTMS parameters and timing of stimulation is essential to allow for study replication and data interpretation. Similarly, therapy-related specifications must be clearly reported and standardized. In order to determine optimal combined therapy, larger sample sizes and randomized, controlled clinical trials are needed to account for variability among individuals and conditions.

AUTHOR CONTRIBUTIONS

KT contributed the acquisition of data and drafting of manuscript. DL and DE contributed study conception and design, as well as critical revision.

ACKNOWLEDGMENTS

The authors would like to acknowledge Daniel Press MD for insight in psychiatric application of rTMS, and Gary Thickbroom Ph.D. for helpful comments during manuscript development.

REFERENCES

Abo, M., Kakuda, W., Watanabe, M., Morooka, A., Kawakami, K., and Senoo, A. (2012). Effectiveness of low-frequency rTMS and intensive speech therapy in poststroke patients with aphasia: a pilot study based on evaluation of fMRI in relation to type of aphasia. *Eur. Neurol.* 68, 199–208. doi: 10.1159/000338773

Amassian, V., and Maccabee, P. (2006). "Transcranial magnetic stimulation," in *Proceeding of the 28th Annual International Conference of the IEEE Engineering in Medicine and Biology Society, 2006,* New York, NY, 1620–1623. doi 10.1109/IEMBS.2006.259398.

Avenanti, A., Coccia, M., Ladavas, E., Provinciali, L., and Ceravolo, M. G. (2012). Low-frequency rTMS promotes use-dependent motor plasticity in chronic stroke: a randomized trial. *Neurology* 78, 256–264. doi: 10.1212/WNL.0b013e3182436558

Barros Galvao, S., dos Santos, R. B., dos Santos, P., Cabral, M. E., and Monte-Silva, K. (2014). Efficacy of coupling repetitive transcranial magnetic stimulation and physical therapy to reduce upper-limb spasticity in patients with stroke: a randomized controlled trial. *Arch. Phys. Med. Rehabil.* 95, 222–229. doi: 10.1016/j.apmr.2013.10.023

Baumer, T., Lange, R., Liepert, J., Weiller, C., Siebner, H. R., Rothwell, J. C., et al. (2003). Repeated premotor rTMS leads to cumulative plastic changes of motor cortex excitability in humans. *Neuroimage* 20, 550–560. doi: 10.1016/S1053-8119(03)00310-0

Bentwich, J., Dobronevsky, E., Aichenbaum, S., Shorer, R., Peretz, R., Khaigrekht, M., et al. (2011). Beneficial effect of repetitive transcranial magnetic stimulation combined with cognitive training for the treatment of Alzheimer's disease: a proof of concept study. *J Neural. Transm. (Vienna)* 118, 463–471. doi: 10.1007/s00702-010-0578-1

Brodie, S. M., Meehan, S., Borich, M. R., and Boyd, L. A. (2014). 5 Hz repetitive transcranial magnetic stimulation over the ipsilesional sensory cortex enhances motor learning after stroke. *Front. Hum. Neurosci.* 8:143. doi: 10.3389/fnhum.2014.00143

Buch, E. R., Johnen, V. M., Nelissen, N., O'Shea, J., and Rushworth, M. F. S. (2011). Noninvasive associative plasticity induction in a corticocortical pathway of the human brain. *J. Neurosci.* 31, 17669–17679. doi: 10.1523/JNEUROSCI.1513-11.2011

Butefisch, C., Hummelsheim, H., Denzler, P., and Mauritz, K. (1995). Repetitive training of isolated movements improves the outcome of motor rehabilitation of the centrally paretic hand. *J. Neurol. Sci.* 130, 59–68. doi: 10.1016/0022-510X(95)00003-K

Cha, H. G., and Kim, M. K. (2016). Effects of repetitive transcranial magnetic stimulation on arm function and decreasing unilateral spatial neglect in subacute stroke: a randomized controlled trial. *Clin. Rehabil.* 30, 649–656. doi: 10.1177/0269215515598817

Chang, W. H., Kim, Y., Bang, O., Kim, S. T., Park, Y. H., and Lee, P. K. W. (2010). Long-term effects of rTMS on motor recovery in patients after subacute stroke. *J. Rehabil Med.* 42, 758–764. doi: 10.2340/16501977-0590

Chang, W. H., Kim, Y. H., Yoo, W. K., Goo, K. H., Park, C. H., Kim, S. T., et al. (2012). rTMS with motor training modulates cortico-basal ganglia-thalamocortical circuits in stroke patients. *Restor. Neurol. Neurosci.* 30, 179–189. doi: 10.3233/RNN-2012-110162

Conforto, A. B., Anjos, S. M., Saposnik, G., Mello, E. A., Nagaya, E. M., Santos, W. Jr., et al. (2012). Transcranial magnetic stimulation in mild to severe hemiparesis early after stroke: a proof of principle and novel approach to improve motor function. *J. Neurol.* 259, 1399–1405. doi: 10.1007/s00415-011-6364-7

Cotelli, M., Fertonani, A., Miozzo, A., Rosini, S., Manenti, R., Padovani, A., et al. (2011). Anomia training and brain stimulation in chronic aphasia. *Neuropsychol. Rehabil.* 21, 717–741. doi: 10.1080/09602011.2011.621275

Damoiseaux, J. S., Rombouts, S., Barkof, F., Scheltens, P., Stam, C., Smith, S., et al. (2006). Consistent resting-state networks across healthy subjects. *Proc. Natl. Acad. Sci. U.S.A.* 103, 12848–12853. doi: 10.1073/pnas.0601417103

Daskalakis, Z. J., Moller, B., Christensen, B. K., Fitzgerald, P. B., Gunraj, C., and Chen, R. (2006). The effects of repetitive transcranial magnetic stimulation on cortical inhibition in healthy human subjects. *Exp. Brain Res.* 174, 403–412. doi: 10.1007/s00221-006-0472-0

Emara, T. H., Moustafa, R. R., ElNahas, N. M., ElGanzoury, A. M., Abdo, T. A., Mohamed, S. A., et al. (2010). Repetitive transcranial magnetic stimulation at 1 Hz and 5 Hz produces sustained improvement in motor function and disability after ischaemic stroke. *Eur. J. Neurol.* 17, 1203–1209. doi: 10.1111/j.1468-1331.2010.03000.x

Gillick, B. T., Krach, L. E., Feyma, T., Rich, T. L., Moberg, K., Thomas, W., et al. (2014). Primed low-frequency repetitive transcranial magnetic stimulation and constraint-induced movement therapy in pediatric hemiparesis: a randomized controlled trial. *Dev. Med. Child Neurol.* 56, 44–52. doi: 10.1111/dmcn.12243

Goetz, S. M., Luber, B., Lisanby, S. H., Murphy, D. L., Kozyrkov, I. C., Grill, W. M., et al. (2016). Enhancement of neuromodulation with novel pulse shapes generated by controllable pulse parameter transcranial magnetic stimulation. *Brain Stimul.* 9, 39–47. doi: 10.1016/j.brs.2015.08.013

Gusnard, D. A., and Raichle, M. E. (2001). Searching for a baseline: functional imaging and the resting human brain. *Nat. Rev. Neurosci.* 2, 685–694. doi: 10.1038/35094500

Iyer, M. B., Schleper, N., and Wassermann, E. M. (2003). Priming stimulation enhances depressant effect of low-frequency repetitive transcranial magnetic stimulation. *J. Neurosci.* 23, 10867–10872.

Kakuda, W., Abo, M., Kobayashi, K., Momosaki, R., Yokoi, A., Fukuda, A., et al. (2010). Low-frequency repetitive transcranial magnetic stimulation and intensive occupational therapy for poststroke patients with upper limb hemiparesis: preliminary study of a 15-day protocol. *Int. J. Rehabil. Res.* 33, 339–345. doi: 10.1097/MRR.0b013e32833cdf10

Kakuda, W., Abo, M., Kobayashi, K., Momosaki, R., Yokoi, A., Fakuda, A., et al. (2011). Anti-spastic effect of low-frequency rTMS applied with occupational therapy in post-stroke patients with upper limb hemiparesis. *Brain Inj.* 25, 496–502. doi: 10.3109/02699052.2011.559610

Kakuda, W., Abo, M., Kobayashi, K., Momosaki, R., Yokoi, A., Fukunda, A., et al. (2011). Application of combined 6-Hz primed low frequency rTMS and intensive occupational therapy for upper limb hemiparesis after stroke. *Neurorehabilitation* 29, 365–371. doi: 10.3233/NRE-2011-0714

Kakuda, W., Abo, M., Kobayashi, K., Takagishi, T., Momosaki, R., Yokoi, A., et al. (2011). Baseline severity of upper limb hemiparesis influences the outcome of low-frequency rTMS combined with intensive occupational therapy in patients who have had a stroke. *PM R* 3, 516–522. doi: 10.1016/j.pmrj.2011.02.015

Kakuda, W., Abo, M., Momosaki, R., and Morooka, A. (2011). Therapeutic application of 6 Hz primed low frequency rTMS combined with intensive speech therapy for post-stroke aphasia. *Brain Inj.* 25, 1242–1248. doi: 10.3109/02699052.2011.608212

Kakuda, W., Abo, M., Nobuyoshi, K., Ishikawa, A., Taguchi, K., and Yokoi, A. (2010). Six-day course of repetitive transcranial magnetic stimulation plus occupational therapy for post-stroke patients with upper limb hemiparesis: a case series study. *Disabil. Rehabil.* 32, 801–807. doi: 10.3109/09638280903295474

Kakuda, W., Abo, M., Shimizu, M., Sasanuma, J., Okamoto, T., Yokoi, A., et al. (2012). A multi-center study on low-frequency rTMS combined with intensive occupational therapy for upper limb hemiparesis in post-stroke patients. *J. Neuroeng. Rehabil.* 9:4. doi: 10.1186/1743-0003-9-4

Kakuda, W., Abo, M., Watanabe, S., Momosaki, R., Hashimoto, G., Nakayama, Y., et al. (2013). High-frequency rTMS applied over bilateral leg motor areas combined with mobility training for gait disturbance after stroke: a preliminary study. *Brain Inj.* 27, 1080–1086. doi: 10.3109/02699052.2013.794973

Khedr, E. M., El-Fetoh, N. A., Ali, A. M., El-Hammady, D. H., Khalifa, H., Atta, H., et al. (2014). Dual-hemisphere repetitive transcranial magnetic stimulation for rehabilitation of poststroke aphasia: a randomized, double-blind clinical trial. *Neurorehabil. Neural Repair* 28, 740–750. doi: 10.1177/1545968314521009

Khedr, E. M., Rothwell, J. C., Shawky, O. A., Ahmed, M. A., and Hamdy, A. (2006). Effect of daily repetitive transcranial magnetic stimulation on motor performance in Parkinson's disease. *Mov. Disord.* 21, 2201–2205. doi: 10.1002/mds.21089

Kim, C., Choi, H. E., Jung, H., Lee, B. J., Lee, K. H., and Lim, Y. J. (2014). Comparison of the effects of 1 Hz and 20 Hz rTMS on motor recovery in subacute stroke patients. *Ann. Rehabil. Med.* 38, 585–591. doi: 10.5535/arm.2014.38.5.585

Kim, Y., You, S. H., Ko, M., Park, J., Lee, K., Jang, S. H., et al. (2006). Repetitive transcranial magnetic stimulation-induced corticomotor excitability and associated motor skill acquisition in chronic stroke. *Stroke* 37, 1471–1476. doi: 10.1161/01.STR.0000221233.55497.51

Kimberley, T. J., Schmidt, R. L. S., Chen, M., Dykstra, D. D., and Buetefisch, C. M. (2015). Mixed effectiveness of rTMS and retraining in the treatment of focal hand dystonia. *Front. Hum. Neurosci.* 9:385. doi: 10.3389/fnhum.2015.00385

Koganemaru, S., Sawamoto, N., Aso, T., Sagara, A., Ikkaku, T., Shimada, K., et al. (2015). Task-specific brain reorganization in motor recovery induced by a hybrid-rehabilitation combining training with brain stimulation after stroke. *Neurosci. Res.* 92, 29–38. doi: 10.1016/j.neures.2014.10.004

Kwon, T. G., Kim, Y., Chang, W., Bang, O., and Shin, Y. (2014). Effective method of combining rTMS and motor training in stroke patients. *Restor. Neurol. Neurosci.* 32, 223–232. doi: 10.3233/RNN-130313

Lam, R. W., Chan, P., Wilkins-Ho, M., and Yatham, L. (2008). Repetitive transcranial magnetic stimulation for treatment-resistant depression: a systematic review and metaanalysis. *Can. J. Psychiatry* 53, 621–631.

Lim, J. Y., Kang, E. K., and Paik, N. J. (2010). Repetitive transcranial magnetic stimulation to hemispatial neglect in patients after stroke: an open-label pilot study. *J. Rehabil. Med.* 42, 447–452. doi: 10.2340/16501977-0553

Lomarev, M. P., Kanchana, S., Bara-Jimenez, W., Iyer, M., Wassermann, E. M., and Hallett, M. (2006). Placebo-controlled study of rTMS for the treatment of Parkinson's disease. *Mov. Disord.* 21, 325–331. doi: 10.1002/mds.20713

Malcolm, M. P., Triggs, W. J., Light, K. E., Gonzalez, R., Wu, S., Reid, K., et al. (2007). Repetitive transcranial magnetic stimulation as an adjunct to constraint-induced therapy: an exploratory randomized controlled trial. *Am. J. Phys. Med. Rehabil.* 86, 707–715. doi: 10.1097/PHM.0b013e31813e0de0

Micoulaud-Franchi, J. A., Richieri, R., Lancon, C., and Vion-Dury, J. (2013). [Interactive rTMS protocols in psychiatry]. *Encephale* 39, 426–431. doi: 10.1016/j.encep.2013.04.009

Mills, K. R., and Schubert, M. (1995). Short term synchronization of human motor units and their responses to transcranial magnetic stimulation. *J. Physiol.* 483(Pt. 2), 511–523. doi: 10.1113/jphysiol.1995.sp020602

Momosaki, R., Abo, M., and Kakuda, W. (2014). Bilateral repetitive transcranial magnetic stimulation combined with intensive swallowing rehabilitation for chronic stroke dysphagia: a case series study. *Case Rep. Neurol.* 6, 60–67. doi: 10.1159/000360936

Nexstim Ltd (2015). *Niche Trial: Navigated Inhibitory rTMS to Contralesional Hemisphere Trial.* Available at: https://clinicaltrials.gov/ct2/show/NCT02089464?term=nexstim&rank=1

Nollet, H., Ham, L. V., Deprez, P., and Vanderstraeten, G. (2003). Transcranial magnetic stimulation: review of the technique, basic principles and applications. *Vet. J.* 166, 28–42. doi: 10.1016/S1090-0233(03)00025-X

Nudo, R., Plautz, E., and Frost, S. (2001). Role of adaptive plasticity in recovery of function after damage to motor cortex. *Muscle Nerve* 24, 1000–1019. doi: 10.1002/mus.1104

Park, I., and Yoon, J. (2015). The effect of computer-assisted cognitive rehabilitation and repetitive transcranial magnetic stimulation on cognitive function for stroke patients. *J. Phys. Ther. Sci.* 27, 773–776. doi: 10.1589/jpts.27.773

Pell, G. S., Roth, Y., and Zangen, A. (2011). Modulation of cortical excitability induced by repetitive transcranial magnetic stimulation: influence of timing in geometrical parameters and underlying mechanisms. *Prog. Neurobiol.* 93, 59–98. doi: 10.1016/j.pneurobio.2010.10.003

Rabey, J. M., Dobronevsky, E., Aichenbaum, S., Gonen, O., Marton, R. G., and Khaigrekht, M. (2013). Repetitive transcranial magnetic stimulation combined with cognitive training is a safe and effective modality for the treatment of Alzheimer's disease: a randomized, double-blind study. *J. Neural Transm. (Vienna)* 120, 813–819. doi: 10.1007/s00702-012-0902-z

Rose, D. K., Patten, C., McGuirk, T. E., Lu, X., and Triggs, W. J. (2014). Does inhibitory repetitive transcranial magnetic stimulation augment functional task practice to improve arm recovery in chronic stroke? *Stroke Res. Treat.* 2014, 305236. doi: 10.1155/2014/305236

Rothwell, J. C., Thompson, P. D., Day, B. L., Dick, J. P. R., Kachi, T., Cowan, J. M. A., et al. (1987). Motor cortex stimulation in intact man: 1. General characteristics of EMG responses in different muscles. *Brain* 110(Pt. 5), 1173–1190. doi: 10.1093/brain/110.5.1173

Rubi-Fessen, I., Hartmann, A., Huber, W., Fimm, B., Rommel, T., Thiel, A., et al. (2015). Add-on effects of repetitive transcranial magnetic stimulation on subacute aphasia therapy: enhanced improvement of functional communication and basic linguistic skills: a randomized controlled study. *Arch. Phys. Med. Rehabil.* 96, 1935–1944. doi: 10.1016/j.apmr.2015.06.017

Sanes, J. N., and Donoghue, J. P. (2000). Plasticity and primary motor cortex. *Annu. Rev. Neurosci.* 23, 393–415. doi: 10.1146/annurev.neuro.23.1.393

Seniow, J., Bilik, M., Lesniak, M., Waldowski, K., Iwanski, S., and Czlonkowska, A. (2012). Transcranial magnetic stimulation combined with physiotherapy in rehabilitation of poststroke hemiparesis: a randomized, double blind, placebo-controlled study. *Neurorehabil. Neural Repair* 26, 1072–1079. doi: 10.1177/1545968312445635

Seniow, J., Waldowski, K., Lesniak, M., Iwanski, S., Czepiel, W., and Czlonkowska, A. (2013). Transcranial magnetic stimulation combined with speech and language training in early aphasia rehabilitation: a randomized double-blind controlled pilot study. *Top. Stroke Rehabil.* 20, 20–61. doi: 10.1310/tsr2003-250

Silasi, G., and Murphy, T. H. (2014). Stroke and the connectome: how connectivity guides therapeutic intervention. *Neuron* 83, 1354–1368. doi: 10.1016/j.neuron.2014.08.052

Slotema, C. W., Blom, J. D., Hoek, H. W., and Sommer, I. E. C. (2010). Should we expand the toolbox of psychiatric treatment methods to include repetitive transcranial magnetic stimulation (rTMS)? A meta-analysis of the efficacy of rTMS in psychiatric disorders. *J. Clin. Psychiatry* 71, 873–884. doi: 10.4088/JCP.08m04872gre

Takeuchi, N., Tada, T., Toshima, M., Chuma, T., Matsuo, Y., and Ikoma, K. (2008). Inhibition of the unaffected motor cortex by 1 Hz repetitive transcranial magnetic stimulation enhances motor performance and training effect of the paretic hand in patients with chronic stroke. *J. Rehabil. Med.* 40, 298–303. doi: 10.2340/16501977-0181

Thiel, A., Hartmann, A., Rubi-Fessen, I., Anglade, C., Kracht, L., Weiduschat, N., et al. (2013). Effects of noninvasive brain stimulation on language networks and recovery in early poststroke aphasia. *Stroke* 44, 2240–2246. doi: 10.1161/STROKEAHA.111.000574

Vedeniapin, A., Cheng, L., and George, M. S. (2010). Feasibility of simultaneous cognitive behavioral therapy (CBT) and left prefrontal rTMS for treatment resistant depression. *Brain Stimul.* 3, 207–210. doi: 10.1016/j.brs.2010.03.005

Vongvaivanichakul, P., Tretriluxana, J., Bovonsunthonchai, S., Pakaprot, N., and Laksanakorn, W. (2014). Reach-to-grasp training in individuals with chronic stroke augmented by low-frequency repetitive transcranial magnetic stimulation. *J. Med. Assoc. Thai.* 97(Suppl. 7), S45–S49.

Waldowski, K., Seniow, J., Lesniak, M., Iwanski, S., and Czlonkowska, A. (2012). Effect of low-frequency repetitive transcranial magnetic stimulation on naming abilities in early-stroke aphasic patients: a prospective, randomized, double-blind sham-controlled study. *Sci. World J.* 2012: 518568. doi: 10.1100/2012/518568

Wang, C., Hsieh, C., Tsai, P., Wang, C., Lin, F., and Chan, R. (2014). Efficacy of synchronous verbal training during repetitive transcranial magnetic stimulation in patients with chronic aphasia. *Stroke* 45, 3656–3662. doi: 10.1161/STROKEAHA.114.007058

Wang, R., Tseng, H., Liao, K., Wang, C., Lai, K., and Yang, Y. (2012). rTMS combined with task-oriented training to improve symmetry of interhemispheric corticomotor excitability and gait performance after stroke: a randomized trial. *Neurorehabil. Neural Repair* 26, 222–230. doi: 10.1177/1545968311423265

Weiduschat, N., Thiel, A., Rubi-Fessen, I., Hartmann, A., Kessler, J., Merl, P., et al. (2011). Effects of repetitive transcranial magnetic stimulation in aphasic stroke: a randomized controlled pilot study. *Stroke* 42, 409–415. doi: 10.1161/STROKEAHA.110.597864

Winstein, C. J., Wolf, S. L., Dromerick, A. W., Lane, C. J., Nelsen, M. A., Lewthwaite, R., et al. (2016). Effect of task-oriented rehabilitation program on upper extremity recovery following motor stroke: the ICARE randomized clinical trial. *JAMA* 315, 571–581. doi: 10.1001/jama.2016.0276

Yamada, N., Kakuda, W., Kondo, T., Shimizu, M., Mitani, S., and Abo, M. (2013). Bihemispheric repetitive transcranial magnetic stimulation combined with intensive occupational therapy for upper limb hemiparesis after stroke: a preliminary study. *Int. J. Rehabil. Res.* 36, 323–329. doi: 10.1097/MRR.0b013e3283624907

Yang, Y., Tseng, C., Chiou, S., Liao, K., Cheng, S., Lai, K., et al. (2013). Combination of rTMS and treadmill modulates corticomotor inhibition and improves walking in Parkinson Disease: A Randomized Trial. *Neurorehabil. Neural Repair* 27, 79–86. doi: 10.1177/1545968312451915

Zheng, C., Liao, W., and Xia, W. (2015). Effect of combined low-frequency rTMS and virtual reality training on upper limb function in subacute stroke: a double-blind randomized controlled trial. *J. Huazhong Univ. Sci. Technolog. Med. Sci.* 35, 248–254. doi: 10.1007/s11596-015-1419-0

16

Impact of Short Social Training on Prosocial Behaviors: An fMRI Study

Evgeniya Lukinova[1] and Mikhail Myagkov[2]*

[1] *Skolkovo Institute of Science and Technology, Moscow, Russia,* [2] *Department of Political Science, University of Oregon, Eugene, OR, USA*

Edited by:
Mikhail Lebedev, Duke University, USA

Reviewed by:
Xiaojie Chen, University of Electronic Science and Technology of China, China
Matjaž Perc, University of Maribor, Slovenia

***Correspondence:**
Evgeniya Lukinova
jlukinova@gmail.com

Efficient brain–computer interfaces (BCIs) are in need of knowledge about the human brain and how it interacts, plays games, and socializes with other brains. A breakthrough can be achieved by revealing the microfoundations of sociality, an additional component of the utility function reflecting the value of contributing to group success derived from social identity. Building upon our previous behavioral work, we conduct a series of functional magnetic resonance imaging (fMRI) experiments ($N = 10$ in the Pilot Study and $N = 15$ in the Main Study) to measure whether and how sociality alters the functional activation of and connectivity between specific systems in the brain. The overarching hypothesis of this study is that sociality, even in a minimal form, serves as a natural mechanism of sustainable cooperation by fostering interaction between brain regions associated with social cognition and those related to value calculation. We use group-based manipulations to induce varying levels of sociality and compare behavior in two social dilemmas: Prisoner's Dilemma and variations of Ultimatum Game. We find that activation of the right inferior frontal gyrus, a region previously associated with cognitive control and modulation of the valuation system, is correlated with activity in the medial prefrontal cortex (mPFC) to a greater degree when participants make economic decisions in a game with an acquaintance, high sociality condition, compared to a game with a random individual, low sociality condition. These initial results suggest a specific biological mechanism through which sociality facilitates cooperation, fairness and provision of public goods at the cost of individual gain. Future research should examine neural dynamics in the brain during the computation of utility in the context of strategic games that involve social interaction for a larger sample of subjects.

Keywords: prosocial actions, sociality, value calculation, social cognition, BCI

INTRODUCTION

Daily life confronts us with social situations and interactions on a regular basis. Thus, economic decisions are often embedded in a social context. However, we rarely think of how the brain processes the decisions we make, especially those decisions that affect the outcomes of other people with our decisions. Social factors such as group membership and affiliation motives have powerful effects on a range of behaviors, suggesting that these factors carry substantial decision utility for people. However, this "social utility" is rarely included in the formal models of economic behavior. This paper triangulates the theories of human social behavior from social psychology, decision modeling techniques from behavioral economics, and brain-imaging tools from neuroscience to draw a more precise picture of the mechanisms by which social factors influence economic decisions.

Recent efforts to unite these traditions have proven fruitful in delivering theoretical insights and a model-based precision to the study of economic behavior in a realistic social context (Akerlof and Kranton, 2000, 2010; Perc and Szolnoki, 2010; Perc et al., 2013; Lukinova et al., 2014; Berkman et al., 2015). One behavioral study (Berkman et al., 2015) confirmed that socialization induces prosocial behavior in economic games due to sociality. Participants are introduced in groups creating group differentiation, which easily satisfies the minimal group requirement (Tajfel, 1978). In line with Social Identity Theory we assert some esteem or value is gained by boosting the group (or derogating the outgroup; Tajfel and Turner, 1979) and, in turn, this additional value (Lukinova et al., 2014) plays a decisive role in encouraging prosocial actions. Building upon results of our behavioral work, we now report on a series of functional magnetic resonance imaging (fMRI) experiments that utilize the fMRI technology in combination with socialization and well-known economic games to measure whether and how sociality alters the functional activation of and connectivity between the social cognition network and the valuation network in the brain.

We use experiments in fMRI and laboratory facilities in an attempt to study the neural mechanisms of human social interactions and the microfoundations of prosocial behavior. The main novelty and contribution of this paper is in the reality of social interactions as opposed to artificial social interactions and in the combination of two social dilemmas in the fMRI study. To our knowledge the Prisoner's Dilemma (PD) and various representations (sequential vs. simultaneous; matrix vs. a game tree) of Ultimatum Game (UG) have not appeared together in prior neuroeconomics research. Our study follows pioneer fMRI studies that compare PD to other games (e.g., Stag Hunt; Emonds et al., 2011, 2012). Besides regular UG we use Welfare Game (WG), a novel 2 × 2 simultaneous version of UG that preserves the distributional essence of the game, as well as its antecedent, the UG.

Using fMRI gives us a unique perspective on how sociality works. We examine neural dynamics in specific systems when people compute their utility in the context of strategic games that involve various levels of social interaction. Social science researchers use neuroimaging as the key tool to understand the nature of the various peculiar aspects of human behavior such as "economic irrationality" (Peterson, 2005), altruism and "altruistic punishment" (De Quervain et al., 2004; Waytz et al., 2012), asymmetry between gains and losses (Yacubian et al., 2006), cooperation (Fett et al., 2014; Watanabe et al., 2014), preference of egalitarian outcomes (Sanfey et al., 2003; Tricomi et al., 2010; Dawes et al., 2012; Yamagishi et al., 2012; Osinsky et al., 2013), decision about an unfair split (Güroğlu et al., 2014), and theory of mind (Lee and Harris, 2015; Strombach et al., 2015). If social neuroscience (Cacioppo et al., 2002; Norman et al., 2012) attempts to understand mechanisms that underlie social behavior using a mix of biological and social approaches (Willingham and Dunn, 2003), neuroeconomics opens up the "black box" of the brain by finding neural correlates of choice behavior (Camerer et al., 2005; Lohrenz and Montague, 2008; Glimcher and Fehr, 2013; Lampert et al., 2014; Schroeder and Graziano, 2015) and behavior under risk and uncertainty (Hsu et al., 2005). Unfortunately, current knowledge of neural mechanisms in prosocial decision making is still limited (Fehr and Camerer, 2007; Lee, 2008; Emonds et al., 2011, 2012, 2014; Declerck et al., 2013; Declerck and Boone, 2015; Kuss et al., 2015).

For the purposes of this paper, sociality, or social utility, is defined as an additional component of the utility function reflecting the value of contributing to group success derived from social identity, defined as knowledge, value, and emotional significance for group membership (Tajfel, 1982). In economic terms, social identity may be one of the mechanisms by which sociality comes to have a positive decision utility. There are many ways of manipulating sociality for the purpose of testing its effect on economic decisions and the associated neural systems. To our knowledge, a formal typology of the various kinds of sociality is not currently available, even though such a typology would be quite useful for the present line of research and related efforts. In the course of our behavioral research, we surveyed the relevant literature and identified two broad classes of social manipulations (Low sociality and High sociality). We follow on this distinction in our fMRI study. In particular, during our Pilot fMRI Study we compare playing with humans to playing with computers, whereas in the main study we focus on the difference between the behavior in economic games where the opponent is a random individual or an acquaintance.

We have specific, *a priori* hypotheses about the likely brain regions involved in each of the two target processes (sociality and valuation). A growing body of work implicates the ventral striatal dopamine circuit in the integration and calculation of subjective value or utility, including the ventromedial prefrontal cortex (vmPFC), the ventral aspects of the caudate (vC), and the nucleus accumbens (nAcc; Plassmann et al., 2007; Hare et al., 2008; Ruff and Fehr, 2014). Social cognition, on the other hand reliably recruits activation in a network of brain regions including the dorsomedial prefrontal cortex (dmPFC), the posterior cingulate cortex (PCC), and the temporoparietal junction (TPJ; Amodio and Frith, 2006; Van Overwalle, 2009). Pertinent to the present research, a recent study found that activity in TPJ tracked perceived social distance between an actor and a target, and interacted with the vmPFC, a region involved in value calculation, to modulate the actor's decisions about how to divide up a fixed pot of money to be shared by the actor and the target (Strombach et al., 2015). This study provides proof-of-concept that social cognition regions can interact with valuation regions to influence economic decisions. Existent reviews in neuroeconomics add another neural network that is consistently recruited when people face social dilemmas, i.e., network related to cognitive control (Declerck et al., 2013). Thus, one can formulate a competing hypothesis: the interaction of cognitive control and valuation regions of the brain facilitate prosocial decision making.

Since our experimental design includes two types of economic games we can also examine the question of whether the neural bases of social welfare choices are different from those of collective action. The regions of the brain associated with reward and valuation are under our focus and we hypothesize that these brain regions should be more active during the fair condition than during the unfair condition in the UG. Indeed, the vmPFC is reported to activate during tasks involving inequality in social settings (Fliessbach et al., 2007; Tabibnia et al., 2008; Tricomi et al., 2010; Aoki et al., 2015). Inequality is noticed by participant once reward comparison between the other and herself is accomplished. However, it also hurts when she realizes that she falls behind. We hypothesize that there will be an increased activity in the reward associated brain regions (vmPFC) as well as the brain regions critical for processing emotions, such as amygdala and OFC (Davidson et al., 2000; Dolan, 2002) in variations of UG condition as opposed to the PD game condition.

A more precise understanding of the mechanisms by which sociality affects economic decisions in a collective action situation is the essential next step in improving social brain–computer interfaces (BCIs; Sexton, 2015).

MATERIALS AND METHODS

All participants are recruited through advertisements on campus. All subjects are right handed, healthy, have normal or corrected-to-normal vision, have no history of psychiatric diagnoses, neurological or metabolic illnesses, and are not taking medications that can interfere with the performance of fMRI. Participants can be of any gender and ethnicity, but must be at least 18 years old. The only exclusion criterion is based on MRI safety screening (ferromagnetic metal in the body, e.g., dental braces). The participants in the fMRI experiment can earn $5 just for showing up on the day of experiment and up to $20 more, depending on their decisions throughout the game. During all game conditions the participants earned a number of points that was later transferred to money. Subjects provide written informed consent approved by the University of Oregon Human Studies Committee.

On the day of experiment, four people are invited to the conference room in Lewis Center for neuroimaging (LCNI) that is adjacent to the scanning suite. Thus, in every experiment one participant for the fMRI experiment is paired with three other subjects for the reality of the high sociality conditions: Human and Acquaintance. Before they participate in economic games the subjects have time to get to know each other and engage in an informal conversation, i.e., undergo socialization, the technique adopted from our behavioral research (Berkman et al., 2015). Specifically, the participants are asked to introduce themselves by name to the others and say one exciting thing about themselves. The participants then embark on a 10-min interaction with the goal of creating a list of five attributes they all have in common to report back to the experimenter. Finally, one of the participants is asked to go to the scanning room for fMRI experiment and remaining three participants stay in the conference room and proceed with a computer experiment.

Computer experiment laboratory data ($N = 75$) are collected with the help of the z-Tree (Zurich Toolbox for Readymade Economic Experiments) software package (Fischbacher, 2007). The stimuli presentation is identical to the fMRI experiment, with one row chooser and two column choosers (one of the column choosers plays against a predetermined computer strategy).

Pilot Study

Subjects of the fMRI experiment are 10 UO college students (five females). Stimuli include two sociality conditions (human and computer opponents), two game conditions (PD and WGs), a feedback screen that shows profit of participant based on her decision, and a control condition.

The PD payoff matrix is formed around (1, 2, 4, 6; **Table 1**) values. When one participant defects and the other cooperates, then defector gets the maximum value - 6, and the cooperator receives the minimum payoff of 1. If both cooperate, participants get four each, whereas if both defect, they get two each.

The WG is a novel game not seen in prior research. It resembles a simultaneous version of the UG with an option for an unfair offer. The UG is a game often played in laboratory experiments in which two players interact to decide how to divide a sum of money that is given to them. One of the players proposes how to divide the sum between the two players, and the other can either accept or reject this proposal. If the second player rejects the proposal, none of the players receive anything. However, if the second player accepts, the money is split according to the proposal. Usually the game is played only once or with a randomly chosen partner so that reciprocation is not an issue. For the same reason, players do not change roles within one game. The equilibrium in the UG is not in the favor of the second player. By rejecting the proposal, the second is choosing nothing rather than something. So, for a rational player it would be better to accept any proposal that gives any amount bigger than 0. Contrary to the economic theory of self-interest, multiple studies (Henrich, 2004; Oosterbeek et al., 2004) show that in many cultures people offer (50:50) splits and offers less than 20% are usually rejected.

The WG's payoff structure corresponds to values in PD (1, 2, 4, 6; **Table 1**) Based on the payoffs the row chooser always prefers to choose up. The column chooser's best response to the row chooser's dominant strategy is to choose left. That is why the Nash equilibrium is (2; 6). However, the row chooser always gets a worse payoff than the column chooser. So, if the row chooser prefers egalitarian outcomes, the row player's deviation from the equilibrium can occur and result in either of the two egalitarian options: (1; 1) and (4; 4).

Prior to entering the scanner the subjects complete a series of practice trials of a similar game on paper. This ensures that the

TABLE 1 | Prisoner's dilemma (PD) and Welfare game (WG) payoffs.

	PD			Welfare Game	
	L	R		L	R
U	4, 4	1, 6	U	2, 6	6, 2
D	6, 1	2, 2	D	1, 1	4, 4

PD and WG payoffs are presented in the matrix form. One of the players chooses between rows, i.e., between up (U) and down (D). The other player (randomly paired) chooses between columns, i.e., between left (L) and right (R).

participants understand and are ready for the stimuli presented in the actual experiment. Participants are told on the day of experiment that they will be Row choosers [choosing between up (U) and down (D)] and will maintain the same role for the whole experiment. Subjects are instructed to look at the central plus sign, and had to switch their attention from the central plus sign to the game stimulus (a table 2 × 2 that is centered on the central plus sign) in each trial to determine the their response by pressing either left or right button on the button box in their right hand. Subjects know that by pressing the left button, they choose up (U) and by pressing the right button - down (D). This study uses deception. Participants are told that their opponents in the high sociality condition are humans. In reality, the participant in the fMRI study always plays a computerized strategy with fixed probabilities: for PD game, right (R) with $p = 0.85$, left (L) with $p = 0.15$; for WG, L with $p = 0.85$, R with $p = 0.15$. Feedback collected following the experiment indicates that the deception was effective and that subjects believed that their opponents were human.

In order to answer the research questions the following neural experimental design is used. The experiment consisted of four blocks [Humans + PD (PG1), Humans + WG (PG2), Computers + PD (CG1), Computers + WG (CG2)] with events within each block. To distinguish between blocks the instruction screen in the beginning of each block indicates whether the participant will play a computer or a human. The game condition does not change throughout the block. The blocks are alternated: for half of the participants the order is PG1, PG2, CG1, CG2, for the other half - CG1, CG2, PG1, PG2. We use an event-related fMRI design with a pseudorandom (predetermined unpredictable) order of game and control condition within a block with the same interstimulus and intertrial intervals used in M. Posner attention studies (Flombaum and Posner, 2005; Abdullaev et al., 2010) that approximate an exponential distribution with a certain mean. The jittering of the time intervals between game and feedback and between feedback and the next trial is done in order to separate brain activity to the game and feedback stimuli.

In the game condition (**Figure 1**), the plus sign remains on the center of the screen for 1000 ms. The game stimulus follows after a variable interval ("one of 12 predetermined intervals including three 300 ms intervals, and one each of 550, 800, 1050, 1550, 2300, 3300, 4800, 6550, and 11800 ms, approximating an exponential distribution with a mean interval of 2800 ms;" Abdullaev et al., 2010). The game stimulus stays until response or for 30000 ms. Then a fixation screen is on for 1000 ms followed by another variable intertrial interval (mean of 6000 ms) and finally the feedback screen is on for 2000 ms till the onset of the next trial.

In the control condition, the plus sign remains on the center of the screen for 1000 ms. The control stimulus (each cell in **Figure 1** 2 × 2 table is replaced with "X, X") follows after a variable interval (mean of 2800 ms). The control stimulus stays until response or for 5000 ms. As in the game condition, then fixation screen is on for 1000 ms followed by another variable intertrial interval (mean of 6000 ms) till the onset of the next trial. Four blocks are presented, and each block has 30 trials (20 game condition trials and 10 control condition trials) with a different pseudorandom order of conditions and intervals.

Responses are recorded with two buttons on an MRI-compatible button box. Reaction times (RT) are measured from the game stimulus to the button press. The control trial is constructed in order to isolate the mechanical activity of the finger pressing on the button box. We expected that with each button press, we should see the ipsilateral cerebellum and the contralateral primary motor cortex activation. Also there is a 30 s baseline period in front of each block with no stimuli except a central plus sign for fixation. So that each condition of the task can be compared to the baseline period.

fMRI stimuli are presented for the participant in the MRI scanner and behavioral data are collected using the Presentation program[1] run on a computer. Stimuli are presented with a digital projector/reverse screen display system to the screen at the back end of the MRI scanner bore. Subjects see the screen via a small tilted mirror attached to the birdcage coil in front of their eyes.

Imaging is performed using a 3T Siemens Allegra head-only MRI scanner at Lewis Center for Neuroimaging. A standard birdcage coil is used to acquire data from the entire brain. Subjects wear earplugs and earphones to protect their hearing. Additional soft padding is used between earphones and inside the wall of the head coil to diminish head movements.

For functional MRI, the EP2D-BOLD (Blood oxygen level dependent) sequence is run with repetition time (TR) = 2000 ms, echo time (TE) = 30 ms, flip angle = 90°, Field of View (FOV) = 200 mm. The brain is covered with 32 4 mm thick slices acquired in a custom manner (first even slices and then odd slices). For structural MRI scan, the 3D Magnetization Prepared Rapid Acquisition Gradient Echo (MPRAGE) TR = 2500 ms, TE = 4.3 8ms, flip angle = 8°, FOV = 256, 160 slices is run for 8 min to acquire 1 mm^3 high resolution anatomical scans for registration purposes.

Main Study

Subjects of the fMRI experiment are 15 individuals recruited from the Eugene, OR community, college-aged (eight females). The procedures are nearly identical to the Pilot Study, except for the sociality, game conditions, and fMRI acquisition. Stimuli include two within-subject opponent conditions, Low sociality (Random Individual), and High sociality (Acquaintance), and two within-subject game conditions, PD, UG as responder. Thus, each trial falls into one of four cells, with participants playing anonymously against either someone from the Eugene community who the participant has not met or someone from the socialized group, and playing the PD game, or the UG game as responder. This study uses deception. Although participants believe they are playing with real people (according to participants' feedback), the opponent in all three games is in reality a computer that follows the Nash equilibrium strategy with random noise to reduce suspicion. Following the game phase of each trial, participants are shown a feedback screen displaying the profit the

[1] www.neurobehavioralsystems.com

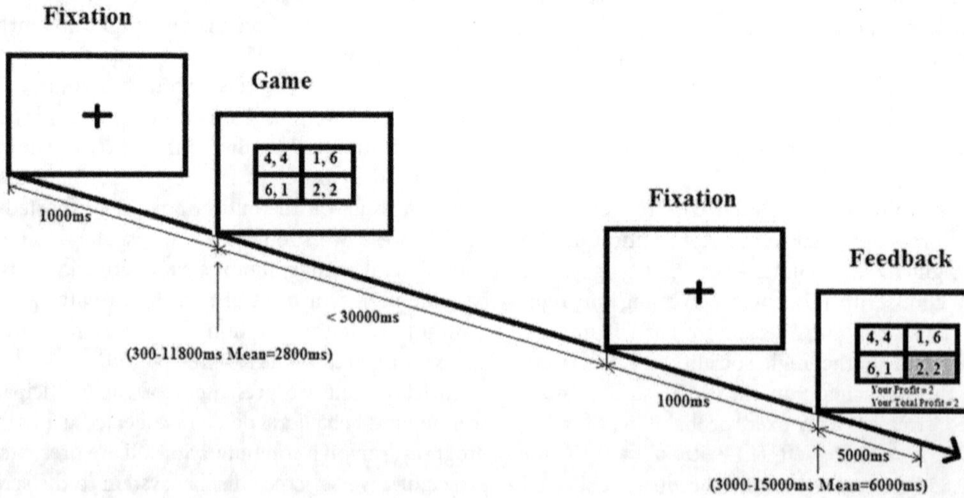

FIGURE 1 | Game condition schedule. Following the fixation cross, there is a game phase for each trial, where participants need to make a choice in a social dilemma. After pressing on the button box, participants are shown a feedback screen displaying the profit the participants earn based on their decision and the decision of their partner.

participant earned based on their decision and the decision of the partner.

Therefore, the experiment consists of four blocks (Acquaintance + PD, Acquaintance + Ultimatum, Random Individual + PD, Random Individual + Ultimatum) with 30 trials within each block (20 experimental and 10 control trials). To distinguish between blocks the instruction screen in the beginning of each block specifies, whether the participant would play against a person from his/her Socialized group (Acquaintance) or against a Random Individual.

The PD game payoffs are the same as in Pilot Study (**Table 1**). The UG is modeled in such a way that a participant always chooses between two options, either accept an unfair offer that corresponds to up (U) or reject the offer pressing down (D). Equally likely are offered (2; 6) and (3; 5) splits, where the lesser value is an offer to a participant.

MR scans are acquired in the Siemens Skyra 3 Tesla scanner at LCNI, a research-dedicated, whole-body system optimized for functional brain imaging. Participants are situated in the scanner by one of LCNI's imaging technicians, who also control the scanner during the session. Experimental stimuli (e.g., images, instructions) are presented using a magnet-compatible, rear-projection system controlled by a PC using Presentation Software. Participant responses (e.g., up/down decisions) are collected on a 10-key button box (only two buttons are used) capable of recording responses to the millisecond level. A shimming protocol maximizes homogeneity in the field, and a 30 s, T2*-weighted scout allows slice prescriptions for all subsequent scans. We acquire a high-resolution anatomical T1-weighted MP-RAGE scan (TR/TE = 2300/2.1 ms, 192 × 192 matrix, 1 mm thick, 160 sagittal slices, FOV = 256), functional images with a T2*-weighted echo-planar scan (33 axial slices, TR/TE = 2000/30 ms, 90-deg flip, 64 × 64 matrix, 4 mm thick, FOV = 200), and in-plane gradient echo field map magnitude and phase images to correct for inhomogeneities in the magnetic field (33 axial slices, TR/TE = 345/8.06 ms, 40-deg flip, 64 × 64 matrix, 4 mm thick, FOV = 200).

Analysis

The epochs used for the analysis are from the game stimulus onset until response.

FSL Procedures

The Pilot Study is first analyzed using General Linear Modeling (GLM) as implemented in the FSL 5.0.2 (FMRIB Software Library). fMRI data is analyzed using FEAT (FMRIB Expert Analysis Tool) available as part of FSL[2] (Smith et al., 2004). Preprocessing includes the default options, such as separating images of brain from the rest of the images of the head, i.e., creating a brain mask, using the Brain Extraction Tool (BET; Smith, 2002), pre-whitening for local autocorrelation correction using FILM (FMRIB Improved Linear Model; Woolrich et al., 2001), motion correction based on rigid-body transformations using MCFLIRT (Motion Correction FMRIB Linear Image Registration Tool; Jenkinson et al., 2002), spatial smoothing using a Gaussian kernel and highpass temporal filtering as implemented in FSL as well as slice timing correction using a customized text file.

The analysis is done in three steps. On the first level we analyze each session's data, i.e., execute time-series analysis of the raw 4D fMRI data. We generate voxel-wise parameter estimates of the hemodynamic (blood-oxygen-level-dependent) responses to the different stimuli we used in the fMRI experiment. These voxel-wise parameter estimates represent the change in the blood-oxygenation level for a given stimulus compared to the baseline neural activation of no stimulus presentation and control stimulus. Modeled regressors include cooperation, i.e., choosing up (U) in PD game both in the human and computer

[2]www.fmrib.ox.ac.uk/fsl

conditions, C_PG1 and C_CG1, respectively; defection, D_PG1 and D_CG1; inequity aversion [down (D) in WG], IA_PG2 and IA_CG2; and inequity tolerance, IT_PG2 and IT_CG2. Each explanatory variable is created by convolving the stimulus actual duration times (from onset of stimulus till response using one of the buttons) within each stimulus with a standard gamma hemodynamic response function using FEAT. Through first-level analysis, we obtain parameter estimates as well as statistical maps for each regressor.

On the second level we combine each subject's activation across several blocks and create contrasts (for human vs. computer conditions: C_PG1 vs. C_CG1, D_PG1 vs. D_CG1, IA_PG2 vs. IA_CG2, IT_PG2 vs. IT_CG2; and WF vs. PD: IA_PG2 vs. C_PG1) using a fixed effects analysis with cluster-level statistical threshold of $Z > 2.3$ and $p < 0.05$. In order to compare human condition to computer condition and inequity aversion in WG to cooperation in PD we subtract one stimulus type (e.g., in Low sociality condition) from another type (e.g., in High sociality condition). The hypothesis of interest here is whether in each voxel the activation to human condition stimuli is greater than in computer condition. We also implement this type of contrast in the opposite direction, i.e., where activation in computer condition is higher than activation in human condition. In result, we generate statistical maps for each of the five contrasts for each subject. These contrast activation maps are registered to each subject's own high-resolution structural image and also to the Montreal Neurological Institute (MNI) 152-standard template.

Finally on the third level, we use FLAME (FMRIB's Local Analysis of Mixed Effects) modeling and one-sample t-test to decide whether the group activates on average. Mixed effects model the subject variability and, therefore, allow making inferences about the wider population from which the subjects are drawn. Each of the contrasts for the group are Gaussianized intro Z-statistical images and thresholded at $Z > 2.3$ with a cluster-corrected significance threshold of $p < 0.05$ (Worsley, 2001). The high resolution structural MRI images of individual subjects are standardized to the MNI space and averaged within the group to create an average structural template.

SPM 12 Procedures

The Main Study is analyzed using identical procedures in SPM12 (Wellcome Department of Cognitive Neurology, London, UK[3]), which includes correction for field inhomogeneities, realignment, and coregistration of functional images to each subject's own high-resolution structural image using a six-parameter rigid body transformation model, reorientation to the plane containing the anterior and posterior commissures, spatial normalization into space compatible with an MNI atlas, and smoothing using a 6 mm^3 FWHM Gaussian kernel. Statistical analyses are implemented in SPM12. For each participant, event-related condition effects are estimated according to the general linear model, using a canonical hemodynamic response function, high-pass filtering (128 s), and a first-order autoregressive error structure. At the individual level, BOLD signal is modeled in a fixed effects analysis with separate regressors modeling each condition of interest during the game presentation period, for the decision making, and feedback periods. Linear contrasts are created for each comparison of interest (e.g., PD + High Sociality vs. UG + High Sociality, PD + Low Sociality vs. UG + Low Sociality, PD + High Sociality vs. PD + Low Sociality, and UG + High Sociality vs. UG + Low Sociality). These contrasts are then imported to group-level random effects analyses for inference to the population. The above-threshold activations table (shown at $P < 0.05$, FWE) is created with WFU_pickatlas[4]. The particular regions reported in the results are visualized using xjView toolbox[5].

PPI in AFNI

Psychophysiological interaction (PPI) analysis is conducted in AFNI[6]. We define the seed region as medial PFC (defined using the Harvard–Oxford structural atlas[7]). The PPI analysis identifies regions showing differential coupling with the mPFC during High Sociality vs. Low Sociality conditions. The mPFC ROI is projected from MNI space to individual subject space, the time series data are extracted from the combined left and right mPFC, and terms associated with the baseline, linear drift, and head motion are removed. These cleaned time series data are deconvolved with an assumed gamma impulse response function, and then multiplied by the High Sociality vs. Low Sociality condition contrast to generate an interaction term. An additional GLM is implemented as before, but with additional regressors corresponding to the deconvolved mPFC time series, the High Sociality vs. Low Sociality condition contrast, and the interaction of these two regressors, which is the key term in the PPI analysis. This final interaction regressor is used to identify brain regions in which functional coupling with the mPFC differs during the interaction with an Acquaintance compared to Random Individual. Beta weights corresponding to this interaction regressor are converted to Z-scores to allow for between-subject comparison.

RESULTS

Behavioral Results

In the PD the trend is typical, with high (moderate) levels of cooperation in the first few rounds devolving into consistent moderate (high) levels of defection. The only difference is witnessed between high sociality (humans, acquaintances) and low sociality (computers, random individuals) conditions (**Table 2**). Playing acquaintances in the Main Study resulted in slightly higher levels of cooperation than those in the Pilot Study for Humans condition. Nevertheless, we observe significant difference between cooperation rates in the PD in the Pilot Study

[3]www.fil.ion.ucl.ac.uk/spm/

[4]http://www.nitrc.org/projects/wfu_pickatlas/

[5]http://www.alivelearn.net/xjview

[6]http://afni.nimh.nih.gov/sscc/gangc/CD-CorrAna.html

[7]http://www.cma.mgh.harvard.edu/

TABLE 2 | Computer experiment behavioral results.

Pilot study conditions	Cooperation in PD	Inequity tolerance in WG	Main study conditions	Cooperation in PD	Inequity tolerance in UG
Human	28%	30%	Acquaintance	49%	76%
Computer	16%	46%	Random individual	18%	66%

Behavioral results of computer experiments for Pilot and Main studies are reported. The percentages of cooperative decisions (choose U or L in the PD) and the frequency of inequity tolerance decisions (choose U in the WG or accepted an unfair offer in the UG) across studies and conditions are listed.

TABLE 3 | fMRI experiment behavioral results.

Pilot study conditions	Cooperation in PD	Inequity tolerance in WG	Main study conditions	Cooperation in PD	Inequity tolerance in UG
Human	26%	40%	Acquaintance	34%	71%
Computer	15%	62%	Random individual	21%	51%

Behavioral results of fMRI experiments for Pilot and Main studies are reported.

(Humans vs. Computers, $N = 30$, p-value $= 0.002$, t-test) and in the Main Study (Acquaintances vs. Random Individuals, $N = 45$, p-value $= 0.0006$, t-test).

Results of the Computer Experiment for Welfare and UGs are puzzling. Whereas for WG the egalitarian outcome (inequity aversion), rather than Nash equilibrium (2; 6) is more likely, for the UG accepting unfair offers (inequity tolerance) is predominant. The difference between sociality conditions is not significant.

For the fMRI portion of the experiment the same pattern remains: rates of cooperation are significantly higher for the high sociality condition than those for the low sociality condition (**Table 3**; Pilot Study: Humans vs. Computers, $N = 10$, p-value $= 0.001$, t-test; Main Study: Acquaintances vs. Random Individuals, $N = 15$, p-value $= 0.02$, t-test). It is important to notice that the cooperation level averages oscillated around the mean till the very last round due to the persistent tests of cooperative strategy by participants that face nasty Nash equilibrium computerized strategy.

We observe significant difference between sociality conditions, for the Welfare and UG (Pilot Study: Humans vs. Computers, $N = 10$, p-value $= 0.05$, t-test; Main Study: Acquaintances vs. Random Individuals, $N = 15$, p-value $= 0.05$, t-test). The directions of the effect are distinct: acceptance of unfair offers is higher for Computers (low sociality) compared to Humans (high sociality) conditions, but is lower for Random Individual (low sociality) compared to Acquaintance (high sociality) conditions, similar to what is seen in the Computer Experiment. The WG is a simultaneous game, whereas the UG is sequential. In the UG the subject accepts or rejects the offer that is presented to her. In the WG she does not know what will be offered, so it is not necessarily inequity aversion, but might be as well risk aversion. In other words in WG the subject provides a hedge against potential inequity by forcing the egalitarian outcome, whereas in the UG it is not possible without losing everything. That is why in UG most of the subjects tolerate inequity.

fMRI Results, Pilot Study

The fMRI analysis of the Pilot Study in FSL focuses on the functional activity pattern associated with social domain and economic games participants play. We determine areas in the brain where the neural activation is higher for subjects playing with humans, than playing with computers in completing several different tasks. We report functional activation in the areas as specified in MNI structural atlas (Mazziotta et al., 2001; Collins et al., 2004) and Talairach Daemon Labels atlas (Lancaster et al., 2000).

Cooperation in the PD game with humans compared to cooperation in PD with computers is associated with a signal increase in dorsolateral prefrontal cortex (DLPFC), Brodmann areas (BA) 8 and 9 (Cooperation contrast: BA 8 [$x = 69$, $y = 69$, $z = 55$ (MNI_152 space coordinates)], Z-score $= 3.01467$). Whereas BA 9 functions include sustaining attention and working memory, BA 8 is even more intriguing, as it is linked to the management of uncertainty (Platt and Huettel, 2008) as well as hopes or high expectations. Many studies see DLPFC as a contributor to rational decision-making in social situations. Although cooperation in the PD game is seen by many as irrational, the theory of sociality (Lukinova et al., 2014; Berkman et al., 2015) provides a rational explanation for such behavior by adding an economic component to the subject's utility function in the social context. Thus, activation in the Cooperation contrast can be attributed to another demonstration of sociality at work, where brain processes cooperation as a rational decision.

Contrast between WG and PD game displays highlight in BA 30 [$x = 36$, $y = 45$, $z = 33$ (MNI_152 space coordinates), Z-score $= 2.55405$] that along with adjacent areas forms posterior cingulate gyrus. Its functions include spatial memory and orientation (Owen et al., 1996), as well as face recognition (Leube et al., 2001). Neither the former, nor the latter directly correspond to the stimuli presented to the subjects. BA 39 [$x = 61$, $y = 33$, $z = 51$ (MNI_152 space coordinates), Z-score $= 2.54531$], located at the middle temporal gyrus, is also involved in calculation (Grabner et al., 2007), as well as in "theory of mind" (Goel et al., 1995), i.e., modeling knowledge, rationality, etc., of another person's mind. Indeed, calculation and "theory of mind" occur in both games (Rilling et al., 2004), however, while the PD game is familiar and is frequently used in multiple courses in college, the WG, as a rare simultaneous version of UG, requires participants to think

TABLE 4 | Above-threshold activations (shown at $P < 0.05$, FWE) are presented for the contrasts of interest.

Contrast	Anatomical region	Coordinates (*x, y, z*)	*T*-statistic	*Z*-statistic	Cluster size
PD > UG					
	L inferior frontal gyrus	(−38, 3, 34)	11.49	4.87	2
	L inferior parietal lobule	(−41, −44, 58)	10.5	4.72	1
UG > PD					
	R superior frontal gyrus	(21, 49, −18)	12.49	4.8	2
High sociality > Low sociality					
	L sub-gyral	(−35, −38, 38)	11.08	4.81	1
	L superior frontal gyrus	(−10, 12, 58)	10.63	4.74	1
	R inferior semi-lunar lobule	(12, −60, −52)	9.28	5.15	6
	L pre-central gyrus	(−36, −12, 58)	8.87	5.07	10
	L post-central gyrus	(−40, −36, 64)	8.81	5.05	7
	R cingulate gyrus	(−42, −24, 40)	8.27	4.91	3
	R superior temporal gyrus	(50, 20, −18)	7.87	4.79	1
Low sociality > High sociality					
	L inferior parietal lobule	(−35, −47, 46)	13.66	5.16	6
	L inferior parietal lobule	(−35, −56, 46)	13.16	5.09	4
	L inferior frontal gyrus	(−50, 9, 34)	13	5.07	2
	L precuneus	(−7, −62, 54)	11.02	4.8	1
	R precuneus	(3, −56, 54)	10.94	4.79	2
	R cingulate gyrus	(18, −38, 38)	8.83	5.06	1
	R parahippocampal gyrus	(38, −22, −18)	8.58	4.99	1

MNI_152 space coordinates are reported.

through other subject's strategy and execute the cost-benefit analysis.

fMRI Results, Main Study

The analysis of neuroimaging data in SPM focuses on the functional activity pattern between games and opponent conditions (**Table 4**; shown at $P < 0.05$, FWE).

One of the goals is to determine brain areas where neural activation is higher in one game or another. In Pilot Study, when participant plays in a PD Game compared to her making decisions in a WG besides significant clusters already identified, activation is higher in vmPFC, Brodmann area 32 (BA 32, $x = 5.70$, $y = 25.53$, $z = 34.81$; T-statistic $= 6.0101$). It is likely that brain activation differences between games, namely WG and UGs, are mainly due to calculation issues and the novelty of WG to college students. It is vital that BA 32 associated with rational thought processes does not appear to be more activated, when comparing PD and UG in the Main Study.

When comparing cooperation decision in PD to acceptance of unfair offers in the UG or agreement to Nash equilibrium in the WG, no significant clusters are found. We assert that in the social setting the neural basis for tolerability to defection (opponent's strategy in PD is nasty) and tolerability to inequity (advantageous position of column chooser in WG and unfair offer in UG) is identical, representing confrontation with the social world that is at times unjust and rough.

Besides the BA 8 and BA 9 activations already identified in the Pilot Study differences between sociality conditions in PD also show higher activations in orbitofrontal area, BA 11 ($x = -28.80$, $y = 50.61$, $z = -9.89$, T-statistic $= 6.0101$; **Figure 2**), known for its connection to planning, reasoning, and decision making. Cooperation in high sociality condition is indeed attributed to a well-planned and a reasonable, if not rational decision. The contrasts between High sociality and Low sociality involve among others the following brain activations: Superior

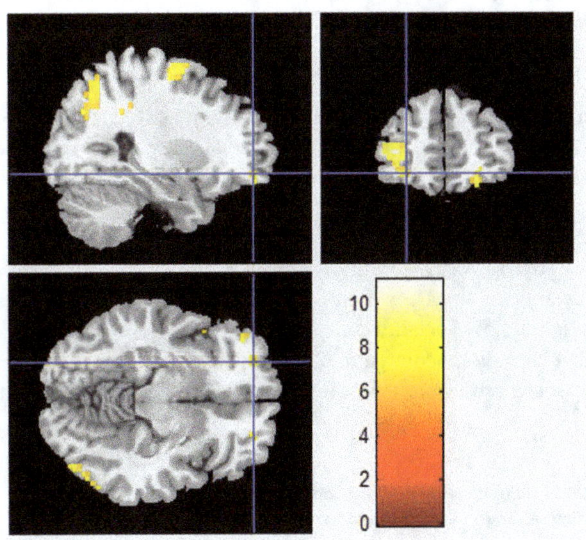

FIGURE 2 | High sociality > Low sociality contrast (BA 11). Contrast between High sociality and low sociality conditions reveals activations in orbitofrontal area, BA 11 ($x = -28.80$, $y = 50.61$, $z = -9.89$). This area is associated with planning, reasoning, and decision making in general.

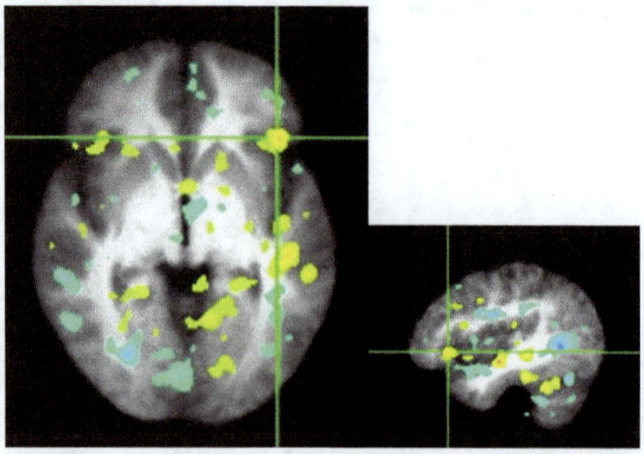

FIGURE 3 | *Z*-scores from the seed to the inferior frontal gyrus in the axial and sagittal views. Functional connectivity of mPFC with the right inferior frontal gyrus, a region previously associated with cognitive control and modulation of the valuation system. Regions depicted are found to correlate with mPFC to a greater degree when participants make economic decisions as they interacted with others in the high sociality condition compared to the low sociality condition.

Frontal Gyri, Inferior Frontal Gyrus, Anterior Cingulate, and Parahippocampal Gyrus.

We conduct preliminary connectivity tests using PPI analysis using the mPFC as a seed, a brain region associated with valuation. The software used for obtaining the activations is Analysis of Functional Neuro-Images (AFNI). The presence of a positive context-dependent interaction in a region (i.e., a PPI) can be interpreted as greater relative connectivity between that region and the seed in one condition compared to another. In this case, the regions depicted in **Figure 3** are found to correlate with mPFC to a greater degree when participants made decision in PD as they interacted with others in the high sociality condition compared to the low sociality condition. **Table 5** shows the correlation coefficients for the areas of interest, i.e., the areas highlighted for the High > Low Sociality contrast.

Several regions emerge that have previously been implicated in prosocial economic choice (e.g., the right inferior frontal gyrus

TABLE 5 | R coefficients with seeded ROI in the medial frontal gyrus (coefficient range −0.0019445 to 0.01676).

	AFNI-r coefficient	# of voxels	% max coefficient
Fusiform gyrus	0.006777	1492	0.4043
Inferior frontal gyrus	0.006322	731	0.3772
Insula	0.006274	509	0.3743
Anterior cingulate	0.006351	381	0.3789
Parahippocampal gyrus	0.005702	306	0.3402

Regions that were significantly positively correlated with medial prefrontal cortex (mPFC) to a greater degree when participants made economic decisions as they interacted with others in the high sociality condition compared to the low sociality condition: r refers to the Pearson correlation coefficient relating neural activity in that cluster and mPFC activation coefficients at the group level.

and the DLPFC; Tabibnia et al., 2008). Notably, these regions modulate activation of the valuation system in cases when self-control is necessary to override impulsive or habitual choices such as selfish economic decisions (Hare et al., 2008). Several small peaks also emerge in the valuation network proper (not shown), but the small sample size prevents strong inferences based on these data.

DISCUSSION

If social cognition constantly results in a different pattern of brain activity than a non-social one and the regions of brain activation during social cognition have a special status (high levels of activity even at rest) in the brain (Adolphs, 2003; Jenkins and Mitchell, 2011), to what extent are brain systems that control social behavior domain specific (Cosmides and Tooby, 1994; Stone et al., 2007)? If evolutionary perspective provides theoretical grounding for domain specificity, neuroscience then gives an opportunity to investigate it.

This paper focuses on the comparison of two sociality conditions. It is the first attempt to find what brain regions correspond to a neural value of sociality and lay a foundation to identify and estimate this neural value. The key is to induce prosocial behaviors in economic games, different in nature, but common in representation. Our findings support the theory of sociality. Indeed, we assert that additional social utility is calculated in the human brain, when a person interacts with someone from the socialized group she identifies herself with. This additional social utility may cause prosocial decisions, such as cooperation in the PD, and may as well appear rational to the brain. A good way of talking about sociality is by illustrating what happens when it is impaired (Edmiston et al., 2015): sociality can be described as the opposite of autism.

Based on our research we propose that economic games, such as PD representing collective action and the UG, the simplest demonstration of bargaining, can be intertwined. We observed that presenting UG and PD together results in higher cooperation rates than when participants deal with the PD only. One explanation is a spillover effect produced during the UG. In the social environment, norms of fairness in the UG may encourage us to be as well fair in the PD, i.e., cooperate. Recent findings, however, do not report any correlation between rejecting unfair offers and prosocial behaviors in other games (Yamagishi et al., 2012). The fact that we did not observe significant differences in activations between the games could be due to highly perplexed cognitive processes involved in these social dilemmas when sociality is induced.

The data collected from the fMRI experiments can serve to answer many more questions, than those raised in this paper. For example, how do subjects perceive outcomes? While in this study, our main focus is on the stimuli from onset till response, next we can take into account the reaction toward the outcome displayed to the participant. How will participants react to unfairness or defection? Or how will participants react and what brain activation will be related to it if they defect, while the opponent cooperated? Why do dopaminergic and subcortical regions show no activation in the task? These research questions: to identify the brain regions that are sensitive to sociality and to test the relative effectiveness of the sociality inductions in altering neural activation in the social cognition and valuation networks and economic decisions - hold promise to advance the social aspects of BCI (Sexton, 2015).

AUTHOR CONTRIBUTIONS

All authors designed the experiments; EL carried out the experiments, programmed the software for the experiment, prepared the data, and conducted the analysis; EL wrote the paper; all authors reviewed the paper and the results.

ACKNOWLEDGMENT

We thank Elliot Berkman for useful suggestions in experimental design and data analysis.

REFERENCES

Abdullaev, Y., Posner, M. I., Nunnally, R., and Dishion, T. J. (2010). Functional MRI evidence for inefficient attentional control in adolescent chronic cannabis abuse. *Behav. Brain Res.* 215, 45–57. doi: 10.1016/j.bbr.2010.06.023

Adolphs, R. (2003). Cognitive neuroscience of human social behaviour. *Nat. Rev. Neurosci.* 4, 165–178. doi: 10.1038/nrn1056

Akerlof, G. A., and Kranton, R. E. (2000). Economics and identity. *Q. J. Econ.* 115, 715–753. doi: 10.1162/003355300554881

Akerlof, G. A., and Kranton, R. E. (2010). *Identity Economics: How Our Identities Shape Our Work, Wages, and Well-Being.* Princeton, NJ: Princeton University Press.

Amodio, D. M., and Frith, C. D. (2006). Meeting of minds: the medial frontal cortex and social cognition. *Nat. Rev. Neurosci.* 7, 268–277. doi: 10.1038/nrn1884

Aoki, R., Yomogida, Y., and Matsumoto, K. (2015). The neural bases for valuing social equality. *Neurosci. Res.* 90, 33–40. doi: 10.1016/j.neures.2014.10.020

Berkman, E. T., Lukinova, E., Menshikov, I., and Myagkov, M. (2015). Sociality as a natural mechanism of public goods provision. *PLoS ONE* 10:e0119685. doi: 10.1371/journal.pone.0119685

Cacioppo, J. T., Berntson, G. G., Adolphs, R., Carter, C. S., Davidson, R. J., Mcclintock, M. K., et al. (2002). *Foundations in Social Neuroscience.* Cambridge, MA: MIT Press.

Camerer, C., Loewenstein, G., and Prelec, D. (2005). Neuroeconomics: how neuroscience can inform economics. *J. Econ. Lit.* 43, 9–64. doi: 10.1257/0022051053737843

Collins, D. L., Holmes, C. J., Peters, T. M., and Evans, A. C. (2004). Automatic 3-D model-based neuroanatomical segmentation. *Hum. Brain Mapp.* 3, 190–208. doi: 10.1002/hbm.460030304

Cosmides, L., and Tooby, J. (1994). "Origins of domain specificity: the evolution of functional organization," in *Mapping the Mind: Domain Specificity in Cognition and Culture*, eds L. Hirschfeld and S. Gelman (New York, NY: Cambridge University Press), 85–116.

Davidson, R. J., Putnam, K. M., and Larson, C. L. (2000). Dysfunction in the neural circuitry of emotion regulation–a possible prelude to violence. *Science* 289, 591–594. doi: 10.1126/science.289.5479.591

Dawes, C. T., Loewen, P. J., Schreiber, D., Simmons, A. N., Flagan, T., McElreath, R., et al. (2012). Neural basis of egalitarian behavior. *Proc. Natl. Acad. Sci. U.S.A.* 109, 6479–6483. doi: 10.1073/pnas.1118653109

De Quervain, D. J. F., Fischbacher, U., Treyer, V., Schellhammer, M., Schnyder, U., Buck, A., et al. (2004). The neural basis of altruistic punishment. *Science* 305, 1254–1258. doi: 10.1126/science.1100735

Declerck, C., and Boone, C. (2015). *Neuroeconomics of Prosocial Behavior: The Compassionate Egoist.* Cambridge, MA: Academic Press.

Declerck, C. H., Boone, C., and Emonds, G. (2013). When do people cooperate? The neuroeconomics of prosocial decision making. *Brain Cogn.* 81, 95–117. doi: 10.1016/j.bandc.2012.09.009

Dolan, R. J. (2002). Emotion, cognition, and behavior. *Science* 298, 1191–1194. doi: 10.1126/science.1076358

Edmiston, E. K., Merkle, K., and Corbett, B. A. (2015). Neural and cortisol responses during play with human and computer partners in children with autism. *Soc. Cogn. Affect. Neurosci.* 10, 1074–1083. doi: 10.1093/scan/nsu159

Emonds, G., Declerck, C. H., Boone, C., Seurinck, R., and Achten, R. (2014). Establishing cooperation in a mixed-motive social dilemma. An fMRI study investigating the role of social value orientation and dispositional trust. *Soc. Neurosci.* 9, 10–22. doi: 10.1080/17470919.2013.858080

Emonds, G., Declerck, C. H., Boone, C., Vandervliet, E. J., and Parizel, P. M. (2012). The cognitive demands on cooperation in social dilemmas: an fMRI study. *Soc. Neurosci.* 7, 494–509. doi: 10.1080/17470919.2012.655426

Emonds, G., Declerck, C. H., Boone, C., Vandervliet, E. J. M., and Parizel, P. M. (2011). Comparing the neural basis of decision making in social dilemmas of people with different social value orientations, a fMRI study. *J. Neurosci. Psychol. Econ.* 4, 11–24. doi: 10.1037/a0020151

Fehr, E., and Camerer, C. F. (2007). Social neuroeconomics: the neural circuitry of social preferences. *Trends Cogn. Sci.* 11, 419–427. doi: 10.1016/j.tics.2007.09.002

Fett, A. K. J., Gromann, P. M., Giampietro, V., Shergill, S. S., and Krabbendam, L. (2014). Default distrust? An fMRI investigation of the neural development of trust and cooperation. *Soc. Cogn. Affect. Neurosci.* 9, 395–402. doi: 10.1093/scan/nss144

Fischbacher, U. (2007). z-Tree: Zurich toolbox for ready-made economic experiments. *Exp. Econ.* 10, 171–178. doi: 10.1007/s10683-006-9159-4

Fliessbach, K., Weber, B., Trautner, P., Dohmen, T., Sunde, U., Elger, C. E., et al. (2007). Social comparison affects reward-related brain activity in the human ventral striatum. *Science* 318, 1305–1308. doi: 10.1126/science.1145876

Flombaum, J. I., and Posner, M. I. (2005). The activation of attentional networks. *Neuroimage* 26, 471–479. doi: 10.1016/j.neuroimage.2005.02.004

Glimcher, P. W., and Fehr, E. (2013). *Neuroeconomics: Decision Making and the Brain.* Cambridge, MA: Academic Press.

Goel, V., Grafman, J., Sadato, N., and Hallett, M. (1995). Modeling other minds. *Neuroreport* 6, 1741–1746. doi: 10.1097/00001756-199509000-00009

Grabner, R. H., Ansari, D., Reishofer, G., Stern, E., Ebner, F., and Neuper, C. (2007). Individual differences in mathematical competence predict parietal brain activation during mental calculation. *Neuroimage* 38, 346–356. doi: 10.1016/j.neuroimage.2007.07.041

Güroğlu, B., Will, G. J., and Crone, E. A. (2014). Neural correlates of advantageous and disadvantageous inequity in sharing decisions. *PLoS ONE* 9:e107996. doi: 10.1371/journal.pone.0107996

Hare, T. A., O'doherty, J., Camerer, C. F., Schultz, W., and Rangel, A. (2008). Dissociating the role of the orbitofrontal cortex and the striatum in the computation of goal values and prediction errors. *J. Neurosci.* 28, 5623–5630. doi: 10.1523/JNEUROSCI.1309-08.2008

Henrich, J. P. (2004). *Foundations of Human Sociality: Economic Experiments and Ethnographic Evidence from Fifteen Small-Scale Societies.* New York, NY: Oxford University Press.

Hsu, M., Bhatt, M., Adolphs, R., Tranel, D., and Camerer, C. F. (2005). Neural systems responding to degrees of uncertainty in human decision-making. *Science* 310, 1680–1683. doi: 10.1126/science.1115327

Jenkins, A. C., and Mitchell, J. P. (2011). "How has cognitive neuroscience contributed to social psychological theory?," in *Social Neuroscience: Toward*

Understanding the Underpinnings of the Social Mind, eds A. Todorov, S. T. Fiske, and D. A. Prentice (Oxford: Oxford University Press).

Jenkinson, M., Bannister, P., Brady, M., and Smith, S. (2002). Improved optimization for the robust and accurate linear registration and motion correction of brain images. *Neuroimage* 17, 825–841. doi: 10.1006/nimg.2002.1132

Kuss, K., Falk, A., Trautner, P., Montag, C., Weber, B., and Fliessbach, K. (2015). Neuronal correlates of social decision making are influenced by social value orientation—an fMRI study. *Front. Behav. Neurosci.* 9:40. doi: 10.3389/fnbeh.2015.00040

Lampert, K., Phelps, E. A., Glimcher, P., and Fehr, E. (2014). "Neuroeconomics of emotion and decision making," in *Neuroeconomics: Decision Making and the Brain*, eds P. W. Glimcher and E. Fehr (Amsterdam: Elsevier Inc.), 219–236.

Lancaster, J. L., Woldorff, M. G., Parsons, L. M., Liotti, M., Freitas, C. S., Rainey, L., et al. (2000). Automated Talairach atlas labels for functional brain mapping. *Hum. Brain Mapp.* 10, 120–131. doi: 10.1002/1097-0193(200007)10:3<120::AID-HBM30>3.0.CO;2-8

Lee, D. (2008). Game theory and neural basis of social decision making. *Nat. Neurosci.* 11, 404–409. doi: 10.1038/nn2065

Lee, V. K., and Harris, L. T. (2015). How social cognition can inform social decision making. *Front. Neurosci.* 7:259. doi: 10.3389/fnins.2013.00259

Leube, D. T., Erb, M., Grodd, W., Bartels, M., and Kircher, T. T. J. (2001). Differential activation in parahippocampal and prefrontal cortex during word and face encoding tasks. *Neuroreport* 12, 2773–2777. doi: 10.1097/00001756-200108280-00035

Lohrenz, T., and Montague, P. R. (2008). "Neuroeconomics: What neuroscience can learn from economics," in *Psychology and Economic Behaviour*, ed. A. Lewis (Cambridge, MA: Cambridge University Press), 457–492.

Lukinova, E., Myagkov, M., and Shishkin, P. (2014). The value of sociality. *Foresight* 16, 309–328. doi: 10.1108/FS-11-2012-0086

Mazziotta, J., Toga, A., Evans, A., Fox, P., Lancaster, J., Zilles, K., et al. (2001). A probabilistic atlas and reference system for the human brain: international Consortium for Brain Mapping (ICBM). *Philos. Trans. R. Soc. Lond. B Biol. Sci.* 356, 1293–1322. doi: 10.1098/rstb.2001.0915

Norman, G. J., Hawkley, L. C., Cole, S. W., Berntson, G. G., and Cacioppo, J. T. (2012). Social neuroscience: the social brain, oxytocin, and health. *Soc. Neurosci.* 7, 18–29. doi: 10.1080/17470919.2011.568702

Oosterbeek, H., Sloof, R., and Van De Kuilen, G. (2004). Cultural differences in ultimatum game experiments: evidence from a meta-analysis. *Exp. Econ.* 7, 171–188. doi: 10.1023/B:EXEC.0000026978.14316.74

Osinsky, R., Mussel, P., Öhrlein, L., and Hewig, J. (2013). A neural signature of the creation of social evaluation. *Soc. Cogn. Affect. Neurosci.* 9, 731–763. doi: 10.1093/scan/nst051

Owen, A. M., Milner, B., Petrides, M., and Evans, A. C. (1996). A specific role for the right parahippocampal gyrus in the retrieval of object-location: a positron emission tomography study. *J. Cogn. Neurosci.* 8, 588–602. doi: 10.1162/jocn.1996.8.6.588

Perc, M., Gómez-Gardeñes, J., Szolnoki, A., Floría, L. M., and Moreno, Y. (2013). Evolutionary dynamics of group interactions on structured populations: a review. *J. R. Soc. Interface* 10:20120997. doi: 10.1098/rsif.2012.0997

Perc, M., and Szolnoki, A. (2010). Coevolutionary games—a mini review. *Biosystems* 99, 109–125. doi: 10.1016/j.biosystems.2009.10.003

Peterson, R. L. (2005). The neuroscience of investing: fMRI of the reward system. *Brain Res. Bull.* 67, 391–397. doi: 10.1016/j.brainresbull.2005.06.015

Plassmann, H., O'doherty, J., and Rangel, A. (2007). Orbitofrontal cortex encodes willingness to pay in everyday economic transactions. *J. Neurosci.* 27, 9984–9988. doi: 10.1523/JNEUROSCI.2131-07.2007

Platt, M. L., and Huettel, S. A. (2008). Risky business: the neuroeconomics of decision making under uncertainty. *Nat. Neurosci.* 11, 398–403. doi: 10.1038/nn2062

Rilling, J. K., Sanfey, A. G., Aronson, J. A., Nystrom, L. E., and Cohen, J. D. (2004). The neural correlates of theory of mind within interpersonal interactions. *Neuroimage* 22, 1694–1703. doi: 10.1016/j.neuroimage.2004.04.015

Ruff, C. C., and Fehr, E. (2014). The neurobiology of rewards and values in social decision making. *Nat. Rev. Neurosci.* 15, 549–562. doi: 10.1038/nrn3776

Sanfey, A. G., Rilling, J. K., Aronson, J. A., Nystrom, L. E., and Cohen, J. D. (2003). The neural basis of economic decision-making in the ultimatum game. *Science* 300, 1755–1758. doi: 10.1126/science.1082976

Schroeder, D. A., and Graziano, W. G. (2015). *The Oxford Handbook of Prosocial Behavior*. New York, NY: Oxford University Press.

Sexton, C. A. (2015). The overlooked potential for social factors to improve effectiveness of brain-computer interfaces. *Front. Syst. Neurosci.* 9:70. doi: 10.3389/fnsys.2015.00070

Smith, S. M. (2002). Fast robust automated brain extraction. *Hum. Brain Mapp.* 17, 143–155. doi: 10.1002/hbm.10062

Smith, S. M., Jenkinson, M., Woolrich, M. W., Beckmann, C. F., Behrens, T., Johansen-Berg, H., et al. (2004). Advances in functional and structural MR image analysis and implementation as FSL. *Neuroimage* 23, S208–S219. doi: 10.1016/j.neuroimage.2004.07.051

Stone, V. E., Winkielman, P., and Harmon-Jones, E. (2007). "An evolutionary perspective on domain specificity in social intelligence," in *Social Neuroscience: Integrating Biological and Psychological Explanations of Social Behavior*, eds E. Harmon-Jones and P. Winkielman (New York, NY: Guilford Press), 316–349.

Strombach, T., Weber, B., Hangebrauk, Z., Kenning, P., Karipidis, I. I., Tobler, P. N., et al. (2015). Social discounting involves modulation of neural value signals by temporoparietal junction. *Proc. Natl. Acad. Sci. U.S.A.* 112, 1619–1624. doi: 10.1073/pnas.1414715112

Tabibnia, G., Satpute, A. B., and Lieberman, M. D. (2008). The sunny side of fairness. *Psychol. Sci.* 19:339–347. doi: 10.1111/j.1467-9280.2008.02091.x

Tajfel, H. (1982). Social psychology of intergroup relations. *Annu. Rev. Psychol.* 33, 1–39. doi: 10.1146/annurev.ps.33.020182.000245

Tajfel, H., and Turner, J. C. (1979). "An integrative theory of intergroup conflict," in *The Social Psychology of Intergroup Relations*, eds W. G. Austin and S. Worchel (Monterey, CA: Brooks-Cole).

Tajfel, H. E. (1978). *Differentiation between Social Groups: Studies in the Social Psychology of Intergroup Relations*. London: Academic Press.

Tricomi, E., Rangel, A., Camerer, C. F., and O'Doherty, J. P. (2010). Neural evidence for inequality-averse social preferences. *Nature* 463, 1089–1091. doi: 10.1038/nature08785

Van Overwalle, F. (2009). Social cognition and the brain: a meta-analysis. *Hum. Brain Mapp.* 30, 829–858. doi: 10.1002/hbm.20547

Watanabe, T., Takezawa, M., Nakawake, Y., Kunimatsu, A., Yamasue, H., Nakamura, M., et al. (2014). Two distinct neural mechanisms underlying indirect reciprocity. *Proc. Natl. Acad. Sci. U.S.A.* 111, 3990–3995. doi: 10.1073/pnas.1318570111

Waytz, A., Zaki, J., and Mitchell, J. P. (2012). Response of dorsomedial prefrontal cortex predicts altruistic behavior. *J. Neurosci.* 32, 7646–7650. doi: 10.1523/JNEUROSCI.6193-11.2012

Willingham, D. T., and Dunn, E. W. (2003). What neuroimaging and brain localization can do, cannot do and should not do for social psychology. *J. Pers. Soc. Psychol.* 85:662–671. doi: 10.1037/0022-3514.85.4.662

Woolrich, M. W., Ripley, B. D., Brady, M., and Smith, S. M. (2001). Temporal autocorrelation in univariate linear modeling of FMRI data. *Neuroimage* 14, 1370–1386. doi: 10.1006/nimg.2001.0931

Worsley, K. J. (2001). "Statistical analysis of activation images," in *Functional MRI: An Introduction to Methods*, eds P. Jezzard, P. M. Matthews, and S. M. Smith (Oxford: Oxford University Press), 251–270.

Yacubian, J., Gläscher, J., Schroeder, K., Sommer, T., Braus, D. F., and Büchel, C. (2006). Dissociable systems for gain- and loss-related value predictions and errors of prediction in the human brain. *J. Neurosci.* 26, 9530–9537. doi: 10.1523/JNEUROSCI.2915-06.2006

Yamagishi, T., Horita, Y., Mifune, N., Hashimoto, H., Li, Y., Shinada, M., et al. (2012). Rejection of unfair offers in the ultimatum game is no evidence of strong reciprocity. *Proc. Natl. Acad. Sci. U.S.A.* 109, 20364–20368. doi: 10.1073/pnas.1212126109

17

An Array of Highly Flexible Electrodes with a Tailored Configuration Locked by Gelatin during Implantation—Initial Evaluation in Cortex Cerebri of Awake Rats

Johan Agorelius[1,2], Fotios Tsanakalis[1], Annika Friberg[1], Palmi T. Thorbergsson[1], Lina M. E. Pettersson[1*†] and Jens Schouenborg[1,2*†]*

[1] *Department of Experimental Medical Science, Neuronano Research Centre, Lund University, Lund, Sweden,* [2] *The Nanometer Structure Consortium, Lund University, Lund, Sweden*

Edited by:
Manuel Fernando Casanova, University of Louisville, USA

Reviewed by:
Jit Muthuswamy, Arizona State University, USA
Ulrich G. Hofmann, Albert-Ludwigs-University Freiburg, Germany

****Correspondence:***
Johan Agorelius, Lina M. E. Pettersson and Jens Schouenborg, Department of Experimental Medical Science, Neuronano Research Center, Lund University, BMC F10, SE-221 84 Lund, Sweden
johan.agorelius@med.lu.se; lina.pettersson@med.lu.se; jens.schouenborg@med.lu.se

† These authors jointly directed this work.

Background: A major challenge in the field of neural interfaces is to overcome the problem of poor stability of neuronal recordings, which impedes long-term studies of individual neurons in the brain. Conceivably, unstable recordings reflect relative movements between electrode and tissue. To address this challenge, we have developed a new ultra-flexible electrode array and evaluated its performance in awake non-restrained animals.

Methods: An array of eight separated gold leads ($4 \times 10\ \mu m$), individually flexible in 3D, were cut from a gold sheet using laser milling and insulated with Parylene C. To provide structural support during implantation into rat cortex, the electrode array was embedded in a hard gelatin based material, which dissolves after implantation. Recordings were made during 3 weeks. At termination, the animals were perfused with fixative and frozen to prevent dislocation of the implanted electrodes. A thick slice of brain tissue, with the electrode array still in situ, was made transparent using methyl salicylate to evaluate the conformation of the implanted electrode array.

Results: Median noise levels and signal/noise remained relatively stable during the 3 week observation period; 4.3–5.9 μV and 2.8–4.2, respectively. The spike amplitudes were often quite stable within recording sessions and for 15% of recordings where single-units were identified, the highest-SNR unit had an amplitude higher than 150 μV. In addition, high correlations (>0.96) between unit waveforms recorded at different time points were obtained for 58% of the electrode sites. The structure of the electrode array was well preserved 3 weeks after implantation.

Conclusions: A new implantable multichannel neural interface, comprising electrodes individually flexible in 3D that retain its architecture and functionality after implantation has been developed. Since the new neural interface design is adaptable, it offers a versatile tool to explore the function of various brain structures.

Keywords: brain machine interface, flexible electronic implant, neural probe, embedding material, brain micro-motions, stable neural recordings, mechanical compliance, neuromodulation

Introduction

A major challenge in the field of Brain-Machine Interfaces (BMIs) is that the stability of neuronal recordings often is insufficient for studies of single neuronal activity over long periods of time. Unstable electrode position in the tissue can occur if the implant is too rigid to follow the movements of the brain during for example the respiratory and cardiac cycles (Britt and Rossi, 1982) but can also be caused by body movements (Jackson and Fetz, 2007; Santhanam et al., 2007). Moreover, the quality, i.e., signal-to-noise ratio, commonly gradually deteriorates over time (Rousche and Normann, 1998; Williams et al., 1999; Polikov et al., 2005). This deterioration may in part also be due to instability, since micro-motions between probe and tissue are likely to cause continuous irritation or indeed injury of the tissue that result in long-term glial activation and unfavorable effects on nearby neurons (Turner et al., 1999; Williams et al., 1999; Szarowski et al., 2003; Biran et al., 2005; Gilletti and Muthuswamy, 2006; Seymour and Kipke, 2007; Thelin et al., 2011; Lind et al., 2013). These glial reactions and effects on nearby neurons are known to impair recording quality (Nolta et al., 2015).

The largest micro-motions occur between the brain and the skull in the awake freely moving animals (Kim et al., 2004; Gilletti and Muthuswamy, 2006; Biran et al., 2007). For this reason, flexible leads on the cortical surface connecting the implanted rather stiff electrodes to the electronics have been developed (Rousche and Normann, 1998; Jackson and Fetz, 2007; Musallam et al., 2007). However, there are also significant micro-motions inside the brain caused by propagating waves of blood inside the vessels (Eide, 2008; Wagshul et al., 2011). The propagating nature of these movements implies that the movements inside the brain are not uniform. On top of these movements, there are movements caused by respiration. If the implanted electrodes cannot follow these tissue movements in all three dimensions, micro-forces/micro-movements between tissue and the recording sites on the electrodes will ensue. Indeed, it is a common experience, when performing acute electrophysiological experiments using stiff microelectrodes for extracellular recordings, that substantial pulsative movements inside the brain can occur as an effect of e.g., heart beats despite stabilization of the surface. As a result, such recordings tend to be short lived if the electrode is too close to the recorded neurons. Hence, to allow close contacts with neurons for longer periods of time, a high degree of mechanical compliance between electrodes and tissue is likely to be beneficial.

To improve mechanical compliance between electrodes and tissue, efforts have been made to increase the flexibility of the implanted electrodes themselves (Rousche et al., 2001; Kipke et al., 2002; Takeuchi et al., 2005; Stice et al., 2007; Bae et al., 2008; Krüger et al., 2010; Andrei et al., 2012; Felix et al., 2012; Lee et al., 2012; Kuo et al., 2013; Ejserholm et al., 2014; Kozai et al., 2014; Sohal et al., 2014). However, some of them are too flexible to be implanted on their own, and thus structural support in the form of a stiff guide or cannula (Kipke et al., 2002; Felix et al., 2012; Kuo et al., 2013; De Faveri et al., 2014; Sohal et al., 2014) has been used. These guides/cannulae cause additional stab wound-like injuries on their own, and on removal risk perturbing the position of the implanted flexible electrodes. Many of these flexible electrodes embed the conductive leads in a polymer sheet. However, this reduces their flexibility to one dimension only, and since the electrode leads are fixed in the polymer they cannot move independently of each other. In addition, such chip-like constructions also permanently split the tissue into two halves, causing an irreversible disruption of communication between neural networks on the two sides and therefore create a less than ideal situation when analyzing the function of neuronal networks. Hence, the challenge of providing an implantable array of independent highly flexible electrodes and that can be provided with an architecture adapted to the target tissue still remains.

The aim of the present project was thus to develop a fully functional and implantable array of ultra-thin electrodes, individually flexible in three dimensions after implantation. We present a new type of array of ultra-flexible electrodes which by being embedded in a hard but dissolvable gelatin based material retains its conformation and arrangement during implantation. Preliminary performance tests in awake rats showed encouraging results.

Materials and Methods

Design and Fabrication of the Electrode Array

We designed an array of eight wavy electrodes, thus flexible/extendable in three dimensions, each equipped with a distal protruding branch from where neuronal recordings could be made (**Figure 1**). The electrode array conformation was designed to allow recordings from different cortical laminae. The design was created using AutoCAD 2011 software and digitally imported into a Laser Machining System (Laser mill 50, standard micro-milling system, Nd:YAG laser system, New Wave Research, Inc., Fremont, CA). A 4 μm-thick sheet of gold foil (Rosenobel-Doppelgold 23 3/4 karat, J.G. Eytzinger GmbH, Germany) was fastened onto a microscope glass slide using polyethylene glycol (Sigma-Aldrich). Gold leads, 10 μm in width were milled under a fixed 20X objective using pulsed green laser light (wavelength 532 nm, energy density 10 J/cm^2).

The glass slide containing the milled electrodes was mounted with silicon (Elastosil A07) and aligned on a metal frame to which a printed circuit board (PCB) was attached. The individual leads were manually soldered to the PCB one by one using a flux mixture solution (62% Sn, 36% Pb, 2% Ag) applied between the electrodes to be soldered and the contacts on the PCB. This process was performed under a stereomicroscope (SMZ1500, Nikon Instruments Europe BV, The Netherlands). To wash away the remaining flux mixture from between the PCB leads and to release the electrode leads from the glass slide, the metal frame was immersed in 70% ethanol, after which the glass slide was carefully removed manually.

An acrylic coating (HumiSeal advanced protective coating for electronics) was applied as protection over the soldered leads and over the bottom part of the PCB. The electrode array, including the PCB, was then coated with Parylene C (4 μm thick) using a Compact Bench Top Coating System (Labtop 3000, Para Tech Coating Inc., CA, US).

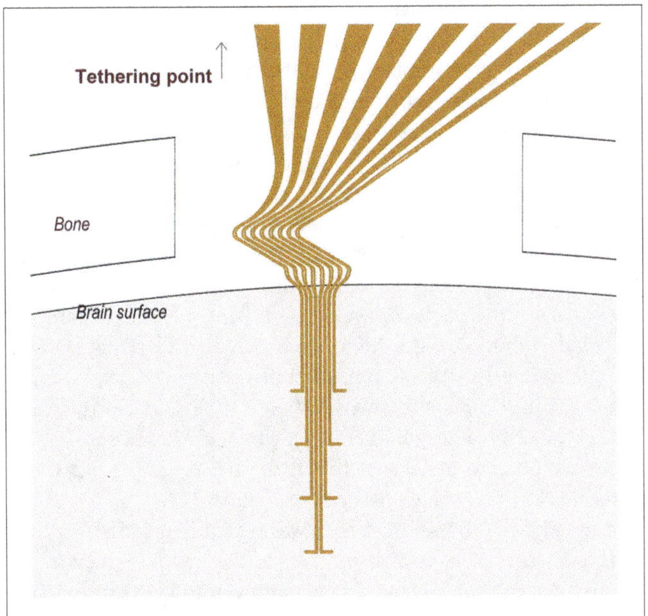

FIGURE 1 | A schematic of the 3D flexible electrode array. Note the Z-shaped proximal part of the electrode array located between the cranium and the brain surface, and the tips (10 μm) of the distal protrusions which serve as recording sites.

There were no obvious inherent strain forces in the construct since the gold electrodes were not displaced after being cut out from the gold sheet and also kept their conformation when insulated with parylene C.

To prepare the active recording sites on the protruding tips, the parylene coating was photo-ablated on both sides, over an area extending 10 μm from each electrode lead tip, using focused UV radiation (wavelength 355 nm, energy density 1.4 J/cm^2) under a 20x objective. The successful exposure of the lead recording sites was monitored in real time during the ablation process and subsequently carefully confirmed with Scanning Electron Microscopy (SEM).

A ∼40 mm long, 150 μm thick, un-insulated silver wire (Advent research Materials Ltd, England) was attached to the chip in the assigned "ground" position in order to be used as animal ground for the recordings. The electrode, connected to the chip, was finally released from the frame.

Impedance Spectroscopy

The electrical properties of each electrode lead were evaluated by impedance spectroscopy (Gamry Instruments, Series G 300, USA). After immersion in 0.9% saline solution, the impedance of the individual channels was measured by applying a 10 mV AC voltage with a frequency of 1 KHz, using a large Pt wire as counter electrode and an Ag/AgCl electrode in phosphate buffer as reference. The mean impedance of the individual channels was 832 kΩ (*SD* = 230 kΩ). It should be noted that repeated impedance measurements did not significantly change the impedance of the electrodes.

Embedding of the Electrodes

The gold electrodes used in this study are highly flexible, for instance they cannot be inserted into water without bending. To provide structural support during implantation, the ultra-flexible electrode array was embedded in a hard, but dissolvable, gelatin B based matrix material. The gelatin matrix was prepared by slowly heating a mixture of 3 g gelatin (Gelatin powder Ph.Eur., 24360.368, WWR International AB, Sweden), 750 mg PEG 400 (81172-1L, Sigma-Aldrich Chemie GmbH, Germany), 150 mg glycerol 98% (GRP Rectapur, 24 387.361, VWR, BDH Prolabo, France), and 7 mL Millipore water (Millipak-20 Filter Unit 0.22 μm 1/4 in), to 70°C, giving a final concentration of 27.5% gelatin, 1.4% glycerol and 6.9% PEG. The mixture was then placed on a hot plate while stirring. The electrode array was placed inside a custom made Poly Methyl Methacrylate (PMMA) mold and the gelatin mixture was injected. The humidity during drying was held at 21%, and the gelatin was dried first 24 h inside the mold, and then 24 h with the top lid of the mold removed. The remaining water content after drying was estimated to be below 4% (by measuring the weight of the probes ($n = 5$) before and after drying). This method enabled production of a probe embedded in a gelatin matrix with a sharp rigid tip that allowed for penetration of the brain tissue (**Figure 3B**).

Finally, a thin coat of a water retardation material was applied in order to delay dissolution of the matrix material until the implant was fully implanted. In short, the gelatin-embedded electrode array was dip-coated in a 5% (w/w) solution of kollicoat (Fluka, Sigma-Aldrich Sweden AB) in 99.7% ethanol, two times with a drying interval of 24 h in between each coat, and at least 1 h between the last coating and implantation.

Animal Surgery

Approval for the experiments was obtained in advance from the Malmö/Lund Animal Ethics Committee on Animal Experiments (ethical permit M60-13) and all experiments in this work conform to the regulatory standards of this approval. All rats had free access to food and water and were kept in a 12-h light/dark cycle at a constant environmental temperature of 21°C and 65% humidity.

Female Sprague-Dawley rats were implanted with the embedded ultra-flexible electrode array in the hind paw area of the primary somatosensory (SI) cortex at the following stereotactic coordinates; 1.5 mm rostral and 2.0 mm lateral from Bregma. The rats weighed 222.5 g (*SD* = 3.8 g) at the time of surgery, corresponding to approximately 9–10 weeks. In short, anesthesia was induced by placing the rat in a chamber of 2% isoflurane (Isoba®vet., Apoteksbolaget, Sweden) with 40% oxygen and 60% nitrous oxide (Granmo et al., 2013). The animal was placed on a heating pad and its body temperature was monitored and kept at a stable level. The head was shaved and the rat was mounted in a stereotactic frame (KOPF Instruments, USA). After disinfection of the skin with 70% ethanol, the skull was exposed with a midline incision. The skin was retracted and the skull was cleaned from connective tissue under a stereomicroscope (Leica Microsystems, M651, Germany). Two holes (0.8 mm) were drilled anterior to bregma and one posterior to the SI cortex using a high-speed stereotaxic drill (Dest 300

IN, model MM 323IN, Silfradent, Italy). Small custom-made titanium screws with a length of 1900 μm were screwed ~570 μm into the holes. The choice of material was based on the fact that titanium is a well-known biocompatible material commonly used in implants and which has the potential to integrate into the bone of the skull, yielding increased screw stability and thus adherence of the implant to the skull. The screws were used as anchoring sites for the dental cement (FujuCEM, GC, Europe, Belgium), which was applied at a later stage to attach the electrode/PCB to the skull. The ground wire was wired around the screw and inserted in a separate hole so as to be in contact with the CSF, see below.

A craniotomy, ~2 mm in the rostro-caudal direction, and ~3.5 mm in the medio-lateral dimension was made in the bone of the skull at the SI cortex coordinates, while leaving the underlying dura mater intact. The hind paw area in the S1 cortex was targeted using stereotactical implantation (Kalliomäki et al., 1993). Onset latencies of tactile response were measured from the stimulation artifact. The hole was rinsed with 0.9 % sterile saline solution to clear away any possible debris and prevent tissues from drying.

The embedded electrode was mounted in a hydraulic micromanipulator (KOPF Instruments, USA) and positioned above the SI cortex coordinates. The dura mater was carefully incised and deflected. Care was taken to always keep a thin layer of saline on the cortical surface to prevent it from drying. The electrode was implanted at the above mentioned coordinates to a depth of 1800 μm with a speed of 50 μm/s. After implantation, the ground wire was looped around one of the screws, and subsequently inserted under the bone on top of the dura on the contralateral side of the skull. A small piece of collagen biomatrix for dura regeneration (TissuDura, Baxter International Inc., USA) was positioned in the hole on top of the animal ground wire. The wire was secured and the hole was protected by application of dental cement. To increase the adherence of the PCB and dental cement to the skull, a primer, RelyX™ Unicem, Aplicap™ (3M, Sollentuna; Sweden) was applied prior to dental cement application.

In order to roughly estimate how long after implantation a neural signal could be obtained from the electrodes, a short-lasting recording was made in the anesthetized animal after implantation. In the three animals used for recordings (on 2–4 out of 8 electrode sites in each animal), neuronal activity was detectable already 30–40 min after implantation.

During surgery, the eyes were shielded with a compress which was continually refreshed with physiological saline. In addition, care was taken to make absolutely sure that ethanol or disinfectant was not applied anywhere in the vicinity of the eyes.

After surgery the rat was given subcutaneous injections of 0.01 mg/kg of temgesic (buprenorfin; Schering-Plough, Belgium) to relieve postoperative pain and animals were monitored during the awakening phase. At the end of the experimental period, (3 weeks post implantation), animals were killed by an intraperitoneal injection overdose of pentobarbital and transcardially perfused with saline (0.9%) followed by ice-cold 4% paraformaldehyde (PF) in 0.1 M phosphate buffer, pH 7.4. The brains were post fixed in PF overnight.

Tissue Clarification

To evaluate how well the flexible electrode array maintains its conformation after implantation, the head and brain with the probe still in situ was sectioned and processed according to the clarification protocol described below.

In short, after fixation, the whole head was snap frozen in isopentane on dry ice and stored at −80°C. This preparation method was developed in order to prevent distortion or removal of the electrode from the brain during sectioning of the skull and brain tissue. The top part of the skull bone including the upper part of the electrode was cut off using a circular diamond saw blade mounted on a high-speed dental drill (Desk 200 In, Silfradent, Italy) at 10,000 rpm. After this, the frozen head was cut in 4.5–5.5 mm thick slices with a tissue-slicing machine (ABW 300 GM, 242 W, Avery Berkel, UK), while still kept deep frozen. Care was taken to make sure that the entire electrode array was contained within a single tissue slice (**Figure 3C**).

For clarification the tissue slice was rinsed in 0.1 M phosphate buffered saline (3 × 5 min) to remove the fixative, dehydrated through ethanol of increased concentration (50, 70, and 99.5%, 3–4 h in each), and finally cleared in increasing concentrations (50, 70 in ethanol and 100%) of methyl salicylate (Sigma-Aldrich, Stockholm, Sweden) at least 5 h in each immersion. The conformation of the electrode within the brain slice was examined after clarification and compared with the conformation of the same gelatin embedded electrode before implantation, using 11.5 × magnification stereo microscope (SMZ 1500, Nikon, Japan) with 0.5x WD 136 objective (Nikon, Japan).

In-vivo Electrophysiology in Awake Animals

To evaluate the functionality and stability of the 3D electrode, *in vivo* recordings of single unit activity were made, in awake and non-restrained animals. Neural recordings were performed 2–5 times a week, starting day 1 (1 day after implantation) up to the end point at day 21.

The *in-vivo* recordings were performed in a faraday cage to eliminate external electromagnetic interference. Rats were briefly anesthetized with isoflurane (as per above) to connect the PCB to a 64 channel Plexon data acquisition system via a 20X head stage, a commutator and pre-amplifier (OmniPlex, Plexon Inc, Texas, USA) with a 60 cm long cable. The anesthetic gas was discontinued and signals were recorded from awake and non-restrained rats enclosed in a cage-like container.

To verify the physiological nature of the recorded activity, tactile stimulations of the glabrous skin of the contralateral hind paw were performed by triggering a tactile stimulator connected to a Master 8 stimulator (A.M.P.I., Jerusalem, Israel). At least one session of tactile stimulations was performed per animal. For each session a minimum of 150 tactile stimulations were performed and event time stamps were registered together with the electrophysiological recordings.

Data Analysis

The performance of the developed electrode arrays was evaluated by analyzing the noise levels, signal-to-noise ratio (SNR), yield (ratio of active electrodes that recorded single units and total number of electrodes) and stability of the neural recordings over a period of 3 weeks.

Recording Parameters

The electrophysiological data were sampled at 16 bit and 40 kHz per channel using a Plexon data acquisition system (Plexon Inc., Texas, USA). The signals were bandpass-filtered (0.25–8 kHz) using a noncausal filter (Quian Quiroga, 2009) and re-referenced using Common Median Referencing (Rolston et al., 2009) to eliminate common-mode artifacts. All post-acquisition analysis was performed automatically using in-house written Matlab (Mathworks Inc.) programs.

Unit-identification

Putative single-units were identified using an unsupervised algorithm consisting of a simple amplitude-threshold detector (Quiroga et al., 2004) and clustering with Gaussian Mixture Models (GMM) (Pouzat et al., 2002; Ludwig et al., 2006). The threshold for spike detection was set as minus four times the estimated noise level (standard deviation of background noise) and spikes were aligned temporally at the point of maximum amplitude of the detected valley (Mitra and Bokil, 2008). The noise level was estimated using the maximum absolute deviation (MAD) estimator for standard deviation (Quiroga et al., 2004), given by:

$$\widehat{\sigma}_N = median\frac{|signal|}{0.6745}. \quad (1)$$

As features for spike sorting, the first six principal component analysis (PCA) weights were used (Lewicki, 1998). To estimate the number of units, the feature-distributions were fitted to GMMs with one to six components and the model for which the Bayesian Information Criterion (BIC) converged (BIC < 10% of the BIC-range for all models) was selected. The spikes were assigned to the unit (mixture-component) according to their maximum posterior membership-probability. Spikes that did not have a posterior membership-probability above 0.8 for any unit were classified as outliers (Ludwig et al., 2006).

Signal-to noise ratio (SNR) of units was defined as:

$$SNR = \frac{s_{pp}}{2 \cdot \sigma_N} \quad (2)$$

where s_{pp} is the peak-to-peak amplitude of the unit-waveform and σ_N is the standard deviation of residuals after subtracting the unit-waveform from each detected spike waveform. ISI (inter-spike interval) violation rate was defined as the percentage of ISIs that were shorter than 1 ms.

An automatic unit-validation procedure largely based on the manual procedure described in Suner et al. (2005) was implemented to identify putative units that could be reasonably assumed to represent neuronal activity. In Suner et al. (2005), this validation was performed by visual inspection of unit-waveforms, and by rejecting units that did not have at least a biphasic component. In order to do this in an objective and consistent manner, we extracted several descriptive features of the unit-waveforms related to this criterion. Those were: (1) polarity of the pre- and post-peak phases of the waveform (identifies strictly monophasic waveforms), (2) the amplitude-difference between waveform endpoints relative to the maximum amplitude (rejecting strongly unbalanced waveforms likely to be artifacts), (3) the number of zero-crossings of pre- and post-peak phases of the waveform (rejecting waveforms with more than 3 zero-crossings in one of the phases) and (4) temporal location of the waveform-peak (rejecting slowly varying waveforms, usually representing artifacts). In addition to these waveshape-related features, we used (5) SNR (rejecting units with SNR < 2 and SNR > 20, representing noise and artifacts, respectively), (6) ISI violation rate (rejecting units with >0.5% ISI violation rate), (7) amplitude-threshold-rate (rejecting units that only marginally crossed the detection threshold), and (8) amplitude (rejecting units with amplitude < 25 uV). The thresholds for the individual metrics were set empirically to obtain consistent rejection of units that would have been likely to be rejected by a manual procedure.

The SNR was further used to classify units as good ($SNR \geq 4$), fair ($2 \leq SNR < 4$), poor ($1 \leq SNR < 2$), and no-signal ($SNR < 1$). In addition to these classes, we introduced a fifth class containing very-high SNR units ($SNR > 6$).

Recording Performance Over Time

To make a preliminary assessment of the recording performance over time, we measured noise level (Equation 1), SNR of valid units (Equation 2), yield, and relative difference in amplitude between units with highly correlated unit-waveforms recorded on the same channel but on different days. When evaluating performance, the SNR of recordings was taken as the SNR of the highest-SNR valid single-unit identified in the recording. Yield was defined as the percentage of electrode-sites on which at least one valid unit with $SNR \geq 2$ (at least fair) or $SNR \geq 4$ (at least good) was identified (Ludwig et al., 2006) and was quantified both on a per-week basis and with all days pooled together. To identify units recorded on the same channel but on different days, that might represent the same neuron, we used a method similar to that described in Fraser and Schwartz (2012) in which both the shapes of unit-waveforms and firing statistics were compared between recording sessions. However, since our experiments were performed mainly during spontaneous behavior, no measures related to firing statistics were included in our procedure. Hence, we emphasize that while suggestive, the analysis applied here does not allow safe conclusion on whether or not pairs of valid units with a high correlation between waveform shapes between different recording sessions indeed represent the same neuron.

For all pairs of valid units with $SNR \geq 2$ (at least fair) identified on different days, the similarity-measure was taken as the Fisher-transformed maximum value of the cross-correlation between the unit-waveforms. The waveform-correlation threshold for what to consider as units with highly similar waveforms was set as the 90th percentile limit of the distribution of Fisher-transformed waveform-correlations for pairs consisting of units from separate animals. This resulted in a waveform-correlation threshold of 0.96. The correlation threshold was then applied to all same-animal, same-channel, different-day unit-pairs, and pairs with correlation above 0.96 were assumed to putatively represent the same neuron. When multiple unit-pairs were found, only the pair with the highest waveform-correlation was considered.

Results

Design Features

The resulting electrode array comprised a Z-shaped suspension in the upper part of the shank designed to absorb the major part of the motions between the brain and the skull (Supplementary Video 1). Each of the electrode leads was equipped with a 100 μm long protrusion perpendicular to the main axis, which served a dual function of adding to the flexibility and anchorage in the tissue close to the recording sites. The electrode array was designed to obtain recordings from four different depths, each 400 μm apart, corresponding to layer IV–VI of the rat primary somatosensory cortex. SEM examination of the probe confirmed that a ~100 μm^2 area of gold surface was de-insulated at the recording sites. To assess the thickness necessary to allow implantation we implanted probes with a thickness of 75 μm (one animal), 100 μm (4 animals), and 125 μm (3 animals). While a thickness of 75–100 μm was deemed to thin to avoid bending during implantation, 125 um thick vehicles did not bend. From these tests we deduced the minimal thickness.

A compression test (Zwick GmbH & Co. KG, Materials Testing Machine with load cell Zwick/Roell KAP-Z (0.04-4N), zero-point deviation 0.02% and pre-load 0.08 N. Acquisition system Zwick/Roell testXpert II) was performed on five gelatin embedded and coated, dummy probes (gold-sheet corresponding to the total area of all 8 leads before individual cut out). The average maximum deformation force (Fmax, force at which the probe begins to bend) was equal to 0.373 N (SD = 0.18). This stiffness combined with a needle shaped tip was enough to allow implantation of the electrodes into the tissue with only minor dimpling of the surface.

The shape of the gelatin matrix after molding resulted in a probe with a needle shaped tip and an oval shank diameter (~400 μm wide and ~130 μm thick). To avoid dimpling of the cortical surface during implantation, a sharp tip angle (mean tip angle 41.3°, SD = 3.2°) and a tapering distal part is important. The shape used here was therefore a trade-off between the need for stabilization during implantation and a need to keep the size of the probe as small as possible.

Evaluation of Implantation and Electrode Conformation

The implantation into rat cortex proved to be smooth, without bleeding (n = 15) or visible conformational changes of the flexible electrode array. The gelatin matrix remained stiff enough to withstand implantation to the intended depth of 1800 μm. To investigate whether any gelatin is likely to remain non-dissolved around the implanted electrode array, gelatin embedded electrode arrays were implanted into the brains of four animals. The brain surface was kept exposed and monitored for 3.5 h. During this time the brain surface was covered by a thin layer of saline to mimic the conditions of the normal implantation procedure in which the skull opening is sealed with dental cement. These experiments showed that the brain surface had contracted around the implant with no visual trace of gelatin in any of the four animals after 3.5 h (**Figure 2**). Clarification of brain tissue slices with the electrode array still in situ (3 rats) confirmed that the electrode array could be implanted into the brain and remain in the brain for 3 weeks with preserved conformation (**Figure 3**).

Quality of Recordings in Non-restrained Awake Animals

Evaluation of electrode functionality showed that single unit activity was readily recorded during the full length of the experiment (3 weeks in 3 rats). Single units often remained quite stable both in amplitude and waveform during individual

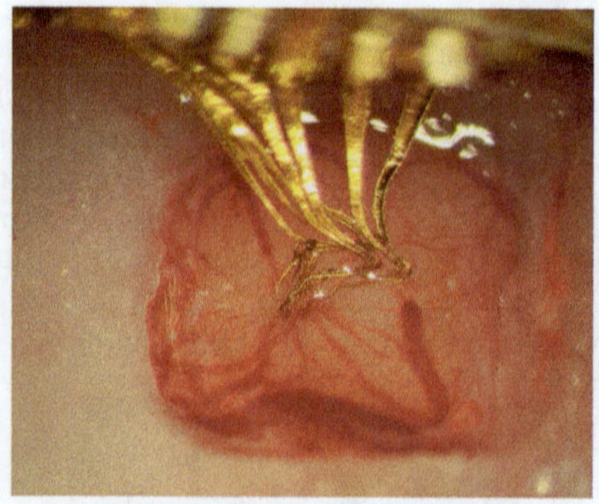

FIGURE 2 | Photograph taken 3.5 h after implantation of the gelatin embedded electrode, showing that the gelatin has dissolved and the brain surface contracted around the electrode array.

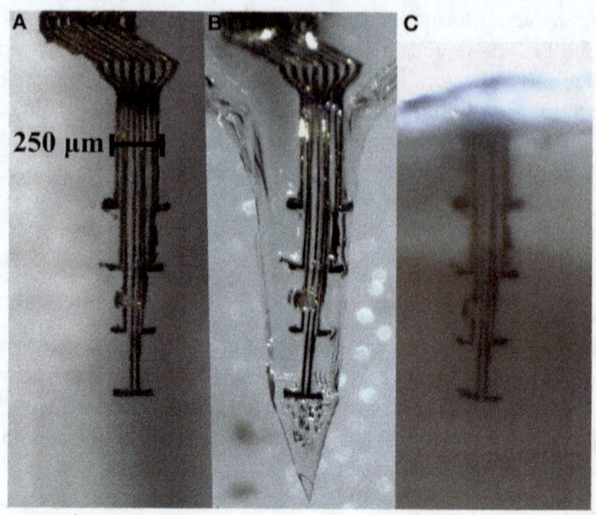

FIGURE 3 | Electrode array comprising eight thin (4 x 10 μm) gold leads insulated with Parylene C, except for an area (10 x 10 μm) at the tip of the 100 μm long protrusions. (A) An electrode array before embedding into a gelatin based matrix. **(B)** The same electrode array after being embedded into a gelatin matrix shaped as a needle, and in **(C)**, same electrode array inside a section of clarified brain tissue 3 weeks post implantation. Note that the conformation of the electrode array is well preserved inside the gelatin matrix as well as after implantation in the brain.

recording sessions (up to 50 min) as shown in **Figure 4**, indicating that the electrode recording sites remained relatively stable in the tissue during the time-course of individual recordings.

In order to verify the physiological nature of the detected spike activity tactile stimulations of the hind paw were performed and correlated to evoked spike activity through the calculation of a peri-stimulus time histogram (PSTH). An example of a single unit with high correlation to tactile stimulation is shown in **Figure 5**.

The signal quality was good throughout the experiment with an overall median noise level of 5.42 μV (IQR[1] = 2.16 μV) and overall median single-unit SNR of 3.30 (IQR = 2.30), respectively. As can be seen in **Figure 6A**, the noise level increased significantly (Mann-Whitney test, $p < 0.001$) between weeks 1 and 2, or from 4.27 to 5.95 μV (median) but remained stable ($p > 0.05$) between weeks 2 and 3. The SNR remained stable ($p > 0.05$) between weeks 1 and 2, but increased significantly ($p < 0.01$) between weeks 2 and 3, from 2.78 to 4.21 (median) (**Figure 6B**). In some cases, units with very high SNR (SNR > 6) were identified, indicating that the corresponding electrode sites in these cases were located very close to active neurons. In many cases, several single units with lower SNR were identified on the same channel, indicating that signals from more distant or electrically isolated neurons were also recorded.

Out of all electrode sites, 87.5% yielded at least one fair unit (SNR > 2), and 29.2% at least one good unit (SNR > 4) at some point in time. Over the course of the experiment, the weekly yield for both good and fair units showed a clear tendency to increase (**Figure 6C**).

On the Stability of Unit Recordings

To assess the positional stability of electrodes within the time-span of individual recording sessions, we measured the variation in mean spike-amplitude for every identified single-unit within a 1-s long moving window applied to the entire recording session. The sliding window was applied in order to diminish the influence of noise on the assessment of amplitude-variation. The amplitude-variation for a given unit was quantified as the standard deviation of relative amplitude deviations across all window positions. This analysis showed that the spike-amplitude remained relatively stable during the time-span of individual recordings, with an overall median standard deviation of 8.65% (IQR = 6.21%) across all identified single-units. Thus, for example, a single-unit with average peak-to-peak amplitude of approximately 130 μV (**Figure 4**) would be expected to vary around 130 μV by approximately 11.2 μV (8.65% of 130 μV).

Single-unit recordings obtained during different recording sessions with a waveform correlation higher than 0.96 [see

[1] IQR = Interquartile-range.

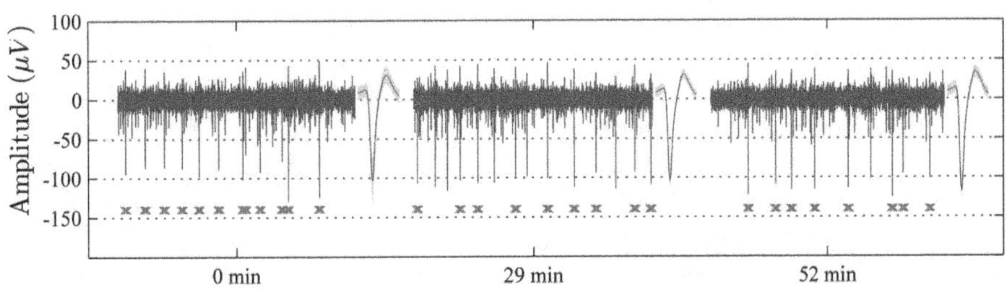

FIGURE 4 | Samples of 1 s long recordings extracted at 0, 29, and 52 min from one electrode channel in an awake non-restrained rat. The unit spike with the highest signal to noise ratio in each segment is shown to the right of respective sample (mean waveform ± standard deviation). Note the high level of stability of the recordings with respect to spike-waveforms (waveform correlation > 0.99 between the indicated unit waveforms of all three segments) and amplitude, as well as the overall recording qualities. The spike-times of the indicated single-unit are marked in red below the sweeps.

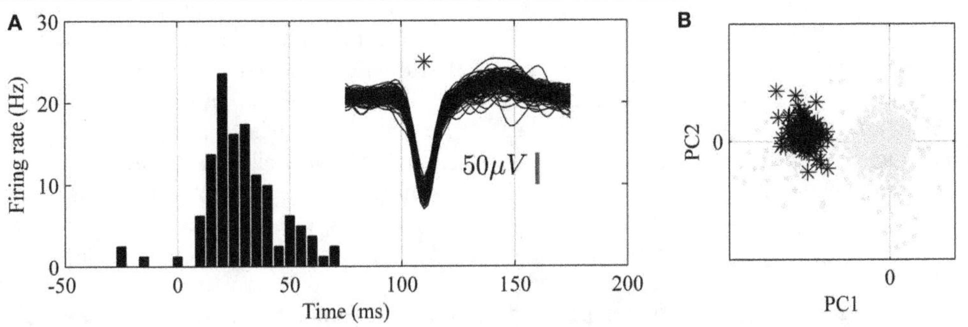

FIGURE 5 | Analysis of unit responses to tactile stimulation of the hind paw in awake, non-restrained rat. (A) Peristimulus-Time-Histogram (PSTH) for an identified single-unit (superimposed 1.6 ms long spike wave-forms for the unit are shown to the right, $n = 150$). **(B)** Principal component analysis (PCA). Note that the single unit (black stars) is well isolated from the background noise (gray dots) in the principal component (PC1 and PC2) feature space.

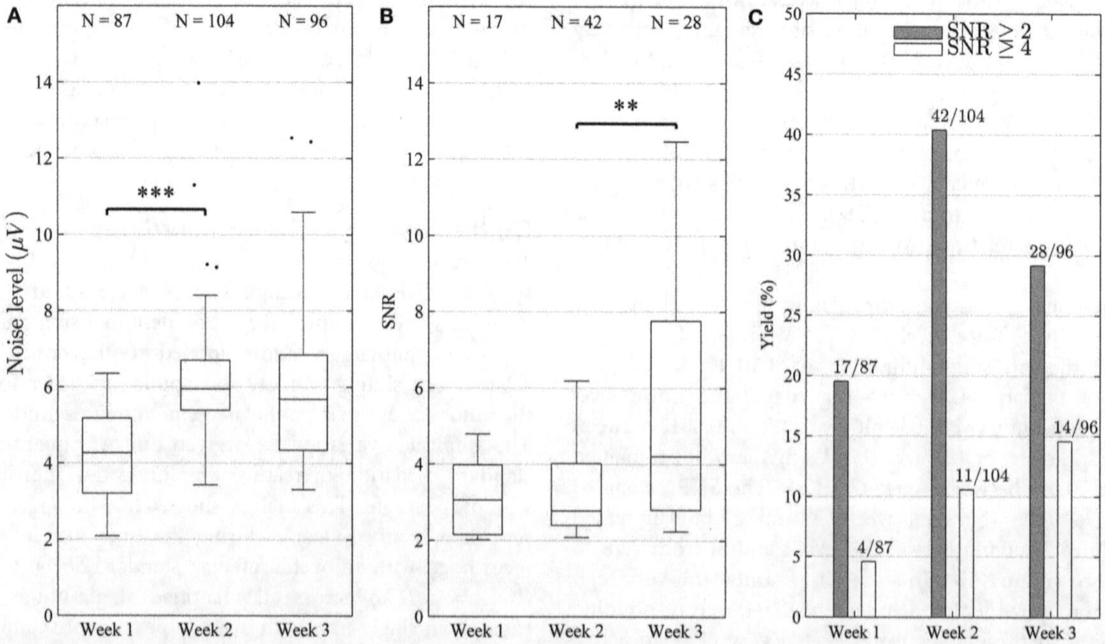

FIGURE 6 | Characterization of electrode performance over time. (A) Noise level estimated by Equation (1) (distributions shown as median and percentiles values) including all electrode channels. The noise increased significantly (***$p < 0.001$) between weeks 1 and 2, but remained stable between weeks 2 and 3 ($p > 0.05$). **(B)** Signal to noise ratio (SNR) of single-units (distribution including all identified units shown as median and percentile values) remained stable ($p > 0.05$) between week 1 and 2, but increased significantly between week 2 and 3 (**$p < 0.01$). This reflects the fact that high amplitude units were added during week 3. The increase in SNR and yield suggest that the overall recording conditions improved during the course of the experiment. **(C)** Bar diagram depicting yield in percentage (number of channels with units divided by number of channels is shown on top of each bar). It can be seen that yield increased for both good (SNR ≥ 4) and fair (SNR ≥ 2) units **(C)**, although the increase was not strictly monotonic for fair units (peaked during week 2).

Section Materials and Methods (subsection Recording Performance Over Time)] were obtained during the larger part of the experimental period in all animals. The relative difference in amplitude for such correlated waveforms was close to 1 (median = 1.22, IQR = 0.72) during the whole experiment (**Figure 7A**). No significant ($p > 0.05$) difference in relative amplitude difference was observed between week 1 and 2, and week 2 and 3. However, the relative difference in amplitude tended to be smaller (closer to 1) between week 2 and 3. Despite this relatively low overall difference in amplitude, we did observe some cases where the amplitude (and thus SNR) differed significantly (up to a factor of around 3) while the waveform remained relatively unchanged (correlation > 0.96) (**Figures 7B,C**).

In 13 out of 87 recordings where single-units were identified, the units with the highest-SNR had amplitudes greater than 150 μV. The maximum amplitude obtained for a unit was 424 uV. When comparing the waveforms of those units only, and with a stricter fixed waveform-correlation threshold of 0.99, 8 putative same-neuron pairs were identified, extending across a period of 1 day to 1 week, all within the period from day 13 and onward. Given that units with spike amplitudes >150 μV are likely to originate from units that are positioned close to the recordings electrodes (Pettersen and Einevoll, 2008; Thorbergsson et al., 2012), the high waveform correlations between recording sessions in these 8 putative same-neuron pairs is consistent with a high level of positional stability between electrode and neuron. It should be kept in mind, however, that when comparing single-units from discontinuous sessions exhibiting a high correlation of waveform shape (even for cases with correlations >0.99), it cannot be excluded that the recordings derive from different neurons since only spontaneous activity was recorded.

Discussion

In the present study, we provide a viable solution to the long-standing problem of how to implant electrode arrays, which are too flexible to be implanted without support, with retained conformation during and after implantation. The advantage of this new method is that it allows a tailored architecture of ultra-thin, and therefore more biocompatible electrodes, to be implanted in the brain. In other words, the electrode array can be designed to match the architecture of the tissue. In addition, electrodes individually flexible in all dimensions are expected to reduce the effects of micromotions/microforces which are likely to trigger tissue reactions. Furthermore, the free space between individual leads allows for electrode-tissue integration and prevents the array from creating a significant diffusion barrier. Preliminary tests in 3 animals also demonstrate that high quality recordings from single neurons can indeed by obtained using these electrodes, which is very encouraging.

We chose a rather simple array design with relatively few curved ultrathin leads as our first version. However, it should

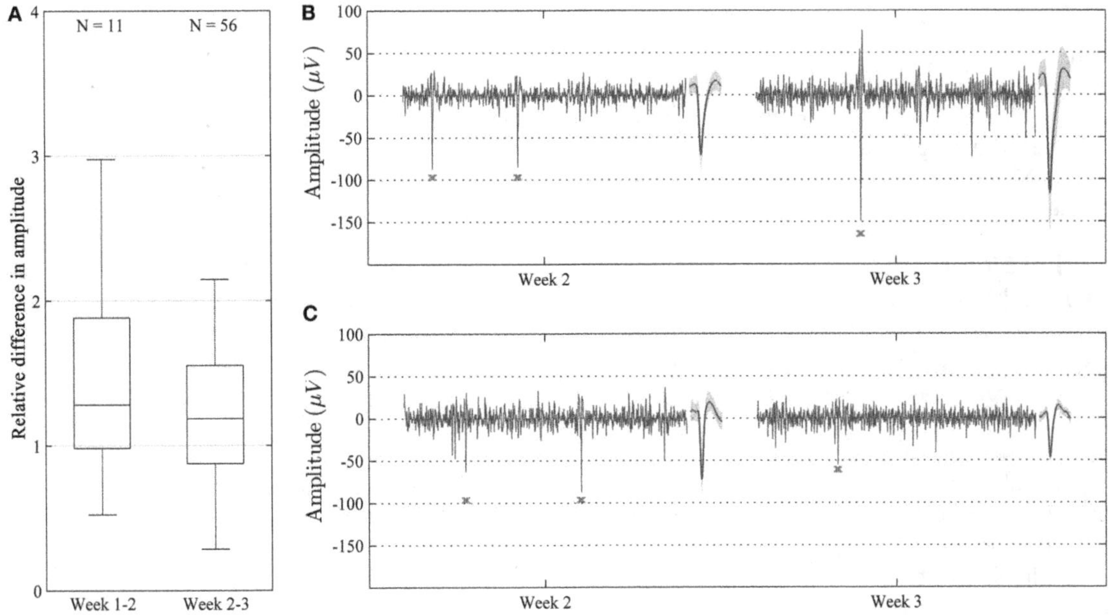

FIGURE 7 | Characterization of relative amplitudes of single unit spikes with high waveform correlation (>0.96) during two consecutive weeks. (A) Relative difference in amplitude shown as median and percentile values. The amplitude of units showed a tendency to increase over time, but this difference was not significant ($p > 0.05$). **(B,C)** Representative recordings (100 ms long) during week 2 and 3 in two different animals. Recordings are made from the same channel and show highly correlated units (waveform correlation > 0.96). Mean waveform ± standard deviation is shown to the right of each recording. In some cases, the amplitude of the units increased from week 2 to 3 **(B)**, whereas in some other cases, the amplitude decreased **(C)**.

be noted that the gelatin based vehicle can harbor practically any design of electrode array, including individual leads in the nanometer scales (Witteveen et al., 2010; Suyatin et al., 2013), as well as a larger number of individual channels. The design of the electrode array and hence relative position of recording sites can be adapted to the anatomical structure of various target areas demonstrating its potential for a wide range of applications in neuroscience research and in the clinic (Schouenborg, 2013).

On the Quality and Stability of the Obtained Recordings

The SNR and noise levels found in the present study appear to be similar to data from other current electrodes (Ludwig et al., 2006). A fair comparison of signal quality with the performance of other electrodes would, however, require standardized conditions (Ward et al., 2009). The SNR (Equation 2) was defined on a per-unit basis, using the noise level estimation for each unit individually and not the recording noise-level as defined by Equation (1). The reason for this choice was to ensure compatibility with the SNR-classes defined in Suner et al. (2005). In general, the noise-level estimate in Equation (2) was higher than that of Equation (1). Also, the factor 2 in the denominator of Equation (2) is based on the assumption of bipolar unit-waveforms with positive and negative phases of equal amplitude. However, this was very seldom the case for the units reported here, also suggesting a general underestimation of SNR. Moreover, the generally small variation in spike amplitude within the recording-sessions shows that good recording stability can be obtained in the freely moving animal.

For the majority of electrode sites, single-units were detected at different points in time that, according to the waveform shape criterion (waveform correlation > 0.96), might represent the same neurons. For all three animals, such units were detected over the major part of the observation-period of 3 weeks. Some of those units had high spike amplitudes (>150 μV) indicating that the de-insulated electrode recording sites were located close to the neurons. These findings are consistent with the assumption that good positional stability can be obtained when electrodes flexible in 3D are used. Note, however, that while a high correlation is a necessary criterion for classifying unit pairs as originating from same neurons it is not a sufficient criterion. Since recordings were discontinued between sessions it is still possible that unit pairs with a high correlation and with small changes in amplitudes could originate from different neurons (Fraser and Schwartz, 2012).

The presence of small amplitude fluctuations of unit spikes during the recording sessions suggests that micro-motions, while presumably being significantly reduced by the flexible design of the neural interface, still remain between electrodes and recorded neurons. Moreover, due to the embedding technology used here, it is expected that displacement of neurons relative to the electrodes will occur during the initial period after implantation when the tissue retracts as the gelatin gel is dissolved. Characterization of gelatin dissolution showed that gelatin dissolved and the brain contracted around the implant within 3.5 h. The inevitable loss of cells during the implantation procedure, as well as accompanying glial activation (Biran et al., 2005; Polikov et al., 2005; Leach et al., 2010) will also cause some displacement of nearby neurons, and thus instability in recordings, during the initial week (Ludwig et al., 2006). The findings that the SNR and yield of neurons recorded per channel in fact increased over time may be related to such structural changes in the tissue. This also suggests that longer periods of stable and high quality recordings from the same neurons are within reach. Nevertheless, this remains to be evaluated in long-term studies.

Gel Embedded Electrode Arrays—Comparison with Chip-based Electrode Arrays

In this study, we demonstrate that the overall configuration of the array was well preserved after implantation. This implies there were no significant inherent strain forces in the electrode construction, which could have resulted in non-intended changes in electrode conformation after dissolution of the gelatin. Importantly, the individually separated channels (as in contrast to electrodes embedded into a sheet of polymer) allow for better diffusion inside the tissue and the opportunity for the tissue to integrate with the implant thereby creating a seamless integration of electronics and neural networks.

Gelatin was chosen as the main embedding material due to its biocompatible properties. For example, it is well known that neurons thrive on gelatin in cultures (Abranches et al., 2009) and cells embedded in gelatin have been implanted with no adverse signs reported in humans (Watts et al., 2003; Stover and Watts, 2008). Gelatin is also known to minimize bleeding, presumably due the hemostatic properties of collagen, which is the main constituent of gelatin (Marieb and Hoehn, 2010). There was no visual bleeding during and after any of the implantations of these electrodes (total number of implantations in this study $n = 15$). Thus, the minimal bleeding observed during implantation in this study could be due to the hemostatic properties of collagen.

Moreover, in a previous study in our lab we found that the brain is capable of eliminating implanted pure gelatin needles without forming a permanent scar (Lind et al., 2010). By contrast, a "stab wound" scar was clearly present after 12 weeks when using a non-gelatin embedded needle. More recently, we also found that gelatin coating of flexible probes not only significantly reduces microglial activation but also appears to preserve a normal neuronal density in the area adjacent to the electrode, i.e., a 50 μm wide zone around flexible probes (Köhler et al., 2015). This is in sharp contrast to previous studies reporting a reduction in neuronal density ranging between 20 and 60% in this inner zone (Biran et al., 2005; McConnell et al., 2009; Winslow and Tresco, 2010).

Limitations and Future Directions

The development of biocompatible neural interfaces is a very time consuming process, involving multiple cycles of design changes followed by *in vivo* testing. In fact, the present study took several years of developmental work. The present work was focused on evaluating the performance *in vivo* during a relatively short period of time. This short-term study shows that the proposed method makes it possible to manufacture and implant arrays of ultra-flexible, individually separated electrodes whose recording quality is improved after 2 weeks. Given these promising results, long-term studies are a logical next step. Such long-term studies are also needed to compare long-term performance with current neural interfaces and to evaluate several potential improvements of the developed neural interface. For example, the exposed de-insulated tips may be provided with surface enlargements to reduce the impedance and thereby the noise level, e.g., by electroplating procedures (Desai et al., 2010; Ludwig et al., 2011; Ejserholm et al., 2014). Also, the flexibility, and thereby presumably stability, can be further improved by e.g., using thinner leads and/or more curvy shapes of the leads. However, thinner electrodes are more prone to break during manufacturing and implantation procedures and this may thus limit the feasibility of such attempts. Notably, the previous assumption that the size of the electrodes *per se* is critical for long-term glial reactions (Stice et al., 2007; Thelin et al., 2011) may however be erroneous since also large implanted probes elicit very small chronic reactions provided they are truly floating in the brain, i.e., that their specific weight is close to that of the tissue (Lind et al., 2013).

While the present results are encouraging, future long-term studies of probe functions would benefit from being performed during well-defined behavioral tasks to permit an analysis of possible probe induced alterations in neuronal activity. Moreover, more frequent recording sessions would make the unit-tracking procedure more reliable due to the possibility to include measures related to firing-characteristics (Fraser and Schwartz, 2012) and facilitate a more precise quantification of the day-to-day changes of the relative position of the electrode.

It should also be noted that, while a primary purpose of embedding the electrodes in a hard but dissolvable matrix material was to provide the necessary support for fragile electrodes during implantation, the possibility of adding drugs to the embedding material could potentially also provide new opportunities in e.g., pharmacology (Ek et al., 2010). Moreover, by incorporating drugs in the embedding matrix material, e.g., neurotrophic factors, which are released locally in the brain during and after the implantation, it may be possible to promote restitution of the neuronal circuits after the injury caused by the implantation (Gámez et al., 2004; Chang, 2009).

Concluding Remarks

While this first design of gelatin embedded electrode arrays most likely can be improved as discussed above, the present results are encouraging since they suggests that stable long-term communications with the same neurons are indeed attainable. From a research perspective, the importance of stable communication lies in that it will open up for an extraordinarily detailed analysis of how the neuronal circuits in the brain functions under physiological and pathological conditions (Schouenborg, 2011). In particular, the identification and analysis of plastic long-term alterations in neural networks, e.g., during learning or during neurodegenerative diseases, would benefit considerably by stable long-term recordings from the same neurons.

From a clinical perspective, stable recordings of neural activity is a prerequisite for developing robust and interactive protocols for enhancing efficacy and safety of stimulation based treatment (for example deep brain stimulation). In addition, the finding that the configuration of the highly flexible electrode array was retained inside the cortex cerebri after 3 weeks, indicate that a seamless integration of electronics and neural circuits is possible in the near future. Such integration, in particular if stability can be achieved over long periods of time, has the potential of enabling highly interesting neuroengineering development in the future, aiming at, for example, restitution of neural circuits after injury.

Acknowledgments

This project was sponsored by a Linnaeus grant (project number 60012701) and project 01013 from the Swedish Research Council, The Knut and Alice Wallenberg Foundation (project number: KAW 2004.0119), grants from Skåne County Council (ALF), 2014/354 and the Nanometer Structure Consortium (nmC@LU) at Lund University. The authors would like to thank Petter Pettersson, Peter Paulander and Suzanne Rosander-Jönsson for their skillful technical assistance.

References

Abranches, E., Silva, M., Pradier, L., Schulz, H., Hummel, O., Henrique, D., et al. (2009). Neural differentiation of embryonic stem cells *in vitro*: a road map to neurogenesis in the embryo. *PLoS ONE* 4:6286. doi: 10.1371/journal.pone.0006286

Andrei, A., Tutunjyan, N., Verbinnen, G., Vanput, S., Krylychkina, O., Eberle, W., et al. (2012). "Fabrication and successful *in-vivo* implantation of a flexible neural implant with a hybrid polyimide-silicon design," in *Proceedings of the Annual International Conference of the IEEE Engineering in Medicine and Biology Society, EMBS* (San Diego, CA), 3890–3893.

Bae, W. J., Ruddy, B. P., Richardson, A. G., Hunter, I. W., and Bizzi, E. (2008). "Cortical recording with polypyrrole microwire electrodes," in *Conference Proceedings?: Annual International Conference of the IEEE Engineering in Medicine and Biology Society* (Vancouver, BC), 5794–5797.

Biran, R., Martin, D. C., and Tresco, P. A. (2005). Neuronal cell loss accompanies the brain tissue response to chronically implanted silicon microelectrode arrays. *Exp. Neurol.* 195, 115–126. doi: 10.1016/j.expneurol.2005.04.020

Biran, R., Martin, D. C., and Tresco, P. A. (2007). The brain tissue response to implanted silicon microelectrode arrays is increased when the device is tethered to the skull. *J. Biomed. Mat. Res. Part A* 82, 169–178. doi: 10.1002/jbm.a.31138

Britt, R. H., and Rossi, G. T. (1982). Quantitative analysis of methods for reducing physiological brain pulsations. *J. Neurosci. Methods* 6, 219–229. doi: 10.1016/0165-0270(82)90085-1

Chang, C.-J. (2009). The effect of pulse-released nerve growth factor from genipin-crosslinked gelatin in schwann cell-seeded polycaprolactone conduits on large-gap peripheral nerve regeneration. *Tissue Eng. Part A*, 15, 547–557. doi: 10.1089/ten.tea.2007.0342

De Faveri, S., Maggiolini, E., Miele, E., De Angelis, F., Cesca, F., Benfenati, F., et al. (2014). Bio-inspired hybrid microelectrodes: a hybrid solution to improve long-term performance of chronic intracortical implants. *Front. Neuroeng.* 7:7. doi: 10.3389/fneng.2014.00007

Desai, S. A., Rolston, J. D., Guo, L., and Potter, S. M. (2010). Improving impedance of implantable microwire multi-electrode arrays by ultrasonic electroplating of durable platinum black. *Front. Neuroeng.* 3:5. doi: 10.3389/fneng.2010.00005

Eide, P. K. (2008). Comparison of simultaneous continuous intracranial pressure (ICP) signals from ICP sensors placed within the brain parenchyma and the epidural space. *Med. Eng. Phys.* 30, 34–40. doi: 10.1016/j.medengphy.2007.01.005

Ejserholm, F., Köhler, P., Granmo, M., Schouenborg, J., and Bengtsson, M., W. L. (2014). μ-Foil polymer electrode array for intracortical neural recordings. *IEEE J. Trans. Eng. Health Med.* 2, 1–7. doi: 10.1109/JTEHM.2014.2326859

Ek, F., Danielsen, N., Eriksson, J., Petersson, P., and Schouenborg, J. (2010). *Microelectrode and multiple microelectrodes.* Patent US 8954142 B2. PCT/SE2010/000152.

Felix, S., Shah, K., George, D., Tolosa, V., Tooker, A., Sheth, H., et al. (2012). "Removable silicon insertion stiffeners for neural probes using polyethylene glycol as a biodissolvable adhesive," in *Proceedings of the Annual International Conference of the IEEE Engineering in Medicine and Biology Society, EMBS* (San Diego, CA), 871–874.

Fraser, G. W., and Schwartz, A. B. (2012). Recording from the same neurons chronically in motor cortex. *J. Neurophysiol.* 107, 1970–1978. doi: 10.1152/jn.01012.2010

Gámez, E., Goto, Y., Nagata, K., Iwaki, T., Sasaki, T., and Matsuda, T. (2004). Photofabricated gelatin-based nerve conduits: nerve tissue regeneration potentials. *Cell Transp.* 13, 549–564. doi: 10.3727/000000004783983639

Gilletti, A., and Muthuswamy, J. (2006). Brain micromotion around implants in the rodent somatosensory cortex. *J. Neural Eng.* 3, 189–195. doi: 10.1088/1741-2560/3/3/001

Granmo, M., Jensen, T., and Schouenborg, J. (2013). Nociceptive transmission to rat primary somatosensory cortex - comparison of sedative and analgesic effects. *PLoS ONE* 8:e53966. doi: 10.1371/journal.pone.0053966

Jackson, A., and Fetz, E. E. (2007). Compact movable microwire array for long-term chronic unit recording in cerebral cortex of primates. *J. Neurophysiol.* 98, 3109–3118. doi: 10.1152/jn.00569.2007

Kalliomäki, J., Weng, H.-R., Nilsson, H.-J., and Schouenborg, J. (1993). Nociceptive C fibre input to the primary somatosensory cortex (SI). A field potential study in the rat. *Brain Res.* 622, 262–270. doi: 10.1016/0006-8993(93)90827-A

Kim, Y. T., Hitchcock, R. W., Bridge, M. J., and Tresco, P. A. (2004). Chronic response of adult rat brain tissue to implants anchored to the skull. *Biomaterials* 25, 2229–2237. doi: 10.1016/j.biomaterials.2003.09.010

Kipke, D. R., Pellinen, D. S., and Vetter, R. J. (2002). "Advanced neural implants using thin-film polymers," in *2002 IEEE International Symposium on Circuits and Systems. Proceedings (Cat. No.02CH37353)* (Phoenix-Scottsdale, AZ), 4.

Köhler, P., Wolff, A., Ejserholm, F., Wallman, L., Schouenborg, J., and Linsmeier, C. E. (2015). Influence of probe flexibility and gelatin embedding on neuronal density and glial responses to brain implants. *PLoS ONE* 10:e0119340. doi: 10.1371/journal.pone.0119340

Kozai, T. D. Y., Gugel, Z., Li, X., Gilgunn, P. J., Khilwani, R., Ozdoganlar, O. B., et al. (2014). Chronic tissue response to carboxymethyl cellulose based dissolvable insertion needle for ultra-small neural probes. *Biomaterials* 35, 9255–9268. doi: 10.1016/j.biomaterials.2014.07.039

Krüger, J., Carulana, F., Volta, R. D., and Rizzolatti, G. (2010). Seven years of recording from monkey cortex with a chronically implanted multiple microelectrode. *Front. Neuroeng.* 3:6. doi: 10.3389/fneng.2010.00006

Kuo, J. T. W., Kim, B. J., Hara, S. A., Lee, C. D., Gutierrez, C. A., Hoang, T. Q., et al. (2013). Novel flexible Parylene neural probe with 3D sheath structure for enhancing tissue integration. *Lab. Chip.* 13, 554–561. doi: 10.1039/c2lc40935f

Leach, J. B., Achyuta, A. K. H., and Murthy, S. K. (2010). Bridging the divide between neuroprosthetic design, tissue engineering and neurobiology. *Front. Neuroeng.* 2:18. doi: 10.3389/neuro.16.018.2009

Lee, S. E., Jun, S. B., Lee, H. J., Kim, J., Lee, S. W., Im, C., et al. (2012). A flexible depth probe using liquid crystal polymer. *IEEE Trans. Biomed. Eng.* 59, 2085–2094. doi: 10.1109/TBME.2012.2196274

Lewicki, M. S. (1998). A review of methods for spike sorting: the detection and classification of neural action potentials. *Netw. (Bristol, England)* 9, R53–R78. Available online at: http://www.ncbi.nlm.nih.gov/pubmed/10221571

Lind, G., Linsmeier, C. E., and Schouenborg, J. (2013). The density difference between tissue and neural probes is a key factor for glial scarring. *Sci. Rep.* 3:2942. doi: 10.1038/srep02942

Lind, G., Linsmeier, C. E., Thelin, J., and Schouenborg, J. (2010). Gelatine-embedded electrodes–a novel biocompatible vehicle allowing implantation of highly flexible microelectrodes. *J. Neural Eng.* 7:046005. doi: 10.1088/1741-2560/7/4/046005

Ludwig, K. A., Langhals, N. B., Joseph, M. D., Richardson-Burns, S. M., Hendricks, J. L., and Kipke, D. R. (2011). Poly(3,4-ethylenedioxythiophene) (PEDOT) polymer coatings facilitate smaller neural recording electrodes. *J. Neural Eng.* 8:014001. doi: 10.1088/1741-2560/8/1/014001

Ludwig, K. A., Uram, J. D., Yang, J., Martin, D. C., and Kipke, D. R. (2006). Chronic neural recordings using silicon microelectrode arrays electrochemically deposited with a poly(3,4-ethylenedioxythiophene) (PEDOT) film. *J. Neural Eng.* 3, 59–70. doi: 10.1088/1741-2560/3/1/007

Marieb, E. N., and Hoehn, K. (2010). Human anatomy and physiology. *Physiology* 7, 664–668. doi: 10.1038/nnano.2011.234

McConnell, G. C., Rees, H. D., Levey, A. I., Gutekunst, C.-A., Gross, R. E., and Bellamkonda, R. V. (2009). Implanted neural electrodes cause chronic, local inflammation that is correlated with local neurodegeneration. *J. Neural Eng.* 6:056003. doi: 10.1088/1741-2560/6/5/056003

Mitra, P., and Bokil, H. (2008). *Observed Brain Dynamics*. Oxford University Press. Available online at: http://www.amazon.com/Observed-Brain-Dynamics-Partha-Mitra/dp/0195178084

Musallam, S., Bak, M. J., Troyk, P. R., and Andersen, R. A. (2007). A floating metal microelectrode array for chronic implantation. *J. Neurosci. Methods* 160, 122–127. doi: 10.1016/j.jneumeth.2006.09.005

Nolta, N. F., Christensen, M. B., Crane, P. D., Skousen, J. L., and Tresco, P. A. (2015). BBB leakage, astrogliosis, and tissue loss correlate with silicon microelectrode array recording performance. *Biomaterials* 53, 753–762. doi: 10.1016/j.biomaterials.2015.02.081

Pettersen, K. H., and Einevoll, G. T. (2008). Amplitude variability and extracellular low-pass filtering of neuronal spikes. *Biophys. J.* 94, 784–802. doi: 10.1529/biophysj.107.111179

Polikov, V. S., Tresco, P. A., and Reichert, W. M. (2005). Response of brain tissue to chronically implanted neural electrodes. *J. Neurosci. Methods* 148, 1–18. doi: 10.1016/j.jneumeth.2005.08.015

Pouzat, C., Mazor, O., and Laurent, G. (2002). Using noise signature to optimize spike-sorting and to assess neuronal classification quality. *J. Neurosci. Methods* 122, 43–57. doi: 10.1016/S0165-0270(02)00276-5

Quian Quiroga, R. (2009). What is the real shape of extracellular spikes? *J. Neurosci. Methods* 177, 194–198. doi: 10.1016/j.jneumeth.2008.09.033

Quiroga, R. Q., Nadasdy, Z., and Ben-Shaul, Y. (2004). Unsupervised spike detection and sorting with wavelets and superparamagnetic clustering. *Neural Comput.* 16, 1661–1687. doi: 10.1162/089976604774201631

Rolston, J. D., Gross, R. E., and Potter, S. M. (2009). "Common median referencing for improved action potential detection with multielectrode arrays," in *Conference Proceedings: Annual International Conference of the IEEE Engineering in Medicine and Biology Society* (Minneapolis, MN), 1604–1607.

Rousche, P. J., and Normann, R. A. (1998). Chronic recording capability of the utah intracortical electrode array in cat sensory cortex. *J. Neurosci. Methods* 82, 1–15. doi: 10.1016/S0165-0270(98)00031-4

Rousche, P. J., Pellinen, D. S., Pivin, D. P. Jr., Williams, J. C., Vetter, R. J., and Kipke, D. R. (2001). Flexible polyimide-based intracortical electrode arrays with bioactive capability. *IEEE Trans. Biomed. Eng.* 48, 361–370. doi: 10.1109/10.914800

Santhanam, G., Linderman, M. D., Gilja, V., Afshar, A., Ryu, S. I., Meng, T. H., et al. (2007). HermesB: A continuous neural recording system for freely behaving primates. *IEEE Trans. Biomed. Eng.* 54, 2037–2050. doi: 10.1109/TBME.2007.895753

Schouenborg, J. (2011). Biocompatible multichannel electrodes for long-term neurophysiological studies and clinical therapy-Novel concepts and design. *Progr. Brain Res.* 194, 61–70. doi: 10.1016/B978-0-444-53815-4.00017-0

Schouenborg, J. (2013). *Medical Electrode, Electrode Bundle and Electrode Bundle Array*. US 8,386,006 B2, Feb 2013.

Seymour, J. P., and Kipke, D. R. (2007). Neural probe design for reduced tissue encapsulation in CNS. *Biomaterials* 28, 3594–3607. doi: 10.1016/j.biomaterials.2007.03.024

Sohal, H. S., Jackson, A., Jackson, R., Clowry, G. J., Vassilevski, K., O'Neill, A., et al. (2014). The sinusoidal probe: a new approach to improve electrode longevity. *Front. Neuroeng.* 7:10. doi: 10.3389/fneng.2014.00010

Stice, P., Gilletti, A., Panitch, A., and Muthuswamy, J. (2007). Thin microelectrodes reduce GFAP expression in the implant site in rodent somatosensory cortex. *J. Neural Eng.* 4, 42–53. doi: 10.1088/1741-2560/4/2/005

Stover, N. P., and Watts, R. L. (2008). Spheramine for treatment of Parkinson's disease. *Neurotherapeutics* 5, 252–259. doi: 10.1016/j.nurt.2008.02.006

Suner, S., Fellows, M. R., Vargas-Irwin, C., Nakata, G. K., and Donoghue, J. P. (2005). Reliability of signals from a chronically implanted, silicon-based electrode array in non-human primate primary motor cortex. *IEEE Trans. Neural Syst. Rehabil. Eng.* 13, 524–541. doi: 10.1109/TNSRE.2005.857687

Suyatin, D. B., Wallman, L., Thelin, J., Prinz, C. N., Jörntell, H., Samuelson, L., et al. (2013). Nanowire-based electrode for acute *in vivo* neural recordings in the brain. *PLoS ONE* 8:56673. doi: 10.1371/journal.pone.0056673

Szarowski, D. H., Andersen, M. D., Retterer, S., Spence, A. J., Isaacson, M., Craighead, H. G., et al. (2003). Brain responses to micro-machined silicon devices. *Brain Res.* 983, 23–35. doi: 10.1016/S0006-8993(03)03023-3

Takeuchi, S., Ziegler, D., Yoshida, Y., Mabuchi, K., and Suzuki, T. (2005). Parylene flexible neural probes integrated with microfluidic channels. *Lab. Chip.* 5, 519–523. doi: 10.1039/b417497f

Thelin, J., Jörntell, H., Psouni, E., Garwicz, M., Schouenborg, J., Danielsen, N., et al. (2011). Implant size and fixation mode strongly influence tissue reactions in the CNS. *PLoS ONE* 6:16267. doi: 10.1371/journal.pone.0016267

Thorbergsson, P. T., Garwicz, M., Schouenborg, J., and Johansson, A. J. (2012). Computationally efficient simulation of extracellular recordings with multielectrode arrays. *J. Neurosci. Methods* 211, 133–144. doi: 10.1016/j.jneumeth.2012.08.011

Turner, J. N., Shain, W., Szarowski, D. H., Andersen, M., Martins, S., Isaacson, M., et al. (1999). Cerebral astrocyte response to micromachined silicon implants. *Exp. Neurol.* 156, 33–49. doi: 10.1006/exnr.1998.6983

Wagshul, M. E., Eide, P. K., and Madsen, J. R. (2011). The pulsating brain: a review of experimental and clinical studies of intracranial pulsatility. *Fluids Barriers CNS* 8:5. doi: 10.1186/2045-8118-8-5

Ward, M. P., Rajdev, P., Ellison, C., and Irazoqui, P. P. (2009). Toward a comparison of microelectrodes for acute and chronic recordings. *Brain Res.* 1282, 183–200. doi: 10.1016/j.brainres.2009.05.052

Watts, R. L., Raiser, C. D., Stover, N. P., Cornfeldt, M. L., Schweikert, A. W., Allen, R. C., et al. (2003). Stereotaxic intrastriatal implantation of human retinal pigment epithelial (hRPE) cells attached to gelatin microcarriers: a potential new cell therapy for Parkinson's disease. *J. Neural Transm. Suppl.* 65, 215–227. doi: 10.1007/978-3-7091-0643-3_14

Williams, J. C., Rennaker, R. L., and Kipke, D. R. (1999). Long-term neural recording characteristics of wire microelectrode arrays implanted in cerebral cortex. *Brain Res. Protoc.* 4, 303–313. doi: 10.1016/S1385-299X(99)00034-3

Winslow, B. D., and Tresco, P. A. (2010). Quantitative analysis of the tissue response to chronically implanted microwire electrodes in rat cortex. *Biomaterials* 31, 1558–1567. doi: 10.1016/j.biomaterials.2009.11.049

Witteveen, J. A., Suyatin, D. B., Gällentoft, L., Schouenborg, J., Danielsen, N., and Prinz, C. N. (2010). Gelatin/glycerol coating to preserve mechanically compliant nanowire electrodes from damage during brain implantation. *J. Vac. Sci. Technol. B* 28, C6K13–C6K16. doi: 10.1116/1.3498764

18

Noninvasive Brain Stimulation for the Treatment of Auditory Verbal Hallucinations in Schizophrenia: Methods, Effects and Challenges

Katharina M. Kubera[1]*, *Anja Barth*[1], *Dusan Hirjak*[1], *Philipp A. Thomann*[1] and *Robert C. Wolf*[1,2]

[1] *Center for Psychosocial Medicine, Department of General Psychiatry, University of Heidelberg, Heidelberg, Germany,*
[2] *Department of Psychiatry, Psychotherapy and Psychosomatics, Saarland University, Homburg, Germany*

Edited by:
Ioan Opris,
Wake Forest University School of Medicine, USA

Reviewed by:
Krystal Lynn Parker,
University of Iowa, USA
Puiu F. Balan,
KU Leuven, Belgium

***Correspondence:**
Katharina M. Kubera,
Center for Psychosocial Medicine, Department of General Psychiatry, University of Heidelberg, Voßstraße 4, 69115 Heidelberg, Germany
katharina.kubera@med.uni-heidelberg.de

This mini-review focuses on noninvasive brain stimulation techniques as an augmentation method for the treatment of persistent auditory verbal hallucinations (AVH) in patients with schizophrenia. Paradigmatically, we place emphasis on transcranial magnetic stimulation (TMS). We specifically discuss rationales of stimulation and consider methodological questions together with issues of phenotypic diversity in individuals with drug-refractory and persistent AVH. Eventually, we provide a brief outlook for future investigations and treatment directions. Taken together, current evidence suggests TMS as a promising method in the treatment of AVH. Low-frequency stimulation of the superior temporal cortex (STC) may reduce symptom severity and frequency. Yet clinical effects are of relatively short duration and effect sizes appear to decrease over time along with publication of larger trials. Apart from considering other innovative stimulation techniques, such as transcranial Direct Current Stimulation (tDCS), and optimizing stimulation protocols, treatment of AVH using noninvasive brain stimulation will essentially rely on accurate identification of potential responders and non-responders for these treatment modalities. In this regard, future studies will need to consider distinct phenotypic presentations of AVH in patients with schizophrenia, together with the putative functional neurocircuitry underlying these phenotypes.

Keywords: transcranial magnetic stimulation, auditory verbal hallucinations, phenotypes, schizophrenia, brain stimulation, brain function

Introduction

Auditory verbal hallucinations (AVH) are defined as auditive perceptions involving a verbal aspect in the absence of a provoking external stimulus (Aleman and de Haan, 1998). They represent a core symptom of schizophrenia and related spectrum disorders, but they also frequently occur in other psychiatric entities and in the non-psychiatric general population. In schizophrenia the term AVH comprises a multi-dimensional and heterogeneous group of symptoms that can be differentiated by certain phenomenological aspects such as subjective loudness, acoustic clarity, location and subjective reality. About 60–80% of patients affected by schizophrenia experience AVH (Aleman and de Haan, 1998; Hugdahl et al., 2008), such as conversing, commenting or imperative spoken speech in distinct voices. These symptoms, especially when the verbal content is experienced as negative, intrusive or persecutory, often induce high levels of distress and lead to significant psychosocial impairment. AVH are a highly relevant feature of schizophrenia that have attracted extensive clinical, phenomenological and neurobiological interest, yet treating these symptoms, especially in persons suffering from persistent AVH which do either not or not sufficiently respond to psychopharmacotherapy, is still a major clinical challenge. In approximately 25% of patients with schizophrenia, AVH are refractory to psychotropic drug treatment and can chronically persist (Shergill et al., 1998). Currently, there are no randomized controlled trials available which specifically investigated effects of psychopharmacotherapy (either monotherapy or combined drug regimes) on AVH severity reduction or full symptom remission. In a recent review (Sommer et al., 2012), data from the European First-Episode Schizophrenia Trial (EUFEST) was used to assess effects of five antipsychotic agents on AVH severity. Superiority of one treatment option against another was not confirmed for AVH severity (Sommer et al., 2012). Clinically, clozapine is still the drug of choice for patients with AVH who are resistant to two other antipsychotic agents. At present, no clinical trial has been published that specifically compares the efficacy of clozapine in comparison to other antipsychotic agents in the treatment of drug-resistant AVH.

Transcranial Magnetic Stimulation

Given the need for effective treatment modalities, it is not surprising to see that over the past decade brain stimulation techniques have been increasingly used to ameliorate symptom burden in patients with schizophrenia suffering from persistent and mostly pharmacorefractory AVH. Among these approaches, a possible augmentation strategy for the treatment of psychiatric disorders (in particular catatonia and severe depression) is elctroconvulsive therapy (ECT). For patients with schizophrenia a meta-analysis of 10 double-blind RCT showed a significant effect for ECT (Tharyan and Adams, 2005), although none of the studies provided any specific details on AVH improvement (Sommer et al., 2012). In a recent review Nieuwdorp and colleagues summarized different stimulation methods including transcranial magnetic stimulation (TMS), ECT and transcranial Direct Current Stimulation (tDCS) in patients with medication-resistant psychosis (Nieuwdorp et al., 2015). The authors concluded that currently there is only weak evidence for stimulation techniques to relieve pharmacorefractory psychosis. Specifically considering AVH, further studies are needed to draw any strong conclusions about ECT as a treatment option for patients presenting with persistent AVH.

In the last decade, TMS has evolved into a therapeutic modality for several psychiatric and neurological symptoms. In particular, TMS is widely used to treat patients with major depression, obsessive-compulsive disorder (OCD) and specific symptoms of schizophrenia (AVH and negative symptoms) (Slotema et al., 2010). Its application as an adjunctive therapy is currently proposed by European specialists with evidence level C (Lefaucheur et al., 2014) taking into account that it is generally regarded as safe. We consider the application of TMS for treating individuals presenting with persistent AVH as paradigmatic. The use of TMS impressively illustrates a translational approach from basic neuroscience/neuroimaging to clinical treatment. However, it also illustrates fundamental methodological, neurobiological and phenomenological questions and challenges, which we will refer to in the following paragraphs.

TMS: Putative Mechanisms of Action

TMS is a technique which allows a non-invasive stimulation of cortical neurons through the scalp. Originally, TMS was implemented as a neurophysiological tool for the study of the human motor system (Barker et al., 1985). Put simply, TMS uses a strong pulse of electrical current in a coil which is placed over the brain generating rapidly pulsating magnetic fields, which pass through the scalp, skull, and meninges, into the brain (Wassermann and Zimmermann, 2012). Thus, changing magnetic fields produce electrical impulses that stimulate superficial cortical neurons 2–3 cm below the device (Wassermann and Zimmermann, 2012). Modern devices can generate a rapid succession of pulses, called repetitive TMS (rTMS) by producing a relatively powerful magnetic field (about 1.5–3T), but only lasting very shortly (ms) (George and Aston-Jones, 2010). Frequencies of 1 Hz or lower are considered to be inhibitory, while frequencies of 5 Hz and higher are considered to be excitatory (Aleman, 2013). The specific topology of the induced electrical field in the brain is a source of uncertainty, because it is influenced by the complex shape and diverse conductivity of the cranial contents (Wassermann and Zimmermann, 2012), e.g., cerebrospinal fluid and foraminas in cranial bone. Long-term potentiation (LTP) and long-term depression (LTD) are believed to be key processes underlying long-term effects of rTMS (Chervyakov et al., 2015). *In vitro* experiments of hippocampal slice cultures suggest that rTMS can alter cortical excitability in terms of LTP of synaptic transmission inducing an increase in synaptic strength and postsynaptic AMPA receptor changes (Vlachos et al., 2012). At the level of functional connectivity, long-lasting enhancement is reflected by increased hippocampal-cortical network coupling after rTMS (Wang and Voss, 2015).

How Effective is rTMS in the Treatment of AVH?

As a target region for rTMS in patients with AVH the superior temporal cortex (STC) is of special interest given converging multimodal imaging evidence suggesting a crucial role in AVH generation and perception (Allen et al., 2008; Waters et al., 2012). The rationale for stimulating this region is to inhibit cortical overactivity and potentially influence generative phenomena (i.e., AVH) which are thought to be closely associated with regionally increased cortical activity. Up to now, several randomized sham-controlled studies targeting the left temporoparietal cortex have been conducted and summarized in seven meta-analyses revealing effect sizes (Hedges' "g") ranging from 0.42 (i.e., a close to moderate effect) to 1.04 (regarded as high effect; Aleman et al., 2007; Tranulis et al., 2008; Freitas et al., 2009; Slotema et al., 2012, 2014). With the inclusion of the studies with larger patient samples, the mean weighted effect size of rTMS directed at the left temporoparietal area for AVH appears to decrease over time, although the effect is still significant (Slotema et al., 2012, 2014; Hoffman et al., 2013). Of note, Slotema and colleagues showed that the effect of rTMS was no longer significant at one month of follow-up revealing a mean weighted effect size of 0.40 (95% confidence interval = −0.23–0.102; Slotema et al., 2012). For a detailed description of the included studies, please see tables provided by Slotema and colleagues. Side effects were mild and the number of dropouts in the real TMS group was not significantly higher than in the sham group. Only few MRI studies investigated other regions than the left temporoparietal area as target regions for rTMS. Abnormal activation of the right hemisphere regions such as the inferior frontal gyrus and the postcentral gyrus is a frequently reported finding in patients who experience persistent AVH (Kuhn and Gallinat, 2012). Activation changes have been most consistently shown for areas of the prefrontal and temporal cortices (Allen et al., 2007; Sommer et al., 2008; Raij et al., 2009). Based on former findings in neuroimaging studies that both the right and the left temporal activation are associated with AVH (Shergill et al., 2000; Sommer et al., 2007) three studies directed rTMS at the right comparing with the left temporoparietal gyrus for the treatment of AVH (Lee et al., 2005; Jandl et al., 2006; Loo et al., 2010). According to these studies, no superior effects of right-sided stimulation (Slotema et al., 2014) were observed. Correspondingly, neither stimulation of Broca's area nor its contralateral homologue was an effective target (Schonfeldt-Lecuona et al., 2004). Overall, these findings support the notion that deficient generation, monitoring and perception of inner speech rather than speech expression are disrupted functions in patients with persistent AVH (Shergill et al., 2000; Wolf et al., 2011). Abnormal STC function clearly plays a critical role in the expression of AVH, especially in those patients presenting with chronic and treatment-refractory symptoms. Recent studies showed that stimulation of this region with low-frequency rTMS may reduce the severity and frequency of AVH in schizophrenia patients, but the duration of the effect of rTMS may be less than one month (Slotema et al., 2012).

Methodological Issues with TMS and the Challenge of Treating Phenotypic Diversity

As briefly discussed in the previous paragraph, it is noteworthy that therapeutic effects of rTMS in AVH patients are not long-lasting, and that along with publication of studies with larger patient populations, the effect size of rTMS over the left temporoparietal area has decreased over time (Slotema et al., 2012, 2014). Several studies published between 2004 and 2014 did not observe beneficial effects of rTMS in the treatment of persistent AVH (Schonfeldt-Lecuona et al., 2004; Slotema et al., 2011; Blumberger et al., 2012; Rosenberg et al., 2012; Bais et al., 2014). Several reasons may account for these phenomena. Two specific aspects of stimulation will be discussed, which may be superior to left sided STC intervention and which may also account for these variable results. Subsequently we will address the problem of the phenotypic diversity which is inherent to AVH both at the neural and phenomenological level.

Is Bilateral Stimulation Superior?

It may be conceivable that bilateral could be superior over unilateral stimulation, especially given known dissociations of left- vs. right-hemispheric function. Up to now, however, only one study examined bilateral rTMS of the TPJ (Bais et al., 2014). The authors suggested that AVH frequency might be one of the most sufficient parameters to measure the responsiveness of left sided rTMS. In comparison, right-sided rTMS allows for a more complete management of AVH in terms of emotional and non-linguistic aspects which are suggested to originate in the right hemisphere. Contrary to their prediction, however, Bais and could not show any beneficial effect of bilateral rTMS in comparison to left sided rTMS and sham in improving AVH (Bais et al., 2014). Neurophysiological aspects such as transcallosal inhibition, and fewer rTMS impulses (50%) in a bilateral design (Thiel et al., 2006; Bais et al., 2014) might account for these negative results.

Is STC stimulation alone sufficient?

The functional dominance of STC stimulation over other brain regions has been questioned by accumulating neuroimaging data acquired in patients with AVH. For instance, an association between AVH-severity and STC gray matter volume loss has been suggested by univariate voxel-based morphometry studies (Modinos et al., 2013). In contrast, using a multivariate statistical approach for structural data analysis, two distinct abnormal structural networks were recently identified in patients with persistent AVH, including a bilateral prefrontal system and a bilateral temporal/medial frontal network (Kubera et al., 2014). The latter structural network also differed between patients with persistent AVH compared to non-hallucinating patients (Kubera et al., 2014). It is possible that unilateral temporoparietal stimulation might not be sufficient to induce a relevant neuronal change in both networks, whose mutual interplay has still to be determined. Also, the relationship between structure and function still remains unresolved, e.g., in individuals with persistent AVH the impact of neural loss to neural network transmission, including effects in more remote neural networks, is unclear.

From a functional point of view, both "symptom capture" (i.e., inferring AVH-related brain activity from symptom occurrence) and "symptom interference" (i.e., inferring AVH-related brain dysfunction from paradigm-driven data) MRI studies have been conducted to investigate neural activation patterns in schizophrenia patients experiencing treatment-resistant AVH (Lawrie et al., 2002; Mechelli et al., 2007; Wolf et al., 2011). The vast majority of these studies focused on brain activity in speech-related pathways (Lavigne et al., 2015), according to the prevailing model of AVH suggesting a link between symptom generation and dysfunctional inner speech perception and monitoring (Hugdahl et al., 2008). From these studies, the left STC emerged as regions linked to AVH and in turn set the rationale for targeted stimulation.

Yet the left temporal cortex, although a crucial neural node for hallucinatory symptom expression, is not the sole region which is thought to be involved in AVH generation and persistence. The prefrontal cortices have been frequently found to exhibit abnormal neural activity in patients with AVH, both at the level of regional function and at the level of functional connectivity (Kuhn and Gallinat, 2012; Alderson-Day et al., 2015). Although the processes subserved by abnormal prefrontal activity in patients experiencing AVH are not fully elucidated at present, several explanations have been put forward, such as deficient attentional and executive control over speech- and self-monitoring relevant brain regions. In addition, converging evidence suggests that AVH are not related to regional brain dysfunction alone, but rather to abnormal neural network coupling in several distinct neural networks including systems engaged in language, attention, executive function, memory and self-referential processing (Stephane et al., 2001; Allen et al., 2008; Wolf et al., 2011; Diederen et al., 2013). Thus, single-site stimulation may not fully cover all key regions involved in AVH pathophysiology. In this regard, bilateral or bifocal stimulation could be a promising approach. Based on the hypothesis of temporal hyperactivity and frontal hypoactivation in schizophrenia patients presenting with AVH, Brunelin and colleagues used a different non-invasive stimulation method, i.e., tDCS (Brunelin et al., 2012). Unlike TMS, in tDCS a weak direct current passes through the brain between two electrodes, i.e., modulation of two spatially remote regions is possible. Brunelin and co-workers used cathodal left temporoparietal junction (TPJ) stimulation and anodal left dorsolateral prefrontal stimulation. After five days of treatment a significant decrease of hallucinatory symptoms was shown, and this effect remained significant three months after stimulation. These findings were recently replicated (Mondino et al., 2015) and provides a promising outlook for further clinical trials. Nevertheless, given that tDCS is a relatively new technique employed in AVH treatment, several stimulation parameters (e.g., electrode placement and stimulation intensity, frequency and duration) have to be investigated in more detail to optimize future treatment options (Koops et al., 2015).

It is noteworthy that although the lateral prefrontal and temporal cortices clearly are involved in AVH generation, there is also good evidence suggesting a role of cortical midline regions in AVH symptom expression. Abnormal cerebral blood flow could also be detected not only in the primary temporal cortex and Broca's area, but also in the cingulate cortex (Wolf et al., 2012; Kindler et al., 2013). In a recent study exploring resting-state functional connectivity of the brain, cross-network abnormalities could be detected between the so called "default mode network" (DMN) and the "salience network," including core midline regions such as the bilateral paracingulate cortex and bilateral anterior cingulate cortex (Alonso-Solís et al., 2015). Of note, DMN subsystems have been essentially involved in self-referential and mnemonic processes (Andrews-Hanna et al., 2010; Sambataro et al., 2013). Abnormal network interactions between the DMN and language-processing and auditory networks could well explain deficient self-monitoring and a lack of self-referential attribution of voices (Northoff and Qin, 2011). This body of evidence indicates important contributions of cortical midline regions to the pathomechanisms of persistent AVH. TMS alone might be insufficient to stimulate these regions in treatment-resistant patients.

The Challenge of Phenotypic Diversity

When treating AVH in patients with schizophrenia using focal stimulation techniques, the clinical endpoint appears to be clearly defined. In the vast majority of cases, this is at least a reduction in overall AVH severity. Yet it should be kept in mind that schizophrenia is a phenomenologically heterogeneous disorder with several distinct phenotypic presentations at both the clinical and neurobiological level, and the very same heterogeneity also applies to persons with chronic AVH. In addition, the multidimensionality of AVH has been long acknowledged by phenomenological research (Kronmüller et al., 2011; McCarthy-Jones et al., 2014), but research has only recently begun to specifically explore therapeutic effects on distinct symptom domains (Leff et al., 2013).

Apart from refining and technically developing stimulation techniques *per se*, a major focus of future research will be the identification of markers which can predict stimulation treatment response. An approach which might prove to be helpful for predicting responders and non-responders in the future is subtyping AVH patients according to both neurobiological and clinical criteria. For instance, it has been attempted, albeit with limited success, to improve responsiveness to rTMS by targeting the site of maximal neural activation associated with the hallucinatory event (Slotema et al., 2011). More recently, Homan and colleagues (Homan et al., 2012) showed that higher resting-brain perfusion as measured with arterial spin labeling in the left STC prior to treatment predicted a clinical response to rTMS (Homan et al., 2012). This marker may guide stratification strategies in future interventional trials. Also, it is important to acknowledge that certain symptom characteristics, such as location of voices in inner our outer space, may map to distinct neural correlates. In this respect, a relationship between white matter volume in the right temporal junction and spatial features such as outer vs. inner location of voices has been identified (Plaze et al., 2011). However, stimulation of the right temporal lobe could not show a superior treatment effect. A possible explanation is that there may well be structural differences between hallucinating characterized by "physical" features with yet unknown consequences for brain function and treatment response. Another explanation for non-response to stimulation could include neural ceiling effects, e.g., related to various degrees of subjective symptom control. Over time, patients with persistent AVH seek for ways of coping with their voices, e.g., by deliberately directing their attentional focus to specific external stimuli (which can be auditory) or by employing individual modes of verbal control. The degree of control over AVH is associated with distinct frontotemporal cortical correlates in contrast to physical or affective symptom dimensions (Wolf et al., 2012). Also, increased frontotemporal connectivity in hallucinating patients is modulated by the degree of control over verbal material (Lavigne et al., 2015). Thus, it is possible that different degrees of control over AVH severity prior to therapeutic stimulation could influence treatment response.

McCarthy-Jones and colleagues proposed different subtypes of AVH, which might respond to different treatment modalities. These subtypes may be identified at the levels phenomenology, cognition, neurology, etiology, treatment response, diagnosis, and voice hearer's own interpretation (McCarthy-Jones et al., 2014). Particularly, an AVH subtype characterized at a neural level by chronic deafferentiation of the auditory cortex is proposed, according to the hypothesis of AVH as misattributed forms of inner speech (Ford and Mathalon, 2005). This subtype might be specifically responsive to focal stimulation treatment, i.e., rTMS or tDCS. Furthermore, specific subtypes might show both common and distinct regions of activation in both "symptom capture" and "symptom interference" studies, so that future neuroimaging studies may consider specific subtypes in their protocol and report details of AVH phenomenology. The majority of functional neuroimaging studies used total severity and frequency scores of hallucinations (Auditory Hallucinations Rating Scale (AHRS), Auditory Hallucinations Subscale/Psychotic Symptom Rating Scale [AHS/PSYRATS]) as main outcome parameters. To discriminate more fine-grained aspects of change in hallucinations, especially in homogenous subgroups, it might be advantageous to describe different phenomenological dimensions before and their changes after focal therapy. The PSYRATS and a 4-dimensional model within the AHS has previous been recommended to integrate into research and clinical applications (Woodward et al., 2014).

Conclusion

In the past decade non-invasive brain stimulation techniques became increasingly relevant for the treatment of drug-refractory AVH. Evidence for ECT for specifically treating AVH is very limited. There is evidence for beneficial effects of rTMS over left temporal and temporoparietal areas, but effect sizes for this treatment modality are moderate, and beneficial long-term effects are unlikely. It has been suggested that rTMS may reduce aberrant internally generated activity associated with AVH at the site of stimulation. Still, the role of rTMS in changing aberrant network function putatively involved in the generation of AVH has to be clarified. A further major challenge for future research is identifying of patients who do respond to treatment and those who do not or only insufficient. Supported by neuroimaging evidence, the magnitude of left STC activity has been promoted as a potential predictor of clinical improvement. Given the phenomenological diversity of schizophrenia and AVH in particular, it is expected that subtyping patients with AVH will essentially contribute to identify responders from non-responders for focal augmentative therapies. In this respect, in accordance with other authors we strongly advocate further development of reliable and valid psychometric assessments and neurobiological markers paralleling the optimization of future stimulation protocols. Other neuromodulatory interventions, such as tDCS provide very promising data as well but larger trials are needed.

References

Alderson-Day, B., McCarthy-Jones, S., and Fernyhough, C. (2015). Hearing voices in the resting brain: A review of intrinsic functional connectivity research on auditory verbal hallucinations. *Neurosci. Biobehav. Rev.* 55, 78–87. doi: 10.1016/j.neubiorev.2015.04.016

Aleman, A. (2013). Use of repetitive transcranial magnetic stimulation for treatment in psychiatry. *Clin. Psychopharmacol. Neurosci.* 11, 53–59. doi: 10.9758/cpn.2013.11.2.53

Aleman, A., and de Haan, E. H. (1998). On redefining hallucination. *Am. J. Orthopsychiatry.* 68, 656–659. doi: 10.1037/h0080376

Aleman, A., Sommer, I. E., and Kahn, R. S. (2007). Efficacy of slow repetitive transcranial magnetic stimulation in the treatment of resistant auditory hallucinations in schizophrenia: a meta-analysis. *J. Clin. Psychiatry.* 68, 416–421. doi: 10.4088/jcp.v68n0310

Allen, P., Aleman, A., and McGuire, P. K. (2007). Inner speech models of auditory verbal hallucinations: evidence from behavioural and neuroimaging studies. *Int. Rev. Psychiatry.* 19, 407–415. doi: 10.1080/09540260701486498

Allen, P., Larøi, F., McGuire, P. K., and Aleman, A. (2008). The hallucinating brain: a review of structural and functional neuroimaging studies of hallucinations. *Neurosci. Biobehav. Rev.* 32, 175–191. doi: 10.1016/j.neubiorev.2007.07.012

Alonso-Solís, A., Vives-Gilabert, Y., Grasa, E., Portella, M. J., Rabella, M., Sauras, R. B., et al. (2015). Resting-state functional connectivity alterations in the default network of schizophrenia patients with persistent auditory verbal hallucinations. *Schizophr. Res.* 161, 261–268. doi: 10.1016/j.schres.2014.10.047

Andrews-Hanna, J. R., Reidler, J. S., Sepulcre, J., Poulin, R., and Buckner, R. L. (2010). Functional-anatomic fractionation of the brain's default network. *Neuron.* 65, 550–562. doi: 10.1016/j.neuron.2010.02.005

Bais, L., Vercammen, A., Stewart, R., van Es, F., Visser, B., Aleman, A., et al. (2014). Short and long term effects of left and bilateral repetitive transcranial magnetic stimulation in schizophrenia patients with auditory verbal hallucinations: a randomized controlled trial. *PLoS One.* 9:e108828. doi: 10.1371/journal.pone.0108828

Barker, A. T., Jalinous, R., and Freeston, I. L. (1985). Non-invasive magnetic stimulation of human motor cortex. *Lancet* 1, 1106–1107. doi: 10.1016/S0140-6736(85)92413-4

Blumberger, D. M., Christensen, B. K., Zipursky, R. B., Moller, B., Chen, R., Fitzgerald, P. B., et al. (2012). MRI-targeted repetitive transcranial magnetic stimulation of Heschl's gyrus for refractory auditory hallucinations. *Brain Stimul.* 5, 577–585. doi: 10.1016/j.brs.2011.12.002

Brunelin, J., Mondino, M., Gassab, L., Haesebaert, F., Gaha, L., Suaud-Chagny, M. F., et al. (2012). Examining transcranial direct-current stimulation (tDCS) as a treatment for hallucinations in schizophrenia. *Am. J. Psychiatry.* 169, 719–724. doi: 10.1176/appi.ajp.2012.11071091

Chervyakov, A. V., Chernyavsky, A. Y., Sinitsyn, D. O., and Piradov, M. A. (2015). Possible Mechanisms Underlying the Therapeutic Effects of Transcranial Magnetic Stimulation. *Front. Hum. Neurosci.* 9:303. doi: 10.3389/fnhum.2015.00303

Diederen, K. M., Neggers, S. F., de Weijer, A. D., van Lutterveld, R., Daalman, K., Eickhoff, S. B., et al. (2013). Aberrant resting-state connectivity in non-psychotic individuals with auditory hallucinations. *Psychol. Med.* 43, 1685–1696. doi: 10.1017/s0033291712002541

Ford, J. M., and Mathalon, D. H. (2005). Corollary discharge dysfunction in schizophrenia: can it explain auditory hallucinations? *Int. J. Psychophysiol.* 58, 179–189. doi: 10.1016/j.ijpsycho.2005.01.014

Freitas, C., Fregni, F., and Pascual-Leone, A. (2009). Meta-analysis of the effects of repetitive transcranial magnetic stimulation (rTMS) on negative and positive symptoms in schizophrenia. *Schizophrenia Research.* 108, 11–24. doi: 10.1016/j.schres.2008.11.027

George, M. S., and Aston-Jones, G. (2010). Noninvasive techniques for probing neurocircuitry and treating illness: vagus nerve stimulation (VNS), transcranial magnetic stimulation (TMS) and transcranial direct current stimulation (tDCS). *Neuropsychopharmacology.* 35, 301–316. doi: 10.1038/npp.2009.87

Hoffman, R. E., Wu, K., Pittman, B., Cahill, J. D., Hawkins, K. A., Fernandez, T., et al. (2013). Transcranial magnetic stimulation of Wernicke's and Right homologous sites to curtail "voices": a randomized trial. *Biol. Psychiatry.* 73, 1008–1014. doi: 10.1016/j.biopsych.2013.01.016

Homan, P., Kindler, J., Hauf, M., Hubl, D., and Dierks, T. (2012). Cerebral blood flow identifies responders to transcranial magnetic stimulation in auditory verbal hallucinations. *Transl. Psychiatry.* 2:e189. doi: 10.1038/tp.2012.114

Hugdahl, K., Løberg, E. M., Specht, K., Steen, V. M., van Wageningen, H., and Jørgensen, H. A. (2008). Auditory hallucinations in schizophrenia: the role of cognitive, brain structural and genetic disturbances in the left temporal lobe. *Front. Hum. Neurosci.* 1:6. doi: 10.3389/neuro.09.006.2007

Jandl, M., Steyer, J., Weber, M., Linden, D. E., Rothmeier, J., Maurer, K., et al. (2006). Treating auditory hallucinations by transcranial magnetic stimulation: a randomized controlled cross-over trial. *Neuropsychobiology.* 53, 63–69. doi: 10.1159/000091721

Kindler, J., Homan, P., Jann, K., Federspiel, A., Flury, R., Hauf, M., et al. (2013). Reduced neuronal activity in language-related regions after transcranial magnetic stimulation therapy for auditory verbal hallucinations. *Biological Psychiatry.* 73, 518–524. doi: 10.1016/j.biopsych.2012.06.019

Koops, S., van den Brink, H., and Sommer, I. E. (2015). Transcranial direct current stimulation as a treatment for auditory hallucinations. *Front. Psychol.* 6:244. doi: 10.3389/fpsyg.2015.00244

Kronmüller, K. T., von Bock, A., Grupe, S., Büche, L., Gentner, N. C., Rückl, S., et al. (2011). Psychometric evaluation of the Psychotic Symptom Rating Scales. *Compr. Psychiatry.* 52, 102–108. doi: 10.1016/j.comppsych.2010.04.014

Kubera, K. M., Sambataro, F., Vasic, N., Wolf, N. D., Frasch, K., Hirjak, D., et al. (2014). Source-based morphometry of gray matter volume in patients with schizophrenia who have persistent auditory verbal hallucinations. *Prog. Neuropsychopharmacol. Biol. Psychiatry.* 50, 102–109. doi: 10.1016/j.pnpbp.2013.11.015

Kuhn, S., and Gallinat, J. (2012). Quantitative meta-analysis on state and trait aspects of auditory verbal hallucinations in schizophrenia. *Schizophr. Bull.* 38, 779–786. doi: 10.1093/schbul/sbq152

Lavigne, K. M., Rapin, L. A., Metzak, P. D., Whitman, J. C., Jung, K., Dohen, M., et al. (2015). Left-dominant temporal-frontal hypercoupling in schizophrenia patients with hallucinations during speech perception. *Schizophr. Bull.* 41, 259–567. doi: 10.1093/schbul/sbu004

Lawrie, S. M., Buechel, C., Whalley, H. C., Frith, C. D., Friston, K. J., and Johnstone, E. C. (2002). Reduced frontotemporal functional connectivity in schizophrenia associated with auditory hallucinations. *Biol. Psychiatry.* 51, 1008–1011. doi: 10.1016/s0006-3223(02)01316-1

Lee, S. H., Kim, W., Chung, Y. C., Jung, K. H., Bahk, W. M., Jun, T. Y., et al. (2005). A double blind study showing that two weeks of daily repetitive TMS over the left or right temporoparietal cortex reduces symptoms in patients with schizophrenia who are having treatment-refractory auditory hallucinations. *Neurosci. Lett.* 376, 177–181. doi: 10.1016/j.neulet.2004.11.048

Lefaucheur, J. P., Andre-Obadia, N., Antal, A., Ayache, S. S., Baeken, C., Benninger, D. H., et al. (2014). Evidence-based guidelines on the therapeutic use of repetitive transcranial magnetic stimulation (rTMS). *Clin. Neurophysiol.* 125, 2150–2206. doi: 10.1016/j.clinph.2014.05.021

Leff, J., Williams, G., Huckvale, M. A., Arbuthnot, M., and Leff, A. P. (2013). Computer-assisted therapy for medication-resistant auditory hallucinations: proof-of-concept study. *Br. J. Psychiatry.* 202, 428–433. doi: 10.1192/bjp.bp.112.124883

Loo, C. K., Sainsbury, K., Mitchell, P., Hadzi-Pavlovic, D., and Sachdev, P. S. (2010). A sham-controlled trial of left and right temporal rTMS for the treatment of auditory hallucinations. *Psychol. Med.* 40, 541–546. doi: 10.1017/s0033291709990900

McCarthy-Jones, S., Thomas, N., Strauss, C., Dodgson, G., Jones, N., Woods, A., et al. (2014). Better than mermaids and stray dogs? Subtyping auditory verbal hallucinations and its implications for research and practice. *Schizophr. Bull.* 4, S275–S284. doi: 10.1093/schbul/sbu018

Mechelli, A., Allen, P., Amaro, E., Jr., Fu, C. H., Williams, S. C., Brammer, M. J., et al. (2007). Misattribution of speech and impaired connectivity in patients with auditory verbal hallucinations. *Hum. Brain Mapp.* 28, 1213–1222. doi: 10.1002/hbm.20341

Modinos, G., Costafreda, S. G., van Tol, M. J., McGuire, P. K., Aleman, A., and Allen, P. (2013). Neuroanatomy of auditory verbal hallucinations in schizophrenia: a quantitative meta-analysis of voxel-based morphometry studies. *Cortex.* 49, 1046–1055. doi: 10.1016/j.cortex.2012.01.009

Mondino, M., Haesebaert, F., Poulet, E., Suaud-Chagny, M. F., and Brunelin, J. (2015). Fronto-temporal transcranial Direct Current Stimulation (tDCS) reduces source-monitoring deficits and auditory hallucinations in patients with schizophrenia. *Schizophr. Res.* 161, 515–516. doi: 10.1016/j.schres.2014.10.054

Nieuwdorp, W., Koops, S., Somers, M., and Sommer, I. E. (2015). Transcranial magnetic stimulation, transcranial direct current stimulation and electroconvulsive therapy for medication-resistant psychosis of schizophrenia. *Curr. Opin. Psychiatry.* 28, 222–228. doi: 10.1097/yco.0000000000000156

Northoff, G., and Qin, P. (2011). How can the brain's resting state activity generate hallucinations? A 'resting state hypothesis' of auditory verbal hallucinations. *Schizophr. Res.* 127, 202–214. doi: 10.1016/j.schres.2010.11.009

Plaze, M., Paillere-Martinot, M. L., Penttila, J., Januel, D., de Beaurepaire, R., Bellivier, F., et al. (2011). "Where do auditory hallucinations come from?"—a brain morphometry study of schizophrenia patients with inner or outer space hallucinations. *Schizophr. Bull.* 37, 212–221. doi: 10.1093/schbul/sbp081

Raij, T. T., Valkonen-Korhonen, M., Holi, M., Therman, S., Lehtonen, J., and Hari, R. (2009). Reality of auditory verbal hallucinations. *Brain.* 132, 2994–3001. doi: 10.1093/brain/awp186

Rosenberg, O., Gersner, R., Klein, L. D., Kotler, M., Zangen, A., and Dannon, P. (2012). Deep transcranial magnetic stimulation add-on for the treatment of auditory hallucinations: a double-blind study. *Ann. Gen. Psychiatry.* 11:13. doi: 10.1186/1744-859x-11-13

Sambataro, F., Wolf, N. D., Pennuto, M., Vasic, N., and Wolf, R. C. (2013). Revisiting default mode network function in major depression: evidence for disrupted subsystem connectivity. *Psychol. Med.* 44, 2041–2051. doi: 10.1017/s0033291713002596

Schonfeldt-Lecuona, C., Grön, G., Walter, H., Büchler, N., Wunderlich, A., Spitzer, M., et al. (2004). Stereotaxic rTMS for the treatment of auditory hallucinations in schizophrenia. *Neuroreport.* 15, 1669–1673. doi: 10.1097/01.wnr.0000126504.89983.ec

Shergill, S. S., Bullmore, E., Simmons, A., Murray, R., and McGuire, P. (2000). Functional anatomy of auditory verbal imagery in schizophrenic patients with auditory hallucinations. *Am. J. Psychiatry.* 157, 1691–1693. doi: 10.1176/appi.ajp.157.10.1691

Shergill, S. S., Murray, R. M., and McGuire, P. K. (1998). Auditory hallucinations: a review of psychological treatments. *Schizophr. Res.* 32, 137–150. doi: 10.1016/s0920-9964(98)00052-8

Slotema, C. W., Aleman, A., Daskalakis, Z. J., and Sommer, I. E. (2012). Meta-analysis of repetitive transcranial magnetic stimulation in the treatment of auditory verbal hallucinations: update and effects after one month. *Schizophr. Res.* 142, 40–45. doi: 10.1016/j.schres.2012.08.025

Slotema, C. W., Blom, J. D., de Weijer, A. D., Diederen, K. M., Goekoop, R., Looijestijn, J., et al. (2011). Can low-frequency repetitive transcranial magnetic stimulation really relieve medication-resistant auditory verbal hallucinations? Negative results from a large randomized controlled trial. *Biol. Psychiatry.* 69, 450–456. doi: 10.1016/j.biopsych.2010.09.051

Slotema, C. W., Blom, J. D., Hoek, H. W., and Sommer, I. E. (2010). Should we expand the toolbox of psychiatric treatment methods to include Repetitive Transcranial Magnetic Stimulation (rTMS)? A meta-analysis of the efficacy of rTMS in psychiatric disorders. *J. Clin. Psychiatry.* 71, 873–884. doi: 10.4088/jcp.08m04872gre

Slotema, C. W., Blom, J. D., van Lutterveld, R., Hoek, H. W., and Sommer, I. E. (2014). Review of the efficacy of transcranial magnetic stimulation for auditory verbal hallucinations. *Biol. Psychiatry.* 76, 101–110. doi: 10.1016/j.biopsych.2013.09.038

Sommer, I. E., de Weijer, A. D., Daalman, K., Neggers, S. F., Somers, M., Kahn, R. S., et al. (2007). Can fMRI-guidance improve the efficacy of rTMS treatment for auditory verbal hallucinations? *Schizophr. Res.* 93, 406–408. doi: 10.1016/j.schres.2007.03.020

Sommer, I. E., Diederen, K. M., Blom, J. D., Willems, A., Kushan, L., Slotema, K., et al. (2008). Auditory verbal hallucinations predominantly activate the right inferior frontal area. *Brain.* 131, 3169–3177. doi: 10.1093/brain/awn251

Sommer, I. E., Slotema, C. W., Daskalakis, Z. J., Derks, E. M., Blom, J. D., and van der Gaag, M. (2012). The treatment of hallucinations in schizophrenia spectrum disorders. *Schizophr. Bull.* 38, 704–714. doi: 10.1093/schbul/sbs034

Stephane, M., Barton, S., and Boutros, N. N. (2001). Auditory verbal hallucinations and dysfunction of the neural substrates of speech. *Schizophr. Res.* 50, 61–78. doi: 10.1016/s0920-9964(00)00150-x

Tharyan, P., and Adams, C. E. (2005). Electroconvulsive therapy for schizophrenia. *Cochrane Database Syst. Rev.* 18:CD000076. doi: 10.1002/9780470987353.ch27

Thiel, A., Schumacher, B., Wienhard, K., Gairing, S., Kracht, L. W., Wagner, R., et al. (2006). Direct demonstration of transcallosal disinhibition in language networks. *J. Cereb. Blood Flow Metab.* 26, 1122–1127. doi: 10.1038/sj.jcbfm.9600350

Tranulis, C., Sepehry, A. A., Galinowski, A., and Stip, E. (2008). Should we treat auditory hallucinations with repetitive transcranial magnetic stimulation? A metaanalysis. *Can. J. Psychiatry.* 53, 577–586.

Vlachos, A., Muller-Dahlhaus, F., Rosskopp, J., Lenz, M., Ziemann, U., and Deller, T. (2012). Repetitive magnetic stimulation induces functional and structural plasticity of excitatory postsynapses in mouse organotypic hippocampal slice cultures. *J. Neurosci.* 32, 17514–17523. doi: 10.1523/jneurosci.0409-12.2012

Wang, J. X., and Voss, J. L. (2015). Long-lasting enhancements of memory and hippocampal-cortical functional connectivity following multiple-day targeted noninvasive stimulation. *Hippocampus.* 25, 877–883. doi: 10.1002/hipo.22416

Wassermann, E. M., and Zimmermann, T.. (2012). Transcranial magnetic brain stimulation: therapeutic promises and scientific gaps. *Pharmacol. Ther.* 133, 98–107. doi: 10.1016/j.pharmthera.2011.09.003

Waters, F., Allen, P., Aleman, A., Fernyhough, C., Woodward, T. S., Badcock, J. C., et al. (2012). Auditory hallucinations in schizophrenia and nonschizophrenia populations: a review and integrated model of cognitive mechanisms. *Schizophr. Bull.* 38, 683–693. doi: 10.1093/schbul/sbs045

Wolf, N. D., Grön, G., Sambataro, F., Vasic, N., Frasch, K., Schmid, M., et al. (2012). Magnetic resonance perfusion imaging of auditory verbal hallucinations in patients with schizophrenia. *Schizophr. Res.* 134, 285–287. doi: 10.1016/j.schres.2011.11.018

Wolf, N. D., Sambataro, F., Vasic, N., Frasch, K., Schmid, M., Schönfeldt-Lecuona, C., et al. (2011). Dysconnectivity of multiple resting-state networks in patients with schizophrenia who have persistent auditory verbal hallucinations. *J. Psychiatry. Neurosci.* 36, 366–374. doi: 10.1503/jpn.110008

Woodward, T. S., Jung, K., Hwang, H., Yin, J., Taylor, L., Menon, M., et al. (2014). Symptom dimensions of the psychotic symptom rating scales in psychosis: a multisite study. *Schizophr. Bull.* 4, S265–S274. doi: 10.1093/schbul/sbu014

19

Control Capabilities of Myoelectric Robotic Prostheses by Hand Amputees: A Scientific Research and Market Overview

Manfredo Atzori and Henning Müller*

Information Systems Institute, University of Applied Sciences Western Switzerland (HES-SO Valais), Sierre, Switzerland

Edited by:
Mikhail Lebedev, Duke University, USA

Reviewed by:
Ning Jiang, University of Waterloo, Canada
Kianoush Nazarpour, Newcastle University, UK
Agamemnon Krasoulis, University of Edinburgh, UK

***Correspondence:**
Manfredo Atzori
manfredo.atzori@hevs.ch

Hand amputation can dramatically affect the capabilities of a person. Cortical reorganization occurs in the brain, but the motor and somatosensorial cortex can interact with the remnant muscles of the missing hand even many years after the amputation, leading to the possibility to restore the capabilities of hand amputees through myoelectric prostheses. Myoelectric hand prostheses with many degrees of freedom are commercially available and recent advances in rehabilitation robotics suggest that their natural control can be performed in real life. The first commercial products exploiting pattern recognition to recognize the movements have recently been released, however the most common control systems are still usually unnatural and must be learned through long training. Dexterous and naturally controlled robotic prostheses can become reality in the everyday life of amputees but the path still requires many steps. This mini-review aims to improve the situation by giving an overview of the advancements in the commercial and scientific domains in order to outline the current and future chances in this field and to foster the integration between market and scientific research.

Keywords: electromyography, prosthetics, rehabilitation robotics, machine learning

INTRODUCTION

It is estimated that 41,000 persons were living with a major loss of an upper limb in 2005 (Ziegler-Graham et al., 2008). A hand amputation is one of the most impairing injuries and it can dramatically affect the capabilities of a person. Recent scientific and commercial advances in man-machine interfaces are promising and suggest that dexterous, naturally controlled, proportional and simultaneous robotic prostheses could be reality in the future of amputees. Nevertheless, the outline of the situation in the market and scientific field is complex and the path to naturally controlled prostheses still requires several steps.

Man-machine interfaces have been developed to control hand prostheses via the brain (Lebedev and Nicolelis, 2006), peripheral nerves (Navarro et al., 2005) or the muscles (Cipriani et al., 2011). The first two methods are promising but they usually require invasive procedures to obtain robust performance, thus they are currently applied only in scientific research. The third method (surface electromyography, sEMG) is probably the most widely used both in commercial settings and in scientific research.

Myoelectric hand prostheses with many degrees of freedom and very good mechanical capabilities are now commercially available. However, prosthetics companies target most of their communication efforts to end users. Thus they highlight the practical capabilities of the hands, but they usually do not provide information regarding the technical functionalities and specifications of the prostheses that can be exploitable by academic researchers. Previous papers presented some hand prostheses in detail (Belter et al., 2013) but the market changes quickly.

The scientific research field is even more complex and quickly changing. Many papers have been written in scientific research about the natural control of robotic hands by intact and transradial hand amputated subjects. Most of the methods rely on the use of sEMG and of pattern recognition or proportional control algorithms. The first commercial products exploiting pattern recognition to recognize the movements have recently been released. Targeted muscle reinnervation (TMR) can allow the exploitation of these methods even on subjects with above-elbow amputations. Benchmark databases to compare the performance of different methods and setups have been released (Atzori et al., 2014a). However, several steps are still required to obtain proportional, naturally controlled, robust and usable robotic hand prostheses (bionic hands).

Since the market and the scientific field are so complex and changing so quickly, it can be difficult to have a complete overview of them and to remain constantly updated in both fields. This mini-review aims to be a resource for young and experienced researchers in academia and prosthetic companies by providing a synthetic but complete overview of the current level of advancement in the commercial and scientific reality.

MARKET OUTLINE

A relatively wide choice of devices is available to restore the capabilities of hand amputees by myoelectric robotic prostheses. Such devices are continuously evolving according to technology, scientific research, market needs and user requirements. The devices usually include two main parts: prosthetic hands and control systems.

Prosthetic Hands

Currently, hand prostheses include cosmetic prostheses, kinematic prostheses and myoelectric prostheses. Cosmetic prostheses offer esthetical and psychological support. Kinematic prostheses also have functional capabilities, since the user can control the opening and closing of a gripper hand through the motion of the shoulder. Myoelectric prosthesis users can control a battery-powered hand through the electrical signal emitted by the remnant muscles, usually located in the forearm.

The continuous improvements in the field and the different targets and aims of the papers published by the companies can make it difficult for researchers to remain updated with the capabilities of available prostheses. For example, Belter et al. (2013) performed a very thorough description of the mechanical properties of prosthetic hands produced by four companies, but in less than 2 years several companies produced new versions or made substantial changes to the products from a mechanical or electronic point of view. Thus, the market and research achievements often remain disconnected.

Many prosthetic hands are commercially available. However, few have the capability to reproduce many movements. The following selection represents some of the currently most advanced hand prostheses and gives a representation of different companies and approaches: (1) Touch Bionics i-limb Quantum; (2) Otto Bock Michelangelo; (3) Steeper Bebionic v3; and (4) Vincent hand Evolution 2. **Table 1** summarizes the most important features that can be useful in a laboratory. The features are grouped into the following four categories: general technical data, dexterity related features, force related features and control related features.

Control Systems

Usually two or three sEMG electrodes are located in the socket in correspondence to specific muscles (**Figure 1**). A myoelectric impulse (i.e., an increase in the amplitude of the electrical signal emitted by the muscles) is used to open and close the prosthetic hand. The number of movements can be increased employing specific (e.g., sequential) control strategies. Such control strategies are usually still far from being natural, thus controlling prostheses requires a high level of skill and a training procedure. Control problems contribute to the scarce capabilities and acceptance of sEMG prostheses (Atkins et al., 1996), but they are likely promising for improvements in a near future.

In **Table 1** we summarize some of the most important control related features for the considered prosthetic hands including: number of electrodes, movement control type, movement command and particular features of each control system. As can be noticed in **Table 1**, despite the mechanical characteristics of the prosthesis allowing to reproduce up to 24 hand movements, the control systems rely in most cases on few (1–3) electrodes and on sequential control strategies or on specific movement triggers (in some cases tunable through a mobile app or other strategies). In sequential control strategies, a specific signal (for example, a simultaneous activation of two sEMG electrodes, usually called co-contraction) is used to switch between a set of predefined movements. In movement triggers on the other hand specific patterns of electrode activation are related to specific movements of the prosthesis. The mentioned methods are not natural, in the sense that they do not correspond to the movement that the subject would have thought to do before the amputation. However, they offer robust results, which is one of the main needs in real life.

Several of the considered prostheses include external sources of information as well. In particular, Touch Bionics i-limb Quantum recently introduced gesture control (recorded via gyroscope, accelerometer and magnetometer) and grip chips (that use blue-tooth chips attached to specific objects) to perform movement selection, while Steeper Bebionic exploits finger position encoders to perform falling object prevention. Sometimes research achievements translate to clinical practice too. In 2013 a pattern recognition system similar to the ones described in the scientific literature was made commercially available (http://www.coaptengineering.com/).

TABLE 1 | Characteristics of the examined prosthetic hands.

	Company name Prosthesis model	Touch Bionics i-limb Quantum	Otto Bock Michelangelo with Axon Bus Technology	Steeper Bebionic v3	Vincent GmbH Evolution 2
General technical data	Weight (without battery)	474–515 g	~510 g	550–598 g (365–390 g small hand)	380–410g
	Operating voltage	7.4 V	11.1 V	7.4 V	6–8 V
	Battery type	Lithium polymer	Li-Ion	Li-Ion	Li-Pol
	Battery capacity	1300–2400 mAh	1500 mAh	1300–2200 mAh	1300–2600 mAh
	Number of actuators	6	2	5	6
Dexterity	Active fingers	5 independent	3	5 independent	5 (+12 *active joints*)
	Thumb rotation	Powered	Powered	Manual	Powered
	Total number of grip patterns	24	7	14	20
	Grip patterns available at any moment	7	7	11	20
	Flexible wrist	Available	Included	Available	Available
	Rotating wrist	Available	Available	Available	Available
	Rotating wrist	*(active or passive)*	*(active or passive)*	*(active or passive)*	*(only passive)*
	Full closing time	0.8 s (0.7 s small hand)	0.37 s	0.5–1 s	0.8 s
	Finger position encoders	No	*2 motor position encoders*	5 *(one in each actuator)*	2 *(in thumb actuators)*
Force	Power grip	100–136 N	~70 N	140.1 N (280 N small hand)	60 N
	Lateral pinch	40 N (60 N small hand)	~60 N	26.5 N (53 N small hand)	15 N
	Adaptive Grip	Yes	Yes	Yes	Yes
	Falling object prevention	Active *(auto-grasp, based on accidental sEMG signal detection)*	No	Active *(auto-grip, based on finger position encoders)*	Passive *(spring load)*
	Proportional control	Yes	Yes	Yes	Yes
	N° of electrodes	1–2	1–2–3	1–2	1–2 wired
Control	Movement control type	Movement triggers, mobile app, bluetooth grip chips, favorite environment, gesture control	Sequential, 4-channel control	Sequential, Morph RFId GRIP selection compatible	Single trigger or Vincent Morse code
	Movement command	Hold open, double impulse, triple impulse, co-contraction	Different switching modes available, fast and high signal controls rotation in 4-channel control	Co-contraction/ open-open signal	Hold signal (opening or closing), double signal, co-contraction, alternating signal
	Particular features	Various control methods thumb rotating manually and automatically	Sensor hand speed *(stiff and harder finger tips)*; Fragile objects grasping	Fully free flexing fingers	Very low weight
	Feedback	No	No	Audible beeps and/or vibration *(grip changes)*	Vibration *(force detected via motor current and DMS sensors)*

The Coapt system can include up to eight sEMG electrodes. It is generic and it is typically set up to control the number of powered DOFs the patient's prosthesis has. That is, if a powered elbow, wrist, and terminal device are built into the prosthesis then the Coapt system is set to control these. If, however the prosthesis only has a powered terminal device and/or wrist, the Coapt system is set up for those DOFs. Wherever possible, Coapt performs natural control. The technician is encouraged to work with the patient to determine which are the most physiological, repeatable, consistent, and intuitive movements to use for control. Slight variations can be attempted if necessary, also through re-calibration procedures. The number of natural grasping patterns that can be achieved varies. According to Coapt, typically users can select between 3–6 naturally. It should be noted that the physical interconnection of the Coapt system and several prostheses has yet to be implemented. An example of movement-triggered control that we received by Coapt is the following one:

1. Hand closing: closing prosthesis.
2. Hand opening: opening prosthesis.
3. Wrist clockwise/counterclockwise rotation: powered wrist clockwise/counterclockwise rotation.
4. Double impulse of natural hand opening: grip A.
5. Triple impulse of natural hand opening: grip B.
6. Holding the hand open: grip C.
7. Single impulse of natural hand opening: grip D.

SCIENTIFIC RESEARCH OUTLINE

Many papers have been written in scientific research about the control of robotic hands and prostheses by intact and hand amputated subjects.

Usually several electrodes are placed on the forearm of the subject to record the myoelectric signals (**Figure 1**) with a dense sampling approach (Fukuda et al., 2003; Tenore et al., 2009; Li et al., 2010) or a precise anatomical positioning strategy (De Luca, 1997; Castellini et al., 2009a). The most common control procedures can be subdivided into pattern recognition or proportional control approaches, which can be applied to sEMG and multimodal signals.

Pattern recognition algorithms are used to classify the movement that the subject aims to perform according to a label (Scheme and Englehart, 2011). Pattern recognition results provided in several cases classification accuracy over 90–95% on less than 10 classes (e.g., Castellini et al., 2009b), however average results are usually below 80–90% (Peerdeman et al., 2011). Movement classification methods require movement labeling and they are restricted to a predetermined set of hand movements. Simultaneous pattern recognition has been studied recently (Jiang et al., 2013b; Ortiz-Catalan et al., 2013; Young et al., 2013), however usually such procedures consider simultaneous motions as new classes, thus they can reduce the robustness of the classifier.

Proportional and simultaneous control of a large number of degrees of freedom of the prosthesis can allow achieving more natural and dexterous control using unsupervised or supervised methods (Fougner et al., 2012; Farina et al., 2014). Unsupervised methods are usually based on signal factorization (e.g., through Non-Negative Matrix Factorization, NMF), they require a short calibration phase and they are relatively independent on the number and exact location of the electrodes (Jiang et al., 2009, 2014a,b; Muceli et al., 2014). Supervised methods (Nielsen et al., 2011; Muceli and Farina, 2012; Ameri et al., 2014a,b; Gijsberts et al., 2014b; Hahne et al., 2014) are usually based on regression techniques (e.g., Linear Regression, LR, Artificial Neural Networks, ANN, Support Vector Machines, SVM) that require a reliable ground truth for hand kinematics. This is easy for intact subjects (e.g., using data gloves), but it can be difficult for amputees, for whom the ground truth can be acquired only via bilateral mirrored contractions (Nielsen et al., 2011) or via visual cues (Ameri et al., 2014a,b). Recently, semi-supervised methods (NMF) and supervised methods (LR, ANN) were compared to evaluate the impact of precise kinematics estimation for accurately completing goal-directed tasks (Jiang et al., 2014b). The results showed that, although the three algorithms' mapping accuracies were significantly different, their online performance was similar. These results underline the hypothesis that good proportional myoelectric control can be achieved by the interaction and adaptation of the user with the myoelectric controller through closed-loop feedback. The same hypothesis is also demonstrated in other recent papers on multiple degrees of freedom for intact subjects (Pistohl et al., 2013; Antuvan et al., 2014) and hand amputees (Jiang et al., 2014a). Despite most of the proportional studies concentrating on full hand movements (e.g., hand supination, pronation, rotation, flexion, extension), proportional and simultaneous control has a strong potential for decoding finger kinematics as well. In particular, recent work described average correlation coefficients of up to 0.9 for the estimation of single finger movements (Smith et al., 2008) and 0.8 for the estimation of simultaneous and complex movements (Ngeo et al., 2014).

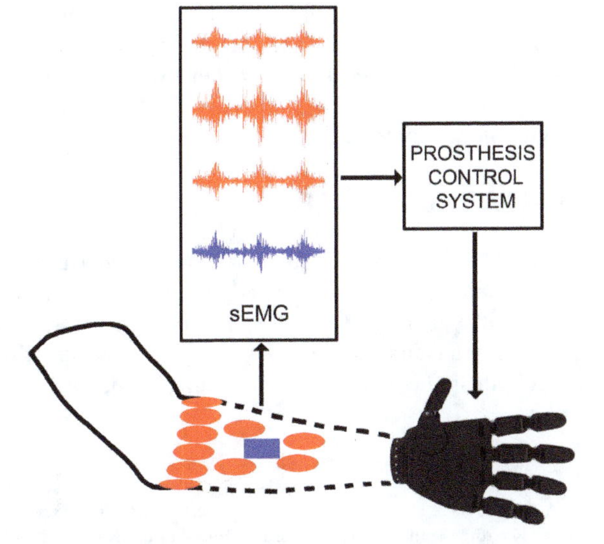

FIGURE 1 | Scheme of a generic myoelectric control system: (i) for commercial prosthesis without pattern recognition (blue rectangle); and (ii) for research (or control system with pattern recognition; red ellipses). The same architecture is assumed in the external forearm.

Also in scientific research, additional sources of information can be used to improve the performance of myoelectric control. Computer vision has been integrated to predetermine the type and size of the required grasp in relation to the object (Došen et al., 2010; Markovic et al., 2014). Accelerometers showed excellent capabilities to recognize hand movements using pattern recognition and regression methods, both alone and in combination with sEMG electrodes (Atzori et al., 2014b; Gijsberts et al., 2014a; Krasoulis et al., 2015).

A common problem in the field is that often the studies are highly specific and they are not directly comparable, due to different acquisition setups, protocols and analysis pipelines. Moreover, often the datasets are not publicly available. The NinaPro project (Atzori et al., 2015) released a publicly available benchmark with EMG, kinematic and dynamic data sources from intact and amputated subjects to help the scientific community to overcome control problems (http://ninaweb.hevs.ch/). Ninapro was recently used to evaluate regression methods for the continuous decoding of finger movements from sEMG and accelerometry (Krasoulis et al., 2015), to apply Dynamic time warping (DTW) in the context of myoelectric control (AbdelMaseeh et al., 2015) and to present the *Movement Error Rate*, an alternative to the standard window-based accuracy in pattern recognition (Gijsberts et al., 2014a).

Many factors can theoretically influence sEMG controlled prosthesis, including anatomical characteristics of the subjects

(Farina et al., 2002), training in using myoelectric prostheses (Cipriani et al., 2011), clinical parameters of the subjects (e.g., level of the amputation, phantom limb sensation intensity; Atzori et al., in press), fatigue, sweating, changes in electrode or arm positioning, surgical procedures used during the amputation and even cortical reorganization. However, few studies addressed these effects.

Implanting intramuscular EMG-recording devices reduces the number of parameters affecting the EMG signal and it can improve simultaneous control of multi-DOF prosthetic wrist and hand (Smith et al., 2014, 2015).

TMR is a surgical procedure that redirects the nerves that used to control the muscles of the hand to innervate accessory muscles from which surface sEMG is recorded. Impressive results have been obtained with this method, especially in persons with above-elbow or shoulder amputations (Kuiken et al., 2009). The same technique has also been applied on muscles transferred to the forearm to better integrate with traditional commercial prostheses (Aszmann et al., 2015).

The opposite neural direction, i.e., transferring information from the hand prosthesis to the brain, has been studied in several papers as well. Several attempts have been performed using non-invasive or invasive methods. Electrocutaneous and vibratory stimulation channels have been extensively studied in the past Szeto and Saunders (1982). TMR represents a promising solution also in this case, since it theoretically allows a certain amount of sensory feedback (Marasco et al., 2009). However, to date, the only example of real-time use of neural interfaces for the effective bidirectional control of dexterous prosthetic hands performing different grasping tasks is given by Raspopovic et al. (2014).

Despite the achievements described in this article, there are still several challenges before amputees can benefit from the mentioned signal processing developments (Jiang et al., 2012). First, robustness is probably the most important and challenging problem, in particular for simultaneous and proportional control. Second, the sensory-motor loop should be closed with proper feedback systems, thus opening new possibilities for effective and intuitive prosthetic control. Third, most of the studies are performed in controlled laboratory conditions with non-amputated subjects, which do not adapt to several different real life conditions of amputees (Fougner et al., 2011; Jiang et al., 2013a; He et al., 2015a,b).

CONCLUSIONS

Hand amputation can dramatically affect the capabilities of a person. The augmentation of the functionalities of the nervous and muscular system through external devices can already improve the situation of amputees. The market and the scientific field are complex and changing quickly, thus it is often difficult for young researchers to have a complete overview of them, as well as for experienced researchers to remain constantly updated in both the fields. In this mini review, we provide a synthetic but complete overview of the current level of advancement in the commercial and scientific reality, addressing each field in a specific section.

The commercial outline highlights the existence of very advanced prosthetic hands and control systems. Four of the most advanced prosthetic hands were analyzed, showing important mechanical and control differences. In particular, the number of actuators ranges between 2 (Otto Bock Michelangelo), 5 (Steeper Bebionic 3) and 6 (Touch Bionics i-limb Quantum and Vincent Evolution 2) while the number of finger position encoders ranges between 0 (Touch Bionics i-limb Quantum), 2 (Otto Bock Michelangelo, Vincent Evolution 2) and 5 (Steeper Bebionic 3). The first commercial control system based on pattern recognition has been released and it seems a great advancement with respect to previous ones. However natural, proportional and simultaneous control of a large number of degrees of freedom is currently not available.

The scientific research outline shows a large variety of control methods and several possible improvements. Pattern recognition, proportional control and TMR are extremely promising. Common sEMG data resources and benchmarks have been proposed recently to compare different sEMG analysis methods. Most of the factors that can theoretically affect the control of myoelectric prostheses, such as clinical data (e.g., level of the amputation, phantom limb sensation intensity) were recently studied. Finally sensorial feedback recently showed very promising advancements.

In conclusion, the path to proportional, naturally controlled, robust and usable robotic hand prostheses with sensorial feedback (bionic hands) seems to be well initiated and extremely promising for the coming years even though it is still a challenging work in progress.

ACKNOWLEDGMENTS

We would like to thank Valentina Baruchello and Hugh Gill at Touch Bionics, Bruce Rattray at Steeper, Stefan Schultz at Vincent, Blair Lock at Coapt Engineering, Martin Wehrle, Amsüss Sebastian and Karsten Ley at Otto Bock, and their teams for their helpfulness in providing information for this study.

REFERENCES

AbdelMaseeh, M., Chen, T.-W., and Stashuk, D. (2015). Extraction and classification of multichannel electromyographic activation trajectories for hand movement recognition. *IEEE Trans. Neural Syst. Rehabil. Eng.* doi: 10.1109/tnsre.2015.2447217 [Epub ahead of print].

Ameri, A., Kamavuako, E. N., Scheme, E. J., Englehart, K. B., and Parker, P. A. (2014a). Real-time, simultaneous Myoelectric control using visual target-based training paradigm. *Biomed. Signal Process. Control* 13, 8–14. doi: 10.1016/j.bspc.2014.03.006

Ameri, A., Kamavuako, E. N., Scheme, E. J., Englehart, K. B., and Parker, P. (2014b). Support vector regression for improved real-time, simultaneous

Myoelectric control. *IEEE Trans. Neural Syst. Rehabil. Eng.* 22, 1198–1209. doi: 10.1109/TNSRE.2014.2323576

Antuvan, C. W., Ison, M., and Artemiadis, P. (2014). Embedded human control of robots using Myoelectric interfaces. *IEEE Trans. Neural Syst. Rehabil. Eng.* 22, 820–827. doi: 10.1109/TNSRE.2014.2302212

Aszmann, O. C., Roche, A. D., Salminger, S., Paternostro-Sluga, T., Herceg, M., Sturma, A., et al. (2015). Bionic reconstruction to restore hand function after brachial plexus injury: a case series of three patients. *Lancet* 385, 2183–2189. doi: 10.1016/s0140-6736(14)61776-1

Atkins, D. J., Heard, D. C. Y., and Donovan, W. H. (1996). Epidemiologic overview of individuals with upper-limb loss and their reported research priorities. *J. Prosthet. Orthot.* 8, 2–11. doi: 10.1097/00008526-199600810-00003

Atzori, M., Gijsberts, A., Castellini, C., Caputo, B., Hager, A.-G. M., Elsig, S., et al. (2014a). Electromyography data for non-invasive naturally-controlled Robotic hand prostheses. *Sci. Data* 1:140053. doi: 10.1038/sdata.2014.53

Atzori, M., Gijsberts, A., Müller, H., and Caputo, B. (2014b). Classification of hand movements in amputated subjects by sEMG and accelerometers, in *Annual International Conference of the IEEE Engineering in Medicine and Biology Society (EMBC)* (Chicago, IL: IEEE), 3545–3549.

Atzori, M., Gijsberts, A., Castellini, C., Caputo, B., Mittaz Hager, A.-G., Elsig, S., et al. (in press). Clinical parameter effect on the capability to control Myoelectric Robotic prosthetic hands. *J. Rehabil. Res. Dev.* [Epub ahead of print].

Atzori, M., Gijsberts, A., Kuzborskij, I., Elsig, S., Mittaz Hager, A.-G., Deriaz, O., et al. (2015). Characterization of a benchmark database for Myoelectric movement classification. *IEEE Trans. Neural Syst. Rehabil. Eng.* 23, 73–83. doi: 10.1109/TNSRE.2014.2328495

Belter, J. T., Segil, J. L., Dollar, A. M., and Weir, R. F. (2013). Mechanical design and performance specifications of anthropomorphic prosthetic hands: a review. *J. Rehabil. Res. Dev.* 50, 599–618. doi: 10.1682/jrrd.2011.10.0188

Castellini, C., Fiorilla, A. E., and Sandini, G. (2009a). Multi-subject/daily-life activity EMG-based control of mechanical hands. *J. Neuroeng. Rehabil.* 6:41. doi: 10.1186/1743-0003-6-41

Castellini, C., Gruppioni, E., Davalli, A., and Sandini, G. (2009b). Fine detection of grasp force and posture by amputees via surface electromyography. *J. Physiol. Paris* 103, 255–262. doi: 10.1016/j.jphysparis.2009.08.008

Cipriani, C., Antfolk, C., Controzzi, M., Lundborg, G., Rosen, B., Carrozza, M. C., et al. (2011). Online Myoelectric control of a dexterous hand prosthesis by transradial amputees. *IEEE Trans. Neural Syst. Rehabil. Eng.* 19, 260–270. doi: 10.1109/TNSRE.2011.2108667

De Luca, C. J. (1997). The use of surface electromyography in biomechanics. *J. Appl. Biomech.* 13, 135–163.

Došen, S., Cipriani, C., Kostić, M., Controzzi, M., Carrozza, M. C., and Popović, D. B. (2010). Cognitive vision system for control of dexterous prosthetic hands: experimental evaluation. *J. Neuroeng. Rehabil.* 7:42. doi: 10.1186/1743-0003-7-42

Farina, D., Cescon, C., and Merletti, R. (2002). Influence of anatomical, physical and detection-system parameters on surface EMG. *Biol. Cybern.* 86, 445–456. doi: 10.1007/s00422-002-0309-2

Farina, D., Jiang, N., Rehbaum, H., Holobar, A., Graimann, B., Dietl, H., et al. (2014). The extraction of neural information from the surface EMG for the control of upper-limb prostheses: emerging avenues and challenges. *IEEE Trans. Neural Syst. Rehabil. Eng.* 22, 797–809. doi: 10.1109/TNSRE.2014.2305111

Fougner, A., Scheme, E., Chan, A. D. C., Englehart, K., and Stavdahl, O. (2011). Resolving the limb position effect in Myoelectric pattern recognition. *IEEE Trans. Neural Syst. Rehabil. Eng.* 19, 644–651. doi: 10.1109/TNSRE.2011.2163529

Fougner, A., Stavdahl, Ø., Kyberd, P. J., Losier, Y. G., and Parker, P. A. (2012). Control of upper limb prostheses: terminology and proportional Myoelectric control-a review. *IEEE Trans. Neural Syst. Rehabil. Eng.* 20, 663–677. doi: 10.1109/TNSRE.2012.2196711

Fukuda, O., Tsuji, T., Kaneko, M., Otsuka, A., and Tsuji, O. F. T. (2003). A human-assisting manipulator teleoperated by EMG signals and arm motions. *IEEE Trans. Robot. Autom.* 19, 210–222. doi: 10.1109/tra.2003.808873

Gijsberts, A., Atzori, M., Castellini, C., Muller, H., and Caputo, B. (2014a). The movement error rate for evaluation of machine learning methods for sEMG-based hand movement classification. *IEEE Trans. Neural Syst. Rehabil. Eng.* 22, 735–744. doi: 10.1109/TNSRE.2014.2303394

Gijsberts, A., Bohra, R., González, D. S., Werner, A., Nowak, M., Caputo, B., et al. (2014b). Stable Myoelectric control of a hand prosthesis using non-linear incremental learning. *Front. Neurorobot.* 8:8. doi: 10.3389/fnbot.2014.00008

Hahne, J. M., Bießmann, F., Jiang, N., Rehbaum, H., Farina, D., Meinecke, F. C., et al. (2014). Linear and nonlinear regression techniques for simultaneous and proportional Myoelectric control. *IEEE Trans. Neural Syst. Rehabil. Eng.* 22, 269–279. doi: 10.1109/TNSRE.2014.2305520

He, J., Zhang, D., Jiang, N., Sheng, X., Farina, D., and Zhu, X. (2015a). User adaptation in long-term, open-loop Myoelectric training: implications for EMG pattern recognition in prosthesis control. *J. Neural Eng.* 12:046005. doi: 10.1088/1741-2560/12/4/046005

He, J., Zhang, D., Sheng, X., Li, S., and Zhu, X. (2015b). Invariant surface EMG feature against varying contraction level for Myoelectric control based on muscle coordination. *IEEE J. Biomed. Health Inform.* 19, 874–882. doi: 10.1109/JBHI.2014.2330356

Jiang, N., Dosen, S., Muller, K., and Farina, D. (2012). Myoelectric control of artificial limbs-is there a need to change focus? *IEEE Signal Process. Mag.* 29, 150–152. doi: 10.1109/msp.2012.2203480

Jiang, N., Englehart, K. B., Parker, P. A., and Englehart, K. B. (2009). Extracting simultaneous and proportional neural control information for multiple degree of freedom prostheses from the surface electromyographic signal. *IEEE Trans. Biomed. Eng.* 56, 1070–1080. doi: 10.1109/TBME.2008.2007967

Jiang, N., Muceli, S., Graimann, B., and Farina, D. (2013a). Effect of arm position on the prediction of kinematics from EMG in amputees. *Med. Biol. Eng. Comput.* 51, 143–151. doi: 10.1007/s11517-012-0979-4

Jiang, N., Tian, L., Fang, P., Dai, Y., and Li, G. (2013b). Motion recognition for simultaneous control of multifunctional transradial prostheses, in *Engineering in Medicine and Biology Society (EMBC), 2013 35th Annual International Conference of the IEEE* (Osaka: IEEE), 1603–1606.

Jiang, N., Rehbaum, H., Vujaklija, I., Graimann, B., and Farina, D. (2014a). Intuitive, online, simultaneous and proportional Myoelectric control over two degrees-of-freedom in upper limb amputees. *IEEE Trans. Neural Syst. Rehabil. Eng.* 22, 501–510. doi: 10.1109/TNSRE.2013.2278411

Jiang, N., Vujaklija, I., Rehbaum, H., Graimann, B., and Farina, D. (2014b). Is accurate mapping of EMG signals on kinematics needed for precise online Myoelectric control? *IEEE Trans. Neural Syst. Rehabil. Eng.* 22, 549–558. doi: 10.1109/tnsre.2013.2287383

Krasoulis, A., Vijayakumar, S., and Nazarpour, K. (2015). Evaluation of regression methods for the continuous decoding of finger movement from surface EMG and accelerometry, in *Neural Engineering (NER), 2015 7th International IEEE/EMBS Conference on* (Montpellier: IEEE), 631–634.

Kuiken, T. A., Li, G., Lock, B. A., Lipschutz, R. D., Miller, L. A., Stubblefield, K. A., et al. (2009). Targeted muscle reinnervation for real-time Myoelectric control of multifunction artificial arms. *JAMA* 301, 619–628. doi: 10.1001/jama.2009.116

Lebedev, M. A., and Nicolelis, M. A. L. (2006). Brain-machine interfaces: past, present and future. *Trends Neurosci.* 29, 536–546. doi: 10.1016/j.tins.2006.07.004

Li, G., Schultz, A. E., and Kuiken, T. A. (2010). Quantifying pattern recognition-based Myoelectric control of multifunctional transradial prostheses. *IEEE Trans. Neural Syst. Rehabil. Eng.* 18, 185–192. doi: 10.1109/TNSRE.2009.2039619

Marasco, P. D., Schultz, A. E., and Kuiken, T. A. (2009). Sensory capacity of reinnervated skin after redirection of amputated upper limb nerves to the chest. *Brain* 132, 1441–1448. doi: 10.1093/brain/awp082

Markovic, M., Dosen, S., Cipriani, C., Popovic, D., and Farina, D. (2014). Stereovision and augmented reality for closed-loop control of grasping in hand prostheses. *J. Neural Eng.* 11:046001. doi: 10.1088/1741-2560/11/4/046001

Muceli, S., and Farina, D. (2012). Simultaneous and proportional estimation of hand kinematics from EMG during mirrored movements at multiple degrees-of-freedom. *IEEE Trans. Neural Syst. Rehabil. Eng.* 20, 371–378. doi: 10.1109/TNSRE.2011.2178039

Muceli, S., Jiang, N., and Farina, D. (2014). Extracting signals robust to electrode number and shift for online simultaneous and proportional Myoelectric control by factorization algorithms. *IEEE Trans. Neural Syst. Rehabil. Eng.* 22, 623–633. doi: 10.1109/TNSRE.2013.2282898

Navarro, X., Krueger, T. B., Lago, N., Micera, S., Stieglitz, T., and Dario, P. (2005). A critical review of interfaces with the peripheral nervous system for the control of neuroprostheses and hybrid bionic systems. *J. Peripher. Nerv. Syst.* 10, 229–258. doi: 10.1111/j.1085-9489.2005.10303.x

Ngeo, J. G., Tamei, T., and Shibata, T. (2014). Continuous and simultaneous estimation of finger kinematics using inputs from an EMG-to-muscle activation model. *J. Neuroeng. Rehabil.* 11:122. doi: 10.1186/1743-0003-11-122

Nielsen, J. L. G., Holmgaard, S., Jiang, N., Englehart, K. B., Farina, D., and Parker, P. A. (2011). Simultaneous and proportional force estimation for multifunction Myoelectric prostheses using mirrored bilateral training. *IEEE Trans. Biomed. Eng.* 58, 681–688. doi: 10.1109/TBME.2010.2068298

Ortiz-Catalan, M., Branemark, R., and Hakansson, B. (2013). Evaluation of classifier topologies for the real-time classification of simultaneous limb motions. *Conf. Proc. IEEE Eng. Med. Biol. Soc.* 2013, 6651–6654. doi: 10.1109/EMBC.2013.6611081

Peerdeman, B., Boere, D., Witteveen, H., Huis in 't Veld, R., Hermens, H., Stramigioli, S., et al. (2011). Myoelectric forearm prostheses: state of the art from a user-centered perspective. *J. Rehabil. Res. Dev.* 48, 719–738. doi: 10.1682/jrrd.2010.08.0161

Pistohl, T., Cipriani, C., Jackson, A., and Nazarpour, K. (2013). Abstract and proportional Myoelectric control for multi-fingered hand prostheses. *Ann. Biomed. Eng.* 41, 2687–2698. doi: 10.1007/s10439-013-0876-5

Raspopovic, S., Capogrosso, M., Petrini, F. M., Bonizzato, M., Rigosa, J., Di Pino, G., et al. (2014). Restoring natural sensory feedback in real-time bidirectional hand prostheses. *Sci. Transl. Med.* 6:222ra19. doi: 10.1126/scitranslmed.3006820

Scheme, E., and Englehart, K. (2011). Electromyogram pattern recognition for control of powered upper-limb prostheses: state of the art and challenges for clinical use. *J. Rehabil. Res. Dev.* 48, 643–659. doi: 10.1682/jrrd.2010.09.0177

Smith, L. H., Kuiken, T. A., and Hargrove, L. J. (2014). Real-time simultaneous and proportional Myoelectric control using intramuscular EMG. *J. Neural Eng.* 11:066013. doi: 10.1088/1741-2560/11/6/066013

Smith, L. H., Kuiken, T. A., and Hargrove, L. J. (2015). Linear regression using intramuscular EMG for simultaneous Myoelectric control of a wrist and hand system, in *Neural Engineering (NER), 2015 7th International IEEE/EMBS Conference on* (Montpellier: IEEE), 619–622.

Smith, R. J., Tenore, F., Huberdeau, D., Cummings, R. E., and Thakor, N. V. (2008). Continuous decoding of finger position from surface EMG signals for the control of powered prostheses. *Conf. Proc. IEEE Eng. Med. Biol. Soc.* 2008, 197–200. doi: 10.1109/IEMBS.2008.4649124

Szeto, A. Y. J., and Saunders, F. A. (1982). Electrocutaneous stimulation for sensory communication in rehabilitation engineering. *IEEE Trans. Biomed. Eng.* 4, 300–308. doi: 10.1109/tbme.1982.324948

Tenore, F. V. G., Ramos, A., Fahmy, A., Acharya, S., Etienne-Cummings, R., and Thakor, N. V. (2009). Decoding of individuated finger movements using surface electromyography. *IEEE Trans. Biomed. Eng.* 56, 1427–1434. doi: 10.1109/TBME.2008.2005485

Young, A. J., Smith, L. H., Rouse, E. J., and Hargrove, L. J. (2013). Classification of simultaneous movements using surface EMG pattern recognition. *IEEE Trans. Biomed. Eng.* 60, 1250–1258. doi: 10.1109/TBME.2012.2232293

Ziegler-Graham, K., MacKenzie, E. J., Ephraim, P. L., Travison, T. G., and Brookmeyer, R. (2008). Estimating the prevalence of limb loss in the United States: 2005 to 2050. *Arch. Phys. Med. Rehabil.* 89, 422–429. doi: 10.1016/j.apmr.2007.11.005

20

^{123}I-FP-CIT SPECT Imaging in Early Diagnosis of Dementia in Patients with and without a Vascular Component

Marina Garriga[1,2], *Marta Milà*[1], *Manzoor Mir*[3], *Raid Al-Baradie*[3], *Sonia Huertas*[1], *Cesar Castejon*[1], *Laura Casas*[1], *Dolors Badenes*[1], *Nuria Giménez*[4], *M. Angels Font*[4], *Jose M. Gonzalez*[5], *Maria Ysamat*[5], *Miguel Aguilar*[1], *Mark Slevin*[6] *and Jerzy Krupinski*[1,6]*

[1] Neurology Unit, Hospital Universitari Mútua Terrassa, Terrassa, Spain, [2] Psychiatric Unit, Hospital Universitari Mútua Terrassa, Terrassa, Spain, [3] College of Applied Medical Sciences, Majmaah University Almajmaah, Al Majmaah, Saudi Arabia, [4] Research Unit, Research Foundation Mútua Terrassa, Universitat de Barcelona, Barcelona, Spain, [5] Cetir-Grup Medic, CTD, Hospital Universitari Mútua de Terrassa, Terrassa, Spain, [6] School of Healthcare Science, Manchester Metropolitan University, Manchester, UK

Edited by:
Mikhail Lebedev,
Duke University, USA

Reviewed by:
Juan C. Rivas,
Universidad del Valle, Colombia
Mengchao Cui,
Beijing Normal University, China

***Correspondence:**
Jerzy Krupinski,
Neurology Unit, Hospital Universitari
Mútua Terrassa, Plaça Dr. Robert,
5 08221 Terrassa, Catalonia, Spain
jkrupinski@mutuaterrassa.es

Alzheimer's disease (AD) and vascular dementia (VaD) are the most common cause of dementia. Cerebral ischemia is a major risk factor for development of dementia. ^{123}I-FP-CIT SPECT (DaTScan) is a complementary tool in the differential diagnoses of patients with incomplete or uncertain Parkinsonism. Additional application of DaTScan enables the categorization of Parkinsonian disease with dementia (PDD), and its differentiation from pure AD, and may further contribute to change the therapeutic decision. The aim of this study was to analyze the vascular contribution towards dementia and mild cognitive impairment (MCI). We evaluated the utility of DaTScan for the early diagnosis of dementia in patients with and without a clinical vascular component, and the association between neuropsychological function, vascular component and dopaminergic function on DaTScan. One-hundred and five patients with MCI or the initial phases of dementia were studied prospectively. We developed an initial assessment using neurologic examination, blood tests, cognitive function tests, structural neuroimaging and DaTScan. The vascular component was later quantified in two ways: clinically, according to the Framingham Risk Score (FRS) and by structural neuroimaging using Wahlund Scale Total Score (WSTS). Early diagnosis of dementia was associated with an abnormal DaTScan. A significant association was found between a high WSTS and an abnormal DaTScan ($p < 0.01$). Mixed AD was the group with the highest vascular component, followed by the VaD group, while MCI and pure AD showed similar WSTS. No significant associations were found between neuropsychological impairment and DaTScan independently of associated vascular component. DaTScan seems to be a good tool to discriminate, in a first clinical assessment, patients with MCI from those with established dementia. There was bigger general vascular affectation observable in MRI or CT in patients with abnormal dopaminergic uptake seen on DaTScan.

Keywords: dementia, mild cognitive impairment, Framingham risk score, ^{123}I-FP-CIT SPECT

Introduction

Dementia is a chronic brain syndrome which affects 35.6 million people worldwide and this number is expected to triple by 2050 (115.4 million). Thus, it has an enormous impact on health care provision currently costing the world more than US$ 604 billion per year (Wimo et al., 2013).

The most frequent cause of dementia in the elderly is Alzheimer's disease (AD), followed by vascular dementia (VaD), Parkinson disease with dementia (PDD) and Lewy Body dementia (LBD). Together these account for over 90% of cases of dementia in the elderly (Albanese et al., 2007).

Although they have distinct features, the different types of dementia overlap clinically and pathologically, especially in the early stages and particularly in regards to the contribution of brain ischemia (Iadecola and Gorelick, 2003). Increasing evidence demonstrates that ischemia is not only an additive cause of brain damage in all types of dementia but also contributes specifically to the underlying disease processes (Niwa et al., 2002; Iadecola and Gorelick, 2003) Many cardiovascular risk factors (CVRF), such as hypertension, diabetes, dyslipidemia, and smoking increase the risk of AD, suggesting a vascular contribution to the etiology of AD. Ischemia upregulates and deregulates the entire amyloidogenic cascade. Within the framework of the neurovascular unit, vascular dysfunction may reduce the clearance of β-amyloid (Aβ) via the blood brain barrier or indirectly increase Aβ deposition. Amyloid deposition is considered the pivotal event in the AD pathological cascade, but whether the accumulation is accelerated by CVRF remains unclear (Breteler, 2000; Purnell et al., 2009; **Figure 1**). The evidence is stronger for VaD and AD, but there is a lack of research into the potential contribution of ischemia to LBD or PDD.

Other studies showed that most CVRF also increase the risk for AD (Tatemichi et al., 1994; Tanimukai et al., 1998; Kalaria, 2012). In large epidemiological studies, the prevalence of AD is reported to increase with the severity of atherosclerosis, the presence of atrial fibrillation, hypertension, diabetes mellitus, hyperinsulinemia and insulin resistance, and a previous stroke (Skoog et al., 1996; Leibson et al., 1997; Ott et al., 1997). Antihypertensive treatments can prevent stroke and also the risk of dementia (Sörös et al., 2013). Further, abnormalities in the cerebral white matter thought to be ischemic in nature are more common in AD than controls, and its severity correlates with mild cognitive impairment (MCI) progression to AD (Scheltens et al., 1992; Eckerström et al., 2011).

The occurrence of both AD pathology and vascular brain injury is very common, especially amongst the oldest of old and can be classified as mixed AD. Although epidemiologic studies report that vascular risk factors for arteriosclerosis increase the risk of incident AD, both autopsy, MRI and amyloid positron emission tomography (PET) studies indicate that AD and vascular lesions contribute additively, but independently, to the risk of dementia. The literature confirms the malignancy of AD and highlights the adverse effects of microinfarcts on cognitive function. For the clinical diagnosis of mixed AD, the presence of AD can be recognized by neuropsychological profile, structural imaging, cerebrospinal fluid biomarkers, and glucose PET and amyloid PET imaging. The diagnosis of mixed AD, however, still hinges predominantly on the structural MRI findings (Chui and Ramirez-Gomez, 2015). Studies on neuroimaging have reported that over 70% of patients consulting for neurodegenerative disease have abnormal MRI findings suggestive of a vascular component (Mills et al., 2007). White matter hyperintensities (WMHs) on brain MRI reflect cardiovascular risk profiles, and greater WMH volume is associated with cerebral hypometabolism and cognitive decline, particularly in tests of executive function (DeCarli et al., 1995; Jeerakathil et al., 2004; Carmichael et al., 2010). These structural and cognitive changes were associated with CVRF. The Framingham Stroke Risk Profile score, a composite risk score of CVRF that measures 10-year probability of stroke, was negatively associated with total cerebral brain volume and positively related to prevalent WMHs. The association between multiple CVRF was examined by a number of studies using the Framingham Stroke Risk Profile. High Framingham scores correlate with poor cognitive performance (Wolf et al., 1991; Elias et al., 2004; Jeerakathil et al., 2004). These results confirm that ischemia is a major risk factor for dementia. In fact, 10% of stroke patients develop dementia shortly after their first stroke and more than a third develop dementia after recurrent strokes. Subjects not developing dementia as a direct consequence of a stroke have a 10-fold increase in the risk of dementia over the next 5 years (Pendlebury and Rothwell, 2009).

Neuroimaging techniques play a major role as diagnostic instruments (Visser et al., 2012). In particular, emission tomography (single photon emission computed tomography, SPECT and PET) provides a unique tool to investigate functional and neurochemical changes, both in those with established dementia and at risk of subsequent cognitive decline (de Souza et al., 2012; Herholz, 2012).

AD is characterized by bilateral temporoparietal hypoperfusion on SPECT and hypometabolism on PET, which may precede the onset of clinical dementia. Similar changes can be demonstrated in those with MCI and in those genetically at risk of developing AD (Brun and Englund, 1986; Vanitallie, 2013). In turn, VaD is related to multiple, asymmetric, perfusion deficits secondary to brain multi infarction (Chen et al., 2013).

In contrast, in LBD medial parietal and occipital perfusion deficits are seen together with mainly pre-synaptic dopaminergic changes, most commonly a reduction in the striatal pre-synaptic dopamine transporter (DAT) which can be visualized using appropriate tracers [e.g., ^{123}I-N-3-fluoropropyl-2beta-carbomethoxy-3beta-4-iodophenyl tropane (^{123}I-FP-CIT SPECT); McKeith et al., 2005; Cummings et al., 2011].

Thus, advanced functional imaging has a promising potential in supporting dementia diagnosis. Indeed, imaging of the DAT defines integrity of the dopaminergic system, and hence its degeneration *in vivo* (Varrone and Halldin, 2010). Its main clinical application is in patients with mild, incomplete, or uncertain Parkinsonism (Weng et al., 2004; Tolosa et al., 2007; Eshuis et al., 2006). That is, striatal uptake correlating with

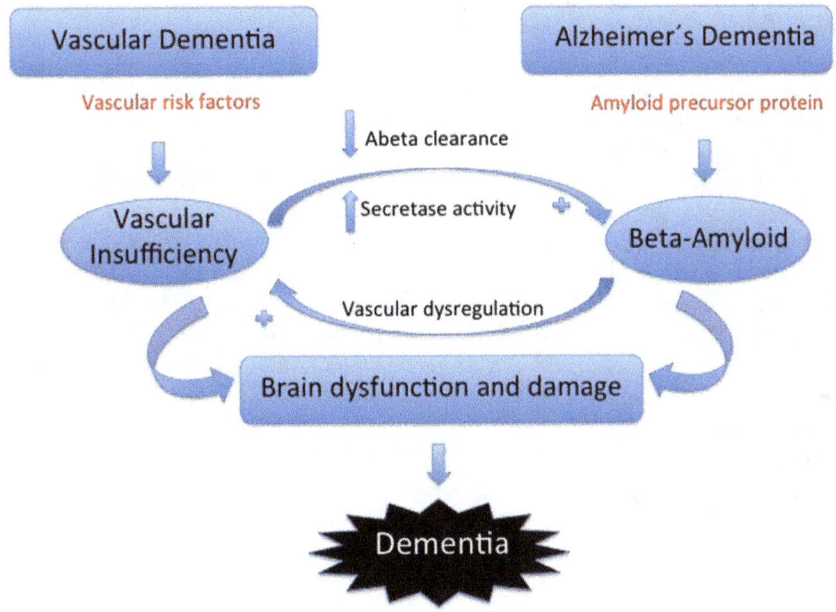

FIGURE 1 | In VaD, cerebrovascular risk factors induce neurovascular dysfunction leading to brain dysfunction and damage. In Alzheimer's disease (AD), cleavage of amyloid precursor protein by by β- and γ-secretases leads to Aβ accumulation, which also causes brain dysfunction and damage. Although individually these pathways are capable of inducing cognitive impairment, their interaction enhances their pathogenic effects. Thus, Aβ induces vascular dysregulation and aggravates vascular insufficiency, thereby enhancing the brain dysfunction and damage associated with vascular risk factors. In addition, the hypoxia-ischemia resulting from the vascular insufficiency increases Aβ cleavage from APP and reduces Aβ clearance through the cerebral vasculature, promoting Aβ accumulation and the attendant deleterious effects on the brain (Iadecola, 2010).

disease severity, in particular bradykinesia and rigidity. Also, it is a useful tool in the monitoring of progression in clinical trials of potential neuroprotective drugs and in differentiating juvenile-onset Parkinson's disease (abnormal ^{123}I-FP-CIT SPECT) from dopa-responsive dystonia (normal ^{123}I-FP-CIT SPECT; Marshall and Grosset, 2003).

Dopamine loss is seen even in the earliest clinical presentations of true Parkinsonism; a normal scan suggests an alternative diagnosis such as essential tremor, drug-induced Parkinsonism, or psychogenic Parkinsonism (Cummings et al., 2011). Congruence between working clinical diagnosis and DAT imaging increases over time in favor of baseline ^{123}I-FP-CIT SPECT imaging results. Additional applications, especially accurate when combining with other neuroimaging tools such as FDG-PET, characterize dementia with Parkinsonian features (Cummings et al., 2011; Garibotto et al., 2013). Furthermore, it is possible to differentiate AD from LBD [normal tracer uptake in AD and abnormal in dementia with Lewy bodies (DLB) with sensitivity and specificity of 78–88% and 94–100%, respectively; McKeith et al., 2005].

Regarding the vascular component involved in dementia, the role of nuclear medicine imaging in the diagnosis of vascular Parkinsonism (VP) or VaD has been addressed by only a few studies up to now and with non-definitive results. Some of these suggest normal ^{123}I-FP-CIT SPECT (Gerschlager et al., 2002; Lorberboym et al., 2004; García Vicente et al., 2005) in VP while others suggest reduced ^{123}I-FP-CIT binding as well as a lower mean asymmetry index than Parkinson's disease (Zijlmans et al., 2007). In general more studies reported higher percentage of normal FP-CIT SPECT in VP patients (Bouwmans et al., 2013).

The aim of this study was to analyze the vascular contribution towards dementia and MCI. We evaluated the utility of FP-CIT SPECT for the early diagnosis of dementia in patients with and without a clinical vascular component, and the association between neuropsychological function, vascular component and dopaminergic function on FP-CIT SPECT.

Materials and Methods

Subjects

The study population included 105 patients. They were recruited prospectively from the outpatient Dementia and Stroke Unit. We included patients with clinical diagnosis of MCI (n = 50), probable dementia (AD and VaD, n = 37), and Parkinson disease with dementia (PDD and DLB, n = 18; **Table 1**).

TABLE 1 | Distribution of different diagnoses in our study group.

	N	Age	Sex M:F
Mild cognitive impairment (MCI)	50	72 ± 8	26:24
Alzheimer's disease (AD)	31	76 ± 7	12:19
Parkinson disease with dementia (PDD)	12	77 ± 6	10:2
Vascular dementia (VaD)	6	73 ± 9	3:3
Lewy body dementia (LBD)	6	73 ± 11	3:3

Data are presented as mean (±SD) or number.

Dementia was diagnosed according to the *Diagnostic and Statistical Manual of Mental Disorders*, fourth edition (DSM-IV), and AD based on the criteria of the *National Institute of Neurological and Communicative Disorders and Stroke* and the *Alzheimer's Disease and Related Disorders Association* for definite, probable, or possible. Independently, two trained neurologists made the diagnosis and the final diagnosis was established by consensus. Patients with hemispheric vascular accident or severe isolated aphasia were not included. Also, patients with prior cranial trauma, severe heart, kidney or liver disease, cancer or infection signs were excluded from our study.

Baseline Assessment

Demographic and Clinical Variables and Cardiovascular Risk Profile

Demographic data included age and gender. We also recorded medical history including data such as CVRF and psychiatric disorders. CVRF were extracted from the medical history: hypertension, dyslipidemia, Diabetes Mellitus, smoke habit, family history of dementia or cardiovascular disease, presence of peripheral vascular disease (PVD), coronary artery disease (CAD) or prior stroke. Cardiovascular risk score was calculated using the recently developed Framingham General Cardiovascular Disease Risk from the Framingham Heart Study (Wolf et al., 1991; D'Agostino et al., 2008). Framingham Risk Score (FRS) was estimated in all patients according to age, gender, total cholesterol levels, HDL levels, systolic blood pressure, hypertension treatment, smoking habit, diabetic status, and vascular disease (CAD, PVD, stroke). Those patients presenting moderate or high FRS were categorized as having a clinical vascular component, while all the rest were considered as not having it.

Data were provided by the patient and/or caregiver or extracted from medical reports if available.

Physical Examination

Neurological clinical examination was performed. Assessments were undertaken according to the local practice. The Mini-Mental State Examination (MMSE) was administered as a cognitive screening test. The effect of cognitive impairment on global functioning was measured with the Clinical Dementia Rating Scale (CDR) and the Global Deterioration Scale (GDS). Instrumental activities of daily living (IADL) and ADL functions were measured with the Blessed Dementia Rating Scale (BDRS), the Bayer ADL or self-rating Bayer ADL scale.

Motor sub-scale of the Unified Parkinson's Disease Rating (UPDRS- III) was used as a measure to help in the description of the extrapyramidal symptoms (EPS). Neuropsychiatric symptoms were measured with the Neuropsychiatric Inventory (NPI) and depression rates on the elderly were measured with the Yesavage scale.

Neuropsychological Battery

A standardized protocol was administered by a trained neuropsychologist. We selected a short version of the Barcelona test. The domains tested were orientation, attention, immediate and differed memory, language, praxis, gnosis, executive functions and working memory. Neuropsychologists were also asked to give a GDS of the cognitive impairment evaluated.

Complementary Physical Examinations

General blood tests were realized including lipid profile. According to our laboratory criteria, lipid abnormal profile was defined as cholesterol levels higher than 200 mg/dl, high density lipoprotein cholesterol (HDL) lower than 56 mg/dL if men and lower than 65 mg/dL if women, low density lipoprotein (LDL) cholesterol higher than 100 mg/dl and triglycerides higher than 190 mg/dL.

Neuroimaging Study

In addition to the clinical vascular component defined using FRS, the vascular contribution in each group of patients was also quantified from WMHs on anatomic neuroimaging.

MRI and CT imaging

MRI was used preferentially, if not available CT was used. MRI was performed on a Symphony MR A-35 1.5 T scanner and processed using MR 2004 A Syngo software. CT imaging was performed on Siemens Sensation Somaton E scanner and processed using the software CT 2007 -S 16 C. Axial CT or T2 weighted MRI images were used for the quantification of the vascular component using a validated score according to Wahlund scale (from 0 to 3; Wahlund et al., 2001). The Wahlund scale was used in the analyses of WMHs in five cerebral areas in both hemispheres: frontal, parieto-occipital, temporal lobes, infratentorial area and basal ganglia. WMHs on MRI were defined as ill-defined hyperintensities >5 mm on T2 images, and on CT as ill-defined and moderately hypodense areas of >5 mm. Lacunes were described as well-defined areas of >2 mm with attenuation (on CT) or signal characteristics (on MRI) the same as cerebrospinal fluid. If lesions with these characteristics were <2 mm, they were considered perivascular spaces. Changes in the basal ganglia were rated in the same way and considered WMHs even if located in the gray matter nuclei, which contains a small amount of white matter. The Total Score of the Wahlund Scale (WSTS) was finally quantified as the mean value of the five cerebral areas analyzed.

Molecular imaging of dopaminergic activity by ^{123}I-FP-CIT SPECT

SPECT images were acquired on a 2 headed gamma camera hybrid SPECT-TC Infinia HW4 General Electronic with a high resolution collimator. Images were acquired 3 h after a single intravenous injection of 5 mCi (111–185 MBq) of the radiotracer ^{123}I Ioflupane. Subjects underwent standard thyroid blocking with potassium iodide oral administration (120 mg) 1–4 h before and 12–24 h after the radiotracer injection. Images were assessed using a dichotomous division of normal (0) *vs.* lower uptake (1).

Statistical Analyses

Demographic parameters were expressed as absolute values and percentages for the qualitative variables and by mean and standard deviation for the quantitative variables.

In bivariate analysis, qualitative variables were compared using the χ^2 test or Fisher exact probability Test, when appropriated. To complete the comparison between qualitative and quantitative variables Student's t-test was carried out. For the mean comparisons ANOVA test was used. Finally, Pearson correlation coefficients were used to examine the relationship between quantitative variables. A two-sided P value of <0.05 was used to assess statistical significance. For significant variables, 95% confidence intervals (CI) were established.

Statistical analyses were performed using the Statistical Package for the Social Sciences SPSS 17.0 (SPSS Inc., Chicago, IL, USA).

Ethical Considerations

This study was done in accordance with the Review Board and Ethics Committee of our center. Written informed consent was always obtained from patients.

Results

Subject Demographics

Subject's demographic characteristics, CVRF, results of neurological, neuropsychological and neuroimaging examination frequencies of MCI group compared to the dementia group are shown in **Table 2**. In **Table 3** the same features are described as N(%) for each dementia type and also MCI.

TABLE 2 | Subject's demographic characteristics, distributions of CVRF, results of neurological, neuropsychological and neuroimaging examination in MCI group compared to the dementia group.

N (%)	MCI	Dementia
Sex M:F	26 (52):24 (48)	29 (53):26 (47)
Age	72 ± 8	75 ± 8
Vascular component	14 (29)	14 (26)
EPS	0 (0)	17 (31)
Hypertension	29 (62)	31 (66)
Dyslipidemia	16 (34)	17 (36)
Diabetes mellitus	12 (26)	15 (32)
Smoking or ex-smoking	10 (21)	10 (21)
PVD	2 (5)	3 (7)
CAD	4 (10)	6 (14)
Prior stroke	15 (37)	11 (26)
Total cholesterol	194 ± 40	190 ± 47
HDL cholesterol	50 ± 18	51 ± 21
LDL cholesterol	108 ± 63	103 ± 55
Triglycerides♯	137 ± 100	171 ± 59
HACHINSKI	4 ± 3	4 ± 3
GDS *fast*	3 ± 1	4 ± 1
MMSE♯	25 ± 4	21 ± 5
UPDRS-III *motorsub-scale*♯	9 ± 9	37 ± 15*
WSTS♯	0.5 ± 0.4	0.7 ± 0.6
^{123}I-FP-CIT SPECT decrease uptake♯	7 (21)	14 (45)

Numbers and % are presented for each group. ♯$p < 0.05$; **This refers only to PDD group.*

Vascular History and Risk Factors

Within clinically diagnosed AD, 7 out of 31 patients had vascular lesions on imaging and were classified as mixed AD. However, none of the CVRF studied was associated with dementia. Similar frequencies of hypertension were seen in MCI and dementia (62 *vs.* 66%, respectively). The same smoking habit frequency was found in MCI compared to dementia (21%). Zero percent smokers were found in the VaD group and the highest frequency existed in DLB (40% smokers).

HDL levels were normal for all the different subtypes of dementia except DLB and PDD, which presented with lower levels (36 ± 22 mg/dL and 47 ± 13 mg/dL, respectively). Elevated LDL levels were found in AD (136 ± 48 mg/dL). Overall dementia presented with general abnormal triglycerides levels (171 ± 59 mg/dL).

Regarding the clinical component according to FRS, no significant association was found with dementia compared to MCI (frequencies of 64% and 63%, respectively). When studying the different types of cognitive impairment separately, PDD showed the highest frequency (92%) followed by VaD (67%), MCI (63%), DLB (60%) and AD (53.6%).

Related to the presence of PVD this showed the highest frequency within the VaD group (20%) and no significant differences were observed between MCI (5%) and overall dementia (7%). The dementia group presented with higher frequency (14 *vs.* 10% in MCI) of CAD, and similar frequencies were seen in AD, VaD, PDD (13, 20 and 22% respectively). MCI patients had more prior strokes than dementia patients (37 *vs.* 26%). When ischemic lesions were examined according to Hachinski ischemic scale, VaD had the highest score (6 ± 5 total score).

Parkinsonism Features

The presence of extrapyramidal signs (EPS) was measured with UPDRS III (motor subscale) test. In our sample, 17 patients presented with EPS, corresponding to all patients with PDD and DLB. UPDRS III scores were higher in PDD than in MCI (mean values of 37 *vs.* 9 in a 0–108 scale).

Cognitive Test Function and Neuropsychological Battery

Our population of probable dementia patients did not show significant differences regarding MMSE scores among dementia subtypes (mean MMSE score for probable dementia and MCI was 21 and 25, respectively).

A significant association was found between dementia and the global neuropsychological function, measured as a summary of the different affected areas ($p = 0.025$).

When we analyzed each neuropsychological area separately, patients with overall dementia (regardless of dementia subtype) had a higher frequency of affectation of the orientation domain compared to those with MCI (35% in MCI and 58% in dementia,

TABLE 3 | Subject's demographic characteristics, CVRF, results of neurological, neuropsychological and neuroimaging examination in different dementia subtypes and in MCI patients.

N (%)	AD	VaD	PDD	LBD	MCI
Vascular component	7 (23)	5 (83)	2 (17)	0	14 (28)
EPS	0	0	12 (100)	6 (100)	0 (0)
Hypertension	18 (67)	4 (80)	8 (80)	1 (17)	29 (62)
Dyslipidaemia	9 (33)	2 (40)	4 (40)	2 (33)	16 (34)
Diabetes mellitus	6 (22)	2 (40)	4 (40)	3 (50)	12 (26)
Smoking or ex-smoker	6 (22)	0	2 (20)	2 (33)	10 (21)
PVD	1 (4)	1 (20)	1 (11)	0	2 (5)
CAD	3 (13)	1 (20)	2 (22)	0	4 (10)
Prior stroke	5 (21)	3 (60)	2 (22)	1 (17)	15 (37)
Total cholesterol	205 ± 49	165 ± 39	172 ± 34	186 ± 62	194 ± 4
HDL cholesterol	56 ± 17	66 ± 30	36 ± 22	47 ± 14	50 ± 18
LDL cholesterol	136 ± 48	83 ± 22	82 ± 56	74	108 ± 63
Triglycerides	144 ± 65	84 ± 31	97 ± 46	117 ± 68	137 ± 100
HACHINSKI	4 ± 3	6 ± 5	5 ± 3	2 ± 2	4 ± 4
GDS *fast*	4 ± 1	NA	4 ± 1	NA	3 ± 1
MMSE	22 ± 5	22 ± 6	19 ± 3	19 ± 6	25 ± 4
UPDRS-III *motor sub-scale*	NA	NA	38 ± 17	33 ± 4	9 ± 9
WSTS	0.6 ± 0.5	0.7 ± 0.6	0.8 ± 0.5	0.3 ± 0.4	0.5 ± 0.4
^{123}I-FP-CIT SPECT lower uptake	3 (23)	0 (0)	7 (78)	4 (80)	7 (21)

Numbers and percentage are presented.

$p < 0.05$). Speech was also more affected in dementia (16% in MCI and 39% in dementia, $p < 0.05$) and gnosis alterations was not found in MCI (0%) while 13% of patients with dementia presented with gnosis alterations ($p < 0.05$). No significant differences were found in relation to the other tested functions (memory, working memory, attention, praxis).

Association Between Vascular Component and WSTS

We used the WSTS to quantify the vascular lesions observed either in MRI or CT and then studied their association with the qualitatively established clinical vascular component.

An association was found between the presenting clinical vascular component according to FRS and WSTS calculated using MRI and CT images. Patients presenting with a clinical vascular component showed a higher mean WSTS (mean WSTS 0.7 *vs.* 0.4, $p < 0.05$ respectively).

We also found significant association regarding frontal, basal ganglia, infratentorial and Wahlund Scores with vascular component according to FRS ($p < 0.05$).

Association Between WSTS and Clinical Diagnoses: Mixed AD has Higher WSTS than Other Dementia Types or MCI

One of our aims was to study the contribution of the clinical vascular component towards brain damage and dementia. Hence, after seeing association between clinical vascular component according to FRS and WSTS, we wanted to look at the association between having a high WSTS and the clinical diagnoses of either dementia or MCI. Although not being statistically significant, the highest mean WSTS was found in the PDD group of patients. Moreover, when AD patients with clinical vascular component (mixed AD, 7/31 patients) were separated from the pure AD they appeared to have the highest WSTS. In contrary, pure AD showed a lower WSTS, even lower than that observed in MCI (**Figure 2**).

Association between area-specific WSTS and clinical diagnosis was only found in infratentorial WSTS, which is linked to PDD ($p < 0.05$).

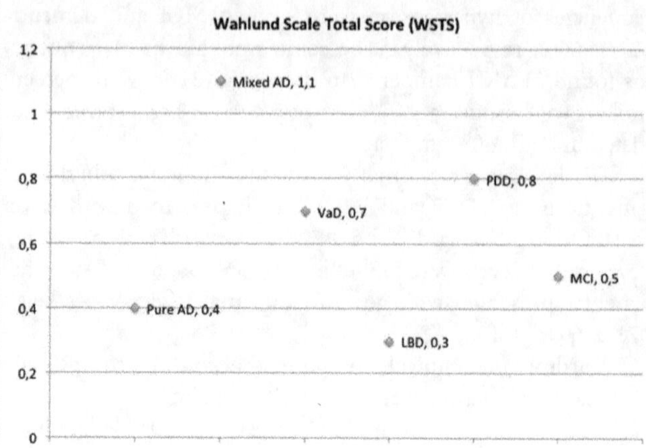

FIGURE 2 | Mean values of wahlund scale total score (WSTS) measured on MRI/CT for each patient group. AD patients with clinical vascular component (mixed AD) have the highest score, followed by VaD and PDD. DLB showed the lowest score, while mild cognitive impairment (MCI) and pure AD presented with comparable values.

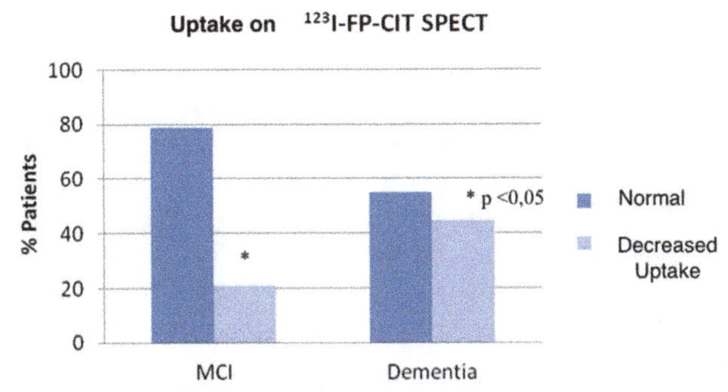

FIGURE 3 | Dopaminergic uptake distribution observed on ^{123}I-FP-CIT SPECT for MCI and dementia group.

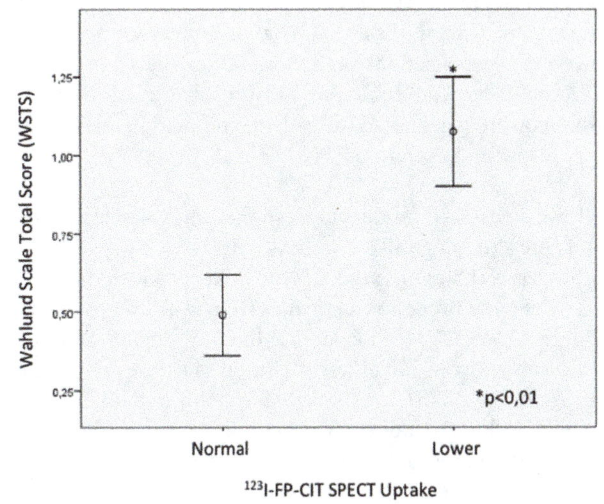

FIGURE 4 | Association between WSTS and abnormal dopaminergic uptake in ^{123}I-FP-CIT SPECT (p < 0.01).

Association Between Clinical Diagnoses and Uptake in ^{123}I-FP-CIT SPECT

^{123}I-FP-CIT SPECT was available in 33 MCI and 31 dementia patients (13/31 AD, 4/6 VaD, 9/12 PDD, 5/6 LBD, respectively), a total of 61% of studied population. A significantly higher frequency of decreased uptake in ^{123}I-FP-CIT SPECT was found in patients with dementia compared to MCI (21% patients with decreased uptake in MCI *vs.* 45% patients in dementia group, $p < 0.05$; **Figure 3**; **Table 2**). As expected, patients with Parkinsonism (DLB and PDD) showed the highest frequency of decreased dopaminergic uptake (80% in DLB and 78% in PDD; **Table 3**).

Association Between WSTS and Dopaminergic Uptake in ^{123}I-FP-CIT SPECT

A significant association was found between dopaminergic uptake seen on ^{123}I-FP-CIT SPECT and the vascular component quantified using WSTS ($p < 0.01$; **Figure 4**). Thus, patients presenting higher WSTS more frequently showed an abnormal ^{123}I-FP-CIT SPECT image ($p < 0.01$; **Figure 5**).

Nevertheless, no significant association was found between an abnormal ^{123}I-FP CIT SPECT image and the vascular component according to FRS.

No Association Between Dopaminergic Uptake ^{123}I-FP-CIT SPECT nor WSTS and Neuropsychological Function

In relation to the association between dopaminergic uptake observed in ^{123}I-FP-CIT SPECT and the neuropsychological function examined by an ordinary test battery. No significant results have been obtained when studying each neusopsychological function separately, and neither with the overall performance on neuropsycological tests. No relationship was found between neuropsychological function and the clinical vascular component measured using WSTS.

Discussion

In this study we aimed to analyze the contribution of vascular component (assessed clinically and on neuroimaging) to clinical diagnoses of the common types of dementia and MCI. We tested the potential application of ^{123}I-CIT-SPECT imaging in dementia, particularly when the vascular component is present. We looked at the association between having vascular component and presenting an abnormal ^{123}I-CIT-SPECT. Finally, we studied the association between neuropsychological function and vascular component or abnormal ^{123}I-CIT-SPECT. A better understanding of the association between these variables could help providing new tools for a more accurate and early diagnoses of common types of dementia.

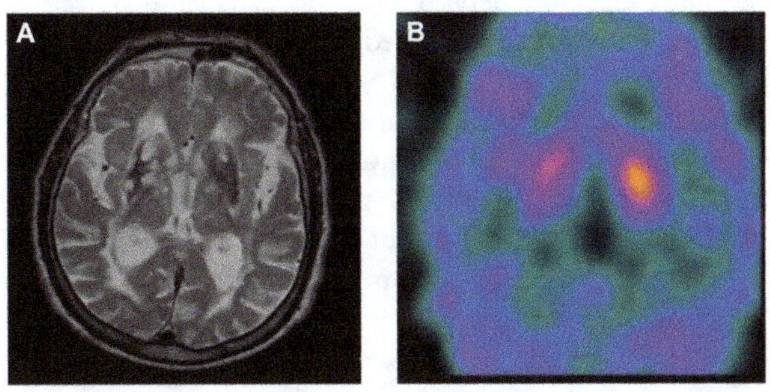

FIGURE 5 | MRI and ^{123}I-FP-CIT SPECT Images from a representative patient to show relation existing between abnormal MRI and uptake on ^{123}I-FP-CIT SPECT. (A) MRI T2-potentiated showing diffuse cerebral atrophy with increased size and depth of cerebral grooves and ventricular supratentorial enlargement. Multiple lacunar chronic infarctions, some of those were hemeorrhagic in the lenticular and head of caudate nuclei. Chronic periventricular ischemia leucoencephalopaty and focal hyperintensities in parietal frontal and temporal bilateral white matter WSTS = 1.6.
(B) ^{123}I-FP-CIT SPECT from the same subject showing detectable decreased uptake in right putamen.

Our results showed an association between clinical vascular component according to FRS and quantification of the vascular component using WSTS on MRI and CT images. These results are in line with what would be expected and confirm the reliability of the quantification of WMHs lesions using Wahlund scale in our population (Wahlund et al., 2001). Further, it confirms that it was a well selected population. The association between WMHs for each brain area separately was significantly different in frontal, basal ganglia and infratentorial areas. However, no association was found within the temporal area, which actually would be the most likely, considering that most frequent types of AD-like dementia are characterized by temporo-parietal alterations (Fischer et al., 1990; Jabłoński et al., 2011; Marchesi, 2011).

It was observed in previous studies that vascular lesions contribute to cognitive decline. It was suggested that cerebrovascular lesions induce amyloid deposition perhaps accelerating the process of dementia (Garcia-Alloza et al., 2011; Pluta et al., 2013). Although, we did not find a significant association between the different clinical diagnoses of cognitive impairment and WSTS, we have observed a notable frequency of the vascular component on neuroimaging within the AD group. The later group probably was formed by mixed AD population. These findings confirmed the fact that vascular accident history contributes to the etiology and/or progression of dementia. Patients with mixed AD and PDD had a high WSTS, even higher than in patients with VaD. Although not being statistically significant, these results are in line with the association between AD or PDD and WMHs. No conclusions can be drawn related to overall dementia and MCI WSTS.

In relation to the particular areas affected by ischemic lesions and each diagnoses, we only found a significant association relating to the infratentorial region in PDD. This could be explained by the fact that in our PDD group there was a high frequency of VP, as this group presented with a high mean of WSTS (0.8 ± 0.5) with 92% frequency of clinical vascular component according to FRS. Further, the non-association of VaD and any specific brain region could be due to a diffuse pattern of this type of dementia, unusual low FRS of this group and/or the few number of patients in this group.

Furthermore, we evaluated the potential utility of ^{123}I-FP-CIT SPECT as a diagnostic tool to discriminate dementia from MCI, and differentiate among different dementia types, emphasizing on dementia with a vascular component. Our study showed that ^{123}I-FP-CIT SPECT is a useful tool to discriminate MCI from overall dementia subtypes. This is a promising observation, since it is a major clinical priority to be able to more accurately confirm dementia diagnoses and predict MCI progression. However, in our study we could not demonstrate the utility of ^{123}I-FP-CIT SPECT to discriminate among different dementia types.

As expected, most of patients with PDD and all but one of those with LBD showed an abnormal ^{123}I-FP-CIT SPECT. Nevertheless, three patients with PD did not show an abnormal ^{123}I-FP-CIT SPECT, suggestive of possible iatrogenic Parkinsonism. We hypothesized that patients with VaD could show an abnormal ^{123}I-FP-CIT SPECT if ischemic lesions affected directly or indirectly the dopaminergic control of cortical-striatal circuits. This was not seen in our study probably because of the small number of patients with VaD (n = 6), none of which showed abnormal ^{123}I-FP-CIT SPECT.

Once we had demonstrated the utility of ^{123}I-FP-CIT SPECT to differentiate dementia *vs.* MCI, we then studied the association between abnormal ^{123}I-FP-CIT SPECT and presence of the vascular component clinically assessed with the FRS and quantified on neuroimaging using WSTS. An association between the vascular component according to FRS and abnormal ^{123}I-FP-CIT SPECT was not found, but the association between dopaminergic function and WSTS was statistically significant. Thus, our results showed that ^{123}I-FP-CIT SPECT discriminates between vascular risk factors load and vascular component quantified using WSTS and that neuroimaging of vascular lesions is indeed important. Wahlund scale criteria thus being more accurate in analysing the grade of vascular component observable than classical FRS. It is interesting that WSTS, as a global brain WMHs score, rather than basal ganglia sub-score, is associated with an abnormal ^{123}I-FP-CIT SPECT imaging. This suggests that this technique can reflect vascular alterations other than those affecting basal ganglia. The association observed between abnormal ^{123}I-FP-CIT SPECT and the vascular component quantified by WSTS could be justified because dementia patients have a significantly higher frequency of abnormal ^{123}I-FP-CIT SPECT, in particular, the PDD group seems to be the responsible for this finding. PDD and LBD had the highest frequency of abnormal ^{123}I-FP-CIT SPECT and PDD showed the second highest WSTS after mixed AD. Moreover, AD showed a high vascular contribution (high mean WSTS) and the frequency of abnormal ^{123}I-FP-CIT SPECT was higher (23%) than expected according to previous reports that confirm the utility of ^{123}I-FP-CIT SPECT in the differentiation of PDD/LBD from AD (O'Brien et al., 2009; Cummings et al., 2011). Some studies reported that approximately 5–10% of ^{123}I-FP-CIT SPECT in patients with clinical dementia showed intermediate scans. Thus, abnormal images within AD group may represent mixed LBD/AD disease (Kemp and Holmes, 2007).

In conclusion, our study supports the utility of ^{123}I-FP-CIT SPECT to detect abnormal dopaminergic function in those patients that showed a high WSTS corresponding to a high grade of generalized ischemic brain lesions. This decrease uptake could be due to the loss of dopaminergic innervation in the striatum as a consequence of ischemia or the alteration of dopaminergic system because of abnormal cell functionality, characteristic of oxidative stress that could precede cell death in dementia or MCI (Kim et al., 2012).

There is growing evidence demonstrating that the vascular component has an active role in dementia mechanisms and its progress and is probably involved in most dementia subtypes which share similar physiopathological features (Iadecola and Gorelick, 2003). Therefore, it is not surprising that an abnormal ^{123}I-FP-CIT SPECT is associated with cerebrovascular lesions related to dementia, but cannot differentiate among dementia subtypes that have an important vascular component, such as mixed AD, VaD or VP.

It is known that ^{123}I-FP-CIT SPECT is useful to discriminate AD from PDD/LBD, and hence to distinguish patients in whom dopaminergic therapy may be beneficial (Varrone and Halldin, 2010; Cummings et al., 2011). Therefore, an abnormal scan suggests underlying neurodegeneration, supportive of a diagnosis of Parkinson's disease, or atypical parkinsonism, LBD and even VP if the nigrostriatal system is affected. Conversely, a normal dopaminergic imaging supports an alternative diagnosis such as AD, essential tremor or iatrogenic parkinsonism. In our study, we demonstrated that ^{123}I-FP-CIT SPECT could be also useful to confirm diagnosis of dementia among those patients with MCI.

Recent studies have demonstrated a 6–8% decline of DAT per decade (Erixon-Lindroth et al., 2005), suggesting DAT binding is a powerful mediator of age-related cognitive changes. These findings should be taken under consideration when designing and interpreting *in vivo* imaging studies.

Finally, this study did not find a significant association between neuropsychological function and abnormal ^{123}I-FP-CIT SPECT nor high WSTS. This suggests that neither measurement of vascular component score nor the functionality of dopaminergic system can detect degree of cognitive decline in our sample.

Limitations

It is important to note that patients with VaD in our sample had lower FRS scores than expected; the distribution of CVRF was low and they did not appear to have the highest WSTS-being lower than those observed in AD, where cholesterol levels seemed to be a risk factor to develop AD. This fact could be due to the small number of patients in our sample, especially in the VaD group. Another limitation of our study was the use of clinical diagnosis as the gold standard, which may not always be accurate.

Further studies are needed to better elucidate the potential role of dopaminergic transporter imaging on detecting vascular brain damage and its association with clinical dementia.

Conclusion

In agreement with previous reports ^{123}I-FP-CIT SPECT imaging is abnormal in patients with extrapyramidal signs (PDD and DLB). Interestingly, around 20% of patients with pure AD or MCI had abnormal SPECT. The new finding is that on initial visit ^{123}I-FP-CIT SPECT can differentiate severity in terms of classification between MCI and dementia, thus helping establish more accurately initial diagnosis and maybe providing a useful tool to discriminate MCI from overall dementia at clinical practice. Furthermore, in our sample, the vascular contribution is shown to be relevant and present among AD and PDD patients, in line with previously reported data and in addition, there is a good correlation between uptake on ^{123}I-FP-CIT SPECT and ischemic score on MRI or CT.

Author Contributions

All authors contributed to work. Marta Milà and Marina Garriga participated in patients selection, screening and follow up. Manzoor Mir and Raid Al-Baradie helped with analysis of data, Sonia Huertas, Cesar Castejon, Miguel Aguilar, Jerzy Krupinski evaluated patients, helped with manuscript, Laura Casas and Dolors Badenes performed neuropsychological tests. Marta Milà, Raid Al-Baradie, Manzoor Mir analyzed molecular images, Marta Milà and Marina Garriga quantified MRIs. All authors contributed to the final version of the manuscript.

Acknowledgments

This work was supported by SATSC 2014-03, Stroke-Chair grant form Saudi Arabia and unrestricted grant from GE Healthcare, beca Fundació Mútua Terrassa to JK.

References

Albanese, E., Banerjee, S., Dhanasiri, S., Fernandez, J. L., Ferri, C., Knapp, M., et al. (2007). *A Report to the Alzheimer's Society on the Prevalence and Ecnonomic Cost of Dementia in the UK.* Dementia UK: King's College London and London School of Economics.

Bouwmans, A. E., Vlaar, A. M., Mess, W. H., Kessels, A., and Weber, W. E. (2013). Specificity and sensitivity of transcranial sonography of the substantia nigra in the diagnosis of Parkinson's disease: prospective cohort study in 196 patients. *BMJ Open* 3:e002613. doi: 10.1136/bmjopen-2013-002613

Breteler, M. M. (2000). Vascular risk factors for Alzheimer's disease: an epidemiologic perspective. *Neurobiol. Aging* 21, 153–160. doi: 10.1016/S0197-4580(99)00110-4

Brun, A., and Englund, E. (1986). Brain changes in dementia of Alzheimer's type relevant to new imaging diagnostic methods. *Prog. Neuropsychopharmacol. Biol. Psychiatry* 10, 297–308. doi: 10.1016/0278-5846(86)90009-6

Carmichael, O., Schwarz, C., Drucker, D., Fletcher, E., Harvey, D., Beckett, L., et al. (2010). Longitudinal changes in white matter disease and cognition in the first year of the Alzheimer disease neuroimaging initiative. *Arch. Neurol.* 67, 1370–1378. doi: 10.1001/archneurol.2010.284

Chen, Y. J., Deutsch, G., Satya, R., Liu, H. G., and Mountz, J. M. (2013). A semi-quantitative method for correlating brain disease groups with normal controls using SPECT: Alzheimer's disease versus vascular dementia. *Comput. Med. Imaging Graph.* 37, 40–47. doi: 10.1016/j.compmedimag.2012.11.001

Chui, H. C., and Ramirez-Gomez, L. (2015). Clinical and imaging features of mixed Alzheimer and vascular pathologies. *Alzheimers Res. Ther.* 7:21. doi: 10.1186/s13195-015-0104-7

Cummings, J. L., Henchcliffe, C., Schaier, S., Simuni, T., Waxman, A., and Kemp, P. (2011). The role of dopaminergic imaging in patients with symptoms of dopaminergic system neurodegeneration. *Brain* 134(Pt. 11), 3146–3166. doi: 10.1093/brain/awr177

D'Agostino, R. B. Sr., Vasan, R. S., Pencina, M. J., Wolf, P. A., Cobain, M., Massaro, J. M., et al. (2008). General cardiovascular risk profile for use in primary care: the Framingham heart study. *Circulation* 117, 743–753. doi: 10.1161/CIRCULATIONAHA.107.699579

DeCarli, C., Murphy, D. G., Tranh, M., Grady, C. L., Haxby, J. V., Gillette, J. A., et al. (1995). The effect of white matter hyperintensity volume on brain structure, cognitive performance and cerebral metabolism of glucose in 51 healthy adults. *Neurology* 45, 2077–2084. doi: 10.1212/wnl.45.11.2077

de Souza, L. C., Lehéricy, S., Dubois, B., Stella, F., and Sarazin, M. (2012). Neuroimaging in dementias. *Curr. Opin. Psychiatry* 25, 473–479. doi: 10.1097/YCO.0b013e328357b9ab

Eckerström, C., Olsson, E., Klasson, N., Bjerke, M., Göthlin, M., Jonsson, M., et al. (2011). High white matter lesion load is associated with hippocampal atrophy in mild cognitive impairment. *Dement. Geriatr. Cogn. Disord.* 31, 132–138. doi: 10.1159/000323014

Elias, M. F., Sullivan, L. M., D'Agostino, R. B., Elias, P. K., Beiser, A., Au, R., et al. (2004). Framingham stroke risk profile and lowered cognitive performance. *Stroke* 35, 404–409. doi: 10.1161/01.str.0000103141.82869.77

Erixon-Lindroth, N., Farde, L., Wahlin, T. B., Sovago, J., Halldin, C., and Bäckman, L. (2005). The role of the striatal dopamine transporter in cognitive aging. *Psychiatry Res.* 138, 1–12. doi: 10.1016/j.pscychresns.2004.09.005

Eshuis, S. A., Maguire, R. P., Leenders, K. L., Jonkman, S., and Jager, P. L. (2006). Comparison of FP-CIT SPECT with F-DOPA PET in patients with de novo and advanced Parkinson's disease. *Eur. J. Nucl. Med. Mol. Imaging* 33, 200–209. doi: 10.1007/s00259-005-1904-y

Fischer, V. W., Siddiqi, A., and Yusufaly, Y. (1990). Altered angioarchitecture in selected areas of brains with Alzheimer's disease. *Acta Neuropathol.* 79, 672–679. doi: 10.1007/bf00294246

Garcia-Alloza, M., Gregory, J., Kuchibhotla, K. V., Fine, S., Wei, Y., Ayata, C., et al. (2011). Cerebrovascular lesions induce transient β-amyloid deposition. *Brain* 134(Pt 12), 3697–3707. doi: 10.1093/brain/awr300

García Vicente, A. M., Vaamonde Cano, J., Soriano Castrejón, A., Martínez Delgado, C., Talavera Rubio, P., Poblete García, V. M., et al. (2005). Utility of 123-I ioflupane SPECT in the assessment of patients with Parkinsonian syndrome and cerebral vasculopathy. *Rev. Esp. Med. Nucl.* 24, 392–403. doi: 10.1016/S0212-6982(05)74184-7

Garibotto, V., Montandon, M. L., Viaud, C. T., Allaoua, M., Assal, F., Burkhard, P. R., et al. (2013). Regions of interest-based discriminant analysis of DaTSCAN SPECT and FDG-PET for the classification of dementia. *Clin. Nucl. Med.* 38, e112–e117. doi: 10.1097/rlu.0b013e318279b991

Gerschlager, W., Bencsits, G., Pirker, W., Bloem, B. R., Asenbaum, S., Prayer, D., et al. (2002). ^{123}Ibeta-CIT SPECT distinguishes vascular parkinsonism from Parkinson's disease. *Mov. Disord.* 17, 518–523. doi: 10.1002/mds.10092

Herholz, K. (2012). Use of FDG PET as an imaging biomarker in clinical trials of Alzheimer's disease. *Biomark. Med.* 6, 431–439. doi: 10.2217/bmm.12.51

Iadecola, C. (2010). The overlap between neurodegenerative and vascular factors in the pathogenesis of dementia. *Acta Neuropathol.* 120, 287–296. doi: 10.1007/s00401-010-0718-6

Iadecola, C., and Gorelick, P. B. (2003). Converging pathogenic mechanisms in vascular and neurodegenerative dementia. *Stroke* 34, 335–337. doi: 10.1161/01.str.0000054050.51530.76

Jabłoński, M., Maciejewski, R., Januszewski, S., Ułamek, M., and Pluta, R. (2011). One year follow up in ischemic brain injury and the role of Alzheimer factors. *Physiol. Res.* 60(Suppl. 1), S113–S119.

Jeerakathil, T., Wolf, P. A., Beiser, A., Massaro, J., Seshadri, S., D'Agostino, R. B., et al. (2004). Stroke risk profile predicts white matter hyperintensity volume: the Framingham study. *Stroke* 35, 1857–1861. doi: 10.1161/01.str.0000135226.53499.85

Kalaria, R. N. (2012). Risk factors and neurodegenerative mechanisms in stroke related dementia. *Panminerva Med.* 54, 139–148.

Kemp, P. M., and Holmes, C. (2007). Imaging in dementia with Lewy bodies: a review. *Nucl. Med. Commun.* 28, 511–519. Review. doi: 10.1097/mnm.0b013e3281e20a12

Kim, H. A., Miller, A. A., Drummond, G. R., Thrift, A. G., Arumugam, T. V., Phan, T. G., et al. (2012). Vascular cognitive impairment and Alzheimer's disease: role of cerebral hypoperfusion and oxidative stress. *Naunyn Schmiedebergs Arch. Pharmacol.* 385, 953–959. doi: 10.1007/s00210-012-0790-7

Leibson, C. L., Rocca, W. A., Hanson, V. A., Cha, R., Kokmen, E., O'Brien, P. C., et al. (1997). The risk of dementia among persons with diabetes mellitus: a population-based cohort study. *Ann. N Y Acad. Sci.* 826, 422–427. doi: 10.1111/j.1749-6632.1997.tb48496.x

Lorberboym, M., Djaldetti, R., Melamed, E., Sadeh, M., and Lampl, Y. (2004). ^{123}I-FP-CIT SPECT imaging of dopamine transporters in patients with cerebrovascular disease and clinical diagnosis of vascular parkinsonism. *J. Nucl. Med.* 45, 1688–1693.

Marchesi, V. T. (2011). Alzheimer's dementia begins as a disease of small blood vessels, damaged by oxidative-induced inflammation and dysregulated amyloid metabolism: implications for early detection and therapy. *FASEB J.* 25, 5–13. doi: 10.1096/fj.11-0102ufm

Marshall, V., and Grosset, D. (2003). Role of dopamine transporter imaging in routine clinical practice. *Mov. Disord.* 18, 1415–1423. doi: 10.1002/mds.10592

McKeith, I. G., Dickson, D. W., Lowe, J., Emre, M., O'Brien, J. T., Feldman, H., et al. (2005). Diagnosis and management of dementia with Lewy bodies: third report of the DLB consortium. *Neurology* 65, 1863–1872. doi: 10.1212/01.wnl.0000187889.17253.b1

Mills, S., Cain, J., Purandare, N., and Jackson, A. (2007). Biomarkers of cerebrovascular disease in dementia. *Br. J. Radiol.* 80 Spec. No. 2, S128–S145. doi: 10.1259/bjr/79217686

Niwa, K., Kazama, K., Younkin, L., Younkin, S. G., Carlson, G. A., and Iadecola, C. (2002). Cerebrovascular autoregulation is profoundly impaired in mice overexpressing amyloid precursor protein. *Am. J. Physiol. Heart Circ. Physiol.* 283, H315–H323. doi: 10.1152/ajpheart.00022.2002

O'Brien, J. T., McKeith, I. G., Walker, Z., Tatsch, K., Booij, J., Darcourt, J., et al. (2009). Diagnostic accuracy of ^{123}I-FP-CIT SPECT in possible dementia with Lewy bodies. *Br. J. Psychiatry* 194, 34–39. doi: 10.1192/bjp.bp.108.052050

Ott, A., Breteler, M. M., de Bruyne, M. C., van Harskamp, F., Grobbee, D. E., and Hofman, A. (1997). Atrial fibrillation and dementia in a population-based study. The Rotterdam study. *Stroke* 28, 316–321. doi: 10.1161/01.str.28.2.316

Pendlebury, S. T., and Rothwell, P. M. (2009). Prevalence, incidence and factors associated with pre-stroke and post-stroke dementia: a systematic review and meta-analysis. *Lancet Neurol.* 8, 1006–1018. doi: 10.1016/s1474-4422(09)70236-4

Pluta, R., Furmaga-Jabłońska, W., Maciejewski, R., Ułamek-Kozioł, M., and Jabłoński, M. (2013). Brain ischemia activates β- and γ-secretase cleavage of amyloid precursor protein: significance in sporadic Alzheimer's disease. *Mol. Neurobiol.* 47, 425–434. doi: 10.1007/s12035-012-8360-z

Purnell, C., Gao, S., Callahan, C. M., and Hendrie, H. C. (2009). Cardiovascular risk factors and incident Alzheimer disease: a systematic review of the literature. *Alzheimer Dis. Assoc. Disord.* 23, 1–10. doi: 10.1097/WAD.0b013e318187541c

Scheltens, P., Barkhof, F., Valk, J., Algra, P. R., van der Hoop, R. G., Nauta, J., et al. (1992). White matter lesions on magnetic resonance imaging in clinically diagnosed Alzheimer's disease. Evidence for heterogeneity. *Brain* 115(Pt. 3), 735–748. doi: 10.1093/brain/115.3.735

Skoog, I., Lernfelt, B., Landahl, S., Palmertz, B., Andreasson, L. A., Nilsson, L., et al. (1996). 15-year longitudinal study of blood pressure and dementia. *Lancet* 347, 1141–1145. doi: 10.1016/s0140-6736(96)90608-x

Sörös, P., Whitehead, S., Spence, J. D., and Hachinski, V. (2013). Antihypertensive treatment can prevent stroke and cognitive decline. *Nat. Rev. Neurol.* 9, 174–178. doi: 10.1038/nrneurol.2012.255

Tanimukai, H., Imaizumi, K., Kudo, T., Katayama, T., Tsuda, M., Takagi, T., et al. (1998). Alzheimer-associated presenilin-1 gene is induced in gerbil hippocampus after transient ischemia. *Brain Res. Mol. Brain Res.* 54, 212–218. doi: 10.1016/s0169-328x(97)00337-9

Tatemichi, T. K., Paik, M., Bagiella, E., Desmond, D. W., Stern, Y., Sano, M., et al. (1994). Risk of dementia after stroke in a hospitalized cohort: results of a longitudinal study. *Neurology* 44, 1885–1891. doi: 10.1212/wnl.44.10.1885

Tolosa, E., Borght, T. V., Moreno, E., and DaTSCAN Clinically Uncertain Parkinsonian Syndromes Study Group. (2007). Accuracy of DaTSCAN (^{123}I-Ioflupane) SPECT in diagnosis of patients with clinically uncertain parkinsonism: 2-year follow-up of an open-label study. *Mov. Disord.* 22, 2346–2351. doi: 10.1002/mds.21710

Vanitallie, T. B. (2013). Preclinical sporadic Alzheimer's disease: target for personalized diagnosis and preventive intervention. *Metabolism* 62(Suppl. 1), S30–S33. doi: 10.1016/j.metabol.2012.08.024

Varrone, A., and Halldin, C. (2010). Molecular imaging of the dopamine transporter. *J. Nucl. Med.* 51, 1331–1334. doi: 10.2967/jnumed.109.065656

Visser, P. J., Wolf, H., Frisoni, G., and Gertz, H. J. (2012). Disclosure of Alzheimer's disease biomarker status in subjects with mild cognitive impairment. *Biomark. Med.* 6, 365–368. doi: 10.2217/bmm.12.58

Wahlund, L. O., Barkhof, F., Fazekas, F., Bronge, L., Augustin, M., Sjögre, M., et al. (2001). A new rating scale for age-related white matter changes applicable to MRI and CT. *Stroke* 32, 1318–1322. doi: 10.1161/01.STR.32.6.1318

Weng, Y. H., Yen, T. C., Chen, M. C., Kao, P. F., Tzen, K. Y., Chen, R. S., et al. (2004). Sensitivity and specificity of 99mTc-TRODAT-1 SPECT imaging in differentiating patients with idiopathic Parkinson's disease from healthy subjects. *J. Nucl. Med.* 45, 393–401.

Wimo, A., Jönsson, L., Bond, J., Prince, M., Winblad, B., and Alzheimer Disease International. (2013). The worldwide economic impact of dementia 2010. *Alzheimers Dement.* 9, 1–11.e3. doi: 10.1016/j.jalz.2012.11.006

Wolf, P. A., D'Agostino, R. B., Belanger, A. J., and Kannel, W. B. (1991). Probability of stroke: a risk profile from the Framingham study. *Stroke* 22, 312–318. doi: 10.1161/01.str.22.3.312

21

Comparison of Haptic Guidance and Error Amplification Robotic Trainings for the Learning of a Timing-Based Motor Task by Healthy Seniors

*Amy E. Bouchard, Hélène Corriveau and Marie-Hélène Milot**

Centre de Recherche sur le Vieillissement, Université de Sherbrooke, Sherbrooke, QC, Canada

Edited by:
Mikhail Lebedev, Duke University, USA

Reviewed by:
Herbert Heuer, Leibniz Research Centre for Working Environment and Human Factors, Germany
Andrea Cristina De Lima-Pardini, University of São Paulo, Brazil
Jon Doan, University of Lethbridge, Canada

***Correspondence:**
Marie-Helene Milot, Centre de Recherche sur le Vieillissement, Université de Sherbrooke, 1036 Belvédère sud, Sherbrooke, QC J1H 4C4, Canada
marie-helene.milot@usherbrooke.ca

With age, a decline in the temporal aspect of movement is observed such as a longer movement execution time and a decreased timing accuracy. Robotic training can represent an interesting approach to help improve movement timing among the elderly. Two types of robotic training—haptic guidance (HG; demonstrating the correct movement for a better movement planning and improved execution of movement) and error amplification (EA; exaggerating movement errors to have a more rapid and complete learning) have been positively used in young healthy subjects to boost timing accuracy. For healthy seniors, only HG training has been used so far where significant and positive timing gains have been obtained. The goal of the study was to evaluate and compare the impact of both HG and EA robotic trainings on the improvement of seniors' movement timing. Thirty-two healthy seniors (mean age 68 ± 4 years) learned to play a pinball-like game by triggering a one-degree-of-freedom hand robot at the proper time to make a flipper move and direct a falling ball toward a randomly positioned target. During HG and EA robotic trainings, the subjects' timing errors were decreased and increased, respectively, based on the subjects' timing errors in initiating a movement. Results showed that only HG training benefited learning, but the improvement did not generalize to untrained targets. Also, age had no influence on the efficacy of HG robotic training, meaning that the oldest subjects did not benefit more from HG training than the younger senior subjects. Using HG to teach the correct timing of movement seems to be a good strategy to improve motor learning for the elderly as for younger people. However, more studies are needed to assess the long-term impact of HG robotic training on improvement in movement timing.

Keywords: haptic guidance, error amplification, timing, aging, learning

Introduction

Movements are made up of spatial (e.g., direction of movement) and temporal (e.g., reaction time and timing of muscle activation) aspects, which can be controlled separately depending on the task that is to be performed (Georgopoulos, 2002). The temporal aspect of movement plays an important role in the accomplishment of many everyday activities like playing tennis (Marchal-Crespo et al., 2013) or using a motorized wheelchair (Marchal Crespo and Reinkensmeyer, 2008). With age, and as compared to younger individuals, a decline in the temporal aspect of movement occurs, translating into a slowing of internalized timing processes, as highlighted by the synchronization-continuation paradigm, and by deficits in temporal predictions for accurate movement production (Carnahan et al., 1996; Wishart et al., 2000; McAuley et al., 2006; van Dijk et al., 2007; Marchal-Crespo et al., 2010; Seidler et al., 2010; Pietschmann et al., 2011; Turgeon and Wing, 2012; Hoogendam et al., 2014), negatively impacting daily activities. Explanations for this age-related timing deficit may be explained by changes in the nervous system (Seidler et al., 2010). For example, a decrease in the nigrostriatal region's dopamine (DA) functioning, important for motor learning, is observed with age (van Dijk et al., 2007). In fact, van Dijk et al. (2007) found that the availability of the DA transporters (DAT) was negatively correlated ($r = -0.40$) with older individuals' reaction times; in other words, the slower the reaction time, the higher the deficiency in DAT. Other studies have also found significant relations between decreased functional performance found with aging and decreased fractional anisotropy, a measure of fiber density (Zahr et al., 2009), or decreased volume in the cerebellum, which plays an essential role in movement timing (Raz et al., 2005; Seidler et al., 2010). In addition, it is suggested that elders strategically prioritize the spatial aspects of movement over the temporal aspects, in other words favoring a better control of movements over their speed in order to achieve a required task (Seidler-Dobrin et al., 1998).

Despite these drawbacks, seniors can still learn new motor skills (Voelcker-Rehage, 2008), although often at a significantly slower pace (Marchal-Crespo et al., 2010; Pietschmann et al., 2011). The fact that they have the potential for motor learning is important because the elderly population needs to be able to learn new timing tasks like driving a powered wheelchair, or playing sports such as golf in order to maintain a good quality of life as they age (Carnahan et al., 1996; Wishart et al., 2000; Marchal-Crespo et al., 2010). Yet, few studies have attempted to improve elderly movement timing.

One solution is robotic training (Patton and Mussa-Ivaldi, 2004; Marchal Crespo and Reinkensmeyer, 2008; Marchal-Crespo et al., 2010, 2013; Milot et al., 2010; Luttgen and Heuer, 2013). Two emerging types of robotic training, haptic guidance (HG) and error amplification (EA), are increasingly used as effective training methods for improving movement execution in both healthy persons and those having a pathology (Liu et al., 2006; Patton et al., 2006a,b; Cesqui et al., 2008; Marchal Crespo and Reinkensmeyer, 2008; Marchal-Crespo et al., 2010, 2013, 2014; Milot et al., 2010; Luttgen and Heuer, 2013). HG is based on the principle that guiding the person to make the correct movement would provide the nervous system with additional proprioceptive and somatosensory cues to allow for a better planning of movement and thus reducing timing errors and improving movement execution (Marchal-Crespo et al., 2010; Milot et al., 2010; Luttgen and Heuer, 2013). EA, on the other hand, is based on the theory that error is an essential neural signal for motor adaptation (Thoroughman and Shadmehr, 2000), where the nervous system detects and corrects these errors for future movements (Milot et al., 2010). By artificially increasing movement errors, EA training would then allow a faster and more complete learning (Emken and Reinkensmeyer, 2005). In a previous study, we evaluated and compared the immediate impact of HG and EA robotic trainings on movement timing for 20 young healthy participants, while they played a computerized pinball-like game (Milot et al., 2010). The results showed that both EA and HG training were effective in improving timing accuracy so that it was appropriate for hitting a target with the pinball. Moreover, the effectiveness of the robotic trainings was dependent on the participant's initial skill level, where less-skilled participants seemed to benefit more from HG and better-skilled participants from EA. The results of our study further supported studies that used HG or EA robotic trainings, where faster execution times (Feygin et al., 2002; Bluteau et al., 2008) and improved timed movement for the task (Marchal Crespo and Reinkensmeyer, 2008; Luttgen and Heuer, 2013; Marchal-Crespo et al., 2013, 2014) were noted following HG or EA training. However, these studies were conducted on young and healthy individuals. Very few studies have compared the effectiveness of both EA and HG to improve movement timing in the elderly, despite there being a negative impact of aging on movement timing. Only one study by Marchal-Crespo et al. (2010) trained elders with HG on a computerized steering task. The authors found that after receiving HG training, elders improved their timing by straightening their wheel faster after having just coming out of turns.

With respect to the benefits of HG and EA robotic training on the performance of timed movement in young healthy individuals, the goal of the study was to directly compare and evaluate the impact of both types of robotic trainings on improving movement timing accuracy in elders. Since learning can still take place with age (Carnahan et al., 1996; Wishart et al., 2000; Marchal-Crespo et al., 2010; Pietschmann et al., 2011) and following our previous results on young healthy individuals (Milot et al., 2010) which showed that timing error can be improved using HG and EA robotic trainings, we expected both EA and HG to be equally effective in improving seniors' timing errors. However, knowing that there is a decrease in motor skill observed with older age (Hoogendam et al., 2014), we hypothesized that our oldest senior participants would more likely have a poorer task performance and would thus benefit the most from HG, whereas our younger senior participants would not necessarily be bad performers and would therefore benefit more from EA.

Materials and Methods

Participants

Thirty-two healthy participants (10 male; 22 female) between the ages of 61 and 75 (mean age 68 ± 4 years) took part in the study. In order to participate in the study, individuals had to meet the following criteria: (1) be at least 60 years of age, (2) be right-handed [*Edinburgh Handedness Inventory* (Oldfield, 1971)], and (3) be able to flex the right wrist by at least 10° without any pain. The exclusion criteria were: having a cognitive impairment as evaluated by the *Montreal Cognitive Assessment* exam [score < 26 on the Version 7.3 (Gluhm et al., 2013)]; having an active neurological (e.g., stroke) or orthopedic (e.g., fracture) problem in the right upper limb; having a visual problem (e.g., a cataract) that was non-corrected and would prevent the proper viewing of a computer screen. This project was approved by the CSSS-IUGS ethics board and all participants signed the consent form.

Timing Exerciser Orthosis (TEO)

Timing exerciser orthosis (TEO) is a modified version of TAPPER, which was used in a previous study (Milot et al., 2010). TEO is a one degree of freedom robot that allows 10° of wrist flexion of both the left and right hands. It is mounted on an aluminum frame and is mechanically actuated by a Dynamixel MX-106 servomotor (*Robotis Inc*, USA), sampled at 1,000 Hz for the recording of the servomotor's torque and position data. A forearm brace also ensures the participant's comfort and safety. A button, placed on the frame, allows the participants to experience sensory feedback during each trial but pressing the button did not play a role in triggering the sequence of the timing task (see **Figure 1**).

Since the task was time dependent, a photodiode (*BPW21R*, Vishay, Germany), placed at the bottom right corner of the computer screen, was used as a time reference in order to detect the start of the task. This was done by the appearance of a luminous white dot at the bottom right corner of the computer screen, which was read by the photodiode, as a red ball appeared at the top of the computer screen simultaneously. This photodiode and TEO were plugged into a USB-6008 data acquisition card (*National Instruments*, USA), sampled at 5,000 Hz. This acquisition card allowed the synchronization between the photodiode and the servomotor for the timing task.

Pinball Simulation Game

The pinball-like game is similar to the one used in a previous study [for more details see (Milot et al., 2010)]. In sum, the goal of the game was to hit targets to earn as many points as possible. A total of five colored-targets located at specific positions across the computer screen were randomly presented to the participants. A red ball that fell toward a flipper could be seen on the computer screen during each trial. In order to hit a specific target, participants had to activate TEO with the correct timing (with a timing accuracy of 4 ms) so the flipper could rotate and have the ball to bounce upward toward the target. TEO was activated when the participants flexed their wrists at a torque ≥ 0.5 Nm. One out of three feedback messages were provided during each trial, depending on the participant's timing accuracy ("Wow! Just on time!," "Too early! Hit later!," and "Too late! Hit sooner!"). The pinball simulator was created using LabVIEW™ 2013 software.

Haptic Guidance and Error Amplification Algorithms

The algorithms were slightly modified from those that we used in a previous study (Milot et al., 2010). To decrease participants' timing errors during HG, we wanted to delay or speed up the start of the robot when the participants initiated wrist movement too early or too late, respectively. The exact opposite was done to increase errors during EA. More specifically, $t = 0$ was defined as the time in which the ball began to fall toward the flipper. Tbp was defined as the time in which TEO was activated. So:

$$\text{Tbp} = \text{Tip} + \text{Dc} \quad (1)$$

where Tip was the time in which the motor sensors detected the initiation of the participant's wrist flexion and Dc was defined as the programmed delay in which the participant initiated movement and TEO was commanded to move. The values that ensured success for hitting each target were defined as Tbd and Tid, therefore:

$$\text{Tbd} = \text{Tid} + \text{Dcd} \quad (2)$$

where Tbd was defined as the time in which TEO needed to move in order for the ball to bounce back in time to hit the target, Tid was the desired time in which the participant should have initiated movement, and Dcd was a constant (0.5 s).

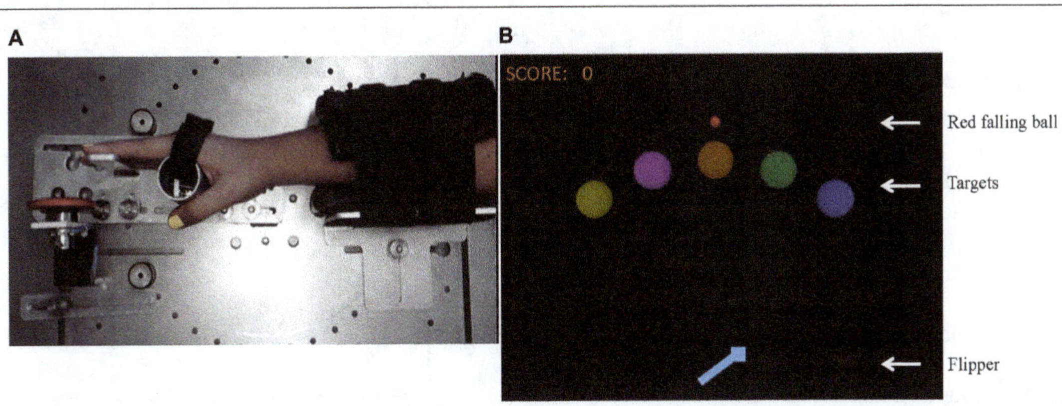

FIGURE 1 | (A) The Timing Exerciser Orthosis (TEO) robot; **(B)** Description of the computerized pinball-like game: a red ball appears at the top of the screen and falls toward the virtual flipper. Subjects flex their right wrist to activate TEO. TEO moves the wrist at an angle of 10°, allowing the subject's fingers to touch the button while rotating the flipper. The ball touches the flipper, and then bounces toward the target.

Next, Ep was defined as the timing error in which the participant initiated movement, thus:

$$\text{Ep} = \text{Tip} - \text{Tid} \tag{3}$$

Furthermore, Eb represented TEO's timing error, where:

$$\text{Eb} = \text{Tbp} - \text{Tbd} = \text{Ep} + \text{Dc} - \text{Dcd} \tag{4}$$

We wanted Eb to be proportional to Ep, so:

$$\text{Eb} = k\text{Ep} \tag{5}$$

where k was defined as the EA gain. By substituting equation 4 into equation 5 and solving for Dc, we obtained the following equation for the programmed delay:

$$\text{Dc} = \text{Dcd} + \text{Ep}(k - 1) \tag{6}$$

Equation 6 was used to establish the delay between when the participant initiated wrist movement, and when TEO began to move, in order to proportionally decrease or increase the participant's timing errors. Note that no HG or EA trainings were provided when $k = 1$, where a $k > 1$ caused an increase in timing errors and a $k < 1$ resulted in a decrease in timing errors.

Furthermore, knowing that baseline skill level can influence motor learning during HG or EA (Milot et al., 2010), we wanted to adjust each participant's k-value to his own skill level. We did so during a 39-trial baseline adjustment phase (B2), where participants played at a constant game difficulty ($k = 0.4$). When the B2 phase was completed, we classified each participant's timing errors in an ascending order and chose the 12th *Ep*-value. This 12th *Ep*-value was chosen based on the fact that we wanted subjects to experience at least a 30% rate of success in the subsequent baseline (B3) and retention conditions (RCs). Afterward, taking the upper limit of timing accuracy in order to ensure a successful hit, that is 4 ms (corresponding to Eb), we calculated each participant's final k-value using equation 5.

$$k = 4/12^{\text{th}}\text{Ep} \tag{7}$$

The choice of a $k = 0.4$ was driven by our previous study, where the maximum k-value reached among the young participants was 0.27. It was reasonable to think that seniors would not reach a k-value higher than 0.27 at the end of the B2 adjustment phase. Thus, the robot was providing some help during B2 but to a much lower level than what the subjects really needed to be successful at least 30% of the time, just like during B3 and the RCs.

For each condition, the k-value was increased or decreased by 90%, in EA and HG, respectively, to increase and decrease the participant's timing errors. This 90% change in the k-value was sufficient to significantly produce a difference in error between both HG and EA training conditions (Milot et al., 2010).

Study Design

Participants were randomly assigned to the two testing conditions; those in Condition 1 experienced the EA training first and the HG second, whereas those in Condition 2 received the HG training first followed by EA (see **Figure 2**).

Before each condition, participants played a Baseline (B1) phase to gain familiarity with the task to be played. B1 was set at a fixed k-value of 1, meaning that no HG or EA trainings were provided for 40 trials. Next, a 39-trial adjustment phase (B2) served to determine each participant's k-value. After, participants played a B3 phase according to their k-value determined in B2, for 40 trials. Afterward, participants received the training phase (EA or HG), depending on which condition they were in. Each training phase had 75 trials and a 60 s pause after the first 40 trials. During both HG and EA, 20% of the trials were catch trials, meaning that the k-value unexpectedly returned to baseline to ensure that the participants would remain watchful throughout the training, especially during HG. A RC equal to B3 followed each training session to allow evaluating the impact of HG or EA robotic training. During HG and EA, three targets (yellow, orange, blue) were presented one at the time to the subjects whereas during B3 and the RC conditions, the two remaining targets were shown along with the three trained targets to assess generalization of the task to untrained targets.

Statistical Analysis

Subjects' timing errors were calculated for each trial of each condition. Then, for each subject, two values were computed: (1) mean absolute timing errors and (2) related SDs. Afterward, across subjects, the mean and SD of values #1 and #2 were computed and retained for analysis. The normality of data was assessed using Shapiro–Wilk W-test, where non-parametric statistical methods were used for non-normally distributed data that could not be transformed. An independent t-test was used to assess if the two groups (EA1 and HG1) were comparable at baseline in regards to age and baseline timing errors during B3. Also, Wilcoxon signed-rank tests were used to evaluate the stability of the learning curve for the timing task (comparison of the mean of the first and last 10 trials of B3 for the entire group of subjects) and introduction to HG and EA training (comparison of the last 10 trials of B3 to the first 10 trials of HG or EA for each training group). Next, a paired t-test was used to determine the efficacy of each training type (EA1–B3 and HG1–B3) on the improvement of the timing task, not taking into account the crossover study design, as well as a Wilcoxon signed-rank test to look at the SD of the absolute timing errors. The Hill–Armitage approach (Senn, 2002) to crossover study analysis was used to

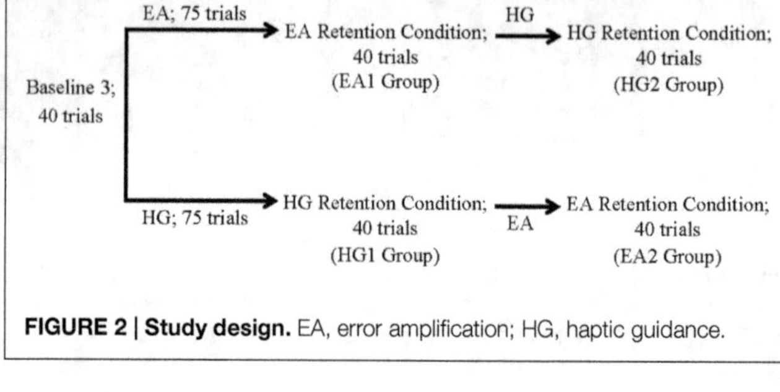

FIGURE 2 | Study design. EA, error amplification; HG, haptic guidance.

evaluate: (1) the difference in efficiency between the two types of trainings, by comparing the mean change (EA1 − HG2) of the EA1 group with that of the HG1 group (HG1 − EA2), and (2) whether there was no influence of training order administration, by comparing the mean of the sums (EA1 + HG2) and (HG1 + EA2) between groups. Finally, to evaluate the impact of age on the improvement in timing errors, two approaches were used. First, for each training group, a Pearson product moment correlation was performed to evaluate the relation between age and the change in absolute timing score following HG and EA, respectively. Second, following Senn (2002) procedure, a cross-over difference (mean change in absolute timing errors between the RCs of HG and EA, regardless of treatment order) was calculated and put in relation to age, using a Pearson product moment correlation. One-tailed tests were used and the significance level was set at 0.05. All statistical analyses were performed using IBM SPSS® software version 18.

Results

Success Rate, Learning Stability, and Baseline Group Comparison

At B1, where no robotic assistance was provided, the mean success rate of the entire group of subjects reached 2 ± 2%. However, at B3, when the game difficulty was adjusted to each subject's skill level, the overall mean success rate reached 25 ± 13%; confirming that the adjustment phase worked properly.

Also, when comparing the first and last 10 trials of B3 for the entire group, no difference in the subjects' absolute timing errors was noted (11.2 ± 5.6 ms vs. 10.1 ± 4.4 ms; $z = -0.88$; $p = 0.19$), meaning that a learning stability of the task has been reached before HG or EA trainings were introduced.

Finally, when comparing HG1 and EA1 training groups, no significant difference was noted in regards to age (68 ± 4 years vs. 68 ± 3 years, $t(30) = 0.24$; $p = 0.41$), and overall mean absolute timing errors at B3 (11.7 ± 4.3 ms vs. 9.8 ± 3.8 ms, $t(30) = -1.33$; $p = 0.10$).

Introduction to HG and EA

When introduced to HG, a significant decrease in the subjects' absolute timing errors was noted as compared to the last 10 trials of B3 (10.5 ± 4.8 ms vs. 1.4 ± 0.84 ms, $z = -3.52$; $p < 0.05$). On the contrary, when introduced to EA, a significant increase in the subjects' absolute timing errors was noted when comparing the last 10 trials of B3 to the first 10 trials of EA (9.8 ± 4.2 ms vs. 18.7 ± 6.5 ms, $z = -3.52$; $p < 0.05$). This means that HG and EA robotic training adequately decreased and increased subjects' timing errors, respectively.

Impact of Each Training Type on Timing Errors

When comparing the subjects' baseline performance on trained targets to that of their RC following HG training, a significant decrease in absolute timing errors was noted (11.7 ± 4.4 ms vs. 9.7 ± 3.4 ms, $t(15) = 1.76$; $p = 0.049$). At the same time, subjects were less variable in their timing errors as a significant improvement in the SD of their absolute timing errors was noted when comparing the value of B3 to that of the HG RC (9.5 ± 3.6 ms vs. 7.4 ± 3.2 ms; $z = -2.17$; $p = 0.01$; see **Figure 3**). In addition, when comparing the subjects' performance on untrained targets between B3 and HG RC, a trend toward a generalization of learning to untrained targets occurred with HG training (11.6 ± 3.2 ms vs. 10.4 ± 3.9 ms; $t(15) = 1.35$; $p = 0.09$). Further analysis also showed that during HG training, the subjects remained alert throughout the training, even though the robot provided them help, since no difference between the absolute timing errors of HG catch trials and B3 was observed (11.0 ± 3.9 ms vs. 11.7 ± 4.4 ms; $t(15) = 0.68$; $p = 0.25$).

Following training with EA, no difference in the subjects' absolute timing errors on trained targets was observed when comparing timing errors of B3 to that of the EA RC (9.8 ± 3.8 ms vs. 11.4 ± 5.9 ms; $t(15) = -1.16$; $p = 0.13$). In addition, a trend toward a worsening in the variability of the absolute timing errors was observed (7.9 ± 4.9 ms vs. 9.5 ± 7.2 ms; $z = -1.5$; $p = 0.07$; see **Figure 3**) as well as no generalization to untrained targets (10.6 ± 5.1 ms vs. 11.7 ± 5.6 ms; $t(15) = -1.08$; $p = 0.15$). Finally, like HG training, no difference between the subjects baseline performance at B3 and the one during EA catch trials was noted (9.8 ± 0.94 ms vs. 10.7 ± 5.3 ms; $t(15) = -1.02$; $p = 0.16$).

Finally, when comparing the change in absolute timing errors between HG1 and EA1 groups, a significant difference was noted (1.9 ± 4.5 ms vs. −1.6 ± 5.3 ms; $t(30) = -2.02$; $p = 0.03$). In other words, training with HG was more beneficial to learning the timed-based task than training with EA.

Comparison of the Efficacy of HG and EA Robotic Training on Improvement of Timing Errors and the Impact of Age

When looking at the subjects' absolute timing error on trained targets, the Hill–Armitage statistical analysis revealed no difference in the efficacy between HG and EA robotic trainings ($U = 102$; $p = 0.17$) and no effect of training order administration on the learning of the timing task ($U = 109$; $p = 0.25$). Although no significant difference in efficiency between the two types of training was noted, when looking at the change in absolute timing errors between RCs of both training groups (HG1/EA2 vs. and EA1/HG2), we performed further analyses by comparing the absolute timing errors of B3 to those of EA2 and HG2. Thus, if looking at the absolute timing errors of B3 to that of EA2, for the group that trained first with HG, a significant improvement in timing errors was noted (11.7 ± 4.4 ms vs. 9.9 ± 4.3 ms; $t(15) = 2.01$; $p = 0.03$). In addition, no difference in absolute timing errors between HG1 and EA2 was noted (9.7 ± 3.4 ms vs. 9.9 ± 4.3 ms; $t(15) = 0.14$; $p = 0.44$). This means that if training first with HG, no worsening in the subjects' performance occurred after training with EA. On the other hand, when looking at the absolute timing errors between B3 and HG2, for the group that trained first with EA, a trend toward a worsening in timing errors was noted (9.8 ± 3.8 ms vs. 11.7 ± 4.4 ms; $t(15) = -1.5$; $p = 0.08$). In addition, no difference between the absolute timing errors of EA1 and HG2 was observed (11.7 ± 4.4 ms vs.

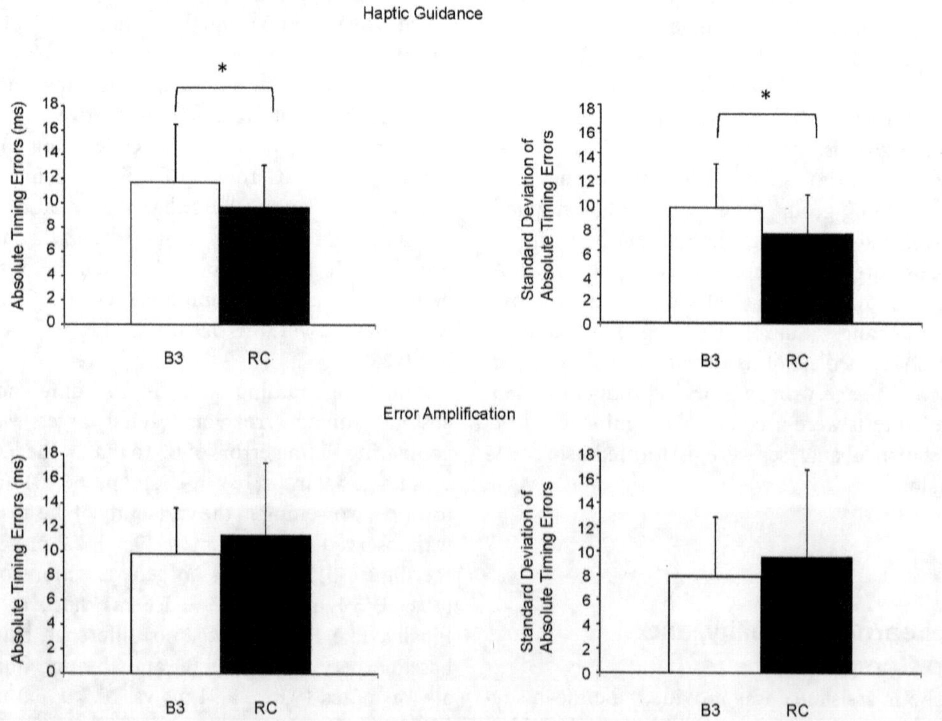

FIGURE 3 | Improvement in absolute timing errors and related SD following HG and EA robotic trainings. B3, baseline 3; RC, retention condition, $^*p < 0.05$.

12.6 ± 7.7ms; $t(15) = 0.81$; $p = 0.22$). This means that HG training was not effective, if given after EA training.

When looking at the impact of age on the subjects' absolute timing errors for each training group, no significant relation was found for the HG1 group ($r = 0.12$; $p = 0.33$). On the other hand, a significant relationship was obtained for the EA1 group ($r = -0.59$; $p = 0.008$); meaning that for the oldest subjects, training with EA was even more detrimental to learning. In addition, age was not related to the change in subjects' performance from HG RC to EA RC ($r = 0.04$, $p = 0.41$; see **Figure 4**).

Discussion

The results of the current study showed that a robotic hand device aimed at reducing healthy seniors timing errors was effective in improving learning a timing-based task, regardless of age. However, improved learning was mostly limited to trained targets. On the other hand, artificially increasing seniors' timing errors with the use of the robotic device did not promote learning and its generalization. It actually worsened performance with increasing age.

The fact that HG training did improve subjects' performance further supports the use of HG training for learning time-based tasks (Marchal-Crespo et al., 2010, 2013; Milot et al., 2010; Luttgen and Heuer, 2013). For example, the study of Marchal-Crespo et al. (2010) obtained a significant improvement in steering timing when healthy seniors trained with HG as compared to no guidance. Likewise, in our previous study on healthy young subjects using a similar pinball-like task (Milot et al., 2010), for subjects less-skilled at the task, that is having a k-value < 0.1, HG seemed to benefit learning more. Looking at the mean k-value of the current subjects (mean k-value of 0.06), they did fall within this less-skilled subcategory. As mentioned by Luttgen and Heuer (2013), if a task's characteristic is difficult to demonstrate either visually or verbally, such as the timing of a task, robotic guidance may provide a helpful role, especially for subjects who struggle with the task.

However, HG training did not translate into generalization of performance, although a trend was noted. Lack of generalization following HG training has been found in several other studies using a variety of tasks (Marchal Crespo and Reinkensmeyer, 2008; Marchal-Crespo et al., 2013). As mentioned by Marchal Crespo and Reinkensmeyer (2008), it could be thought that the current subjects relied too much on the robotic assistance during training with HG, hindering generalization of learning to other targets. Yet, this is not the case as the subjects' timing errors during HG catch trials did not increase when the robotic assistance was unexpectedly removed as compared to their B3 timing errors. Another explanation could come from the formation of an internal model of the task by the motor system. Indeed, formation of an internal model of the task is important to allow generalization of performance beyond the position (Grafton et al., 2008) or timing (Milot et al., 2010) of trained targets. In young healthy subjects, it was demonstrated that the

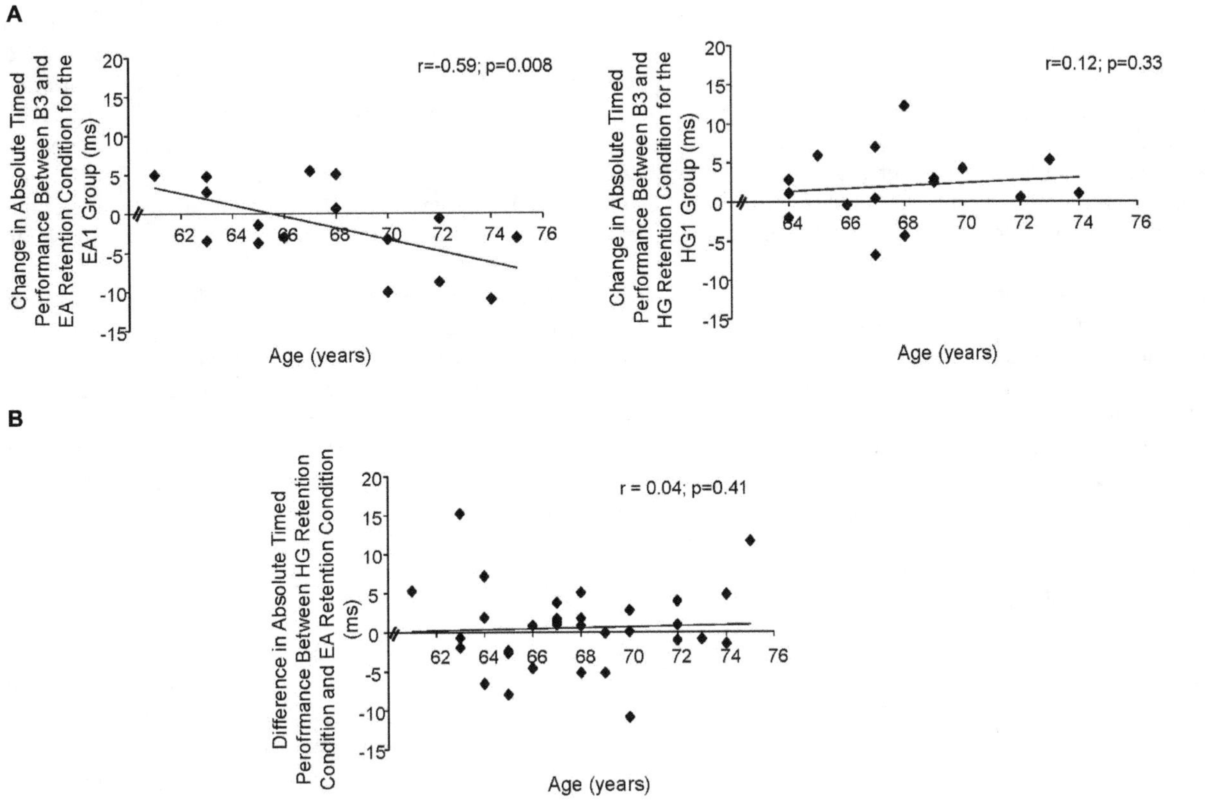

FIGURE 4 | Correlation between age and: (A) the change in absolute timed performance for EA1 group and HG1 group. Note that a negative value means a worsening of performance; **(B)** the cross-over difference between the absolute timing errors of the HG RC, and EA RC, $p < 0.05$.

motor system does indeed create an internal model of timing that can serve for generalization (Milot et al., 2010). However, the creation of an internal model is driven by errors (Thoroughman and Shadmehr, 2000) and because our subjects' k-values were small, they experienced a reduced range of timing errors (Marchal Crespo and Reinkensmeyer, 2008). This might have prevented the motor system to form an adequate internal model of the timing task to allow generalization of performance to untrained targets.

The fact that the subjects' timing errors decreased after HG training suggest that as one ages, learning can still occur, supporting results of previous studies on seniors' ability to learn new tasks (van Dijk et al., 2007; Marchal-Crespo et al., 2010; Pietschmann et al., 2011). Knowing that with age, motor performance usually worsens (Hoogendam et al., 2014) it was expected that HG would have been more beneficial for the oldest subjects. However, no relation with age and the change in timing errors following HG was obtained. Further looking at the data, no relation between age and k-value was also noted (data not shown); meaning that our oldest subjects did not systematically perform worst at the task to begin with and thus did not necessarily need more help from the robot while playing. To support, Marchal-Crespo et al. (2010) did not find an age dependent relation with motor performance while training with HG on their timing task. Age became an important factor when looking at the long-term retention of the learned task, which was not assessed in the current study.

When looking at the impact of EA training on improvement in timing errors, no significant change in either the absolute timing errors or related SDs was noted. This is not in line with studies on young healthy subjects where EA training translated into a significant improvement in learning various tasks (Patton and Mussa-Ivaldi, 2004; Milot et al., 2010; Marchal-Crespo et al., 2014). Consequently, it seems that exaggerating timing errors in the course of learning for individuals that are more prone to present baseline timing deficits because of normal aging might not be a good strategy to boost learning as for young individuals. Contrarily, following the results of our previous study, for young subjects that were less-skilled at the timing task, EA training did not improve learning (Milot et al., 2010). Explanation of this result was based on the challenge-point theory (Guadagnoli and Lee, 2004), which suggests that learning is a function of both skill level and task difficulty. Thus, for the less-skilled subgroup of young healthy subjects, it was thought that EA training was too challenging for their skill level, overwhelming the motor system with too much information to process and thus hindering any learning. This could be especially true for the current senior subjects knowing that slowness in information processing is observed in the elderly as compared to young individuals due to changes in structural and functional features of the nervous system (Seidler et al., 2010). This is supported also by the significant negative relation found between age and deterioration of timing accuracy following EA training. Thus, with age, EA training could have a more pronounced detrimental effect on learning. On the other hand, it seems that if EA training is given after HG training, no worsening of performance occurs. It is possible that teaching seniors how to perform a timing-task first allows them to improve their skill level and thus makes EA training less challenging.

Although age had a significant negative impact on learning for the EA training group, it did not play an important role when related to the change in score between HG and EA RCs when taking into account all subjects. This could be related to the fact that even though HG training significantly improved subjects' timing errors, its efficacy was not superior to EA training, when looking at the mean change in absolute timing errors of the RCs between the two groups. The high variability in training responses, often observed with aging (Seidler-Dobrin et al., 1998; Marchal-Crespo et al., 2010), could have prevented the detection of the superiority of HG robotic training over EA when taking into account all subjects, and in parallel precluded to a significant impact of age on the change in score between both types of training.

Limits

Even though the task that was practiced in this study was similar to the one used in a previous study on young healthy subjects, it was difficult to directly compare the results of both studies since the robots, as well as the determination of each subject's skill level, differed. The inclusion of a control group with young healthy individuals in the current study would have helped to better interpret the impact of aging on the learning of movement timing. However, when looking at the *k*-value of both studies, representing each subject's baseline skill level, it is noticeable that the senior subjects did have on average lower *k*-values than young subjects (0.06 vs. 0.15), possibly suggesting a decline in motor timing ability with age. In addition, since no *k*-values reached a value greater than 1 during EA, one could say that no true EA was provided during EA. This fact was also acknowledged in a previous study with young healthy subjects, where it was hypothesized that providing true EA could have been too demanding and thus detrimental to learning. This is even truer with the elderly subjects of this study since, as opposed to young healthy subjects, no learning occurred with EA when the error gains were smaller than 1. Nevertheless, our elderly subjects experienced a significant increase in their timing errors when comparing their baseline performances to their performances when being introduced to EA. Also, one could ask about the relevance of using a pinball-like game to assess timing performance of seniors instead of a more meaningful timing task. The rationale behind the choice of this task was based on the study by Wishart et al. (2000) which suggested that to better evaluate the impact of age on learning, the task should be an unfamiliar one, requiring effortful processing, as opposed to a task that is automatic, involving almost unconscious processing. Thus, by choosing a pinball-like game, we thought that this task was unfamiliar enough to the subjects to properly assess the effect of age on learning. Finally, the long-term retention as well as the clinical importance of a 2-ms improvement in timing following HG training were not established in the current study. Was the improvement in timing maintained over time? Was the change in timing important enough to positively impact seniors' performance in their everyday activities? Because studies on motor timing in the elderly are scarce, these questions are yet to be answered and more studies are needed to explore these questions. Nevertheless, knowing that the current robotic training significantly and positively helped improve elderly timing, its use with neurologically impaired individuals, where timing deficits can be even more substantial, is worth evaluating. A study is underway to assess the impact of both HG and EA robotic trainings on timing improvement for post-stroke individuals.

Conclusion

This study evaluated the impact of both HG and EA robotic trainings on the improvement of motor timing in healthy seniors. The results showed that HG was beneficial to learning, with subjects improving their timing accuracy regardless of age. However, learning was restricted to the targets in which practice occurred. No improvement in seniors' timing errors was noted following EA training. Moreover, a worsening of performance was noted with age after EA training, suggesting that this type of training can be detrimental to learning as one age. Future research should look at the long-term impacts of HG and EA robotic trainings as well as the effects of these robotic trainings on the performance of daily activities to validate their clinical usefulness, particularly with impaired populations.

Authors Contributions

Conception and design the experiment: MHM, HC
Collection of data: AB
Analysis and interpretation: MHM
Writing of the manuscript: MHM, AB
Revising the manuscript: MHM, AB, HC

Acknowledgments

The authors would like to thank Mathieu Hamel and Antoine Guillerand for their technical support as well as Prof. David J. Reinkensmeyer for his input on the manuscript. The project was conducted at the Technological Innovations Lab at the Research Center on Aging of the CSSS-IUGS, Sherbrooke, Qc, Canada with the help of M-HM's start-up funds from the Faculté de médecine et des sciences de la santé of the Université de Sherbrooke.

References

Bluteau, J., Coquillart, S., Payan, Y., and Gentaz, E. (2008). Haptic guidance improves the visuo-manual tracking of trajectories. *PLoS ONE* 3:e1775. doi: 10.1371/journal.pone.0001775

Carnahan, H., Vandervoort, A. A., and Swanson, L. R. (1996). The influence of summary knowledge of results and aging on motor learning. *Res. Q. Exerc. Sport* 67, 280–287. doi: 10.1080/02701367.1996.10607955

Cesqui, B., Aliboni, S., Mazzoleni, S., Corrozza, M. C., Postoraro, F., and Micero, S. (2008). "On the use of divergent force fields in robot-mediated neurorehabilitation," in *Proceedings of the 2nd Biennial IEEE/RAS-EMBS International Conference on Biomedical Robotics and Biomechatronics*, Scottsdale, AZ.

Emken, J. L., and Reinkensmeyer, D. J. (2005). Robot-enhanced motor learning: accelerating internal model formation during locomotion by transient dynamic amplification. *IEEE Trans. Neural. Syst. Rehabil. Eng.* 13, 33–39. doi: 10.1109/TNSRE.2004.843173

Feygin, D., Keehner, M., and Tendick, F. (2002). "Haptic guidance: experimental evaluation of a haptic training method for a perceptual motor skill," in *Proceedings of the 10th Symp. On Haptic Interfaces For Virtual Environment and Teleoperator System. (HAPTICS'02)*, Orlando, FL.

Georgopoulos, A. P. (2002). Cognitive motor control: spatial and temporal aspects. *Curr. Opin. Neurobiol.* 12, 678–683. doi: 10.1016/S0959-4388(02)00382-3

Gluhm, S., Goldstein, J., Loc, K., Colt, A., Liew, C. V., and Corey-Bloom, J. (2013). Cognitive performance on the mini-mental state examination and the montreal cognitive assessment across the healthy adult lifespan. *Cogn. Behav. Neurol.* 26, 1–5. doi: 10.1097/WNN.0b013e31828b7d26

Grafton, S. T., and Schmitt, P., Van Horn, J., Diedrichsen, J. (2008). Neural substrates of visuomotor learning based on improved feedback control and prediction. *Neuroimage* 39, 1383–1395. doi: 10.1016/j.neuroimage.2007.09.062

Guadagnoli, M. A., and Lee, T. D. (2004). Challenge point: a framework for conceptualizing the effects of various practice conditions in motor learning. *J. Mot. Behav.* 36, 212–224. doi: 10.3200/JMBR.36.2.212-224

Hoogendam, Y. Y., van der Lijn, F., Vernooij, M. W., Hofman, A., Niessen, W. J., van der Lugt, A., et al. (2014). Older age relates to worsening of fine motor skills: a population-based study of middle-aged and elderly persons. *Front. Aging Neurosci.* 6:259. doi: 10.3389/fnagi.2014.00259

Liu, J., Cramer, S. C., and Reinkensmeyer, D. J. (2006). Learning to perform a new movement with robotic assistance: comparison of haptic guidance and visual demonstration. *J. Neuroeng. Rehabil.* 3, 20. doi: 10.1186/1743-0003-3-20

Luttgen, J., and Heuer, H. (2013). The influence of robotic guidance on different types of motor timing. *J. Mot. Behav.* 45, 249–258. doi: 10.1080/00222895.2013.785926

Marchal-Crespo, L., McHughen, S., Cramer, S. C., and Reinkensmeyer, D. J. (2010). The effect of haptic guidance, aging, and initial skill level on motor learning of a steering task. *Exp. Brain Res.* 201, 209–220. doi: 10.1007/s00221-009-2026-8

Marchal Crespo, L., and Reinkensmeyer, D. J. (2008). Haptic guidance can enhance motor learning of a steering task. *J. Mot. Behav.* 40, 545–556. doi: 10.3200/JMBR.40.6.545-557

Marchal-Crespo, L., Schneider, J., Jaeger, L., and Riener, R. (2014). Learning a locomotor task: with or without errors? *J. Neuroeng. Rehabil.* 11, 25. doi: 10.1186/1743-0003-11-25

Marchal-Crespo, L., van Raai, M., Rauter, G., Wolf, P., and Riener, R. (2013). The effect of haptic guidance and visual feedback on learning a complex tennis task. *Exp. Brain Res.* 231, 277–291. doi: 10.1007/s00221-013-3690-2

McAuley, J. D., Jones, M. R., Holub, S., Johnston, H. M., and Miller, N. S. (2006). The time of our lives: life span development of timing and event tracking. *J. Exp. Psychol. Gen.* 135, 348–367. doi: 10.1037/0096-3445.135.3.348

Milot, M. H., Marchal-Crespo, L., Green, C. S., Cramer, S. C., and Reinkensmeyer, D. J. (2010). Comparison of error-amplification and haptic-guidance training techniques for learning of a timing-based motor task by healthy individuals. *Exp. Brain Res.* 201, 119–131. doi: 10.1007/s00221-009-2014-z

Oldfield, R. C. (1971). The assessment and analysis of handedness: the Edinburgh inventory. *Neuropsychologia* 9, 97–113. doi: 10.1016/0028-3932(71)90067-4

Patton, J. L., Kovic, M., and Mussa-Ivaldi, F. A. (2006a). Custom-designed haptic training for restoring reaching ability to individuals with poststroke hemiparesis. *J. Rehabil. Res. Dev.* 43, 643–656. doi: 10.1682/JRRD.2005.05.0088

Patton, J. L., Stoykov, M. E., Kovic, M., and Mussa-Ivaldi, F. A. (2006b). Evaluation of robotic training forces that either enhance or reduce error in chronic hemiparetic stroke survivors. *Exp. Brain Res.* 168, 368–383. doi: 10.1007/s00221-005-0097-8

Patton, J. L., and Mussa-Ivaldi, F. A. (2004). Robot-assisted adaptive training: custom force fields for teaching movement patterns. *IEEE Trans. Biomed. Eng.* 51, 636–646. doi: 10.1109/TBME.2003.821035

Pietschmann, M., Endrass, T., and Kathmann, N. (2011). Age-related alterations in performance monitoring during and after learning. *Neurobiol. Aging* 32, 1320–1330. doi: 10.1016/j.neurobiolaging.2009.07.016

Raz, N., Lindenberger, U., Rodrigue, K. M., Kennedy, K. M., Head, D., Williamson A., et al. (2005). Regional brain changes in aging healthy adults: general trends, individual differences and modifiers. *Cereb. Cortex* 15, 1676–1689. doi: 10.1093/cercor/bhi044

Seidler, R. D., Bernard, J. A., Burutolu, T. B., Fling, B. W., Gordon, M. T., Gwin, J. T., et al. (2010). Motor control and aging: links to age-related brain structural, functional, and biochemical effects. *Neurosci. Biobehav. Rev.* 34, 721–733. doi: 10.1016/j.neubiorev.2009.10.005

Seidler-Dobrin, R. D., He, J., and Stelmach, G. E. (1998). Coactivation to reduce variability in the elderly. *Motor. Control.* 2, 314–330.

Senn, S. (2002). *Cross-over Trials in Clinical Research.* Hoboken: John Wiley & Sons Ltd. doi: 10.1002/0470854596

Thoroughman, K. A., and Shadmehr, R. (2000). Learning of action through adaptive combination of motor primitives. *Nature* 407, 742–747. doi: 10.1038/35037588

Turgeon, M., and Wing, A. M. (2012). Late onset of age-related difference in unpaced tapping with no age-related difference in phase-shift error detection and correction. *Psychol. Aging* 27, 1152–1163. doi: 10.1037/a0029925

van Dijk, H., Mulder, T., and Hermens, H. J. (2007). Effects of age and content of augmented feedback on learning an isometric force-production task. *Exp. Aging Res.* 33, 341–353. doi: 10.1080/03610730701319194

Voelcker-Rehage, C. (2008). Motor-skill learning in older adults-a review of studies on age-related differences. *Eur. Rev. Aging Phys. Act.* 5, 5–16. doi: 10.1007/s11556-008-0030-9

Wishart, L. R., Lee, T. D., Murdoch, J. E., and Hodges, N. J. (2000). Effects of aging on automatic and effortful processes in bimanual coordination. *J. Gerontol. B Psychol. Sci. Soc. Sci.* 55, 85–94. doi: 10.1093/geronb/55.2.P85

Zahr, N. M., Rohlfing, T., Pfefferbaum, A., and Sullivan, E. V. (2009). Problem solving, working memory, and motor correlates of association and commissural fiber bundles in normal aging: a quantitative fiber tracking study. *Neuroimage* 44, 1050–1062. doi: 10.1016/j.neuroimage.2008.09.046

22

Hearing Colors: An Example of Brain Plasticity

Arantxa Alfaro[1,2], *Ángela Bernabeu*[3], *Carlos Agulló*[3], *Jaime Parra*[4] *and Eduardo Fernández*[1,5*]

[1] CIBER-BBN, Madrid, Spain, [2] Hospital Vega Baja, Orihuela, Spain, [3] Department of Magnetic Resonance, INSCANER S.L., Alicante, Spain, [4] Hospital San Rafael, Madrid, Spain, [5] Institute of Bioengineering, Universidad Miguel Hernández, Elche, Spain

Edited by:
Ioan Opris,
Wake Forest University School of Medicine, USA

Reviewed by:
Jitendra Sharma,
Massachusetts Institute of Technology, USA
Preston E. Garraghty,
Indiana University, USA

***Correspondence:**
Eduardo Fernández,
Institute of Bioengineering,
Universidad Miguel Hernández, Avda.
Universidad s/n, Elche 03202
Alicante, Spain

Sensory substitution devices (SSDs) are providing new ways for improving or replacing sensory abilities that have been lost due to disease or injury, and at the same time offer unprecedented opportunities to address how the nervous system could lead to an augmentation of its capacities. In this work we have evaluated a color-blind subject using a new visual-to-auditory SSD device called "Eyeborg", that allows colors to be perceived as sounds. We used a combination of neuroimaging techniques including Functional Magnetic Resonance Imaging (fMRI), Diffusion Tensor Imaging (DTI) and proton Magnetic Resonance Spectroscopy (^{1}H-MRS) to study potential brain plasticity in this subject. Our results suggest that after 8 years of continuous use of this device there could be significant adaptive and compensatory changes within the brain. In particular, we found changes in functional neural patterns, structural connectivity and cortical topography at the visual and auditive cortex of the Eyeborg user in comparison with a control population. Although at the moment we cannot claim that the continuous use of the Eyeborg is the only reason for these findings, our results may shed further light on potential brain changes associated with the use of other SSDs. This could help to better understand how the brain adapts to several pathologies and uncover adaptive resources such as cross-modal representations. We expect that the precise understanding of these changes will have clear implications for rehabilitative training, device development and for more efficient programs for people with disabilities.

Keywords: functional magnetic resonance imaging (fMRI), diffusion tensor imaging (DTI), magnetic resonance spectroscopy, sensory substitution device (SSD), neuroplasticity, blindness, visual cortex

Introduction

Neuroplasticity is an intrinsic property of the brain, which allows us to adapt to environmental pressures, physiologic changes and experiences by dynamic shifts in the strength of pre-existing connections or by establishing new networks in response to changes in afferent inputs or efferent demands (Pascual-Leone et al., 2005). Consequently, the adult brain has a remarkable capacity to change and adapt throughout the development of lifetime, requiring changes at different levels (genes, molecules, synapses, etc.), and is associated with structural and functional reorganization of the brain (Cramer et al., 2011).

Plasticity can occur during development, learning, in response to the environment or disease, or in relation to therapy. As we interact with a rich multisensory world, our sensory experiences are the product of extensive and dynamic neural connections, which are highly influenced by our experiences and developmental constraints. Such ability can be viewed as adaptivewhen associated with a gain in function (Cohen et al., 1997) or as maladaptive when linked to negative consequences such as loss of function or increased injury (Nudo, 2006). Consequently, the understanding of the nature of these changes is important not only in terms of establishing the brain's true adaptive potential but also in guiding future rehabilitation strategies (Merabet and Pascual-Leone, 2010).

Sensory substitution devices (SSDs) in people with severe visual impairment offer amazing opportunities to study how the nervous system reorganizes its structure, function and connections when one sensory modality is supplied by another modality. Efficient use of SSDs is based on the brain's ability to reorganize itself and it depends on the possibility of teaching the brain new complex perceptual skills as well as a different way to process sensory information (Proulx et al., 2014). Although, the most common modality to replace sight is touch, several authors proposed special devices for visual substitution by the auditory pathway in the context of real time reactivity (Meijer, 1992; Capelle et al., 1998; Cronly-Dillon et al., 1999; Striem-Amit et al., 2012; Abboud et al., 2014; Maidenbaum et al., 2014). Sound spatialization consists of virtually creating a three-dimensional auditory environment, where sound sources can be positioned all around the listener. However, these devices often generate unpleasant sensations and lack color information. This motivated the creation of new SSDs that encode color information such as Soundview (Nie et al., 2009), Haptic-Color Glove (Kahol et al., 2006), SeeColOr (Bologna et al., 2009) and EyeMusic (Abboud et al., 2014).

In this framework, our group has had the opportunity to evaluate the brain changes related to the continued use of a visual-to-auditory prosthetic device called *Eyeborg* specifically designed to help color-blind people. This device was developed by Neil Harbisson and Adam Montandon in 2003 and allows colors to be perceived as sound (Eyeborg, 2015). Briefly, it consists of a small video sensor placed at eye level of the head that transmits color information to a computer chip. Electromagnetic light waves are turned into sound frequencies that are heard as musical notes with distinct pitches in real-time (high frequency colors have high notes and low frequency colors have low notes). The computer chip is resting on the back of the head so the sound is heard through vibrations that are directly transmitted into the skull by bone conduction. It is thought that a proficient user of *Eyeborg* could perceive 360 different hues, one for each degree on the color wheel. Each hue is assigned to an audible frequency between 384 and 718 Hz, which allows differentiation between brighter and darker variations as well as color saturation (due to lighting conditions and the environment) and the recognition of the similarities and differences between hues.

In this work, we introduce the potential adaptive and compensatory changes within the brain associated with the continuous use of Eyeborg in a subject with achromatopsia (an irreversible visual impairment characterized by the inability to perceive colors). Our results suggest that after 8 years of continuous use of this device there could be significant changes in functional neural patterns, structural connectivity and cortical topography. Although there is still a lot of work to be done and we cannot claim that the continuous use of the Eyeborg is the only reason for these findings, our study offers the amazing opportunity to delve into the brain's potential for change by using SSDs. Moreover, it could contribute to a better understanding of the functional and crossmodal organization that supports the neuroenhancement.

Materials and Methods

Participants

Five non-synesthete adults (mean 32.2 ± 2.38 years old; males 3, females 2; 4 right handed, 1 left handed) participated in this study. All were enrolled as part of a broader study examining brain plasticity. One of them (the main subject of this study) had difficulty distinguishing colors from childhood and was diagnosed of achromatopsia when he was 11 years old. He is a proficient Eyeborg user that had been using the device, intensively, throughout the whole day during the past 8 years. The control group was an age matched population of healthy volunteers. None of them had absolute pitch. The protocol was approved by the institutional review board and all volunteers gave their written informed consent prior to entering the study.

Neuroimage Studies

All neuroimaging studies were performed in a Philips Achieva 3T (Philips Medical Systems, Netherlands) with a SENSE Neurovascular coil (18 elements) supplied by the manufacturer. No sedation or contrast agent was given. The protocol included a high-resolution T1-weighted gradient-echo scan: 212 slices, 0.8 mm isotropic voxels, field of view 250 × 250 mm, TR 11 ms and TE 4.9 ms. After the structural data was acquired, functional magnetic resonance (fMRI), diffusion tensor imaging (DTI) and single voxel MR Spectroscopy (^{1}H-MRS) studies were carried out.

Functional Magnetic Resonance Imaging (fMRI)

For the fMRI experiments four different block paradigms were carried out. The visual and auditive stimuli were presented with a special compatible system (VisuaStim Digital Glasses; Resonance Technology, Northridge, CA, USA). Subjects were instructed to keep their gaze fixed on the screen. The tasks were performed in the same order in all the subjects to reduce task interaction effects. No oral output was required avoiding overt movement. fMRI experiment were carried out in the dark.

For the first two paradigms retinotopic mapping stimuli were carried out following conventional procedures based on previously published studies (Engel et al., 1994). The stimuli consisted of high-contrast checkerboards in a rotating wedge and expanding ring. Both stimuli moved in a periodic pattern and completed a full cycle in 24 s with a total of 5 cycles per scanning run. Images were acquired throughout a blood oxygenation level-dependent (BOLD) sensitive T2-weighted multi-slice gradient echo EPI sequence (TE = 35 ms, TR = 2500 ms, FOV = 230 × 230, 64 × 64 matrix). Twentytwo contiguous 4-mm thick axial slices were prescribed parallel to the AC–PC ensuring a full coverage of the occipital lobe. A total of 160 whole brain volumes were collected.

The third paradigm was a color test based on previously published studies (Beauchamp et al., 1999). The stimuli consisted of five wedges arranged around a central fixation bar, extending from one to four degrees of eccentricity. In the chromatic trials subjects were instructed to decide if the colors in the intervening wedges formed an orderly sequence or not. During achromatic trials, wedges of different luminance were presented and subjects decided if the sequence presented a regular luminance sequence or didn't. The functional scan parameters were as follows: TR = 3000 ms, TE = 35 ms, FOV: 230 × 230, 64 × 64 matrix. Thirty contiguous 4-mm thick axial slices were prescribed parallel to the AC–PC with a total of 84 whole brain volumes collected.

Finally, the forth paradigm consisted of studies where images and sounds were presented simultaneously (Tregellas et al., 2009). The subjects were instructed to look at the images and pay attention to their accompanying sounds, thinking about a putative color that could be assigned to the sound. To encode the sound we used specific algorithms provided by the *Eyeborg* designers. Therefore, we tried to simulate the usage of the Eyeborg inside the environment of the MRI machine. The test presented two condition blocks with a duration of 14 s for each condition. The functional scan parameters were as follows: time repetition = 2000 ms, time echo = 35 ms, FOV: 230 × 230, 64 × 64 matrix. Thirty contiguous 4-mm thick axial slices were prescribed parallel to the AC–PC with a total of 210 whole brain volumes collected.

For the fMRI data analysis, we used SPM8 (The Wellcome Trust Center for Neuroimaging)[1] implemented in MATLAB 2010a (MathWorks, Inc., Massachusetts). We initially performed motion correction, normalization to the Montreal Neurological Institute (MNI) template, and spatial smoothing (8 mm). After the realignment processes, we checked the head-movement parameters which were not used as covariates in the analyses. The task-related activation was evaluated statistically on a voxel-by-voxel basis using a general linear model at the individual level to generate contrast images, which then were incorporated into analysis at the group level. Statistically significant clusters of activity were recorded for each condition. Only those clusters with a corrected P value of 0.05 or less and clusters of 10 voxels or greater are reported. The coordinates reported by SPM (which were in "MNI space") were transformed to the stereotaxic coordinate frame developed by Talairach and Tournoux (available at http://macdownload.informer.com/talairach-client) and thus enabled comparison to a reference atlas for appropriate neuroanatomical localization. In order to test whether results obtained for our single subject are valid at the population level, we performed a random effects group analysis (RFX) with the help of BrainVoyager QX (Goebel et al., 2006). This neuroimaging software package was also used in same cases for visualization of anatomical and functional data sets.

Diffusion Tensor Imaging (DTI)

DTI-MR was performed in transversal slice orientation, using a single-shot EPI sequence with diffusion encoding in 32 directions (values 0 and 800 s/mm^2). The acquired voxel size was 2 × 2 × 2 mm^3 in 60 slices, with a SENSE factor of 1.9. The diffusion-weighted data were transferred to a workstation for analysis. Before DTI analysis eddy current compensation was applied by affine registration to B0 image. Tractography was then performed using the PRIDE fiber-tracking tool supplied by Philips Medical Systems, as described previously (Nilsson et al., 2007). The ROIs were drawn manually based on the anatomical images and on previously published atlases (Wakana et al., 2004). Tractography was performed based on the connection between two regions of interest (ROI) in order to minimize the risk of including other tracts. Fibers running through the 2 ROIs were computed automatically by the software taking into account a minimum fractional anisotropy value (FA) of 0.3, maximum fiber angle between fibers of 27° and minimum fiber length of 10 mm as stopping criteria.

Magnetic Resonance Spectroscopy (^{1}H-MRS)

For the ^{1}H-MRS study the volume of interest was placed based on anatomical structures. The aim was to get an overall spectroscopic representation of different areas within the visual cortex (V1, V2 and V4) avoiding contamination of the surrounding tissues. The resulted volume size was 14 cm^3 for V1, 12 cm^3 for V2 and 7 cm^3 for V4. Shimming and tuning were achieved with automated procedures before acquisition. Water signal was suppressed with selective water signal inversion. For the spectroscopic measurements a standard short-echo-time acquisition mode sequence (TR/TE/averages = 2000/32/128) was used. A total of 512 data points were collected over a spectral width of 1000 Hz. Assignment of the resonances of interest included N-acetylaspartate and other N-acetyl-containing compounds (NAA) at 2.02 ppm, glutamate and glutamine (Glx) at 2.35 ppm, creatine plus phosphocreatine (Cr) at 3.03 ppm, choline and other trimethylamine-containing compounds (Cho) at 3.20 ppm, and myo-inositol (mIno) at 3.55 ppm (Haga et al., 2009). Spectrum analysis was performed off-line with the help of jMRUI 3.0 package (Naressi et al., 2001) available through the MRUI Project[2] as documented in previous studies (Bernabeu et al., 2009; Poveda et al., 2010).

Results

All the subjects of the study presented normal MRI images of the brain with neither detectable degenerative changes nor any brain lesions.

Functional Magnetic Resonance Imaging (fMRI)

Basic visual retinotopic fMRI paradigms showed brain activation in the corresponding visual areas (BA17, BA18 and BA19) in all the subjects studied. No significant differences in the brain

[1] http://www.fil.ion.ucl.ac.uk/spm

[2] www.mrui.uab.es/mrui

activation pattern were observed between the Eyeborg user and the control subjects (data not shown).

The analysis of the color paradigm showed clear differences between the activated areas of the Eyeborg user and the controls. Particularly, during the chromatic phase of the test, the Eyeborg user showed activation in V1 (BA17) and other small clusters of activation located mainly in the left V2 (BA18). However, the control group showed strong bilateral activation with a great number of other brain areas involved (**Figure 1**). Thus the color-selective activation in the control group (chromatic blocks vs. fixation) was situated in occipital, temporal, parietal and frontal cortex. More specifically, these areas were located in: (1) occipital lobe (areas BA18 and BA19); (2) temporal lobe related to object and face recognition (BA37), language and auditory processing (BA21, BA22, BA42), memory (BA38) and high level object representation (visual stream BA20); and (3) parietal lobe related to stimulation and texture discrimination tasks (BA40), visuo-motor coordination (BA7, BA6, BA4), and somatosensory functions (BA2); and (4) prefrontal cortex, related with executive functions (BA9, BA10, BA11, 46) and semantic tasks (45, 44). During the achromatic stimulation blocks there was a significant decrease in the number of brain-activated areas in all subjects. In the Eyeborg user we only found activation in areas BA17 and left BA18. In contrast, the control group presented during this achromatic

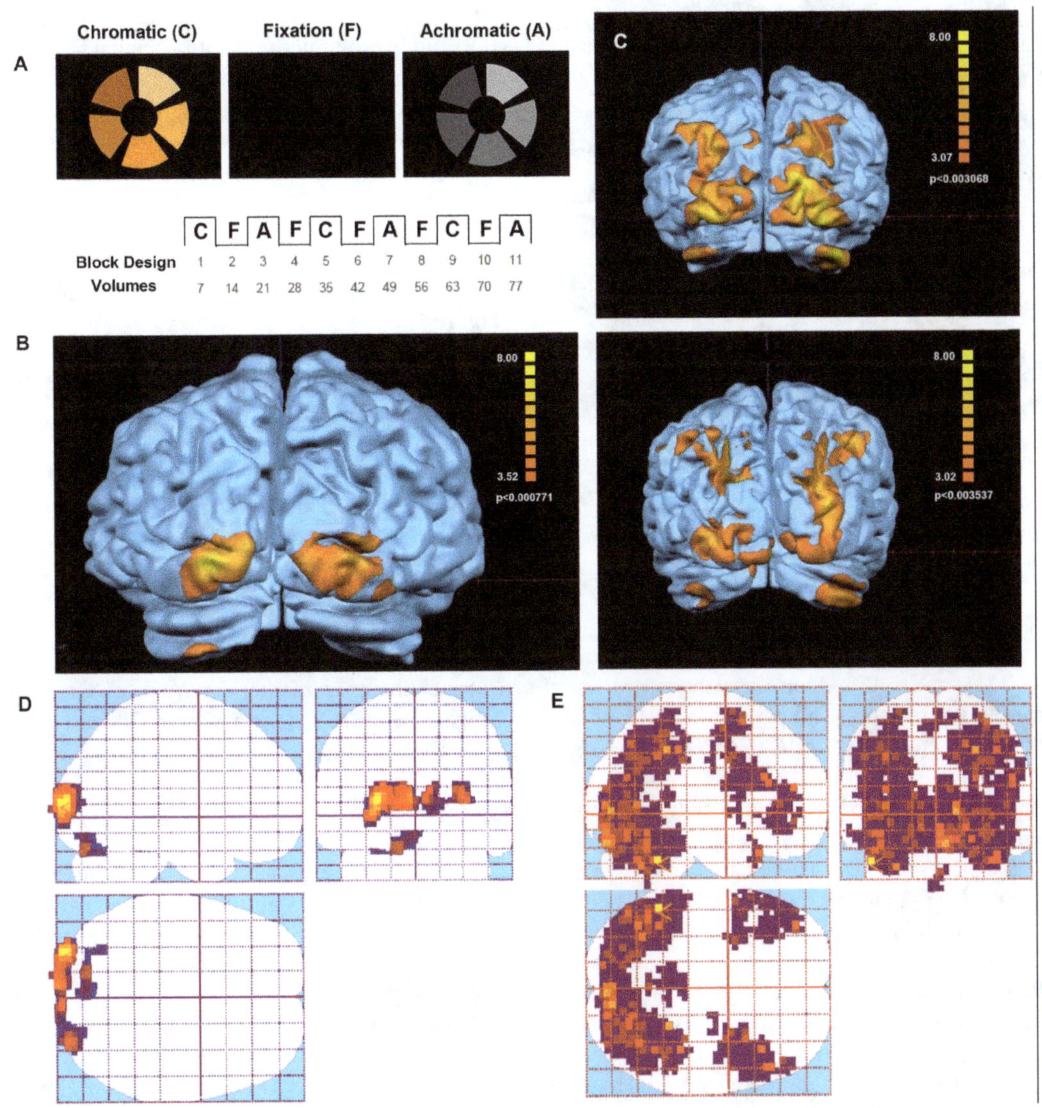

FIGURE 1 | Visual stimulus and Functional Magnetic Resonance Imaging (fMRI) activation in the Eyeborg user and the control group. **(A)** Protocol of the Farnsworth-Munsell test. Within each scan series, the stimulus alternated between blocks of chromatic or achromatic discrimination trials and fixation. **(B)** Areas showing a significant response to chromatic stimulation in the Eyeborg user. **(C)** Areas showing a significant response to chromatic stimulation in two representative controls (single subjects). **(D)** Statistical parametric maps of the Eyeborg user are shown in standard anatomical space. **(E)** Statistical parametric maps of the whole control population in standard anatomical space.

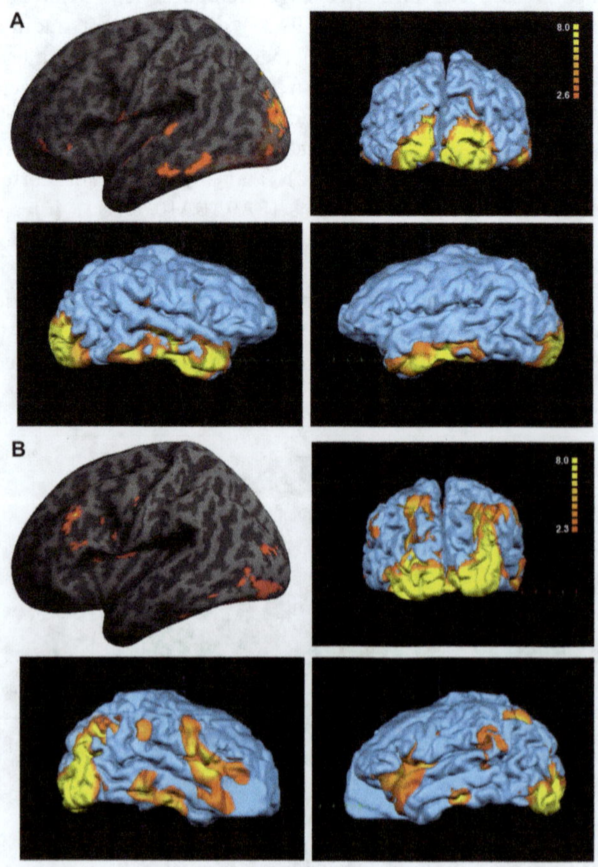

FIGURE 2 | Analysis of the paradigm involving the presentation of simultaneously visual and auditory stimulation. (A) Data corresponding to the Eyeborg user (single subject analysis) showing a strong effect on temporal and occipital cortex. **(B)** Averaged activation of the control group in response to the same paradigm of stimulation.

stimulation a higher number of occipital areas activated such as BA17, BA18 and BA19. Moreover, there was brain activation located in the temporal and parietal lobes (BA7 and BA37) and within the entorhinal cortex (BA28) of the right hemisphere.

The paradigm that comprised visual and auditory stimuli showed interesting and significant differences between the Eyeborg user and the controls. Particularly, the Eyeborg user displayed a wider brain activation of the auditory pathway and also involved frontal, temporal and occipital areas (**Figure 2**; **Table 1**). The frontal activated areas were mainly BA6, BA10 and BA11, which are related to motor and executive functions. The temporal activation was in primary auditory cortex (BA42) and also in areas related to language and auditory processing (BA21) and memory and emotion (BA38). Furthermore, in the Eyeborg user there was a robust activation located in the left BA22 area, which contains Wernicke's area, and bilateral activation in BA13 (located in the insula) when we presented simultaneously visual and auditory stimuli that were previously encoded by the Eyeborg algorithms.

Diffusion Tensor Imaging (DTI)

We used DTI to trace the microstructure of the main white matter tracts between the brain areas dedicated to auditory and visual processing (temporal and occipital cortices, respectively). By measuring diffusivity in multiple directions, we estimate the FA value. FA is a normalized measure used in diffusion neuroimaging studies which reflects fiber density, axonal diameter, and myelination in white matter (Yoshida et al., 2013). The more aligned fibers are within a tract, the higher the tract or regional FA value, therefore FA differences between groups can be regarded as a surrogate marker of structural adaptation in the white matter (Fabri et al., 2014; Kantarci, 2014).

When we compared the fiber tracts between the Eyeborg user and the controls we found higher FA values in the Eyeborg user in the corpus callosum (CC), and also (although they were not statistically significant) in both inferior longitudinal fasciculus (ILF) and in both inferior fronto-occipital fasciculus (IFOF) (see **Table 2**). Neither differences nor interhemispheric asymmetry in the FA or in the apparent diffusion coefficient (ADC) values were observed between groups (data not). In addition to this, by comparing the relative positions and properties of the estimated tracts we found more estimated fiber tracks in the temporal-callosal connections of the Eyeborg user. Furthermore, the IFOF of the Eyeborg user presented a region located in the temporal-basal area with a higher white matter density (**Figure 3**).

Magnetic Resonance Spectroscopy (^{1}H-MRS)

The mean values and the corresponding standard deviations of the estimated metabolite ratios for the Eyeborg user and the controls are reported in **Table 3**. There were some differences between the metabolite ratios mIno/Cr, NAA/Cr and Glx/Cr in the visual areas of the Eyeborg user when compared to controls although they were not statistically significant. Specifically, there was an increase in the levels of mIno, a putative marker of glia, in V4 which is the area involved in visual color processing. Furthermore, the Eyeborg user showed an increase in the neuronal integrity marker NAA (NAA/Cr ratio) in V2 and a higher Glx/Cr (Glutamate plus Glutamine) proportion in V1 and V2.

Discussion

This study represents the first attempt to directly assess the structural adjustments and neuroplastic changes related to the chronic use of the *Eyeborg*, an electronic device that allows colors to be perceived as sounds. This offers the amazing opportunity to investigate the link between brain activity, conscious perception and technological devices. Our results suggest that after 8 years of continuous use of this device, there could be some adaptive and compensatory changes within the brain. However, we should take into account that this is a very preliminary investigation that needs to be confirmed by further studies with a larger sample size. Thus, some of these changes could exist before the use of the Eyeborg and therefore we cannot claim that the continuous use of the Eyeborg is the only reason of these findings. Nonetheless, several studies have looked into differential activation before and

TABLE 1 | Talairach coordinates and Z-scores of the maximally activated voxels associated with the presentation of simultaneously visual and auditory stimulation.

	Left Hemisphere					Right Hemisphere				
	x	*y*	*z*	*T* value	Brodman Area	*x*	*y*	*z*	*T* value	Brodman Area
Eyeborg user	−9.59	−97.6	18.39	19.4	18	12	−94	22	25	19
	−63.59	−11.2	3.99	15.62	22	33.6	−79.6	−21.2	18.8	18
	−52.79	−0.4	−10.4	11.11	38	69.6	−14.8	0.39	22.58	21
	−34.79	−36.4	18.39	10.09	13	58.8	13.99	−6.8	15.65	38
	−34.79	57.2	−6.8	5.71	10	66	−18.4	18.4	14.69	42
	−27.6	57.2	−3.2	5.53	10	48	−36.4	25.6	8.8	13
						30	50	−14	7.55	11
						22.8	60.79	−6.8	4.74	10
						48	6.79	43.6	6.92	6
						48	3.2	36.4	5.54	6
Controls	−38.39	−35.59	−6.8	31.76	47	44.4	−32.8	3.9	181	41
	−45.6	−35.6	14.79	17.99	46	26.4	−79.6	−10.4	169.13	18
	−23.99	17.6	57.9	29.35	6	44.4	3.2	25.6	29.5	9
	−38.4	3.2	54.4	23.45	6	37.2	6.79	25.6	20.74	9
	−16.8	39.2	50.8	19.04	8	44.4	−4	29.2	7.96	6
	−34.79	13	29	24.2	9	40.8	35.6	−14	27	11
	−31.2	−0.4	18.4	16.93	13	44.4	42.79	−3.2	22.3	10
	−42	6	22	20.04	9	66	−40	−14	12.42	21
	−49.2	−54	43.6	9.37	40	48	−29.2	50.8	8.98	40
	−34.8	−54.4	54.4	3.23	7	55.2	−22	36.4	5.47	2
	−49.2	−4	36.4	8.85	6	48	−25	36	5.04	2
	−49.2	−11.2	47.2	6.21	4	33.6	3.2	−17.6	5.62	38
	−42	−7.6	43.6	5.78	6	40.8	28.4	22	7.78	46
	−49.2	28.4	32.8	6.25	9					
	−49.2	21.2	36.4	6.08	9					
	−52.79	13.99	32.79	3.5	9					

Specification of active clusters at $p < 0.001$ (cluster criterion: 10 voxels).

TABLE 2 | Diffusion Tensor Imaging results for white selected white matter tracts in the Eyeborg user and controls.

		FA value	ADC value (10^{-3}MM^2/S)
Corpus callosum	Eyeborg user	0.57 ± 0.02*	0.92 ± 0.03
	Controls	0.52 ± 0.03	0.88 ± 0.02
Inferior longitudinal fasciculus			
Left	Eyeborg user	0.53 ± 0.01	0.85 ± 0.02
	Controls	0.49 ± 0.03	0.84 ± 0.04
Right	Eyeborg user	0.51 ± 0.01	0.86 ± 0.02
	Controls	0.48 ± 0.02	0.82 ± 0.04
Inferior fronto-occipital fasciculus			
Left	Eyeborg user	0.51 ± 0.06	0.82 ± 0.02
	Controls	0.45 ± 0.08	0.85 ± 0.09
Right	Eyeborg user	0.50 ± 0.07	0.83 ± 0.01
	Controls	0.48 ± 0.01	0.89 ± 0.02

*FA = fractional anisotropy value; ADC = apparent diffusion coefficient; *$p < 0.05$. Diffusion Tensor Imaging results for white selected white matter tracts in the Eyeborg user and controls.*

after learning how to use a specific SSD (Ptito et al., 2005; Amedi et al., 2007; Poirier et al., 2007; Connell and Merabet, 2014) showing similar cognitive and neural changes.

The fMRI version of the Farnsworth-Munsell 100 Hue test, requires the use of color information to make perceptual decisions about the sequencing of colors and is able to circumvent the difficulties found in previous studies of color processing areas using passive viewing of colors or simple color discrimination (Beauchamp et al., 1999). Our results showed that the activation in our subject during both, the chromatic and achromatic phases in the color test paradigm, were very similar and constrained to V1 (BA17) and the left V2 area (BA18). This finding fits perfectly with his difficulty for distinguishing between colors and his vision in shades of gray and confirms the usefulness of this test for studying the organization of color-selective areas in normal subjects and in persons with achromatopsia.

The paradigm that comprised visual-auditory stimuli also displayed significant differences in the brain activation pattern of the Eyeborg user. Thus when we presented simultaneously visual images and their correspondent sounds encoded by the Eyeborg algorithms, the activated areas involved the temporal lobe and included the auditory cortex (BA42), Wernicke's area (BA22) and the rostral part of the superior and middle temporal gyri (BA38), which has been recently related to color and structural judgments of familiar objects (Kellenbach et al., 2005). A particular point of interest is the bilateral activation of BA13 in the Eyeborg user. This finding was not present in any of the control subjects. BA13 is located in the posterior insular cortex and several studies relate this area with phonation, pitch judgment and melodic perception (Zatorre et al., 1994; Kikuta et al., 2006). Moreover, there were

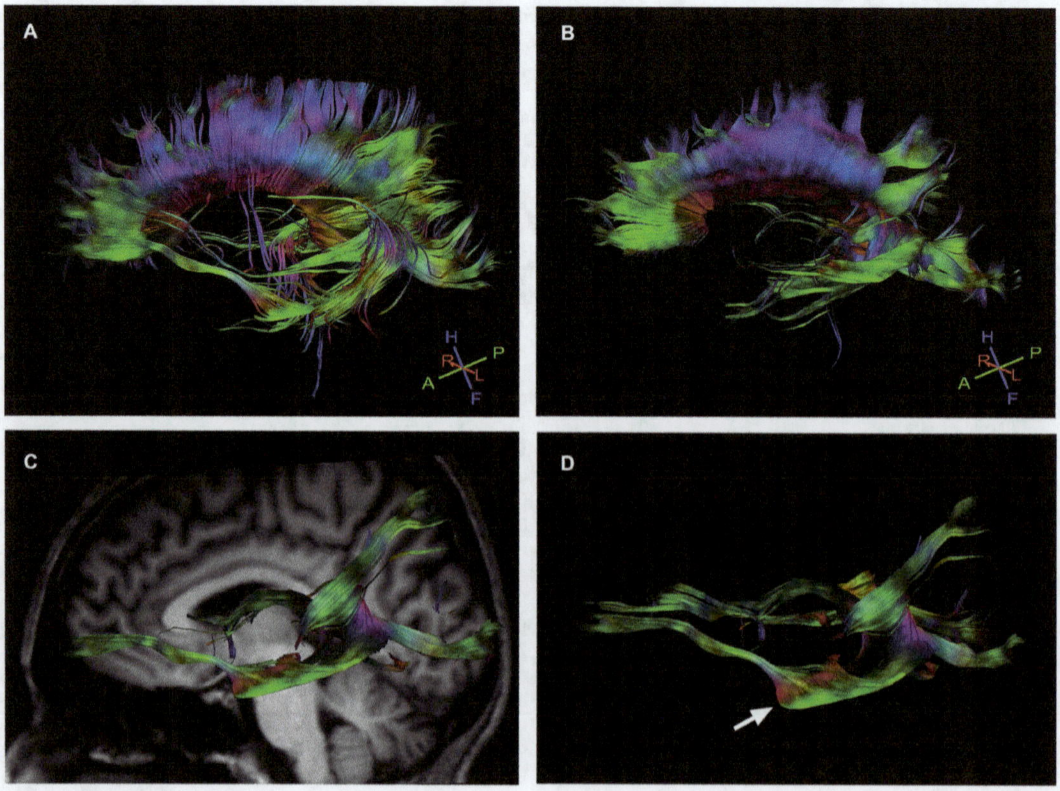

FIGURE 3 | Tractography results. (A) Callosal fiber tracks in the Eyeborg user. **(B)** Callosal fiber tracks in a representative control subject (matched in age and sex). **(C)** Left inferior fronto-occipital fasciculus (IFOF), which connects the ventral occipital lobe and the orbitofrontal cortex, in the Eyeborg user. **(D)** Enlargement of the IFOF displayed in panel **(C)**. The arrow points the region with increased myelin density related to the temporal lobe.

robust activations in prefrontal, orbito-frontal, premotor and supplementary motor cortex (BA10, BA11 and BA6). We think that the activation of the orbito-frontal cortex is highly relevant due to its robust connections not only with limbic and olfactory systems but also with the ventral visual pathways involved in the analysis of form and color of the visual information. However, it is also possible that it can be related to some ectopic changes due to other adaptive processes or even to some other preexisting anomalous connections in this particular subject.

The individual variability observed in functional imaging studies may also be related to underlying anatomical patterns that can be studied thanks to recent methodological advances in DTI and fiber tractography (DTI). Our results showed an enhanced structural connectivity between frontal lobe and auditory and visual association areas in the Eyeborg user. Thus, compared to controls, the Eyeborg user has an increased myelin density, which is probably related to a greater number of axons in the IFOF. This is a ventral associative bundle that connects the ventral occipital lobe and the orbitofrontal cortex. Furthermore, IFOF also constitutes one of the major efferent and afferent neuronal projections between the prefrontal cortex, auditory and visual association cortex (Catani et al., 2003; Catani and Mesulam, 2008).

As our subject reports seeing colors upon hearing sounds by using the *Eyeborg*, we hypothesized that the increased FA in IFOF might be related with a pattern of functional connectivity between frontal, auditory and visual association areas and could be involved in enhanced cross-modal associations to process the new information. In support of this idea, an increased structural connectivity in the right IFOF in people with color-music synesthesia has been recently described. This suggests that this perceptual experience could be linked to higher white matter connectivity in this pathway (Zamm et al., 2013). Presently, it

TABLE 3 | ^{1}H-MRS results showing the metabolite ratios for the Eyeborg user and the control subjects.

	Metabolite ratios			
Voxel Location	**NAA/Cr**	**Glx/Cr**	**Cho/Cr**	**mIno/Cr**
V1				
Eyeborg user	1.53	1.74	0.46	0.42
Controls	1.45 ± 0.12	1.33 ± 0.31	0.52 ± 0.06	0.55 ± 0.09
V2				
Eyeborg user	1.63	1.27	0.56	0.57
Controls	1.41 ± 0.12	1.05 ± 0.30	0.44 ± 0.01	0.58 ± 0.12
V4				
Eyeborg user	1.48	0.93	0.43	0.8
Controls	1.44 ± 0.10	1.07 ± 0.17	0.64 ± 0.18	0.62 ± 0.11

(NAA), N-acetylaspartate and other N-acetyl-containing compounds. (Glx), Glutamate and Glutamine. (Cr), Creatine. (Cho), Choline. (mIno), Myo-inositol. Data obtained at ^{1}H MR spectroscopy.

remains an open question as to whether, sensory substitution and synesthesia share similar neural mechanisms. In fact, some authors point out that sensory substitution shows properties of synesthesia, as both are associated with atypical perceptual experiences elicited by the processing of a qualitatively different stimulus to that which normally gives rise to that experience (Zamm et al., 2013). In this context, results from the current study seem to suggest that color-sound synesthesia as well as the continued use of the *Eyeborg* could potentially share a common underlying neuroanatomical basis where IFOF has a major role. Another important finding is the higher FA values in ILF in the Eyeborg user. ILF is a direct connection from the occipital cortex to the anterior part of the temporal lobe, running laterally and inferiorly above optic radiation fibers. However, it is important to note that in contrast to IFOF, which is known as a direct pathway (one that connects the occipital, posterior temporal, and the orbito-frontal areas), the ILF is considered to be an indirect pathway that essentially connects similar brain locations. This leads us to believe that IFOF and ILF are probably enhancing similar perceptive processes in our subject, which could be represented by a functional heightened network between frontal, auditory and visual association areas.

The DTI also reveals other structural differences in the Eyeborg user such as an increase of white matter tracts in the CC. The CC is the largest bundle of the human brain and connects left and right cerebral hemispheres. It allows the transfer of inputs from one hemisphere to the other and is involved in several motor, perceptual and cognitive functions (Catani and Thiebaut de Schotten, 2008). In the case of our subject, increased connectivity in CC could be ascribed to the use of *Eyeborg*, however future work will be needed to determine the exact meaning and repeatability of these connectivity changes.

On the other hand, the magnetic resonance spectroscopy (^{1}H-MRS) also revealed some changes in metabolic levels of mIno, NAA and Glx in the visual brain areas of the Eyeborg user. Myo-inositol is the most common biological stereoisomer of inositol, a sugar-like molecule synthesized mainly within astrocytes, which has been proposed as a marker of remodeling and plays an essential role in the mechanisms of brain adaptation and plasticity (Bernabeu et al., 2009; Weaver et al., 2013). Specifically, we found an increase in the levels of mIno/Cr in V4, which is mostly involved in color constancy and responds according to perceptual color space. Furthermore, we also found an increase in the NAA/Cr ratio in V2, that is particularly localized within neurons and considered as a major marker for neural integrity. This could reflect not only a higher neuronal and axonal density but also compensatory adjustments in which neurons could be actively implicated. Likewise, there is an increase in the Glx/Cr (Glutamate plus Glutamine) ratio in V1 and V2, in the Eyeborg user which could reflect changes in excitatory biochemical pathways in these areas and a higher synaptic activity (Hensch and Fagiolini, 2005; Bavelier et al., 2010). Taken together all these findings might suggest, the existence of an interconnected network in which glia and neurons work together to process and adapt to the novel sensory experience. In support of this idea, it has been recently proposed (Weaver et al., 2013) that continued use of SSDs might have an effect analogous to the environmental enrichment, resulting in an increase in the astrocyte population and its excitatory synapses that might lead to functional changes in brain activity.

In conclusion, we have tried to present some cues about the possible brain changes associated with the use of the Eyeborg. Our results suggest that there are metabolic, structural and functional changes, particularly in visual and auditive cortices, following the continuous use of this specific SSD device. However, we should emphasize that this is a preliminary work and that further studies, including the analysis of the same subjects before and after the continuous use of a SSD device such as the Eyeborg should be performed. We expect that the precise understanding of these plastic changes will have clear implications for new device development and for more efficient rehabilitative programs for people with disabilities. Furthermore, they could also be helpful in the framework of other approaches for restoring lost neural functions such as innovative artificial vision systems or novel cochlear implants (Fernández et al., 2005; Fernandez and Merabet, 2011).

Acknowledgments

We are very grateful to all our volunteers for their time and their help in supporting this study. This work has been supported in part by grant MAT2012-39290-C02-01, by the Bidons Egara Research Chair of the University Miguel Hernández and by a research grant of the Spanish Blind Organization (ONCE).

References

Abboud, S., Hanassy, S., Levy-Tzedek, S., Maidenbaum, S., and Amedi, A. (2014). EyeMusic: introducing a "visual" colorful experience for the blind using auditory sensory substitution. *Restor. Neurol Neurosci.* 32, 247–257. doi: 10.3233/RNN-130338

Amedi, A., Stern, W. M., Camprodon, J. A., Bermpohl, F., Merabet, L., Rotman, S., et al. (2007). Shape conveyed by visual-to-auditory sensory substitution activates the lateral occipital complex. *Nat. Neurosci.* 10, 687–689. doi: 10.1038/nn1912

Bavelier, D., Levi, D. M., Li, R. W., Dan, Y., and Hensch, T. K. (2010). Removing brakes on adult brain plasticity: from molecular to behavioral interventions. *J. Neurosci.* 30, 14964–14971. doi: 10.1523/JNEUROSCI.4812-10.2010

Beauchamp, M. S., Haxby, J. V., Jennings, J. E., and DeYoe, E. A. (1999). An fMRI version of the Farnsworth-Munsell 100-Hue test reveals multiple color-selective areas in human ventral occipitotemporal cortex. *Cereb. Cortex* 9, 257–263. doi: 10.1093/cercor/9.3.257

Bernabeu, A., Alfaro, A., García, M., and Fernández, E. (2009). Proton magnetic resonance spectroscopy (^{1}H-MRS) reveals the presence of elevated myo-inositol in the occipital cortex of blind subjects. *Neuroimage* 47, 1172–1176. doi: 10.1016/j.neuroimage.2009.04.080

Bologna, G., Deville, B., and Pun, T. (2009). On the use of the auditory pathway to represent image scenes in real-time. *Neurocomputing* 72, 839–849. doi: 10.1016/j.neucom.2008.06.020

Capelle, C., Trullemans, C., Arno, P., and Veraart, C. (1998). A real-time experimental prototype for enhancement of vision rehabilitation using auditory substitution. *IEEE Trans. Biomed. Eng.* 45, 1279–1293. doi: 10.1109/10.720206

Catani, M., Jones, D. K., Donato, R., and Ffytche, D. H. (2003). Occipito-temporal connections in the human brain. *Brain* 126, 2093–2107. doi: 10.1093/brain/awg203

Catani, M., and Mesulam, M. (2008). The arcuate fasciculus and the disconnection theme in language and aphasia: history and current state. *Cortex* 44, 953–961. doi: 10.1016/j.cortex.2008.04.002

Catani, M., and Thiebaut de Schotten, M. (2008). A diffusion tensor imaging tractography atlas for virtual *in vivo* dissections. *Cortex* 44, 1105–1132. doi: 10.1016/j.cortex.2008.05.004

Cohen, L. G., Celnik, P., Pascual-Leone, A., Corwell, B., Falz, L., Dambrosia, J., et al. (1997). Functional relevance of cross-modal plasticity in blind humans. *Nature* 389, 180–183. doi: 10.1038/38278

Connell, N., and Merabet, L. B. (2014). Uncovering the connectivity of the brain in relation to novel vision rehabilitation strategies. *Neurology* 83, 484–485. doi: 10.1212/WNL.0000000000000664

Cramer, S. C., Sur, M., Dobkin, B. H., O'Brien, C., Sanger, T. D., Trojanowski, J. Q., et al. (2011). Harnessing neuroplasticity for clinical applications. *Brain* 134, 1591–1609. doi: 10.1093/brain/awr039

Cronly-Dillon, J., Persaud, K., and Gregory, R. P. (1999). The perception of visual images encoded in musical form: a study in cross-modality information transfer. *Proc. Biol. Sci.* 266, 2427–2433. doi: 10.1098/rspb.1999.0942

Engel, S. A., Rumelhart, D. E., Wandell, B. A., Lee, A. T., Glover, G. H., Chichilnisky, E. J., et al. (1994). fMRI of human visual cortex. *Nature* 369:525. doi: 10.1038/369525a0

Eyeborg. (2015). Available online at: http://en.wikipedia.org/wiki/Eyeborg. Accessed on 2015.

Fabri, M., Pierpaoli, C., Barbaresi, P., and Polonara, G. (2014). Functional topography of the corpus callosum investigated by DTI and fMRI. *World J. Radiol.* 6, 895–906. doi: 10.4329/wjr.v6.i12.895

Fernandez, E., and Merabet, L. B. (2011). "Cortical plasticity and reorganization in severe vision loss," in *Visual Prosthetics*, ed G. Dagnelie (New York, NY: Springer), 77–92.

Fernández, E., Pelayo, F., Romero, S., Bongard, M., Marin, C., Alfaro, A., et al. (2005). Development of a cortical visual neuroprosthesis for the blind: the relevance of neuroplasticity. *J. Neural Eng.* 2, R1–R12. doi: 10.1088/1741-2560/2/4/r01

Goebel, R., Esposito, F., and Formisano, E. (2006). Analysis of functional image analysis contest (FIAC) data with brainvoyager QX: from single-subject to cortically aligned group general linear model analysis and self-organizing group independent component analysis. *Hum. Brain Mapp.* 27, 392–401. doi: 10.1002/hbm.20249

Haga, K. K., Khor, Y. P., Farrall, A., and Wardlaw, J. M. (2009). A systematic review of brain metabolite changes, measured with 1H magnetic resonance spectroscopy, in healthy aging. *Neurobiol. Aging* 30, 353–363. doi: 10.1016/j.neurobiolaging.2007.07.005

Hensch, T. K., and Fagiolini, M. (2005). Excitatory-inhibitory balance and critical period plasticity in developing visual cortex. *Prog. Brain Res.* 147, 115–124. doi: 10.1016/s0079-6123(04)47009-5

Kahol, K., French, J., Bratton, L., and Panchanathan, S. (2006). Learning and perceiving colors haptically. *Proc. ASSETS* 173–180. doi: 10.1145/1168987.1169017

Kantarci, K. (2014). Fractional anisotropy of the fornix and hippocampal atrophy in Alzheimer's disease. *Front. Aging Neurosci.* 6:316. doi: 10.3389/fnagi.2014.00316

Kellenbach, M. L., Hovius, M., and Patterson, K. (2005). A pet study of visual and semantic knowledge about objects. *Cortex* 41, 121–132. doi: 10.1016/s0010-9452(08)70887-6

Kikuta, K., Takagi, Y., Nozaki, K., Hanakawa, T., Okada, T., Miki, Y., et al. (2006). Early experience with 3-T magnetic resonance tractography in the surgery of cerebral arteriovenous malformations in and around the visual pathway. *Neurosurgery* 58, 331–337; discussion 331–337. doi: 10.1227/01.neu.0000195017.82776.90

Maidenbaum, S., Abboud, S., and Amedi, A. (2014). Sensory substitution: closing the gap between basic research and widespread practical visual rehabilitation. *Neurosci. Biobehav. Rev.* 41, 3–15. doi: 10.1016/j.neubiorev.2013.11.007

Meijer, P. B. (1992). An experimental system for auditory image representations. *IEEE Trans. Biomed. Eng.* 39, 112–121. doi: 10.1109/10.121642

Merabet, L. B., and Pascual-Leone, A. (2010). Neural reorganization following sensory loss: the opportunity of change. *Nat. Rev. Neurosci.* 11, 44–52. doi: 10.1038/nrn2758

Naressi, A., Couturier, C., Castang, I., de Beer, R., and Graveron-Demilly, D. (2001). Java-based graphical user interface for MRUI, a software package for quantitation of *in vivo*/medical magnetic resonance spectroscopy signals. *Comput. Biol. Med.* 31, 269–286. doi: 10.1016/s0010-4825(01)00006-3

Nie, M., Ren, J., Li, Z., Niu, J., Qiu, Y., Zhu, Y., et al. (2009). SoundView: an auditory guidance system based on environment understanding for the visually impaired people. *Conf. Proc. IEEE Eng. Med. Biol. Soc.* 2009, 7240–7243. doi: 10.1109/IEMBS.2009.5334754

Nilsson, C., Markenroth Bloch, K., Brockstedt, S., Lätt, J., Widner, H., and Larsson, E. M. (2007). Tracking the neurodegeneration of parkinsonian disorders–a pilot study. *Neuroradiology* 49, 111–119. doi: 10.1007/s00234-006-0165-1

Nudo, R. J. (2006). Plasticity. *NeuroRx* 3, 420–427. doi: 10.1016/j.nurx.2006.07.006

Pascual-Leone, A., Amedi, A., Fregni, F., and Merabet, L. B. (2005). The plastic human brain cortex. *Annu. Rev. Neurosci.* 28, 377–401. doi: 10.1146/annurev.neuro.27.070203.144216

Poirier, C., De Volder, A., Tranduy, D., and Scheiber, C. (2007). Pattern recognition using a device substituting audition for vision in blindfolded sighted subjects. *Neuropsychologia* 45, 1108–1121. doi: 10.1016/j.neuropsychologia.2006.09.018

Poveda, M. J., Bernabeu, A., Concepción, L., Roa, E., de Madaria, E., Zapater, P., et al. (2010). Brain edema dynamics in patients with overt hepatic encephalopathy a magnetic resonance imaging study. *Neuroimage* 52, 481–487. doi: 10.1016/j.neuroimage.2010.04.260

Proulx, M. J., Ptito, M., and Amedi, A. (2014). Multisensory integration, sensory substitution and visual rehabilitation. *Neurosci. Biobehav. Rev.* 41, 1–2. doi: 10.1016/j.neubiorev.2014.03.004

Ptito, M., Moesgaard, S. M., Gjedde, A., and Kupers, R. (2005). Cross-modal plasticity revealed by electrotactile stimulation of the tongue in the congenitally blind. *Brain* 128, 606–614. doi: 10.1093/brain/awh380

Striem-Amit, E., Guendelman, M., and Amedi, A. (2012). 'Visual' acuity of the congenitally blind using visual-to-auditory sensory substitution. *PLoS One* 7:e33136. doi: 10.1371/journal.pone.0033136

Tregellas, J. R., Ellis, J., Shatti, S., Du, Y. P., and Rojas, D. C. (2009). Increased hippocampal, thalamic and prefrontal hemodynamic response to an urban noise stimulus in schizophrenia. *Am. J. Psychiatry* 166, 354–360. doi: 10.1176/appi.ajp.2008.08030411

Wakana, S., Jiang, H., Nagae-Poetscher, L. M., van Zijl, P. C., and Mori, S. (2004). Fiber tract-based atlas of human white matter anatomy. *Radiology* 230, 77–87. doi: 10.1148/radiol.2301021640

Weaver, K. E., Richards, T. L., Saenz, M., Petropoulos, H., and Fine, I. (2013). Neurochemical changes within human early blind occipital cortex. *Neuroscience* 252, 222–233. doi: 10.1016/j.neuroscience.2013.08.004

Yoshida, S., Oishi, K., Faria, A. V., and Mori, S. (2013). Diffusion tensor imaging of normal brain development. *Pediatr. Radiol.* 43, 15–27. doi: 10.1007/s00247-012-2496-x

Zamm, A., Schlaug, G., Eagleman, D. M., and Loui, P. (2013). Pathways to seeing music: enhanced structural connectivity in colored-music synesthesia. *Neuroimage* 74, 359–366. doi: 10.1016/j.neuroimage.2013.02.024

Zatorre, R. J., Evans, A. C., and Meyer, E. (1994). Neural mechanisms underlying melodic perception and memory for pitch. *J. Neurosci.* 14, 1908–1919.

23

Weighing the Cost and Benefit of Transcranial Direct Current Stimulation on Different Reading Subskills

Jessica W. Younger[1,2]*, *Melissa Randazzo Wagner*[1,3] *and James R. Booth*[1,2]

[1] *Department of Communication Sciences and Disorders, Northwestern University, Evanston, IL, USA,* [2] *Department of Communication Sciences and Disorders, University of Texas at Austin, Austin, TX, USA,* [3] *Department of Communication Sciences and Disorders, Teachers College, Columbia University, New York, NY, USA*

Edited by:
Manuel Fernando Casanova, University of Louisville, USA

Reviewed by:
Gabriele Miceli, University of Trento, Italy
Deniz Doruk, Harvard Medical School, USA

***Correspondence:**
Jessica W. Younger
jrwise@utexas.edu

Adults struggling with low reading skills are underserved by limited available treatments. While brain stimulation techniques such as transcranial direct current stimulation (tDCS) has the potential to improve a variety of cognitive functions, little work has been done examining its potential to treat reading disabilities. Research on the effects of tDCS on reading abilities has been somewhat inconsistent perhaps in part due to discrepancies between studies in the nature of the tasks. In the current study, we examined the effect of tDCS to the left inferior parietal lobe (L IPL) on two reading tasks in low-to-average readers. We compared performance on a sight word efficiency (SWE) task and a rhyme judgment task before and after either stimulation to the L IPL, right superior parietal lobe (R SPL), or sham stimulation. Readers who received stimulation to the L IPL showed greater improvements on the SWE task, but less improvement on the rhyme judgment task compared to the R SPL and sham groups. This study demonstrates for the first time both a positive and negative effect of stimulation under the same stimulation parameters within the same participants. The results highlight the need to consider multiple tasks when assessing the potential of using tDCS as a treatment.

Keywords: reading intervention, transcranial direct current stimulation, parietal lobes, sight word efficiency, rhyming

INTRODUCTION

Over the last decade, interest in using brain stimulation techniques as a therapeutic tool to treat cognitive impairment in adults has received increasing attention (Dubljević et al., 2014). Brain stimulation is a non-invasive method using electrical currents to alter the firing potential of neurons in the affected area. While there are a variety of techniques that can be used to stimulate the brain, two primary techniques are transcranial magnetic stimulation (TMS) and transcranial direct current stimulation (tDCS). TMS delivers a larger current and is thought to cause neurons to fire (Ridding and Rothwell, 2007) while tDCS delivers a much smaller current and is believed to change the membrane potential of neurons (Nitsche et al., 2008; Priori et al., 2009) Both techniques have been used to enhance performance on tasks involved in a variety of cognitive processes in healthy and impaired adults (Miniussi et al., 2008; Nitsche et al., 2008; Williams et al., 2009; Nitsche and Paulus, 2011; Krause and Cohen Kadosh, 2013). While the evidence for brain stimulation improving function in healthy adults has been somewhat controversial (see Horvath et al., 2015 but also Price et al., 2015), its use as a treatment in patient populations with brain injury has been promising (Fregni and Pascual-Leone, 2007; Miniussi et al., 2008; Wong and Tsang, 2013).

More recently, research using brain stimulation to treat learning disorders, such as dyslexia and dyscalculia, has been called for (Cohen Kadosh et al., 2013; Krause and Cohen Kadosh, 2013; Vicario and Nitsche, 2013). While those with learning disorders do not have frank insult to the brain, they are believed to have altered brain activation in key brain regions when compared to typical adults (Pugh et al., 2001; Price and Ansari, 2013; Norton et al., 2014; Kucian and von Aster, 2015). The case for using neuromodulation to treat learning disorders is thus conceptually straightforward; stimulation to modify the activity in a brain region shown to be integral to the cognitive process of interest and differentially activated in the disordered population should normalize activation in that region and therefore normalize performance. However, identifying the brain regions integral to the process is not trivial, particularly in the case of reading.

Neuroimaging research has identified several brain regions that show altered function in individuals with dyslexia that may serve as potential targets of brain stimulation. Three brain areas in particular have consistently shown altered functionality compared to typical readers—the inferior frontal gyrus (IFG), temporo-parietal areas, and occipito-temporal areas (Richlan et al., 2009, 2011). Meta-analysis of neuroimaging studies suggest the IFG may be hyperactive in adults with dyslexia as a compensatory region, while temporo-parietal and occipito-temporal areas may be hypoactive, reflecting impaired processing during reading. Brain stimulation could be used to either enhance potential compensatory regions in an attempt to strengthen these networks or enhance areas that are consistently underactive in people with dyslexia in an attempt to normalize their function.

So far, neuromodulation studies examining the tool's potential to improve reading ability have stimulated regions shown to be underactivated in poor readers, and all have had some success (Costanzo et al., 2012, 2013; Turkeltaub et al., 2012; Heth and Lavidor, 2015; Thomson et al., 2015). However, the exact nature of the reading improvements has been somewhat inconsistent across studies. Turkeltaub et al. (2012) first demonstrated the potential for tDCS to be used as a treatment for low-to-average readers by showing improved reading fluency after stimulation to the left superior temporal gyrus (STG) compared to sham stimulation. These findings were corroborated by Costanzo et al.'s TMS studies (Costanzo et al., 2012, 2013) that found TMS to the left STG increased real word reading speed and text reading accuracy in both dyslexic and average readers. However, a later tDCS study by Thomson et al. (2015) was inconsistent with the findings of Turkeltaub et al. (2012). Thomson et al. (2015) stimulated an overlapping, but slightly superior region to that stimulated in Turkeltaub et al. (2012) in average readers and found that right hemisphere stimulation led to improvements on real word reading ability, not left hemisphere.

The Costanzo et al.'s TMS studies (Costanzo et al., 2012, 2013) showed that the particular section of the temporo-parietal region that is stimulated leads to specific results. In contrast to the increases in real word reading following STG stimulation mentioned above, stimulation to the more superior temporo-parietal cortex, specifically, the left inferior parietal lobe (L IPL), led to increases in pseudoword reading. While the lack of improvements in real word reading, the ultimate goal of reading therapy, is discouraging, stimulation to the IPL and surrounding areas merits further investigation. In particular, tDCS to the more superior aspects of the temporo-parietal cortex may lead to greater gains in reading ability compared to the precisely targeted stimulation of TMS given the diffusivity of tDCS. The superior portion of the temporo-parietal cortex including not just IPL, but also the angular gyrus (AG) and supramarginal gyrus (SMG), have been specifically related to smaller-grained grapheme-to-phoneme mapping (Pugh et al., 2000; Simos et al., 2001; Booth et al., 2003; Jobard et al., 2003; Cao et al., 2006; Bitan et al., 2007b; He et al., 2013), which developmental and cross-linguistic studies of reading suggest is important for the initial development of the reading network (Pugh et al., 2000; Cao et al., 2006, 2015; Richlan et al., 2011; Martin et al., 2015). Therefore, we propose that facilitation of small-grain grapheme-to-phoneme processing via modulation of activation in superior portions of the temporo-parietal cortex may lead to gains in multiple aspects of reading ability including reading fluency and improved grapheme-phoneme mappings in low-to-average ability adults.

This hypothesis is supported by second language learning studies with adults (Hashimoto and Sakai, 2004; Mei et al., 2014) and reading remediation studies with children (Temple et al., 2003; Simos et al., 2007; Meyler et al., 2008; Rezaie et al., 2011b) and adults (Eden et al., 2004) that show greater ability related gains in superior vs. inferior temporo-parietal cortex. Further, functional connectivity between the IPL in particular and regions involved in orthographic processing such as the fusiform gyrus (FG) has been demonstrated to be related to word reading ability (Koyama et al., 2011; Simon et al., 2013). Developmental studies have suggested that the strength of the connection between grapheme-to-phoneme processing regions such as the IPL and the orthographic processing regions such as the FG may be critical for the specialization of these orthographic processing regions, in line with interactive specialization models of development that have been extended to reading (Johnson, 2001; Schlaggar and McCandliss, 2007; Price and Devlin, 2011). Indeed, dyslexic readers tend to have reduced connectivity between these two regions compared to controls. In contrast, there is little evidence suggesting the connectivity between the STG and FG is crucial for reading ability (Horwitz et al., 1998; Pugh et al., 2000; Booth et al., 2008; Cao et al., 2008; Quaglino et al., 2008; van der Mark et al., 2011; Finn et al., 2014).

In order to test the hypothesis that tDCS to superior portions of the temporo-parietal cortex will lead to reading improvement for low ability readers, we stimulated the left IPL in low-to-average readers and measured their improvement on two reading tasks; single word reading efficiency and a rhyme judgment task. Both require the use of phonological and orthographic information, but in different ways. Single word reading efficiency requires articulating the phonological output from orthographic input. This skill has been shown to be related to both overall word reading ability and the ability to decode words based on grapheme-to-phoneme mappings (Adlof et al., 2006; Vellutino et al., 2007; Barth et al., 2009). Despite the orthographic processing component, neuroimaging studies have suggested that this skill is most related to parietal areas including the IPL and AG (He et al., 2013) typically implicated in grapheme-phoneme mappings, compared to areas involved in whole-word orthographic mappings. Further, training studies have shown that instruction in grapheme-to-phoneme mapping results in improvement in single word reading fluency (Ashmore et al., 2002; Simos et al., 2007) and these gains are related to activation in parietal areas (Rezaie et al., 2011a,b). The rhyme judgment task, in contrast, does not require articulation. Rather it requires the activation and memory of phonological representations, sometimes in the face of conflicting orthographic information. For this reason, this task is a measure of phonological working memory and the strength of the grapheme-to-phoneme maps needed to be activated to complete the task accurately. Behavioral studies have shown the rhyming task to be related to reading ability (Maclean et al., 1987; Ziegler and Goswami, 2005; Kovelman et al., 2012) and neuroimaging studies have shown activation in the left IPL to be related to ability on this task (Booth et al., 2003; Hoeft et al., 2006; Bitan et al., 2007a). Together, both tasks provide measures of orthographic and phonological processing that are related to activation in the left IPL. By using these two tasks, we can address how tDCS affects both the mental manipulation and articulation of phonological representation and therefore have a broader picture of what abilities can be impacted by tDCS.

METHODS

This study was carried out in accordance with the recommendations of the University of Texas at Austin Institutional Review Board with written informed consent from all subjects. All subjects gave written informed consent in accordance with the Declaration of Helsinki.

Participants

In total, 100 right-handed 18–35 year-old native English speakers with normal or corrected-to-normal vision were screened for below average reading ability (<100 standard score) as determined by the Sight Word Efficiency (SWE) subtest of the Test of Word Reading Efficiency (TOWRE; Torgesen et al., 1999) in line with Turkeltaub et al. (2012). All participants reported no history of neurological disorder, psychiatric disorder, significant head trauma, hearing loss, substance abuse, seizure or migraine, metal implants, and current pregnancy. Of the initial 100, 54 participants scored below average, however, 14 did not complete both days of the experiment, and were therefore not included in the sample. An additional four participants were excluded for scoring <50% accuracy on behavioral measures. The remaining participants had at least average (>80 standard score) intelligence as measured by the Wechsler Abbreviated Scale of Intelligence (WASI; Wechsler, 2008). Scores on the SWE ranged from 74 to 99 pre-stimulation (within two standard deviations of 50th percentile performance of 100). Participants were randomly assigned to one of three groups, L IPL, right superior parietal lobe (R SPL), or Sham. Assignment to the R SPL group was done as part of an additional experiment not reported here. For the current experiment, the R SPL group served as a stimulation control condition in which participants received stimulation to a non-target region which complemented the no stimulation control condition fulfilled by the Sham group.

Of those who met all performance criteria, 11 (7 female) received real stimulation to the L IPL, 14 (6 female) received sham stimulation, and 11 (9 female) received real stimulation to the R SPL. Due to an imbalance in the run orders in the sham group, four participants were randomly eliminated for a final sample of 10 (4 female). One-way ANOVAs revealed no significant effects of group on all group characteristics and baseline measures as reported in **Table 1**.

Procedure

Participants took part in a single-blind, sham and stimulation controlled study comparing pre- and post-stimulation performance on two measures of reading ability: single word reading efficiency and rhyme judgment. Participants completed two sessions that took place 3–5 days apart. During the first session, participants completed standardized tests and baseline assessments of reading ability. During the second session, participants received either sham or real stimulation for 20 min, after which they completed an alternate form of the reading ability measures using different sets of stimuli. Alternate forms of the tasks were counterbalanced across participants.

Transcranial Direct Current Stimulation

Direct current was administered using a battery-driven DC stimulator device (NeuroConn) via two saline-soaked electrodes (5 × 5 cm; 25 cm^2). The anode electrode was placed over either the L IPL (P3) or R SPL (CP4) according to the international 10–20 system for electroencephalography (EEG) electrode placement (Herwig et al., 2003). The cathode (return) electrode was placed over the contralateral supraorbital frontal region. This montage allows the source of effects of stimulation to be more reliably attributed to the anodal stimulation of the target site instead of the cathodal stimulation of the reference site, as suggested by Turkeltaub et al. (2012). During real stimulation, 1.5 mA

TABLE 1 | Participant demographics and mean (SD) for performance for each participant group.

	L IPL	R SPL	Sham
Age (years)	26.8 (5.5)	25.2 (3.5)	26.2 (4.9)
Gender (f)	7	8	4
IQ	112.1 (10.9)	111.0 (11.70)	109.3 (9.9)
Pre-single word reading	88.5 (8.4)	88.1 (7.6)	89.2 (7.9)
Pre-rhyme judgment RT (ms)	854 (124)	972 (147)	998 (193)
Pre-rhyme judgment accuracy (%)	91.6 (7.0)	88.4 (9.5)	87.9 (12.0)

IQ measured by Wechsler Abbreviated Scale of Intelligence. Single Word Reading was measured by the Sight Word Efficiency subscale of the Test of Word Reading Efficiency. IQ and Single Word Reading have $\mu = 100$, $\sigma = 15$.

of current (current density 0.06 mA/cm2) was delivered for 20 min. During sham stimulation, the machine ramped up to 1.5 mA for 30 s, then extinguished over a 5 s fade-out. Using this procedure allows participants to feel the initial sensations (e.g., tingling or itching) associated with stimulation without any after-effects of stimulation being induced (Nitsche and Paulus, 2000). These stimulation parameters replicate the parameters used in Turkeltaub et al. (2012) and are within the safety limits established in prior studies on humans and animals (Iyer et al., 2005; Nitsche et al., 2008; Bikson et al., 2009).

Experimental Tasks

Single Word Reading Efficiency

Word reading efficiency was measured via the SWE subtest of the TOWRE. This test is a measure of ability to read real words accurately and quickly. Participants were given 45 s to read aloud as many of 104 words as possible. A standard score is determined by the number of words read correctly within 45 s, and this score was used as the metric of single word reading efficiency.

Rhyme Judgment Task

The ability to map orthography to phonology and phonological working memory were assessed with a rhyme judgment task in which participants were presented with a series of visual word pairs and asked to indicate whether the words rhymed or not. Word pairs were designed to manipulate orthographic and phonological similarity to ensure participants could not rely on orthography alone and phonological representations had to be used to accurately complete the task. There were two congruent conditions in which word pairs had either similar orthography and phonology (e.g., CAGE-RAGE) or not (e.g., TRIAL-FALL), and two incongruent conditions in which word pairs had either similar orthography but dissimilar phonology (e.g., PINT-MINT) or dissimilar orthography but similar phonology (e.g., GRADE-PAID) pairs. Each condition had 12 trials for a total of 48 trials in each session.

All words were monosyllabic, having neither homophones nor homographs and were matched across condition for written word frequency in children (Zeno, 1995) and the sum of written bigram frequency (Balota et al., 2007). Stimuli used in each version of the task were matched on average stimuli length, frequency, number of orthographic neighbors, and number of phonological neighbors (Balota et al., 2007).

Participants were asked to respond as quickly and as accurately as possible. The first word was presented for 800 ms followed by a 200 ms inter-stimulus interval and the presentation of the second word. Participants could respond as soon as the second word was presented up to 2500 ms after the onset of the word. After the participant responded, a red fixation cross appeared signaling the inter-trial interval. The task was self-paced and participants were able to control when the next trial began. Average reaction times (RT) to correct trials trimmed to include only responses within 2.5 standard deviations from an individual's average reaction time were used as the metric of rhyme judgment ability due to ceiling effects on accuracy.

Analysis

Performance on each experimental task was submitted to a 3 (Stimulation group; L IPL, Sham, R SPL) × 2 (Time; Session 1, Session 2) mixed-model ANOVA in order to determine whether a measure showed a Group × Time interaction. Planned follow-up tests were conducted using separate 2 (Stimulation group; L IPL, Sham or R SPL) × 2 (Time; Session 1, Session 2) mixed-model ANOVAs to examine potential Group × Time interactions for the L IPL group compared to the two control groups (Sham, R SPL) separately.

RESULTS

Single Word Reading

The 3 × 2 ANOVA revealed a significant main effect of Time [$F_{(1, 29)} = 24.68$, $p < 0.001$] and significant Group × Time interaction [$F_{(2, 29)} = 4.41$, $p = 0.021$], indicating that although all groups showed changes in their performance over time, the groups differed in the magnitude of these changes. Follow-up tests revealed the L IPL group showed significantly greater improvement compared to the Sham group [$F_{(1, 19)} = 7$, $p = 0.016$] and a trend toward greater improvement compared to the R SPL group [$F_{(1, 20)} = 4.22$, $p = 0.053$]. One sample t-tests indicated that the L IPL and R SPL groups' improvement was significantly greater than 0 [L IPL: $t_{(10)} = 4.17$, $p < 0.005$; R SPL: $t_{(10)} = 2.37$, $p < 0.05$], while the Sham group did not show improvement [$t_{(9)} = 1.72$, $p > 0.1$] see **Table 2** and **Figure 1**. The results of the current study result in an effect size (Cohen's d) of 1.57 for L IPL stimulation, greater than the 0.46 for left STG stimulation found by Turkeltaub et al. (2012).

Rhyme Judgment

All participants performed well on the rhyme judgment task as indicated by high accuracy at Time 1 and Time 2. A 3 × 3 ANOVA did not reveal a main effect of Time or any Group × Time interactions ($p > 0.1$). One sample t-tests for each group individually showed that no group's gain in accuracy was significantly greater than 0 ($p > 0.1$). These findings indicate that there was neither a practice effect nor an effect of stimulation on accuracy, possibly due to ceiling effects.

The 3 × 2 ANOVA again revealed a significant main effect of Time [$F_{(1, 29)} = 28.9$, $p < 0.001$] and significant Group × Time interaction [$F_{(2, 29)} = 4.13$, $p = 0.026$], indicating a change over time, but a group difference in the magnitude of the change. Follow-up tests showed the Sham group experienced significantly greater improvements in RT compared to the L IPL group [$F_{(1, 19)} = 7.27, p = 0.014$]. However, the R SPL group was not significantly different from either the Sham group [$F_{(1, 19)} = 2.62, p > 0.1$] or the L IPL group [$F_{(1, 20)} = 1.69, p > 0.1$]. *Post-hoc* one-sample t-tests, though, indicate that both the Sham and R SPL groups' improvement was significantly greater than 0 while the L IPL group did not improve [Sham: $t_{(9)} = 2.54, p = 0.006$; R SPL: $t_{(10)} = 2.31, p = 0.044$; L IPL: $t_{(10)} = 1.74, p > 0.1$] see **Table 2** and **Figure 2.**

TABLE 2 | Mean (SD) on reading measures pre- and post-stimulation.

	L IPL		R SPL		Sham	
	Pre	**Post**	**Pre**	**Post**	**Pre**	**Post**
Single word reading	88.5 (8.4)	98.8 (14.3)	88.1 (7.6)	92.2 (8.3)	89.2 (7.9)	91.7 (8.2)
Rhyme judgment RT (ms)	854 (124)	811 (142)	972 (147)	885 (141)	998 (193)	820 (99)
Rhyme judgment accuracy (%)	91.7 (7.0)	94.7 (7.5)	88.4 (9.5)	89.6 (10.6)	87.9 (12.1)	90.0 (9.0)

Single Word Reading has $\mu = 100$, $\sigma = 15$.

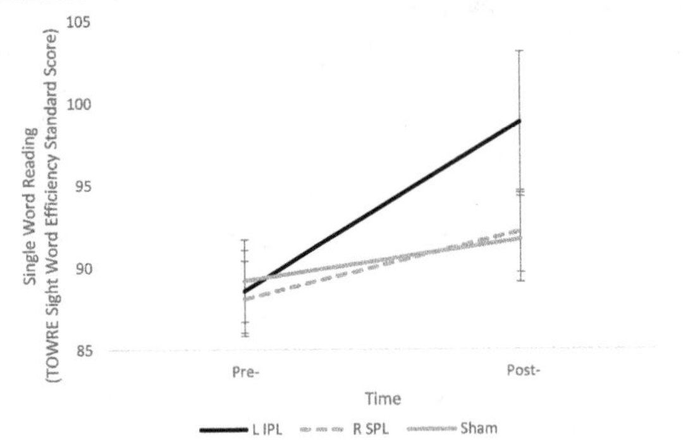

FIGURE 1 | Change in Single Word Reading Efficiency pre- and post-stimulation for each group. A significant Group × Time interaction indicates the L IPL group showed significantly greater improvement than the R SPL and Sham groups. Error bars indicate one standard deviation.

DISCUSSION

The goal of the current study was to assess whether stimulation of the L IPL improves multiple aspect of reading for low-to-average readers by measuring its impact on two tasks that tap into different subskills of reading. While L IPL stimulation did result in gains in single word reading efficiency, it resulted in relative impairment on the rhyme judgment task, demonstrating for the first time a significant positive and negative effect on two different tasks with the same stimulation parameters within the same group of participants. Although our results indicate stimulation to the L IPL may be a good site for improving reading fluency for low-to-average readers, the lack of improvement on the rhyme judgment task warrants caution in advocating the left IPL as a site to improve several aspects of reading.

The positive influence of L IPL stimulation on reading fluency measures for low-to-average readers was consistent with our hypothesis. Although there was a main effect of time, indicating there was a general practice effect for all groups, the L IPL stimulation resulted in greater improvement than the Sham or R SPL stimulation. Our finding that stimulation to the IPL led to greater improvements for low-to-average readers than previous reports of stimulation to the STG (Turkeltaub et al., 2012) are in line with studies indicating that single word reading fluency abilities depend on grapheme-to-phoneme mapping skills supported by the superior aspects of the temporo-parietal cortex (Ashmore et al., 2002; Simos et al., 2007; Rezaie et al., 2011a,b; He et al., 2013). This finding suggests that improvements in single word reading can result from increased grapheme-to-phoneme mapping abilities, even in adults. However, it should be noted that montage differences between the current study and that by Turkeltaub et al. (2012) could also account for the difference in effect size between the two studies. Turkeltaub et al. (2012) used a bilateral montage, meaning that the cathode or reference electrode was placed on the contralateral hemisphere (i.e., right STG). The results of that study cannot be attributed solely to facilitation of the left hemisphere, and the effects could have been due to alteration in the balance between the two hemispheres or even to inhibition of the right hemisphere. In contrast, in the current study, the cathode electrode was placed on the contralateral forehead. While we cannot rule out that the effects in the current study were due to inhibition of the frontal lobe, it is more reasonable to conclude that the effects are due to the modulation of activation in the stimulation site and surrounding areas. As Turkeltaub et al. (2012) themselves point out, it could be that unilateral stimulation may be more beneficial than bilateral stimulation. Further research should explore how montage affects the behavioral consequences of stimulation.

Our results that left hemisphere stimulation leads to improvement in SWE is in contrast to Thomson et al. (2015) who found that right, but not left, hemisphere stimulation led to behavioral improvements. These conflicting results are likely due to the difference in populations used in each study. In keeping with the Turkeltaub et al. (2012) findings that stimulation only led to improvements in low-to-average readers, the current study only used readers who had below average performance on the TOWRE. However, Thomson et al. (2015) used participants with a wide range of reading abilities. Because individual differences in skill have been shown to have an effect on the behavioral changes induced by tDCS, including individuals with a large range of reading ability may have diluted the effects for the left hemisphere stimulation in the Thomson et al. (2015) study. Future research should examine how individual differences in reading ability affect the impact of tDCS on behavioral performance.

In contrast to the expected results of tDCS on the SWE, the negative effect of L IPL stimulation on improvement on the rhyming judgment task in low-to-average readers was unexpected. Previous neuroimaging work with both children and adults has shown that increases in activation in the left IPL are associated with better performance on the rhyming task (Hoeft et al., 2006; Bitan et al., 2007a; Cao et al., 2015). If anodal stimulation to the L IPL did increase activation in that area as hypothesized, the stimulation group should have

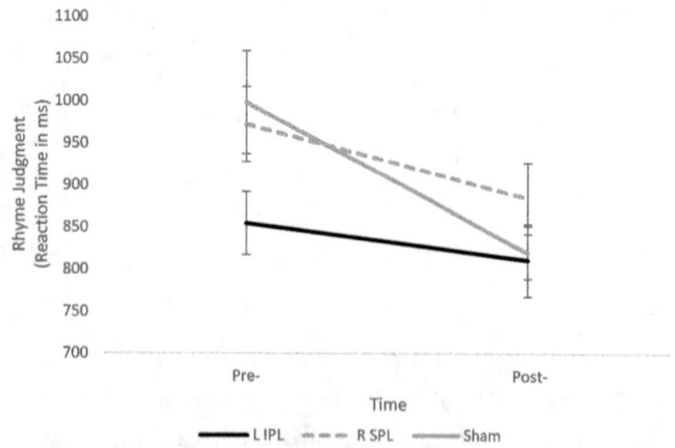

FIGURE 2 | Change in Rhyme Judgment performance pre- and post-stimulation for each group. A significant Group × Time interaction indicates the Sham group showed significantly greater improvement than the L IPL and R SPL groups. Error bars indicate one standard deviation.

shown increases in performance following stimulation. However, research with anodal stimulation to the IPL in the context of working memory has shown that stimulation actually impairs performance relative to sham, particularly in low performers (Jones and Berryhill, 2012; Sandrini et al., 2012). Specifically, Sandrini et al. (2012) showed that anodal stimulation abolished practice effects on a working memory task. These findings are in line with the results of the current study; while the L IPL stimulation group did not perform worse after stimulation, they did not demonstrate practice effects as seen in the sham group. The rhyming task involves phonological working memory when the phonological representation of the first word must be held in mind until the second word is presented and the two phonological representations can be compared to make a rhyme decision. Therefore, the effects of stimulation on working memory abilities may have prevented improvements on the task. Previous work examining the effect of stimulation to the parietal lobes has suggested that stimulation interferes with working memory by creating an imbalance of activation between the two hemispheres and interfering with the natural inter-hemispheric inhibition that occurs in the absence of stimulation (Sparing et al., 2009; Sandrini et al., 2012; Park and Friston, 2013; Krause and Cohen Kadosh, 2014). Inter-hemispheric inhibition may explain the seemingly contradictory results of the current study. As reading skills develop, activation during reading becomes more lateralized to the left hemisphere with the right hemisphere playing a decreasing role in reading (Turkeltaub et al., 2003; Eden et al., 2004; Shaywitz et al., 2004). Simulation causing disruptions to inter-hemispheric inhibition may thus be less likely to affect single word reading abilities, and therefore, we can expect improvements on single word reading tasks such as those seen in the current study. However, previous research has shown that low-to-average and dyslexic readers tend to have more bilateral activation during reading tasks with a phonological working memory component (Milne et al., 2002; Illingworth and Bishop, 2009; Xu et al., 2015). Given that the subjects in the current study were all low-to-average readers, it could be the case that the disruption to inter-hemispheric inhibition in the parietal lobes was particularly detrimental to their phonological working memory abilities, preventing the expected practice effects on the rhyming task. Our findings highlight the importance of considering the impact that individual differences may have on neural processing and subsequently the effects of tDCS.

From a clinical perspective, perhaps the most important finding from the current study is that tDCS can positively impact one skill while negatively impacting another. Our results underscore the importance of including multiple tasks that potentially tap into different underlying cognitive processes in order to assess whether the potential costs of stimulation outweigh the potential gains. Assessing multiple tasks becomes especially important when considering whether tDCS should be recommended as a treatment. In the current study, the cost in practice effect on speed during a rhyme judgment task is probably worth the gains seen in single word reading for low-to-average readers; accuracy was not affected and speed did not decrease after stimulation. However, this population was low-to-average in skill, not impaired. The cost to benefit ratio may increase as reading skill decreases. Further studies examining how individual differences impact the effects of tDCS on multiple reading tasks are needed before being able to advocate for tDCS as a treatment for reading disabilities.

Further, our findings that tDCS had a differential effect on two aspects of reading in low-to-average readers has implications for the design of future tDCS studies. In the current study, both tasks were reading-related, but the differences between tasks in the working memory component are in line with the literature that anodal tDCS does not have the expected positive effect on working memory abilities. These results support the idea that tDCS can affect cognitive processes differently, depending on how the target or surrounding brain area is involved in a given cognitive process. Future research is still needed to determine the circumstances in which the conventional idea that anodal stimulation leads to enhancement of activation and behavior while cathodal stimulation leads to inhibition of activation and behavior holds true (De Berker et al., 2013; Bestmann et al., 2015). When selecting target sites, the areas' involvement in multiple cognitive processes should be considered. The impact of stimulation on each of these processes should then be examined so that we might better understand whether tDCS can influence cognitive processes differently.

Limitations

The current study used a between subjects design, meaning that the different stimulation groups were composed of different individuals. While the groups were equated on task behavioral abilities, it is virtually impossible to equate them on all factors that could potentially impact the effects of stimulation. For example, other research groups have shown that individual differences in physiological measures such as skull thickness, and levels of certain hormones and neurotransmitters such as GABA, can affect the way stimulation affects an individual (Krause and Cohen Kadosh, 2014). Additionally, measures of non-reading related neurocognitive abilities were not collected. It is possible that differences in other cognitive processes between the two groups may have affected results. While the current study did not control for such measures, the use of random assignment to group and ensuring the group was matched on task performance should minimize potential confounds from these factors.

Finally, as with all tDCS studies, without the use of neuroimaging techniques such as structural or functional magnetic resonance imaging (fMRI), we are unable to confirm that the stimulated area was in fact the targeted area. Individual differences in anatomy may have led to differences in how well the stimulation site aligned with the brain regions that are actually used to perform the tasks. Similarly, due to the distributed effects of tDCS we cannot make strong conclusions about whether the results are due to stimulation to the targeted region or surrounding and connected regions without neuroimaging measures. Future research with tDCS would benefit from using neuroimaging methods to have more precisely located targets and a better understanding of the locations that were actually affected in order to develop the most effective treatment methods.

CONCLUSIONS

Our study provides important cautionary evidence for the use of tDCS as a treatment for low reading ability. Although stimulation to the left IPL led to greater improvements in reading fluency than those previously demonstrated with a different stimulation site (2012), we also found a negative effect on another subcomponent of reading in low-to-average readers, i.e., rhyming two visually presented words. These positive and negative effects on two different subcomponents of reading were demonstrated using the same stimulation parameters within the same participants. These results stress the need for further research examining the effect of a set of stimulation parameters on complementary skills so that potential users of tDCS as a therapy can accurately weigh the costs and benefits of the treatment.

AUTHOR CONTRIBUTIONS

MR and JB conceived and designed the experiments. MR and JY performed the experiments. JY and JB analyzed and interpreted the data. JY drafted the manuscript. JY, MR, and JB performed a critical review of the manuscript. All the authors read and approved the final version of the manuscript.

ACKNOWLEDGMENTS

This research was supported by the University of Texas at Austin. The authors would also like to thank the numerous research assistants who assisted in data collection throughout the study.

REFERENCES

Adlof, S. M., Catts, H. W., and Little, T. D. (2006). Should the simple view of reading include a fluency component? *Read. Writ.* 19, 933–958. doi: 10.1007/s11145-006-9024-z

Ashmore, R. A., Farrier, M. J., Paulson, L. H., and Chu, X. (2002). *The Effects of Phonemic Awareness Drills on Phonological Awareness and Word Reading Performance in a Later Learned Alphabetic Script*. Available online at: http://eric.ed.gov/?id=ED471632 (Accessed November 12, 2015).

Balota, D. A., Yap, M. J., Hutchison, K. A., Cortese, M. J., Kessler, B., Loftis, B., et al. (2007). The english lexicon project. *Behav. Res. Methods* 39, 445–459. doi: 10.3758/BF03193014

Barth, A. E., Catts, H. W., and Anthony, J. L. (2009). The component skills underlying reading fluency in adolescent readers: a latent variable analysis. *Read. Writ.* 22, 567–590. doi: 10.1007/s11145-008-9125-y

Bestmann, S., de Berker, A. O., and Bonaiuto, J. (2015). Understanding the behavioural consequences of noninvasive brain stimulation. *Trends Cogn. Sci.* 19, 13–20. doi: 10.1016/j.tics.2014.10.003

Bikson, M., Datta, A., and Elwassif, M. (2009). Establishing safety limits for transcranial direct current stimulation. *Clin. Neurophysiol.* 120, 1033–1034. doi: 10.1016/j.clinph.2009.03.018

Bitan, T., Burman, D. D., Chou, T.-L., Lu, D., Cone, N. E., Cao, F., et al. (2007a). The interaction between orthographic and phonological information in children: an fMRI study. *Hum. Brain Mapp.* 28, 880–891. doi: 10.1002/hbm.20313

Bitan, T., Cheon, J., Lu, D., Burman, D. D., Gitelman, D. R., Mesulam, M.-M., et al. (2007b). Developmental changes in activation and effective connectivity in phonological processing. *Neuroimage* 38, 564–575. doi: 10.1016/j.neuroimage.2007.07.048

Booth, J. R., Burman, D. D., Meyer, J. R., Gitelman, D. R., Parrish, T. B., and Mesulam, M. M. (2003). Relation between brain activation and lexical performance. *Hum. Brain Mapp.* 19, 155–169. doi: 10.1002/hbm.10111

Booth, J. R., Mehdiratta, N., Burman, D. D., and Bitan, T. (2008). Developmental increases in effective connectivity to brain regions involved in phonological processing during tasks with orthographic demands. *Brain Res.* 1189, 78–89. doi: 10.1016/j.brainres.2007.10.080

Cao, F., Bitan, T., and Booth, J. R. (2008). Effective brain connectivity in children with reading difficulties during phonological processing. *Brain Lang.* 107, 91–101. doi: 10.1016/j.bandl.2007.12.009

Cao, F., Bitan, T., Chou, T.-L., Burman, D. D., and Booth, J. R. (2006). Deficient orthographic and phonological representations in children with dyslexia revealed by brain activation patterns. *J. Child Psychol. Psychiatry* 47, 1041–1050. doi: 10.1111/j.1469-7610.2006.01684.x

Cao, F., Brennan, C., and Booth, J. R. (2015). The brain adapts to orthography with experience: evidence from English and Chinese. *Dev. Sci.* 18, 785–798. doi: 10.1111/desc.12245

Cohen Kadosh, R., Dowker, A., Heine, A., Kaufmann, L., and Kucian, K. (2013). Interventions for improving numerical abilities: present and future. *Trends Neurosci. Educ.* 2, 85–93. doi: 10.1016/j.tine.2013.04.001

Costanzo, F., Menghini, D., Caltagirone, C., Oliveri, M., and Vicari, S. (2012). High frequency rTMS over the left parietal lobule increases non-word reading accuracy. *Neuropsychologia* 50, 2645–2651. doi: 10.1016/j.neuropsychologia.2012.07.017

Costanzo, F., Menghini, D., Caltagirone, C., Oliveri, M., and Vicari, S. (2013). How to improve reading skills in dyslexics: the effect of high frequency rTMS. *Neuropsychologia* 51, 2953–2959. doi: 10.1016/j.neuropsychologia.2013.10.018

De Berker, A. O., Bikson, M., and Bestmann, S. (2013). Predicting the behavioral impact of transcranial direct current stimulation: issues and limitations. *Front. Hum. Neurosci.* 7:613. doi: 10.3389/fnhum.2013.00613

Dubljević, V., Saigle, V., and Racine, E. (2014). The rising tide of tDCS in the media and academic literature. *Neuron* 82, 731–736. doi: 10.1016/j.neuron.2014.05.003

Eden, G. F., Jones, K. M., Cappell, K., Gareau, L., Wood, F. B., Zeffiro, T. A., et al. (2004). Neural changes following remediation in adult developmental dyslexia. *Neuron* 44, 411–422. doi: 10.1016/j.neuron.2004.10.019

Finn, E. S., Shen, X., Holahan, J. M., Scheinost, D., Lacadie, C., Papademetris, X., et al. (2014). Disruption of functional networks in dyslexia: a whole-brain, data-driven analysis of connectivity. *Biol. Psychiatry* 76, 397–404. doi: 10.1016/j.biopsych.2013.08.031

Fregni, F., and Pascual-Leone, A. (2007). Technology insight: noninvasive brain stimulation in neurology-perspectives on the therapeutic potential of rTMS and tDCS. *Nat. Clin. Pract. Neurol.* 3, 383–393. doi: 10.1038/ncpneuro0530

Hashimoto, R., and Sakai, K. L. (2004). Learning letters in adulthood. *Neuron* 42, 311–322. doi: 10.1016/S0896-6273(04)00196-5

He, Q., Xue, G., Chen, C., Chen, C., Lu, Z.-L., and Dong, Q. (2013). Decoding the neuroanatomical basis of reading ability: a multivoxel morphometric study. *J. Neurosci.* 33, 12835–12843. doi: 10.1523/JNEUROSCI.0449-13.2013

Herwig, U., Satrapi, P., and Schönfeldt-Lecuona, C. (2003). Using the international 10-20 EEG system for positioning of transcranial magnetic stimulation. *Brain Topogr.* 16, 95–99. doi: 10.1023/B:BRAT.0000006333.93597.9d

Heth, I., and Lavidor, M. (2015). Improved reading measures in adults with dyslexia following transcranial direct current stimulation treatment. *Neuropsychologia* 70, 107–113. doi: 10.1016/j.neuropsychologia.2015.02.022

Hoeft, F., Hernandez, A., McMillon, G., Taylor-Hill, H., Martindale, J. L., Meyler, A., et al. (2006). Neural basis of dyslexia: a comparison between dyslexic and nondyslexic children equated for reading ability. *J. Neurosci.* 26, 10700–10708. doi: 10.1523/JNEUROSCI.4931-05.2006

Horvath, J. C., Forte, J. D., and Carter, O. (2015). Quantitative review finds no evidence of cognitive effects in healthy populations from single-session Transcranial Direct Current Stimulation (tDCS). *Brain Stimul.* 8, 535–550. doi: 10.1016/j.brs.2015.01.400

Horwitz, B., Rumsey, J. M., and Donohue, B. C. (1998). Functional connectivity of the angular gyrus in normal reading and dyslexia. *Proc. Natl. Acad. Sci. U.S.A.* 95, 8939–8944.

Illingworth, S., and Bishop, D. V. M. (2009). Atypical cerebral lateralisation in adults with compensated developmental dyslexia demonstrated using functional transcranial Doppler ultrasound. *Brain Lang.* 111, 61–65. doi: 10.1016/j.bandl.2009.05.002

Iyer, M. B., Mattu, U., Grafman, J., Lomarev, M., Sato, S., and Wassermann, E. M. (2005). Safety and cognitive effect of frontal DC brain polarization in healthy individuals. *Neurology* 64, 872–875. doi: 10.1212/01.WNL.0000152986.07469.E9

Jobard, G., Crivello, F., and Tzourio-Mazoyer, N. (2003). Evaluation of the dual route theory of reading: a metanalysis of 35 neuroimaging studies. *Neuroimage* 20, 693–712. doi: 10.1016/S1053-8119(03)00343-4

Johnson, M. H. (2001). Functional brain development in humans. *Nat. Rev. Neurosci.* 2, 475–483. doi: 10.1038/35081509

Jones, K. T., and Berryhill, M. E. (2012). Parietal contributions to visual working memory depend on task difficulty. *Front. psychiatry* 3:81. doi: 10.3389/fpsyt.2012.00081

Kovelman, I., Norton, E. S., Christodoulou, J. A., Gaab, N., Lieberman, D. A., Triantafyllou, C., et al. (2012). Brain basis of phonological awareness for spoken language in children and its disruption in dyslexia. *Cereb. Cortex* 22, 754–764. doi: 10.1093/cercor/bhr094

Koyama, M. S., Di Martino, A., Zuo, X.-N., Kelly, C., Mennes, M., Jutagir, D. R., et al. (2011). Resting-state functional connectivity indexes reading competence in children and adults. *J. Neurosci.* 31, 8617–8624. doi: 10.1523/JNEUROSCI.4865-10.2011

Krause, B., and Cohen Kadosh, R. (2013). Can transcranial electrical stimulation improve learning difficulties in atypical brain development? A future possibility for cognitive training. *Dev. Cogn. Neurosci.* 6, 176–194. doi: 10.1016/j.dcn.2013.04.001

Krause, B., and Cohen Kadosh, R. (2014). Not all brains are created equal: the relevance of individual differences in responsiveness to transcranial electrical stimulation. *Front. Syst. Neurosci.* 8:25. doi: 10.3389/fnsys.2014.00025

Kucian, K., and von Aster, M. (2015). Developmental dyscalculia. *Eur. J. Pediatr.*. 174, 1–13. doi: 10.1007/s00431-014-2455-7

Maclean, M., Bryant, P., and Bradley, L. (1987). Rhymes, nursery rhymes, and reading in early childhood. *Merril-Palmer Q.* 33, 255–281.

Martin, A., Schurz, M., Kronbichler, M., and Richlan, F. (2015). Reading in the brain of children and adults: a meta-analysis of 40 functional magnetic resonance imaging studies. *Hum. Brain Mapp.* 36, 1963–1981. doi: 10.1002/hbm.22749

Mei, L., Xue, G., Lu, Z.-L., He, Q., Zhang, M., Wei, M., et al. (2014). Artificial language training reveals the neural substrates underlying addressed and assembled phonologies. *PLoS ONE* 9:e93548. doi: 10.1371/journal.pone.0093548

Meyler, A., Keller, T. A., Cherkassky, V. L., Gabrieli, J. D. E., and Just, M. A. (2008). Modifying the brain activation of poor readers during sentence comprehension with extended remedial instruction: a longitudinal study of neuroplasticity. *Neuropsychologia* 46, 2580–2592. doi: 10.1016/j.neuropsychologia.2008.03.012

Milne, R. D., Syngeniotis, A., Jackson, G., and Corballis, M. C. (2002). Mixed lateralization of phonological assembly in developmental dyslexia. *Neurocase* 8, 205–209. doi: 10.1093/neucas/8.3.205

Miniussi, C., Cappa, S. F., Cohen, L. G., Floel, A., Fregni, F., Nitsche, M. A., et al. (2008). Efficacy of repetitive transcranial magnetic stimulation/transcranial direct current stimulation in cognitive neurorehabilitation. *Brain Stimul.* 1, 326–336. doi: 10.1016/j.brs.2008.07.002

Nitsche, M. A., Cohen, L. G., Wassermann, E. M., Priori, A., Lang, N., Antal, A., et al. (2008). Transcranial direct current stimulation: state of the art 2008. *Brain Stimul.* 1, 206–223. doi: 10.1016/j.brs.2008.06.004

Nitsche, M. A., and Paulus, W. (2000). Excitability changes induced in the human motor cortex by weak transcranial direct current stimulation. *J. Physiol.* 527, 633–639. doi: 10.1111/j.1469-7793.2000.t01-1-00633.x

Nitsche, M. A., and Paulus, W. (2011). Transcranial direct current stimulation–update 2011. *Restor. Neurol. Neurosci.* 29, 463–492. doi: 10.3233/RNN-2011-0618

Norton, E. S., Beach, S. D., and de Gabrieli, J. (2014). Neurobiology of dyslexia. *Curr. Opin. Neurobiol.* 30C, 73–78. doi: 10.1016/j.conb.2014.09.007

Park, H.-J., and Friston, K. (2013). Structural and functional brain networks: from connections to cognition. *Science* 342:1238411. doi: 10.1126/science.1238411

Price, A. R., McAdams, H., Grossman, M., and Hamilton, R. H. (2015). A meta-analysis of transcranial direct current stimulation studies examining the reliability of effects on language measures. *Brain Stimul.* 8, 1093–1100. doi: 10.1016/j.brs.2015.06.013

Price, C. J., and Devlin, J. T. (2011). The interactive account of ventral occipitotemporal contributions to reading. *Trends Cogn. Sci.* 15, 246–253. doi: 10.1016/j.tics.2011.04.001

Price, G. R., and Ansari, D. (2013). Dyscalculia: characteristics, causes, and treatments. *Numeracy* 6, 1–18. doi: 10.5038/1936-4660.6.1.2

Priori, A., Hallett, M., and Rothwell, J. C. (2009). Repetitive transcranial magnetic stimulation or transcranial direct current stimulation? *Brain Stimul.* 2, 241–245. doi: 10.1016/j.brs.2009.02.004

Pugh, K. R., Mencl, W. E., Jenner, A. R., Katz, L., Frost, S. J., Lee, J. R., et al. (2001). Neurobiological studies of reading and reading disability. *J. Commun. Disord.* 34, 479–492. doi: 10.1016/S0021-9924(01)00060-0

Pugh, K. R., Mencl, W. E., Shaywitz, B. A., Shaywitz, S. E., Fulbright, R. K., Constable, R., et al. (2000). The angular gyrus in developmental dyslexia: task-specific differences in functional connectivity within posterior cortex. *Psychol. Sci.* 11, 51–56. doi: 10.1111/1467-9280.00214

Quaglino, V., Bourdin, B., Czternasty, G., Vrignaud, P., Fall, S., Meyer, M. E., et al. (2008). Differences in effective connectivity between dyslexic children and normal readers during a pseudoword reading task: an fMRI study. *Neurophysiol. Clin.* 38, 73–82. doi: 10.1016/j.neucli.2007.12.007

Rezaie, R., Simos, P. G., Fletcher, J. M., Cirino, P. T., Vaughn, S., and Papanicolaou, A. C. (2011a). Engagement of temporal lobe regions predicts response to educational interventions in adolescent struggling readers. *Dev. Neuropsychol.* 36, 869–888. doi: 10.1080/87565641.2011.606404

Rezaie, R., Simos, P. G., Fletcher, J. M., Cirino, P. T., Vaughn, S., and Papanicolaou, A. C. (2011b). Temporo-parietal brain activity as a longitudinal predictor of response to educational interventions among middle school struggling readers. *J. Int. Neuropsychol. Soc.* 17, 875–885. doi: 10.1017/S1355617711000890

Richlan, F., Kronbichler, M., and Wimmer, H. (2009). Functional abnormalities in the dyslexic brain: a quantitative meta-analysis of neuroimaging studies. *Hum. Brain Mapp.* 30, 3299–3308. doi: 10.1002/hbm.20752

Richlan, F., Kronbichler, M., and Wimmer, H. (2011). Meta-analyzing brain dysfunctions in dyslexic children and adults. *Neuroimage* 56, 1735–1742. doi: 10.1016/j.neuroimage.2011.02.040

Ridding, M. C., and Rothwell, J. C. (2007). Is there a future for therapeutic use of transcranial magnetic stimulation? *Nat. Rev. Neurosci.* 8, 559–567. doi: 10.1038/nrn2169

Sandrini, M., Fertonani, A., Cohen, L. G., and Miniussi, C. (2012). Double dissociation of working memory load effects induced by bilateral parietal modulation. *Neuropsychologia* 50, 396–402. doi: 10.1016/j.neuropsychologia.2011.12.011

Schlaggar, B. L., and McCandliss, B. D. (2007). Development of neural systems for reading. *Annu. Rev. Neurosci.* 30, 475–503. doi: 10.1146/annurev.neuro.28.061604.135645

Shaywitz, B. A., Shaywitz, S. E., Blachman, B. A., Pugh, K. R., Fulbright, R. K., Skudlarski, P., et al. (2004). Development of left occipitotemporal systems for skilled reading in children after a phonologically- based intervention. *Biol. Psychiatry* 55, 926–933. doi: 10.1016/j.biopsych.2003.12.019

Simon, G., Lanoë, C., Poirel, N., Rossi, S., Lubin, A., Pineau, A., et al. (2013). Dynamics of the anatomical changes that occur in the brains of schoolchildren as they learn to read. *PLoS ONE* 8:e81789. doi: 10.1371/journal.pone.0081789

Simos, P. G., Breier, J. I., and Jack, M. (2001). Age-related changes in regional brain activation during phonological decoding and printed word recognition. *Dev. Neuropsychol.* 19, 37–41. doi: 10.1207/S15326942DN1902

Simos, P. G., Fletcher, J. M., Sarkari, S., Billingsley, R. L., Denton, C., and Papanicolaou, A. C. (2007). Altering the brain circuits for reading through intervention: a magnetic source imaging study. *Neuropsychology* 21, 485–496. doi: 10.1037/0894-4105.21.4.485

Sparing, R., Thimm, M., Hesse, M. D., Küst, J., Karbe, H., and Fink, G. R. (2009). Bidirectional alterations of interhemispheric parietal balance by non-invasive cortical stimulation. *Brain* 132, 3011–3020. doi: 10.1093/brain/awp154

Temple, E., Deutsch, G. K., Poldrack, R. A., Miller, S. L., Tallal, P., Merzenich, M. M., et al. (2003). Neural deficits in children with dyslexia ameliorated by behavioral remediation: evidence from functional MRI. *Proc. Natl. Acad. Sci. U.S.A.* 100, 2860–2865. doi: 10.1073/pnas.0030098100

Thomson, J. M., Doruk, D., Mascio, B., Fregni, F., and Cerruti, C. (2015). Transcranial direct current stimulation modulates efficiency of reading processes. *Front. Hum. Neurosci.* 9:114. doi: 10.3389/fnhum.2015.00114

Torgesen, J., Wagner, R., and Rashotte, C. (1999). *TOWRE–2 Test of Word Reading Efficiency.* Austin, TX: Pro-Ed. Available online at: http://www.mindresources.com/pdfs/SR2011/pages/PAGE_202.pdf (Accessed January 15, 2016).

Turkeltaub, P. E., Benson, J., Hamilton, R. H., Datta, A., Bikson, M., and Coslett, H. B. (2012). Left lateralizing transcranial direct current stimulation improves reading efficiency. *Brain Stimul.* 5, 201–207. doi: 10.1016/j.brs.2011.04.002

Turkeltaub, P. E., Gareau, L., Flowers, D. L., Zeffiro, T. A., and Eden, G. F. (2003). Development of neural mechanisms for reading. *Nat. Neurosci.* 6, 767–773. doi: 10.1038/nn1065

van der Mark, S., Klaver, P., Bucher, K., Maurer, U., Schulz, E., Brem, S., et al. (2011). The left occipitotemporal system in reading: disruption of focal fMRI connectivity to left inferior frontal and inferior parietal language areas in children with dyslexia. *Neuroimage* 54, 2426–2436. doi: 10.1016/j.neuroimage.2010.10.002

Vellutino, F. R., Tunmer, W. E., Jaccard, J. J., and Chen, R. (2007). Components of reading ability: multivariate evidence for a convergent skills model of reading development. *Sci. Stud. Read.* 11, 3–32. doi: 10.1080/10888430709336632

Vicario, C. M., and Nitsche, M. A. (2013). Transcranial direct current stimulation: a remediation tool for the treatment of childhood congenital dyslexia? *Front. Hum. Neurosci.* 7:139. doi: 10.3389/fnhum.2013.00139

Wechsler, D. (2008). *Wechsler Adult Intelligence Scale–Fourth Edition (WAIS–IV).* San Antonio, TX: NCS Pearson. Available online.at: http://www.statisticssolutions.com/academic-solutions/resources/directory-of-survey-instruments/wechsler-adult-intelligence-scale-fourth-edition-wais-iv/ (Accessed January 15, 2016).

Williams, J. A., Imamura, M., and Fregni, F. (2009). Updates on the use of non-invasive brain stimulation in physical and rehabilitation medicine. *J. Rehabil. Med.* 41, 305–311. doi: 10.2340/16501977-0356

Wong, I. S. Y., and Tsang, H. W. H. (2013). A review on the effectiveness of repetitive transcranial magnetic stimulation (rTMS) on post-stroke aphasia. *Rev. Neurosci.* 24, 105–114. doi: 10.1515/revneuro-2012-0072

Xu, M., Yang, J., Siok, W. T., and Tan, L. H. (2015). Atypical lateralization of phonological working memory in developmental dyslexia. *J. Neurolinguist.* 33, 67–77. doi: 10.1016/j.jneuroling.2014.07.004

Zeno, S. (1995). *The Educator's Word Frequency Guide.* Touchstone Applied Science Associates. Available online at: https://scholar.google.com/scholar?q=zeno$+$1995&btnG=&hl=en&as_sdt=0%2C44#0 (Accessed January 15, 2016).

Ziegler, J. C., and Goswami, U. (2005). Reading acquisition, developmental dyslexia, and skilled reading across languages: a psycholinguistic grain size theory. *Psychol. Bull.* 131, 3–29. doi: 10.1037/0033-2909.131.1.3

Transfer of Training from One Working Memory Task to Another: Behavioural and Neural Evidence

Erin L. Beatty[1], Marie-Eve Jobidon[1], Fethi Bouak[1], Ann Nakashima[1], Ingrid Smith[1], Quan Lam[1], Kristen Blackler[1], Bob Cheung[1] and Oshin Vartanian[1,2]*

[1] Defence Research and Development Canada – Toronto Research Centre, Toronto, ON, Canada, [2] Department of Psychology, University of Toronto Scarborough, Toronto, ON, Canada

Edited by:
Mikhail Lebedev,
Duke University, USA

Reviewed by:
Erika K. Hussey,
University of Illinois, USA
Tilo Strobach,
Medical School Hamburg, Germany
Mary M. Torregrossa,
University of Pittsburgh, USA

***Correspondence:**
Erin L. Beatty,
Defence Research and Development Canada – Toronto Research Centre,
1133 Sheppard Avenue West,
Toronto, ON M3K 2C9, Canada
erin.beatty@drdc-rddc.gc.ca

N-back working memory (WM) tasks necessitate the maintenance and updating of dynamic rehearsal sets during performance. The delayed matching-to-sample (dMTS) task is another WM task, which in turn involves the encoding, maintenance, and retrieval of stimulus representations in sequential order. Because both n-back and dMTS engage WM function, we hypothesized that compared to a control task not taxing WM, training on the n-back task would be associated with better performance on dMTS by virtue of training a shared mental capacity. We tested this hypothesis by randomly assigning subjects ($N = 43$) to train on either the n-back (including 2-back and 3-back levels) or an active control task. Following training, dMTS was administered in the fMRI scanner. The n-back group performed marginally better than the active control group on dMTS. In addition, although the n-back group improved more on the less difficult 2-back level than the more difficult 3-back level across training sessions, it was improvement on the 3-back level that accounted for 21% of the variance in dMTS performance. For the control group, improvement in training across sessions was unrelated to dMTS performance. At the neural level, greater activation in the left inferior frontal gyrus, right posterior parietal cortex, and the cerebellum distinguished the n-back group from the control group in the maintenance phase of dMTS. Degree of improvement on the 3-back level across training sessions was correlated with activation in right lateral prefrontal and motor cortices in the maintenance phase of dMTS. Our results suggest that although n-back training is more likely to improve performance in easier blocks, it is improvement in more difficult blocks that is predictive of performance on a target task drawing on WM. In addition, the extent to which training on a task can transfer to another task is likely due to the engagement of shared cognitive capacities and underlying neural substrates—in this case WM.

Keywords: working memory, n-back, cognitive training, delayed matching-to-sample, prefrontal cortex

Introduction

Working memory (WM) can be defined as "a multicomponent system for active maintenance of information in the face of ongoing processing and/or distraction" (Conway et al., 2005, p. 770). Recently, there has been great theoretical and applied interest in the prospects of WM training for improving cognition. This interest stems from the possibility that improvements in WM performance as a function of training might be transferable to other mental activities similarly drawing on WM capacity (Klingberg, 2010; Morrison and Chein, 2011; Buschkuehl et al., 2012). Although there is evidence to show that WM training can produce improvements in verbal as well as visuospatial WM, reliable evidence regarding far transfer to untrained tasks is presently lacking (for review see Melby-Lervåg and Hulme, 2013).

An important factor that might affect transfer is the goodness-of-fit between the specific capacity enhanced during training and the cognitive requirements of the untrained activity. For example, Harrison et al. (2013) showed that training on simple and complex WM span tasks led to improved performance on similar tasks (i.e., reading span and rotation span), despite the use of material with different surface features. Thus, structural and functional similarities between the trained and untrained tasks (e.g., both necessitate the suppression of distractors) appear to increase likelihood of transfer. The same conclusion can be drawn from the study conducted by Dahlin et al. (2008) who demonstrated transfer to a test of WM (i.e., letter memory) after 5 weeks of training in a specific aspect of WM—updating. The control group did not receive any training or specific activity. Importantly, using functional magnetic resonance imaging (fMRI), the researchers were also able to determine that the transfer effect was based on a joint training-related increase in brain activation in the trained and target tasks in the striatum. No transfer was observed to the Stroop task—a task that does not involve updating, and does not typically engage the striatum. Dahlin et al.'s (2008) results suggest that to obtain transfer, it is necessary to train specific aspects of WM (e.g., updating) that are functionally shared by the trained and target tasks. In turn, likelihood of transfer is increased to the extent that training-related changes in neural function occur in the same brain region recruited in relation to the trained process (e.g., updating) in both tasks.

Consistent with these process-specific findings, Salminen et al. (2012) examined transfer effects from WM training to executive functions. Importantly, they mapped particular cognitive processes engaged by their WM training task (i.e., dual n-back) to four aspects of executive functions, and measured transfer effects separately for each of those four processes: updating, coordination of concurrent performance, task switching, and attention. Their results demonstrated transfer from WM training to all aspects of executive function except coordination of concurrent performance, which the authors attributed to a "lack of commonalities" between the trained and target tasks (e.g., differences in the extent to which speeded processing was necessary for optimal performance). Salminen et al.'s (2012) results reinforce the notion that transfer effects depend on specific cognitive processes shared by the WM training and target tasks (see also Persson et al., 2007; Karbach and Kray, 2009; Sprenger et al., 2013; Salminen et al., 2015).

Building on the idea that shared capacities increase the likelihood of transfer of training, we conducted a study to test the hypothesis that training on one WM task would be more strongly associated with better performance on another WM task than training on a task that does not tax WM function. Our training task consisted of the n-back task—one of the most commonly used tasks to assess WM performance in the cognitive neuroscience literature (Kane and Engle, 2002). The n-back task requires that participants decide, on a trial-by-trial basis, whether a stimulus presented in the current trial matches a target stimulus presented a specific number of trials earlier in the sequence. The letter *n* denotes the specific number of trials that separate the current trial from the target trial. This task necessitates both maintenance and updating of dynamic rehearsal sets during performance (Kane et al., 2007). In contrast, participants in the active control group completed the 4-choice reaction time (RT) task (Dollins et al., 1993), which consists of pressing one of four buttons as quickly as possible when one of four target locations on a screen is highlighted (each target being matched to a given button). This task is not hypothesized to tax WM function.

Our target WM task consisted of the delayed matching-to-sample (dMTS) task, a classic measure of short-term visual WM from the animal learning and WM literatures (Miller et al., 1996). dMTS involves the encoding, maintenance, and retrieval of stimulus representations in sequential order (see **Figure 1**). Specifically, during *encoding* participants memorize the stimulus, during *maintenance* they maintain the stimulus in WM, and during *retrieval* they press the button corresponding to the stimulus that matches the stimulus presented during *encoding*. Importantly, both n-back and dMTS are considered to be WM tasks (Rottschy et al., 2012), although as noted above they include different sub-processes. An analysis of n-back and dMTS demonstrates that both engage the maintenance function of WM. Specifically, the n-back task necessitates that stimuli be maintained in WM across presentations so that decisions (match vs. no match) can be made. In turn, in dMTS a stimulus must be maintained for specific delay durations in WM to enable subsequent recognition among the available candidates. We therefore hypothesized that training the maintenance function of WM during n-back would confer an advantage to dMTS performance by virtue of influencing its maintenance phase, because that phase necessitates the maintenance of visual representations in WM.

Importantly, n-back training could also impact the encoding and/or retrieval phases of dMTS because both tasks likely share those sub-processes beyond maintenance alone. For example, although there are explicit and compartmentalized encoding and maintenance phases within dMTS, the updating function inherent in the n-back very likely requires the encoding of memory representations as well as their retrieval for making matching decisions.

In order to pinpoint the locus of transfer-related brain activity, we used fMRI to determine the phase within dMTS wherein activation would distinguish the experimental and control groups. Specifically, if as hypothesized training on the n-back task were to confer an advantage to dMTS performance by virtue of improving the maintenance function within WM, then one should observe a neural difference between the two groups in the maintenance phase. Furthermore, the differences between the two groups during the maintenance phase should be apparent in regions known to underlie delay-period maintenance in

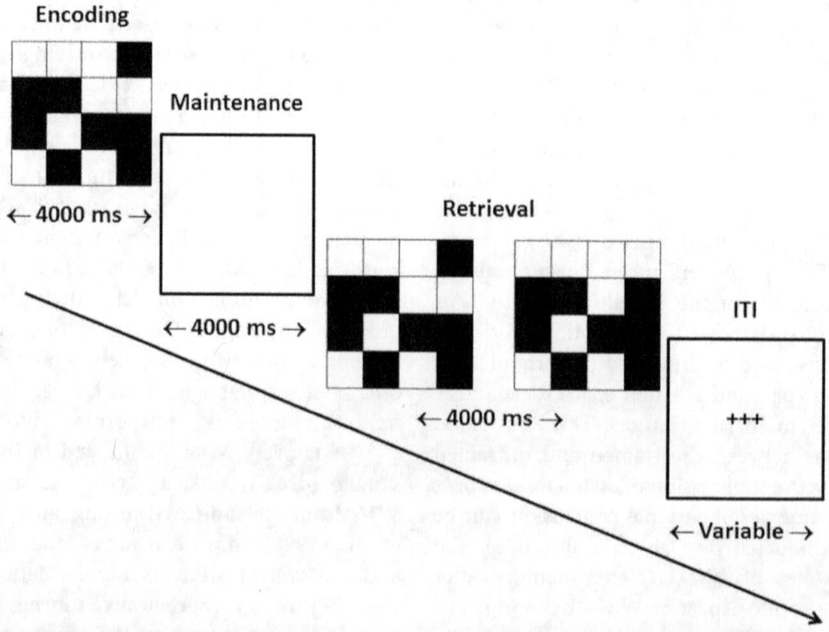

FIGURE 1 | Trial structure of dMTS. dMTS, delayed Matching-to-Sample Task. Participants completed 40 trials of identical structure. During *encoding* participants memorized the stimulus. During *maintenance* participants maintained the stimulus in working memory. During *retrieval* participants pressed the button corresponding to the stimulus (left, right) that matched the stimulus presented during *encoding*. The location (left, right) of the matching stimulus was counterbalanced across trials. The ITI varied randomly between 4,000 and 6,000 ms. ITI, inter-trial interval. Arrow indicates direction of trial.

visual WM, including primarily the dorsolateral and ventrolateral prefrontal cortex (PFC; BAs 9, 44, 45, and 47), the inferior parietal lobule (BA 40) and adjacent parietal regions (see de Zubicaray et al., 2001; Ranganath et al., 2004). Consistent with the idea that training on the n-back could also be related to variation in brain function in the encoding and retrieval phases of dMTS, we also compared the effect of training (i.e., n-back vs. 4-choice RT) within those two phases.

Materials and Methods

Participants

Our protocol was approved by Defence Research and Development Canada's Human Research Ethics Committee. The 43 participants (35 males, eight females) were neurologically healthy right-handed (Oldfield, 1971) volunteers ($M = 30.76$ years, $SD = 9.71$) with normal or corrected-to-normal vision. They were assigned randomly to the experimental ($N = 22$) or active control group ($N = 21$). To ensure similar expectations and motivations, participants were not informed about the existence of the two training conditions, or our hypotheses about the differential effects of training on outcome measures of interest (see Boot et al., 2011). There was no significant difference between the two groups in sex [$\chi^2 (1) = 0.01, p = 0.94$], age [$t(36) = 0.33, p = 0.74$], or fluid intelligence [$t(41) = 0.16, p = 0.87$]—assessed by administering the 18 even or odd items of *Raven's Advanced Progressive Matrices* (Raven et al., 1998) within a time limit of 10 min (see Jaeggi et al., 2008).

Materials and Procedure

Cognitive Training

All participants completed three 20-min training sessions on separate days, administered using the *Cognitive Test Software* (Grushcow, 2008). Average lag time between successive sessions was 1.21 days ($SD = 0.55$). Durations and frequencies in WM training studies have varied greatly, ranging from a single 20-min session to 20 h spread over 10 weeks (see Buschkuehl et al., 2012, Table 1; Klingberg, 2010, Table 2). We focused on a short and concentrated training regimen specifically because we were interested in assessing its feasibility as an intervention strategy in applied professional and educational settings.

n-back

Participants in the experimental group completed the n-back task. Each session consisted of four blocks—two blocks of 2-back and two blocks of 3-back—administered in alternating order and always starting with 2-back. The stimuli in our variant of the n-back were letters. No vowels were used in the task, and we only used a subset of consonants (X, G, H, K, P, Q, S, and W). We did not control for interference lures. Each block contained 150 trials. On 50 trials within each block the presented letter matched the target letter presented two or three positions earlier in the sequence (depending on the block), whereas on the remaining 100 trials it did not. Each letter was presented for 500 ms. Inter-stimulus interval (ISI) was a blank screen presented for 2500 ms. Participants pressed the spacebar when they detected a match.

4-choice RT

Participants in the active control group completed the 4-choice RT task (Dollins et al., 1993). On each trial of this task, one of four adjacent locations on the computer screen was highlighted randomly. Participants pressed one of four keys corresponding to the highlighted location. We selected this task to control for task engagement not involving a WM task. Participants completed 420 trials per session. Based on normative data collected in our lab from the same population using the same task (Nakashima et al., 2011), we expected accuracy to be at ceiling across the three sessions.

dMTS

Participants completed the dMTS in the fMRI scanner 3.29 days (SD = 1.11) after the last training session (see **Figure 1**).

fMRI Acquisition

A 3-Tesla MR scanner with an 8-channel head coil (Discovery MR750, 22.0 software, GE Healthcare, Waukesha, WI, USA) was used to acquire T1 anatomical volume images (0.86 mm × 0.86 mm × 1.0 mm voxels). For functional imaging, T2*-weighted gradient echo spiral-in/out acquisitions were used to produce 26 contiguous 5 mm thick axial slices [repetition time (TR) = 2000 ms; echo time (TE) = 30 ms; flip angle (FA) = 70°; field of view (FOV) = 200 mm; 64 × 64 matrix; voxel dimensions = 3.1 mm × 3.1 mm × 5.0 mm], positioned to cover the whole brain. The first five volumes were discarded to allow for T1 equilibration effects. The number of volumes acquired was 354.

fMRI Analysis

Data were analyzed using Statistical Parametric Mapping (SPM8). Head movement was less than 2 mm. All functional volumes were spatially realigned to the first volume. A mean image created from realigned volumes was spatially normalized to the MNI EPI brain template using non-linear basis functions. The derived spatial transformation was applied to the realigned T2* volumes, and spatially smoothed with an 8 mm full-width at half-maximum isotropic Gaussian kernel. Time series across each voxel were high-pass filtered with a cut-off of 128 s, using cosine functions to remove section-specific low frequency drifts in the BOLD signal. Condition effects at each voxel were estimated according to the GLM and regionally specific effects compared using linear contrasts. The BOLD signal was modeled as a box-car, convolved with a canonical hemodynamic response function.

We applied a combination of voxel-height and cluster extent correction for multiple comparisons using AlphaSim (http://afni.nimh.nih.gov/pub/dist/doc/manual/AlphaSim.pdf) incorporated in REST (Song et al., 2011). Whereas originally AlphaSim was developed for use within the Analysis of Functional Neuroimages (AFNI) software (Cox, 1996), REST enables one to conduct the same analysis on a Windows platform using SPM masks. AlphaSim takes into account the size of the search space and the estimated smoothness, and using Monte Carlo simulations generates probability estimates of a random field of noise, producing a cluster of voxels of a given size for a set of voxels passing a given voxel-wise p-value threshold. Using a random-effects analysis, we report activations that survived $p < 0.05$—corrected for multiple comparisons (FWE) within the avg152T2.nii whole-brain mask from the SPM toolbox. The real smoothness in the three directions was estimated from the residuals (FWHMx = 11.699 mm, FWHMy = 11.869 mm, FWHMz = 10.992 mm). Within our mask, the Monte Carlo simulations determined that a FWE-corrected false-positive probability of $p < 0.05$ was achieved using a voxel-wise threshold of $p < 0.005$ combined with a spatial extent threshold of 249 voxels.

Results

Cognitive Training

For the experimental group we conducted a repeated-measures ANOVA with session (1, 2, and 3) and level (2-back, 3-back) as within-subjects variables. The key dependent variable was d' (sensitivity; Stanislaw and Todorov, 1999; see Kane et al., 2007). When d' is positive (and high), participants are considered to display good sensitivity, whereas when d' is negative participants are incorrectly judging matches as mismatches and vice versa. In addition, we also investigated the effects of the two independent variables on the criterion—defined as the value of the decision variable deemed sufficiently high to determine that there is a match. A liberal value for the criterion biases the participant toward responding that there is a match, whereas a conservative value biases the participant toward responding that there is no match.

For the experimental group, there was a main effect for session, demonstrating that d' improved across sessions, $F(2,42) = 10.50$, $p < 0.001$, $\eta_p^2 = 0.33$. Paired comparisons demonstrated that compared to session 1, d' was higher at sessions 2 and 3. There was no difference between sessions 2 and 3 ($p = 0.10$). There was also a main effect for level, demonstrating that d' was greater on 2-back than 3-back, $F(1,21) = 25.05$, $p < 0.001$, $\eta_p^2 = 0.54$. In addition, there was a session × level interaction such that across three sessions d' improved more for 2-back than 3-back, $F(2,42) = 5.90$, $p < 0.01$, $\eta_p^2 = 0.22$ (**Figure 2**). In contrast, when we focused on the criterion as the dependent variable, the effects of session, level and the session × level interaction were not significant (all $ps \geq 0.99$).

For the active control group we conducted an ANOVA with session (1, 2, and 3) as the within-subjects variable, and accuracy as the dependent variable. As predicted (see Nakashima et al., 2011), performance was at ceiling across sessions 1 ($M = 96.57\%$, SD = 3.10), 2 ($M = 95.93\%$, SD = 4.14), and 3 ($M = 96.86\%$, SD = 2.24), $F(2,38) = 1.48$, $p = 0.25$, $\eta_p^2 = 0.07$. We conducted an additional ANOVA with session (1, 2, and 3) as the within-subjects variable, and RT as the dependent variable. There was a main effect such that RT decreased across the first ($M = 0.45$ s, SD = 0.06), second ($M = 0.42$ s, SD = 0.05) and third sessions ($M = 0.41$ s, SD = 0.05), $F(2,38) = 15.13$, $p = < 0.001$, $\eta_p^2 = 0.44$.

dMTS

The experimental group ($M = 96.70\%$, SD = 4.72) performed marginally better than the active control group ($M = 93.81\%$,

SD = 5.22) on dMTS, $t(41) = 1.91$, $p = 0.06$, Cohen's $d = 0.58$. To directly test whether performance on dMTS would be a function of improvement in training on the n-back, for the experimental group we computed a new variable that was the difference in d' between session 1 and session 3 ($d'_{\text{difference}} = d'_{\text{session 3}} - d'_{\text{session 1}}$)—separately for 2-back and 3-back. Next, we regressed accuracy (%) in dMTS performance onto $d'_{\text{difference}}$. The results demonstrated that degree of improvement in 2-back was unrelated to dMTS performance, $\beta = 0.31, p = 0.16$. In contrast, degree of improvement in 3-back predicted variation in dMTS performance, $\beta = 0.46, p = < 0.05$. This result demonstrates that the degree of improvement in 3-back is a significant factor in dMTS performance. In fact, improvement in 3-back performance during training accounted for 21% of the variance in dMTS performance (**Figure 3A**).

To determine whether the degree of improvement in 4-choice RT was predictive of dMTS performance amongst participants in the control group, we computed a new variable that was the difference in RT between session 1 and session 3 ($RT_{\text{difference}} = RT_{\text{session 3}} - RT_{\text{session 1}}$). Next, we regressed accuracy (%) in dMTS performance onto $RT_{\text{difference}}$. Importantly, only 19 data points (rather than 21) were included in this analysis because one participant failed to complete the third session of training, and another data point was excluded because it was an outlier—determined by its deviation from the means of both distributions by approximately 3 SDs (see Wainer, 1976). Degree of improvement in RT was unrelated to dMTS performance, $\beta = -0.30, p = 0.21$ (**Figure 3B**).

fMRI

Using an event-related design, we specified six regressors corresponding to (1) encoding, (2) maintenance, (3) retrieval, (4) ISI, (5) ITI, and (6) motor response. ISI and motor response were modeled out of the analyses by assigning weights of 0 to their corresponding regressors in all analyses. **Table 1** lists the regions activated in the encoding (−ITI), maintenance (−ITI), and retrieval (−ITI) phases of dMTS *across all participants*. An independent-samples t-test demonstrated greater activation in the n-back than active control group in the maintenance phase in the left inferior frontal gyrus (IFG; $T = 3.97$, $k_E = 389$, $x = -44$, $y = 22$, $z = 16$), the right posterior parietal cortex (PPC; $T = 3.30$, $k_E = 299$, $x = 32$, $y = -74$, $z = 36$), and the cerebellum ($T = 3.56$, $k_E = 277$, $x = -10$, $y = -68$, $z = -42$; **Figure 4**). Neither the reverse contrast nor the contrasts in either direction involving the encoding or retrieval phase revealed any significant difference between the two groups. In other words, the difference in brain activation between the n-back and active control groups was limited exclusively to the maintenance phase of dMTS.

TABLE 1 | Coordinates for the observed activations in the encoding, maintenance, and retrieval phases of delayed matching-to-sample task (dMTS; vs. rest) across all participants.

Contrast	Structure	*x*	*y*	*z*	*T-score*
Encoding−ITI	Precuneus	−16	−68	50	13.52
	Precuneus	24	−68	46	11.89
	Precentral gyrus	−46	−6	46	12.27
	Parahippocampus	38	−14	−30	4.90
Maintenance−ITI	Precuneus	−24	−64	50	13.25
	Inferior parietal lobe	−36	−44	40	12.81
	Superior parietal lobe	12	−64	62	11.70
Retrieval−ITI	Anterior insula	32	26	−2	11.52
	Anterior insula	−28	24	0	9.68
	Cerebellum	0	−50	−36	5.87

The coordinates are reported in MNI space. All reported activation survived whole-brain family-wise error (FWE) correction (p < 0.05) as implemented by AlphaSim in REST (Song et al., 2011).

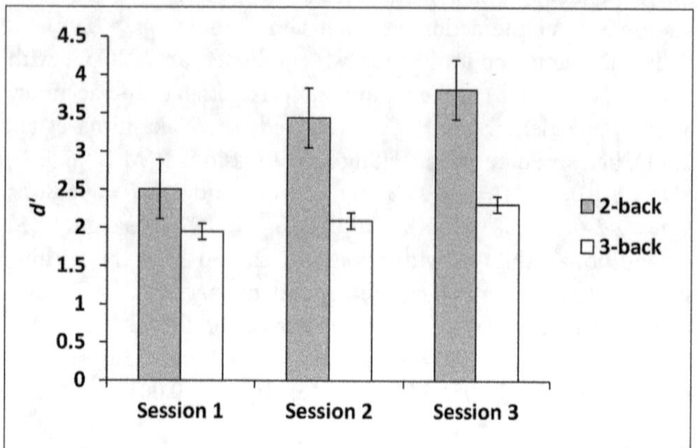

FIGURE 2 | The effects of session and level on n-back performance during training.

The analysis of our behavioral data had demonstrated that improvement in 3-back performance during training accounted for 21% of the variance in dMTS performance (**Figure 3A**). To explore this effect at the neural level, we conducted three separate regression analyses to see whether difference in d' for 3-back ($d'_{\text{difference}} = d'_{\text{session 3}} - d'_{\text{session 1}}$) would covary with brain activation during (1) encoding, (2) maintenance, and (3) retrieval. The results demonstrated that brain activation did not covary in relation to $d'_{\text{difference}}$ during encoding or retrieval. In contrast, during the maintenance phase brain activation in right lateral PFC ($T = 3.68$, $k_E = 260$, $x = 56$, $y = 16$, $z = 10$) and motor cortex ($T = 3.78$, $k_E = 421$, $x = 46$, $y = -22$, $z = 44$) covaried with $d'_{\text{difference}}$ (**Figure 5**).

Although our behavioral data had demonstrated that for the experimental group improvement in 2-back performance was unrelated to dMTS performance, we nevertheless explored this effect at the neural level. As with 3-back, we conducted three separate regression analyses to see whether difference in d' for 2-back ($d'_{\text{difference}} = d'_{\text{session 3}} - d'_{\text{session 1}}$) would covary with brain activation during (1) encoding, (2) maintenance, and (3) retrieval. Demonstrating a pattern similar to 3-back, brain activation did not covary in relation to $d'_{\text{difference}}$ during encoding or retrieval. However, during the maintenance phase $d'_{\text{difference}}$ covaried with activation in a distributed network in the brain, including three locations in right ($T = 6.18$, $k_E = 2164$, $x = 44$, $y = 4$, $z = 28$), left ($T = 4.66$, $k_E = 2161$, $x = -42$, $y = 2$, $z = 16$), and medial ($T = 5.51$, $k_E = 982$, $x = -8$, $y = 14$, $z = 52$)

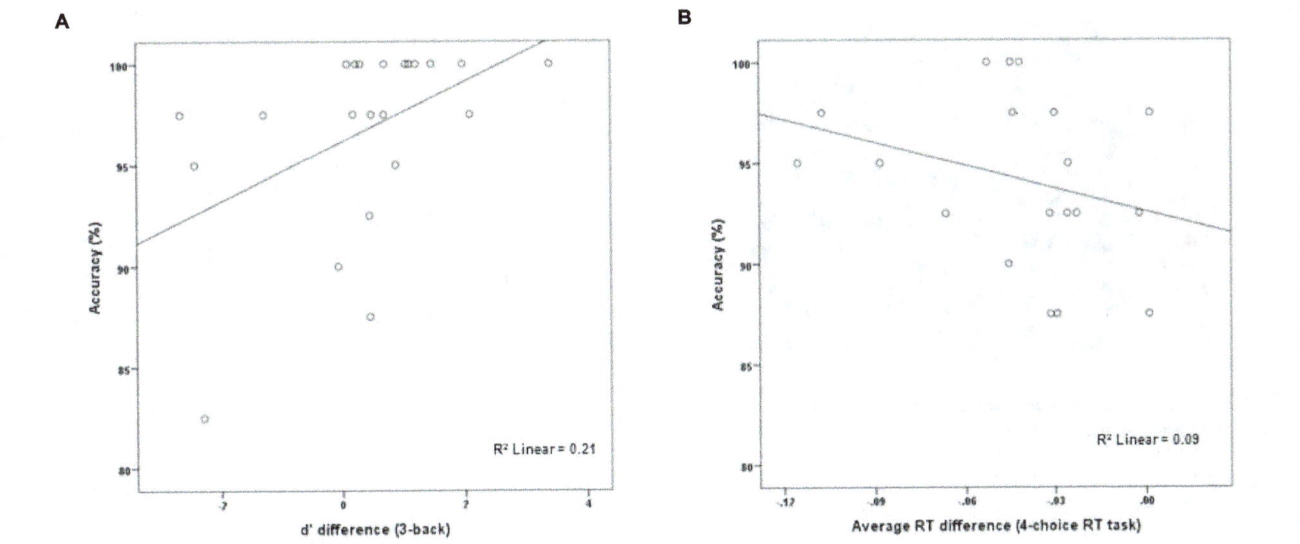

FIGURE 3 | The relationship between degree of training-related improvement in (A) n-back and (B) 4-choice RT and dMTS performance. Whereas the degree of training-related improvement in n-back predicted dMTS performance, degree of improvement in 4-choice RT did not (see text).

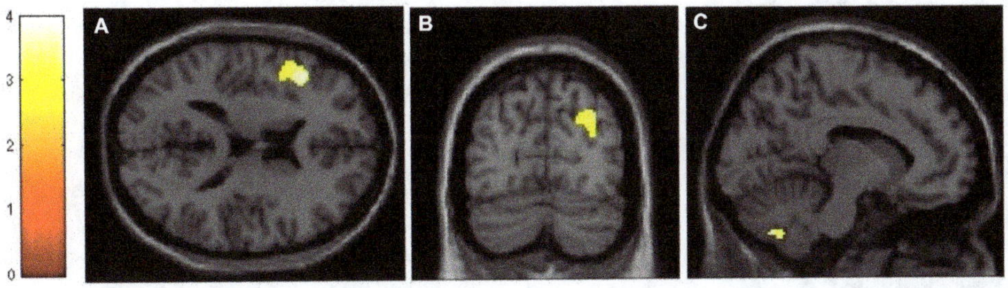

FIGURE 4 | Neural differences between experimental and control conditions during the maintenance phase of dMTS. There was greater activation in left IFG **(A)**, right PPC **(B)**, and cerebellum **(C)** in the experimental than control group during maintenance. SPMs rendered into standard stereotactic space and superimposed on to transverse **(A)**, coronal **(B)**, and saggital **(C)** MRI in standard space. Bar represents the corresponding *T*-score. dMTS, delayed Matching-to-Sample Task, IFG, inferior frontal gyrus, PPC, posterior parietal cortex.

middle frontal gyrus (BA 6), left lateral PFC ($T = 4.62$, $k_E = 940$, $x = -42$, $y = 24$, $z = 6$), right superior parietal lobule ($T = 5.06$, $k_E = 765$, $x = 36$, $y = -56$, $z = 54$), right cingulate ($T = 4.57$, $k_E = 358$, $x = 12$, $y = -10$, $z = 36$), right extrastriate cortex ($T = 4.68$, $k_E = 669$, $x = 36$, $y = -76$, $z = 20$), and three locations in left ($T = 5.52$, $k_E = 2059$, $x = -18$, $y = -74$, $z = -18$; $T = 4.60$, $k_E = 1263$, $x = -10$, $y = -50$, $z = -48$) and right ($T = 3.80$, $k_E = 504$, $x = 28$, $y = -54$, $z = -32$) cerebellum (**Figure 6**).

Finally, although our behavioral data had demonstrated that for the control group improvement in the 4-choice RT task was unrelated to dMTS performance, we nevertheless explored this effect at the neural level as well. Specifically, we conducted three separate regression analyses to see whether difference in RT in the 4-choice RT task ($RT_{difference} = RT_{session\ 3} - RT_{session\ 1}$) would covary with brain activation during (1) encoding, (2) maintenance, and (3) retrieval. Our results demonstrated that there was no relationship between brain activation and $RT_{difference}$ during encoding, maintenance or the retrieval phase.

Discussion

The n-back group performed marginally better than the active control group on dMTS, registering a medium effect size (Cohen, 1988). Importantly, although participants in the experimental condition were more likely to exhibit improvement across the three training sessions in the 2-back level than the 3-back level (**Figure 2**), it was their degree of improvement in the 3-back level that predicted variation in dMTS performance, accounting for 21% of the observed variance in dMTS performance (**Figure 3A**). Critically, degree of improvement in the 4-choice RT task in the control condition was unrelated to dMTS performance or its neural correlates, despite the fact that both are visuospatial tasks. These results demonstrate a dissociation between how training-related improvement in a WM task vs. a non-WM task is related to a target WM task. More specifically, they suggest that although performance on relatively easier levels of n-back is more likely to improve within three brief practice sessions, it is improvement in the more difficult levels that is more likely to be positively

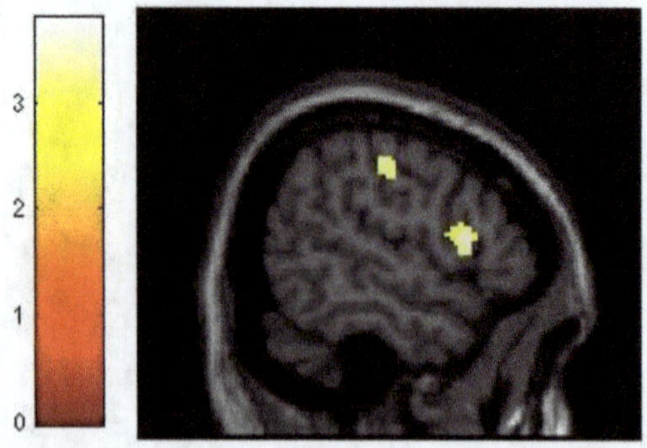

FIGURE 5 | Relationship between training-related improvement in 3-back and brain activation in the maintenance phase of dMTS. Activation in right lateral PFC and motor cortex covaried with degree of training-related improvement in 3-back. SPM rendered into standard stereotactic space and superimposed on saggital MRI in standard space. Bar represents the corresponding *T*-score. dMTS, delayed Matching-to-Sample Task.

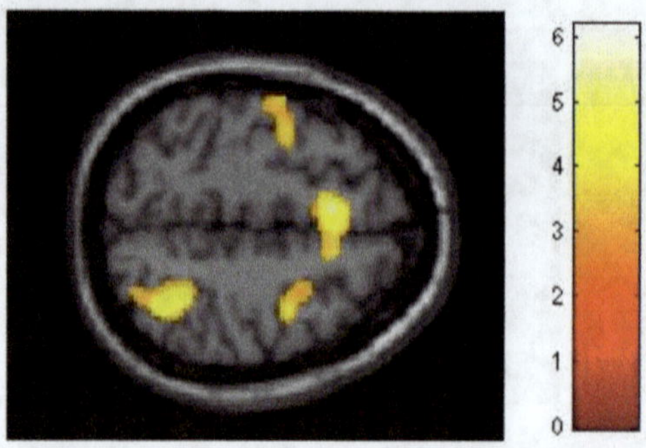

FIGURE 6 | Relationship between training-related improvement in 2-back and brain activation in the maintenance phase of dMTS. Activation in a distributed network including the superior parietal lobe and middle frontal gyrus (left, right, medial) covaried with degree of training-related improvement in 2-back. SPM rendered into standard stereotactic space and superimposed on transverse MRI in standard space. Bar represents the corresponding *T*-score. dMTS, delayed Matching-to-Sample Task.

related to performance on target tasks drawing on the same capacity.

In addition, the neural difference between the two groups was only apparent during the maintenance phase of dMTS, and localized to the left IFG, right PPC and the cerebellum. Sustained activation in the PFC has been related to maintenance in memory (Fuster, 1991). Indeed, IFG activation has been shown to be involved in the maintenance phase of the delayed non-matching-to-sample task (de Zubicaray et al., 2001). This is consistent with the involvement of the ventrolateral regions of the left PFC in delay-period maintenance in visual WM tasks (Ranganath et al., 2004). In addition, posterior parietal regions have been shown to contribute to various aspects of visual short-term mnemonic function including maintenance (Munk et al., 2002) and active maintenance of information in WM (Cohen et al., 1997). In fact, PPC activity has been shown to predict individual differences in visual short-term memory capacity (Todd and Marois, 2005; see also Todd and Marois, 2004). Our neural results suggest that the effects of n-back training on transfer-related brain function in dMTS are likely to be observed in regions that underlie capacities enhanced during training, and subsequently recruited by the untrained task. Our behavioral task analysis had led us to believe that n-back training would likely benefit dMTS performance because both tasks tax the maintenance function in WM, among others. Our neural results are generally consistent with this idea, although further experimentation is needed to determine that the regions distinguishing the two groups during maintenance indeed underlie transfer from n-back to dMTS.

Because training-related improvement in 3-back predicted dMTS performance (**Figure 3A**), we explored this effect at the neural level. Our results revealed that during the maintenance phase of dMTS, brain activation in right lateral PFC and motor cortex covaried with training-related improvement in 3-back (**Figure 5**). This region of the lateral PFC corresponds to Brodmann Area 44, and has been shown to be involved in both the storage and manipulation aspects of WM (see Wager and Smith, 2003). Our results suggest that this region is sensitive to training-related changes in relation to 3-back, and could be a region shared by both the n-back and dMTS for maintenance in WM.

In addition, although behaviourally training-related improvement in 2-back was unrelated to dMTS performance, our analyses of fMRI data demonstrated that during the maintenance phase of dMTS brain activation in a distributed network including the middle frontal gyrus, lateral PFC, superior parietal lobule, cingulate, extrastriate cortex, and the cerebellum covaried with training-related improvement in 2-back (**Figure 6**). Within this network, the frontal and parietal regions represent well-established nodes in the fronto-parietal WM network (Petrides, 2005; D'Esposito, 2008). Although these results demonstrate that brain activation during the maintenance phase of dMTS was modulated by the degree of training-related improvement in 2-back, care must be exercised in interpreting this finding given the absence of a corresponding behavioral effect (**Figure 3B**).

Limitations

Our results must be considered preliminary because our study had a number of limitations. First, our design involved randomly assigning participants to two treatment conditions, and subsequently measuring differences between the two groups on an outcome measure (i.e., dMTS) following training. As such, our results are correlational, and we cannot draw causal inferences. In addition, although the degree of training-related improvement in 3-back predicted and accounted for 21% of the variance in dMTS performance (**Figure 3A**), gain data alone cannot be used as evidence for inferring transfer effects (Tidwell et al., 2014). Rather, there is reason to further explore the possibility of a causal link between n-back training and performance on other WM tasks, including dMTS.

Second, our active control condition was meant to control for task engagement only—defined by identical frequency and duration of training. Although in WM training studies active control conditions are preferable to passive control conditions (Shipstead et al., 2010), it would be better still to include both types of control conditions in a given design. Particularly desirable would be to use control conditions that enable one to isolate specific components of training that are believed to be related to transfer to dMTS performance (e.g., updating, maintenance, etc.). The present results lay the groundwork for implementing such a design feature in future studies, perhaps comparing different types of WM training that tax different aspects of WM function.

Third, although the durations and frequencies of training sessions in WM training studies have ranged greatly in the past, ranging from one 20- or 30-min session to 20 h spread over 10 weeks (see Buschkuehl et al., 2012, Table 1; Klingberg, 2010, Table 2), our WM training intervention was relatively short and involved a non-adaptive WM task. Future studies would benefit from implementing an adaptive WM task, possibly administered in the context of more frequent training sessions.

Fourth, it is likely that there was a ceiling effect associated with our outcome measure (dMTS). In turn, this might have made it more difficult to observe differences between the two training conditions on this task, given that there was less room for improvement. There are at least two ways to increase the difficulty level on dMTS. First, on each trial we used a stimulus consisting of a 4 × 4 matrix (**Figure 1**). Doubling the matrix dimensions (i.e., 8 × 8) reduces average accuracy rates to around 70% (Nakashima et al., 2011). Second, whereas we used a fixed delay period, dMTS paradigms can incorporate variable delay periods. This will enable one to analyze differences in performance as a function of varying delay periods. These modifications can be incorporated in future studies.

Conclusion

Our results demonstrated that a group training on the n-back task performed marginally better than an active control group on dMTS. Although the n-back group improved more on 2-back than 3-back across three training sessions, it was improvement in 3-back that predicted and accounted for 21% of the variance in dMTS performance. There was no relationship between training-related gains and dMTS performance in the control group. At the neural level, the n-back group exhibited greater activation in the left IFG, right PPC and the cerebellum during the maintenance phase within dMTS. In addition, degree of improvement in 3-back covaried with brain activation in the right lateral prefrontal and motor cortices during the maintenance phase of dMTS, as did the degree of improvement in 2-back and activation in a distributed network including fronto-parietal WM nodes. In contrast, in the control group no relationship was observed between degree of improvement on the 4-choice RT task and dMTS performance. Combined, our results suggest that n-back training is more closely associated with dMTS performance than training on a task that does not tax WM.

Acknowledgments

We thank Ruby Endre, Garry Detzler and Fred Tam for assistance with data collection, and Chao-Gan Yan for help with running AlphaSim in REST. This work was supported by a Department of National Defence *Applied Research Project* under the direction of the last author. Portions of this work were presented at the annual meeting of the Association for Psychological Science, held in San Francisco, CA, USA, May 2014.

References

Boot, W. R., Blakely, D. P., and Simons, D. J. (2011). Do action video games improve perception and cognition? *Front. Psychol.* 2:226. doi: 10.3389/fpsyg.2011.00226

Buschkuehl, M., Jaeggi, S. M., and Jonides, J. (2012). Neuronal effects following working memory training. *Dev. Cogn. Neurosci.* 2(Suppl. 1), S167–S179. doi: 10.1016/j.dcn.2011.10.001

Cohen, J. (1988). *Statistical Power Analysis for the Behavioral Sciences.* Hillsdale, NJ: Lawrence Erlbaum Associates.

Cohen, J. D., Perlstein, W. M., Braver, T. S., Nystrom, L. E., Noll, D. C., Jonides, J., et al. (1997). Temporal dynamics of brain activation during a working memory task. *Nature* 386, 604–608. doi: 10.1038/386604a0

Conway, A. R., Kane, M. J., Bunting, M. F., Hambrick, D. Z., Wilhelm, O., and Engle, R. W. (2005). Working memory span tasks: a methodological review and user's guide. *Psychon. Bull. Rev.* 12, 769–786. doi: 10.3758/BF03196772

Cox, R. W. (1996). AFNI: software for analysis and visualization of functional magnetic resonance neuroimages. *Comput. Biomed. Res.* 29, 162–173. doi: 10.1006/cbmr.1996.0014

Dahlin, E., Neely, A. S., Larsson, A., Backman, L., and Nyberg, L. (2008). Transfer of learning after updating training mediated by the striatum. *Science* 320, 1510–1512. doi: 10.1126/science.1155466

D'Esposito, M. (2008). "Working memory," in *Handbook of Clinical Neurology: Neuropsychology and Behavioral Neurology*, eds G. Goldenberg and B. Miller (Amsterdam: Elsevier), 237–247.

de Zubicaray, G. I., Mcmahon, K., Wilson, S. J., and Muthiah, S. (2001). Brain activity during the encoding, retention, and retrieval of stimulus representations. *Learn. Mem.* 8, 243–251. doi: 10.1101/lm.40301

Dollins, A. B., Lynch, H. J., Wurtman, R. J., Deng, M. H., Kischka, K. U., Gleason, R. E., et al. (1993). Effect of pharmacological daytime doses of melatonin on human mood and performance. *Psychopharmacology (Berl.)* 112, 490–496. doi: 10.1007/BF02244899

Fuster, J. M. (1991). The prefrontal cortex and its relation to behavior. *Prog. Brain Res.* 87, 201–211. doi: 10.1016/j.pscychresns.2009.03.012

Grushcow, M. (2008). *Cognitive Test Software [Computer Software]*. North York, ON: NTT Systems Inc.

Harrison, T. L., Shipstead, Z., Hicks, K. L., Hambrick, D. Z., Redick, T. S., and Engle, R. W. (2013). Working memory training may increase working memory capacity but not fluid intelligence. *Psychol. Sci.* 24, 2409–2419. doi: 10.1177/0956797613492984

Jaeggi, S. M., Buschkuehl, M., Jonides, J., and Perrig, W. J. (2008). Improving fluid intelligence with training on working memory. *Proc. Natl. Acad. Sci. U.S.A.* 105, 6829–6833. doi: 10.1073/pnas.0801268105

Kane, M. J., Conway, A. R., Miura, T. K., and Colflesh, G. J. (2007). Working memory, attention control, and the N-back task: a question of construct validity. *J. Exp. Psychol. Learn. Mem. Cogn.* 33, 615–622. doi: 10.1037/0278-7393.33.3.615

Kane, M. J., and Engle, R. W. (2002). The role of prefrontal cortex in working-memory capacity, executive attention, and general fluid intelligence:

an individual-differences perspective. *Psychon. Bull. Rev.* 9, 637–671. doi: 10.3758/BF03196323

Karbach, J., and Kray, J. (2009). How useful is executive control training? Age differences in near and far transfer of task-switching training. *Dev. Sci.* 12, 978–990. doi: 10.1111/j.1467-7687.2009.00846.x

Klingberg, T. (2010). Training and plasticity of working memory. *Trends Cogn. Sci.* 14, 317–324. doi: 10.1016/j.tics.2010.05.002

Melby-Lervåg, M., and Hulme, C. (2013). Is working memory training effective? A meta-analytic review. *Dev. Psychol.* 49, 270–291. doi: 10.1037/a0028228

Miller, E. K., Erickson, C. A., and Desimone, R. (1996). Neural mechanisms of visual working memory in prefrontal cortex of the macaque. *J. Neurosci.* 16, 5154–5167.

Morrison, A. B., and Chein, J. M. (2011). Does working memory training work? The promise and challenges of enhancing cognition by training working memory. *Psychon. Bull. Rev.* 18, 46–60. doi: 10.3758/s13423-010-0034-30

Munk, M. H., Linden, D. E., Muckli, L., Lanfermann, H., Zanella, F. E., Singer, W., et al. (2002). Distributed cortical systems in visual short-term memory revealed by event-related functional magnetic resonance imaging. *Cereb. Cortex* 12, 866–876. doi: 10.1093/cercor/12.8.866

Nakashima, A., Vartanian, O., Bouak, F., Hofer, K., and Cheung, B. (2011). "A test battery for the assessment of psychological and physiological performance following primary blast wave exposure," in *Proceedings of the Military and Veterans Health Research Forum*, eds A. B. Aiken and S. A. H. Bélanger (Kingston, ON: Canadian Defence Academy Press), 134–153.

Oldfield, R. C. (1971). The assessment and analysis of handedness: the Edinburgh inventory. *Neuropsychologia* 9, 97–113. doi: 10.1016/0028-3932(71)90067-4

Persson, J., Welsh, K. M., Jonides, J., and Reuter-Lorenz, P. A. (2007). Cognitive fatigue of executive processes: interaction between interference resolution tasks. *Neuropsychologia* 45, 1571–1579. doi: 10.1016/j.neuropsychologia.2006.12.007

Petrides, M. (2005). Lateral prefrontal cortex: architectonic and functional organization. *Philos. Trans. R. Soc. Lond. B Biol. Sci.* 360, 781–795. doi: 10.1098/rstb.2005.1631

Ranganath, C., Cohen, M. X., Dam, C., and D'esposito, M. (2004). Inferior temporal, prefrontal, and hippocampal contributions to visual working memory maintenance and associative memory retrieval. *J. Neurosci.* 24, 3917–3925. doi: 10.1523/JNEUROSCI.5053-03.2004

Raven, J., Raven, J. C., and Court, J. H. (1998). *Raven Manual: Section 4. Advanced Progressive Matrices.* Oxford: Oxford Psychologists Press.

Rottschy, C., Langner, R., Dogan, I., Reetz, K., Laird, A. R., Schulz, J. B., et al. (2012). Modelling neural correlates of working memory: a coordinate-based meta-analysis. *Neuroimage* 60, 830–846. doi: 10.1016/j.neuroimage.2011.11.050

Salminen, T., Frensch, P., Strobach, T., and Schubert, T. (2015). Age-specific differences of dual n-back training. *Neuropsychol. Dev. Cogn. B Aging Neuropsychol. Cogn.* 1–22. doi: 10.1080/13825585.2015.1031723 [Epub ahead of print].

Salminen, T., Strobach, T., and Schubert, T. (2012). On the impacts of working memory training on executive functioning. *Front. Hum. Neurosci.* 6:166. doi: 10.3389/fnhum.2012.00166

Shipstead, Z., Redick, T. S., and Engle, R. W. (2010). Does working memory training generalize? *Psychol. Belg.* 50, 245–276. doi: 10.5334/pb-50-3-4-245

Song, X. W., Dong, Z. Y., Long, X. Y., Li, S. F., Zuo, X. N., Zhu, C. Z., et al. (2011). REST: a toolkit for resting-state functional magnetic resonance imaging data processing. *PLoS ONE* 6:e25031. doi: 10.1371/journal.pone.0025031

Sprenger, A. M., Atkins, S. M., Bolger, D. J., Harbison, J. I., Novick, J. M., Chrabaszcz, J. S., et al. (2013). Training working memory: limits of transfer. *Intelligence* 41, 638–663. doi: 10.1016/j.intell.2013.07.013

Stanislaw, H., and Todorov, N. (1999). Calculation of signal detection theory measures. *Behav. Res. Methods Instrum. Comput.* 31, 137–149. doi: 10.3758/bf03207704

Tidwell, J. W., Dougherty, M. R., Chrabaszcz, J. R., Thomas, R. P., and Mendoza, J. L. (2014). What counts as evidence for working memory training? Problems with correlated gains and dichotomization. *Psychon. Bull. Rev.* 21, 620–628. doi: 10.3758/s13423-013-0560-567

Todd, J. J., and Marois, R. (2004). Capacity limit of visual short-term memory in human posterior parietal cortex. *Nature* 428, 751–754. doi: 10.1038/nature02466

Todd, J. J., and Marois, R. (2005). Posterior parietal cortex activity predicts individual differences in visual short-term memory capacity. *Cogn. Affect. Behav. Neurosci.* 5, 144–155. doi: 10.3758/cabn.5.2.144

Wager, T. D., and Smith, E. E. (2003). Neuroimaging studies of working memory: a meta-analysis. *Cogn. Affect. Behav. Neurosci.* 3, 255–274. doi: 10.3758/CABN.3.4.255

Wainer, H. (1976). Robust statistics: a survey and some prescriptions. *J. Educ. Stat.* 1, 285–312. doi: 10.2307/1164985

25

Compensation or Restoration: Closed-Loop Feedback of Movement Quality for Assisted Reach-to-Grasp Exercises with a Multi-Joint Arm Exoskeleton

Florian Grimm, Georgios Naros and Alireza Gharabaghi*

Division of Functional and Restorative Neurosurgery, and Centre for Integrative Neuroscience, Eberhard Karls University, Tuebingen, Germany

Edited by:
Mikhail Lebedev,
Duke University, USA

Reviewed by:
Arturo Forner-Cordero,
University of São Paulo, Brazil
Wiktor Sieklicki,
Gdansk University of Technology, Poland
Ilya Boristchev,
IT Universe, Russia

****Correspondence:***
Alireza Gharabaghi
alireza.gharabaghi@uni-tuebingen.de

Assistive technology allows for intensive practice and kinematic measurements during rehabilitation exercises. More recent approaches attach a gravity-compensating multi-joint exoskeleton to the upper extremity to facilitate task-oriented training in three-dimensional space with virtual reality feedback. The movement quality, however, is mostly captured through end-point measures that lack information on proximal inter-joint coordination. This limits the differentiation between compensation strategies and genuine restoration both during the exercise and in the course of rehabilitation. We extended in this proof-of-concept study a commercially available seven degree-of-freedom arm exoskeleton by using the real-time sensor data to display a three-dimensional multi-joint visualization of the user's arm. Ten healthy subjects and three severely affected chronic stroke patients performed reach-to-grasp exercises resembling activities of daily living assisted by the attached exoskeleton and received closed-loop online feedback of the three-dimensional movement in virtual reality. Patients in this pilot study differed significantly with regard to motor performance (accuracy, temporal efficiency, range of motion) and movement quality (proximal inter-joint coordination) from the healthy control group. In the course of 20 training and feedback sessions over 4 weeks, these pathological measures improved significantly toward the reference parameters of healthy participants. It was moreover feasible to capture the evolution of movement pattern kinematics of the shoulder and elbow and to quantify the individual degree of natural movement restoration for each patient. The virtual reality visualization and closed-loop feedback of joint-specific movement kinematics makes it possible to detect compensation strategies and may provide a tool to achieve the rehabilitation goals in accordance with the individual capacity for genuine functional restoration; a proposal that warrants further investigation in controlled studies with a larger cohort of stroke patients.

Keywords: robot-assisted rehabilitation, stroke rehabilitation, hemiparesis, motor recovery, upper-limb outcome assessment

INTRODUCTION

Assistive rehabilitation technology allows an increase and standardization in the amount of upper limb movement therapy after stroke, potentially resulting in improved arm/hand function and muscle strength, albeit respective trials have, as yet, provided only low-quality evidence (Kwakkel et al., 2008; Mehrholz et al., 2015). In clinical settings, therapists often provide the patient with feedback on the movement quality to encourage relearning of premorbid movement patterns (Cirstea and Levin, 2007). Particularly in patients with severe impairment, deficits in the range and coordination of elbow and shoulder movements might interfere with reaching performance (Cirstea and Levin, 2000; Cirstea et al., 2003). Moreover, motor compensation could limit gains in motor function by learned non-use and lead to pain and joint contractures in the long run (Cirstea and Levin, 2007). However, although robot-assisted therapy focuses on task performance, it usually does not differentiate between compensation strategies and genuine motor restoration despite being capable of objective movement evaluation (Kwakkel et al., 2008). Although kinematic parameters would be particularly suitable for assessing movement quality during rehabilitation exercises, current robotic devices tend to capture end-point measures that lack information on proximal interjoint coordination (Nordin et al., 2014) which would be necessary to differentiate recovery from compensation. In this context, a gravity-compensating multi-joint exoskeleton could not only support reach-to grasp movements in severely affected stroke patients but also provide closed-loop virtual reality feedback of movement quality during task-oriented training. This pilot study intended to explore the methodological feasibility and clinical validity of virtual reality visualization and closed-loop feedback of joint-specific movement kinematics to capture the evolution of upper extremity movement patterns in severely affected stroke patients. We furthermore wanted to quantify the individual degree of natural movement restoration or compensation for each patient. When a proof-of-concept is demonstrated here, such an approach would provide a tool to follow rehabilitation goals in accordance with the individual capacity for genuine functional restoration, a strategy that could then be verified by further investigations in controlled studies.

MATERIALS AND METHODS

We recruited ten right-handed healthy subjects (6 males, mean age: 29 ± 4 [24 39] years) and three right-handed stroke patients (all male, mean age: 62 ± 6 [56 68] years). The patients were in the chronic phase after stroke (57 ± 22 [34 78] months) and presented with a severe and persistent hemiparesis of the left side. To ensure that our results were comparable to earlier studies, *coordination*, *speed* and *reflexes* were not taken into account. This resulted in a modified upper extremity Fugl-Meyer-Assessment scores (UE-FMA) of 12, 12, and 25, respectively. This study was in accordance with the guidelines of the ethic committee of the local medical faculty. Participants performed either a single session (healthy control group) or 20 sessions in the course of 4 weeks (patients) of reach-to-grasp training with a multi-joint exoskeleton attached to the left arm. The orthosis was calibrated according to the individual anatomy (e.g., shoulder position, forearm/upper arm length) of each patient. This setup and calibration of the system before every session took about 5 min per patient. Each session lasted approximately 30 min and consisted of 150 trials. The general experimental setup has already been described in detail elsewhere (Grimm and Gharabaghi, 2016; Grimm et al., under review) and is cited here when applied in the same way.

Exoskeleton and Virtual Reality

We used a commercially available (Armeo Spring, Hocoma, Volketswil, Switzerland) rehabilitation exoskeleton for shoulder, elbow and wrist joints with seven axes (i.e., degrees of freedom) providing antigravity support for the paretic arm and registration of movement kinematics and grip force. This device allowed individual adjustments e.g., of gravity compensation, thereby supporting patients with severe impairment in performing task-oriented practice within a motivating virtual environment. Kinematic sensor data was provided by 7 built-in angle sensors (sensor resolution <0.2°) for shoulder flexion/abduction (1 sensor), shoulder rotation (2 sensors), elbow flexion/extension (1 sensor for horizontal registration, 1 sensor for vertical registration), forearm pronation/supination (1 sensor) and wrist flexion/extension (1 sensor). The shoulder rotation was calculated as the sum of the two sensors. The upper arm movement was calculated as the angle between forearm and upper-arm in three-dimensional space. The sensors were placed directly in the movement axis of the exoskeleton within the joints, allowing an accurate registration of the actual joint position of the upper arm, forearm and hand (**Figure 1**). Kinematic data of hand closure/opening could not be captured directly with this set up. We therefore estimated the hand function indirectly by registering the grip force. Grip force has previously been shown to correlate with motor function in chronic stroke patients (Boissy et al., 1999) and was captured with an in build mid-palmar grip pressure sensor in the present study.

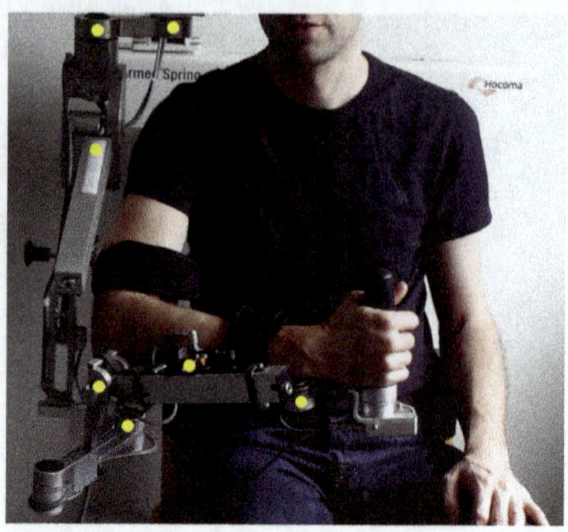

FIGURE 1 | Exoskelleton setup and location of angle sensors within the device (yellow dots).

Thereby, a complete real-time registration of the subject's kinematic reach-to-grasp movement could be performed with the orthosis. We extended these features in-house by using the real-time sensor data of the exoskeleton to display a three-dimensional multi-joint visualization of the user's arm in virtual reality (**Figure 2A**). The exercises where displayed to the subjects on a monitor in front of the setup. For this purpose, we captured the angles of all arm joints and the grip force from a shared memory block using a file mapping communication protocol. The virtual arm engine was programmed in a Microsoft XNA^{TM} framework. The arm model utilized by the engine was constructed as a meshed bone-skin combination with 54 bones (3Ds Max 2010^{TM}, Autodesk). The measured joint angles and grip forces of the device were used to modify the bone-vectors of the meshed model according to the movements of the user thereby providing online closed-loop feedback. The kinematic data and the 3D virtual representation were updated in 20 ms intervals. The joint angles of the exoskeleton were directly represented in virtual reality, whereas the grip forces were augmented to feedback natural hand function. Prior to each session, participants were instructed to perform a natural reach-to-grasp movement during the task by using distal (elbow) rather than proximal (shoulder) movements. The participants were moreover encouraged to track and adjust their movements accordingly with the information provided by the virtual environment. Furthermore, they were informed that their movement quality would be captured and evaluated afterwards. This preparation was intended to prime the participants to exploit the information provided by the virtual feedback. The three-dimensional visualization of the arm was then applied during each task as an implicit online feedback of movement quality, since explicit information can disrupt motor learning in stroke patients (Boyd and Winstein, 2004; Cirstea and Levin, 2007). Various virtual training paradigms were designed to allow for different rehabilitation exercises resembling activities of daily living.

Task Design

In this study, participants performed a reach-to-grasp movement toward a ball which changed its position in virtual space after each trial, necessitating three-dimensional transfer movements. The ball had to be grasped, carried to a distant basket and then released again (**Figure 2B**). The virtual hand could interact with the ball as soon as it entered a defined range around the latter. The ball changed its color according to the hand position (white: out of range, green: possible to grasp, yellow: possible to transfer, red: possible to release). The grasping and releasing of the virtual ball was performed by applying force to the grip sensor and opening the hand, respectively, while the threshold was adjusted to the individual strength of the user. No other support was provided during the exercises. The level of orthotic assistance remained constant in the course of the 20 sessions.

Outcome Measures

The kinematic assessment included both motor performance and movement quality (Nordin et al., 2014). The motor performance was estimated with regard to accuracy, temporal efficiency and range of motion. Movement accuracy, more specifically the decrease of inaccuracy, was captured by calculating changes of movement direction along an optimal path toward the targets, by estimating the distance function between the hand-position and the final endpoint, and by calculating the second derivative of the function to acquire the number of turning points for each task (Cirstea et al., 2006). Temporal efficiency was captured as the mean velocity of the hand between the targets while calculating their distance for X-, Y- and Z-directions in virtual units (vu). The range of motion of each joint was measured according to the orthosis and displayed in degrees along with the mean change in grip pressure. Movement quality of proximal inter-joint coordination was defined as the amount of compensatory shoulder inward rotation during the task and quantified by a shoulder/elbow index, i.e., the degree of inward rotation of the shoulder in relation to the degree of elbow movement. More specifically, a larger proportion of shoulder movement would indicate compensation, while a larger proportion of elbow movement for the same task would indicate a rather natural movement.

Statistics

Statistical analysis was performed on a Matlab 2010b Engine. Data was tested for linear distribution using the Lilliefors-test (2-sided goodness-of-fit test). The non-parametric Kruskal–Wallis was used for group comparisons. To estimate the evolution of parameters during training, a robust multilinear regression model was fitted. Although the Lilliefors-test revealed normality of the data, a robust multilinear regression analysis was applied in order to minimize the impact of outliers. The fitting function was

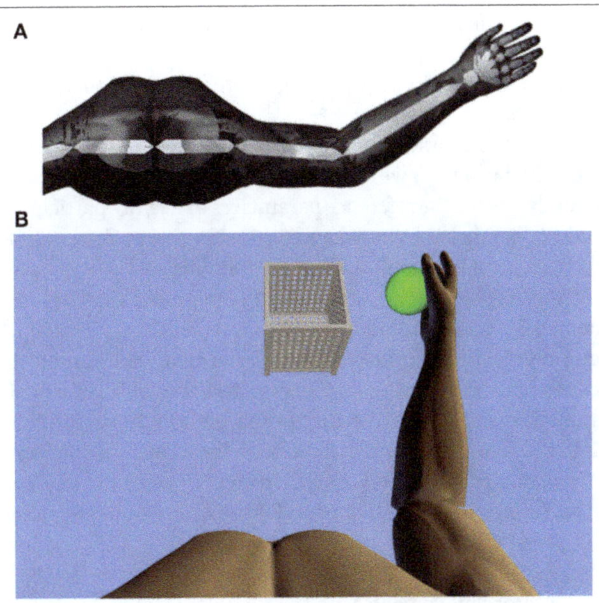

FIGURE 2 | (A) Bone architecture of the three-dimensional multi-joint visualization of the user's arm in virtual reality. **(B)** Virtual training environment for reach-to-grasp movements toward a ball which changes its position in space after each trial. The ball has to be grasped, carried to a distant basket and then released again.

TABLE 1 | Overview of kinematic data for subjects and patients, respectively.

Parameter	Subjects	Patients	*p*-value
Inaccuracy, number of turning points	4.20 ± 0.42 [4.00 5.00]	8.75 ± 2.51 [6.00 13.00]	<0.001
Average velocity (distance/time) (vu/s)	13.86 ± 2.17 [11.31 17.53]	3.89 ± 1.85 [0.90 8.04]	<0.001
Grip pressure	0.45 ± 0.19 [0.14 0.69]	0.684 ± 0.27371 [0.22 1.04]	<0.001
Shoulder movement, angle in degrees (°)	32.90 ± 8.03 [21.81 44.42]	22.00 ± 12.48 [11.93 35.97]	<0.001
Elbow movement, angle in degrees (°)	36.83 ± 7.65 [19.65 44.79]	19.18 ± 5.03 [6.94 28.87]	<0.001
Shoulder/elbow index	0.78 ± 0.05 [0.71 0.88]	1.36 ± 0.30 [1.0 1.58]	<0.001

TABLE 2 | Individual slopes of robust multilinear regression models of kinematic changes in the three stroke patients (n.s.: not significant).

Parameter	Patient 1	Patient 2	Patient 3
Inaccuracy, turning points	−0.24, $p = 0.26$ (n.s.)	−0.14, $p = 0.02$	−0,06, $p < 0.001$
Average velocity (distance/time) (vu/s)	+ 0.14e-3, $p < 0.001$	+ 0.13e-3, $p < 0.001$	+ 0.17e-3, $p < 0.001$
Grip pressure	+1.1e-3, $p = 0.08$ (n.s.)	+4.4e-3, $p < 0.001$	+8.4e-3, $p < 0.001$
Shoulder movement, angle in degrees (°)	+0.14, $p = 0.45$ (n.s.)	+0.4, $p = 0.01$	+1.2, $p < 0.001$
Elbow movement, angle in degrees (°)	+0.49, $p = 0.01$	+0.36, $p = 0.01$	+0.36, $p < 0.001$
Shoulder/elbow index	−27e-3, $p = 0.007$	−15e-3, $p = 0.05$	−6e-3, $p = 0.46$ (n.s.)

based on an iteratively reweighted least squares algorithm. The weights of each iteration were calculated by applying a bisquared function to the residuals of the previous iteration. For every fitting function the slope *b* of coefficient estimates was presented. The significance level was set to $p = 0.05$ for all tests.

RESULTS

Patients differed significantly with regard to motor performance (accuracy, temporal efficiency, range of motion) and movement quality (proximal inter-joint coordination) from the healthy control group (**Table 1**). Most notably, they applied compensatory strategies by using more shoulder than elbow movements.

However, the patients showed motor learning in the course of the training program with significant changes in most kinematic measures toward the reference parameters of healthy participants (**Table 2**) paralleled by improved FMA-UA scores (+1, +2, +5 points, respectively) in the end of the training.

Most importantly, the evolution of movement pattern kinematics of the shoulder and elbow enabled us to quantify the individual degree of natural movement restoration for each patient: Patient 1 had the lowest scores in all kinematic parameters and also showed the poorest motor performance (**Figure 3**). However, he presented with the steepest evolution of movement quality and was the only patient to reach the reference parameter of healthy participants (**Figure 4**). By contrast, patient 3 showed the highest kinematic parameters, i.e., the best motor performance (**Figure 3**), but also revealed the strongest compensatory movements with the shoulder (**Figure 4**).

DISCUSSION

Rehabilitation devices with a gravity-compensating arm exoskeleton provide assistance for intensive exercises in severely affected stroke patients and may thereby improve motor performance in the course of a training intervention (Housman et al., 2009). However, functional gains in hemiparetic patients are often achieved by non-physiologic movements with a disturbed shoulder-arm inter-joint coordination (Levin, 1996; Levin et al., 2002). Although these compensatory strategies might be efficient in short-term task accomplishment, they may lead to long-term complications such as pain and joint-contracture (Cirstea and Levin, 2007). Movement pattern kinematics may provide accurate, valid, reproducible and predictive measures of the impairment severity in chronic stroke (Subramanian et al., 2010) and of atypical movement patterns that aim to compensate the diminished range of motion of the affected limb (Cirstea and Levin, 2000). In this context, providing detailed information about how the movement is carried out, i.e., the movement quality regarding inter-joint coordination, is more liable to recover premorbid movement patters and to avoid compensatory movements than to provide information about movement outcome, i.e., end-point based accuracy information, only (Cirstea et al., 2006; Cirstea and Levin, 2007). When this feedback is administered during virtual reality training, even less compensation was achieved in the moderate-to-severe group (Subramanian et al., 2013). However, in these previous studies, information on movement quality was provided *explicitly* to the patients via auditory feedback. Moreover, all patients who received this feedback on their movement pattern kinematics were *mildly or moderately-to-severely* affected and were able to perform reach-to-grasp movements without assistance.

In the present feasibility study, we extended this line of research by incorporating information on movement quality as *implicit* closed-loop feedback in the virtual environment of an exoskeleton-based rehabilitation device suitable for *severely affected* stroke patients who require gravity-support to perform activities of daily living such as reach-to-grasp exercises. Notably, antigravity-support did not interfere with the

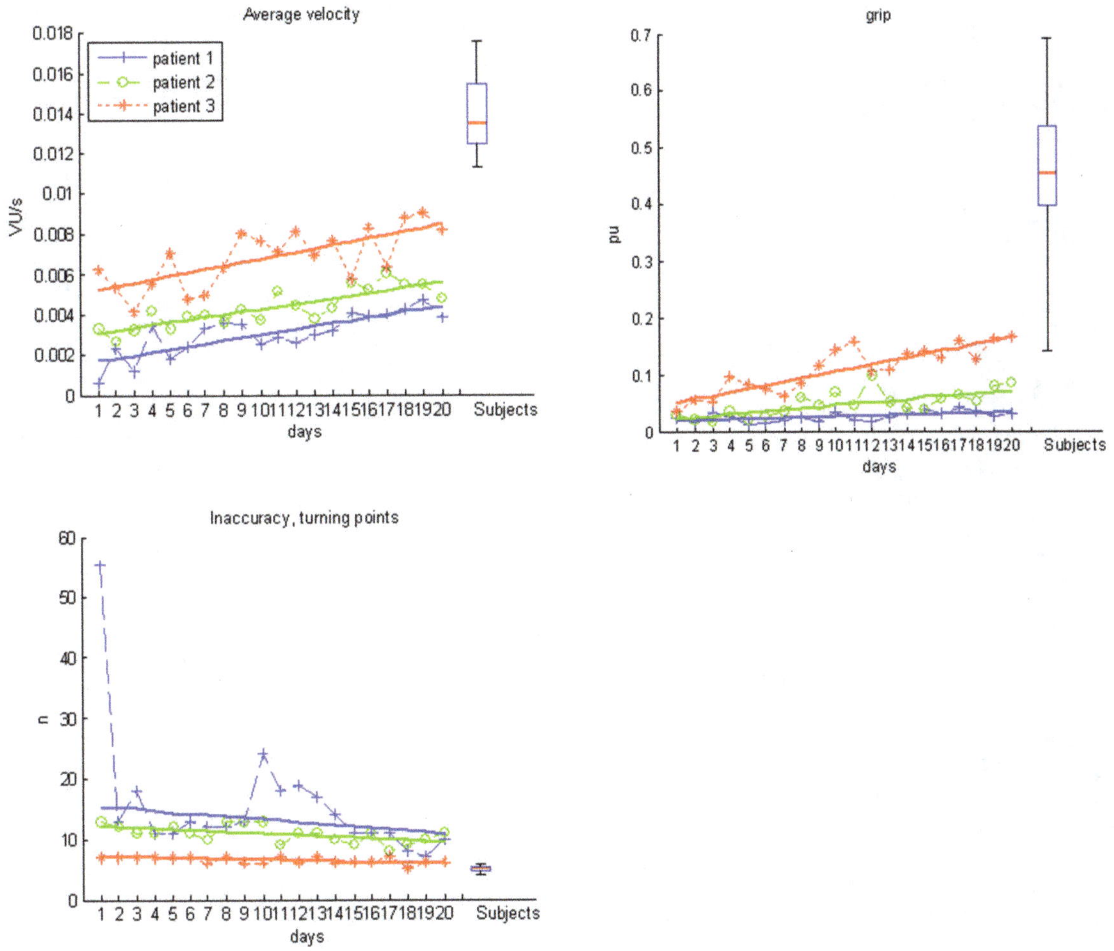

FIGURE 3 | Motor performance data for subjects (boxplots) and individual patients over the time course of training.

kinematic evaluation of proximal inter-joint coordination. By contrast, this approach allowed disentangling in patients with severe impairments whether improved motor performance was achieved by compensation or by functional restoration. Notably, improvement in kinematic measures may be misleading since driven by compensatory strategies. The observations of this study highlighted that these measures were not sufficient to fully assess the evolution during motor rehabilitation thereby supporting the analysis of multi-joint information along the movement trajectory. Moreover, the continuous visual feedback of the whole arm kinematics allowed the patients to adjust their movement quality online during each task; an approach closely resembling natural motor learning. Although pathological measures improved significantly toward the reference parameters of healthy participants, this study did not provide evidence for the specificity of these effects to the implemented setup, i.e., feedback modality. Future studies need therefore to address this question by directly comparing multi-joint with end-effector feedback in controlled trials with long-term follow up evaluation, before conclusions about the therapeutic superiority of the presented approach can be drawn. In any case, however, the diagnostic advantage of detecting compensatory strategies (i.e., use of proximal instead of distal joints in a reach-to-grasp task) with the help of the multi-joint orthosis remains evident.

Future studies may explore the additional effects of brain stimulation on movement quality for assisted reach-to-grasp exercises: a recent study which applied bilateral transcranial direct current stimulation has demonstrated improved motor performance beyond the natural learning curve while using the very same multi-joint arm exoskeleton studied in the present work (Naros et al., 2016a). Moreover, brain state-dependent transcranial magnetic stimulation has been demonstrated to induce robust increases of corticospinal excitability (Kraus et al., 2016b) and may thereby amplify use-dependent plasticity when applied in conjunction with orthotic rehabilitation devices (Gharabaghi, 2015). Future approaches may also address patients with even more limited residual motor function as well (which might not benefit from the presented approach) by providing closed-loop feedback with a *robotic* multi-joint exoskeleton during brain-states in which both the participant's effort to move and the responsiveness of the brain for peripheral input are reflected (Brauchle et al., 2015). In such a restorative framework,

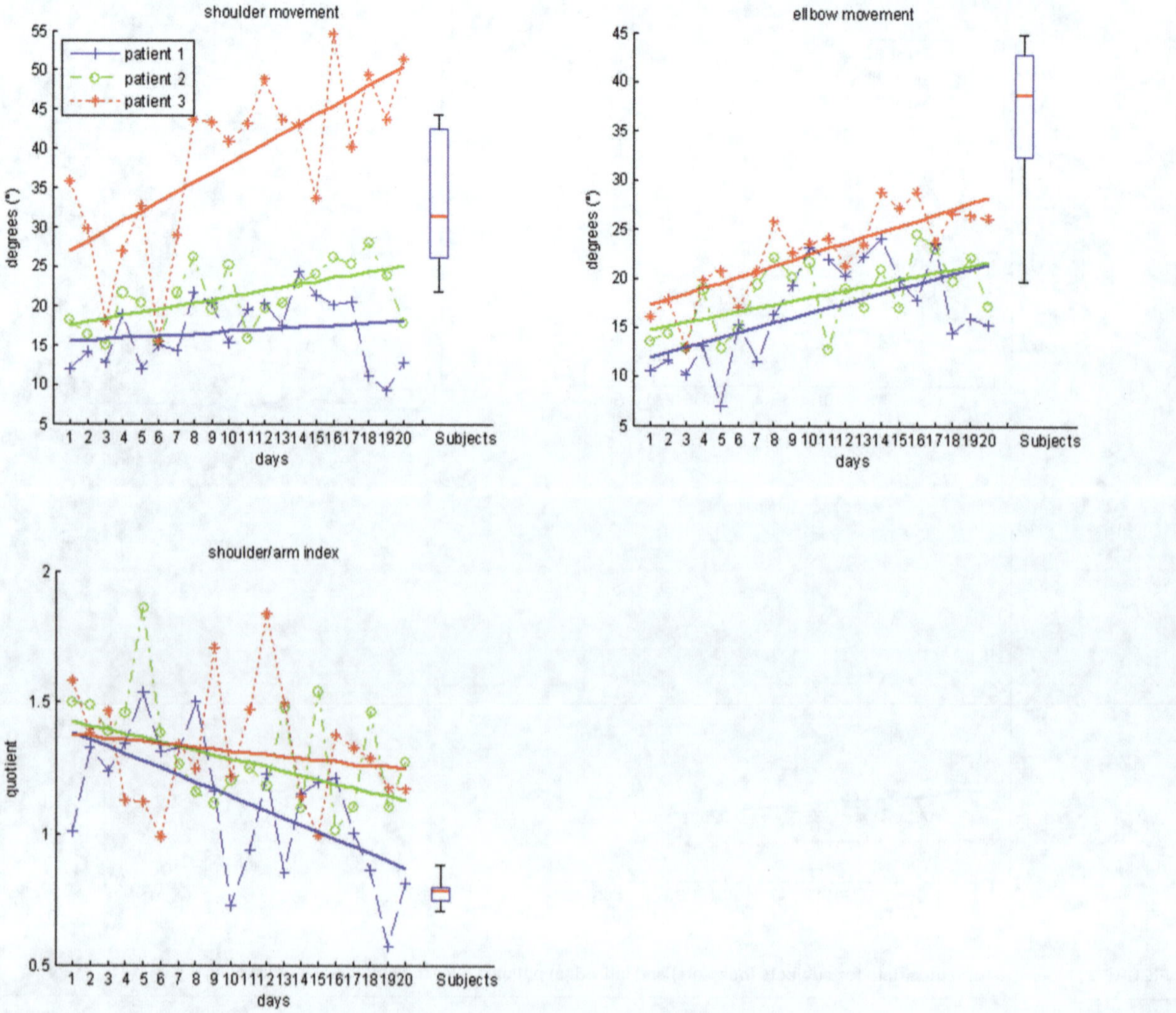

FIGURE 4 | Movement quality data for subjects (boxplots) and individual patients over the time course of training.

closed-loop interfaces follow an operant conditioning rationale, providing contingent feedback to facilitate self-regulation of specific brain activity which is considered to be beneficial for recovery and might ultimately lead to functional gains (Bauer and Gharabaghi, 2015a). Accordingly, these brain-robot interfaces were found to constitute a back-door to the motor system (Bauer et al., 2015; Gharabaghi et al., 2014a), since this type of feedback training may result in connectivity changes of cortico-spinal (Kraus et al., 2016a) and cortico-cortical motor networks (Vukelić et al., 2014; Vukelić and Gharabaghi, 2015a,b) and thereby lead to behavioral gains after the intervention (Naros et al., 2016b). Recently, pilot data has suggested that such restorative brain-robot interfaces may even lead to task-specific motor improvement in chronic stroke (Naros and Gharabaghi, 2015).

Problematic for restorative approaches is, however, that the considerable challenge of these devices (Bauer and Gharabaghi, 2015b; Fels et al., 2015) might condition the patients to explore alternative, i.e., therapeutically non-desired, strategies (Gharabaghi et al., 2014b). Particularly in patients with severe impairments, motor compensation could limit genuine motor restoration. In this context, detection and closed-loop feedback of movement quality during rehabilitation exercises would allow differentiating recovery from compensation and thus encourage the relearning of premorbid movement patterns. For those patients, however, who benefit less from the implicit closed-loop information provided in the presented set-up (e.g., patient 3) more explicit feedback or even segmental movement restriction by the orthosis might be necessary to reinforce the targeted movement pattern.

In conclusion, virtual reality visualization and feedback of joint-specific movement kinematics facilitates to monitor the evolution of upper extremity movement kinematics and to quantify the individual degree of natural movement restoration in the course of rehabilitation training of severely motor impaired patients; controlled studies with a larger cohort of stroke patients need to investigate whether this approach also allows to achieve the rehabilitation goals in accordance with the individual capacity for functional recovery.

AUTHOR CONTRIBUTIONS

FG participated in the study design and software development, supervised the measurement sessions and carried the data analysis. GN supervised the measurement sessions. AG participated in the study design and data analysis. Authors jointly drafted and approved the final manuscript.

ACKNOWLEDGMENTS

AG was supported by grants from the German Research Council [DFG EC 307], and from the Federal Ministry for Education and Research [BFNT 01GQ0761, BMBF 16SV3783, BMBF 0316064B, BMBF16SV5824].

REFERENCES

Bauer, R., and Gharabaghi, A. (2015a). Reinforcement learning for adaptive threshold control of restorative brain-computer interfaces: a Bayesian simulation. *Front. Neurosci.* 9:36. doi: 10.3389/fnins.2015.00036

Bauer, R., and Gharabaghi, A. (2015b). Estimating cognitive load during self-regulation of brain activity and neurofeedback with therapeutic brain-computer interfaces. *Front. Behav. Neurosci.* 9:21. doi: 10.3389/fnbeh.2015.00021

Bauer, R., Fels, M., Vukelić, M., Ziemann, U., and Gharabaghi, A. (2015). Bridging the gap between motor imagery and motor execution with a brain-robot interface. *Neuroimage*. 108, 319–327. doi: 10.1016/j.neuroimage.2014.12.026

Boissy, P., Bourbonnais, D., Carlotti, M. M., Gravel, D., and Arsenault, B. A. (1999). Maximal grip force in chronic stroke subjects and its relationship to global upper extremity function. *Clin. Rehabil.* 13, 354–362. doi: 10.1191/026921599676433080

Boyd, L. A., and Winstein, C. J. (2004). Providing explicit information disrupts implicit motor learning after basal ganglia stroke. *Learn. Mem.* 11, 388–396. doi: 10.1101/lm.80104

Brauchle, D., Vukelić, M., Bauer, R., and Gharabaghi, A. (2015). Brain state-dependent robotic reaching movement with a multi-joint arm exoskeleton: combining brain-machine interfacing and robotic rehabilitation. *Front. Hum. Neurosci.* 9:564. doi: 10.3389/fnhum.2015.00564

Cirstea, C. M., Ptito, A., and Levin, M. F. (2006). Feedback and cognition in arm motor skill reacquisition after stroke. *Stroke* 37, 1237–1242. doi: 10.1161/01.STR.0000217417.89347.63

Cirstea, M. C., and Levin, M. F. (2000). Compensatory strategies for reaching in stroke. *Brain* 123 (Pt 5), 940–953. doi: 10.1093/brain/123.5.940

Cirstea, M. C., and Levin, M. F. (2007). Improvement of arm movement patterns and endpoint control depends on type of feedback during practice in stroke survivors. *Neurorehabil. Neural. Repair* 21, 398–411. doi: 10.1177/1545968306298414

Cirstea, M. C., Ptito, A., and Levin, M. F. (2003). Arm reaching improvements with short-term practice depend on the severity of the motor deficit in stroke. *Exp. Brain Res.* 152, 476–488. doi: 10.1007/s00221-003-1568-4

Fels, M., Bauer, R., and Gharabaghi, A. (2015). Predicting workload profiles of brain–robot interface and electromygraphic neurofeedback with cortical resting-state networks: personal trait or task-specific challenge? *J. Neural. Eng.* 12:046029. doi: 10.1088/1741-2560/12/4/046029

Gharabaghi, A. (2015). Activity-dependent brain stimulation and robot-assisted movements for use-dependent plasticity. *Clin. Neurophysiol.* 126, 853–854. doi: 10.1016/j.clinph.2014.09.004

Gharabaghi, A., Kraus, D., Leão, M. T., Spüler, M., Walter, A., Bogdan, M., et al. (2014a). Coupling brain-machine interfaces with cortical stimulation for brain-state dependent stimulation: enhancing motor cortex excitability for neurorehabilitation. *Front. Hum. Neurosci.* 8:122. doi: 10.3389/fnhum.2014.00122

Gharabaghi, A., Naros, G., Khademi, F., Jesser, J., Spüler, M., Walter, A., et al. (2014b). Learned self-regulation of the lesioned brain with epidural electrocorticography. *Front. Behav. Neurosci.* 8:429. doi: 10.3389/fnbeh.2014.00429

Grimm, F., and Gharabaghi, A. (2016). Closed-loop neuroprosthesis for reach-to-grasp assistance: combining adaptive multi-channel neuromuscular stimulation with a multi-joint arm exoskeleton. *Front. Neurosci.* 10:284. doi: 10.3389/fnins.2016.00284

Housman, S. J., Scott, K. M., and Reinkensmeyer, D. J. (2009). A randomized controlled trial of gravity-supported, computer-enhanced arm exercise for individuals with severe hemiparesis. *Neurorehabil. Neural. Repair* 23, 505–514. doi: 10.1177/1545968308331148

Kraus, D., Naros, G., Bauer, R., Khademi, F., Leão, M. T., Ziemann, U., et al. (2016b). Brain state-dependent transcranial magnetic closed-loop stimulation controlled by sensorimotor desynchronization induces robust increase of corticospinal excitability. *Brain Stimul.* 9, 415–424. doi: 10.1016/j.brs.2016.02.007

Kraus, D., Naros, G., Bauer, R., Leão, M. T., Ziemann, U., and Gharabaghi, A. (2016a). Brain-robot interface driven plasticity: distributed modulation of corticospinal excitability. *Neuroimage* 15, 522–532. doi: 10.1016/j.neuroimage.2015.09.074

Kwakkel, G., Kollen, B. J., and Krebs, H. I. (2008). Effects of robot-assisted therapy on upper limb recovery after stroke: a systematic review. *Neurorehabil. Neural. Repair* 22, 111–121. doi: 10.1177/1545968307305457

Levin, M. F. (1996). Interjoint coordination during pointing movements is disrupted in spastic hemiparesis. *Brain* 119 (Pt 1), 281–293. doi: 10.1093/brain/119.1.281

Levin, M. F., Michaelsen, S. M., Cirstea, C. M., and Roby-Brami, A. (2002). Use of the trunk for reaching targets placed within and beyond the reach in adult hemiparesis. *Exp. Brain Res.* 143, 171–180. doi: 10.1007/s00221-001-0976-6

Mehrholz, J., Pohl, M., Platz, T., Kugler, J., and Elsner, B. (2015). Electromechanical and robot-assisted arm training for improving activities of daily living, arm function, and arm muscle strength after stroke. *Cochrane Database Syst. Rev.* 11:CD006876. doi: 10.1002/14651858.CD006876.pub4

Naros, G., and Gharabaghi, A. (2015). Reinforcement learning of self-regulated β-oscillations for motor restoration in chronic stroke. *Front. Hum. Neurosci.* 9:391. doi: 10.3389/fnhum.2015.00391

Naros, G., Geyer, M., Koch, S., Mayr, L., Ellinger, T., Grimm, F., et al. (2016a). Enhanced motor learning with bilateral transcranial direct current stimulation: Impact of polarity or current flow direction? *Clin. Neurophysiol.* 127, 2119–2126. doi: 10.1016/j.clinph.2015.12.020

Naros, G., Naros, I., Grimm, F., Ziemann, U., and Gharabaghi, A. (2016b). Reinforcement learning of self-regulated sensorimotor β-oscillations improves motor performance. *Neuroimage*. 134, 142–152. doi: 10.1016/j.neuroimage.2016.03.016

Nordin, N., Xie, S. Q., and Wunsche, B. (2014). Assessment of movement quality in robot- assisted upper limb rehabilitation after stroke: a review. *J. Neuroeng. Rehabil.* 11:137. doi: 10.1186/1743-0003-11-137

Subramanian, S. K., Lourenco, C. B., Chilingaryan, G., Sveistrup, H., and Levin, M. F. (2013). Arm motor recovery using a virtual reality intervention in chronic stroke: randomized control trial. *Neurorehabil. Neural. Repair* 27, 13–23. doi: 10.1177/1545968312449695

Subramanian, S. K., Yamanaka, J., Chilingaryan, G., and Levin, M. F. (2010). Validity of movement pattern kinematics as measures of arm motor impairment poststroke. *Stroke* 41, 2303–2308. doi: 10.1161/STROKEAHA.110.593368

Vukelić, M., Bauer, R., Naros, G., Naros, I., Braun, C., and Gharabaghi, A. (2014). Lateralized alpha-band cortical networks regulate volitional modulation of beta-band sensorimotor oscillations. *Neuroimage* 87, 147–153. doi: 10.1016/j.neuroimage.2013.10.003

Vukelić, M., and Gharabaghi, A. (2015a). Oscillatory entrainment of the motor cortical network during motor imagery is modulated by the feedback modality. *Neuroimage* 111, 1–11. doi: 10.1016/j.neuroimage.2015.01.058

Vukelić, M., and Gharabaghi, A. (2015b). Self-regulation of circumscribed brain activity modulates spatially selective and frequency specific connectivity of distributed resting state networks. *Front. Behav. Neurosci.* 9:181. doi: 10.3389/fnbeh.2015.00181

26

Clinical Application of the Hybrid Assistive Limb (HAL) for Gait Training

Anneli Wall[1,2], Jörgen Borg[1,2] and Susanne Palmcrantz[1,2]*

[1] Department of Rehabilitation Medicine, Danderyd University Hospital, Stockholm, Sweden, [2] Department of Clinical Sciences, Karolinska Institute, Stockholm, Sweden

Edited by:
Mikhail Lebedev,
Duke University, USA

Reviewed by:
Jun Morimoto,
ATR Computational Neuroscience Labs, Japan
Mukul Talaty,
Moss, USA
Antoinette Domingo,
San Diego State University, USA

***Correspondence:**
Anneli Wall,
Department of Rehabilitation Medicine, Danderyd University Hospital, Danderyds Sjukhus, Rehabiliteringsmedicinska Universitetskliniken, Hus 39, plan 3, Stockholm 18288, Sweden
anneli.wall@ds.se

Objective: The aim of this study was to review the literature on clinical applications of the Hybrid Assistive Limb system for gait training.

Methods: A systematic literature search was conducted using Web of Science, PubMed, CINAHL and clinicaltrials.gov and additional search was made using reference lists in identified reports. Abstracts were screened, relevant articles were reviewed and subject to quality assessment.

Results: Out of 37 studies, 7 studies fulfilled inclusion criteria. Six studies were single group studies and 1 was an explorative randomized controlled trial. In total, these studies involved 140 participants of whom 118 completed the interventions and 107 used HAL for gait training. Five studies concerned gait training after stroke, 1 after spinal cord injury (SCI) and 1 study after stroke, SCI or other diseases affecting walking ability. Minor and transient side effects occurred but no serious adverse events were reported in the studies. Beneficial effects on gait function variables and independence in walking were observed.

Conclusions: The accumulated findings demonstrate that the HAL system is feasible when used for gait training of patients with lower extremity paresis in a professional setting. Beneficial effects on gait function and independence in walking were observed but data do not allow conclusions. Further controlled studies are recommended.

Keywords: rehabilitation, robotics, gait, walking, locomotion, paresis, review, gait machine

Background

Normal gait depends on the functional integrity and interactions in sensory-motor neural networks at spinal and supraspinal levels (Bowden et al., 2013). This complex system may be disturbed in many neurological conditions such as stroke or spinal cord injury (SCI) resulting in limited mobility and impaired gait function, which are major challenges in neuro rehabilitation. Intensive, repetitive task specific training may drive beneficial neuroplasticity, enhance functional restitution and improve final outcome (Kwakkel et al., 2004; Langhorne et al., 2009, 2011; Peurala et al., 2014). However, there is a need for further development of training methods in response to an increasing understanding of the individual capacity for regaining functioning (Krakauer et al., 2012; Bowden et al., 2013).

Approaches to improve gait function after stroke and SCI include treadmill training with or without use of partial body weight support (BWS), yet the evidence to support this is inconclusive (Schwartz and Meiner, 2013; Dobkin et al., 2014). Gait machines (GM) may allow more reproducible gait movements compared to conventional training and reduce the burden on the therapist. GM work according to the end-effector principle (foot plates move the feet in a controlled gait pattern) or as exoskeletons, which have joints matching the limb joints and motors that drive movements over these joints to assist, e.g., leg movements (Hesse et al., 2010). A recent Cochrane review concluded that electromechanically assisted gait training in combination with physiotherapy after stroke increases the odds of achieving independent walking and most so when applied for severely impaired patients in the first 3 months after stroke (Mehrholz et al., 2013) but less clear after SCI (Mehrholz et al., 2012).

The importance of incorporating more active participation than allowed by gait machines to enhance training effects and the need for new concepts and devices are recognized (Dobkin, 2009; Pennycott et al., 2012). One new approach is represented by the Hybrid Assistive Limb system (HAL). HAL is an exoskeleton with a hybrid system allowing both a voluntary and an autonomous mode of action to support training of gait. HAL comprises a control algorithm and supporting devices, where each knee and hip joint can be controlled separately. Key features of the HAL system have been reported in detail (Kawamoto, 2002; Suzuki et al., 2007; Kawamoto et al., 2010). Movements are triggered by use of either the "Cybernic Voluntary Control" (CVC), which is based on the users voluntary activation of gait muscles as recorded by surface electromyography (EMG), or by the "Cybernic Autonomous Control" (CAC), which is based on the users weight shifting and input from force pressure sensors in the shoes. The CVC mode allows the operator to adjust the degree of support for each joint and reduce the support as training progress and to adjust settings to achieve a gait pattern that is as close as possible to normal gait. In case of complete loss of voluntary activation of gait muscles the CAC mode may be used. Gait is then initiated and sustained by input from force-pressure sensors in the shoes. HAL is manufactured in single-leg and double-leg versions and training with HAL may be performed with or without BWS.

A number of clinical studies with HAL have been conducted and there is a need for an evaluation of available data to guide further trials. The aim of this report was to provide a systematic review in order to evaluate current evidence with regard to feasibility (i.e., usability and safety) and effects and to make recommendations for further studies.

Methods

A systematic search of the literature was conducted using the databases Web of Science, PubMed, and CINAHL. Both MeSH (Medical Subject Headings for Medline) terms and free text relevant for the subject were used and detected synonyms were added to the search. Search terms were (MeSH terms in bold): ((((robot OR robots OR robotic OR robotics OR robot-assisted OR exoskeleton OR machine-assisted OR electro-mechanic OR DGO OR "driven gait orthosis"))) AND (gait OR gaits OR walking OR walk OR walks OR locomotion OR "motor activity")) AND (HAL OR "hybrid assistive limb" OR "wearable robot"). Search limitations were "Humans" and "English," while publication date was unlimited. Using the same search terms, a search was also performed at clinicaltrials.gov, in order to identify ongoing studies and/or unpublished papers (Clinicaltrials, online). Abstracts identified were screened and studies were considered relevant if they addressed any clinical application of the HAL system regardless of study design. If needed the full text article was retrieved and assessed. Relevant studies were exported to EndNote where duplicates were identified and removed. Reference lists of these studies were manually searched for further articles. Studies were included if they were primary research articles, concerned gait training with the Hybrid Assistive Limb. Studies only reporting technology data, including only healthy subjects, single subjects or reviews were excluded. Thirty-seven articles were identified, 20 were retrieved in full text for assessment of eligibility and 13 of these did not fulfill inclusion criteria (see **Figure 1**). Overall 7 studies met the inclusion criteria and were subject to data extraction and analyses (Maeshima et al., 2011; Kawamoto et al., 2013; Kubota et al., 2013; Ueba et al., 2013; Aach et al., 2014; Nilsson et al., 2014; Watanabe et al., 2014). Included studies were subject to critical review by two independent reviewers.

The quality of the included studies, regarding risk of confounding and bias, was evaluated in accordance with the Scottish Intercollegiate Guidelines Network (SIGN) criteria (SIGN, online[1]). According to SIGN the methodological quality can be coded (++) meaning *all or most of criteria fulfilled*, (+) *some of the criteria fulfilled* or (−) *few or no criteria fulfilled*. The evaluation was performed independently by two investigators and in case of disagreement, a third reviewer was consulted. Since two investigators are authors of one of the included studies (Nilsson et al., 2014) this study was assessed by a fourth investigator.

Data extraction was performed by one investigator and checked by the two additional investigators. The extracted data comprised; characteristics of participants, intervention protocols and settings, outcome measures and effects and feasibility.

Results

The 7 studies included 8–38 participants each, 6 were single group studies and 1 was a randomized controlled trial (RCT). In total, the studies involved 140 participants of whom 118 completed the intervention protocols and 107 used HAL for gait training. Extracted study data and results of the quality evaluation are presented in the **Table 1**. All included studies were found to have a high risk of bias and confounding according to the SIGN criteria and do not provide data for a meta-analysis.

Characteristics of Participants Included in the Studies

The most frequent diagnosis reported was stroke ($n = 106$) followed by complete or incomplete SCI ($n = 16$) and other disorders ($n = 18$). Five of the studies included solely persons with stroke, 1 study included solely persons with SCI (Aach et al., 2014) and 1 study included persons with stroke ($n = 12$) and SCI

[1]SIGN. Scottish Intercollegiate Guidelines Network. Available online at: http://www.sign.ac.uk/methodology/checklists.html [Accessed Dec 2014].

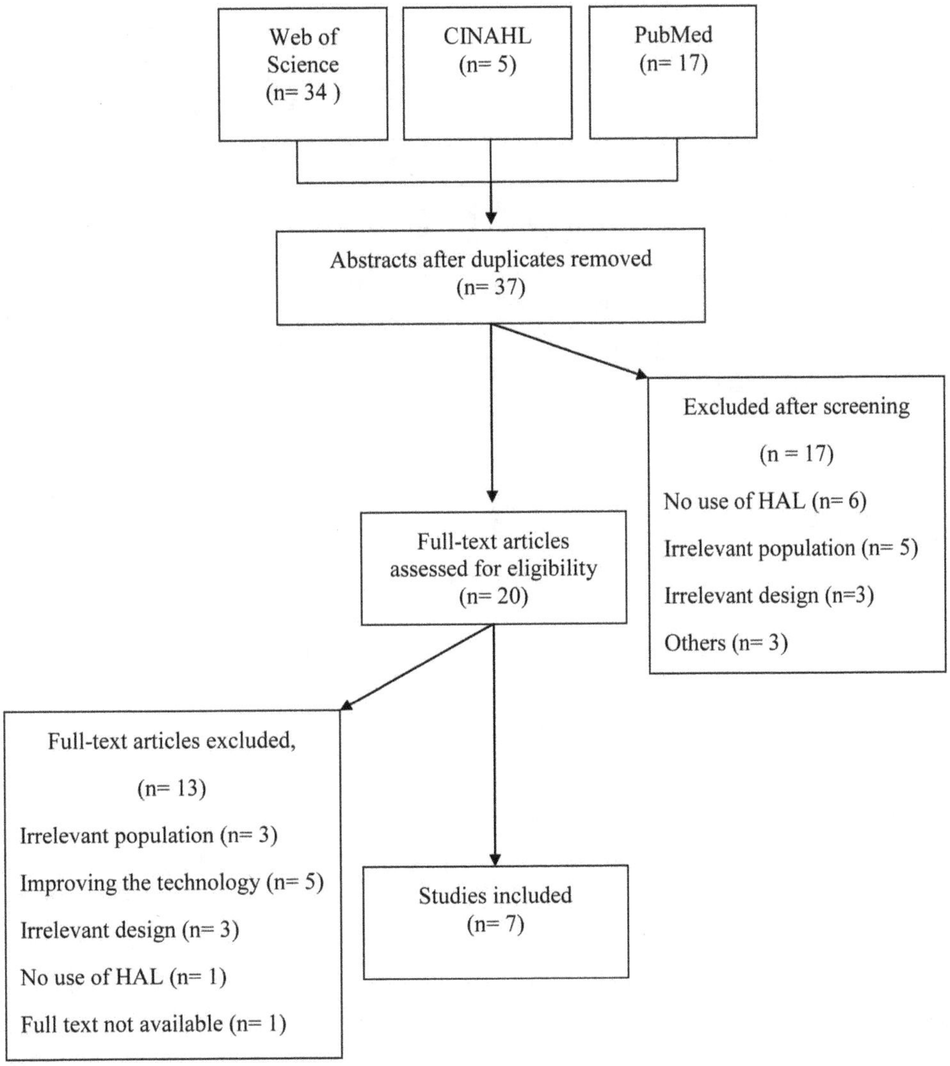

FIGURE 1 | Presentation of the results of the systematic search of the literature.

(n = 8) as well as other disorders (n = 18) (Kubota et al., 2013). Mean age of the participants ranged from 48 to 67 years with a total range of 18–90 years.

In 6 of the included studies a total of 65.7% (n = 67) of the participants who completed the study intervention were men and 34.3% (n = 35) were women. Ueba et al. (2013) did not report gender for participants completing the study but among the included 32% (n = 7) were men and 68% (n = 15) were women.

The total time from disease onset to inclusion ranged from 6 days to 54 years. For persons with SCI the time from injury ranged from 1 to 19 years and for persons with stroke this time ranged from approximately 6 days to 16 years. Three studies (Maeshima et al., 2011; Nilsson et al., 2014; Watanabe et al., 2014) included persons early after stroke, with a mean range of 31–59 days since stroke onset. Two other studies included persons later than 1 year and up to 16 years after stroke onset (Kawamoto et al., 2013; Kubota et al., 2013).

The number of reported dropouts during the study interventions ranged from 6 to 10 and was 22, in total (18 with stroke, 1 with SCI and 3 participants with other diagnosis,). Reported reasons for dropouts were medical (n = 5), technical (n = 1), discharge (n = 2), personal (n = 4) and withdrawal of consent (n = 4). Another 6 participants dropped out due to inappropriate size of shoes, lumbar spondylosis which prevented correct fitting and/or depressive status.

Intervention Protocols and Settings

All except 1 (Ueba et al., 2013) of the 7 studies specifically addressed gait training. The HAL training protocols showed a great variation with regard to frequency, intensity and number of sessions performed. Most studies applied HAL training ≥2 times per week during ≥4 weeks with durations of ≥20 min per session. In the studies involving persons with stroke, the total number of sessions per participant training with HAL ranged from 1 (Maeshima et al., 2011) to 31 (Nilsson et al., 2014). In studies

TABLE 1 | Extracted study data.

First author	Kawamoto et al., 2013	Maeshima et al., 2011	Nilsson et al., 2014	Ueba et al., 2013	Watanabe et al., 2014	Aach et al., 2014	Kubota et al., 2013
Aim	To investigate the feasibility of locomotor training with the HAL in chronic stroke patients and to examine differences between two functional ambulation subgroups	To evaluate the effects of the HAL suit on the gait of stroke patients undergoing rehabilitation	To explore the safety and feasibility of the HAL system when used for early onset, intensive gait training as part of an inpatient rehabilitation program for patients with hemiparetic stroke	To investigate the feasibility and safety of the HAL suit in the rehabilitation of patients in the acute phase after stroke	To examine the effects of gait rehabilitation using the HAL for patients in the recovery phase of stroke to test the feasibility of intervention and outcome assessment protocols for a future randomized controlled trial on a larger scale	To evaluate the possibilities of exoskeletal locomotor training with HAL under voluntary control and identify beneficial effects on functional mobility of the patients Hypothesis: that exoskeleton treadmill training is feasible and safe in application and capable of improving ambulatory mobility in chronic SCI patients	To investigate the feasibility of 16-session (8 week) HAL rehabilitation training for patients with limited mobility
Study design and setting	Single group study Out-patient setting	Single group study Inpatient rehabilitation setting	Single group study Inpatient rehabilitation setting	Single group study Inpatient rehabilitation setting	Randomized controlled study (outcome assessment not blinded) Inpatient rehabilitation setting	Single group study Out-patient setting	Single group study Out-patient setting
Inclusion criteria	1. Requirement of physical assistance or assistive devices for standing up sitting down, and/or walking; 2. Understanding study protocol and expressing voluntary consent 3. A body shape that could fit in the robotic suit HAL 4. Concurrent use of physical and occupational therapies	Not reported	1. <7 weeks since stroke 2. Able to sit 5 min 3. Unable to walk due to paresis 4. Postural control to allow standing with assistance 5. Understand instructions 6. Express informed consent 7. Body size that fits HAL	1. Hemiplegi or ataxia after stroke 2. Height >120 cm weight <100 kg 3. Glascow coma scale >9 4. Systolic BP 100–160 mmHg 5. Saturation > 90% 6. Heart rate between 40 and 120 beats/min 7. Body temperature <37.5°C	1. Hemiparesis from unilateral ischemic/hemorrhagic stroke 2. Time since onset <6 months	1. Traumatic SCI with cronic incomplete or complete paraplegia 2. Present motor functions of hip and knee extensor and flexor muscle groups	1. Musculoskeletal disability affecting ambulation 2. Physical assistance or assistive devices in at least one of following daily activities: standing up, sitting down, and walking 3. Ability to understand study and to express consent 4. Body size that fit HAL 5. Ability to undergo usual physical and occupational therapies
Diagnosis and number of patients	Stroke Divided into two subgroups based on FAC-score FAC 2–3 (dependent ambulatory) FAC 4–5 (independent ambulatory) Included $n = 16$ Completed $n = 16$	Stroke Patients were divided in 3 groups: 1. Assisted group 2. Handrail group 3. Quad cane group included $n = 16$ completed $n = 16$	Stroke Included $n = 8$ Completed $n = 8$	Stroke Included $n = 22$ Completed $n = 16$	Stroke Included $n = 32$ Completed $n = 22$ (11 in each group)	SCI Included $n = 8$ Completed $n = 8$	Stroke $n = 12$ SCI $n = 8$ Musculoskeletal diseases $n = 4$ Other diseases $n = 14$ Included $n = 38$ Completed $n = 32$

(Continued)

TABLE 1 | Continued

First author	Kawamoto et al., 2013	Maeshima et al., 2011	Nilsson et al., 2014	Ueba et al., 2013	Watanabe et al., 2014	Aach et al., 2014	Kubota et al., 2013
Time since event/disease onset	Months, mean: 47.1 ± 37.6 Months, range: 13–132	Days, mean: 52 Days, range: 29–116	Days, range: 6–46	Days, mean: Group 1: 12.7 ± 7.6 Group 2: 9.5 ± 2.4 (divided into two groups based on occurrence of orthostatic hypotension)	Days, mean: HAL group 58.9 ± 46.5 Control group 50.6 ± 33.8	Months, mean: 97.2 ± 88.4 Years, range: 1–19	Years, range: 1–54
Age	Years, mean: 61 Years, range: 18–84	Years, mean: 63 Years, range: 53–78	Years, mean: 53 Years, range: 39–64	Years, mean: 66.6 Years, range: ?-90 (min not reported)	Years, mean: HAL group 67 Control group 75.6 Years, range: not reported	Years, mean: 48 Years, range: 36–63	Years, mean: 53.2 Years, range: 18–81
Gender	Men $n = 12$ Women $n = 4$	Men $n = 9$ Women $n = 7$	Men $n = 8$ Women $n = 0$	Men $n = 7$ Women $n = 15$ (included, completed not reported)	Men $n = 11$ Women $n = 11$ HAL group, men $n = 7$, women $n = 4$ Control group, men $n = 4$, women $n = 7$	Men $n = 6$ Women $n = 2$	Men $n = 21$ Women $n = 11$
Intervention	HAL-training: with use of mobile suspension system and harness. Sit-to-stand and walking No of sessions: $n = 16$ Times/week: approximately $n = 2$ (individualized) Duration, weeks, mean: 10.8 ± 3.5 HAL version: double leg Training lasted 90 min/session HAL training was 20–30 min/session	HAL-training: walking (overground), stair climbing No of sessions: $n = 1$ Times/week: NA Duration: NA HAL version: double leg	HAL-training: with use of treadmill and body weight support No of sessions: median 16, range 6–31 Times/week: $n = 5$ Duration, weeks: approximately $n = 3$ (individualized) HAL version: double leg Training lasted 90 min/session, max 60 min (effective time)	HAL-training: not reported No of sessions, mean: 3.8 ± 3.1 Times/week: not reported Duration, days, mean: 12.1 ± 7 HAL version: double leg	HAL training: with use of mobile suspension system and harness if necessary HAL group: no of sessions: $n = 12$ Times/week: $n = 3$ Duration, weeks: $n = 4$ HAL version: single leg Control group receiving conventional training: no of sessions: $n = 12$ Times/week: $n = 3$ Duration, weeks: $n = 4$ Training lasted 20 min per session	HAL-training: with use of treadmill and body weight support. Included some regular physiotherapy No of sessions, mean: 51.75 ± 5.6 Times/week: $n = 5$ Duration, days: $n = 90$ HAL version: double leg Training lasted 90 min/session	HAL-training: with use of mobile suspension system and harness, or treadmill and body weight support No of sessions: $n = 16$ Times/week: $n = 2$ Duration, weeks: $n = 8$ HAL version: double leg Training lasted 90-min/session (including all). Net walking time was approximately 20 min
Assessments	10 m walk test* (walk speed, number of steps, cadence) Timed up and go Berg balance scale	10 m walk test (stride length, speed) Physiological cost index Assessed before, during, after HAL training and the next day	10 m walk test Timed up and go Berg balance scale Functional ambulation categories NIH stroke scale Fugl-Meyer-LE Clinical outcome variable scale Falls-efficacy scale Barthel index Functional independence measure EQ-5D	Orthostatic hypotension and several medical and functional variables were assessed	10 m walk test (Max walking speed) Timed up and go Functional ambulation categories* 6 min walk test Fugl-Meyer-LE Short physical performance battery Isometric muscle strength	10 m walk test (time, number of steps, assistance) Timed up and go 6 min walk test Walking index for SCI II (WISCI II) Lower extremity motor score Muscle volume ASIA impairment scale	10 m walk test* Timed up and go* Berg balance scale*

(Continued)

TABLE 1 | Continued

First author	Kawamoto et al., 2013	Maeshima et al., 2011	Nilsson et al., 2014	Ueba et al., 2013	Watanabe et al., 2014	Aach et al., 2014	Kubota et al., 2013
Results	Dependent ambulators: improvements in 10 m walk test (speed, cadence and number of steps) and berg balance scale. statistically significant differences ($p < 0.05$) Independent ambulators: improvements in Berg Balance Scale. Statistically significant differences ($p < 0.05$) Whole group: improvements in 10 m walk test and berg balance scale. Statistically significant differences ($p < 0.05$) Adverse events reported as: no training-related serious adverse events were observed	During HAL training physiological cost index (PCI) increased in $n = 11$ participants. PCI was associated with ability to ambulate ($p < 0.05$) Walking speed decreased during training in $n = 12$ participants. Speed was associated with ability to ambulate ($p < 0.05$) Stride length increased during training in $n = 4$ participants. Stride length was not associated with ability to ambulate (p-value not reported) Adverse events: not reported	Improvements in FAC, Fugl-Meyer-LE, 10 m walk test, and berg balance scale Statistically significant differences: not reported Adverse events reported as: no serious adverse events occurred	Improved walking and torso posture $n = 2$ Standing with HAL $n = 12$ No change $n = 2$ Withdrew $n = 6$ Statistically significant differences ($p < 0.05$): not reported Adverse events reported as: orthostatic hypotension ($n = 4$)	HAL group: improvements in independent walking (FAC), walking speed, timed up and go, 6 min walk test and Fugl-Meyer LE. Statistically significant differences ($p < 0.05$) Control group: improvements in independent walking (FAC), short physical performance and timed Up and go. Statistically significant differences ($p < 0.05$) Between groups: improvements in independent walking (FAC) greater in HAL group. Statistically significant differences ($p < 0.04$) Adverse events reported as: no participants withdrew because of adverse effects	All patients improved in treadmill training with HAL. Mean walking speed and average walking time increased Improvements in 10 m walk test (gait speed, number of steps), lower extremity motor score, timed up and go, 6 min walk test statistically significant differences ($p < 0.05$) Improvements in walking index for SCI II. No statistically significant differences ($p < 0.05$) Adverse events reported as: neither adverse nor severe adverse events occurred during the intervention	Improvements in gait speed, steps and cadence based on 10 m walk test, (27 participants) Statistically significant differences ($p < 0.05$) Improvements according to timed up and go and berg balance scale. No statistically significant differences ($p < 0.05$) Adverse events reported as: no serious training-related adverse events
Quality according to SIGN criteria	(–)	(–)	(–)	(–)	(–)	(–)	(–)

Indicated as the primary outcome in the study.

involving persons with SCI, Aach et al. (2014) used a mean of 51.75 sessions while the number of sessions for persons with SCI in the study by Kubota et al. (2013) was 16. Data on the use of the active CVC mode and the autonomous CAC mode was not consistently reported. Based on the information provided, we anticipate that 6 of the studies used the CVC mode during training but the extent is not clear. One study (Ueba et al., 2013) did not report on modes used. Four studies reported the total length of each training sessions to be approximately 90 min including assessments, donning, doffing and effective walking time. The effective training time in these studies was approximately 20–30 min per session. Training with HAL was performed by use of BWS and/or a mobile suspension system in 5 studies, by over ground training in 1 study and was not defined in 1 study. Four studies were conducted in inpatient rehabilitation settings and 3 in out-patient care (see **Table 1**).

Outcome Measures and Effects

All assessments were performed without wearing HAL except for one study (Maeshima et al., 2011) where measurements were performed both with and without HAL. Outcome measures mainly related to walking ability. Most frequently used were the 10 m walking test ($n = 6$) (Wade et al., 1987), Timed up and Go ($n = 5$) (Podsiadlo and Richardson, 1991), and Berg Balance Scale ($n = 3$) (Berg et al., 1992). Assessments performed at baseline and after the training period were reported in all studies except 1 (Ueba et al., 2013). No study reported on a long-term follow up. The explorative RCT (Watanabe et al., 2014) compared the effect of HAL-training to the effect of conventional training in the subacute phase after stroke and included 11 participants in each group. The study shows a significant differences ($p = 0.04$) according to the Functional Ambulation Categories (FAC) (Holden et al., 1984) between groups, in favor for the HAL training group. This study has several limitations with regard to study sample size, varying time after stroke and lack of blinding of outcome assessments, as recognized by the authors. One other study (Nilsson et al., 2014) also used FAC and observed improvements suggesting a beneficial effect in a single group. Other studies also report on varying effects such as improvements in walking- and torso posture, gait speed, number of steps and cadence, functional ambulation/independent walking, motor function in lower extremity, activity performance and/or balance (see **Table 1**).

Adverse Events

All studies except 1 (Maeshima et al., 2011) explicitly reported on adverse events. Except for transient complaints related to pressure of the suit, irritated skin, training related pain etc., no adverse events during training with HAL were reported.

Discussion

The aim of this review was to explore existing evidence regarding gait training with the exoskeleton HAL (Hybrid Assistive Limb). We included 7 studies, each with small study samples but comprising a total of 140 patients. Of these, 118 completed the intervention and 107 used HAL. Studies differed in terms of aim, design, duration of intervention, patients/diagnosis, setting and participant characteristics as well as allocation, randomization, blinding and outcome measures. Only 1 study compared training with HAL with other training (Watanabe et al., 2014) but outcome assessment in that study was not blinded. Although no study provides conclusive data on the effects of gait training with HAL as compared to other training and the risk of confounding and bias was considered high, the experiences of training with HAL and the responses that were observed will be useful in the design of further studies.

Feasibility

In total, adult subjects within a broad age range (18–90 years) participated. Both genders were represented, however two thirds were men. Since the majority of subjects had a stroke diagnosis and gender proportions are fairly similar in this diagnostic group, the uneven distribution is surprising but only scarcely commented on in the studies.

Study participants in both post-acute and long-term after stroke onset were represented and 88 out of 106 included subjects completed the study interventions. One small experimental study included subjects with paraplegia 1–19 years after spinal cord injury where all completed the intervention (Aach et al., 2014) while no study addressed effects of training with HAL in the post-acute phase after SCI. The severity of paresis and gait problems varied both within and between the included studies, from severe (only able to maintain sitting balance) to moderate (independent walkers) and a corresponding use of HAL mode and BWS. Reasons for training of independent walkers were not stated or discussed in the included studies although plausible beneficial effects may be, e.g., an increase in walking speed and/or distance or level of independence. The reported numbers of dropouts were low and a total of 107 participants, representing a broad spectrum of motor impairments completed >1500 training sessions with the HAL system without any reported serious adverse events.

Thus, the accumulated results of the included studies demonstrate that training with the HAL system is feasible when applied in professional settings, irrespective of the patients age and sex and the severity of the lower extremity paresis. The feasibility of training with HAL in the post-acute phase after SCI will need to be explored further.

Intervention Protocols and Settings

Even though not stated, the variability in applied frequency, intensity and duration of the reported training sessions and evaluations of outcome, probably reflect both theoretical and practical considerations of, e.g., training needed to achieve significant effects, participants' functional level and study resources. Reasonably, the optimal design would allow training programs to be on the edge for each participant's capacity with regard to the intensity and length of each training session. The intensity and length of the training periods must also consider the patient's functional level as well as the capacity and aims with regard to, e.g., on neuroplasticity, musculoskeletal function, cardiovascular function, gait pattern or independence in walking. Three or more sessions weekly during the training period would probably be justified from a neuroplasticity and relearning perspective (Bowden et al., 2013).

Both single- and double-leg versions of HAL were used even though not specified in all studies. Reasonably the double-leg version is most relevant for subjects with paraparesis and the single-leg version most often appropriate for subjects with one sided paresis.

Only 2 of the studies included patients early after stroke when the potential to utilize beneficial neuroplasticity processes is higher (Bowden et al., 2013) and there is a need for controlled HAL studies in this area. Post-acute studies are more challenging as they have to consider both the impact of spontaneous recovery early after the event as well as other post-acute health problems.

Outcome Measures and Effects

Outcome measures in the included studies primarily relate to aspects of gait function and walking. Most frequently used was the 10 m walking test, which is a measure of over ground walking speed. Six studies report a positive impact on gait function after HAL training, 5 of these specifically on walking speed and 2 studies report increased level of independence in walking according to the FAC (Nilsson et al., 2014; Watanabe et al., 2014). FAC is the most commonly used outcome measure in studies of walking after robotic training for patients with severe to moderate walking limitations in both the acute and chronic phase after stroke (Geroin et al., 2013). FAC takes the persons level of independence and amount of personal assistance required into account, which from the individuals' perspective is more important than walking speed. However, gait speed may be associated with functional ambulation ability (Perry et al., 1995; Dobkin et al., 2014) and a gait speed improvement may generate improved function and quality of life (Schmid et al., 2007). Therefore, we suggest both the FAC and the 10 m walking test to be used in further studies. In studies including participants with severely impaired gait function at baseline and who are unable to walk 10 m, the 2 min walk test (Kosak and Smith, 2005) is an option to be considered in order to achieve baseline data also when participants cannot walk (i.e., 0 m in 2 min). The potential effect of HAL training on movement related function such as gait pattern is poorly addressed in the included studies. Future studies should consider using assessments that cover also these aspects, for example by use of 3-dimensional motion analysis.

Data on self-perceived aspects of the training were scarce and we found no data on perceived activity performance, participation in everyday life, health or cost-effectiveness that need to be approached in future studies. Further, no study reported on potential effects on cardiovascular, metabolic, emotional or cognitive functions of training with the HAL system. The possible additional value of training with HAL in these areas should be of interest in future studies.

Further, controlled studies should compare training with the HAL system with the most relevant alternative training method. As pointed out, gait machines such as the Lokomat differs from the HAL system in terms of the degree of active patient participation. Comparison studies of these gait machines would be of interest. However, until now, studies using Lokomat have not consistently demonstrated effects, regarding sensory-motor function, gait speed, balance and/or mobility, that are superior to those achieved with conventional training (Swinnen et al., 2010; Ucar et al., 2014; van Nunen et al., 2014) although there might be other advantages such as less therapist burden. Thus, further studies that compare the effects of training with the HAL system to the effects of well designed "conventional training" are justified. Moreover, studies combining robotics with other therapeutic interventions with increasing evidence support, such as Fluoxetine (Chollet et al., 2011), BMI (Brain-Machine Interface) (Shindo et al., 2011; Noda et al., 2012) or brain stimulation (Liew et al., 2014) are also of great interest.

Currently, there are a number of exoskeletons at various stages of development or clinical applications. In addition to differences in mechanical design and control strategies existing exoskeletons uses different activation systems to produce movement of the limb. The most common are hydraulic, pneumatic, and electric motor actuator. In a recent review by Chen et al. (2013) focused on lower extremity robots, the authors divides exoskeletons in different subgroups depending on their functioning and design and conclude that real-time control strategies with timely assistance are a new promising area in rehabilitation therapy. The importance of incorporating more active participation in electromechanical gait training (Dobkin, 2009; Pennycott et al., 2012) as well as of allowing variation of the task during training to promote adequate motor learning (Hidler and Sainburg, 2011) has also been addressed previously.

Some recently developed designs of exoskeletons have taken this into account by establishing intention-based control strategies. In the Ekso (Ekso Bionics, online[2]), ReWalk (Rewalk, online[3]), and in Indego (Indego, online[4]) stepping is initiated by shifting of bodyweight. In Indego, shifting of body weight is used in combination with functional electric stimulation (FES). Another exoskeleton the MINDWALKER (Mindwalker, online[5]) uses EEG and EMG based control.

Recent studies using Ekso for patients in different stages after SCI conclude that the system is safe and show improvements in walking while wearing Ekso (Ekso Clinical Research, online[6]). For inpatient rehabilitation after stroke the authors find Ekso safe to use and indicate that the training may have an effect on cadence as a result of training with Ekso (Ekso Clinical Research, online). However, the number of participant in these studies are limited and do not allow any further conclusions. Ongoing studies after both SCI and severe stroke (Clinicaltrials, online) will evaluate potential effects on ambulation and mobility.

Indego has been introduces in single-subject clinical trials in SCI patients (Quintero et al., 2011; Farris et al., 2014). An ongoing study will evaluate the safety and effectiveness of using Indego

[2]Ekso Bionics. Available online at: http://intl.eksobionics.com/ekso. [Accessed March 2015].

[3]ReWalk. Available online at: http://www.rewalk.com/products/rewalk-rehabilitation/. [Accessed March 2015].

[4]Indego. Available online at: http://www.indego.com/indego/en/home. [Accessed March 2015].

[5]Mindwalker. Available online at: https://mindwalker-project.eu/. [Accessed March 2015].

[6]Ekso Clinical Research, Summary of Findings. Available online at: http://intl.eksobionics.com/clinical-research-summary-download. [Accessed March 2015].

for non-ambulatory or poorly ambulatory SCI patients during standing and walking (Clinicaltrials, online[7]).

In a study by Zeilig et al. (2012) ReWalk was found to be well tolerated and did not cause any adverse events among persons with SCI. This was repeated in a study by Spungen et al. (ReWalk Peer Reviewed Publications, online[8]) where persons with motor-complete paraplegia performed different community-based activities while wearing ReWalk. Several ongoing studies where ReWalk is used after SCI are registered at Clinicaltrials.gov.

Like the HAL, exoskeletons such as the powered knee-ankle-foot-orthosis (KAFO) (Sawicki and Ferris, 2009) and NEUROExos (Cain et al., 2007) use EMG activity to detect a person's intended movement. In both KAFO and NEUROExos EMG activity is used to control the activation of a pneumatic power system to provide torque over the ankle and/or knee joint. In HAL the wearer's joint torque is estimated from the EMG signals on both hip and knee muscles and an electrical motor actuator is used to generate power over these joints (Suzuki et al., 2007).

[7]Clinicaltrials.gov. Available online at: https://www.clinicaltrials.gov/ [Accessed Dec 2014].

[8]ReWalk, Peer Reviewed Publications. Available online at: http://www.rewalk.com/technology/peer-reviewed-publications-copy/. [Accessed March 2015].

This brief survey of other exoskeletons points to a general need for randomized controlled studies where exoskeletons that allow active participation are compared to other types of interventions as well as for studies with larger study populations.

Study Limitations

Since the Hybrid Assistive Limb was developed and is most frequently used in Japan there might be studies published in Japanese journals that were not included in this review. Of note, in 6 of the included studies, the inventor and CEO of the company, Professor Y. Sankai, behind the Hybrid Assistive Limb system is one co-author. No studies using qualitative approach were discovered, which could have been due to the search strategy used. However, even when a broader search was performed, no qualitative studies appeared.

Conclusions and Recommendations

This review identified consistent evidence that the use of the HAL system is feasible when used for gait training in hospital and rehabilitation settings. Data suggest that such training may have beneficial effects on gait function and independence in walking after stroke and after spinal cord injury, but do not allow any conclusions in this respect. Further, well designed controlled studies in these areas are recommended to explore effect sizes and to be followed by larger, confirmatory studies.

References

Aach, M., Cruciger, O., Sczesny-Kaiser, M., Hoffken, O., Meindl, R. C., Tegenthoff, M., et al. (2014). Voluntary driven exoskeleton as a new tool for rehabilitation inchronicspinal cord injury: a pilot study. *Spine J.* 14, 2847–2853. doi: 10.1016/j.spinee.2014.03.042

Berg, K. O., Maki, B. E., Williams, J. I., Holliday, P. J., and Wood-Dauphinee, S. L. (1992). Clinical and laboratory measures of postural balance in an elderly population. *Arch. Phys. Med. Rehabil.* 73, 1073–1080.

Bowden, M. G., Woodbury, M. L., and Duncan, P. W. (2013). Promoting neuroplasticity and recovery after stroke: future directions for rehabilitation clinical trials. *Curr. Opin. Neurol.* 26, 37–42. doi: 10.1097/WCO.0b013e32835c5ba0

Cain, S. M., Gordon, K. E., and Ferris, D. P. (2007). Locomotor adaptation to a powered ankle-foot orthosis depends on control method. *J. Neuroeng. Rehabil.* 4:48. doi: 10.1186/1743-0003-4-48

Chen, G., Chan, C. K., Guo, Z., and Yu, H. (2013). A review of lower extremity assistive robotic exoskeletons in rehabilitation therapy. *Crit. Rev. Biomed. Eng.* 41, 343–363. doi: 10.1615/CritRevBiomedEng.2014010453

Chollet, F., Tardy, J., Albucher, J. F., Thalamas, C., Berard, E., Lamy, C., et al. (2011). Fluoxetine for motor recovery after acute ischaemic stroke (FLAME): a randomised placebo-controlled trial. *Lancet Neurol.* 10, 123–130. doi: 10.1016/S1474-4422(10)70314-8

Dobkin, B. H. (2009). Motor rehabilitation after stroke, traumatic brain, and spinal cord injury: common denominators within recent clinical trials. *Curr. Opin. Neurol.* 22, 563–569. doi: 10.1097/WCO.0b013e3283314b11

Dobkin, B. H., Nadeau, S. E., Behrman, A. L., Wu, S. S., Rose, D. K., Bowden, M., et al. (2014). Prediction of responders for outcome measures of locomotor Experience Applied Post Stroke trial. *J. Rehabil. Res. Dev.* 51, 39–50. doi: 10.1682/JRRD.2013.04.0080

Farris, R. J., Quintero, H. A., Murray, S. A., Ha, K. H., Hartigan, C., and Goldfarb, M. (2014). A preliminary assessment of legged mobility provided by a lower limb exoskeleton for persons with paraplegia. *IEEE Trans. Neural Syst. Rehabil. Eng.* 22, 482–490. doi: 10.1109/TNSRE.2013.2268320

Geroin, C., Mazzoleni, S., Smania, N., Gandolfi, M., Bonaiuti, D., Gasperini, G., et al. (2013). Systematic review of outcome measures of walking training using electromechanical and robotic devices in patients with stroke. *J. Rehabil. Med.* 45, 987–996. doi: 10.2340/16501977-1234

Hesse, S., Waldner, A., and Tomelleri, C. (2010). Innovative gait robot for the repetitive practice of floor walking and stair climbing up and down in stroke patients. *J. Neuroeng. Rehabil.* 7:30. doi: 10.1186/1743-0003-7-30

Hidler, J., and Sainburg, R. (2011). Role of Robotics in Neurorehabilitation. *Top. Spinal Cord Inj. Rehabil.* 17, 42–49. doi: 10.1310/sci1701-42

Holden, M. K., Gill, K. M., Magliozzi, M. R., Nathan, J., and Piehl-Baker, L. (1984). Clinical gait assessment in the neurologically impaired. Reliability and meaningfulness. *Phys. Ther.* 64, 35–40.

Kawamoto, H. (2002). "Power assist system HAL-3 for gait disorder person," in *Lecture Notes in Computer Science, ICCHP 2002, LNCS 2398*, eds K. Miesenberger, J. Klaus, and W. Zagler (Berlin; Heidelberg: Springer-Verlag), 196–203.

Kawamoto, H., Kamibayashi, K., Nakata, Y., Yamawaki, K., Ariyasu, R., Sankai, Y., et al. (2013). Pilot study of locomotion improvement using hybrid assistive limb in chronic stroke patients. *BMC Neurol.* 13:141. doi: 10.1186/1471-2377-13-141

Kawamoto, H., Taal, S., Niniss, H., Hayashi, T., Kamibayashi, K., Eguchi, K., et al. (2010). "Voluntary motion support control of Robot Suit HAL triggered by bioelectrical signal for hemiplegia," in *Conference Proceedings:Annual International Conference of the IEEE Engineering in Medicine and Biology Society. IEEE Engineering in Medicine and Biology Society. Annual Conference* (Buenos Aires), 462–466.

Kosak, M., and Smith, T. (2005). Comparison of the 2-, 6-, and 12-minute walk tests in patients with stroke. *J. Rehabil. Res. Dev.* 42, 103–107. doi: 10.1682/JRRD.2003.11.0171

Krakauer, J. W., Carmichael, S. T., Corbett, D., and Wittenberg, G. F. (2012). Getting neurorehabilitation right: what can be learned from animal models? *Neurorehabil. Neural Repair* 26, 923–931. doi: 10.1177/1545968312440745

Kubota, S., Nakata, Y., Eguchi, K., Kawamoto, H., Kamibayashi, K., Sakane, M., et al. (2013). Feasibility of rehabilitation training with a newly developed wearable robot for patients with limited mobility. *Arch. Phys. Med. Rehabil.* 94, 1080–1087. doi: 10.1016/j.apmr.2012.12.020

Kwakkel, G., van Peppen, R., Wagenaar, R. C., Wood Dauphinee, S., Richards, C., Ashburn, A., et al. (2004). Effects of augmented exercise therapy time after stroke: a meta-analysis. *Stroke* 35, 2529–2539. doi: 10.1161/01.STR.0000143153.76460.7d

Langhorne, P., Bernhardt, J., and Kwakkel, G. (2011). Stroke rehabilitation. *Lancet* 377, 1693–1702. doi: 10.1016/S0140-6736(11)60325-5

Langhorne, P., Coupar, F., and Pollock, A. (2009). Motor recovery after stroke: a systematic review. *Lancet Neurol.* 8, 741–754. doi: 10.1016/S1474-4422(09)70150-4

Liew, S. L., Santarnecchi, E., Buch, E. R., and Cohen, L. G. (2014). Non-invasive brain stimulation in neurorehabilitation: local and distant effects for motor recovery. *Front. Hum. Neurosci.* 8:378. doi: 10.3389/fnhum.2014.00378

Maeshima, S., Osawa, A., Nishio, D., Hirano, Y., Takeda, K., Kigawa, H., et al. (2011). Efficacy of a hybrid assistive limb in post-stroke hemiplegic patients: a preliminary report. *BMC Neurol.* 11:116. doi: 10.1186/1471-2377-11-116

Mehrholz, J., Elsner, B., Werner, C., Kugler, J., and Pohl, M. (2013). Electromechanical-assisted training for walking after stroke: updated evidence. *Stroke* 44, e127–e128. doi: 10.1161/STROKEAHA.113.003061

Mehrholz, J., Kugler, J., and Pohl, M. (2012). Locomotor training for walking after spinal cord injury. *Cochrane Database Syst. Rev.* 11:CD006676. doi: 10.1002/14651858.CD006676.pub3

Nilsson, A., Vreede, K. S., Haglund, V., Kawamoto, H., Sankai, Y., and Borg, J. (2014). Gait training early after stroke with a new exoskeleton—the hybrid assistive limb: a study of safety and feasibility. *J. Neuroeng. Rehabil.* 11:92. doi: 10.1186/1743-0003-11-92

Noda, T., Sugimoto, N., Furukawa, J., Sato, M., Sang-Ho, H., and Morimoto, J. (2012). "Brain-controlled exoskeleton robot for BMI rehabilitation. Humanoid Robots (Humanoids)," in *12th IEEE-RAS International Conference* (Osaka), 21–27. doi: 10.1109/HUMANOIDS.2012.6651494

Pennycott, A., Wyss, D., Vallery, H., Klamroth-Marganska, V., and Riener, R. (2012). Towards more effective robotic gait training for stroke rehabilitation: a review. *J. Neuroeng. Rehabil.* 9:65. doi: 10.1186/1743-0003-9-65

Perry, J., Garrett, M., Gronley, J. K., and Mulroy, S. J. (1995). Classification of walking handicap in the stroke population. *Stroke* 26, 982–989. doi: 10.1161/01.STR.26.6.982

Peurala, S. H., Karttunen, A. H., Sjogren, T., Paltamaa, J., and Heinonen, A. (2014). Evidence for the effectiveness of walking training on walking and self-care after stroke: a systematic review and meta-analysis of randomized controlled trials. *J. Rehabil. Med.* 46, 387–399. doi: 10.2340/16501977-1805

Podsiadlo, D., and Richardson, S. (1991). The timed "Up & Go": a test of basic functional mobility for frail elderly persons. *J. Am. Geriatr. Soc.* 39, 142–148.

Quintero, H. A., Farris, R. J., Hartigan, C., Clesson, I., and Goldfarb, M. (2011). A powered lower limb orthosis for providing legged mobility in paraplegic individuals. *Top Spinal Cord Inj. Rehabil.* 17, 25–33. doi: 10.1310/sci1701-25

Sawicki, G. S., and Ferris, D. P. (2009). A pneumatically powered knee-ankle-foot orthosis (KAFO) with myoelectric activation and inhibition. *J. Neuroeng. Rehabil.* 6:23. doi: 10.1186/1743-0003-6-23

Schmid, A., Duncan, P. W., Studenski, S., Lai, S. M., Richards, L., Perera, S., et al. (2007). Improvements in speed-based gait classifications are meaningful. *Stroke* 38, 2096–2100. doi: 10.1161/STROKEAHA.106.475921

Schwartz, I., and Meiner, Z. (2013). The influence of locomotor treatment using robotic body-weight-supported treadmill training on rehabilitation outcome of patients suffering from neurological disorders. *Harefuah* 152, 166–171, 182, 181.

Shindo, K., Kawashima, K., Ushiba, J., Ota, N., Ito, M., Ota, T., et al. (2011). Effects of neurofeedback training with an electroencephalogram-based brain-computer interface for hand paralysis in patients with chronic stroke: a preliminary case series study. *J. Rehabil. Med.* 43, 951–957. doi: 10.2340/16501977-0859

Suzuki, K., Mito, G., Kawamoto, H., Hasegawa, Y., and Sankai, Y. (2007). Intention-based walking support for paraplegia patients with Robot Suit HAL. *Adv. Robot.* 21, 1441–1469. doi: 10.1163/156855307781746061

Swinnen, E., Duerinck, S., Baeyens, J. P., Meeusen, R., and Kerckhofs, E. (2010). Effectiveness of robot-assisted gait training in persons with spinal cord injury: a systematic review. *J. Rehabil. Med.* 42, 520–526. doi: 10.2340/16501977-0538

Ucar, D. E., Paker, N., and Bugdayci, D. (2014). Lokomat: a therapeutic chance for patients with chronic hemiplegia. *NeuroRehabilitation* 34, 447–453. doi: 10.3233/NRE-141054

Ueba, T., Hamada, O., Ogata, T., Inoue, T., Shiota, E., and Sankai, Y. (2013). Feasibility and safety of acute phase rehabilitation after stroke using the hybrid assistive limb robot suit. *Neurol. Med. Chir. (Tokyo)* 53, 287–290. doi: 10.2176/nmc.53.287

van Nunen, M. P., Gerrits, K. H., Konijnenbelt, M., Janssen, T. W., and De Haan, A. (2014). Recovery of walking ability using a robotic device in subacute stroke patients: a randomized controlled study. *Disabil. Rehabil. Assist. Technol.* 10, 141–148. doi: 10.3109/17483107.2013.873489

Wade, D. T., Wood, V. A., Heller, A., Maggs, J., and Langton Hewer, R. (1987). Walking after stroke. Measurement and recovery over the first 3 months. *Scand. J. Rehabil. Med.* 19, 25–30.

Watanabe, H., Tanaka, N., Inuta, T., Saitou, H., and Yanagi, H. (2014). Locomotion improvement using a hybrid assistive limb in recovery phase stroke patients: a randomized controlled pilot study. *Arch. Phys. Med. Rehabil.* 95, 2006–2012. doi: 10.1016/j.apmr.2014.07.002

Zeilig, G., Weingarden, H., Zwecker, M., Dudkiewicz, I., Bloch, A., and Esquenazi, A. (2012). Safety and tolerance of the ReWalk™ exoskeleton suit for ambulation by people with complete spinal cord injury: a pilot study. *J. Spinal Cord Med.* 35, 96–101. doi: 10.1179/2045772312Y.0000000003

Permissions

All chapters in this book were first published in Journal of Allergy, by Hindawi Publishing Corporation; hereby published with permission under the Creative Commons Attribution License or equivalent. Every chapter published in this book has been scrutinized by our experts. Their significance has been extensively debated. The topics covered herein carry significant findings which will fuel the growth of the discipline. They may even be implemented as practical applications or may be referred to as a beginning point for another development.

The contributors of this book come from diverse backgrounds, making this book a truly international effort. This book will bring forth new frontiers with its revolutionizing research information and detailed analysis of the nascent developments around the world.

We would like to thank all the contributing authors for lending their expertise to make the book truly unique. They have played a crucial role in the development of this book. Without their invaluable contributions this book wouldn't have been possible. They have made vital efforts to compile up to date information on the varied aspects of this subject to make this book a valuable addition to the collection of many professionals and students.

This book was conceptualized with the vision of imparting up-to-date information and advanced data in this field. To ensure the same, a matchless editorial board was set up. Every individual on the board went through rigorous rounds of assessment to prove their worth. After which they invested a large part of their time researching and compiling the most relevant data for our readers.

The editorial board has been involved in producing this book since its inception. They have spent rigorous hours researching and exploring the diverse topics which have resulted in the successful publishing of this book. They have passed on their knowledge of decades through this book. To expedite this challenging task, the publisher supported the team at every step. A small team of assistant editors was also appointed to further simplify the editing procedure and attain best results for the readers.

Apart from the editorial board, the designing team has also invested a significant amount of their time in understanding the subject and creating the most relevant covers. They scrutinized every image to scout for the most suitable representation of the subject and create an appropriate cover for the book.

The publishing team has been an ardent support to the editorial, designing and production team. Their endless efforts to recruit the best for this project, has resulted in the accomplishment of this book. They are a veteran in the field of academics and their pool of knowledge is as vast as their experience in printing. Their expertise and guidance has proved useful at every step. Their uncompromising quality standards have made this book an exceptional effort. Their encouragement from time to time has been an inspiration for everyone.

The publisher and the editorial board hope that this book will prove to be a valuable piece of knowledge for researchers, students, practitioners and scholars across the globe.

List of Contributors

Vera Talis and Alexander Grishin
Institute for Information Transmission Problems, Moscow, Russia

Yves Ballay
Institut National de la Santé et de la Recherche Médicale, U1093, Cognition Action Plasticité Sensorimotrice, Dijon, France

Thierry Pozzo
Institut National de la Santé et de la Recherche Médicale, U1093, Cognition Action Plasticité Sensorimotrice, Dijon, France
Department of Robotics, Brain and Cognitive Sciences, Istituto Italiano di Tecnologia, Genova, Italy
Université de Bourgogne, UFR STAPS (Sciences du Sport), Dijon, France

Mehdi Ordikhani-Seyedlar, Helge B. D. Sorensen and Sadasivan Puthusserypady
Division of Biomedical Engineering, Department of Electrical Engineering, Technical University of Denmark, Lyngby, Denmark

Mikhail A. Lebedev
Department of Neurobiology, Duke University, Durham, NC, USA
Center for Neuroengineering, Duke University, Durham, NC, USA

Johannes Mallow
Institute for Biometry and Medical Informatics, Medical Faculty, Otto-von-Guericke University, Magdeburg, Germany

Johannes Bernarding
Institute for Biometry and Medical Informatics, Medical Faculty, Otto-von-Guericke University, Magdeburg, Germany
Center for Behavioural Brain Sciences, Otto-von-Guericke University, Magdeburg, Germany

Michael Luchtmann
University Clinic for Neurosurgery, Otto-von-Guericke University, Magdeburg, Germany

Anja Bethmann and André Brechmann
Special-Lab Non-Invasive Brain Imaging, Leibniz Institute for Neurobiology, Magdeburg, Germany

Stefano Vassanelli and Mufti Mahmud
NeuroChip Laboratory, Department of Biomedical Sciences, University of Padova, Padova, Italy

Yang Bai
Department of Automation, Institute of Electrical Engineering, Yanshan University, Qinhuangdao, China,

Xiaoyu Xia
Department of Neurosurgery, PLA Army General Hospital, Beijing, China
Department of Biomedical Engineering, Medical School, Tsinghua University, Beijing, China

Jiannan Kang
Department of Biomedical Engineering, Institute of Electronic Information Engineering, Hebei University, Baoding, China

Xiaoxiao Yin, Yi Yang and Jianghong He
Department of Neurosurgery, PLA Army General Hospital, Beijing, China

Xiaoli Li
State Key Laboratory of Cognitive Neuroscience and Learning & IDG/McGovern Institute for Brain Research, Beijing Normal University, Beijing, China
Center for Collaboration and Innovation in Brain and Learning Sciences, Beijing Normal University, Beijing, China

Stephan Waldert
Sobell Department of Motor Neuroscience and Movement Disorders, University College London Institute of Neurology, University College London, London, UK

Fumihiko Taya, Yu Sun and Anastasios Bezerianos
Centre for Life Sciences, Singapore Institute for Neurotechnology (SINAPSE), National University of Singapore, Singapore, Singapore

Fabio Babiloni
Department of Molecular Medicine, University "Sapienza" of Rome, Rome, Italy

Nitish Thakor
Centre for Life Sciences, Singapore Institute for Neurotechnology (SINAPSE), National University of Singapore, Singapore, Singapore
Department of Electrical and Computer Engineering, National University of Singapore, Singapore, Singapore

Department of Biomedical Engineering, Johns Hopkins University, Baltimore, MD, USA

Sarah Jarvis and Simon R. Schultz
Centre for Neurotechnology and Department of Bioengineering, Imperial College London, London, UK

Ioan Opris
Miami Project, University of Florida, Miami, FL, USA

Mikhail A. Lebedev
Department of Neurobiology, Duke University, Durham, NC, USA

Randall J. Nelson
Department of Anatomy and Neurobiology, The University of Tennessee Health Science Center, Memphis, TN, USA

Leigh E. Charvet and Margaret Kasschau
Department of Neurology, Stony Brook Medicine, Stony Brook, NY, USA

Abhishek Datta
Soterix Medical Inc., NY, USA

Helena Knotkova
MJHS Institute for Innovation in Palliative Care, NY, USA

Michael C. Stevens
Olin Neuropsychiatry Research Center, Yale University School of Medicine, New Haven, CT, USA

Angelo Alonzo and Colleen Loo
School of Psychiatry, University of New South Wales, Black Dog Institute, Randwick, Australia,

Kevin R. Krull
Department of Epidemiology and Cancer Control, St. Jude Children's Research Hospital, Memphis, Tennessee, USA

Marom Bikson
Department of Biomedical Engineering, The City College of New York of CUNY, NY, USA

Shirley Telles, Nilkamal Singh and Acharya Balkrishna
Patanjali Research Foundation, Haridwar, India

Anirban Dutta
INRIA (Sophia Antipolis) - CNRS: UMR5506 - Université Montpellier, Montpellier, France
Laboratoire d'Informatique de Robotique et de Microélectronique de Montpellier (LIRMM), CNRS: UMR5506 - Université Montpellier, Montpellier, France

Iyad Obeid and Joseph Picone
Electrical and Computer Engineering, Temple University, Philadelphia, PA, USA

Antonio G. Zippo and Gabriele E. M. Biella
Institute of Molecular Bioimaging and Physiology, National Research Council, Segrate, Italy

Pantaleo Romanelli
Ab Medica, Lainate, Italy,

Napoleon R. Torres Martinez and Alim L. Benabid
Commissariat à l'Energie Atomique et aux Energies Alternatives, Laboratoire d' Électronique des Technologies de l'Information, CLINATEC, Grenoble, France

Gian C. Caramenti
Institute of Biomedical Technology, Segrate, Italy

K. Zoe Tsagaris
Non-Invasive Brain Stimulation and Human Motor Control Laboratory, Burke Medical Research Institute, White Plains, NY, USA

Douglas R. Labar and Dylan J. Edwards
Non-Invasive Brain Stimulation and Human Motor Control Laboratory, Burke Medical Research Institute, White Plains, NY, USA
Department of Neurology, New York Presbyterian, Weill Cornell Medicine, New York, NY, USA

Evgeniya Lukinova
Skolkovo Institute of Science and Technology, Moscow, Russia,

Mikhail Myagkov
Department of Political Science, University of Oregon, Eugene, OR, USA

Johan Agorelius and Jens Schouenborg
Department of Experimental Medical Science, Neuronano Research Centre, Lund University, Lund, Sweden
The Nanometer Structure Consortium, Lund University, Lund, Sweden

Fotios Tsanakalis, Annika Friberg, Palmi T. Thorbergsson and Lina M. E. Pettersson
Department of Experimental Medical Science, Neuronano Research Centre, Lund University, Lund, Sweden

Katharina M. Kubera, Anja Barth, Dusan Hirjak and Philipp A. Thomann
Center for Psychosocial Medicine, Department of General Psychiatry, University of Heidelberg, Heidelberg, Germany

Robert C. Wolf
Department of Psychiatry, Psychotherapy and Psychosomatics, Saarland University, Homburg, Germany

Manfredo Atzori and Henning Müller
Information Systems Institute, University of Applied Sciences Western Switzerland (HES-SO Valais), Sierre, Switzerland

Marina Garriga
Neurology Unit, Hospital Universitari Mútua Terrassa, Terrassa, Spain
Psychiatric Unit, Hospital Universitari Mútua Terrassa, Terrassa, Spain

Marta Milà, Sonia Huertas, Cesar Castejon, Laura Casas, Dolors Badenes and Miguel Aguilar
Neurology Unit, Hospital Universitari Mútua Terrassa, Terrassa, Spain

Manzoor Mir and Raid Al-Baradie
College of Applied Medical Sciences, Majmaah University Almajmaah, Al Majmaah, Saudi Arabia,

Nuria Giménez and M. Angels Font
Research Unit, Research Foundation Mútua Terrassa, Universitat de Barcelona, Barcelona, Spain

Jose M. Gonzalez and Maria Ysamat
Cetir-Grup Medic, CTD, Hospital Universitari Mútua de Terrassa, Terrassa, Spain

Mark Slevin
School of Healthcare Science, Manchester Metropolitan University, Manchester, UK

Jerzy Krupinski
Neurology Unit, Hospital Universitari Mútua Terrassa, Terrassa, Spain
School of Healthcare Science, Manchester Metropolitan University, Manchester, UK

Amy E. Bouchard, Hélène Corriveau and Marie-Hélène Milot
Centre de Recherche sur le Vieillissement, Université de Sherbrooke, Sherbrooke, QC, Canada

Arantxa Alfaro
CIBER-BBN, Madrid, Spain
Hospital Vega Baja, Orihuela, Spain

Ángela Bernabeu and Carlos Agulló
Department of Magnetic Resonance, INSCANER S.L., Alicante, Spain

Jaime Parra
Hospital San Rafael, Madrid, Spain

Eduardo Fernández
Institute of Bioengineering, Universidad Miguel Hernández, Elche, Spain

Jessica W. Younger and James R. Booth
Department of Communication Sciences and Disorders, Northwestern University, Evanston, IL, USA
Department of Communication Sciences and Disorders, University of Texas at Austin, Austin, TX, USA
Department of Communication Sciences and Disorders, Teachers College, Columbia University, New York, NY, USA

Melissa Randazzo Wagner
Department of Communication Sciences and Disorders, Northwestern University, Evanston, IL, USA
Department of Communication Sciences and Disorders, Teachers College, Columbia University, New York, NY, USA

Erin L. Beatty1, Marie-Eve Jobidon, Fethi Bouak, Ann Nakashima, IngridSmith, Quan Lam, Kristen Blackler and Bob Cheung
Defence Research and Development Canada - Toronto Research Centre, Toronto, ON, Canada

Oshin Vartanian
Defence Research and Development Canada - Toronto Research Centre, Toronto, ON, Canada
Department of Psychology, University of Toronto Scarborough, Toronto, ON, Canada

Florian Grimm, Georgios Naros and Alireza Gharabaghi
Division of Functional and Restorative Neurosurgery and Centre for Integrative Neuroscience, Eberhard Karls University, Tuebingen, Germany

Anneli Wall, Jörgen Borg and Susanne Palmcrantz
Department of Rehabilitation Medicine, Danderyd University Hospital, Stockholm, Sweden
Department of Clinical Sciences, Karolinska Institute, Stockholm, Sweden

Index

www.ingramcontent.com/pod-product-compliance
Lightning Source LLC
LaVergne TN
LVHW080925210926
848485LV00004B/734
* 9 7 8 1 6 3 9 8 9 0 8 7 3 *

Frailty and Sarcopenia: Current Issues and Research

Frailty and Sarcopenia: Current Issues and Research

Edited by Kylen Mitchell

STATES
ACADEMIC PRESS
www.statesacademicpress.com

States Academic Press,
109 South 5th Street,
Brooklyn, NY 11249, USA

Visit us on the World Wide Web at:
www.statesacademicpress.com

ISBN: 978-1-63989-219-8

Cataloging-in-Publication Data

Frailty and sarcopenia : current issues and research / edited by Kylen Mitchell.
p. cm.
Includes bibliographical references and index.
ISBN 978-1-63989-219-8
1. Musculoskeletal system--Diseases. 2. Musculoskeletal system--Abnormalities.
3. Musculoskeletal system--Wounds and injuries. I. Mitchell, Kylen.

RC925 .F73 2022
616.74--dc23

Table of Contents

Preface

This book has been an outcome of determined endeavour from a group of educationists in the field. The primary objective was to involve a broad spectrum of professionals from diverse cultural background involved in the field for developing new researches. The book not only targets students but also scholars pursuing higher research for further enhancement of the theoretical and practical applications of the subject.

Frailty is a clinically recognizable syndrome associated with aging and an increased risk of catastrophic decline in the health of elderly people. Muscles start degenerating with age which results in weakness, decreased energy, slowing, lower activity and severe unintended weight loss. Sarcopenia can be a cause of frailty. It is the degenerative loss of skeletal muscle strength, quality and mass with age. The rate of muscle loss depends on several factors such as nutrition, exercise level and co-morbidities. Sarcopenia leads to reduced functional status and can cause significant disability from increased weakness. Muscle loss within this disease occurs due to changes in muscle synthesis signaling pathways. This book provides significant information of this discipline to help develop a good understanding of frailty and sarcopenia. Also included herein is a detailed explanation of the current issues and research on these medical conditions. This book is appropriate for students seeking detailed information in this area as well as for experts.

It was an honour to edit such a profound book and also a challenging task to compile and examine all the relevant data for accuracy and originality. I wish to acknowledge the efforts of the contributors for submitting such brilliant and diverse chapters in the field and for endlessly working for the completion of the book. Last, but not the least; I thank my family for being a constant source of support in all my research endeavours.

Editor

1

Epidemiology of Sarcopenia and Frailty

Harnish P Patel, Esther Clift, Lucy Lewis and
Cyrus Cooper

Abstract

Sarcopenia and frailty are common in older persons and pose particular challenges for health and social care systems especially in the context of global population ageing. Sarcopenia, the loss of skeletal muscle mass, strength and function with age is associated with adverse individual physical and metabolic changes contributing to morbidity and mortality. The health and socioeconomic implications of sarcopenia are also considerable. Sarcopenia is a core component of physical frailty that together impact negatively on an individual's capability to live independently. Frailty is a biological syndrome of low reserve and resistance to stressors resulting from cumulative declines across multiple physiological systems that collectively predispose an individual to adverse outcomes. Frailty develops along a continuum from independence through to death as physiological reserves progressively diminish an individual's capacity to recover from an acute insult or illness. Managing sarcopenia and frailty involves the multidisciplinary led completion of a comprehensive care plan that is patient centred, responsive to the needs of the patient and adaptable therefore enabling an individual to maintain their independence.

Keywords: Sarcopenia, frail, epidemiology, Comprehensive Geriatric Assessment

1. Introduction

Over the past two centuries, there has been a demographic transformation across the world and people are living longer [1]. For the first time in history, people can expect to live beyond their 60th birthday. In fact, survival to age 80 is anticipated to be the norm for all of today's young people. People aged 60 or over are set to increase from 841 million to more than 2 billion between 2013 and 2050. This equates to 21.1% of the world's population [1]. Globally, the number of people aged 80 years or over, the "oldest-old", is growing even faster. In 2000, there were 71 million people aged 80 or over worldwide. Since then, the number of oldest-old has grown by 77% to 125 million in 2015, and it is projected to increase by 61% over the next 15 years, reaching nearly 202 million in 2030. Projections indicate that in 2050 the oldest-old will number 434 million globally, having more than tripled in number since 2015 [2]. These demographic changes are largely due to the advances in public health and modern medicine that have reduced early life mortality, reduced the rate of infectious diseases [3] and have allowed people to live with one or more long-term conditions. Whilst this is a cause for celebration, these cumulative changes pose significant challenges for delivering health and social care to older people in all nations concerned.

The situation within the UK is no different. Medical and technological advances in the treatment of illnesses and diseases have improved mortality rates in the oldest age groups. In 2013–2015, a UK male aged 85 could expect to live to age 90.8 years and a female to 91.8 years. Life expectancy at birth has increased throughout England, Scotland, Wales and Northern Ireland due to improvements in mortality in older age. Life expectancy is highest in England with Scotland having the lowest of the four UK constituent countries (Office of National Statistics 2016, *ONS.gov.uk*).

However, numerous people who are living longer in the UK do so with one or more long-term medical conditions and many are living with frailty. The clinical conditions of sarcopenia and frailty are particularly complex expressions of ageing that impact a range of health and social care settings [4, 5]. Sarcopenia is associated with adverse individual physical and metabolic changes contributing to morbidity and mortality, whilst frailty is defined as a state of increased vulnerability as a consequence of cumulative physiological decline across multiple systems predisposing to poor resolution of homeostasis after a stressor event, which increases the risk of adverse outcomes [4, 6]. In this chapter, we will review the epidemiology, pathogenesis, diagnosis of sarcopenia and frailty as well as give an overview of Comprehensive Geriatric Assessment (CGA) as a method of systematically evaluating an older person's treatment, management and long-term follow-up needs.

2. Skeletal muscle and sarcopenia

Skeletal muscle comprises approximately 40% of total body mass and therefore constitutes one of the largest organ systems of the body [7]. Skeletal muscle plays an essential role in both physical, for example, locomotion and metabolic functioning, for example, thermoregulation, metabolism of glucose and amino acids. Muscle is also a reservoir for proteins and energy that can be utilised in periods of stress or undernutrition, for example, acute deterioration in health and hospitalisation.

2.1. Diagnosing sarcopenia

Sarcopenia has previously been defined based solely on lean mass as a function of height (appendicular lean mass [ALM] is measured by dual-energy X-ray absorptiometry [DXA] divided by height squared) where sarcopenia was diagnosed −1 to −2 SD below gender-specific mean values of a younger control group [8]. However, direct proportionality between loss of muscle mass and impaired strength/function cannot be inferred as longitudinal as well as cross-sectional studies show that younger individuals can be stronger and older individuals are weaker than would be predicted by their muscle mass [9, 10]. Therefore muscle quality or force generated per unit area is important and the definition of sarcopenia now extends to encompass loss of strength and or physical performance [6, 10]. Sarcopenia, is the progressive and generalised loss of skeletal muscle mass, strength and physical performance with age and as such it is a core component of physical frailty [6, 11, 12]. Sarcopenia is associated with a broad array of adverse physical and metabolic outcomes including falls [13], disability, hospitalisation, diabetes [14], osteoporosis [15] and also mortality [16]. The economic costs associated with 'sarcopenia' in the year 2000 were estimated to be $18.5 billion in the USA alone [17].

Recent diagnostic algorithms include those proposed by EWGSOP [6], The International working group (IWG) on sarcopenia [18], The Foundation for the National Health Institutes of Health (FNIH) Sarcopenia Project [11] and the Asian Working Group for Sarcopenia (AWGS) [19]; the later driven by the need to account for ethnic variations in body composition and muscle function in order to further research sarcopenia in the Asian subcontinent.

The EWGSOP definition requires the presence of slower walk speed (<0.8 m/s) [20] or weaker strength (grip <30 kg for men, <20 kg for women) [21] in combination with low muscle mass (defined as ALM/ht^2 ≤7.23 kg/m^2 for men and ≤5.67 kg/m^2 for women). The International Working Group (IWG) on sarcopenia included impaired physical performance in addition to slow walk speed before measuring muscle mass in their working definition for the diagnosis of sarcopenia. The Foundations of National Institutes of Health (FNIH) sarcopenia project based in the USA incorporated clinically relevant cut points of low muscle mass and strength (grip strength <26 kg for men and <16 kg for women and ALM adjusted for BMI <0.789 for men and <0.512 for women) [11]. Similarly, the AWGS included gait speed <0.8 mm/s, ALM/ht^2 <7.0 m^2 in men and <5.4 kg/m^2 in women and grip strength <26 kg for men and <18 kg in women [19] in their working definition of sarcopenia. From a clinical point of view, these algorithms enable case finding for sarcopenia and conceptually identify stages of sarcopenia that allow intervention. For example, the pre-sarcopenia stage is characteristic of low muscle mass without impact on muscle strength or physical performance, the sarcopenia stage is characterised by low muscle mass, low muscle strength or poorer physical performance, whilst severe sarcopenia is when all three criteria within the algorithm are met [6].

2.2. Prevalence of sarcopenia

The prevalence of sarcopenia increases with age but figures are influenced by the diagnostic algorithm used, ethnic population studied, cut-off values for lean mass and function and the health care setting, that is, community versus in hospital [22]. For example, a recent systematic review reported that the prevalence rates differed for community-dwelling older people aged ≥60 years (up to 29%), in long-term care age >70 years (up to 33%) and in an acute care hospitals, age ≥ 65 years (up to 10%) [23].

2.3. Measuring muscle mass

The commonest approach to measuring muscle mass is through bioimpedance analysis (BIA) and where available, dual-energy X-ray absorptiometry (DXA) scanning. Computerised tomography (CT) and magnetic resonance imaging (MRI) can also be used [24]. The approach that is undertaken to measure muscle mass is dependent on feasibility, access, costs and sample size. For example, BIA utilises portable equipment and can be used across a range of health care settings and calculates fat-free mass rather than true muscle mass based on the electrical conductivity of various body tissues. Whole body DXA will enable the calculation of total and appendicular lean mass but may overestimate lean mass values in those with extracellular fluid accumulation. Computerised tomography (CT) and magnetic resonance imaging (MRI) can differentiate fat from muscle, which can be useful to make assumptions on muscle quality. However, high operational costs and radiation, in the case for CT, limits their use in the diagnosis of sarcopenia.

2.4. Measuring muscle strength

Grip strength measured using hand-held dynamometry, has gained wide acceptance as a reliable and valid measure of muscle strength across health care settings and is an integral component in the international diagnostic algorithms for sarcopenia [25–27]. Other methods to measure muscle 'strength' include ascertainment of knee extensor power, isometric knee strength and quadriceps torque but these require static and bulky equipment that are not readily portable and can be impractical in routine clinical practice as well as in epidemiological studies.

2.5. Measuring physical performance

Slower gait speed is associated with risk of future morbidity and mortality and is therefore suitable for inclusion in diagnostic algorithms for sarcopenia [28]. Other objectively measured physical performance measures such as chair rise time; time taken to complete five sit to stand actions and standing balance; and the time for sustaining balance on one leg have also been associated with higher risk of all-cause mortality in older people [16, 29]. Gait speed requires intact coordination, neural and joint control so may not be practical in context of acutely unwell hospitalised older people. Grip strength measurements in this situation may have better predictive value and be more feasible [25–27, 30].

2.6. Questionnaires to aid the diagnosis of sarcopenia

The SARC-F questionnaire was developed to predict poor muscle function [31, 32] and is based on five questions that ascertain how much difficulty an individual has performing the following parameters: ability to rise from a chair, walk assisted or unassisted, climb stairs, carry heavy loads (as a measure of strength) and ascertainment on the number of falls a person has had in the last year.

Each parameter is assigned a score: 0 (none); 1(some) or 2 (a lot); the falls parameter (none = 0, 1–3 = 1, 4 or more = 2). A total score of ≥4 (scale 0–10) suggests that the subject is symptomatic of sarcopenia. The SARC-F questionnaire has been shown to have excellent specificity but poor sensitivity for sarcopenia based on the consensus criteria from the IWG, EWGSOP and AWG. However, it has been shown to predict physical limitation over a four-year follow-up and may be useful for case identification and subsequent diagnostic evaluation for sarcopenia in community based but not hospital or care home-based settings [33].

Despite the recent progress in refining and implementing diagnostic criteria for sarcopenia over the past decade, there is no consensus on global diagnostic criteria for sarcopenia based on cut-off values for skeletal muscle mass indices, grip strength and walking speed. In fact, the variance in the criteria indicate that ethnic, gender and cultural differences dictate population-specific criteria are required in order to account for the genome/environment interactions that contribute to sarcopenia, thus influencing the design of both observational and intervention studies [24, 34].

2.7. Pathogenesis of sarcopenia

In sarcopenic muscle, the rate of muscle injury (from normal contraction) exceeds that of repair and regeneration. There may also be decreased satellite cell (muscle stem cell), proliferative capability and renewal [35, 36] in combination with altered inter- and intracellular environments that favour catabolism. This increase in catabolism is associated with a decrease in growth factors such as circulating insulin, growth hormone and testosterone and muscle-specific IGF-1 levels [37]. Furthermore, the production of reactive oxygen species and oxidative stress can lead to mitochondrial DNA damage and a progressive decline in mitochondrial function and energy depletion [38]. At a tissue level, skeletal muscle is continuously remodelled in response to workload, tension, nutrition and anabolic stimulation. The cues associated with the age-related decline in muscle mass and strength include behavioural (i.e. decrease in physical activity/sedentary lifestyle), extrinsic (i.e. undernutrition) and intrinsic factors (i.e. hormonal changes, inflammation, oxidative stress and denervation) [39] (**Figure 1**).

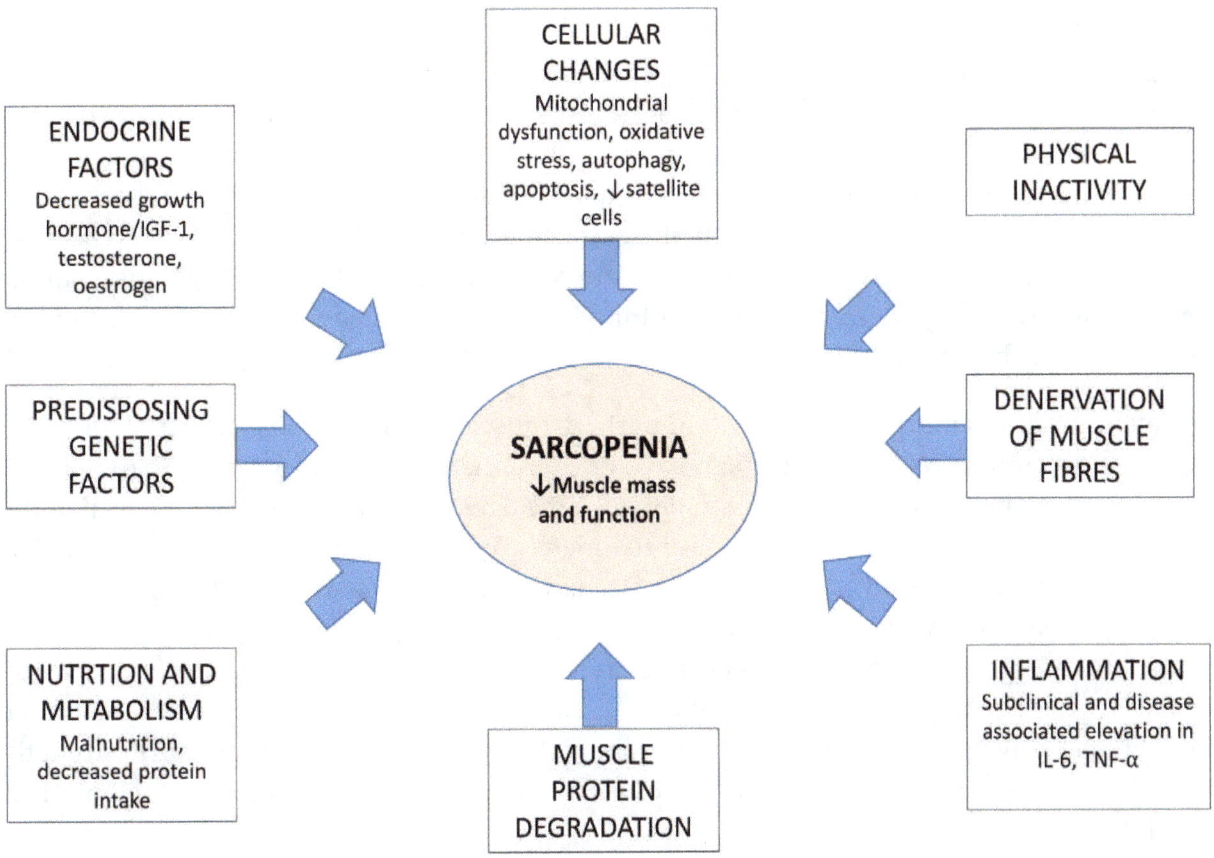

Figure 1. The main mechanisms involved in the aetiology of sarcopenia.

The complex dynamic genome/environment interplay involved in the balancing of muscle synthesis and breakdown is mediated through multiple cell signalling pathways [40] that include IGF-1/AKT/mTOR and NF-κB (nuclear factor-kB). These pathways influence the balance between synthesis and degradation. For example, the IGF-I/AKT/mTOR pathways promote protein synthesis and the maintenance of skeletal muscle mass. By contrast, the activation of NF-kB by inflammatory mediators including tumour necrosis factor (TNF) and interleukin 6 (IL-6) upregulate the E3 ubiquitin ligases MAFbx (atrogin-1) and MURF-1, which signal the muscle atrophic process. Skeletal muscle ageing is also characterised by a continuous cycle of denervation and reinnervation as a consequence of the loss of alpha-motor neurones within the central nervous system (CNS), withdrawal of nerve terminals from the neuromuscular junctions (NMJ) and axonal sprouting from neighbouring neurons collectively giving rise to larger, inefficient motor units.

Remodelling of skeletal muscle tissue through neuropathic, neurohormonal and inflammatory pathways leads to a reduction in muscle cross-sectional area, volume and a reduced rate of force generation. This is characterised by the presence of fewer type I oxidative (slow twitch) and type II glycolytic (fast twitch) myofibres as well as myofibre atrophy. The loss of type II fibres, with concomitant decrease in satellite cells [41], is associated with decreased strength and ability to generate power. Moreover, there is a concurrent increase in non-contractile material within the fascicles that affects muscle quality. Collectively, these processes lead to the reduced muscle functional performance.

2.8. A life course approach to understand the aetiology of sarcopenia

Muscle development in humans begins at 6 weeks of gestation and continues until approximately 24 weeks when the total number of fibres is set. Any subsequent increase in muscle bulk occurs by hypertrophy as evidenced by an increase in fibre cross-sectional area, and not by hyperplasia. Therefore, the number of muscle fibres formed prenatally influences the potential for postnatal hypertrophy [42]. Muscle mass increases during childhood and adolescence until adult muscle cross-sectional areas are reached shortly after puberty. Muscle mass then remains relatively constant in early adulthood until the later part of the 4th decade of life when a decline begins [43].

Skeletal muscle strength is determined, in part, by muscle mass, which is a function of myofibre size and number. On average, men have greater muscle mass and strength than women at any given point in the life course [44]. Between the ages of 20 and 80 years, total lean body mass has been reported to decline by approximately 18% in males and by 27% in females [45]. Therefore, the 'health' of skeletal muscle in an older person is a function of the peak levels attained in early life and the extrinsic and intrinsic changes operating through middle years into old age, for example, physical activity, nutrition, disease and disuse and hormonal changes. There is also robust epidemiological evidence suggesting that low birth weight, a marker of an adverse early intrauterine environment, is associated with a poorer grip strength in older adults and that the mechanism may be driven by myofibre development and number [46, 47].

3. Frailty

Frailty is a common clinical syndrome, which is often seen in older adults, especially in women compared to men and younger aged adults [48–50]. Frailty is distinct from disability and comorbidity and independently carries a high risk for poor health outcomes such as falls, hospitalisation, disability and mortality [51, 52]. Whilst, sarcopenia contributes to and is a core component of physical frailty, the syndrome of frailty is comprised of several interlinked domains that impact on an older person's independence, quality of life and medium- to long-term outcomes. Cognitive frailty refers to progressive cognitive decline in absence of a diagnosis of dementia, social frailty refers to loneliness and the lack of robust social networks as well as poor income whilst psychological frailty refers to the inherent traits in an individual that may predispose an individual to adversity, for example, bereavement, low mood, lack of motivation and labile emotions [53, 54]. Multimorbidity, defined by the UK National Institute for Health and Care Excellence (NICE, guidance 56), is the presence of two or more distinct long-term conditions, is also associated with a higher risk of developing frailty [54, 55]. This conceptual model illustrates that assessing and managing a patient who is living with frailty requires a more holistic approach to manage the cause, or combination of causes that have precipitated acute decompensation [5] (**Figure 2**).

Frailty is best understood as a multisystem disorder, with perhaps both independent and linked mechanisms operating across organ or physiological systems. Accumulating dysregulation across multiple systems can negatively affect previous normal functional homeostatic mechanisms accelerating the development and progression of frailty. This is relevant not only for improved understanding of this syndrome but also because a key implication of loss of reserve across multiple systems is that therapeutic intervention of any single system, that is, endocrine, brain, immune/inflammatory or indeed an individual domain, that is, social, physical or cognitive, is unlikely to ameliorate the abnormal health state of frailty. For those living with frailty, even a minor insult such as a minor infection or change in medication can lead to a large disproportionate change in an individual's health and social care state that inevitably results in an acute hospital admission (**Figure 2**).

Older people living with frailty do so as a consequence of accelerated loss of biological reserves across multiple systems over a lifetime and individuals experience frequent transitions between frailty states over time. Using the life course approach to conceptualise frailty is worth considering as this broadens the window of opportunity to identify markers and mechanisms contributing to frailty with a view to intervention [56] (**Figure 2**). For example, the presence of weight loss or weakness earlier in the life course, that is, slow walk speed and exhaustion may identify people at especially high risk of rapid decline [57].

3.1. Identification of frailty

Detection of frailty should be an essential part of assessment of older people and the identification of reliable tools to determine frailty within acute and community settings is currently a research and clinical priority. Recognising and identifying people who are living with frailty not only enables clinicians and health care professionals to respond quickly and

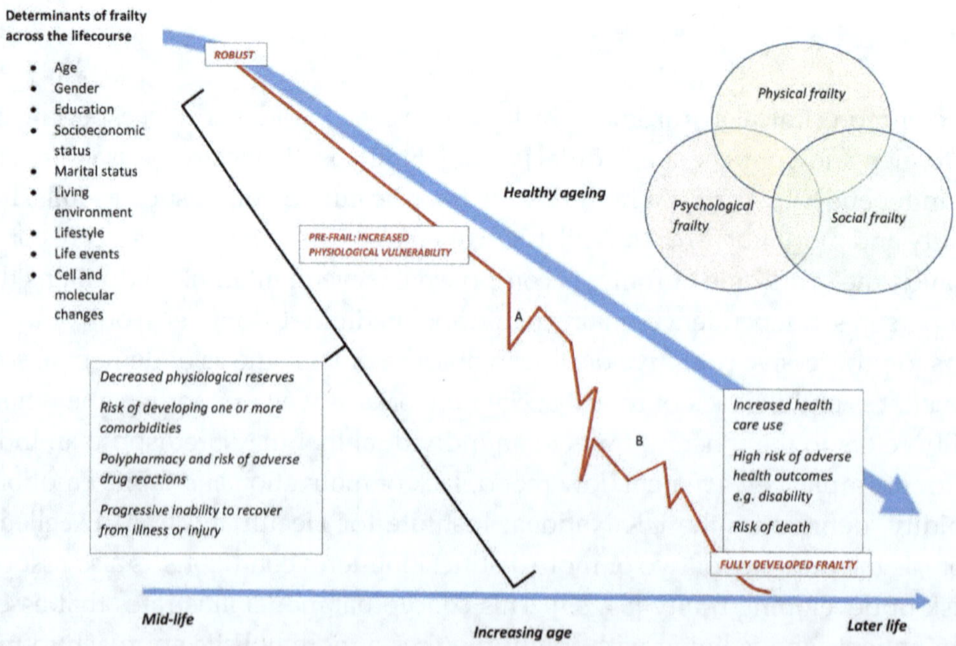

Figure 2. Healthy ageing is depicted by the blue solid line. Frailty (red line) develops as a continuum from being physiologically robust and independent to being at high risk of hospitalisation, institutionalisation and death. In more physiologically robust individuals, full recovery is likely after an insult, for example, infection (A), but later in the time course, moderate to severe frailty predisposes to recurrent hospital admissions as a consequence of a disproportionate deterioration in health and social and/or psychological health from a relatively minor insult or stress (B). The recovery from subsequent insults takes longer as physiological reserves are depleted until the individual cannot compensate adequately, and the ability to perform daily activities diminishes leading to dependency and disability.

appropriately to minimise exposures that may not be beneficial or could be harmful, that is, polypharmacy, invasive investigations, but also anticipate and prevent functional decline and potentially reverse the state of frailty with appropriate interventions.

The two established international models of frailty are the phenotype model and the cumulative deficit model. The phenotype model developed by Fried identifies frailty by the presence of at least three of five physical characteristics: weight loss, exhaustion, low energy expenditure, slow walking speed and low handgrip strength [51]. The cumulative deficit model developed by Rockwood et al. identifies frailty on the basis of the accumulation of a range of 'deficits', which can be symptoms, sensory deficits, clinical signs, diseases, disabilities and abnormal laboratory test results that then allow an index to be calculated. The frailty index is a function of the number of deficits present in an individual divided by the total number of deficits possible within the population sample [58]. The number of deficits measures accumulated vulnerability, which is related to adverse outcomes. In this regard, a frailty index will range from 0 to 1, with values over 0.67 identifying a level of frailty beyond which accumulation of further deficits is not sustainable with life [59]. Despite the difference in approaches to measuring frailty, both tools are able to predict adverse outcome, which provides support for the notion of frailty as a unified construct [60]. In clinical practice, identification of frailty using the Clinical Frailty Scale (CFS), a visual tool based on a comprehensive clinical assessment of a patient, enables assignment of a frailty category [58]. There are seven CFS categories ranging from 1 (fit) to 7 (severe frailty) and increasing CFS frailty has been demonstrated to have predictive validity for adverse outcomes of institutionalisation and mortality. In outpatient settings, The PRISMA-7 questionnaire, can be used to identify persons who are living with frailty and disability. These questions are:

1. Are you more than 85 years? Yes = 1 point
2. Male? Yes = 1 point
3. In general, do you have any health problems that require you to limit your activities? Yes = 1 point
4. Do you need someone to help you on a regular basis? Yes = 1 point
5. In general, do you have any health problems that require you to stay at home? Yes = 1 point
6. In case of need, can you count on someone close to you? No = 1 point
7. Do you regularly use a stick, walker or wheelchair to get about? Yes = 1 point

A score of > 3 can be used to identify frailty.

A further important concept of frailty as a syndrome is that individuals may have previously unrecognised and inadequately addressed conditions that do not characteristically fall into a single organ category but can have a major impact on quality of life. Identification of these 'frailty syndromes' can help health care professionals manage and potentially delay their complications. These, often inter-related syndromes, include but are not limited to falls, delirium, weight loss and malnutrition, fluctuating disability, polypharmacy, social isolation, fragility fracture(s) and recurrent hospital admissions (**Figure 3**).

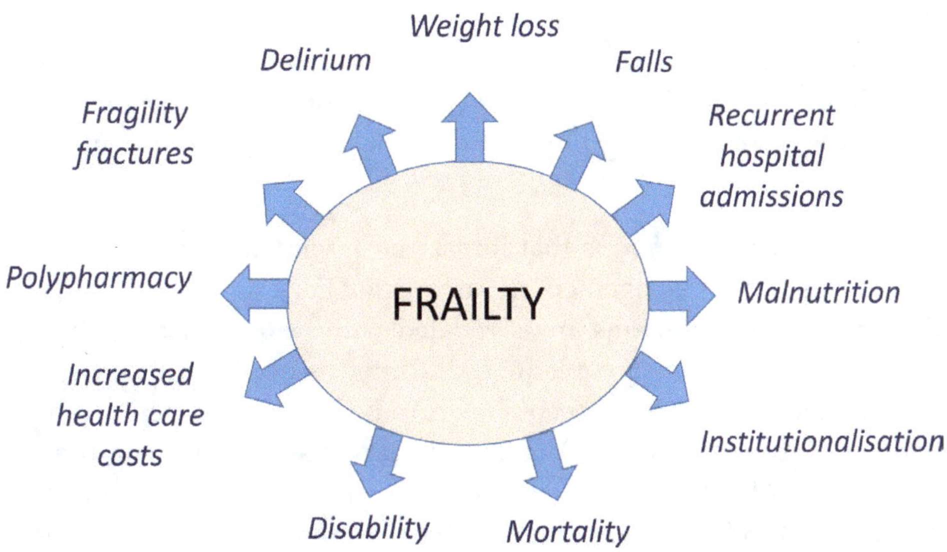

Figure 3. Consequences of living with frailty.

3.2. Prevalence of frailty

Given poor outcomes relating to morbidity, mortality and disability, it is useful to understand the prevalence of frailty to inform the provision of appropriate health and social care interventions. Prevalence figures have been well documented in many OECD (Convention of the Organisation for Economic Cooperation and Development) countries such a USA, Canada, Netherlands and the UK but data on relative incidence in developing countries is sparse [49]. Prevalence estimates based on 21 cohorts of 61,500 community-dwelling older adults across mainly developed countries estimated frailty prevalence between 4 and 59% and varied according to the operational definitions, for example, the physical phenotype versus frailty index-based models. However, there was general agreement that frailty increases with age and is higher in women than in men. In populations aged 80–84, the pooled prevalence rate was reported to be 15.7% whilst in those over 85 the prevalence increased to 26% [49]. This figure may be substantially higher in institutionalised older people. In an analysis of the Study on health, Ageing and Retirement in Europe, SHARE (n = 18,566) and Study on global AGEing and adult health, SAGE (n = 161,542), two large international data sets of adults over 50 years in which a frailty index was calculated, more women were classed as frail and frailty as a syndrome was distributed along the socioeconomic gradient amongst both higher and lower income countries such that individuals with less education and monetary income were more likely to be frail [48]. Recently, a study of 5450 older people aged 60 and over participating in the English Longitudinal Study of Ageing (ELSA) reported that the prevalence of frailty using the physical frailty phenotype rose from 6.5% in those aged 60–69 to 65% in those over the age of 90, with frail individuals reporting decreased physical function and difficulties in performing activities of daily living [50].

3.3. Interventions for individuals living with sarcopenia and frailty

A multi-dimensional approach to managing sarcopenia and indeed frailty involves promoting physical activity, optimising nutrition/prevention of malnutrition, minimising polypharmacy and attending to and individual's social and psychological aspects of health, that is, care support and home adaptations. Management goals for an older person with sarcopenia or frailty revolve around improving physical function and maintaining independence and well-being.

Exercise and nutritional interventions that impact positively on muscle mass and function play a significant role in the management of sarcopenia. For example, combination physical activity and nutritional interventions are associated with better function, strength and less inflammation in older sarcopenic people [61, 62]. In terms of physical activity, progressive resistance and aerobic exercise have been shown to be the most beneficial for the prevention and 'treatment' of sarcopenia [23, 63–65]. Whilst progressive resistance exercise improves lean mass, strength and function [66], optimising exercise capacity through aerobic activity improves metabolic control, reduces oxidative stress, insulin sensitivity and can stimulate a hypertrophic response on muscle fibres. Despite being shown to be safe and effective in older people [63, 67, 68], implementing progressive exercise in clinical practice is not always readily achievable.

Falls are serious and sometimes fatal complications of sarcopenia. In this regard, a multi-component approach that addresses balance and gait, flexibility and endurance, lower limb strengthening exercises is required to manage fallers. Such approaches are associated with improved reaction time, gait, balance, strength coordination and physical and cognitive function [69, 70]. Group and home-based exercise programmes, which incorporate safety interventions, may reduce the rate and risk of falling [71]. Moreover, targeted home-based or group-based exercise interventions can also improve mobility and functional outcomes for older people with frailty [72, 73].

Intervening earlier in the life course before the onset of sarcopenia may have immense benefits for later skeletal muscle health. For example, increased levels of leisure time physical activity in mid-life were associated with stronger grip strength in both men and women at age 60–64. This is consistent with optimising peak strength earlier in the life course, therefore reducing the impact of sarcopenia. Therefore, regular physical activity in adolescence and adulthood may prevent steep decline in muscle strength in early old age [74].

The synthesis of muscle fibres requires adequate protein substrates. Physiological changes in the gastrointestinal system occur with age and result in older people eating less, having early satiety, losing their sense of taste and having a blunted anabolic response to ingested proteins [75]. As such, older people may require more protein to counteract the inflammatory and catabolic effects of co-existent co morbidities and their exacerbations [76]. Protein supplements vary in their composition and evidence from trials at present is inconstant to develop evidence-based recommendations for protein supplementation in sarcopenia [77]. However, observational evidence suggests essential amino acids, that is, leucine, beta-hydroxy-beta-methylbutyrate (HMB), a bioactive metabolite of leucine, stimulates muscle protein synthesis more than non-essential amino acids and may be useful for maintain lean body mass and improving muscle function [78–82]. A recent consensus statement from the multinational PROT-AGE group recommends protein intake in older people of at least 1.2–1.5 g of protein per body weight (kg) a day to maintain muscle homeostatsis [83]. Nutritional interventions in sarcopenia are covered in more detail elsewhere in this book.

3.4. Possible targets for pharmacological treatment

Observational studies indicate the potential beneficial effects of testosterone on muscle mass and function given the associated anabolic and satellite cell stimulatory activity. Randomised controlled trials of testosterone have not demonstrated benefits on muscle function because of adverse cardiovascular outcomes [34]. Studies of growth hormone (GH) supplementation have shown more harm than benefit in older patients; whilst GH therapy may increase muscle mass, it has not always increased muscle strength or functional performance. Moreover, unwanted side effects precludes GH as a treatment for sarcopenia. These include arthralgia, paraesthesia, fatigue, carpal tunnel syndrome and mortality in some observational human studies [84, 85].

There has been interest in selective androgen receptor modulators (SARMS) for sarcopenia treatment, which stems from the observed anabolic effect of testosterone. SARMS are androgen receptor ligands that display selective activation of androgen signalling in target tissues, for example, skeletal muscle. However, none are in clinical use and trials will be needed on the safety and efficacy of SARMS in improving physical function in older people with sarcopenia [34, 86].

Myostatin, a member of the TGF-β superfamily, is a negative regulator of skeletal muscle growth and is upregulated in many muscle wasting disorders [87]. Based on these observations, myostatin and its receptor activin type IIb pose attractive targets for therapeutic intervention. Though there are currently no anti-myostatin drugs used in clinical practice, myostatin receptor antibodies are currently under review with the focus on older people with lower lean mass [34].

Angiotensin-converting enzyme inhibitor (ACEi), for example, perindopril, use was associated with improvement in 6-m walk tests in older persons with functional impairment but did not show increased benefit with additional exercise training. Whilst ACEi use may have beneficial effects on muscle function [88], a recent meta-analysis of four trials concluded that ACEi did not improve walk distance or age-related strength decline in older people therefore, further evidence from clinical trials are needed [89].

3.5. Comprehensive Geriatric Assessment (CGA)

Frailty is a dynamic process that predisposes an individual to a spiral of decline that leads to increasing frailty and risk of worsening disability, predisposition to falls, hospital as well as care home admission and death [51, 58]. Although current screening for frailty identifies individuals at risk, validated tools do not recommend intervention. It is imperative that when managing frailty, assessments should not only seek to determine and treat specific illnesses, but that they should endeavour to maintain and where possible, improve quality of life. It is clear that older person's needs are more complex and that they often have co-existent functional, psychological and social needs. This predisposes an individual to atypical clinical presentations that can often be misunderstood and which often require a different approach to care that diverts away from an organ specific diagnosis towards a holistic and integrated view of their problems.

Older people and their caregivers should purposefully be involved in making informed decisions relating to health and social care needs as well as advanced care planning. A useful method for planning the care of those living with moderate to severe frailty through a process of assessment, summation, conversation, planning, intervention, monitoring and review is Comprehensive Geriatric Assessment (CGA). CGA is a process, which is patient centred, responsive, adaptable and most effective when disseminated amongst key professionals working across the acute and community sectors. CGA is defined as a *'multidimensional interdisciplinary diagnostic process focused on determining a frail older person's medical, psychological and functional capability in order to develop a coordinated and integrated plan for treatment and long term follow up'* [90].

The purpose of CGA is to improve diagnostic accuracy, optimise treatment and outcomes and crucially, allow effective integrated case management to ensure that the care plan is enacted and remains responsive to the patient's needs over time. CGA requires the systematic evaluation of physical, functional, medical, nutritional, cognitive and social components that influences an older person's health that can also extend to financial, spiritual, psychological and palliative needs (**Figure 4**). How CGA is delivered is variable and very much depends on the care setting, for example, home, hospital, clinic or nursing home but, to be effective, often requires coordination of several inter-professional services that can include clinicians, community nursing, therapy, social services, pharmacy, nutrition and dietetics, optometry and audiology. There are no set universal criteria to identify patients in need for a CGA however, patients who are 'too well' or are 'too sick' are less likely to derive benefit from the process. CGA becomes important for patients who are identified as living with frailty through the use of validated instruments or have one or more of the 'frailty syndromes' previously mentioned. There is evidence from multiple meta-analyses that CGA delivered to patients within the hospital setting as well as in the community is associated with better function and cognition, decrease in mortality, less likelihood of being institutionalised, less likelihood of patients experiencing deterioration in their health [90–93].

A critical component of CGA is a medication review and the STOPP/START approach to polypharmacy is a useful evidence-based tool [94]. The well-being components of the CGA may include the promotion of regular physical activity and exercise delivered through home-based plans [95] or external activity classes, social engagement through day centres and community networks, adaptations to the home environment to assist with falls prevention, caregiver support and nutritional optimisation. By undertaking a CGA with the person and those closest to them, if they wish, individuals are able to identify their own personal goals therefore reclaiming some of the lost independence they may have encountered as a result of living with frailty. Equally, the process will enable appropriate advanced care planning discussions for individuals with severe frailty in conjunction with palliative care support for those who may be entering the terminal phase of their life.

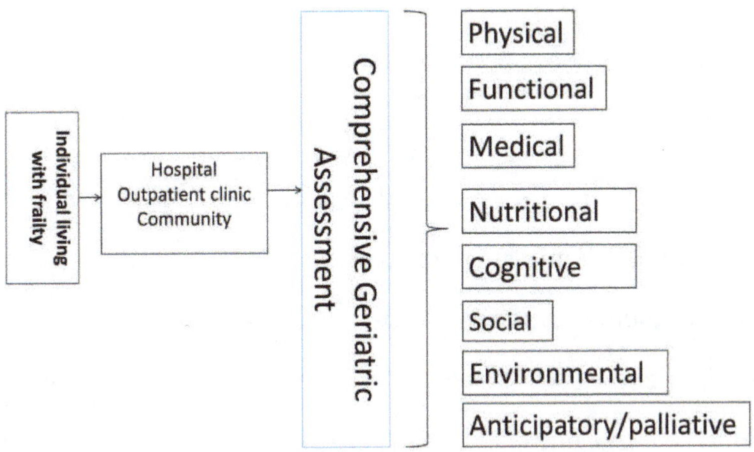

Figure 4. Core components of an inter-professional Comprehensive Geriatric Assessment. The process involves data gathering, multidisciplinary team discussions, development of the plan with the patient and their caregiver, implementation, monitoring and revision of the plan so that it remains responsive to the needs of the patient.

4. Conclusions

Sarcopenia and frailty are inter-related conditions that are common in older age and identify people who have an increased risk of a range of adverse outcomes. Sarcopenia has a complex aetiology involving neurohormonal, immunological and nutritional mechanisms. Frailty is a multisystem disorder, which commonly includes sarcopenia as a core component. Whilst there are clear physiological and pathophysiological explanations for the development and definition of frailty, there is need to understand that frailty as a term can be perceived as a state of dependency, subjugation or defeat; the appearance of being weak in later life. Not all older people are frail. These connotations and negative perceptions need to be challenged through education and training.

There is robust evidence to support the implementation of exercise and activity programmes for older people with sarcopenia and frailty, and that the adverse health trajectories of frailty may be modified through a range of interventions through the process of Comprehensive Geriatric Assessment. Better identification of sarcopenia and frailty in older age enables pro-active targeting of interventions to improve outcomes and modify future health trajectories that benefit older people as well as their caregivers.

Acknowledgements

This work was supported by the NIHR Southampton Biomedical Research Centre, Nutrition, the MRC Lifecourse Epidemiology Unit and the University of Southampton. This report is independent research by the NIHR BRC Funding Scheme. The views expressed in this publication are those of the authors and not necessarily those of the NHS, the NIHR or the Department of Health. HPP is supported by the NIHR Southampton Biomedical Research Centre Nutrition, EC and LL are supported by Health Education England Wessex Consultant Practitioner Trainee scheme. All authors declare they have no conflict of interest.

Author details

Harnish P Patel[1,2,3,4*], Esther Clift[5], Lucy Lewis[5] and Cyrus Cooper[4,6]

*Address all correspondence to: hp@mrc.soton.ac.uk

1 Academic Geriatric Medicine, University Hospital Southampton, UK

2 Department of Medicine for Older People, University Hospital Southampton, UK

3 NIHR Biomedical Research Centre, Southampton, UK

4 MRC Lifecourse Epidemiology Unit, University of Southampton, Southampton, UK

5 Health Education England, Wessex, UK

6 University of Oxford, Oxford, UK

References

[1] Chatterji S, Byles J, Cutler D, Seeman T, Verdes E. Health, functioning, and disability in older adults—present status and future implications. Lancet. 2015;**385**(9967):563-575. DOI: 10.1016/s0140-6736(14)61462-8

[2] World population ageing. United Nations, Department of Economic and Social Affairs, Population Division; 2015. World Population Ageing, United Nations (ST/ESA/SER.A/390)

[3] Willcox DC, Willcox BJ, Poon LW. Centenarian studies: Important contributors to our understanding of the aging process and longevity. Current Gerontology and Geriatrics Research. 2010;**2010**:484529. DOI: 10.1155/2010/484529

[4] Clegg A, Young J, Iliffe S, Rikkert MO, Rockwood K. Frailty in elderly people. Lancet. 2013;**381**(9868):752-762. DOI: 10.1016/s0140-6736(12)62167-9

[5] Turner G, Clegg A. Best practice guidelines for the management of frailty: A British Geriatrics Society, Age UK and Royal College of General Practitioners report. Age and Ageing. 2014;**43**(6):744-747. DOI: 10.1093/ageing/afu138

[6] Cruz-Jentoft AJ, Baeyens JP, Bauer JM, Boirie Y, Cederholm T, Landi F et al. Sarcopenia: European consensus on definition and diagnosis: Report of the European Working Group on Sarcopenia in Older People. Age and Ageing. 2010;**39**(4):412-423

[7] Sender R, Fuchs S, Milo R. Revised estimates for the number of human and bacteria cells in the body. PLoS Biology. 2016;**14**(8):e1002533. DOI: 10.1371/journal.pbio.1002533

[8] Delmonico MJ, Harris TB, Lee JS, Visser M, Nevitt M, Kritchevsky SB et al. Alternative definitions of sarcopenia, lower extremity performance, and functional impairment with aging in older men and women. Journal of the American Geriatrics Society. 2007;**55**(5):769-774. DOI: 10.1111/j.1532-5415.2007.01140.x

[9] Kallman DA, Plato CC, Tobin JD. The role of muscle loss in the age-related decline of grip strength: Cross-sectional and longitudinal perspectives. Journal of Gerontology. 1990;**45**(3):M82-M88

[10] Newman A B, et al. Strength, but not muscle mass is associated with mortality in the health aging and body composition study cohort. Journal of Gerontology: Medical Science. 2006;**61A**(1):72-77

[11] Studenski SA, Peters KW, Alley DE, Cawthon PM, McLean RR, Harris TB et al. The FNIH sarcopenia project: Rationale, study description, conference recommendations, and final estimates. The Journals of Gerontology. Series A, Biological Sciences and Medical Sciences. 2014;**69**(5):547-558. DOI: 10.1093/gerona/glu010

[12] Sayer AA, Robinson SM, Patel HP, Shavlakadze T, Cooper C, Grounds MD. New horizons in the pathogenesis, diagnosis and management of sarcopenia. Age and Ageing. 2013;**42**

[13] Landi F, Liperoti R, Russo A, Giovannini S, Tosato M, Capoluongo E et al. Sarcopenia as a risk factor for falls in elderly individuals: Results from the ilSIRENTE study. Clinical nutrition (Edinburgh, Scotland). 2012;**31**(5):652-658. DOI: 10.1016/j.clnu.2012.02.007

[14] Sayer AA, Dennison EM, Syddall HE, Gilbody HJ, Phillips DI, Cooper C. Type 2 diabetes, muscle strength, and impaired physical function: The tip of the iceberg? Diabetes Care. 2005;**28**(10):2541-2542

[15] Di Monaco M, Vallero F, Di Monaco R, Tappero R. Prevalence of sarcopenia and its association with osteoporosis in 313 older women following a hip fracture. Archives of Gerontology and Geriatrics. 2011;**52**(1):71-74

[16] Cooper R, Kuh D, Hardy R. Objectively measured physical capability levels and mortality: Systematic review and meta-analysis. BMJ. 2010;**341**:c4467. DOI: 10.1136/bmj.c4467

[17] Janssen I, Shepard DS, Katzmarzyk PT, Roubenoff R. The healthcare costs of sarcopenia in the United States. Journal of the American Geriatrics Society. 2004;**52**(1):80-85

[18] Fielding RA, Vellas B, Evans WJ, Bhasin S, Morley JE, Newman AB et al. Sarcopenia: An undiagnosed condition in older adults. Current consensus definition: prevalence, etiology, and consequences. International working group on sarcopenia. Journal of the American Medical Directors Association. 2011;**12**(4):249-256. DOI: 10.1016/j.jamda.2011.01.003

[19] Chen LK, Liu LK, Woo J, Assantachai P, Auyeung TW, Bahyah KS et al. Sarcopenia in Asia: Consensus report of the Asian Working Group for Sarcopenia. Journal of the American Medical Directors Association. 2014;**15**(2):95-101. DOI: 10.1016/j.jamda.2013.11.025

[20] Abellan van Kan G, Rolland Y, Andrieu S, Bauer J, Beauchet O, Bonnefoy M et al. Gait speed at usual pace as a predictor of adverse outcomes in community-dwelling older people an International Academy on Nutrition and Aging (IANA) Task Force. The Journal of Nutrition, Health & Aging. 2009;**13**(10):881-889

[21] Lauretani F, Russo CR, Bandinelli S, Bartali B, Cavazzini C, Di Iorio A et al. Age-associated changes in skeletal muscles and their effect on mobility: An operational diagnosis of sarcopenia. Journal of Applied Physiology. 2003;**95**(5):1851-1860

[22] Patel HP, Syddall HE, Jameson K, Robinson S, Denison H, Roberts HC et al. Prevalence of sarcopenia in community-dwelling older people in the UK using the European Working Group on Sarcopenia in Older People (EWGSOP) definition: Findings from the Hertfordshire Cohort Study (HCS). Age and Ageing. 2013;**42**. Epub ahead of print

[23] Cruz-Jentoft AJ, Landi F, Schneider SM, Zuniga C, Arai H, Boirie Y et al. Prevalence of and interventions for sarcopenia in ageing adults: A systematic review. Report of the International Sarcopenia Initiative (EWGSOP and IWGS). Age and Ageing. 2014;**43**(6):748-759. DOI: 10.1093/ageing/afu115

[24] Cooper C, Dere W, Evans W, Kanis JA, Rizzoli R, Sayer AA et al. Frailty and sarcopenia: definitions and outcome parameters. Osteoporosis International: A Journal Established

As Result of Cooperation Between the European Foundation for Osteoporosis and the National Osteoporosis Foundation of the USA. 2012;**23**(7):1839-1848. DOI: 10.1007/s00198-012-1913-1

[25] Roberts HC, Denison HJ, Martin HJ, Patel HP, Syddall H, Cooper C et al. A review of the measurement of grip strength in clinical and epidemiological studies: Towards a standardised approach. Age and Ageing. 2011;**40**(4):423-429

[26] Roberts HC, Syddall HE, Cooper C, Aihie Sayer A. Is grip strength associated with length of stay in hospitalised older patients admitted for rehabilitation? Findings from the Southampton grip strength study. Age and Ageing. 2012;**41**(5):641-646. DOI: 10.1093/ageing/afs089

[27] Sayer AA, Kirkwood TB. Grip strength and mortality: A biomarker of ageing? Lancet. 2015;**386**(9990):226-227. DOI: 10.1016/s0140-6736(14)62349-7

[28] Vermeulen J, Neyens JC, van Rossum E, Spreeuwenberg MD, de Witte LP. Predicting ADL disability in community-dwelling elderly people using physical frailty indicators: A systematic review. BMC Geriatrics. 2011;**11**:33. DOI: 10.1186/1471-2318-11-33

[29] Mijnarends DM, Meijers JM, Halfens RJ, ter Borg S, Luiking YC, Verlaan S et al. Validity and reliability of tools to measure muscle mass, strength, and physical performance in community-dwelling older people: A systematic review. Journal of the American Medical Directors Association. 2013;**14**(3):170-178. DOI: 10.1016/j.jamda.2012.10.009

[30] Dodds RM, Syddall HE, Cooper R, Benzeval M, Deary IJ, Dennison EM. Grip strength across the life course: Normative data from twelve British studies. PloS One. 2014;**9**. DOI: 10.1371/journal.pone.0113637

[31] Malmstrom TK, Morley JE. SARC-F: A simple questionnaire to rapidly diagnose sarcopenia. Journal of the American Medical Directors Association. 2013;**14**(8):531-532. DOI: 10.1016/j.jamda.2013.05.018

[32] Cao L, Chen S, Zou C, Ding X, Gao L, Liao Z et al. A pilot study of the SARC-F scale on screening sarcopenia and physical disability in the Chinese older people. The Journal of Nutrition, Health & Aging. 2014;**18**(3):277-283. DOI: 10.1007/s12603-013-0410-3

[33] Woo J, Leung J, Morley JE. Validating the SARC-F: A suitable community screening tool for sarcopenia? Journal of the American Medical Directors Association. 2014;**15**(9):630-634. DOI: 10.1016/j.jamda.2014.04.021

[34] Cesari M, Fielding R, Benichou O, Bernabei R, Bhasin S, Guralnik JM et al. Pharmacological interventions in frailty and sarcopenia: Report by the international conference on frailty and sarcopenia research task force. The Journal of Frailty & Aging. 2015;**4**(3):114-120. DOI: 10.14283/jfa.2015.64

[35] Zammit PS, Partridge TA, Yablonka-Reuveni Z. The skeletal muscle satellite cell: The stem cell that came in from the cold. Journal of Histochemistry and Cytochemistry. 2006;**54**(11):1177-1191

[36] Patel HP, White MC, Westbury L, Syddall HE, Stephens PJ, Clough GF et al. Skeletal muscle morphology in sarcopenia defined using the EWGSOP criteria: Findings from the Hertfordshire Sarcopenia Study (HSS). BMC Geriatrics. 2015;**15**:171. DOI: 10.1186/s12877-015-0171-4

[37] Evans WJ, Paolisso G, Abbatecola AM, Corsonello A, Bustacchini S, Strollo F et al. Frailty and muscle metabolism dysregulation in the elderly. Biogerontology. 2010;**11**(5):527-536. DOI: 10.1007/s10522-010-9297-0

[38] Arthur PG, Grounds MD, Shavlakadze T. Oxidative stress as a therapeutic target during muscle wasting: Considering the complex interactions. Current Opinion in Clinical Nutrition and Metabolic Care. 2008;**11**(4):408-416. DOI: 10.1097/MCO.0b013e328302f3fe

[39] Morley JE. Pharmacologic options for the treatment of sarcopenia. Calcif Tissue Int. 2016 Apr;**98**(4):319-33. DOI: 10.1007/s00223-015-0022-5. Epub 2015 Jun 23

[40] Goodman CA, Mayhew DL, Hornberger TA. Recent progress toward understanding the molecular mechanisms that regulate skeletal muscle mass. Cell Signal. 2011;**23**

[41] Verdijk LB, Koopman R, Schaart G, Meijer K, Savelberg HH, van Loon LJ. Satellite cell content is specifically reduced in type II skeletal muscle fibers in the elderly. American Journal of Physiology Endocrinology and Metabolism. 2007;**292**(1):E151-E157. DOI: 10.1152/ajpendo.00278.2006

[42] Maltin CA, Delday MI, Sinclair KD, Steven J, Sneddon AA. Impact of manipulations of myogenesis in utero on the performance of adult skeletal muscle. Reproduction. 2001;**122**(3):359-374

[43] Janssen I. The epidemiology of sarcopenia. Clinics in Geriatric Medicine. 2011;**27**(3):355-363. DOI: 10.1016/j.cger.2011.03.004

[44] Samson MM, Meeuwsen IB, Crowe A, Dessens JA, Duursma SA, Verhaar HJ. Relationships between physical performance measures, age, height and body weight in healthy adults. Age and Ageing. 2000;**29**(3):235-242

[45] Janssen I, Heymsfield SB, Wang ZM, Ross R. Skeletal muscle mass and distribution in 468 men and women aged 18-88 yr. Journal of Applied Physiology. 2000;**89**(1):81-88

[46] Patel HP, Jameson KA, Syddall HE, Martin HJ, Stewart CE, Cooper C et al. Developmental influences, muscle morphology, and sarcopenia in community-dwelling older men. The Journal of Gerontology. Series A, Biological Science and Medical Science. 2012;**67**(1):82-87

[47] Dodds R, Denison HJ, Ntani G, Cooper R, Cooper C, Sayer AA et al. Birth weight and muscle strength: A systematic review and meta-analysis. The Journal of Nutrition, Health & Aging. 2012;**16**(7):609-615

[48] Harttgen K, Kowal P, Strulik H, Chatterji S, Vollmer S. Patterns of frailty in older adults: Comparing results from higher and lower income countries using the Survey of Health, Ageing and Retirement in Europe (SHARE) and the Study on Global AGEing and Adult Health (SAGE). PloS One. 2013;**8**(10):e75847. DOI: 10.1371/journal.pone.0075847

[49] Collard RM, Boter H, Schoevers RA, Oude Voshaar RC. Prevalence of frailty in community-dwelling older persons: A systematic review. Journal of the American Geriatrics Society. 2012;**60**(8):1487-1492. DOI: 10.1111/j.1532-5415.2012.04054.x

[50] Gale CR, Cooper C, Sayer AA. Prevalence of frailty and disability: Findings from the English Longitudinal Study of Ageing. Age and Ageing. 2015;**44**(1):162-165. DOI: 10.1093/ageing/afu148

[51] Fried LP, Tangen CM, Walston J, Newman AB, Hirsch C, Gottdiener J et al. Frailty in older adults: Evidence for a phenotype. The Journal of Gerontology. Series A, Biological Science and Medical Science. 2001;**56**(3):M146-M156

[52] Gill TM, Gahbauer EA, Han L, Allore HG. The relationship between intervening hospitalizations and transitions between frailty states. The Journals of Gerontology. Series A, Biological Sciences and Medical Sciences 2011;**66**(11):1238-1243. DOI: 10.1093/gerona/glr142

[53] Kelaiditi E, Cesari M, Canevelli M, van Kan GA, Ousset PJ, Gillette-Guyonnet S et al. Cognitive frailty: Rational and definition from an (I.A.N.A./I.A.G.G.) international consensus group. The Journal of Nutrition, Health & Aging. 2013;**17**(9):726-734. DOI: 10.1007/s12603-013-0367-2

[54] Gobbens RJ, van Assen MA, Luijkx KG, Schols JM. The predictive validity of the Tilburg Frailty Indicator: Disability, health care utilization, and quality of life in a population at risk. The Gerontologist. 2012;**52**(5):619-631. DOI: 10.1093/geront/gnr135

[55] Farmer C, Fenu E, O'Flynn N, Guthrie B. Clinical assessment and management of multimorbidity: Summary of NICE guidance. BMJ. 2016;**354**:i4843. DOI: 10.1136/bmj.i4843

[56] Gill TM, Gahbauer EA, Allore HG, Ham L. Transitions between frailty states among community-living older persons. Archives of Internal Medicine. 2006;**166**. DOI: 10.1001/archinte.166.4.418

[57] Xue QL, Bandeen-Roche K, Varadhan R, Zhou J, Fried LP. Initial manifestations of frailty criteria and the development of frailty phenotype in the Women's Health and Aging Study II. Journal of Gerontology Series A, Biological Science and Medical Science. 2008;**63**(9):984-990. DOI: 63/9/984 [pii]

[58] Rockwood K, Song X, MacKnight C, Bergman H, Hogan DB, McDowell I et al. A global clinical measure of fitness and frailty in elderly people. CMAJ: Canadian Medical Association Journal = Journal de l'Association Medicale Canadienne. 2005;**173**(5):489-495. DOI: 10.1503/cmaj.050051

[59] Rockwood K, Mitnitski A. Limits to deficit accumulation in elderly people. Mechanisms of Ageing and Development. 2006;**127**. DOI: 10.1016/j.mad.2006.01.002

[60] Rockwood K, Andrew M, Mitnitski A. A comparison of two approaches to measuring frailty in elderly people. The Journals of Gerontology. Series A, Biological Sciences and Medical Sciences 2007;**62**(7):738-743

[61] Rondanelli M, Klersy C, Terracol G, Talluri J, Maugeri R, Guido D et al. Whey protein, amino acids, and vitamin D supplementation with physical activity increases fat-free mass and strength, functionality, and quality of life and decreases inflammation in sarcopenic elderly. The American Journal of Clinical Nutrition. 2016;**103**(3):830-840. DOI: 10.3945/ajcn.115.113357

[62] Churchward-Venne TA, Murphy CH, Longland TM, Phillips SM. Role of protein and amino acids in promoting lean mass accretion with resistance exercise and attenuating lean mass loss during energy deficit in humans. Amino Acids. 2013;**45**(2):231-240. DOI: 10.1007/s00726-013-1506-0

[63] Liu CJ, Latham NK. Progressive resistance strength training for improving physical function in older adults. The Cochrane Database Syst Rev. 2009 Jul **8**;(3):CD002759. DOI: 10.1002/14651858.CD002759.pub2

[64] Pahor M, Guralnik JM, Ambrosius WT, Blair S, Bonds DE, Church TS et al. Effect of structured physical activity on prevention of major mobility disability in older adults: The LIFE study randomized clinical trial. JAMA. 2014;**311**(23):2387-2396. DOI: 10.1001/jama.2014.5616

[65] Valenzuela T. Efficacy of progressive resistance training interventions in older adults in nursing homes: A systematic review. Journal of the American Medical Directors Association. 2012;**13**(5):418-428. DOI: 10.1016/j.jamda.2011.11.001

[66] Peterson MD, Sen A, Gordon PM. Influence of resistance exercise on lean body mass in aging adults: A meta-analysis. Medicine and Science in Sports and Exercise. 2011;**43**(2):249-258. DOI: 10.1249/MSS.0b013e3181eb6265

[67] Fiatarone MA, O'Neill EF, Ryan ND, Clements KM, Solares GR, Nelson ME et al. Exercise training and nutritional supplementation for physical frailty in very elderly people. The New England Journal of Medicine. 1994;**330**(25):1769-1775

[68] Vincent KR, Braith RW, Feldman RA, Magyari PM, Cutler RB, Persin SA et al. Resistance exercise and physical performance in adults aged 60 to 83. Journal of the American Geriatrics Society. 2002;**50**(6):1100-1107

[69] El-Khoury F, Cassou B, Charles MA, Dargent-Molina P. The effect of fall prevention exercise programmes on fall induced injuries in community dwelling older adults: Systematic review and meta-analysis of randomised controlled trials. BMJ 2013;**347**:f6234. DOI: 10.1136/bmj.f6234

[70] Stubbs B, Brefka S, Denkinger MD. What works to prevent falls in community-dwelling older adults? Umbrella review of meta-analyses of randomized controlled trials. Physical Therapy. 2015;**95**(8):1095-1110. DOI: 10.2522/ptj.20140461

[71] Robertson MC, Gillespie LD. Fall prevention in community-dwelling older adults. JAMA. 2013;**309**(13):1406-1407. DOI: 10.1001/jama.2013.3130

[72] Clegg A, Barber S, Young J, Forster A, Iliffe S. Do home-based exercise interventions improve outcomes for frail older people? Findings from a systematic review. Reviews in Clinical Gerontology. 2012;**22**(1):68-78

[73] Theou O, Stathokostas L, Roland KP, Jakobi JM, Patterson C, Vandervoort AA et al. The effectiveness of exercise interventions for the management of frailty: A systematic review. Journal of Aging Research. 2011;**2011**:569194. DOI: 10.4061/2011/569194

[74] Dodds R, Kuh D, Aihie Sayer A, Cooper R. Physical activity levels across adult life and grip strength in early old age: Updating findings from a British birth cohort. Age and Ageing. 2013;**42**(6):794-798. DOI: 10.1093/ageing/aft124

[75] Robinson S, Cooper C, Aihie SA. Nutrition and sarcopenia: A review of the evidence and implications for preventive strategies. Journal of Aging Research. 2012;**2012**:510801. Epub;%2012 Mar 15.:510801

[76] Wandrag L, Brett SJ, Frost G, Hickson M. Impact of supplementation with amino acids or their metabolites on muscle wasting in patients with critical illness or other muscle wasting illness: a systematic review. Journal of Human Nutrition and Dietetics: The Official Journal of the British Dietetic Association. 2015;**28**(4):313-330. DOI: 10.1111/jhn.12238

[77] Hickson M. Nutritional interventions in sarcopenia: A critical review. The Proceedings of the Nutrition Society. 2015;**74**(4):378-386. DOI: 10.1017/s0029665115002049

[78] Deutz NE, Pereira SL, Hays NP, Oliver JS, Edens NK, Evans CM et al. Effect of beta-hydroxy-beta-methylbutyrate (HMB) on lean body mass during 10 days of bed rest in older adults. Clinical Nutrition (Edinburgh, Scotland). 2013;**32**(5):704-712. DOI: 10.1016/j.clnu.2013.02.011

[79] Paddon-Jones D, Sheffield-Moore M, Zhang XJ, Volpi E, Wolf SE, Aarsland A et al. Amino acid ingestion improves muscle protein synthesis in the young and elderly. American Journal of Physiology Endocrinology and Metabolism. 2004;**286**(3):E321-E328

[80] Wu H, Xia Y, Jiang J, Du H, Guo X, Liu X et al. Effect of beta-hydroxy-beta-methylbutyrate supplementation on muscle loss in older adults: A systematic review and meta-analysis. Archives of Gerontology and Geriatrics. 2015;**61**(2):168-175. DOI: 10.1016/j.archger.2015.06.020

[81] Flakoll P, Sharp R, Baier S, Levenhagen D, Carr C, Nissen S. Effect of beta-hydroxy-beta-methylbutyrate, arginine, and lysine supplementation on strength, functionality, body composition, and protein metabolism in elderly women. Nutrition. 2004;**20**(5):445-451. DOI: 10.1016/j.nut.2004.01.009

[82] Stout JR, Smith-Ryan AE, Fukuda DH, Kendall KL, Moon JR, Hoffman JR et al. Effect of calcium beta-hydroxy-beta-methylbutyrate (CaHMB) with and without resistance training in men and women 65+yrs: A randomized, double-blind pilot trial. Experimental Gerontology. 2013;**48**(11):1303-1310. DOI: 10.1016/j.exger.2013.08.007

[83] Bauer J, Biolo G, Cederholm T, Cesari M, Cruz-Jentoft AJ, Morley JE et al. Evidence-based recommendations for optimal dietary protein intake in older people: A position paper from the PROT-AGE Study Group. Journal of the American Medical Directors Association. 2013;**14**(8):542-559. DOI: 10.1016/j.jamda.2013.05.021

[84] Ali S, Garcia JM. Sarcopenia, cachexia and aging: Diagnosis, mechanisms and therapeutic options - a mini-review. Gerontology. 2014;**60**(4):294-305. DOI: 10.1159/000356760

[85] Giannoulis MG, Martin FC, Nair KS, Umpleby AM, Sonksen P. Hormone replacement therapy and physical function in healthy older men. Time to talk hormones? Endocrine Reviews. 2012;**33**(3):314-377. DOI: 10.1210/er.2012-1002

[86] Cohen S, Nathan JA, Goldberg AL. Muscle wasting in disease: Molecular mechanisms and promising therapies. Nature Reviews Drug Discovery. 2015;**14**(1):58-74. DOI: 10.1038/nrd4467

[87] Huang Z, Chen X, Chen D. Myostatin: A novel insight into its role in metabolism, signal pathways, and expression regulation. Cellular Signalling. 2011;**23**(9):1441-1446. DOI: 10.1016/j.cellsig.2011.05.003

[88] Sumukadas D, Witham MD, Struthers AD, McMurdo ME. Ace inhibitors as a therapy for sarcopenia—Evidence and possible mechanisms. The Journal of Nutrition, Health and Aging. 2008;**12**(7):480-485

[89] Zhou LS, Xu LJ, Wang XQ, Huang YH, Xiao Q. Effect of angiotensin-converting enzyme inhibitors on physical function in elderly subjects: A systematic review and meta-analysis. Drugs & Aging. 2015;**32**(9):727-735. DOI: 10.1007/s40266-015-0288-3

[90] Ellis G, Whitehead MA, O'Neill D, Langhorne P, Robinson D. Comprehensive geriatric assessment for older adults admitted to hospital. The Cochrane Database Syst Rev. 2011 Jul **6**;(7):CD006211. DOI: 10.1002/14651858.CD006211.pub2

[91] Stuck AE, Egger M, Hammer A, Minder CE, Beck JC. Home visits to prevent nursing home admission and functional decline in elderly people: Systematic review and meta-regression analysis. JAMA. 2002;**287**(8):1022-1028

[92] Cameron ID, Fairhall N, Langron C, Lockwood K, Monaghan N, Aggar C et al. A multifactorial interdisciplinary intervention reduces frailty in older people: Randomized trial. BMC Medicine. 2013;**11**:65. DOI: 10.1186/1741-7015-11-65

[93] Huss A, Stuck AE, Rubenstein LZ, Egger M, Clough-Gorr KM. Multidimensional preventive home visit programs for community-dwelling older adults: A systematic review and meta-analysis of randomized controlled trials. The Journals of Gerontology. Series A, Biological Sciences and Medical Sciences 2008;**63**(3):298-307

[94] O'Mahony D, O'Sullivan D, Byrne S, O'Connor MN, Ryan C, Gallagher P. STOPP/START criteria for potentially inappropriate prescribing in older people: Version 2. Age and Ageing. 2015;**44**(2):213-218. DOI: 10.1093/ageing/afu145

[95] Clegg A, Barber S, Young J, Iliffe S, Forster A. The Home-based Older People's Exercise (HOPE) trial: A pilot randomised controlled trial of a home-based exercise intervention for older people with frailty. Age and Ageing. 2014;**43**(5):687-695. DOI: 10.1093/ageing/afu033

2

Sarcopenia in the Context of Skeletal Muscle Function Deficit (SMFD)[1]

Rosaly Correa-de-Araujo

Abstract

Evidence shows that not only changes in skeletal muscle mass but changes in strength and other factors underpinning muscle quality play a role in muscle function decline and impaired mobility associated with aging. Changes in both strength and quality may precede loss of muscle mass. Skeletal muscle function deficit (SMFD) is a terminology that embraces this evolving conceptualization of sarcopenia and age-related muscle dysfunctions. This chapter provides a discussion on sarcopenia in the context of SMFD, including operational definitions and methodological challenges associated with their establishment; integration of muscle quality into SMFD; efforts to identify diagnostic cutoff values for low muscle mass and weakness and their predictive validity to mobility disability; need for standardized muscle quality assessment; clinical and public health relevance and research opportunities. Changes in muscle composition, based on excessive levels of inter- and intramuscular or intramyocellular fat are striking features increasingly addressed in the literature, found to affect muscle metabolism and peak force generation. Methods to easily and rapidly assess muscle composition in multiple clinical settings and with minimal patient burden are needed. Further characterization of SMFD should emphasize integration of muscle quality and factors behind changes in quality, as well as associated clinical and research implications.

Keywords: skeletal muscle function deficit, sarcopenia, reduced muscle mass, low muscle mass, low muscle strength, muscle quality, biomarkers, outcomes

[1]The views expressed in this chapter are those of the author and do not necessarily represent the views of the National Institute of Health, National Institute on Aging, the U.S. Department of Health and Human Services (HHS), or the U.S. Federal Government.

1. Introduction

Numerous efforts around the definition of sarcopenia and its better characterization through biomarkers including cutoff values for muscle mass, muscle strength (weakness), and performance measures, as well as the identification of outcomes of clinical and investigational significance have evolved in the past many years and continue to be heavily investigated. Since 1989, when sarcopenia was first defined as an age-related reduction in muscle mass [1] and the association of low muscle mass and functional impairment was demonstrated [2], scientific and technological advances have helped us improve our understanding of the mechanisms underlying age-related alterations in muscle mass, muscle strength, and muscle quality. Substantial attention has also been given to investigate the relationships of these alterations to mobility impairment, disability, fatigue, risk of metabolic disorders, falls, and mortality in older adults [3]. This ongoing work responds to the need to identify preventive and therapeutic interventions that can delay, improve, revert, or eliminate the changes in muscle mass, strength, and quality. The scientific community, including regulatory scientists, and practicing health care professionals recognize that "a more specific definition of sarcopenia may not only be necessary to align it with new scientific advances, but it is highly desirable on practical grounds because specific criteria are critical for identifying candidate patients for clinical trials that test therapies aimed at reversing or alleviating the complications of sarcopenia and its associated manifestations [4]."

It is estimated that by 2050, 2 billion people worldwide will be age ≥65 years. Preserving mobility and quality of life into old age will be a challenge because impaired mobility is often a precursor of functional decline, disability, and loss of independence. Evidence now shows that not only changes in muscle mass, but other factors underpinning muscle quality also play a role in the decline in muscle function and impaired mobility associated with aging. Changes in muscle quality may precede loss of muscle mass. This provides new opportunities for the assessment of muscle mass, strength, and quality particularly to detect who could benefit from interventions to prevent decline or improve muscle function [5].

The purpose of this chapter is to provide basic science, clinical researchers and expert clinicians with a review of the literature on key efforts to establish clinically meaningful diagnostic cutoff values for low muscle mass and low muscle strength, integrate muscle quality into these efforts, discuss the clinical and public health relevance, and highlight research opportunities for sarcopenia in the context of skeletal muscle function deficit. The new terminology "skeletal muscle function deficit" was coined in 2014 to embrace the evolving concepts of sarcopenia and other aging-related muscle dysfunctions that contribute to clinically meaningful mobility impairments [6].

1.1. Terminology and nosology issues: sarcopenia in the context of skeletal muscle function deficit

Sarcopenia is a condition with a complex multifactorial etiology, which is summarized in **Table 1** [7]. Age-related decreases in muscle performance associated with physical impairment are only partially explained by reduction in muscle mass, with many other pathophysiologic factors contributing to age-related impairments in muscle performance. Based on these facts, decreases in muscle performance and in muscle mass require independent evaluation. The importance of assessing muscle quality, currently defined as strength per unit of appendicular skeletal muscle mass, also continues to be highly emphasized.

Although consensus groups noted below have incorporated the criterion of impaired physical and/or muscle performance into their recommended definitions of sarcopenia, they have not addressed the issue of specific diagnostic terminologies. The lack of sufficient specificity resulting from the use of "sarcopenia," an anatomic term currently used to define a functional condition with which it is imperfectly correlated, and for which nonanatomic contributory factors have been identified, generates confusion. Some of this confusion originates from the fact that reduced muscle mass *per se* is a feature of several other conditions in both older and younger people. Adopting a nosology that accommodates the literal concept of sarcopenia—reduced muscle mass—while applying other diagnostic terms for other age-related muscular conditions that contribute to impaired physical performance seems to hold a valuable clinical approach. "Skeletal muscle function deficit" (SMFD) fits this purpose well. The term indicates a shortfall in function that can evolve to more significant impairment and mobility-disability. The diagnostic criteria for "SMFD" can, then, include: (A) Measures of muscle performance and strength that provide effective cutoff values for identifying those whose mobility disability is related to impairments. Muscle performance is the capacity of a muscle or a group of muscles to generate forces to produce, maintain, sustain, and modify postures and movements that are required for functional activity. Strength is the muscle force exerted to overcome resistance under a specific set of circumstances. Power is the work produced per unit of time or the product of strength and speed. (B) Measures of muscle mass (e.g., "sarcopenic SMFD"), and (C) Measures of muscle quality. Factors impacting muscle quality can be described using measures of muscle composition or myosteatosis (fat infiltration of muscles) as these are very relevant to mobility outcomes and to the identification of effective preventative and therapeutic interventions in older adults. Muscle quality is also largely impacted by intricate intramuscular ultrastructure and morphology of contractile tissue, as well as the relationship between structure and function [6, 8].

A variety of known and putative muscular pathologies can be evaluated as their contribution to SMFD, including newly identified contributory pathologies. This approach also specifies other already recognized conditions that can lead to "SMFD" (e.g., diabetic polyneuropathy or secondary malnutrition), which can be distinguished from age-related conditions contributing to "SMFD" with etiology not yet well established. Further, it accommodates future knowledge in diagnostic specificity based on improved understanding of the mechanisms of aging and disease. Specific neurogenic factors, intrinsic muscle factors, or systemic factors may lead to the characterization of specific subtypes of age-related sarcopenia, to methods for diagnosing them, and to the identification of new therapeutic targets. In sum, the broad concept of "SMFD" comprising a variety of contributory etiologies provides a framework for developing diagnostic categories that are useful for both clinical practice and research. This approach has been successfully implemented with conditions that are clinically manifested as impaired physiologic functions (e.g., congestive heart failure, chronic obstructive pulmonary disease) and have multiple contributory factors [6].

Age-related

- Reduced physical activity
- Mitochondrial dysfunction
- Anorexia of aging
- Apoptosis
- Hormones
- Low levels of testosterone
- Low levels of growth hormone
- Low levels of insulin-like growth factor (IGF)-1
- Elevated levels of cortisol
- Low levels of vitamin D

Proinflammatory cytokines

- Interleukin-1
- Interleukin-6
- Tumor necrosis factor (TNF)-alpha
- Neuronal
- Loss of motor endplates
- Peripheral neuropathy

Vascular

- Peripheral vascular disease
- Reduced capillary function

Weight loss

- Dieting
- Malabsorption
- Disease-related

Hormones

- Low levels of testosterone
- Low levels of growth hormone
- Low levels of insulin-like growth factor (IGF)-1
- Elevated levels of cortisol
- Low levels of vitamin D

Neuronal

- Loss of motor endplates
- Peripheral neuropathy

Table 1. Multifactorial etiology for sarcopenia [7].

2. Operational definitions for sarcopenia

Several operational definitions have emphasized that sarcopenia should now be defined as a loss of muscle function associated with a loss of muscle mass [9–18]. This change in definition from the original meaning of sarcopenia [1] is justified by some experts as necessary due to current knowledge that muscle quality and muscle performance do not directly relate to muscle mass [19, 20]. Two very important factors are thought to be responsible for this knowledge: the compromise of neuromuscular junctions in sarcopenia and the myosteatosis accompanying the aging process [21–24]. Below is a brief description of these operational definitions published by key consensus groups. It should be highlighted that a quantitative definition of sarcopenia that characterizes this condition in terms of rationally-defined cutoff values for lean body mass and muscle strength is comparable to the evolution of the operational definition of osteoporosis in terms of bone mineral density to detect individuals at increased risk for fractures. Efforts to identify an operational definition for sarcopenia include those:

- Based on muscle mass in relationship to the range of muscle mass within a reference population;
- Essentially based on expert opinion, but considering muscle mass and performance criteria;
- Essentially based on expert opinion, but considering muscle mass, muscle strength and physical performance; and
- Evidence-based, data-driven, considering muscle mass, muscle strength, and their predictive validity to mobility disability.

Table 2 summarizes in a comparative way, the currently available operational definitions for sarcopenia. While they might involve similar criteria, marked variations in cutoff values exist as alluded below.

Working group/target population	**Screening**	**Operational definition**	
		Muscle mass	**Muscle strength/ function**
EWGSOP – European Working Group on Sarcopenia in Older People [9]*All person ≥ 65 years*	Gait speed. If gait speed is ≤0.8 m/s, proceed to body composition evaluation. If gait speed >0.8 m/s, measure hand grip strength; if low muscle strength (weakness) is detected, proceed to body composition evaluation	Low muscle mass in patients with gait speed ≤0.8 m/s or normal gait speed but low muscle strength.DXA ASM/height^2 ≤7.23 kg/m^2 for men; ≤5.67 kg/m^2 for women	Low grip strength <30 kg for men; <20 kg for womenorgait speed <0.8 m/s
IWGS/IANA - International Working Group on Sarcopenia Task Force/ International Academy on Nutrition and Aging [11] *Persons with clinical declines in physical function, strength, or health status*	Physical function (4-m gait speed). If gait speed < 1.0 m/s, proceed to body composition evaluation	Low appendicular lean mass/height^2 (assessed by DXA):≤7.23 kg/m^2 for men; ≤5.67 kg/m^2 for women	Poor functioning, gait speed

Working group/target population	Screening	Operational definition	
		Muscle mass	Muscle strength/ function
SIG- Special Interest Group: Cachexia-Anorexia in Chronic Wasting Diseases [12]*Older persons*	–	Low muscle mass (≥2 standard deviations below the mean measured in young adults of same sex and ethnic background)	Low usual gait speed (<0.8 m/s in the 4-m walking speed).Gait speed test can be replaced by other physical performance measures
SCWD - Sarcopenia with Limited Mobility [10]*Persons >60 years with clinical declines in physical function, strength, or health status. Exclude specific muscle diseases, peripheral vascular disease with intermittent claudication, central and peripheral nervous system disorders and cachexia*	Distance walked during a 6-min walk test (cutoff value 400 m) or gait speed <1.0 m/s (4- to 6-m track length)	Low appendicular lean mass/height^2 (≥2 standard deviations below the mean measured in healthy persons aged 20–30 years old from the same ethnic group)	Poor functioning, 6-m walk or gait speed
AWGS -Asian Working Group for Sarcopenia [15]*Community-dwelling persons 60 or ≥ 65 years, according to the definitions of elderly in each individual country.Persons with specific clinical conditions in all health care settings.*	Screening in community settings—people aged 60 or ≥65 years (according to definitions of elderly in each individual country) living in communities.Specific clinical conditions in all health care settings—presence of recent functional decline or functional impairment; unintentional body weight loss for over 5% in a month; depressive mood or cognitive impairment; repeated falls; undernutrition; chronic conditions (e.g., chronic heart failure; chronic obstructive pulmonary disease, diabetes mellitus, chronic kidney disease, connective tissue disease, tuberculosis infection, and other chronic wasting conditions)	2-standard deviations below the mean muscle mass of young reference group or the lower quintile as the cutoff value determination.Low appendicular lean mass/ height^2:<7.0 kg/m^2 for men and <5.4 kg/m^2 for women, using DXA.<7.0 kg/m^2 for men and <5.7kg/m^2 for women, using BIA	Gait speed ≤ 0.8 m/s as the cutoff value for low physical performance.Lower 20th percentile of handgrip as strength as cutoff value for low muscle strength before outcome-based data are available.Low handgrip strength is suggested to be defined as < 26 kg for men and < 18 kg for women.
FNIH - Foundation for the National Institutes of Health, Sarcopenia Project [14]	Patient presents with poor physical function. If weakness is present, proceed to evaluate for low muscle mass; if low muscle mass is detected, it is possible it might be the cause of weakness. If weakness is not present or if low muscle mass is not detected, proceed to investigate for other causes of poor physical performance.	Recommended cutoff value:Appendicular lean mass adjusted to BMI (ALM_{BMI}) <0.789 for men and <0.512 for women.Alternate cutoff value:ALM <19.75 kg for men and <15.02 kg for women.	Gait speed < 0.8 m/ sRecommended cutoff value:Grip strength (GS Max) <26 kg for men and <16 kg for women.Alternate cutoff value:GS adjusted to BMI ($GSMax_{BMI}$) <1.0 for men and <0.56 for women.

Table 2. Comparative summary of sarcopenia definitions.

Muscle mass in relationship to the range of muscle mass within a reference population. The first definition of sarcopenia included the relative muscle mass 2 standard deviations (SDs) below the mean of a large sex-specific reference population 18–40 years old [2]. This definition used a measure of relative muscle mass obtained by dividing absolute muscle mass estimated by dual energy x-ray absorptiometry (DXA) by height squared. Following, sarcopenia was classified per its severity as: (1) Class I sarcopenia (skeletal muscle index between 1 and 2 SDs below the young adult values) and (2) Class II sarcopenia (skeletal muscle index above 2 SDs below the young adult reference). Skeletal muscle index was calculated by dividing total muscle mass by total body mass, with muscle mass evaluated by bioelectrical impedance analysis (BIA) [25].

Essentially expert opinion, but considering muscle mass and performance criteria. Numerous recommendations for a definition of sarcopenia consider muscle mass and performance criteria. The European Working Group on Sarcopenia in Older People (EWGSOP) proposed a diagnosis for sarcopenia that requires low muscle mass (estimated by the ratio of appendicular lean mass (ALM) over height squared, $\leq$7.23 kg/ht^2 for men and $\leq$5.67 kg/ht^2 for women) accompanied by either low muscle strength (measured by grip strength <30 kg for men and <20 kg for women) or low physical performance (measured by gait speed <0.8 m/s). The group defined three stages for the condition: (1) Presarcopenia (loss of muscle mass); (2) sarcopenia (loss of muscle mass accompanied by either loss of strength or physical performance); and (3) severe sarcopenia, with all three aspects present [9]. The definition of sarcopenia by the International Working Group on Sarcopenia (IWGS)/International Academy on Nutrition and Aging (IANA) [11], the European Society for Clinical Nutrition and Metabolism Special Interest Group on cachexia-anorexia in chronic wasting diseases and nutrition in geriatrics [12], and the Society of Sarcopenia, Cachexia, and Wasting Disorders (SCWA) [10], require that both lean mass and gait speed be included in the diagnostic criteria for the condition.

Essentially expert opinion, but considering muscle mass, muscle strength, and physical performance. The Asian Working Group for Sarcopenia (AWGS) decided to take a similar approach for the diagnosis of sarcopenia, but unlike the EWGSOP, it recommends measuring both muscle strength (handgrip strength) and physical performance (usual gait speed) as the screening test [15]. The group also recommends using 60 or 65 years as the age for sarcopenia diagnosis per the definitions of older adults in each Asian country. The group, though, supports using BIA for sarcopenia diagnosis and evaluation of effects. It recommends: (A) Using 2 standard deviations below the mean muscle mass of young reference groups or lower quintile as the cutoff value determination; height-adjusted skeletal muscle mass; for using DXA, cutoff values include 7kg/m^2 in men and 5.4 kg/m^2 in women; for BIA, cutoff values include 7kg/m^2 in men and 5.7 kg/m^2 in women, defined by appendicular skeletal muscle mass/height^2. (B) Using the lower 20th percentile of handgrip strength of a study population before outcomes data are available; low handgrip strength defined as <26 kg for men and <18kg for women. (C) Using $\leq$0.8m/s as the cutoff value for low physical performance.

Evidence-based, data-driven, considering muscle mass, muscle strength, and predictive validity to mobility disability. The studies supported by the National Institute on Aging and the Foundation for the National Institutes of Health (FNIH) Sarcopenia Project utilized a data-driven analysis of a large pool of data (>26,000) from studies on aging (epidemiologic and clinical trials) to identify criteria for clinically relevant low muscle strength (weakness) and low lean mass [17]. By addressing the relationship between mobility impairment (defined as gait speed ≤0.8 m/s) and muscle strength (measured by handgrip strength), strength cutoff values (<26 kg for men and <16 kg for women) were determined below where low strength (weakness) is likely to contribute to slow gait [26]. By relating these strength cutoff values to muscle mass (estimated by appendicular lean mass adjusted to body mass index [ALM/BMI]), additional cutoff values were determined (<0.789 for men, <0.512 for women), below which low lean mass is likely to contribute to low muscle strength [27]. The cutoff values resulting from these analyses were also found to have a predictive significance on incident mobility impairment over 3 years of follow-up. This two-step analyses that links a clinical condition (mobility impairment) to a functional test result (weakness), which is in turn linked to a potential therapeutic target (muscle atrophy) is useful for establishing participant selection criteria and outcome measures for trials of pharmaceutical or other interventions [14, 17, 28]. These studies, however, were conducted in relatively heathy community-dwelling older adults. In addition, harmonization of DXA data was not conducted prior to pooling data from all studies for analysis. Therefore, additional research is ongoing to validate the findings above by analysing harmonized pooled data from well-designed observational and interventional studies from populations of older adults with high prevalence of mobility disability (see RFA-AG-15-013 http://grants.nih.gov/grants/guide/rfa-files/RFA-AG-15-013.html). The main goal is to develop and assess differing diagnostic cutoff values with regard to properties such as sensitivity, specificity, and positive predictive value. Because the populations involved display a variety of chronic conditions, it is possible that differing criteria might be needed to identify population subgroups. The extent to which lack of harmonization of DXA data significantly compromised the reliability of previously established cutoff values is to be seen.

2.1. Validation of the different definitions of sarcopenia

Validation of the different definitions of sarcopenia is ongoing. Using the criteria recommended by the IWGS/IANA, the prevalence of sarcopenia was slightly less compared to the EWGSOP criteria [29]. Using the EWGSOP criteria, 4.6% of males and 7.9% of females in Hertfordshire were found to have sarcopenia [30]; Japanese men and women age 65–80 years were found to have sarcopenia at a rate of 21.8 and 22.99%, respectively [31]; among people 80 years and older, sarcopenia was present in 12.5% [32]; and in nursing homes, 32.8% of the residents had sarcopenia [33]. Still using the EWGSOP criteria, sarcopenia was found to be highly predictive of earlier mortality in nursing home residents [34], in community-dwelling older Korean men [35], and in older adults admitted to acute care [36]. Sarcopenia assessed with the EWGSOP criteria has also been associated with a greater increase in falls [37, 38] and has been shown to predict mobility and instrumental activities of daily living disability [39]. Similarly, the SCWD criteria have been found to predict ADL and IADL difficulties, frailty and mortality in a longitudinal study [40].

Because the FNIH criteria were based on developing cutoffs using a variety of large epidemiological studies [14], these criteria are more restrictive with only 1.3% of men and 2.3% of women being defined as having sarcopenia. While a strong negative percent agreement has been reported with EWGSOP, the positive percent concurrences are generally low (5–32%). Additional comparative studies are needed, particularly to evaluate best predictive ability.

2.2. Methodological challenges in establishing diagnostic cutoff values

Analyses of pooled data from large studies on aging with measures of muscle mass, and strength still face numerous challenges including different follow-up intervals, use of more than one brand and/or generation of devices to measure body composition, use of more than one type of handgrip dynamometer, use of more than one distance to calculate gait speed, and data harmonization issues [17]. Cutoff values for measurements of muscle mass, muscle strength, and physical performance for the diagnosis of sarcopenia may also differ across populations due to a series of factors including race and ethnicity, body size, lifestyle, and cultural backgrounds. Cutoff values established for Caucasians may not be applicable to Africans, Asians, or Hispanics. For example, as acknowledged by the AWGS, the Asian continent has a rapidly growing population with a wide range of ethnicities, cultural, social, religious backgrounds, and lifestyles [15]. In addition, Asia's aging population status and economic development varies significantly across Asian countries. Moreover, the age cutoff that defines the population of older adults may differ not only among Asian countries, but also around the world. The lack or paucity of outcomes-based studies is another factor presenting a challenge to the assessment of sarcopenia.

The discussion in this section focuses on key methodological issues associated with the body composition assessment and the need to establish a standardized approach to develop and apply diagnostic cutoff values. Assessments of body composition vary in precision and in the target tissue. The use of anthropometric methods does not allow tissue-specific inferences. BMI, a descriptive index encompassing both the lean and fat mass, is expressed as weight divided by stature squared (kg/m^2). The availability of extensive national reference data and their established relationships with levels of body fat, morbidity, and mortality in adults is an advantage to the use of BMI. However, the use of BMI alone to evaluate athletes and persons with conditions such as sarcopenia where body weight may be altered considerably by changing proportions of muscle and fat masses is cautioned [41].

BIA produces estimates of total body water, fat-free mass, and fat mass by measuring the resistance of the body as a conductor to a very small alternating electrical current. This is not a direct measure of skeletal muscle. Measurements can be easily altered by fluid retention and health status, providing inaccurate results that limit considerably the clinical application. BIA was developed to mainly determine the volume of body fat and muscle mass, but not specific appendicular muscle mass. While validation studies have been reported on BIA's accuracy in the diagnosis of sarcopenia, results also strongly depend on the accuracy of the equation of the equipment and the conditions associated with the assessment (e.g., temperature, humidity, skin condition, and others) [42–45]. New BIA equipment models will likely provide more precise measurements of appendicular muscle mass [24, 46]. Portability, reasonable cost, fast processing, noninvasiveness, radiation-free functions, and convenience of use are advantages to BIA suitability for sarcopenia assessment in the community. Despite recommendations by EWGSOP on the use of BIA validated equations in sarcopenia research, its use has been discouraged by others [10, 47]. Moreover, BIA equipment in Western countries is not derived from populations from other regions of the world and, therefore, results are unlikely to be able to be extrapolated to particular populations [15].

Currently, the precision of devices to measure body composition such as DXA, computed tomography (CT), and magnetic resonance imaging (MRI) has been well recognized [47]. DXA is currently the most widely employed method for muscle mass measurement in sarcopenia research. It is commonly available in both clinical and research settings, is relatively inexpensive, and provides sufficiently precise results [41, 47, 48]. DXA is considered a suitable alternative to distinguish between fat, bone mineral, and lean tissues, it leads to minimal radiation exposure. However, its use in community screening is still challenging. In 2008, the Center for Disease Control and Prevention (CDC), National Center for Health Statistics (NCHS) released a DXA whole body dataset from the National Health and Nutrition Examination Survey (NHANES) population-based sample acquired with modern fan bean scanners in 15 counties across the United States from 1999 through 2004 [49]. The reference dataset was partitioned by gender and ethnicity and DXA whole body measures of %fat, fat mass/height^2, lean mass/height^2, appendicular lean mass/height^2, %fat trunk/%fat legs ratio, trunk/limb fat mass ratio of fat, bone mineral content (BMC), and bone mineral density (BMD) were analysed to provide reference values for subjects 8–85 years old. DXA reference values for adults were normalized to age; reference values for children included total and subtotal whole body results and were normalized to age, height, or lean mass.

The estimation of fat and lean tissue by DXA is based on assumptions regarding levels of hydration, potassium content, or tissue density, and these assumptions vary with manufacturer. Some analytical differences across manufacturers and models, and the risk of generating biased results due to the low differentiation between water and bone-free lean tissue are among limitations with DXA [48]. Estimates of body composition are also affected by differences in software employed, methodological issues, and intra- and intermachine differences. Testing of specific manufacturers and models revealed that overestimations of fat-free mass may occur. DXA systems are currently capable of scanning a very broad range of weights (neonates to morbidly obese). Repeatability is also very high for all reported total body measures, with the percent fat measures typically better than 1% (standard deviation) and 2% (coefficient of variation) for total fat and lean mass measures. Whole-body DXA scans can be subdivided into arms, legs, trunk, head, and android/gynoid soft tissue regions to report all bone and soft tissue measures within a region. While work is ongoing, there is not yet a reliable phantom that can be used to cross-calibrate DXA systems between manufacturers or a standard of accuracy of percent fat. Some success at representing muscle mass as appendicular lean mass in just the legs and arms has been achieved, but it has yet to be shown as a reasonable surrogate of muscle strength or function. Further work with DXA machines will lead to the development of more refined models of visceral and muscle fat [47].

Despite being considered gold standards for the evaluation of body composition, the use of computed tomography (CT) and magnetic resonance imaging/spectroscopy (MRI)/(MRS) has been impacted by their high cost, CT-generated radiation exposure, and inconvenience for use in community screening. Both are techniques relevant to body composition assessment requiring additional time and software to provide whole body quantities of fat and lean tissue. CT can distinguish body tissues based on a technique helpful to assess nonfat tissue or the fatty infiltration of skeletal muscles. It accurately measures a direct physical property of the muscle (e.g., cross-sectional area and volume). It allows the evaluation of muscle density (a parameter related to intramyocellular adipose tissue deposit) as well as subcutaneous and intramuscular adipose tissue deposition [48].

MRI/MRS has been increasingly used to study body composition in related physiological and pathological conditions. MRI can be used for whole body assessment in normal or moderately overweight people (limitations exist in accommodating very obese people) and measure the volume of body components (e.g., fat tissue, skeletal muscle, organs, and bone). Recent advances suggest that fat tissue is not a homogeneous depot but contains distinct components with different metabolic activities. MRI provides similar measures as CT, with the additional capacity of multiple slice acquisition and 3D volumetric estimates, and no radiation exposure. Quantification of subregions of fat depots such as visceral (i.e., omental, mesenteric, and extraperitoneal), intermuscular, and bone marrow is possible with DXA. A single slice in the upper abdomen has been shown not only to provide the best representation of total volume of visceral fat, but also to correlate with health risks even more closely than the traditionally used slice located at the L4–L5 level. When fat infiltration is increased, MRS imaging allows a more accurate measurement of intramyocellular fat [41, 47]. High technical complexity and costs, as well as inapplicability to persons with older models of implanted medical devices (e.g., joint prostheses) are among the limitations associated with MRI.

2.2.1. *Harmonization of DXA data from multiple studies*

Studies focusing on the development of cutoff values for low muscle mass and low muscle strength frequently use appendicular lean mass (ALM) as a primary independent variable, obtained by DXA. Because these studies generally combine data from many different cohorts to measure ALM, it is critical that DXA measurements be compatible across studies. Owing to the variation between the manufacturers' (Hologic and GE Lunar) designs and systematic improvements in hardware and software instituted over time within each machine type, DXA values obtained for a given individual may vary across machines. It is necessary, therefore, to implement a quantitative adjustment to harmonize or put all measurements on the same theoretical scaling. This harmonization process may require a few steps including the harmonization of DXA values within manufacturer's systems and harmonization between different manufacturers. Studies have been conducted to address standardization and cross-calibration of body composition using GE Healthcare Lunar and Hologic DXA systems. Equations developed are facilitating the combination of results in clinical and epidemiological studies [50–52].

2.3. Sarcopenia diagnosed without measurements

Fracture risk can be determined almost accurately by FRAX questions as by measuring bone mineral density [53]. Because muscle function is more noticeable than bone function, the idea of developing and adopting a simple questionnaire to identify individuals with sarcopenia was realized with the development of the SARC-F scale. This simple and rapid questionnaire to assess the presence of sarcopenia is illustrated in **Table 3** [54]. Robust validation, indicating that SARC-F performed at similar level to the EWSGSOP and AWGS definitions of sarcopenia has been reported, with suggestions that sarcopenia can be screened for without a need to measure muscle mass or to directly measure muscle function [55].

2.4. Sarcopenia and the FY2017 United States Update of the International Statistical Classification of Diseases and Related Health Problems, 10th Revision, Clinical Modifications (ICD-10-CM)

Effective October 1, 2016, the U.S. Department of Health and Human Services (HHS) Centers for Disease Control and Prevention (CDC) has established an ICD-10-CM code for "sarcopenia" (M62.84) for use by the medical community in the United States [56]. For that purpose, sarcopenia is defined as a combination of low muscle mass and weakness in older adults that leads to functional deficits. The new code designation for the condition has the potential to affect the clinical assessment and management of sarcopenia, as well as facilitate data collection and impact sarcopenia research. Because sarcopenia is a condition that can lead to serious adverse outcomes (e.g., mobility impairment, falls, disability, and death) [25, 57–61], the creation of an ICD10-CM code emphasizes the importance of recognizing and treating the condition. The availability of an ICD-10-CM code for sarcopenia has the potential to facilitate recognition of the condition and the future establishment of guidelines for the clinical diagnosis and management of sarcopenia; support requests for tests and referrals, and the development of educational materials targeting potential prevention and management of sarcopenia. It can serve as a stimulus to advance research including new drug development and new indications by the HHS Food and Drug Administration (FDA) for the treatment of sarcopenia. It can certainly contribute to easier access to more reliable data collection on the condition by a variety of system data sources (e.g., electronic medical records, death certificates). Despite these potential advantages, challenges are faced with the need to increase awareness of the availability of such code and, most importantly, how to use it in face of the current lack of a standardized clinical/diagnostic assessment of sarcopenia.

Evaluation component	Questions	Scoring
Strength	How much difficulty do you have in lifting and carrying 10 pounds?	None = 0Some = 1A lot or unable = 2
Assistance with walking	How much difficulty do you have walking across a room?	None = 0Some = 1A lot, use aids, or unable = 2
Rising from a chair	How much difficulty do you have transferring from a chair or bed?	None = 0Some = 1A lot or unable without help = 2
Climbing stairs	How much difficulty do you have climbing a flight of 10 stairs?	None = 0Some = 1A lot or unable = 2
Falls	How many times have you fallen in the past year?	None = 01 to 3 falls = 14 or more falls = 2

Table 3. SARC-F scale: scores of 4 or more indicate sarcopenia [54].

2.5. Biomarkers and outcomes for sarcopenia

The most basic biomarkers (functional, biological, or imaging-related) that can be utilized in clinical trials of sarcopenia and considered the most reliable and promising to evaluate age-related changes of skeletal muscle have been discussed and recommended. **Table 4** summarizes information on these proposed biomarkers for sarcopenia research. In addition, the measurement of motor unit number index, which can be used to assess the number and the size of the motor units is a very important biomarker as loss of motor unit input to muscle is a significant cause of sarcopenia in at least half of older individuals [22, 48, 62].

In view of the molecular mechanisms involved in the pathogenesis of sarcopenia, potential emerging sarcopenia biomarkers have been discussed. Normal muscle mass and function maintenance are thought to be dependent on the dynamic balance between the positive regulators of muscle growth such as bone morphogenetic proteins (BMPs), brain-derived neurotrophic factor (BDNF), follistatin (FST) and irisin, and negative regulators including TGFβ, myostatin, activins A and B, and growth and differentiation factor-15 (GDF-15). The authors hypothesized that the shift in this balance to muscle growth inhibitors, along with increased expression of the C-terminal agrin fragment (CAF) associated with age-dependent neuromuscular junction (NMJ) dysfunction, as well as skeletal muscle-specific troponin T (sTnT), a key component of contractile structure, is a main mechanism underlying sarcopenia pathogenesis. Based on these facts, the molecular elements mentioned above are proposed as emerging sarcopenia biomarkers [63].

As indicated previously the EWGSOP recommends the use of physical performance, muscle strength, and muscle mass as the primary treatment outcome indicators for sarcopenia intervention trials. Activities of daily living, quality of life, metabolic and biochemical markers, inflammatory markers, global impression of change by subject or physician, falls, admission to nursing home or hospital, social support, and mortality are recommended by that group as secondary outcome indicators [9].

The AWGS recommends the following approach in outcome indicators assessment for sarcopenia research. This approach targets the measurement of changes in two ways over a period. The AWGS also recommends the use of fear of falling and incontinence as outcome indicators for sarcopenia research [15]:

- **a.** Static approach: Activities of daily living, quality of life, inflammatory markers, falls, frailty issues, mobility disorders, admission to hospitals, admission to long-term care facilities, and mortality.
- **b.** Dynamic approach: Changes in muscle mass, muscle strength, physical performance, frailty status, instrumental activities of daily living, and activities of daily living.

Finally, the importance of tapping into the patient experience, identifying the linkage between clinical measures and patient reports, and building self-report into submissions for drug

		Inclusion-exclusion criteria	Baseline evaluation	Endpoint assessment
Muscle function	Physical performance measures	+++	+++	+++
	Muscle strength measures	+++	+++	+++
	Disability	+++	+++	+++
Muscle mass	Anthropometry	+	-	-
	Bioelectrical impedance analysis	+	-	-
	Dual energy X-ray absorptiometry	+++	++	++
	Computerized tomography	++	+++	+++
	Magnetic resonance imaging	++	+++	+++
	Echography	++	++	++
	Electrical impedance myography	+	++	++
Biological confounders (mechanisms) Note: The importance of all these biomarkers in the evaluation of sarcopenia will largely depend on the study hypotheses, the specific aims, and/or the target population	Inflammation	++	++	++
	Oxidative damage	++	++	++
	Antioxidants	++	++	++
	Apoptosis	+	++	++
	Nutritional parameters (albumin, hemoglobin, urinary creatinine, others)	+++	++	++
	Hormones (dehydroepiandrosterone, testosterone, insulin-like growth factor-1, others)	++	++	++

- not recommended for this use; + may be of use; but severely limited; ++ suitable for this use; +++ recommended for this use.

Table 4. Potential biomarkers for clinical trials on sarcopenia [48].

approval to the HHS FDA have been a matter of discussion among experts. Work is ongoing with questionnaires focusing on patient-reported outcome measures in sarcopenia, but validation is pending [64]. In addition, the HHS FDA conducted on April 06, 2017, a public meeting on patient-focused drug development for sarcopenia. The HHS FDA is interested in obtaining patient perspectives on the impact of sarcopenia on daily life and patient views on treatment approaches.

3. Integrating muscle quality in efforts to define sarcopenia and muscle quality in the context of skeletal muscle function deficit

Aging is associated with significant changes in body composition, gradual increase in total body fat during adulthood followed by a loss later in life, and remodeling of fat distribution. The latter involves an increase in inter/intramuscular and visceral fat, and a gradual loss of subcutaneous fat. Weight gain and weight loss overtime have been linked with preserved muscle mass and accelerated muscle atrophy, respectively. Both, however, are associated with increased fat infiltration of muscles. Adverse health and functional outcomes including the development of insulin resistance and impaired mechanical muscle function seem to be concurrently or independently associated with the aging changes mentioned above. Evidence suggests that the correlation between "muscle quantity" and "muscle function" (e.g., muscle strength) is relatively weak, and in contrast to muscle strength, muscle mass has been demonstrated to be a poor predictor of functional limitation, gait speed, and even mortality. It is, in fact, becoming increasingly clear that muscle quality (force per unit of muscle mass) and neural function play a key role in the development of mobility disability and that a new endpoint incorporating these aspects in addition to muscle mass and strength might be useful.

3.1. Defining muscle quality: the need for a standardized assessment

Multiple factors are known to underpin muscle quality and determine the changes in muscle function and mobility later in life. Those who conduct sarcopenia-related research have usually used relative force production (ratio of peak force and a measure of body size, regional lean body mass, or cross-sectional area) as the favored approach to characterizing muscle quality [65, 66]. Emerging definitions of muscle quality, however, call for its expansion to include muscle composition, metabolism, aerobic capacity, insulin resistance, fat infiltration, fibrosis, and neural activation [67], all of which easily correlate with the concept of SMFD. The term muscle quality allows investigators to explore aspects of SMFD beyond the construct of age-related decline of lean body mass [6]. While the meaning of muscle quality is linked to the primary functions of the skeletal muscle, it can be expanded to include both physiology and pathophysiology [8]. There is also a need to develop and adopt a standardized assessment of muscle quality. In doing so, it is essential to consider the complexity of the skeletal muscle tissue and its physiologic roles that include not only movement via force production, but also metabolism through its maintenance of glucose/insulin homeostasis and amino acid storage, thermoregulation, and autocrine/paracrine/endocrine signaling via myokine production. This expanded view of muscle quality is essential to improve our understanding of SMFD [8].

A preliminary conceptual model for the assessment of muscle quality has been proposed, built on skeletal muscle primary physiologic functions. This conceptual model is categorized in domains that have both clinical and research applications. The domains are the following: (A) force production; (B) metabolism (endocrine, neurologic, orthopedic); (C) thermoregulation; and (D) signalling/myokine production. No endpoint(s) have been identified as best to establish the quantitative profile of muscle quality. Similarly, no standardized approaches to endpoint measures have been recommended that can be linked to any of the domains above. None have been identified as the most strongly associated with mechanisms controlling muscle function or with predicting mobility status and mortality in older adults. Muscle quality seen under this perspective provides the advantage of going beyond the strict lean body mass-driven assessment approach to sarcopenia research. Ongoing research focusing on the local and systemic effects of fat infiltration of muscles and on the emerging methods to quantify changes in muscle composition and function is reflecting this perspective [8].

3.2. Factors underpinning muscle quality

Below is a brief discussion on the multiple factors underpinning muscle quality, all of which fall under the proposed domains for assessing muscle quality. The concept of muscle quality cannot be represented by a single endpoint measure, but the factors that affect muscle quality are frequent targets of measurement used to characterize skeletal muscle. The discussion provided in this section does not enclose every assessment target, but addresses common examples of factors that may serve as measures for basic, translational, and clinical trials related to muscle quality and sarcopenia or muscle quality in the context of SMFD. Factors intrinsic to skeletal muscles are crucial for function and homeostasis. Factors extrinsic to skeletal muscles considerably impact muscle activity and muscle mass building and maintenance. Both intrinsic and extrinsic factors affect net force production.

3.2.1. Muscle characteristics/architecture

Muscle characteristics include size, fiber type, and contractile components. Fiber type and number determine muscle size. Muscle cross-sectional area has a positive relationship with muscle strength in young lean individuals, while smaller and weaker muscles are usually seen in older adults. Muscle cross-sectional area and lower limb skeletal muscle volume are associated with greater fat mass in both men and women [68], likely due to intermuscular lipid or noncontractile components. There are three types of muscle fibers as identified in **Table 5** [68]. The loss of types I and IIb muscle fibers associated with aging is attributed to changes in activity and consequent disuse and denervation. Conflicting literature demonstrates no link at all or a link between advanced age and changes in muscle fiber composition with gradual loss of type IIb muscle fibers [69]. Conflicting limited evidence is also seen in older adults in relation to changes in muscle fiber type, muscle cross-sectional area, and strength. Contractile properties of types I and II muscle fibers at the single fiber level seem to be maintained independent of the presence of mobility limitation [70], but again, evidence is conflicting. It has been suggested that maximal shortening velocity is lower in single fibers from older adults because of changes in myosin heavy chain isoform distribution to a more hybrid pattern. A

Type I	Type IIa	Type IIb
Predominantly generate energy via oxidative pathways for prolonged low force production.Relatively small cross-sectional area compared to type IIb fibers, but have greater oxidative capacity.Recruited during low intensity activities of daily living (e.g., walking)	Capable of generating energy via oxidative and nonoxidative pathways	Predominantly generate energy via nonoxidative pathways for rapid high force production.Recruited during high intensity activity

Table 5. Types and functions of skeletal muscle fibers [68].

lower maximal shortening velocity in myosin heavy chain has been observed in types I and IIa fiber of older adults including those who are very active. The evidence, however, is debatable because of limitations with study power and potential confounding with physical activity. Preservation of single muscle fiber contractile properties with age is thought to imply that differences in skeletal muscle function are related to quantitative changes in muscle fiber size or number rather than qualitative changes in the muscle's contractile properties [68].

Fiber arrangement within a muscle (e.g., parallel or pennation pattern) will determine fascicle length, pennation angle, and cross-sectional area, all of which can change with age. Older adults 70–81 years of age are reported to have smaller fascicle length and pennation angle (compared to younger adults 27–42 years) of the gastrocnemius medialis [71], but several weeks of bed rest have not resulted in changes in the pennation angle of the vastus lateralis muscle. Nevertheless, modest improvements in muscle architecture are reported to be possible with 4–5 weeks of resistance training. Changes in muscle architecture also appear to precede changes in muscle size in young healthy adults.

Cross-sectional assessment of skeletal muscles provides relevant information on muscle function because both individual muscle fiber diameter and cross-sectional diameter of the whole muscle are associated with strength. Force production is related to the architectural characteristics of the skeletal muscle including muscle fiber length and arrangement in relation to the direction of the force produced by the whole muscle. Thus, both cross-sectional and longitudinal orientation of measures of skeletal muscles are valuable in the assessment of the size-strength relationship and the identification of age-related differences in muscle strength per size. Sarcomeric changes in myofibrillar disorder, Z-line streaming, and dilatation in aged skeletal muscle have been observed in electron microscopic analysis. The characteristics/architectural changes highlighted above have been combined in a composite measure—physiological cross-sectional area (PCSA)—to reflect both strength and change in strength in leg extension [8].

Muscle weakness is attributed to changes in muscle composition, muscle contractile quality, and neural activation [72]. However, measures of muscle composition, size, and architecture generally do not consider the neural input into fibers, which dictate contraction potential and force production. Strength measures are an important indicator of muscle performance and show the ability to change in response to a variety of interventions to tackle sarcopenia and frailty in older women with clinically relevant muscle weakness independent of the presence of low muscle mass [73]. Muscle strength and size have been used as a single measure of muscle quality known as "relative strength," reflecting the expression of muscle force production relative to muscle or body size. It has been suggested that strength per unit of muscle tissue may serve as a better indicator of age-related differences in muscle quality prior to changes in lean tissue mass [74]. A novel functional metric—muscle quality index—estimates muscle power from body anthropometrics and timed chair raises; it has been found to have higher reliability and greater responsiveness following a resistance exercise regimen in older adults, compared to other functional measures (e.g., gait speed, grip strength, the get-up and go test, etc.) [75].

3.2.2. *Muscle aerobic capacity*

Muscle quality and function in both middle-aged and older adults are determined by metabolic characteristics of the muscle. Aerobic capacity reflects the maximal ability to use oxygen (cardiovascular adaptation to transport oxygen; within skeletal muscle adaptation to use oxygen) in response to energy demands of physical activity. Evidence shows that aerobic capacity declines at an accelerated rate after age 50, and is a strong predictor of mobility assessed by gait speed in older adults. Evidence from cross-sectional muscle analyses from healthy men and women (18–90 years) reveals that mitochondrial DNA, mRNA abundance, and energy (ATP) production diminishes with age. Both skeletal muscle mitochondrial capacity and efficiency, and whole body peak aerobic capacity have been linked to gait speed [68, 76, 77].

The progressive decline in mitochondrial function observed in aging results in the accumulation of reactive oxygen species (ROS) generated by the incorporation of a single electron to the oxygen molecule. Specifically, ROS negatively impact muscle quality, playing an extremely important role in all muscle functions, muscle aging, contraction, fatigue, dystrophy or waste [78–80]. Mitochondria are the major producers of ROS, which damage DNA, proteins, and lipids. Animal and human studies have typically shown that aging changes in mitochondria can be reflected by increased mutations in mitochondrial DNA, decreased activity of some mitochondrial enzymes, altered respiration with reduced maximal capacity at least in sedentary individuals, and reduced total mitochondrial content with increased morphological changes. With mitochondrial dynamics altered (e.g., fusion and fission rates, mitochondrially induced apoptosis), net muscle fiber loss and age-related sarcopenia may ensue. Strategies such as exercise and caloric restriction that reduce oxidative damage can improve mitochondrial function. While these strategies may not completely prevent the primary effects of aging, they may help to attenuate the rate of decline [81, 82].

It is also well established that contracting muscles produce both ROS and nitrogen species. Although the sources of oxidant production during exercise continue to be debated, growing evidence suggests that mitochondria are not the dominant source [83]. Regardless of the sources of oxidants in contracting muscles, intense and prolonged exercise can result in oxidative damage to both proteins and lipids in the contracting myocytes. Further, oxidants regulate numerous cell signaling pathways and modulate the expression of many genes. There has been much controversy about measurements of mitochondrial energy production. These controversies may be explained by differences in methodological approaches and whether physical activity is controlled for.

Age-related changes in skeletal muscle mass and composition can result in increased insulin resistance and later to reduced capacity for insulin-mediated glucose disposal. Relative muscle mass in healthy nondiabetic older adults is inversely linked to glucose tolerance and insulin resistance [84]. Muscle strength adjusted for BMI, however, has been reported to be negatively associated with insulin resistance in a large population based study of older women, but not men, after adjustment for confounders. No association between muscle leg strength and insulin resistance in men or women >50 years has been observed in an analysis of the National Health and Nutrition Examination Survey (NHANES) [85]. In some studies, gait speed assessments are found to be inversely associated with insulin resistance, suggesting that insulin resistance may serve as an indicator of poor muscle quality underpinning low levels of physical fitness and poor scores on gait speed tests. Improvement in glucose disposal and skeletal muscle metabolism in older overweight or obese men has been observed over 6 months of both regular aerobic and resistance exercise. Fat infiltration of muscles is also associated with insulin resistance.

3.2.3. *Myosteatosis*

Myosteatosis refers to fat infiltration in skeletal muscle that can lead to large negative clinical effects including poor metabolic and skeletal muscle health, accelerated aging, and impaired longevity. This ectopic fat tissue has become an important factor behind muscle quality and may serve as a predictor of muscle function in older adults. Two modalities of myosteatosis are identified: (1) intermuscular fat, which represents the visible extracellular adipose tissue located beneath the muscle and between and within muscle groups; (2) intramuscular fat or intramyocellular lipids, which represents infiltration within myocytes, i.e., the presence of microscopic lipid droplets used as energy within the muscle. This ectopic fat infiltration increases with aging, seems to act synergistically with sarcopenia and is also present in muscular dystrophies. The biological mechanism underlying increases in myosteatosis with aging in humans remain largely under investigated, with the need to identify and better understand regulatory factors including evidence of senescent cells and cultured cells developing into preadipocytes and fat cells. This is an opportunity for future development of therapies to preserve skeletal muscle health [8, 86, 87].

Individuals with comparable thigh circumference may have distinct muscle function due to the proportion of fat infiltration to contractile elements. In older adults with multimorbidity, intermuscular adipose tissue evaluated by MRI was reported as the strongest predictor of mobility, but strength and quadriceps lean tissue explicated some of the variation in mobility in this study [88]. Increased mobility loss, reflected by decreased six-minute walk distance, decreased gait speed, decreased physical performance, difficulty with repeated chair stands, and slower stair descent and timed get-up and go tests have been reported as the result of myosteatosis effects on muscle metabolism and function [8]. In young healthy persons with 30 days of leg disuse by suspension, myosteatosis was found to increase by 15–20% and exceeded the loss of lean muscles (calf and thigh) [89]. Myosteatosis is also known to lead to the transition of muscle fibers from type II to type I, which result in muscles with impaired contractile capacity and decreased power [90, 91]. It is also suggested that myostetatosis may harm muscle and mobility because fat infiltration leads to changes in muscle fiber orientation.

Proinflammatory cytokines secreted by fat tissue in the skeletal muscle microenvironment may also lead to proteolysis and muscle catabolism [8].

Fat storage and infiltration into muscle may be a marker of metabolic profile. In older adults, intermuscular adipose tissue was found to positively correlate with higher fasting plasma glucose and lower glucose tolerance [92]. Myosteatosis has been linked to insulin resistance and an increased risk of developing type-2 diabetes, hypertension, and dyslipidemia, independent of total body adiposity (measured by BMI or DXA whole body fat). Further investigation, however is still needed on the association of myosteatosis and metabolic disease independent of visceral fat. The metabolic consequences of myosteatosis depend on age, race/ethnicity, aerobic conditioning, sensitivity to insulin, amount of physical activity, and anatomic region. Further investigations are necessary to verify whether myosteatosis acts as a marker of metabolic dysfunction or may have an intermediary modifying role in insulin resistance [8].

Physical activity seems to be able to revert intermuscular fat infiltration. In men 60 years old, six months of aerobic exercise and weight loss decreased intermuscular adipose tissue of the leg and improved fasting plasma glucose and glucose tolerance. Four weeks of an imposed decrease in physical activity due to unilateral lower limb suspension resulted in 15–20% increase in the intermuscular adipose tissue in the thigh and calf, respectively. Strength loss was associated with the increase in the intermuscular adipose tissue, after adjustment for loss of muscle mass and considering initial baseline values.

3.2.4. Muscle fibrosis

Impairment in the muscle repair process can lead to muscle fibrosis, which involves the deposition of collagen and extracellular matrix proteins instead of proteins necessary to repair and restore tissue function. Fibrosis is also seen in different tissues because of extra fat accumulation. The presence of fibrosis in the skeletal muscle of older adults is hypothetical at this point, and further studies are needed to investigate how or whether fibrosis is a factor in muscle quality. Evidence, however, is available indicating that progressive intermuscular adipose tissue infiltration in middle aged or older adults may lead to fibrosis and impairment of muscle function and mobility [68].

3.2.5. Motor units and neuromuscular activation

Other potential factors related to muscle quality in middle and old age include components of the neuromuscular system and neuromuscular activation. Skeletal muscle fibers are organized in bundles of motor units. Each motor unit is innervated by a motor nerve, which connects to an alpha motor-neuron in the spinal cord. Across the lifespan, motor units go through remodeling, denervation and reinnervation. These units are reported to be decreased in the tibialis anterior muscle of men 65 years old and those >80 years compared to younger men (25 years), but the reduced motor unit number was only related to strength in men >80 years [93].

Neuromuscular activation has been proposed as another measure of muscle quality. Impairments in neuromuscular activation affect the rate of force development and muscle power needed for dynamic movements. Improvements in neuromuscular activation generally precede increases in muscle mass in response to resistance training. Neuromuscular activity and acceleration was impaired during dynamic leg extensions in mobility-limited older adults compared to mobile older adults [94]. The rate of neuromuscular activation was significantly associated with physical function scores. Among middle-aged and older adults without mobility limitations, no significant differences in measures of neuromuscular activation were detected. However, whether neuromuscular impairment precedes the development of mobility limitations is still unclear.

3.3. Emerging alternative clinical imaging and other measures of muscle quality

Relatively high costs, limitations with access, and the testing burden associated with invasive techniques are barriers to standardized assessment of muscle quality. The use of routine tissue composition analysis is hampered by the need for further demonstration of its diagnostic value and contribution to both diagnostic and therapeutic decision making. The emerging literature on the effects of age-related increases in intramuscular adipose tissue on muscle performance and metabolism, has led to the development of alternative assessment. Methodological approaches ranging from multifrequency electrical impedance analysis to quantitative diagnostic sonography have been used to characterize skeletal muscle mass and quality in older adults and in those with muscle disease [95]. Noninvasive, high precision, imaging modalities such as MRI has been used to diagnose and assess progression of a number of neuromuscular conditions. Quantitative musculoskeletal diagnostic ultrasound has been proposed as a clinically feasible means of characterizing muscle structure. Ultrasound has been shown to be highly reliable for assessing cross-sectional areas of large individual human muscle and particularly useful in mobility-impaired individuals who cannot be easily transported to scanners (CT, MRI) [48].

Electrical impedance myography (EIM) is another promising technique based on the surface application and measurement of a high frequency, low intensity electrical current applied to specific muscles. It detects changes in the conductivity and permittivity of skeletal muscles caused by alterations in muscle composition and structure. It has been found repeatable and sensitive to skeletal muscle changes in persons with amyotrophic lateral sclerosis. Mass isopotomer distribution analysis based on the evaluation of protein and proteome synthesis rate is obtained by heavy water labelling; it is a very promising approach due to the wide spectrum of proteins analysed [48].

The success of emerging alternative imaging measures of muscle quality relies on their easy-to-use in diverse clinical settings and ability to discriminate between older adults with and without sarcopenia, identify those at risk for impaired muscle performance, and those who can benefit from preventive and therapeutic interventions. A symposium report on "The Need for Standardized Assessment of Muscle Quality in Skeletal Muscle Function Deficit and Other Aging-Related Muscle Dysfunctions" provides a good insight on these emerging approaches [8].

4. Conclusion: clinical relevance and research opportunities

Aging muscles and other aging-related muscle dysfunctions present with a functional deficit in one or more elements or components of SMFD involving muscle mass, muscle strength or muscle quality. To further characterize SMFD, additional investigation and understanding of the factors behind changes in muscle quality with aging are needed. The concept of muscle quality is critical and should be expanded beyond muscle strength or power per unit of muscle mass, to encompass muscle aerobic capacity and other key factors which closely relate to mobility and other important activities of daily living. Assessment or diagnostics tools sensitive to small changes within skeletal muscle that precede a decline in mass, strength and function can enable preventative steps to maintain healthy muscles. Diagnostic ultrasound and other assessment methods continue to be developed for characterizing muscle pathology, and enhanced sonography using sensors to provide user feedback and improve reliability is currently the subject of ongoing investigation and development. Measures of relative muscle force (e.g., specific force or grip strength adjusted for body size) have been proposed as methods to assess changes in muscle quality. Performance-based assessments of muscle power via timed tests of function and body size estimates are associated with lower extremity muscle strength and may be responsive to age-related changes in muscle quality. The challenge remains to reach a consensus on diagnostic criteria, tools, and consistent methodological approaches for assessing or measuring components of SMFD that are practical in a community or clinical setting. These should be considered priority for the scientific community and health care providers.

To date, no studies have assessed exclusively and concurrently aging-related changes in muscle mass, muscle strength, muscle function, and muscle quality. Analyses of pooled data from large studies on aging with measures of muscle mass and strength still face numerous methodological challenges. As highlighted by experts in the field, future well-designed large prospective studies of interventions to improve muscle mass, muscle strength, muscle function, and muscle quality can observe age-related changes in skeletal muscles over time and generate the evidence to help identify individuals that will benefit from interventions to prevent or treat these changes.

From the public health perspective, further characterization of SMFD is very relevant to several ongoing therapeutic developments. For example, we already know that resistance exercise is the primary therapeutic strategy to prevent and reverse sarcopenia; aerobic exercise also has a therapeutic role, as demonstrated by the Lifestyle Interventions and Independence for Elders (LIFE); vitamin D has been shown to enhance muscle function in persons with low muscle function; and evidence that leucine-enriched essential amino acid supplementation will increase muscle mass and potentially function. Limited evidence, however, suggests that testosterone increases muscle mass and strength, and potentially function in older adults with hypogonadism, but its safety remains unclear. Drug development efforts with selective androgen receptor modulators (SARMs) are promising in increasing muscle mass and stair climbing. Ongoing research is also investigating numerous antibodies that modulate myostatin and the activin II receptor, as well as ghrelin agonists, which increase food intake and release growth hormone [7].

The potential impact of clearly addressing SMFD and properly integrating muscle mass, muscle strength, and muscle quality is critical to future therapeutic development to help older adults with muscle dysfunctions maintain independence and quality of life.

Author details

Rosaly Correa-de-Araujo

Address all correspondence to: rosaly.correa-de-araujo@nih.gov

Division of Geriatrics and Clinical Gerontology, National Institute on Aging, National Institutes of Health, U.S. Department of Health and Human Services, Bethesda, MD, USA

References

[1] Rosenberg I. Summary comments: Epidemiological and methodological problems in determining nutritional status of older persons. American Journal of Clinical Nutrition. 1989;**50**:1231-1233

[2] Baumgartner RN, Koehler KM, Gallagher D, et al. Epidemiology of sarcopenia among the elderly in New Mexico. American Journal of Epidemiology. 1998;**17**:755-763

[3] Mitchell WK, Williams J, Atherton P, Larvin W, Land J, Narici M. Sarcopenia, dynapenia, and the impact of advancing age on human skeletal muscle size and strength: A quantitative review. Frontiers in Physiology. 2012;**3**:260. DOI: 10.3389/fphys.2012.00260

[4] Roman D, Mahoney K, Mohamadi A. Sarcopenia: What's in a name? Journal of the American Medical Directors Association. 2013;**14**:80-82.

[5] Correa-de-Araujo R. Skeletal muscle function deficit. In Update in Gerontology and Geriatrics. All India Institute of Medical Science (AIIMS). BUKPRINT. New Delhi, India. pp 106-113. 2015.

[6] Correa-de-Araujo R, Hadley E. Skeletal muscle function deficit: A new terminology to embrace the evolving concepts of sarcopenia and age-related muscle dysfunction. Journals of Gerontology. Series A: Biological Sciences and Medical Sciences. 2014;**5**:591-594

[7] Morley JE, Anker SD. Prevalence, incidence, and clinical impact of sarcopenia: Facts, numbers, and epidemiology—Update 2014. Journal of Cachexia, Sarcopenia and Muscle. 2014;**3**:253-259

[8] Correa-De-Araujo R, Harris-Love MO, Miljkovic I, Fragala MS, Anthony BW, Manini TM. The need for standardized assessment of muscle quality in skeletal muscle function deficit and other aging-related muscle dysfunctions: A symposium report. Frontiers in Physiology. 2017;**8**:87. DOI: 10.3389/fphys.2017.00087

[9] Cruz-Jentoft AJ, Baeyens JP, Bauer JM, et al. Sarcopenia: European consensus on definition and diagnosis: Report of the European Working Group on Sarcopenia in Older People. Age Ageing. 2010;**39**:412-423

[10] Morley JE, Abbatecola AM, Argiles JM, et al. Sarcopenia with limited mobility: An international consensus. Journal of the American Medical Directors Association. 2011;**12**:403-409

[11] Fielding RA, Vellas B, Evans WJ, et al. Sarcopenia: An undiagnosed condition in older adults. Current consensus definition: Prevalence, etiology, and consequences. International Working Group on Sarcopenia. Journal of the American Medical Directors Association. 2011;**12**:249-256

[12] Muscaritoli M, Anker SD, Argiles J, et al. Consensus definition of sarcopenia, cachexia and pre-cachexia: Joint document elaborated by Special Interest Groups (SIG) "cachexia-anorexia in chronic wasting diseases" and "nutrition in geriatrics." Clinical Nutrition. 2010;**29**:154-159

[13] Morley JE. Frailty: A time for action. European Geriatric Medicine. 2013;**4**:215-216

[14] Dam TT, Peters KW, Fragala M, Cawthon PM, Harris TB, McLean R, Shardell M,Alley DE, Kenny A, Ferrucci L, Guralnik J, Kiel DP, Kritchevsky S, Vassileva MT, Studenski S. An evidence-based comparison of operational criteria for the presence of sarcopenia. Journals of Gerontology. Series A: Biological Sciences and Medical Sciences. 2014;**69**(5):584-590

[15] Chen LK, Liu LK, Woo J, Assantachai P, Auyeung TW, Bahyah KS, et al. Sarcopenia in Asia: Consensus report of the Asian Working Group for Sarcopenia. Journal of the American Medical Directors Association. 2014;**15**:95-101

[16] Michel JP. Sarcopenia: There is a need for some steps forward. Journal of the American Medical Directors Association. 2014;**15**:379-380

[17] Studenski et al. The FNIH Sarcopenia Project: Rationale, study description, conference recommendations, and final estimates. Journal of Gerontology. Series A: Biological Sciences and Medical. 2014;**5**:547-558

[18] Cederholm T, Morley JE. Sarcopenia: The new definitions. Current Opinion in Clinical Nutrition & Metabolic Care. 2015;**18**:1-4

[19] Barbat-Artigas S, Rolland Y, Vellas B, Aubertin-Leheudre M. Muscle quantity is not synonymous with muscle quality. Journal of the American Medical Directors Association. 2013;**14**:852.e1-852.e7

[20] Morley JE, Cao L. Rapid screening for sarcopenia. Journal of Cachexia, Sarcopenia and Muscle. 2015;**6**:312-314

[21] Alchin DR. Sarcopenia: Describing rather than defining a condition. Journal of Cachexia, Sarcopenia and Muscle. 2014;**5**:265-268

[22] Drey M, Krieger B, Sieber CC, Bauer JM, Hettwer S, Bertsch T, et al. Motoneuron loss is associated with sarcopenia. Journal of the American Medical Directors Association. 2014;**15**:435-439

[23] Barbat-Artigas S, Pion CH, Leduc-Gaudet JP, Rolland Y, Aubertin-Leheudre M. Exploring the role of muscle mass, obesity, and age in the relationship between muscle quality and physical function. Journal of the American Medical Directors Association. 2014;**15:**303.e13-303.e 20

[24] Kim M, Kim H. Accuracy of segmental multi-frequency bioelectrical impedance analysis for assessing whole-body and appendicular fat mass and lean soft tissue mass in frail women aged 75 years and older. European Journal of Clinical Nutrition. 2013;**67**:395e400

[25] Janssen I, Heymsfield SB, Ross R. Low relative skeletal muscle mass (sarcopenia) in older persons is associated with functional impairment and physical disability. Journal of the American Geriatrics Society. 2002;**50**:889-896

[26] Alley DE, Shardell MD, Peters KW, McLean RR, Dam TT, Kenny AM, Fragala MS,Harris TB, Kiel DP, Guralnik JM, Ferrucci L, Kritchevsky SB, Studenski SA,Vassileva MT, Cawthon PM. Grip strength cutpoints for the identification of clinically relevant weakness. Journal of Gerontology. Series A: Biological Sciences and Medical Sciences. 2014;**69**(5):559-566

[27] Cawthon PM, Peters KW, Shardell MD, McLean RR, Dam TT, Kenny AM, Fragala MS,Harris TB, Kiel DP, Guralnik JM, Ferrucci L, Kritchevsky SB, Vassileva MT,Studenski SA, Alley DE. Cutpoints for low appendicular lean mass that identify older adults with clinically significant weakness. Journal of Gerontology. Series A: Biological Sciences and Medical Sciences. 2014;**69**(5):567-575

[28] McLean RR, Shardell MD, Alley DE, et al. Criteria for clinically relevant weakness and low lean mass and their longitudinal association with incident mobility impairment and mortality: The Foundation for the National Institutes of Health (FNIH) Sarcopenia Project. Journal of Gerontology. Series A: Biological Sciences and Medical Sciences. 2014;**5**:576-583

[29] Lee WJ, Liu LK, Peng LN, Lin MH, Chen LK, ILAS Research Group. Comparisons of sarcopenia defined by IWGS and EWGSOP criteria among older people: Results from the I-Lan longitudinal aging study. Journal of the American Medical Directors Association. 2013;**14**:528.e1-528.e7

[30] Patel HP, Al-Shanti N, Davies LC, Barton SJ, Grounds MD, Tellam RL, et al. Lean mass, muscle strength and gene expression in community dwelling older men: Findings from the Hertfordshire sarcopenia study (HSS). Calcified Tissue International. 2014;**95**(4):308-316

[31] Yamada M, Nishiguchi S, Fukutani N, Tanigawa T, Yukutake T, Kayama H, et al. Prevalence of sarcopenia in community-dwelling Japanese older adults. Journal of the American Medical Directors Association. 2013;**14**:911-915

[32] Legrand D, Vaes B, Matheï C, Swine C, Degryse JM. The prevalence of sarcopenia in very old individuals according to the European consensus definition: Insights from the BELFRAIL study. Age Ageing. 2013;**42**:727-734

[33] Landi F, Liperoti R, Fusco D, Mastropaolo S, Quattrociocchi D, Proia A, et al. Prevalence and risk factors of sarcopenia among nursing home older residents. Journals of Gerontology. Series A: Biological Sciences and Medical Sciences. 2012;**67**:48-55

[34] Landi F, Liperoti R, Fusco D, Mastropaolo S, Quattrociocchi D, Proia A, et al. Sarcopenia and mortality among older nursing home residents. Journal of the American Medical Directors Association. 2012;**13**:121-126

[35] Kim JH, Lim S, Choi SH, Kim KM, Yoon JW, Kim KW, et al. Sarcopenia: An independent predictor of mortality in community dwelling older Korean men. Journal of Gerontology. Series A: Biological Sciences and Medical Sciences. 2014;**69**(10):1244-1252

[36] Vetrano DL, Landi F, Volpato S, Corsonello A, Meloni E, Bernabei R, et al. Association of sarcopenia with short- and long-term mortality in older adults admitted to acute care wards: Results from the CRIME study. Journal of Gerontology. Series A: Biological Sciences and Medical Sciences. 2014;**69**:1154-1161

[37] Wu IC, Lin CC, Hsiung CA, et al. Epidemiology of sarcopenia among community-dwelling older adults in Taiwan: A pooled analysis for a broader adoption of sarcopenia assessments. Geriatrics & Gerontology International. 2014;**14**(Suppl 1):52-60

[38] Tanimoto Y, Watanabe M, Sun W, Sugiura Y, Hayashida I, Kusabiraki T, et al. Sarcopenia and falls in community-dwelling elderly subjects in Japan: Defining sarcopenia according to criteria of the European Working Group on Sarcopenia in Older People. Journal of the American Medical Directors Association. 2010;**11**:391-396

[39] Da Silva AT, de Oliveira Duarte YA, Ferreira Santos JL, Wong R, Lebrão ML. Sarcopenia according to the European Working Group on Sarcopenia in Older People (EWGSOP) versus dynapenia as a risk factor for disability in the elderly. The Journal of Nutrition Health and Aging. 2014;**18**:547-553

[40] Malmstrom TK, Miller DK, Herning MM, Morley JE. Low appendicular skeletal muscle mass (ASM) with limited mobility and poor health outcomes in middle-aged African Americans. Journal of Cachexia, Sarcopenia and Muscle. 2013;**4**:179-186

[41] Duren DL, Sherwood RJ, Czerwinski SA, Lee M, Choh AC, Siervogel RM, Chumlea WC. Body composition methods: Comparisons and interpretation. Journal of Diabetes Science and Technology. 2008;**2**(6):1139-1146

[42] Janssen I, Heymsfield SB, Baumgartner RN, Ross R. Estimation of skeletal muscle mass by bioelectrical impedance analysis. Journal of Applied Physiology. 2000;**89**:465e471

[43] Chien MY, Huang TY, Wu YT. Prevalence of sarcopenia estimated using a bioelectrical impedance analysis prediction equation in community-dwelling elderly people in Taiwan. Journal of the American Geriatrics Society. 2008;**56**:1710e1715

[44] Nigam P, Misra A, Colles SL. Comparison of DEXA-derived body fat measurement to two race-specific bioelectrical impedance equations in healthy Indians. Diabetology & Metabolic Syndrome. 2013;**7**:72-77

[45] Mijnarends DM, Meijers JM, Halfens RJ, et al. Validity and reliability of tools tomeasure muscle mass, strength, and physical performance in community dwelling older people: A systematic review. Journal of the American Medical Directors Association. 2013;**14**:170-178

[46] Yamada Y, Watanabe Y, Ikenaga M, et al. Comparison of single- or multi-frequency bioelectrical impedance analysis and spectroscopy for assessment of appendicular skeletal muscle in the elderly. Journal of Applied Physiology. 2013;**115**:812-818

[47] Baracos V, Caserotti P, Earthman CP, Fields D, Gallagher D, Hall KD, Heymsfield SB, Muller MJ, Rose AN, Pichard C, Redman LM, Shen W, Shepherd JA, Thomas D. Advances in the science and application of body composition. Journal of Parenteral and Enteral Nutrition. 2012;**36**(1):96-107

[48] Cesari M, Fielding RA, Pahor M, Goodpaster B, Hellerstein M, van Kan GA, et al. Biomarkers of sarcopenia in clinical trials recommendations from the International Working Group on Sarcopenia. Journal of Cachexia, Sarcopenia and Muscle. 2012;**3**:181-190

[49] Kelly TL, Wilson KER, Heymsfield SB. Dual X-ray absorptiometry body composition reference values from NHANES. PLoS One. 2009;**4**(9):e7038

[50] Shepherd JA, Fan B, Lu Y, Wu XP, Wacker WK, Ergun DL, Levine MA. A multinational study to develop universal standardization of whole-body bone density and composition using GE Healthcare Lunar and Hologic DXA systems. Journal of Bone and Mineral Research. 2012;**27**(10):2208-2216

[51] Malouf J, DiGregorio S, Del Rio L, Torres F, Marin AM, Farrerons J, Herrera S, Domingo P. Fat tissue measurements by dual-energy X-ray absorptiometry: Cross-calibration of 3 different fan-bean instruments. Journal of Clinical Densitometry: Assessment of Musculoskeletal Health. 2013;**16**(2):212-222

[52] Fan B, Shepherd JA, Levine MA, Steinberg D, Wacker W, Barden HS, Ergun D, Wu XP. National Health and Nutrition Examination Survey whole-body dual-energy X-ray absorptiometry reference data for GE lunar systems. Journal of Clinical Densitometry: Assessment of Musculoskeletal Health. 2014;**17**(3):344-377

[53] Kanis JA, McCloskey E, Johansson H, oden A, Leslie WD. FRAX® with and without bone mineral density. Calcified Tissue International. 2012;**90**:1-13

[54] Malmstrom TK, Morley JE. SARC-F: A simple questionnaire to rapidly diagnose sarcopenia. Journal of the American Medical Directors Association. 2013;**14**:531-532

[55] Morley JE, Malmstrom TK. Can sarcopenia be diagnosed without measurements? European Geriatric Medicine. 2014;**5**:291-293

[56] Alliance for Aging Research. Available from: http://aginginmotion.org/news/2388-2/ [Accessed: January 23, 2017]

[57] Rantanen T, Guralnik JM, Foley D, Masaki K, Leveille S, Curb JD, et al. Midlife hand grip strength as a predictor of old age disability. Journal of the American Medical Association. 1999;**281**:558-560

[58] Szulc P, Beck TJ, Marchand F, Delmas PD. Low skeletal muscle mass is associated with poor structural parameters of bone and impaired balance in elderly men—The MINOS study. Journal of Bone and Mineral Research. 2005;**20**:721-721

[59] Ling CH, Taekema D, deCraen AJ, Gussekloo J, Westendorp RG, Maier AB. Handgrip strength and mortality in the oldest old population: The Leiden 85-plus study. Canadian Medical Association Journal. 2010;**182**:429-435

[60] Landi F, Liperoti R, Russo A, Giovannini S, Tosato M, Capoluongo E, et al. Sarcopenia as a risk factor for falls in elderly individuals: Results from the ilSIRENTE study. Clinical Nutrition. 2012;**31**:652-658

[61] Landi F, Cruz-Jentoft AJ, Liperoti R, Russo A, Giovannini S, Tosato M, et al. Sarcopenia and mortality risk in frail older persons aged 80 years and older: Results from ilSIR-ENTE study. Age Ageing. 2013;**42**:203-209

[62] Scharf G, Heineke J. Finding good biomarkers for sarcopenia. Journal of Cachexia, Sarcopenia and Muscle. 2012;**3**:145-148

[63] Kalinkovich A, Livshits G. Sarcopenia—The search for emerging biomarkers. Ageing Research Reviews. 2015;**22**:58-71

[64] Evans CJ, Chiou CF, Fitzgerald KA, William WJ, Ferral BR, Dale W, et al. Development of a new patient-reported outcome measure in sarcopenia. Journal of the American Medical Directors Association. 2011;**12**:226-233

[65] Cawthon PM, Fox KM, Gandra SR, Delmonico MJ, Chiou C-F, Anthony MS, et al. Do muscle mass, muscle density, strength, and physical function similarly influence risk of hospitalization in older adults? Journal of the American Geriatrics Society. 2009;**57**:1411-1419. DOI: 10.1111/j.1532-5415.2009.02366.x

[66] Kennis E, Verschueren S, Van Roie E, Thomis M, Lefevre J, Delecluse C. Longitudinal impact of aging on muscle quality in middle-aged men. Age **(Dordrecht, Netherlands)**. 2014;**36**:9689. DOI: 10.1007/s11357-014-9689-1

[67] Lafortuna Cl, Tresoldi D, Rizzo G. Influence of body adiposity on structural characteristics of skeletal muscle in men and women. Clinical Physiology and Functional Imaging. 2014;**34**:47-55

[68] McGregor RA, Cameron-Smith D, Poppitt SD. It is not just muscle mass: A review of muscle quality, composition and metabolism during ageing as determinants of muscle function and mobility later in life. Longevity & Healthspan. 2014;**3**:9

[69] Verdjik LB, Snijders T, Beelen M, Savelberg HHCM, Meijer K, Kuipers H, Van Loon LIC. Characteristics of muscle fiber type are predictive of skeletal muscle mass and strength in elderly men. Journal of the American Geriatrics Society. 2010;**58**:2069-2075

[70] Reid KF, Pasha E, Doros G, Clark DI, Patten C, Phillips EM, Frontera WH, Fielding RA. Longitudinal decline of lower extremity muscle power in healthy and mobility limited older adults: Influence of muscle mass, strength, composition, neuromuscular activation and single fiber contractile properties. European Journal of Applied Physiology. 2014;**114**:29-39

[71] Stenroth L, Peitonen J, Cronin NJ, Sipila S, Finni T. Age-related differences in Achilles tendon properties and triceps surae muscle architecture in vivo. Journal of Applied Physiology. 2012;**113**:1537-1544

[72] Clark BC, Manini TM. Functional consequences of sarcopenia and dynapenia in the elderly. Current Opinion in Clinical Nutrition & Metabolic Care. 2010;**13**:271-276. DOI: 10.1097/MCO.0b013e328337819e

[73] Fragala MS, Dam TTL,Barber V, Judge JO, Studenski SA, Cawthon PM et al. Strength and function response to clinical interventions of older women categorized by weakness and low lean mass using classifications from the Foundation for the National Institutes of Health sarcopenia project. The Journal of Gerontology. Series A, Biological Sciences and Medical Sciences. 2015;**70**:202-209. DOI: 10.1093/Gerona/glu110

[74] Francis P, Toomey C, McCormack W, Lyons M, Jakeman P. Measurement of maximal isometric torque and muscle quality of the knee extensors and flexors in healthy 50-70-year-old women. Clinical Physiology and Functional Imaging. 2016 Jan 7. doi:10.1111/cpf.12332. [Epub ahead of print] PubMed PMID: 26749301

[75] Fragala MS, Fukuda DH, Stout JR, Townsend JR, Emerson NS, Boone CH et al. Muscle quality index improves with resistance exercise training in older adults. Experimental Gerontology. 2014;**53**:1-6. DOI: 10.1016/j.exger.2014.01.037

[76] Fiser WM, Hays NP, Rogers SC, Kajkenowa O, Williams AE, Evans CM, Evan WJ. Energetics of walking in elderly people: Factors related to gait speed. The Journal of Gerontology. Series A, Biological Sciences and Medical Sciences. 2010;**65**:1332-1337

[77] Coen PM, Jubrias SA, Distefano G, Amati F, Mackey DC, Glynn NW, Manini TM, Wohigemuth SE, Leeuwenburgh C, Cummings SR, Newman AB, Ferruci L, Toledo FGS, Shankland E, Conley KE, Goodpaster BH. Skeletal muscle mitochondrial energetics are associated with maximal aerobic capacity and walking speed in older adults. The Journal of Gerontology. Series A, Biological Sciences and Medical Sciences. 2013;**68**:447-455

[78] Zuo L, Hallman AH, Yousif M K, Chien MT. Oxidative stress, respiratory muscle dysfunction, and potential therapeutics in chronic obstructive pulmonary disease. Frontiers in Biology. 2012;**7**:506-513. DOI: 10.1007/s11515-012-1251-x

[79] Zuo L, Shiah A, Roberts WJ, Chien MT, Wagner PD, Hogan MC. Low PO_2 conditions induce reactive oxygen species formation during contractions in single skeletal muscle fibers. AJP Regulatory Integrative and Comparative Physiology. 2013;**304**:R1009-R1016. DOI: 10.1152/ajpregu.00563.2012

[80] Zuo L, Best T M, Roberts W J, Diaz PT, Wagner PD. Characterization of reactive oxygen species in diaphragm. Acta Physiology. 2015;**213**:700-710. doi:10.1111/apha.12410.

[81] Seo SY, Lee SR, Kim N, Ko KS, Rhee BD, Han J. Age-related changes in skeletal muscle mitochondria: The role of exercise. Integrative Medicine Research. 2016;**5**:182-186

[82] Peterson CM, Johansen DL, Ravussin E. Skeletal muscle mitochondria and aging: A review. Journal of Aging Research. 2012. article ID 194821, DOI: 10.1155/2012/194821

[83] Powers SK, Ji LL, Kavaziz AN, Jackson MJ. Reactive oxygen species: Impact on skeletal muscle. Comprehensive Physiology. 2011;**1**(2):941-969

[84] Bijlsma AY, Meskers CGM, van Heemst D, Westendorp RGJ, de Craen AJM, Maier AB. Diagnostic criteria for sarcopenia relate differently to insulin resistance. Age. 2013;**35**:2367-2375

[85] Kuo C-K, Lin L-Y, Yu Y-H, Wu K-H, Kuo H-K. Inverse association between insulin resistance and gait speed in nondiabetic older men: Results from the U.S. National Health and Nutrition Examination Survey (NHANES) 1999-2002. BMC Geriatrics. 2009;**9**:49

[86] Miljkovic I, Zmuda JM. Epidemiology of myosteatosis. Current Opinion in Clinical Nutrition & Metabolic Care. 2010;**13**:260-264. DOI: 10.1097/MCO.0b013e328337d826

[87] Beavers KM, Beavers DP, Houston DK, Harris TB, Hue TF, Koster A, Newman AB, Simonsick EM, Studenski SA, Nicklas BJ, Kritchevsky SB. Associations between body composition and gait-speed decline: Results from the health, aging, and body composition study. American Journal of Clinical Nutrition. 2013;**97**:552-560

[88] Marcus RL, Addison O, Dibble LE, Foreman KB, Morrell G, Lastayo P. Intramuscular adipose tissue, sarcopenia, and mobility function in older individuals. Journal of Aging Research. 2012;629-637

[89] Manini TM, Clark BC, Nalls MA, Goodpaster BH, Ploutz-Snyder LL, Harris TB. Reduced physical activity increases intermuscular adipose tissue in healthy young adults. American Journal of Clinical Nutrition. 2007;**85**:377-384

[90] Mastrocola R, Collino M, Nigro D, Chiazza F, D'Antona G, Aragno M, et al. Accumulation of advanced glycation end-products and activation of the SCAP/SREBP Lipogenetic pathway occur in diet-induced obese mouse skeletal muscle. PLoS One. 2015;**10**:e0119587. DOI: 10.1371/journal.pone.0119587

[91] Reid KF, Fielding RA. Skeletal muscle power: A critical determinant of physical functioning in older adults. Exerc. Sport Sciences Reviews. 2012;**40**:4-12. DOI: 10.1097/JES.0b013e31823b5f13

[92] Prior SJ, Joseph LJ, Brandauer J, Katzel LI, Hagberg JM, Ryan AS. Reduction in midthigh low-density muscle with aerobic exercise training and weight loss impacts glucose tolerance in older men. The Journal of Clinical Endocrinology & Metabolism. 2007;**92**:880-886

[93] McNeil CJ, Doherty TJ, Stashuk DW, Rice CL. Motor unit number estimates in the tibialis anterior muscle of young, old, and very old men. Muscle Nerve. 2005;**31**:461-467

[94] Clark DJ, Pojednic RM, Reid KF, Patten C, Pasha EP, Phillips EM, Fielding RA. Longitudinal decline of neuromuscular activation and power in healthy older adults. The Journal of Gerontology. Series A, Biological Sciences and Medical Sciences. 2013;**68**:1419-1425

[95] Harris-Love MO, Monfaredi R, Ismail C, Blackman MR, Cleary K. Quantitative ultrasound: Measurement considerations for the assessment of muscular dystrophy and sarcopenia. Frontiers in Aging Neuroscience. 2014;**6**:1-4. DOI: 10.3389/fnagi.2014.00172

3

From Sarcopenia to Frailty: The Pathophysiological Basis and Potential Target Molecules of Intervention

Zhuowei Yu, Qingwei Ruan, Grazia D'Onofrio and Antonio Greco

Abstract

Skeletal muscle is not only an endocrine organ but also one of core components of musculoskeletal system. Sarcopenia refers to a decline in the skeletal muscle mass and function. The former involves the size and number of changes in two types of myofibers, lower satellite cell density, and regeneration ability. The latter shows a loss of muscle strength. Frailty is a geriatric syndrome with multisystem impairment associated with increased vulnerability to stressors. Sarcopenia increases the risk of frailty and may be one of the major causes of physical frailty phenotype. Sarcopenia is also potentially associated with cognitive frailty phenotype. Aging might be the common underlying pathophysiology of sarcopenia and frailty. Therefore, there are some potential target molecules in aging-related signaling pathways that might be associated with sarcopenia and frailty. Nevertheless, sarcopenia can mediate metabolism and promote accelerate systemic aging, frailty, and age-related diseases by myokines in an endocrine manner. Lifestyle interventions (resistance exercise and dietary restriction) of gerontoscience are effective in the prevention of sarcopenia. Some pharmacological agents are registered in different phases of clinical trials for sarcopenia intervention. Phytochemicals, mTOR inhibitors, metformin and acarbose, NAD precursors, and sirtuin activators demonstrated that multiple target antiaging effects might also have preventive and therapeutic perspectives on sarcopenia and frailty.

Keywords: sarcopenia, physical frailty, cognitive frailty, aging

1. Introduction

Sarcopenia and frailty are two common geriatric conditions that may co-occur within a single individual with aging. Frailty is a heterogeneous clinical condition depended on different domains.

Definitions of frailty includes fried physical frailty phenotype (weight loss, exhaustion, physical inactivity, handgrip strength, and walk time) [1] and frailty index (use of walking aid, activities of daily living, incontinence, cognitive impairment, and multiple other components) [2]. Cognition performance decline is considered as a domain in Frailty index, but as "cognitive frailty" phenotype when physical frailty and potentially reversible cognitive impairment simultaneously occur [3]. Sarcopenia refers to decline in skeletal muscle mass and function, which includes primary sarcopenia, or age-related loss of muscle mass and function decline, and secondary sarcopenia resulting from nutrition, activity, and disease-related loss of muscle mass [4]. Sarcopenia is different from cachexia, which combines the loss of both muscle and fat. Obviously, physical frailty and sarcopenia share the core components, physical function impairment (weakness, slow walking speed, and balance problems), and sarcopenia is considered as the biological substrate and the pathway of physical frailty development [5, 6].

Although it is a controversy, sarcopenia and frailty are two separate conditions based on their definitions, and outpatients with sarcopenia were more likely to be more frail than frail outpatients to be sarcopenic [7]. Skeletal muscle is not only a component of muscloskeletal system but also an endocrine organ. Two components of sarcopenia also obviously contribute to frailty, a geriatric syndrome that has been defined as a multisystem impairment characterized by decreased reserve associated with increased vulnerability to stressors. First, the loss of muscle mass plays a critical role in unintentional weight loss of frailty in the elderly. Second, age-related loss of muscle strength, commonly referred as dynapenia, was associated with both sarcopenia and frailty [8]. Sarcopenia and frailty had the sensitivity and specificity for dynapenia of 33 and 89%, 17 and 98%, respectively. A longitudinal aging study with 731 community-dwelling older people demonstrated that dynapenia was related to the cognitive impairment [9]. Thus, dynapenia is also the important factor responsible for frailty. Moreover, muscle cross-talks with other tissues and organs by myokines in an endocrine manner to mediate metabolism and promote aging, diseases, and frailty. Here, we review the epidemiological evidence and pathophysiological basis of skeletal muscle aging, or primary sarcopenia, that result in frailty and potential target molecules of intervention. Particularly, we focus on the pathophysiological basis of sarcopenia, including age-related changes of nutrient and stress sensors, positive and negative regulators of muscle growth, and the maintenance of muscle mass and function. Moreover, we also summarize the underlying mechanisms of sarcopenia accelerating systemic aging, frailty, and age-related diseases. Finally, we looked for the potential target molecules of intervention of sarcopenia according to the pathophysiological basis and relevant signal pathways.

2. From Sarcopenia to frailty: the pathophysiological basis

2.1. From sarcopenia to physical and cognitive frailty: the epidemiological evidence

Frailty is heterogeneous and contains physical and cognitive multiple domains. In this context, the concept of "Cognitive frailty" becomes essential. It refers to simultaneous presence of physical frailty and potentially reversible cognitive impairment but without dementia [3]. Cognitive frailty includes reversible and potentially reversible subtypes [10] and may represent a precursor of neurodegenerative processes [10]. The link between physical function and cognitive decline provides important targets to develop effective preventive strategies in earlier cognitive impairment stages [3, 11, 12].

Epidemiological studies suggested that sarcopenia increases the risks of both physical frailty and cognitive impairment. Loss of muscle mass and strength is associated with increased dependence, frailty, and mortality. Low appendicular lean mass related to body mass index could detect patients at risk for frailty [13]. A cross-sectional study with small subjects, 273 Japanese community-dwelling older women aged >65 years showed that sarcopenia was related only with prefrailty and frailty, and cognitive decline was related to frailty [14]. However, several studies showed an association between sarcopenia parameters and cognitive impairment. Low handgrip strength was shown to correlate with a decrease in Mini Mental State Examination (MMSE) score [15]. Other studies also reported an association between handgrip strength and the risk of Alzheimer disease and the rate of cognitive decline [16–18]. In prospective studies, a decrease in physical performance in relation to future dementia was demonstrated [19, 20]. Subjects aged >65 years who scored low in a physical performance test had a three-times higher risk of developing dementia at a 6-year follow-up [21]. Recently, the new concept of "Motoric Cognitive Risk (MCR) syndrome" was defined as having mild cognitive impairment (MCI) and slow gait, supporting the common underlying mechanism in physical and cognitive impairment [22]. MCR offered further benefit on predicting dementia than MCI or slow gait alone. A recent study demonstrated an association between increased risk of cognitive impairment, mainly MCI, and poor lower extremity function [21].

2.2. Aging promotes sarcopenia and frailty

Factors relating to skeletal muscle mass and strength changes include the loss of motor units innervating muscle, age-related hormone changes, muscle hypoxia resulting from atherosclerosis and chronic proinflammatory status, decreased physical activity and protein intake, age-related insulin resistance, and mitochondrial dysfunction [23]. Aging leads to a preferential reduction of type II myofiber size. There is a significant loss of type II muscle fibers, lower satellite cell density, and lower satellite cell/fiber ratio in older individuals with sarcopenia [24]. The loss of motor units innervating muscle, especially type II myofibers [25], and the decreased blood flow to muscle [26] results in the loss of muscle mass. Meanwhile, many elderly population with insulin resistance who maintains the sensitivity of glucose metabolism, but not protein synthesis, show age-related anabolic resistance, meaning the reduced muscle protein synthesis [27, 28]. However, muscle of older individuals with type 2 diabetes [29] metabolic syndrome [30] demonstrated a significant low proportion of type I fibers that is positively associated with the severity of insulin resistance. Thus, the loss of muscle mass and the alterations of myofiber type proportion due to insulin resistance could potentially affect whole body glucose homeostasis [31]. Age-related hormone changes, for example, the decline of anabolic hormone testosterone leads to the loss of both muscle mass and strength [32]. The decline in both growth hormone and insulin-like growth factor 1 are related to the loss of muscle mass but not muscle strength [33]. Muscle hypoxia results from atherosclerosis and chronic proinflammatory status leads to the loss of both muscle mass and strength [25]. Other factors, decreased physical activity and protein intake, also involve in the loss of muscle mass.

Age-related decline of the levels of 25(OH) vitamin D due to a decreased production of 25(OH) vitamin D in skin or a decline in vitamin D absorption can result in the decline of muscle function [25]. Age-related insulin resistance causes an increase of fat infiltration into muscle and a decline in muscle strength [34]. Mitochondrial dysfunction in aging skeletal muscle causes oxidative damage and the decline of energy generation to maintain function properly [35].

The biological mechanisms underlying the association between sarcopenia and frailty are uncertain [36]. Any plausible explanations are that physical, motor, and cognitive functions are not causally related but are affected by common underlying pathophysiology [37]. Frailty, cognitive impairment, and sarcopenia share many common risk factors, such as immune or inflammatory response, oxidative stress, and hormonal dysregulation [38, 39]. In view of this, frailty, cognitive impairment, and sarcopenia may be highly interrelated [38, 40]. Inflammatory markers such as C-reactive protein and interleukin-6 concentrations are correlated negatively with muscle strength and physical performance [41, 42]. According to the definition of cognitive frailty, physical factors are the potential causes of cognitive impairment. In a study, high levels of these markers are associated with a 66% increase in cognitive impairment risk at 4-year follow-up in elders with metabolic syndrome [43]. Elevated oxidative stress [44], decreased sex steroid levels [45, 46], and insulin resistance [47, 48] are also involved in the association between physical and cognitive dysfunction.

2.3. The maintenance of muscle mass and function

The maintenance of normal muscle mass and function depends on the dynamic balance between positive and negative regulators of muscle growth. Muscle growth promoters include follustatin (FST), bone morphogenetic proteins (BMPs), brian-derived neurotrophic factor (BDNF), and irisin. Muscle growth suppressors contain myostatin, transforming growth factor beta (TGFβ), activins A and B, growth, and differentiation factor-11 and -15 [49, 50]. Age-related changes of these molecules, together with other factors, such as age-related diseases, chronic low-grade systemic inflammation, insulin resistance, endocrine aging, low physical activity, aging-related impairment of neuromuscular junction dysfunction, and contractile insufficiency because of skeletal muscle-specific troponin T leakage from sarcomere, result in imbalance between positive and negative regulators of muscle growth and sarcopenia development [49]. Muscle growth suppressors through the antibody-coupled, T-cell receptor/anaplastic lymphoma kinase 4,5 (ActR/Alk 4,5), or type I and II TGFβ receptor (TβRI and TβRII), phosphorylate mothers against decapentaplegic homolog 2/3 (SMAD 2/3), then combine SMAD 4 and inhibit the activation of an alternative pathway/mammalian target of rapamycin (Alt/mTOR) signal. TGFβ promotes SMAD3 binding to the promoters of both fibronectin type III domain containing 5 (FNDC5) and procaspase-activating compound 1α (PAC-1α), and suppresses the expression of irisin and PAC-1α [51].The elevated growth differentiation factor 11 (GDF11) increases the risk for age-related frailty and comorbidities [50]. Muscle growth promoters through their receptors phosphorylate SMAD 1/5/8 decrease the inhibition of Alt/mTOR signal and maintain muscle mass and strength. Insulin resistance due to aging, obesity, and diabetes results in the suppression of insulin/insulin-like growth factor-1/phosphatidyl Inositol 3-kinase/protein kinase B (IGF 1/PI3K/AKT)/mTOR, and muscle hypotrophy and dysfunction of metabolism;

the less activated Alk fails to block the nuclear translocation of Foxo 3 to enhance the expression of autophagy-related genes and the consequent protein degradation [31, 52].

2.4. Sarcopenia accelerates systemic aging, frailty, and age-related diseases

Skeletal muscle influence systemic aging and lifespan by nutrient and stress sensors and myokines [53]. DNA damage and mutations are particularly prominent in aging skeletal muscle. Overexpression of phosphoenolpyruvate carboxykinase (PEPCK-C) and mitochondrial uncoupling proteins delays reproductive aging and decreases the incidence of several age-related diseases. Nutrient and stress sensors in sarcopenia include decreased sirturin 1 resulting from low nicotinamide adenine dinucleotide (NAD)+ synthesis and high NAD+ consumption and low adenosine monophosphate-dependent protein kinase (AMPK) activity, which results in the decline of the activity of peroxisome proliferator-activated receptor gamma coactivator-1a (PGC-1a) [54, 55]. The overexpression of AMPK and PGC-1a in muscle not only delays the age-related muscle deterioration but also slows the functional decline of other tissues, delay age-related metabolic defects, including systemic low-grade chronic inflammation, insulin resistance, increase in the stress resistance of the organism and extend lifespan. The other two nutrient sensors, insulin/insulin-like growth factor (IIS) and mTOR signaled nutrient abundance (high fat, amino acids, and sugar diet) and anabolic activity, are major accelerators of aging. mTOR inhibition by rapamycin or mTORC1 activity inhibition by genetical modification, and the downregulation of mTORC1/ribosomal protein S6 kinase beta-1 (S6K1) increases lifespan in mammals [55]. The decrease in regenerative capacity and skeletal muscle loss with age coincides with suppression of IIS pathways which is an attempt to promote longevity of the organism and survival within the tissue [56]. Age-related sarcopenia is associated with an increase in abdominal obesity, which refers to sarcopenic obesity [57]. Sarcopenic obesity leads to the infiltration of fat into the muscle and the accumulation of triglycerides within the cell, which impairs the function of the insulin receptor substrate causing insulin resistance, a lower lipid buffering capacity, and anabolic resistance in muscle [23, 58]. Sarcopenic obesity also results in cognitive impairment because of insulin resistance. In a cohort of 1570 older British men, compared with participants in the normal cognitive aging group, those elder men with severe cognitive impairment were more likely to be sarcopenic, with waist circumference >102 cm, BMI >30 kg/m^2 and to be in the upper quintile of total fat mass, central fat mass, peripheral fat mass, and visceral fat level after age-adjusted multinomial logistic regressions [59]. In experiment animal mouse, obesity in combination with sarcopenia exacerbates blood-brain barrier disruption, neuroinflammation, and oxidative stress of hippocampus, which likely contribute to the remarkable cognitive decline [60]. Calorie restriction and exercise increase the concentrations of metabolic effectors NAD+ and AMP but reduce the concentrations of the hormonal effectors IIS and growth hormone. Meanwhile, these interventions also decrease the levels of glucose, amino acids, and lipids, recover downstream activity, such as DNA repair, mitochondrial biogenesis, and function, promote homeostasis, decrease frailty and comorbidities.

Beyond the profound influence on systemic aging and body metabolism, muscle secrete myokines, which act on muscles and other tissues, such as adipose, bones and brain in an autocrine, paracrine, and endocrine fashion [61]. The metabolites released from muscle and the interactions between muscle and nerve also participate in the systemic effects of muscle on the organism's physiology. Exercise can activate PGC-1α/FNDC5 pathway, promote myokine irisin secretion, induce hippocampal BDNF release, and improve cognitive function [62].

3. From sarcopenia to frailty: the potential target molecules of intervention

The major causes of frailty include chronic diseases, such as congestive heart failure, diabetes, chronic obstructive pulmonary disease (COPD), anemia, polymyalgia rheumatic, and endocrine disorder; decreased nutrient intake because of anorexia resulting from social factors, decline in taste and smell, altered fundal compliance, enhanced release of cholecystokinin, increased leptin and cytokines, sarcopenia, and pain [63]. Treating the chronic diseases can reverse the loss of muscle mass and frailty, such as with angiotensin-converting enzyme inhibitors in some patients with congestive heart failure, both erythropoietin and darbepoietin-α in the individuals with anemia, and vitamin B12 supplementation in acrocytic anemia and related cognitive impairment. Lifestyle interventions play critical roles in the prevention of sarcopenia, frailty, and cognitive impairment. Physical exercise, particularly resistance exercise, can improve muscle mass and strength in the elderly [64, 65] and obese elderly [58]. Individuals with higher initial adiposity experience less improvement in both muscle strength and physical function [66]. Moreover, the addition of caloric restriction during resistance training improves mobility and does not compromise other functional adaptations to resistance training [66]. Resistance training also can increase circulating irisin [67] and improve cognitive performance [62]. In addition, physical exercise and caloric restriction can benefit age-related insulin resistance, reduced mitochondrial biogenesis, and failure of autophagy [68]. However, it is undesirable to use caloric restriction alone in sarcopenic elderly, which results in further loss of lean tissue mass. The oldest olds also with anabolic resistance and frailty find it difficult to perform resistance exercise to achieve benefit effects.

Dietary interventions including protein intake, antioxidants, and vitamin D fortification may benefit the conditions of sarcopenia and frailty. Protein supplies the amino acids, especially leucine, which may activate the signaling pathways required for muscle synthesis. Vitamin D deficiency is common in individuals with sarcopenia, frailty, and cognitive impairment. However, the effects of both protein supplementation and vitamin D intervention on muscle strength and physical performance have mixed results [69]. Although individuals with higher overall antioxidant status have better physical function, such as walking speed [70], antioxidant interventions might not attenuate, and even aggravate sarcopenia due to the health-promoting action of reactive oxygen spices [71].

There are no licensed treatments for sarcopenia and frailty. Pharmacological agents proposed and focused by investigators, with potential for treating sarcopenia include the myostatin signaling pathway and hormone replacement therapy (**Table 1**), currently are at various stages of development [72]. Myostatin, the family member of TGF-β, is a skeletal muscle-specific myokine. Myostain binding with activin type IIB receptor inhibits myoblast proliferation, muscle

Mechanism of action	Drug name	Drug developer	Indication sought	Study phase
I. Myostatin antagonists				
Activin receptor trap	ACE-031	Acceleron	Duchenne muscular dystrophy	Phase 3 (trial terminated early)
Myostatin antibody	REGN-1033	Regeneron/Sanofi	Sarcopenia	Phase 2
	LY-2495655	Eli Lilly	Hip arthroplasty Elderly Fallers Cancer cachexia	Phase 2
	PF-06252616	Pfizer	Inclusion body myositis	Phase 1
Activin receptor inhibitor	Bimagrumab (BMY338)	Novartis	Sarcopenia Hip fracture Cancer and COPD cachexia	Phases 2 and 3 Phase 2
II. Selective androgen receptor modulators	Enobasarm (ostarine)	GTx	Cancer cachexia	Phase 3 (did not meet primary endpoint)
III. Skeletal troponin activators	Tirasemtiv CK-2017357	Cytokinetics	Amyotrophic lateral sclerosis myasthenia gravis	Phases 2 and 3

Table 1. Pharmacological agents in development with potential for treating sarcopenia [72].

strength, and mass by negative regulation of mTOR signaling [73]. Myostatin inhibition by activin receptor trap or inhibitor and myostatin antibody might be useful agent for the treatment of human muscle degenerative diseases (**Table 1**) [72]. Testosterone supplementation is another major focus for drug discovery of sarcopenia. Testosterone could increase both muscle mass and strength in men but are linked to adverse cardiovascular events with short durations of therapy [74, 75]. In order to decrease the side effects of testosterone, the selective androgen receptor molecules, including steroids and nonsteroids, have been developed, and some are at phase 3 (**Table 1**). Tirasemtiv is a fast skeletal troponin activator that sensitizes the sarcomere to calcium and amplifies the function of muscle in neuromuscular diseases, such as Amyotrophic Lateral Sclerosis and myasthenia gravis (**Table 1**) [76, 77].

Age is the greatest risk factor for nearly every major cause of mortality in developed nations [78] and the profound effect of aging on sarcopenia, frailty, and cognitive impairment is often overlooked. A number of aging-associated molecular signals might be the potential target in the prevention and treatment of sarcopenia, frailty, and cognitive impairment. Genetic or pharmacological regulation of NAD+/Sirt1, sestrins/AMPK/PGC1α, IGF-1/Akt/mTOR, TGF-β, myostatin, activins, GDFs /SMAD2/3, BMPs/SMAD1/5/8 signal molecules, myokine irisin and FGF21, the antagonist of myokine myostatin propeptide follistatin or follistatin-like 3, and urocortins can not only improve muscle mass and/or function but also delay frailty and age-related diseases [31, 54, 68]. Besides dietary restriction and exercise, geroscience interventions with translational potential include mTOR inhibitors, metformin and acarbose, NAD precursors and sirtuin activators, modifiers of senescence and telomere dysfunction, hormonal and circulating factors, and mitochondrial-targeted therapeutics [78]. Phytochemicals obviously are ideal geroscience interventions with translational potential. They not only have multiple target molecules in many aging-related signalling pathways, such as sestrins/AMPK/PGC1α, IGF-1/Akt/mTOR, against chronic inflammation and oxidative stress but also have systemic influence with low side effects, including skeletal muscle and other domains of frailty [79, 80].

4. Conclusion and perspective

Sarcopenia is one of the important causes of physical frailty. Frailty contains different phenotypes, such as physical frailty and cognitive frailty or multiple domains in frailty index. Skeletal muscle influences body metabolism, systemic aging, accelerates physical frailty, cognitive impairment, and decrease healthy lifespan. Individuals with primary sarcopenia have an increase in the risk for frailty, cognitive impairment, and age-related diseases. Aging might be the common mechanism of sarcopenia, frailty, and cognitive impairment. Cognitive frailty is an important target of the prevention for both physical and cognitive disability [81]. Although some pharmacological agents are registered in different phases of clinical trials for sarcopenia intervention, no drug is really used for the clinical treatment of sarcopenia. Phytochemicals have effects on multiple targets of aging-related signaling pathways, and other targeted aging molecules, such as mTOR inhibitors, metformin and acarbose, NAD precursors, and sirtuin activators [78, 82], have preventive and therapeutic perspectives on sarcopenia, frailty, and age-related diseases.

Acknowledgements

This work was supported by grants from the Shanghai Hospital Development Center (No. SHDC12014221), Shanghai Municipal Commission of Health and Family Planning, Key developing disciplines (2015ZB0501).

Author details

Zhuowei Yu[1,2], Qingwei Ruan[1,2*], Grazia D'Onofrio[3] and Antonio Greco[3]

*Address all correspondence to: 13661717346@163.com

1 Shanghai Institute of Geriatrics and Gerontology, Shanghai Key Laboratory of Clinical Geriatrics, Huadong Hospital, Shanghai, China

2 Research Center of Aging and Medicine, Shanghai Medical College, Fudan University, Shanghai, China

3 Department of Medical Sciences, Geriatric Unit & Laboratory of Gerontology and Geriatrics, IRCCS "Casa Sollievo della Sofferenza", San Giovanni Rotondo, Foggia, Italy

References

[1] Fried LP, Tangen CM, Walston J, et al. Frailty in older adults evidence for a phenotype. The Journals of Gerontology. Series A, Biological Sciences and Medical Sciences. 2001;**56**:M146eM157

[2] Rockwood K, Stadnyk K, MacKnight C, et al. A brief clinical instrument to classify frailty in elderly people. Lancet. 1999;**353**:205-206

[3] Kelaiditi E, Cesari M, Canevelli M, et al. Cognitive frailty: Rational and definition from an (I.A.N.A./I.A.G.G.) international consensus group. The Journal of Nutrition Health and Aging. 2013;**17**:726-734

[4] Cruz-Jentoft AJ, Baeyens JP, Bauer JM, et al. Sarcopenia: European consensus on definition and diagnosis report of the European working group on sarcopenia in older people. Age Ageing. 2010;**39**:412-423

[5] Bernabei R, Martone AM, Vetrano DL, Calvani R, Landi F, Marzetti E. Frailty, physical frailty, sarcopenia: A new conceptual model. Studies in Health Technology and Informatics. 2014;**203**:78-84

[6] Landi F, Calvani R, Cesari M, Tosato M, Martone AM, Bernabei R, Onder G, Marzetti E. Sarcopenia as the biological substrate of physical frailty. Clinics in Geriatric Medicine. 2015;**31**(3):367-374

[7] Reijnierse EM, Trappenburg MC, Blauw GJ, Verlaan S, de van der Schueren MA, Meskers CG, Maier AB. Common ground? The concordance of sarcopenia and frailty definitions. Journal of American Medical Directors Association. 2016;**17**(4):371.e7-12

[8] Iwamura M, Kanauchi M. A cross-sectional study of the association between dynapenia and higher-level functional capacity in daily living in community-dwelling older adults in Japan. BMC Geriatrics. 2017;**17**:1

[9] Huang CY, Hwang AC, Liu LK, Lee WJ, Chen LY, Peng LN, Lin MH, Chen LK. Association of dynapenia, sarcopenia, and cognitive impairment among community-dwelling older Taiwanese. Rejuvenation Research. 2016;**19**(1):71-78

[10] Ruan Q, Yu Z, Chen M, et al. Cognitive frailty, a novel target for the prevention of elderly dependency. Ageing Research Reviews. 2015;**20**:1-10

[11] Desai AK, Grossberg GT, Chibnall JT. Healthy brain aging: A road map. Clinics in Geriatric Medicine. 2010;**26**:1-16

[12] Ruan Q, D'Onofrio G, Sancarlo D, Greco A, Yu Z. Potential fluid-biomarkers of pathologic brain changes in Alzheimer's disease, implication in the screening of cognitive frailty. Molecular Medicine Report. 2016;**14**(4):3184-3198

[13] Spira D, Buchmann N, Nikolov J, Demuth I, Steinhagen-Thiessen E, Eckardt R, Norman K. Association of low lean mass with frailty and physical performance: A comparison

between two operational definitions of sarcopenia-data from the Berlin Aging Study II (BASE-II). The Journals of Gerontology. Series A, Biological Sciences and Medical Sciences. 2015;**70**(6):779-784

[14] Nishiguchi S, Yamada M, Fukutani N, Adachi D, Tashiro Y, Hotta T, Morino S, Shirooka H, Nozaki Y, Hirata H, Yamaguchi M, Arai H, Tsuboyama T, Aoyama T. Differential association of frailty with cognitive decline and sarcopenia in community-dwelling older adults. Journal of American Medical Directors Association. 2015;**16**(2):120-124

[15] Auyeung TW, Lee JS, Kwok T, Woo J. Physical frailty predicts future cognitive decline-a four-year prospective study in 2737 cognitively normal older adults. The Journal of Nutrition Health and Aging. 2011;**15**:690-769

[16] Alfaro-Acha A, Al Snih S, Raji MA, Kuo YF, Markides KS, Ottenbacher KJ. Handgrip strength and cognitive decline in older Mexican Americans.. The Journals of Gerontology. Series A, Biological Sciences and Medical Sciences. 2006;**61**:859-865

[17] Taekema DG, Gussekloo J, Maier AB, Westendorp RG, de Craen AJ. Handgrip strength as a predictor of functional, psychological and social health. A prospective population-based study among the oldest old. Age Ageing. 2010;**39**:331-337

[18] Boyle PA, Buchman AS, Wilson RS, Leurgans SE, Bennett DA. Association of muscle strength with the risk of Alzheimer disease and the rate of cognitive decline in community-dwelling older persons. Archives of Neurology. 2009;**66**(11):1339-1344

[19] Wang L, Larson EB, Bowen JD, van Belle G. Performance-based physical function and future dementia in older people. Archives of Internal Medicine. 2006;**166**:1115-1120

[20] Camicioli R, Howieson D, Oken B, Sexton G, Kaye J. Motor slowing precedes cognitive impairment in the oldest old. Neurology. 1998;**50**:1496-1498

[21] Moon JH, Moon JH, Kim KM, Choi SH, Lim S, Park KS, Kim KW, Jang HC. Sarcopenia as a predictor of future cognitive impairment in older adults. The Journal of Nutrition Health and Aging. 2016;**20**(5):496-502

[22] Verghese J, Annweiler C, Ayers E, et al. Motoric cognitive risk syndrome: Multicountry prevalence and dementia risk. Neurology. 2014;**83**:718-726

[23] Kalyani RR, Corriere M, Ferrucci L. Age-related and disease-related muscle loss: The effect of diabetes, obesity and other diseases. Lancet Diabetes Endocrinology. 2014;**2**(10):819-829

[24] Purves-Smith FM, Sgarioto N, Hepple RT. Fiber typing in aging muscle. Exercise and Sport Sciences Reviews. 2014;**42**:45-52

[25] Morley JE. Frailty and sarcopenia: The new geriatric giants. Rev Invest Clin. 2016; **68**(2):59-67

[26] Leenders M, Verdijk LB, van der Hoeven L, et al. Patients with type 2 diabetes show a greater decline in muscle mass, muscle strength, and functional capacity with aging. Journal of American Medical Directors Association. 2013;**14**:585-592

[27] Rasmussen BB, Fujita S, Wolfe RR, Mittendorfer B, Roy M, Rowe VL & Volpi E. Insulin resistance of muscle protein metabolism inaging. FASEB Journal. 2006;**20**:768-769

[28] Fujita S, Glynn EL, Timmerman KL, Rasmussen BB & Volpi E. Supraphysiological hyperinsulinaemia is necessary to stimulate skeletal muscle protein anabolism in older adults: Evidence of atrue age-related insulin resistance of muscle protein metabolism. Diabetologia. 2009;**52**:1889-1898

[29] Oberbach A, Bossenz Y, Lehmann S, Niebauer J, Adams V, Paschke R, Schon MR, Bluher M & Punkt K. Altered fiber distribution and fiber-specific glycolytic and oxidative enzyme activity in skeletal muscle of patients with type 2 diabetes. Diabetes Care. 2006;**29**:895-900

[30] Stuart CA, McCurry MP, Marino A, South MA, Howell ME, Layne AS, Ramsey MW & Stone MH. Slow-twitch fiber proportion in skeletal muscle correlates with insulin responsiveness. Journal of Clinical Endocrinology and Metabolism. 2013;**98**:2027-2036

[31] Cleasby ME, Jamieson PM, Atherton PJ. Insulin resistance and sarcopenia: Mechanistic links between common co-morbidities. Journal of Endocrinology. 2016;**229**:R67-R81

[32] Baumgartner RN, Waters DL, Gallagher D, et al. Predictors of skeletal muscle mass in elderly men and women. Mechanisms of Ageing and Development. 1999;**107**:123-136

[33] Morley JE. Scientific overview of hormone treatment used for rejuvenation. Fertility and Sterility. 2013;**99**:1807-1813

[34] Rolland Y, Lauwers-Cances V, Cristini C, et al. Difficulties with physical function associated with obesity, sarcopenia, and sarcopenic-obesity in community-dwelling elderly women: The EPI-DOS study. The American Journal of Clinical Nutrition. 2009;**89**:1895-1900

[35] Hipple RT. Mitochondrial involvement and impact in aging skeletal muscle. Frontiers in Aging Neuroscience. 2014;**6**:211

[36] Clegg A, Young J, Iliffe S, Rikkert, MO, Rockwood K. Frailty in elderly people. Lancet. 2013;**381**(9868):752-762

[37] Hausdorff JM, Buchman AS. What links gait speed and MCI with dementia? A fresh look at the association between motor and cognitive function. The Journals of Gerontology. Series A, Biological Sciences and Medical Sciences. 2013;**68**: 409-411

[38] Fulop T, Larbi A, Witkowski JM, et al. Aging, frailty and age-related diseases. Biogerontology. 2010;**11**(5):547-563

[39] Small GW. The pathogenesis of Alzheimer's disease. Journal of Clinical Psychiatry. 1998;**59**(Suppl 9):7-14

[40] Ruan Q, D'Onofrio G, Sancarlo D, Greco A, Lozupone M, Seripa D, Panza F, Yu Z. Emerging biomarkers and screening for cognitive frailty. Aging Clinical and Experimental Research. 2017. DOI: 10.1007/s40520-017-0741-8 [Epub ahead of print]

[41] Cesari M, Penninx BW, Pahor M, et al. Inflammatory markers and physical performance in older persons: The InCHIANTI study. The Journals of Gerontology. Series A, Biological Sciences and Medical Sciences. 2004;**59**:242-248

[42] Schaap LA, Pluijm SM, Deeg DJ, Visser M. Inflammatory markers and loss of muscle mass (sarcopenia) and strength. American Journal of Medicine. 2006;**119**:526:e529-526. e517

[43] Yaffe K, Kanaya A, Lindquist K, et al. The metabolic syndrome, inflammation, and risk of cognitive decline. Journal of the American Medical Association. 2004;**292**:2237-2242

[44] Berr C, Balansard B, Arnaud J, Roussel A-M, Alpérovitch A. Cognitive decline is associated with systemic oxidative stress: The EVA study. Etude du Vieillissement Arteriel. Journal of American Geriatrics Society. 2000;**48**:1285-1291

[45] Hogervorst E, Bandelow S, Combrinck M, Smith AD. Low free testosterone is an independent risk factor for Alzheimer's disease. Experimental Gerontology. 2004;**39**:1633-1639

[46] Szulc P, Duboeuf F, Marchand F, Delmas PD. Hormonal and lifestyle determinants of appendicular skeletal muscle mass in men: The MINOS study. The American Journal of Clinical Nutrition. 2004;**80**:496-503

[47] Srikanthan P, Karlamangla AS. Relative muscle mass is inversely associated with insulin resistance and pre-diabetes. Findings from the third National Health and Nutrition Examination Survey. The Journal of Clinical Endocrinology & Metabolism. 2011;**96**:2898-2903

[48] Craft S. Insulin resistance and Alzheimer's disease pathogenesis: Potential mechanisms and implications for treatment. Current Alzheimer Research. 2007;**4**:147-152

[49] Kalinkovich A, Livshits G. Sarcopenia—The search for emerging biomarkers. Ageing Research Reviews. 2015;**22**:58-71

[50] Egerman MA, Cadena SM, Gilbert JA, et al. GDF11 increases with age and inhibits skeletal muscle regeneration. Cell Metabolism. 2015;**22**(1):164-174

[51] Tiano JP, Springer DA, Rane SG. SMAD3 negatively regulates serum irisin and skeletal muscle FNDC5 and peroxisome proliferator-activated receptor Y co-activator 1-α during exercise. The Journal of Biological Chemistry. 2015;**290**(12):7671-7684

[52] Sakuma K, Aoi W, Yamaguchi A. Current understanding of sarcopenia: Possible candidates modulating muscle mass. Pflugers Archiv—European Journal of Physiology. 2015;**467**:213-229

[53] Demontis F, Piccirillo R, Goldberg AL, et al. The influence of skeletal muscle on systemic aging and lifespan. Aging Cell. 2013;**12**(6):943-949

[54] Bonkowski MS, Sinclair DA. Slowing ageing by design: The rise of NAD+ and sirtuin-activating compounds. Nature Reviews Molecular Cell Biology. 2016;**17**(11):679-690

[55] López-Otín C, Blasco MA, Partridge L, Serrano M, Kroemer G. The hallmarks of aging. Cell. 2013;**153**(6):1194-1217

[56] Sharples AP, Hughes DC, Deane CS, Saini A, Selman C, Stewart CE. Longevity and skeletal muscle mass: The role of IGF signalling, the sirtuins, dietary restriction and protein intake. Aging Cell. 2015;**14**(4):511-523

[57] Jura M, Kozak LP. Obesity and related consequences to ageing. AGE. 2016;**38**:23

[58] Tardif N, Salles J, Guillet C, Tordjman J, Reggio S, Landrier JF, Giraudet C, Patrac V, Bertrand-Michel J, Migne C, Collin ML, Chardigny JM, Boirie Y, Walrand S. Muscle ectopic fat deposition contributes to anabolic resistance in obese sarcopenic old rats through eIF2α activation. Aging Cell. 2014;**13**(6):1001-1011

[59] Papachristou E, Ramsay SE, Lennon LT, Papacosta O, Iliffe S, Whincup PH, Wannamethee SG. The relationships between body composition characteristics and cognitive functioning in a population-based sample of older British men. BMC Geriatrics. 2015;**15**:172

[60] Tucsek Z, Toth P, Sosnowska D, Gautam T, Mitschelen M, Koller A, Szalai G, Sonntag WE, Ungvari Z, Csiszar A. Obesity in aging exacerbates blood-brain barrier disruption, neuroinflammation, and oxidative stress in the mouse hippocampus: Effects on expression of genes involved in beta-amyloid generation and Alzheimer's disease. The Journals of Gerontology, Series A, Biological Sciences and Medical Sciences. 2014;**69**(10):1212-1226

[61] Ilich JZ, Kelly OJ, Inglis JE, et al. Interrelationship among muscle, fat, and bone: Connecting the dots on cellular, hormonal, and whole body levels. Ageing Research Reviews. 2014;**15**:51-60

[62] Wrann CD, White JP, Salogiannnis J, et al. Exercise induces hippocampal BDNF through a PGC-1α/FNDC5 pathway. Cell Metabolism. 2013;**18**(5):649-659

[63] Sinclair AJ, Morley JE and Vellas B. Pathy's Principles and Practice of Geriatric Medicine. 5th ed. UK: John Wiley & Sons, Ltd; 2012. pp. 1387-1393

[64] Peterson M, Sen A, Gordon P. Influence of resistance exercise on lean body mass in aging adults: A meta-analysis. Medicine & Science in Sports & Exercise. 2012;**43**:249-258

[65] Liu CJ, Latham NK. Progressive resistance strength training for improving physical function in older adults. The Cochrane Database of Systematic Reviews. 2009;(3):CD002759

[66] Nicklas BJ, Chmelo E, Delbono O, Carr JJ, Lyles MF, Marsh AP. Effects of resistance training with and without caloric restriction on physical function and mobility in overweight and obese older adults: A randomized controlled trial. The American Journal of Clinical Nutrition. 2015;**101**(5):991-999

[67] Jedrychowski MP, Wrann CD, Paulo JA, Gerber KK, Szpyt J, Robinson MM, Nair KS, Gygi SP, Spiegelman BM. Detection and quantitation of circulating human irisin by tandem mass spectrometry. Cell Metabolism. 2015;**22**(4):734-740

[68] Sanchis-Gomar F, Pareja-Galeano H, Mayero S, Perez-Quilis C, Lucia A. New molecular targets and lifestyle interventions to delay aging sarcopenia. Front Aging Neuroscience. 2014;**6**:156

[69] Dodds R, Sayer AA. Sarcopenia and frailty: New challenges for clinical practice. Clinical Medicine (London). 2016;**16**(5):455-458

[70] Kaiser M, Bandinelli S, Lunenfeld B. Frailty and the role of nutrition in older people. A review of the current literature. Acta Biomedicine. 2010;**81**(Suppl 1):37-45

[71] Sanchis-Gomar F, and Derbre F. Mitochondrial fission and fusion in human diseases. The New England Journal of Medicine. 2014;**370**:1073-1074

[72] Beaudart C, McCloskey E, Bruyère O, Cesari M, Rolland Y, Rizzoli R, Araujo de Carvalho I, Amuthavalli Thiyagarajan J, Bautmans I, Bertière MC, Brandi ML, Al-Daghri NM, Burlet N, Cavalier E, Cerreta F, Cherubini A, Fielding R, Gielen E, Landi F, Petermans J, Reginster JY, Visser M, Kanis J, Cooper C. Sarcopenia in daily practice: Assessment and management. BMC Geriatrics. 2016;**16**(1):170

[73] Garatachea N, Pinos T, Camara Y, Rodriguez-Romo G, Emanuele E, Ricevuti G, et al. Association of the K153R polymorphism in the myostatin gene and extreme longevity. Age (Dordr). 2013;**35**:2445-2454

[74] Xu L, Freeman G, Cowling BJ, Schooling CM. Testosterone therapy and cardiovascular events among men: A systematic review and meta-analysis of placebo-controlled randomized trials. BMC Medicine. 2013;**11**:108

[75] Wallis CJ, Lo K, Lee Y, Krakowsky Y, Garbens A, Satkunasivam R, Herschorn S, Kodama RT, Cheung P, Narod SA, Nam RK. Survival and cardiovascular events in men treated with testosterone replacement therapy: An intention-to-treat observational cohort study. Lancet Diabetes Endocrinology. 2016;**4**(6):498-506

[76] Sanders DB, Rosenfeld J, Dimachkie MM, Meng L, Malik FI; Tirasemtiv in Myasthenia Gravis Study Group. A double-blinded, randomized, placebo-controlled trial to evaluate efficacy, safety, and tolerability of single doses of tirasemtiv in patients with acetylcholine receptor-binding antibody-positive myasthenia gravis. Neurotherapeutics. 2015;**12**(2):455-460

[77] Russell AJ, Hartman JJ, Hinken AC, Muci AR, Kawas R, Driscoll L, Godinez G, Lee KH, Marquez D, Browne WF 4th, Chen MM, Clarke D, Collibee SE, Garard M, Hansen R, Jia Z, Lu PP, Rodriguez H, Saikali KG, Schaletzky J, Vijayakumar V, Albertus DL, Claflin DR, Morgans DJ, Morgan BP, Malik FI. Activation of fast skeletal muscle troponin as a potential therapeutic approach for treating neuromuscular diseases. Nature Medicine. 2012;**18**(3):452-455

[78] Kaeberlein M, Rabinovitch PS, Martin GM. Healthy aging: The ultimate preventative medicine. Science. 2015;**350**(6265):1191-1193

[79] D'Onofrio G, Sancarlo D, Ruan Q, Yu Z, Panza F, Daniele A, Greco A, Seripa D. Phytochemicals in the treatment of Alzheimer's disease: A systematic review. Current Drug Targets. 2016. [Epub ahead of print]

[80] Corrêa RC, Peralta RM, Haminiuk CW, Maciel GM, Bracht A, Ferreira IC. New phytochemicals as potential human anti-aging compounds: Reality, promise, and challenges. Critical Reviews in Food Science and Nutrition. 2016. [Epub ahead of print]

[81] Panza F, Seripa D, Solfrizzi V, Tortelli R, Greco A, Pilotto A, Logroscino G. Targeting cognitive frailty: Clinical and neurobiological roadmap for a single complex phenotype. Journal of Alzheimer's Disease. 2015;**47**(4):793-813

[82] Verdin E. NAD^+ in aging, metabolism, and neurodegeneration. Science. 2015;**350** (6265):1208-1213

4

Sarcopenia and Malnutrition in the Elderly

Beatriz Lardiés-Sánchez and Alejandro Sanz-París

Abstract

Sarcopenia and malnutrition are both commonly occurring conditions in elderly population. As understood today, sarcopenia is a syndrome characterised by progressive and generalised loss of skeletal muscle mass, physical performance and/or strength, whereas malnutrition has been defined as a condition of an imbalance of energy, protein and other nutrients that can cause measurable negative effects. In many populations, malnutrition and sarcopenia are present simultaneously, and they appear clinically through a combination of decreased body weight and nutrient intake, along with a decrease in muscle mass and function. Moreover, malnutrition is one of the key pathophysiological causes of sarcopenia. Both entities result in numerous and substantial negative outcomes to the patients and the healthcare system, including decreased quality of life and functionality and increased healthcare costs, hospitalisation rates, morbidity and mortality. Early identification of sarcopenia would be of great clinical relevance because the loss of muscle mass and strength with ageing can be largely reversed by proper exercise and nutritional intervention. Clinicians should integrate nutritional assessment with sarcopenia screening for optimal evaluation of these two interrelated issues to help improve clinical outcomes.

Keywords: sarcopenia, malnutrition, muscle, prevalence, elderly people

1. Introduction

The aged population in the developed world is increasing rapidly. Ageing is accompanied by changes in body composition, including a decrease in muscle mass. From the age of 50 years onwards, muscle mass decreases by 1–2% annually and muscle strength is reduced by approximately 1.5% annually between the age of 50 and 60 years [1]. This age-related loss of skeletal muscle mass, resulting in loss of strength and function, is defined as sarcopenia. This geriatric syndrome is associated with an increased risk for adverse outcomes, such as poor quality of life, risk of falls and death. Moreover, it is a major contributing factor of physical disability, frailty and loss of independence in the elderly. It may be thus an important and potentially reversible cause of morbidity and mortality in older persons [2].

On the other hand, malnutrition is described as a chronic or acute condition of the body in which a deficiency or imbalance of energy, protein and other nutrients leads to negative effects on function, clinical outcomes and body composition [3].

Sarcopenia and malnutrition have similar physiological mechanisms and are common and overlapping in older adults. Both entities result in numerous and substantial negative outcomes to the patients and the healthcare system, including decreased quality of life and functionality and increased healthcare costs, hospitalisation rates, morbidity and mortality. Both entities are highly prevalent among population over the age of 65 years and more, especially in those living in nursing homes or hospitalised [4].

Early identification of sarcopenia and malnutrition would seem to be of clinical relevance because the nutritional deficiencies and the loss of muscle mass and strength with ageing can be largely reversed by proper lifelong improvements in nutritional intervention and physical activity. They are probably the most effective intervention to improve physical functioning, prevent falls and disabilities and, consequently, improve the quality of life in the older population. This is especially important given that world is ageing and older adults will utilise healthcare services at an increased rate in the next years [4].

2. Sarcopenia

2.1. Definition, mechanisms, causes and prevalence of sarcopenia

The term sarcopenia is derived from the Greek words 'sarx' (flesh) and 'penia' (loss). Unlike earlier definitions of sarcopenia, focusing on measurements of low muscle mass only, the current definition of sarcopenia according to the European consensus of the EWGSOP (European Working Group on Sarcopenia in Older People) [5] requires the presence of both low muscle mass and low muscle function (muscle strength or physical performance), although they have not achieved consensus on the cut-off points of muscle mass indicating sarcopenia. The International Working Group on Sarcopenia (IWGS) also proposed an operational definition of sarcopenia, which was targeted to individuals with functional decline, mobility-related difficulties, history of recurrent falls, recent unintentional weight loss, post-hospitalisation and chronic conditions [6, 7].

In many older people, sarcopenia is a multifactorial process where several mechanisms can be involved. When the only evident cause of sarcopenia is the ageing, sarcopenia can be considered as primary (or age-related). In fact, malnutrition status is one of the main causes of sarcopenia (protein-poor diet determines a compensatory response characterised by a reduction in lean mass) [8].

Epidemiological data suggest that the prevalence of sarcopenia varies widely, depending on the different populations studied, gender, age, settings, diagnostic criteria used and the cut-off points chosen to define a low muscle mass. In a recent systematic review [9], five European studies were found using EWGSOP criteria to define sarcopenia in ageing people using BIA (bioelectrical impedance analysis) in different settings, with a prevalence of sarcopenia between 7.5 and 77.6%. The highest prevalence was found in people staying in convalescence and rehabilitation units, while community-dwelling older people had the lowest prevalence.

3. Malnutrition

3.1. Definition and aetiology of malnutrition

Malnutrition has been defined as a condition of an imbalance of energy, protein and other nutrients that can cause measurable negative effects on body composition, physical function and clinical outcomes [10].

Older adults are known to be at high risk of malnutrition. Advanced age is an independent risk factor for malnutrition and is associated with a lower body weight, body mass index (BMI) and serum albumin. Malnutrition is not an inevitable side effect of ageing, but many changes associated with the process of ageing can promote a poor nutritional status. The decline in taste acuity and smell, poor dentition and a decreased appetite are some factors that can affect nutrient intake and can lead to malnutrition and its potentially serious consequences. Other factors, such as an increased frequency and severity of acute and chronic medical conditions, multiple medications, social or economic challenges and cognitive decline, all play a role in the aetiology of malnutrition among older adults [11].

3.2. Nutritional assessment in the elderly

The best validated and most widely used test to measure nutritional status of older people is the Mini Nutritional Assessment (MNA). This includes 18 questions regarding weight change, dietary change, gastrointestinal symptoms, mobility, physical assessment and disease and its relationship with nutritional requirements, with a maximum score of 30 points. Patients who score >24 points are considered well nourished, those that score 17–23.5 points are classified as at risk of malnutrition and those who score <17 points are considered malnourished. Using MNA, Guigoz found 5–71% prevalence of malnutrition among 6821 elderly persons after a review of 32 studies and reported that malnutrition risk was higher in those living in nursing homes than in community-dwelling elderly [12].

Another nutritional assessment tool developed for the elderly population is the Nutritional Form for the Elderly (NUFFE). This instrument was designed as a form that contains items that reflect functional, social, nutritional and health-related aspects of nutritional intake [13].

On the other hand, ESPEN (The European Society for Clinical Nutrition and Metabolism) has recently proposed a new consensus definition of malnutrition [14]. According to this definition, individuals identified as 'at risk' of malnutrition proceed in the diagnostic process, with two possible options: body mass index (BMI) <18.5 kg/m^2 or unintentional weight loss (>10% independent of time or >5% in last 3 months), this last option is always combined with either a low BMI <20 kg/m^2 (if <70 years old) or <22 kg/m^2 (if >70 years old) or a low fat-free mass index (FFMI) <15 kg/m^2 (women) and <17 kg/m^2 (men).

3.3. Prevalence of malnutrition

Depending on the method or parameters used for the nutritional assessment, prevalence rates of malnutrition among elderly subjects range between 6.5 and 85%. Early identification of older adults at nutritional risk, followed by adequate nutritional intervention, is expected to contribute to conservation of muscle function and muscle strength, and herewith to maintenance the functional independence, the quality of life and possibly to prolong the survival [15].

The prevalence of malnutrition depends on multiple factors, including the definition and the diagnostic criteria used. This prevalence is greater among older adults in healthcare settings. In fact, in hospital settings, malnutrition is approximately 56% in elderly patients [16].

3.4. Malnutrition-sarcopenia syndrome

Malnutrition is common across varying patient populations, particularly in older adults, and sarcopenia prevalence also increases with age. Moreover, malnutrition is regarded as one important contributing factor in the complex aetiology of sarcopenia, and it may be amenable to intervention. In fact, a diagnostic category of malnutrition-related sarcopenia has been proposed [5]. However, usually older people admitted to nursing homes are screened or assessed for either malnutrition or sarcopenia, but rarely for both conditions concurrently. In several populations, malnutrition and sarcopenia are present simultaneously and manifest clinically through a combination of decreased nutrient intake, decreased body weight, along with a decrease in muscle mass, strength and/or physical function [17].

Vanderwoude et al. [4] proposed the term 'malnutrition-sarcopenia syndrome', which embodies the inherent association of both entities, highlighting their combined impact on clinical outcomes, including increased morbidity, infection and complications (as falls and disability), length of hospital stay and rehospitalisation rates, mortality and healthcare costs, apart from decreased quality of life. Malnutrition and sarcopenia are each independently associated with negative health consequences that impact older adults across healthcare settings [18, 19].

There are few published data demonstrating the co-occurrence of malnutrition and sarcopenia in older adults. In a recent study [20], both entities have been studied in a post-acute care geriatric unit, applying the new ESPEN definition of malnutrition and EWGSOP criteria, assessing the potential clinical relationship between them. The prevalence of malnutrition in this population was 19.3%, and the prevalence of sarcopenia was significantly higher in patients with malnutrition: 82.3 versus 45.1% ($p = 0.03$), which means that most patients with sarcopenia fulfilled the ESPEN criteria for diagnosis of malnutrition. On the other hand, in the study of Senior et al. [21], sarcopenia was defined with EWGSOP criteria and nutritional status was assessed with MNA short-form test. According to these criteria, 14.9% of participants with sarcopenia were malnourished and 48.5% were at risk of malnutrition. The prevalence of malnutrition was higher in subjects with low handgrip strength (62.8%) and in participants with severe sarcopenia (60.8%). Moreover, research has shown that reductions in handgrip strength are common in individuals who have sarcopenia as well as in individuals who are malnourished [5, 22].

4. Screening for malnutrition-sarcopenia

Clinicians should integrate nutrition assessment with sarcopenia screening for optimal evaluation of these two interrelated nutritional issues to help improve patients' clinical outcomes [4].

For sarcopenia screening, a simple clinician tool has been suggested by the EWGSOP [5]. This group has developed an algorithm based on gait speed measurement (a cut-off point of >0.8 m/s identifies risk for sarcopenia) as the easiest and most reliable way to begin sarcopenia screening in clinical practice.

Screening tools for malnutrition are intended for the quick identification of patients at risk of malnutrition, for more in-depth nutritional assessment, or for identifying patients at risk of developing complications or even increased risk of mortality. A variety of malnutrition screening tools are available such as the Malnutrition Screening Tool (MST), Malnutrition Universal Screening Tool (MUST) [23], the short form of the Mini Nutritional Assessment (SF-MNA) [24] and Nutrition Risk Screening-2002 (NRS-2002) [25]. Based on the evidence presented, the combination of screening and assessing for malnutrition and sarcopenia is recommended to screen for the presence of malnutrition-sarcopenia syndrome in at-risk patient populations, particularly older adults in clinical settings [4].

Clinicians are urged to screen, assess and treat these conditions currently. By examining aspects of both conditions, clinicians can more fully assess their patients' clinical and nutritional status and can design targeted therapies to meet their needs and improve outcomes [4].

Examining patient's nutritional and functional status through screening and assessment for both malnutrition and sarcopenia will enable clinical practitioners to determine the presence of both entities in their patients and to target interventions to prevent and avoid them [4].

5. Nutritional interventions to prevent sarcopenia

The relationship between muscle mass, strength, physical function and nutritional status has significant clinical implications regarding the therapeutic approaches [26].

Early identification of sarcopenia would be of great clinical relevance because the loss of muscle mass and strength with ageing can be largely reversed by proper exercise programs and nutritional intervention [27]. Of all the therapeutic options available, lifelong improvements in physical activity and diet are probably the most effective public health intervention and the most important treatment option in nursing home residents for this condition, ongoing independence and autonomy in older people. The Society for Sarcopenia, Cachexia and Wasting Disease developed nutritional recommendations for the prevention and management of sarcopenia, which combined exercise with adequate protein and energy intake [28].

On the other hand, adequate caloric intake has to be considered as an essential requisite for any successful therapeutic approach in the institutionalised elderly participants, in terms of prevention and treatment of sarcopenia. Nutrient intake, especially adequate amounts of high-quality protein and amino acids, is the most important anabolic stimulus of skeletal muscle protein synthesis. Epidemiological studies suggest that a low protein intake is associated with sarcopenia. To prevent it, as optimal dietary protein intake, daily 1.0–1.2 g/kg with an optimal repartition over each daily meal or 25–30 g of high-quality protein per meal are recommended. Specifically, the amino acid leucine and meal-induced insulin, both independently stimulate muscle protein synthesis. It has been demonstrated that exercise and amino acid supplementation (3 g of a leucine-enriched balanced essential amino acid mixture twice a day) together may actually be effective in enhancing muscle strength, variables of muscle mass and walking speed in sarcopenic women [29]. Antioxidants and ω 3-polyunsaturated fatty acids may also contribute to the preservation of muscle function. Low 25-hydroxyvitamin D (25(OH)D) serum level in adults is also a potentially modifiable risk factor for sarcopenia [30]. In fact, nutritional interventions combining adequate amounts of vitamin D and proteins are promising strategies to attenuate sarcopenia development [31]. Some studies have shown the effectiveness of other nutritional factors, such as cheese and milk protein and beta-hydroxy-beta-methylbutyrate (HMB), as a potential supplement to improve muscle quality in sarcopenic elderly people [32, 33].

In a recent study [34], Mediterranean dietary pattern (high in olive, low-fat dairy, vegetable, fish, nut and vegetable oil) has demonstrated a favourable role in the prevention of sarcopenia in postmenopausal women, in comparison with a Western pattern (based on high commercial beverage, sugar and dessert, snacks, solid fat, potato, high-fat dairy, legume, organ meat, fast food and sweets). Another study [35] demonstrated that improvements in clinically relevant measures, such as strength and functionality, could be achieved by supplementation with high-quality oral nutritional supplementation.

Other treatments of sarcopenia currently under investigation include testosterone replacement therapy, oestrogens in women, growth hormone and other behavioural and pharmacological strategies. The main limitation of these treatments is the lack of long-term adherence [8].

Author details

Beatriz Lardiés-Sánchez* and Alejandro Sanz-París

*Address all correspondence to: bealardies@gmail.com

Universitary Hospital Miguel Servet, Zaragoza, Spain

References

[1] Buford TW, Anton SD, Judge AR, Marzetti E, Wohlgemuth SE, Carter CS, et al. Models of accelerated sarcopenia: Critical pieces for solving the puzzle of age-related muscle atrophy. Ageing Research Reviews. 2010;**9**(4):369-383. DOI: 10.1016/j.arr.2010.04.004

[2] Serra Rexach JA. Clinical consequences of sarcopenia. Nutrición Hospitalaria. 2006; **21**(3):46-50

[3] García de Lorenzo A, Álvarez-Hernández J, Planas M, Burgos R, Araujo K. The multidisciplinary consensus work-team on the approach to hospital malnutrition in Spain. Multidisciplinary consensus on the approach to hospital malnutrition in Spain. Nutrición Hospitalaria. 2011;**26**(4):701-710

[4] Vanderwoude MFJ, Alish CJ, Sauer AC, Hegazi RA. Malnutrition-sarcopenia syndrome: Is this the future of nutrition screening and assessment for older adults? Journal of Aging Research. 2012;**2012**:1-8. DOI: 10.1155/2012/651570

[5] Cruz-Jentoft AJ, Baeyens JM, Bauer JM, Boirie Y, Cederholm T, Landi F, et al. Sarcopenia: European consensus on definition and diagnosis: Report of the European Working Group on Sarcopenia in Older People. Age Aging. 2010;**39**:412-423. DOI: 10.1093/ageing/afq034

[6] Fielding RA, Vellas B, Evans WJ, Bhasin S, Morley JE, Newman AB, et al. Sarcopenia: An undiagnosed condition in older adults. Current consensus definition: Prevalence, etiology, and consequences. International Working Group on Sarcopenia. Journal of the American Medical Directors Association. 2011;**12**(4):249-256. DOI: 10.1016/j.jamda.2011.01.003

[7] Visser M, Schaap LA. Consequences of sarcopenia. Clinics in Geriatric Medicine. 2011;**27**:387-399. DOI: 10.1016/j.cger.2011.03.006

[8] Rolland Y, Czerwinski S, Abellan Van Kan G, et al. Sarcopenia: Its assessment, etiology, pathogenesis, consequences and future perspectives. Journal of Nutrition Health and Aging. 2008;**12**:433-450

[9] Lardiés Sánchez B, Sanz-París A, Boj-Carceller D, Cruz-Jentoft AJ. Systematic review: Prevalence of sarcopenia in ageing people using bioelectrical impedance analysis to assess muscle mass. European Geriatric Medicine. 2016;**7**:256-261. DOI: 10.1016/j.eurger.2016.01.014

[10] Sttraton RJ, Green CJ, Elia M. Disease-Related Malnutrition: An Evidence-Based Approach to Treatment. Wallingford, UK; Cambridge, MA: CABI Pub; 2003.

[11] Jensen GL, Mirtallo J, Compher C, Dhaliwal R, Forbes A, Grijalba RF, et al. Adult starvation and disease related malnutrition: A proposal for etiology-based diagnosis in the clinical practice setting from the International Consensus Guideline Committee. Journal of Parenteral and Enteral Nutrition. 2010;**34**(2):156-159

[12] Guigoz Y. The Mini Nutritional Assessment (MNA) review of the literature: What does it tell us? Journal of Nutrition Health and Aging. 2006;**10**(6):466-485

[13] Söderhamn U, Söderhamn O. Reliability and validity of the nutritional form for the elderly (NUFFE). Journal of Advanced Nursing. 2002;**37**(1):28-34

[14] Cederholm T, Bosaeus I, Barazzoni R, Bauer J, Van Gossum A, Klek S, et al. Diagnostic criteria for malnutrition: An ESPEN Consensus Statement Clinical Nutrition. 2015;**34**(3): 335-340. DOI: 10.1016/j.clnu.2015.03.001

[15] Beck AM. Weight loss, mortality and associated potentially modifiable nutritional risk factors among nursing home residents: A Danish follow-up study. Journal of Nutrition Health and Aging. 2015;**19**(1):96-101

[16] Pirlich M, Schütz T, Norman K, et al. The German hospital malnutrition study. Clinical Nutrition. 2006;**25**(4):563-572

[17] Vivanti A, Ward N, Haines T. Nutritional status and associations with falls, balance, mobility and functionality during hospital admission. Journal of Nutrition Health and Aging. 2011;**15**:388-391

[18] Saka B, Ozkaya H, Karisik E, Akin S, Akpinar TS, Tufan F, et al. Malnutrition and sarcopenia are associated with increased mortality rate in nursing home residents: A prospective study. European Geriatric Medicine. 2016;7(3):232-238. DOI: 10.1016/j.eurger.2015.12.010

[19] Landi F, Cruz-Jentoft AJ, Liperoti R, Russo A, Giovanni S, Tosato M, et al. Sarcopenia and mortality risk in frail older persons aged 80 years and older: Results from ilSIR-ENTE study. Age Ageing. 2013;**42**(2):203-209. DOI: 10.1093/ageing/afs194

[20] Sánchez-Rodríguez D, Marco E, Ronquillo-Moreno N, Miralles R, Vázquez-Ibar O, Escalada F. Prevalence of malnutrition and sarcopenia in a post-acute care geriatric unit: Applying the new ESPEN definition and EWGSOP criteria. Clin Nutr. 2016 Sep 9. pii: S0261-5614(16)30233-3. DOI:10.1016/j.clnu.2016.08.024. [Epub ahead of print]

[21] Senior HE, Henwood TR, Beller EM, Mitchell GK, Keogh JW. Prevalence and risk factors of sarcopenia among adults living in nursing homes. Maturitas 2015;**82**(4):418-423. DOI: 10.1016/j.maturitas.2015.08.006

[22] Norman K, Stobäus N, González MC, Schulzke JD, Pirlich M. Hand grip strength: Outcome predictor and marker of nutritional status. Clinical Nutrition. 2006;**30**(2):135-142

[23] Stratton RJ, Hackston A, Longmore D, Dixon R, Price S, Stroud M, King C, Elia M. Malnutrition in hospital outpatients and inpatients: Prevalence, concurrent validity and ease of use of the "malnutrition universal screening tool" (MUST) for adults. British Journal of Nutrition. 2004;**92**(5):799-808

[24] Ranhoff AH, Gjoen AU, Mowé M. Screening for malnutrition in elderly acute medical patients: The usefulness of MNA-SF. Journal of Nutrition Health and Aging. 2005;**9**(4): 221-225

[25] Kondrup J, Rasmussen HH, Hamberg O, Stanga Z, Ad Hoc ESPEN Working Group. Nutritional risk screening (NRS 2002): A new method based on an analysis of controlled clinical trials. Clinical Nutrition. 2003;**22**(3):321-336

[26] Roubenoff R. Sarcopenia: Effects on body composition and function. The Journals of Gerontology. Series A, Biological Sciences and Medical Sciences. 2003;**58**:1012-1017

[27] Malafarina V, Uriz-Otano F, Iniesta R, Gil-Guerrero L. Effectiveness of nutritional supplementation on muscle mass in treatment of sarcopenia in old age: A systematic review. Journal of the American Medical Directors Association. 2013;**14**:10-17. DOI: 10.1016/j.jamda.2012.08.001

[28] Morley JE, Argiles JM, Evans WJ, et al. Nutritional recommendations for the management of sarcopenia. Journal of the American Medical Directors Association. 2010;**11**:391-396

[29] Yanai H. Nutrition for sarcopenia. Journal of Clinical Medicine and Research. 2015;**7**(12):926-931

[30] Visser M, Deeg DJ, Lips P. Longitudinal Aging Study. Low vitamin D and high parathyroid hormone levels as determinants of loss of muscle strength and muscle mass (sarcopenia): The Longitudinal Aging Study Amsterdam. Journal of Clinical Endocrinology and Metabolism. 2003;**88**(12):5766-5772

[31] Verlaan S, Maier AB, Bauer JM, Bautmans I, Brandt K, Donini LM, et al. Sufficient levels of 25-hydroxyvitamin D and protein intake required to increase muscle mass in sarcopenic older adults: The PROVIDE study. Clinical Nutrition. 2017;**pii:S0261-5614**(17):30010-30019. DOI: 10.1016/j.clnu.2017.01.005

[32] Makanae Y, Fujita S. Role of exercise and nutrition in the prevention of sarcopenia. Journal of Nutritional Science and Vitaminology. 2015;**61**:S125-S127

[33] Kim HK, Sazuki T, Saito K, et al. Effects of exercise and amino acid supplementation on body composition and physical function in community-dwelling elderly Japanese sarcopenic women: A randomized controlled trial. Journal of the American Geriatrics Society. 2012;**60**(1):16-23

[34] Mohseni R, Aliakbar S, Abdollahi A, Yekaninejad MS, Maghbooli Z, Mirzaei K. Relationship between major dietary patterns and sarcopenia among menopausal women. Aging Clin Exp Res. 2017 Feb 21. doi:10.1007/s40520-016-0721-4. [Epub ahead of print]

[35] Cramer JT, Cruz-Jentoft AJ, Landi F, Hickson M, Zamboni M, Pereira SL, et al. Impacts of high-protein oral nutritional supplements among malnourished men and women with sarcopenia: A multicenter, randomized, double-blinded, controlled trial. Journal of the American Medical Directors Association. 2016;**17**(11):1044-1055. DOI: 10.1016/j.jamda.2016.08.009

5

Sarcopenic Dysphagia as a New Concept

Kotomi Sakai and Kunihiro Sakuma

Abstract

Dysphagia (swallowing difficulties) is a serious problem associated with malnutrition, dehydration, aspiration pneumonia, and death. Its well-known causes include stroke, neuromuscular disease, and head and neck cancer, and these affect muscles and sensation during deglutition. In recent years, dysphagia due to sarcopenia (i.e. "sarcopenic dysphagia") has been reported as a new concept. Sarcopenic dysphagia results from low swallowing and general skeletal muscle mass and strength. The characteristic changes in swallowing muscles occur primarily in oral and pharyngeal muscles along with other associated factors. With a rapidly aging population, the number of older adults with sarcopenic dysphagia is expected to increase. Therefore, it is necessary to investigate the pathophysiology and treatment strategies for sarcopenic dysphagia. In this chapter, we summarize previous studies related to sarcopenic dysphagia.

Keywords: sarcopenia, deglutition disorders, rehabilitation

1. Introduction

The term "sarcopenia" was first proposed by Rosenberg [1] to describe age-related decrease in muscle mass. In 2010, the European Working Group on Sarcopenia in Older People (EWGSOP) proposed the sarcopenia consensus on definition and diagnostic criteria. The EWGSOP defined sarcopenia as a geriatric syndrome characterized by progressive and generalized loss of muscle mass and strength. In addition, they proposed diagnostic criteria for sarcopenia [2]. Subsequently, the International Working Group on Sarcopenia (IWGS) proposed similar definitions [3]. In 2014, the Asian Working Group for Sarcopenia (AWGS) proposed diagnostic criteria based on data on Asian populations [4]. In 2016, sarcopenia was recognized as an independent condition by an ICD-10-CM code [5]. Currently, sarcopenia is recognized worldwide.

Since sarcopenia is characterized by generalized loss of muscle mass and function, it can involve a concomitant reduction in swallowing muscles mass and function. Swallowing is defined as "the function of clearing food and drink through the oral cavity, pharynx, and esophagus into the stomach at an appropriate rate and speed" by the International Classification of Functioning, Disability and Health [6]. According to medical terminology, "dysphagia" is the symptom (not a disease) characterized by swallowing problems. Dysphagia has been proposed as a geriatric syndrome such as sarcopenia [7]. In 1992, Veldee and Peth indicated that malnutrition affects swallowing muscles; however, the term "sarcopenia" was not coined [8]. In 2005, Robbins et al. used the term "dysphagia due to sarcopenia" in their study [9]. Since then, studies on dysphagia related to sarcopenia have increased drastically. The term "sarcopenic dysphagia" was first used by kuroda in 2012 [10]. Since then, the term "sarcopenic dysphagia" has been used by mainly Japanese researchers [11]. However, this is not a standard medical term. In 2015, Clave and Shaker, worldwide leading researchers in dysphagia, used the term "sarcopenic dysphagia" in a review article [12], wherein sarcopenic dysphagia was introduced as a new concept of dysphagia. To our knowledge, that was the first article that described the term "sarcopenic dysphagia," except those from Japan.

Dysphagia results in serious complications such as aspiration pneumonia, choking, dehydration, malnutrition, and lower quality of life, all of which are potentially lethal. A meta-analysis on aspiration pneumonia in frail older people revealed that dysphagia is a significant risk factor for aspiration pneumonia [13]. Furthermore, dysphagia negatively affects the nationwide cost of medication because of these complications, readmissions, higher drug intake, and prolonged hospitalization [14, 15]. Therefore, dysphagia is a serious problem that should be prevented and treated.

Many studies have been reported on dysphagia due to neurological diseases such as stroke, Parkinson's disease and other forms of dementia, amyotrophic lateral sclerosis, head and neck cancer, and esophageal cancer. However, articles on sarcopenic dysphagia are few because it is a new concept of dysphagia. We described the number of articles about dysphagia based on years of publication in **Table 1**. We used "aging" or "frail" or "sarcopenia" and "dysphagia"

	Total	2016	2015	2014
Stroke	1416	159	145	134
Head and neck cancer	1019	139	141	120
Parkinson's disease	472	50	53	46
Aging	305	31	31	30
Frail	75	8	6	8
Sarcopenia	38	13	11	6

We set the keywords related to sarcopenia (aging, frail, or sarcopenia) and major causes of dysphagia (stroke, head and neck cancer, or Parkinson's disease) for comparison of research interests. We described the number of articles overall and their years of publication in the last three years. Compared to stroke, Parkinson's disease, and head and neck cancer, articles related to sarcopenic dysphagia are less. The articles were accessed on January 7, 2017.

Table 1. Number of articles retrieved for the terms "dysphagia" or "swallowing" and each keyword on PubMed.

or "swallowing" as keywords for retrieving in PubMed. In addition, stroke or Parkinson's disease or head and neck cancer were used as keywords to compare these with the number of articles on dysphagia related to sarcopenia. Since sarcopenia is a geriatric syndrome [2], the number of older adults with sarcopenia would increase with a rapidly aging worldwide population. Similarly, the number of older adults with sarcopenic dysphagia would increase. Thus, it is important to investigate the clinical conditions and treatment strategies for sarcopenic dysphagia. In this chapter, we summarize dysphagia related to sarcopenia based on previous studies on mainly healthy or frail subjects or those with sarcopenia.

2. Epidemiology of sarcopenic dysphagia

2.1. Definition and prevalence

The current definition of sarcopenic dysphagia is "difficulty swallowing due to sarcopenia of general skeletal and swallowing muscles" [7, 12]. Although the diagnostic criteria for sarcopenia are defined by the cutoff value of muscle mass and physical function or muscle strength [2, 16], the diagnostic criteria for sarcopenic dysphagia have not been standardized. However, a few studies have attempted to investigate the prevalence of sarcopenic dysphagia; these included subjects without diseases directly affecting swallowing function, such as stroke, Parkinson's disease, and head and neck cancer. Maeda and Akagi [17, 18] reported its prevalence as 42.3 and 30%, respectively, in acute older inpatients at admission. In addition, in their prospective observational study [19], 26% of acute older inpatients developed sarcopenic dysphagia within 60 days of admission. Their studies mainly included older inpatients with acute internal diseases. For older inpatients, it is easy to develop sarcopenic dysphagia during hospitalization because of rest in bed and anorexia by illness. In our study subjects, from acute hospitals to a rehabilitation hospital [11], 32.2% of older inpatients had sarcopenic dysphagia on admission. Our study included many older inpatients with orthopedic disorders. These findings suggest that the prevalence of sarcopenic dysphagia is approximately 30–40% in older inpatients. In community-dwelling older adults, the review article reported that approximately 15% of them had dysphagia [20]. The risk factors of dysphagia included age, history of clinical disease, and physical frailty, including reduced activities of daily living. However, this review did not have sarcopenic dysphagia as an endpoint. Older inpatients are at a higher risk of sarcopenic dysphagia than community-dwelling older adults. The prevention, assessment, and intervention for sarcopenic dysphagia are important, especially in older inpatients.

2.2. Etiology

Several pathophysiological mechanisms are known for sarcopenia in general skeletal muscles. Sarcopenia is categorized as primary and/or secondary sarcopenia based on etiology [2]. The most prominent cause of primary sarcopenia is aging, while those of secondary sarcopenia are inactivity (bed rest, sedentary lifestyle, deconditioning, or zero-gravity conditions), malnutrition (inadequate dietary intake), and disease (advanced organ failure such as heart, lung, liver, kidney, brain, inflammatory disease, malignancy, or endocrine disease).

Several studies have shown associations of aging, inactivity, malnutrition, and disease with dysphagia [21–23]. The characteristic change in the swallowing mechanism in healthy older adults, because of aging, is referred to as "presbyphagia" [24]. Anatomical and functional changes due to aging render older adults at risk of dysphagia [25, 26]. Though aging causes reduced swallowing function, it does not cause dysphagia. In relation to inactivity, physical inactivity can cause sarcopenic dysphagia [19]. In our study in a rehabilitation hospital [11], physical activity level was independently associated with the functional level of oral intake of food and liquid. In addition, the duration of tentative nil per os (NPO) without dysphagia assessment in patients with aspiration pneumonia resulted in reduced swallowing ability during treatment [27]. Inactivity of swallowing muscles itself can cause disuse of themselves and appendicular skeletal muscles. Aspiration pneumonia in older adults usually results in bedrest and NPO for treatment. Although aspiration pneumonia is known to be caused by dysphagia, it can also cause sacropenic dysphagia because of inactivity and malnutrition with its treatment. In relation to nutritional status, mid-upper arm circumference was associated with swallowing function [10]. In addition, nutritional status was a factor of the prognosis of swallowing ability in older inpatients [19]. In other studies, malnutrition has been suggested to cause dysphagia [8, 28]. Veldee and Peth [8] postulated that swallowing muscles have moderate-to-high percentage of type II fibers because normal swallowing is characterized by rapid contraction of muscles. Furthermore, malnutrition can affect those swallowing muscles because type II fibers are reportedly affected by malnutrition more easily than type I fibers [29–32]. Malnutrition can be one of the main causes of sarcopenic dysphagia.

In relation to the disease, the prevalence of sarcopenia is high among chronically ill patients, ranging from 15 to 50% in patients with cancer and 30 to 45% in patients with liver failure [33]. In addition, cachexia is a metabolic syndrome characterized by loss of muscle mass with or without loss of fat mass, which can cause sarcopenia, and is prevalent in 50 to 80% of cases in several types of cancer [34]. Wakabayashi et al. [23] showed that loss of skeletal muscle mass was related to severe dysphagia in patients with cancer. Patients with chronic progressive diseases such as cancer can develop dysphagia more easily than those with other diseases, owing to sarcopenia. In older adults with Alzheimer's disease, decreased skeletal muscle mass resulted in poor swallowing functions [35]. Dysphagia in neurodegenerative disease can be caused by sarcopenia. Decreased general skeletal muscle mass was considered a risk factor for sarcopenic dysphagia in acute older inpatients [19]. Although the detailed pathophysiological mechanism of sarcopenic dysphagia from decreased general skeletal muscle mass is largely unclear, sarcopenic dysphagia can develop during general sarcopenia.

A high prevalence of sarcopenic dysphagia in older inpatients may be because hospitalization causes further inactivity and/or decrease in nutritional status and leads to severe sarcopenia. Almost all these studies revealed the associations between dysphagia and sarcopenia; however, these are not causal relationships because of the cross-sectional design of these studies. Further studies are required to explore causal relationships. We described the possible pathophysiological mechanism of sarcopenic dysphagia in **Figure 1**.

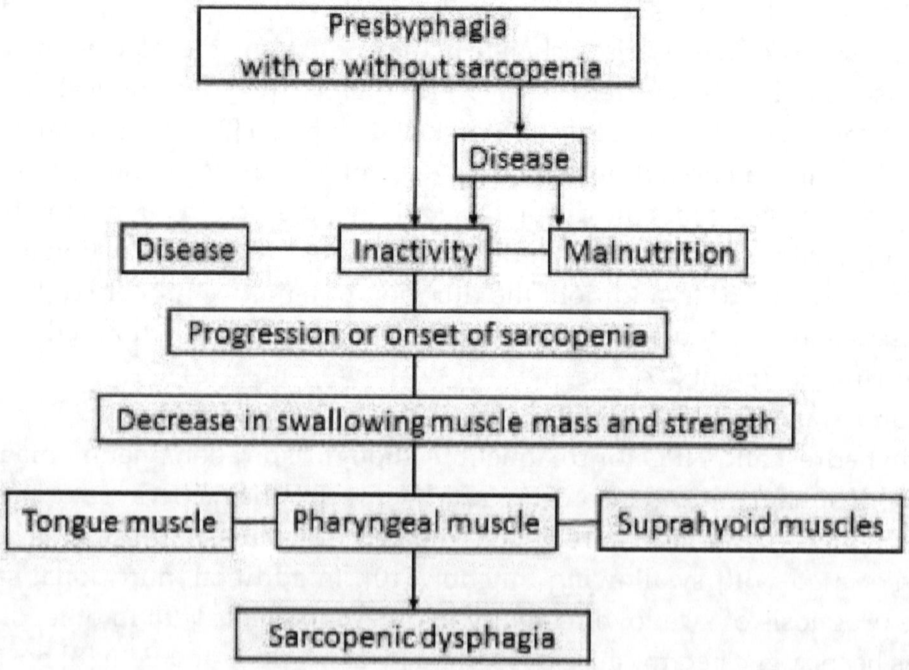

Figure 1. Possible mechanism of sarcopenic dysphagia. Older adults with presbyphagia can develop generalized sarcopenia due to disease, inactivity, or malnutrition. In the progress of generalized sarcopenia, sarcopenic dysphagia can develop due to decreased tongue, pharyngeal, and/or suprahyoid muscle function involved in swallowing.

3. Pathophysiology of sarcopenic dysphagia

3.1. Swallowing process

Swallowing is a complex process involving up to 30 striated muscles [12, 36], although swallowing is a continuous process generally conceptualized as occurring in several discrete phases. The first phase is the "preoral phase" wherein visual and olfactory qualities of food are recognized and they cause salivation, which is needed for bolus preparation [37]. The second phase is the "oral preparatory phase" wherein food is chewed and mixed with saliva to form a bolus that is easily transported to pharynx. The third phase is the "oral transit phase" wherein the tongue begins anterior-to-posterior propulsion of the bolus into pharynx. The fourth phase is the "pharyngeal phase" wherein numerous muscles function in a rapid sequence. The last phase is the "esophageal phase" wherein the bolus enters the esophagus and is transported toward the stomach by peristaltic contractions of the esophagus. Through swallowing, appropriate temporal coordination of feeding and breathing is needed to provide proper nutrition and to prevent aspiration because the pathways for food and air communicate in the pharynx [38].

3.2. Preoral phase to oral transit phase

In the preoral phase, cognitive function is related to dysphagia. In patients with congestive heart failure, cognitive dysfunction is a predictor of dysphagia [39]. In addition, sarcopenia has been independently associated with cognitive impairment in meta-analysis [40]. Thus, cognitive impairment can contribute to development of sarcopenic dysphagia. On transiting from the oral preparatory phase to the pharyngeal phase, several muscles are involved in swallowing, of which the tongue is a major muscle. The previous studies [9, 41] have found that individuals who aspirate have lower tongue strength than those who do not. Thus, tongue strength is a very important factor for swallowing. To our knowledge, Robbins et al. [42] are the first to indicate that tongue strength is affected by sarcopenia. In their study on healthy men, maximal isometric pressures were significantly greater at the tongue blade site in younger subjects, whereas peak swallow pressures remained similar across both young and older subjects. Nicosia et al. [43] also showed the same results in both healthy men and women. However, Robbins and colleagues [44] showed that both maximal isometric pressures and swallow pressures reduced with aging, and differences between maximal isometric pressures and swallow pressures were greater in younger adults than in older ones. Their studies have suggested diminished reserve of tongue strength in older adults. Buehring et al. [45] showed that both anterior and posterior maximum tongue pressure negatively correlated with age among community-dwelling individuals aged ≥ 70 years. Furthermore, Utanohara et al. [46] showed that men aged 20–40 years had higher anterior tongue pressure than the women, and anterior tongue pressure started to decrease from the age of 60 years in men and 70 years in women among healthy older adults. Their study indicated that tongue strength in men reduced with age at a faster rate than it did in women. Collectively, anterior and posterior tongue strength can decrease differently owing to age-related sarcopenia among men and women. Although a standard value of tongue strength in healthy older adults has not been established yet, Robbins et al. [41] considered tongue strength of <40 kPa as low, and Utanohara et al. [46] showed average tongue strength at 60 years of age was 37.6 ± 8.8 and 31.9 ± 8.9 kPa at 70 years of age. These values can be useful references in the clinical settings and in research. However, in our subjects aged ≥ 65 years [11], malnutrition was independently associated with low anterior tongue strength but not with age. Thus, decreased tongue strength in older adults can occur easily owing to malnutrition than because of aging.

The association between tongue strength and grip strength that represents whole body strength has been reported in several studies. Mendes et al. [47] showed that tongue and grip strength were reduced with increasing age. This study indicated that tongue strength was decreased owing to reduction in general muscle strength. Anterior tongue strength was significantly correlated with grip strength [11, 45, 47, 48]. However, Butler et al. [49] reported that posterior tongue strength, not anterior, was correlated with grip strength. The association between general muscle strength and tongue strength, whether anterior or posterior tongue, is under discussion. In addition to the difference of magnitude of tongue strength, Nicosia et al. [43] showed the difference of timing of tongue pressure generation between older and younger healthy adults. Time taken to reach maximal isometric pressure and swallowing pressure for liquids was longer in the older group than in the younger one. The timing of tongue strength generation may be also important in sarcopenic dysphagia.

Regarding tongue composition, a few studies have reported the distribution of tongue adipose tissue. Miller et al. [50] reported greater muscle tissue and correspondingly less adipose tissue in the posterior tongue than in the anterior tongue, whereas Nashi et al. [51] reported greater adipose tissue in the posterior tongue than in the anterior tongue on autopsy. As tongue muscle composition changed, amyloid deposits were found to be higher in older adults [52]. Owing to few studies on the tongue composition change by sarcopenia, further studies are required.

Regarding the association with appendicular skeletal muscle mass and tongue strength, Buehring et al. [45] showed that tongue strength was not significantly different in individuals who did or did not meet skeletal muscle mass criteria for sarcopenia. However, studies in older inpatients [11, 17] found a significant association between appendicular skeletal muscle mass and tongue strength in correlation analyses. In any case, the association between tongue strength and grip strength as one of sarcopenia indices is evident, and decreased tongue strength can be a symptom of sarcopenia and lead to sarcopenic dysphagia. Not only tongue strength but also tongue thickness was related to general muscle mass. Tamura et al. [53] showed that tongue thickness was significantly associated with mid-arm muscle area. Not only appendicular skeletal muscle mass but also tongue muscle mass can be affected by sarcopenia.

3.3. Pharyngeal phase

In the pharyngeal phase of swallowing, decreased pharyngeal strength has been shown to be related to aspiration status [54]. The suprahyoid muscles are important muscles responsible for pharyngeal strength required for swallowing. Feng and colleagues [55] examined the geniohyoid muscle—one of the suprahyoid muscles—using 80 computed tomography scans of the head and neck from healthy older and younger adults and revealed that the geniohyoid muscle atrophies with age in both the midsagittal and anterior coronal planes in men as well as women. In addition, atrophy of the geniohyoid muscle in the midsagittal plane was related to aspiration in men.

The movement of the hyoid bone, which is pulled upward and forward by the suprahyoid muscles, is assessed as an indicator of suprahyoid muscle function in videofluoroscopic swallowing studies (VFSS). VFSS is considered the gold standard examination for assessment of swallowing function because it is the only objective examination that evaluates the oral, palatal, pharyngeal, and pharyngoesophageal components of deglutition, comprehensively. Decreased range of motion and velocity of movement of the hyoid bone is observed more frequently in healthy older men than in younger men [56, 57]. In another study, the elevation of the hyoid was found to be greater in older adults both with and without dysphagia than in younger adults; however, in contrast to older adults without dysphagia, those with dysphagia were unable to use this strategy during deglutition of larger boluses [58]. In another study, the range of motion of the hyoid bone during swallowing was not significantly different between older and younger adults among both men and women. In contrast, the hyoid-larynx distance at rest was greater in both older men and women than in younger ones, and the change between the hyoid-larynx distance at rest and at the maximum approximation during swallowing was greater in older adults than in younger adults (men: mean 1.25 cm in younger men and 1.54 cm in older men; women: 1.07 cm in younger women and 1.19 cm in older women) [59]. The duration of supraglottic closure in VFSS was longer in older healthy adults than in younger healthy adults [60]. In addition, frail older adults showed slower laryngeal closure and upper esophageal sphincter opening and delayed maximal vertical hyoid motion (healthy, 0.310 ± 0.048 s; frail, 0.480 ± 0.055 s) than healthy adults. Tongue bolus propulsion strength measured by means of Newton's second law of motion in the pharyngeal phase in VFSS was 22.16 ± 2.54 mN in healthy older adults; frail older adults exhibited weaker tongue propulsion strength (8.99 ± 1.09 mN), leading to low bolus velocity and less kinetic energy [60]. There have been few studies on kinematic change related to sarcopenic dysphagia based on imaging findings; therefore, further research is warranted to investigate this issue.

In the assessment of dysphagia, jaw-opening strength was proposed as an indicator of suprahyoid muscle strength [61]. Based on measurement of jaw-opening strength in healthy adults, Iida et al. [62] suggested that suprahyoid muscle strength decreases with aging in both men and women. Machida et al. [63] demonstrated that low jaw-opening strength was associated with sarcopenia in older men. Suprahyoid muscle strength may decrease with aging and is further decreased in older men with sarcopenia. Hiramatsu et al. [64] demonstrated that the initiation of saliva swallowing was delayed and the number of saliva swallowings per 30 s decreased after meals in older adults but not in young adults (premeal, mean 7.61 and postmeal 7.30 in younger adults [no significant difference]; premeal, mean 5.35 and postmeal, mean 4.65 in older adults [significant difference, $p < 0.05$]). Their study indicated low endurance of swallowing muscles, including the suprahyoid muscles, in older adults. Low swallowing endurance can be an important component of sarcopenic dysphagia. Compared to studies on tongue muscles related to sarcopenia, fewer studies have been conducted on the suprahyoid muscles in relation to sarcopenia.

Kendall and Leonard [65] demonstrated that elderly patients with dysphagia of unknown etiology had delayed and incomplete pharyngeal constriction compared with both younger and age-matched controls without dysphagia. Leonard et al. [59] investigated spatial displacement variables in adults with no history of dysphagia and swallowing complaints. In their study, older adults with dysphagia exhibited poorer maximal pharyngeal constriction during swallowing as compared to healthy young controls. Dysfunction of pharyngeal constriction can be an important symptom of sarcopenic dysphagia. Based on the MRI scans of the neck in 60 women, Molfenter et al. [66] demonstrated that pharyngeal muscle thickness decreases and the size of the pharyngeal lumen increases with age. Such a structural change in the pharynx can result in incomplete pharyngeal constriction.

As for the sensory impairment associated with dysphagia, silent aspiration is a serious problem. Silent aspiration refers to aspiration before, during, or after swallowing in the absence of cough or visible signs of choking and distress. In a previous study, 32.5% of frail older adults with impaired safety swallow exhibited silent aspiration [60]. In a study on 76 healthy older adults [67], 83% (63/76) and 28% (21/76) exhibited penetration and silent aspiration, respectively. In addition, 85 and 61% of the subjects who exhibited penetration and aspiration, respectively, did not elicit a sensorimotor response. In another study with 56 healthy subjects [68], older adults showed a progressive decline in pharyngeal and supraglottic sensitivity measured using air pulse stimulation; sensory discrimination was 2.07 ± 0.20 mmHg in subjects aged 20–40 years and 2.68 ± 0.63 mmHg in subjects aged 61–90 years. Sarcopenia can lead to sensory decline in the pharynx and larynx and cause silent aspiration.

With regard to the changes in muscle tissue, sarcopenia or fatty degeneration after atrophy of striated muscles was observed to be accompanied by accumulation of macrophages [69, 70]. The numbers of macrophages per striated muscle fiber were 5–6 times greater in the larynx and pharynx than in other parts of the body (e.g. tongue, shoulder, and anus) in old men [71]. This kind of change in muscle tissue can lead to dysfunction of swallowing muscles with age.

3.4. Esophageal phase

Dysphagia caused by problems associated with the esophageal phase of swallowing is termed "esophageal dysphagia". Esophageal dysphagia can occur due to achalasia, diffuse esophageal spasm, nonspecific motor disorders, obstructive lesions such as stenosis or neoplasm, or gastroesophageal reflux disease [72]. Esophageal motility disorder with aging is termed "presbyesophagus" [73]. Neuromuscular dysfunction, decreased resting upper esophageal sphincter (UES) pressure, and delayed relaxation of the UES after swallowing are some age-related changes in swallowing [74, 75]. Sarcopenia can also alter esophageal functions. Sarcopenic esophageal dysphagia may be also important in addition to sarcopenic oropharyngeal dysphagia.

3.5. The coordination of swallowing with respiration

Disturbed respiration can cause aspiration in older adults [76]. The expiration-swallow-expiration (EX/EX) pattern is essential to prevent aspiration [77]. However, the probability of the non-EX/EX respiratory phase pattern has been found to be higher in the middle- and old-age groups than in the young-age group [78]. In addition, older adults had a longer swallowing apnea duration than younger adults for preventing aspiration [78]. Though the coordination of respiration and swallowing is regulated by the central pattern generator center in the brainstem, it can be altered in case of advanced age or disease [79]. This mechanism seems to be related to respiratory function change with age or disease. A few studies showed that respiratory muscle strength was related to sarcopenia [80, 81]. Sarcopenia can affect the safety swallowing respiratory pattern. The relationship between sarcopenic dysphagia and respiratory function should be investigated.

4. Treatment for sarcopenic dysphagia

A systematic review suggested that interventions such as resistance training, compound exercises (a mix of aerobic, flexibility, and/or balance training), and nutritional interventions (protein supplementation, essential amino acid [EAA, mainly leucine] supplementation, β-hydroxy β-methylbutyric acid [HMB; a bioactive metabolite of leucine] supplementation with arginine or alone or fatty acid supplementation) were effective for improvement of generalized muscle mass and strength or functions [82]. Among these interventions, supervised resistance exercise or composite exercise programs for at least 3 months and preferably longer, EAA (with leucine), and HMB were indicated to be more beneficial for improving muscle-related parameters in sarcopenia. In another review, Morley [83] suggested that resistance exercise is the most promising candidate for attenuating sarcopenia. In addition, supplementation with essential amino acids, creatine, vitamin D, or testosterone was also indicated to be effective.

With respect to treatment of dysphagia in relation to sarcopenia, the effectiveness of resistance training intervention to improve tongue muscle function has been demonstrated. Robbins et al. [9] used the Iowa Oral Performance Instrument to examine the effect of an 8-week progressive tongue resistance exercise program consisting of compressing an air-filled bulb between the tongue and hard palate in 10 healthy older adults aged 70–89 years. The frequency of exercise was 30 times in a single session, three times a day, and 3 days a week. The exercise intensity level in that study was 60% of the maximum pressure in the first week and 80% of the maximum pressure in the remaining 7 weeks. In this study, isometric tongue strength (baseline: mean 41 kPa; week 2: 44 kPa [nonsignificant difference]; week 4: 47 kPa [$p = 0.02$ compared to baseline]; week 6: 49 kPa [$p = 0.01$ compared to baseline]), tongue volume (change rate ranges from 2.16 to 10.68% upward), and peak swallowing pressure increased after the intervention. Tongue strength and thickness are decreased in sarcopenia but can have possible reversibility. The method used for measurement of tongue strength is described in **Figure 2**.

The effectiveness of the Shaker Exercise for strengthening the suprahyoid muscles is well-known in the field of dysphagia rehabilitation. The Shaker Exercise consists of an isometric component comprising three head lifts for 60 s each with a 60-s rest period between two consecutive head lifts and an isokinetic component comprising 30 consecutive head lifts at constant velocity (**Figure 3**). Shaker et al. [84] and Easterling [85] examined the effect of this

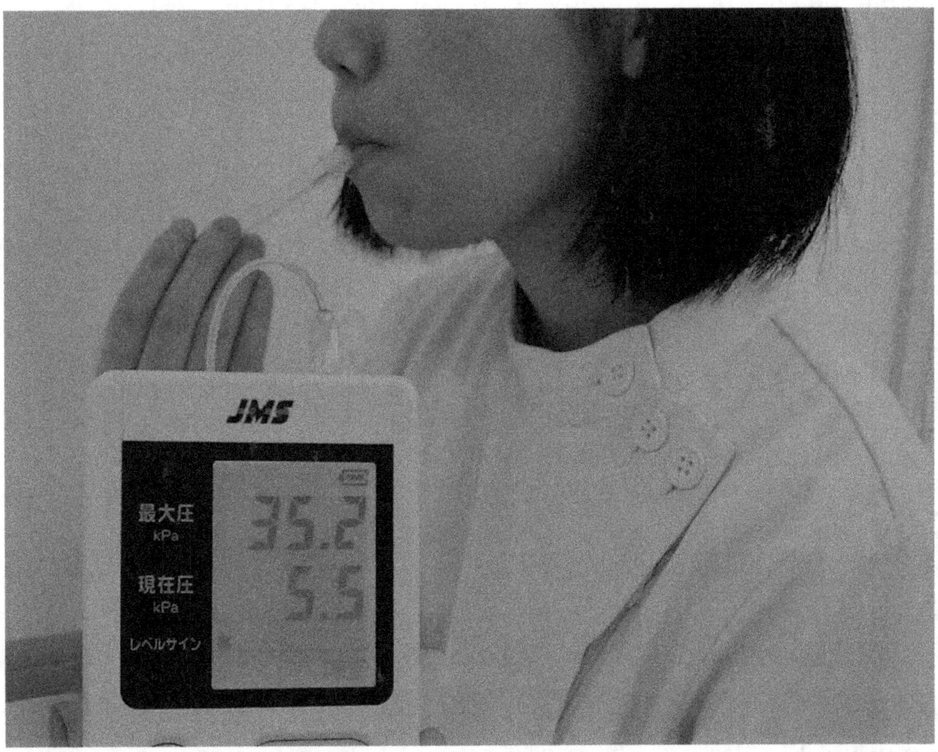

Figure 2. Tongue strength measurement. Compressing an air-filled bulb between the tongue and the hard palate and displaying the maximum tongue strength at the upper row (JMS, Hiroshima, Japan).

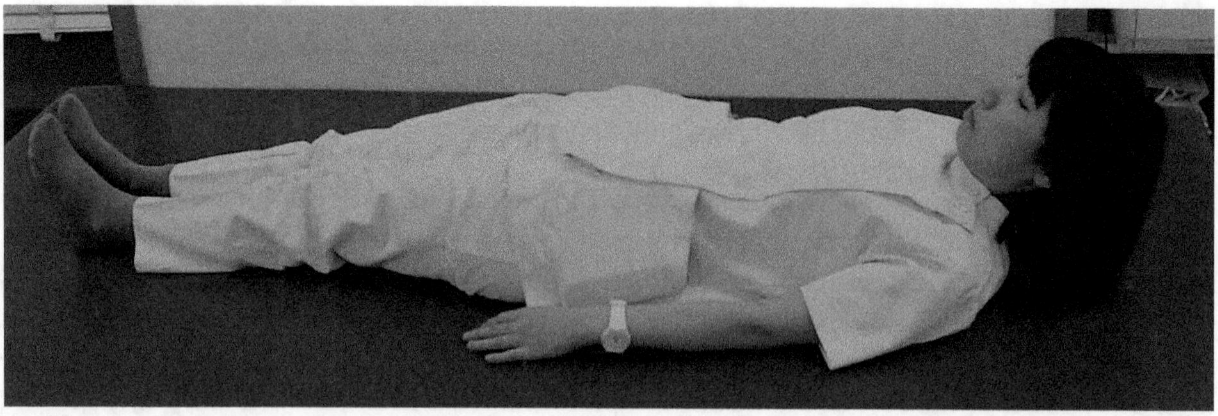

Figure 3. Shaker exercise. Lying on a bed and raising the head without lifting the shoulder, while looking at the toes.

exercise in healthy older adults. They showed that the anterior hyoid and larynx as well as the deglutitive anteroposterior UES opening diameter increased after this exercise was performed three times daily for 6 weeks. Wakabayashi et al. [86] demonstrated that dysphagia with aspiration was independently associated with both malnutrition and low head lifting strength. They suggested head lifting strength as an indicator of the severity of dysphagia in frail older adults. Strengthening the head lifting muscles can be an effective treatment for sarcopenic dysphagia. In recent years, a new method to strengthen the suprahyoid muscles—the Chin Tuck against Resistance (CTAR) exercise—has been developed [87]. This exercise involves squeezing a rubber ball placed between the chin and the manubrium sterni (**Figure 4**). The maximum activation level of the suprahyoid muscles measured using sEMG was significantly greater after this exercise than after both the isometric and isokinetic tasks in the Shaker Exercise; in addition, the CTAR exercise was less strenuous. CTAR was suggested to also be more specific in targeting the suprahyoid muscles than the Shaker exercise [88]. Instead of the rubber ball, a training device named ISO Swallowing Exercise Device (Alternative Speech and Swallowing Solutions, Inc.) was developed in America recently. The CTAR may be more feasible and efficient to improve swallowing function in older adults with sarcopenic dysphagia. The jaw-opening Exercise was developed as another training regimen for improving suprahyoid muscle strength [89]. This exercise is performed by opening the jaw to the maximum extent and maintaining this position for 10 s while feeling a sensation of stretching. This exercise is repeated 5 times with 10 s of rest as 1 set. Two sets of this exercise are needed to be performed daily. After this exercise, the upward movement of the hyoid bone and the opening of the UES significantly increased in all subjects. In addition, the time for pharynx passage also significantly decreased. In this study, among eight subjects with chronic dysphagia, four had dysphagia due to cerebrovascular disease and the remaining four had dysphagia due to possible sarcopenia. Further studies on interventions for people with sarcopenic dysphagia are warranted in the future.

For the treatment of dysphagia and prevention of aspiration pneumonia, compensatory strategies are important [7]. Particularly, modification of the consistency of ingested liquids is commonly used as a compensatory strategy. Rofes et al. [60] demonstrated that the prevalence of penetration and aspiration decreased by increasing the viscosity of ingested liquids

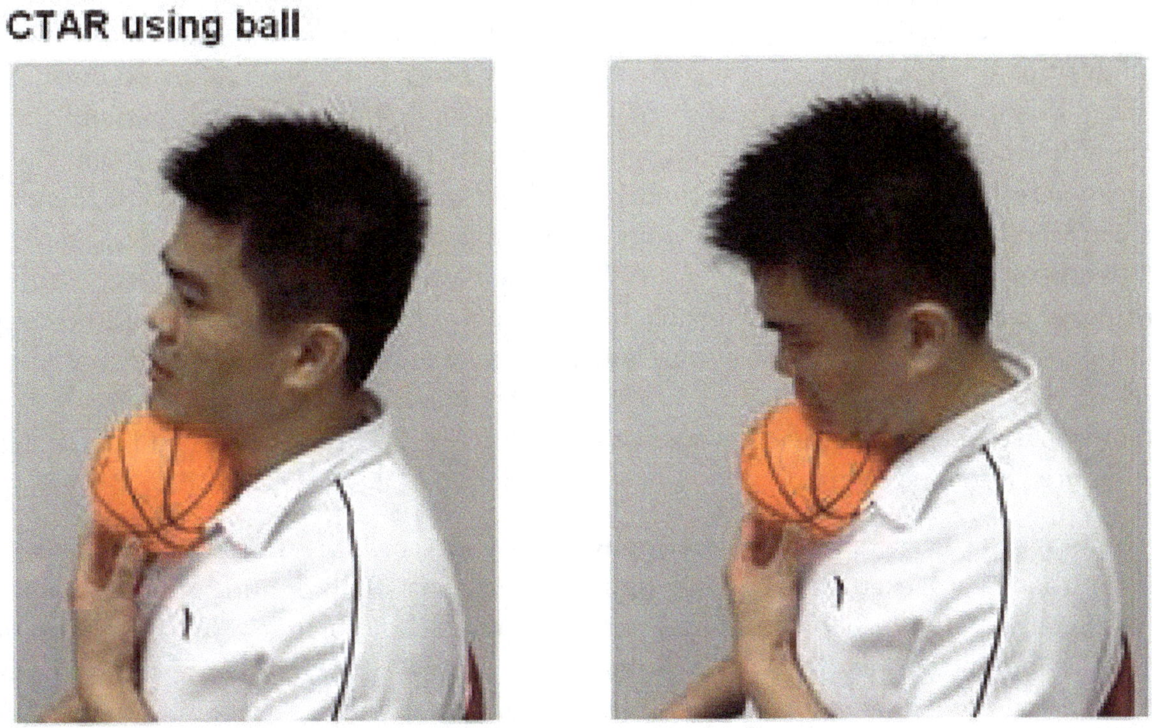

Figure 4. Chin tuck against resistance exercise. Squeezing a rubber ball placed between the chin and the manubrium sterni. Source: http://www.speechtherapyworks.com.sg/blog/new-dysphagia-exercise-chin-tuck-against-resistance-alternative-to-shaker-exercise/.

(liquid, nectar, and pudding viscosity) in frail older patients. In contrast, they also found that the prevalence of oral and pharyngeal residue increased with increase in viscosity. Thus, altering the consistency of ingested liquids can be effective for increasing the safety but not the efficiency of swallowing. The appropriate viscosity level should be determined by objective examination in older adults with sarcopenic dysphagia.

As treatments for sarcopenic dysphagia, nutritional and physical interventions have been indicated to be effective. Maeda and Akagi [90] describes the case of an 80-year-old woman who recovered from sarcopenic dysphagia with aggressive nutritional management and physical therapy in addition to dysphagia therapy. In their nutritional management, the total energy intake increased from 1200 to 1830 kcal/day, and the amount of protein intake increased from 0.84 ideal body weight (IBW)/day to 1.42 g/kg IBW/day. As a result, the oral intake level [91] improved from "nothing by mouth" level to "total oral diet with multiple consistencies, but requiring special preparation or compensations" level. Wakabayashi and Uwano [92] also described the case of a 71-year-old man who recovered from sarcopenic dysphagia with aggressive nutritional management and physical therapy in addition to dysphagia therapy. His energy intake was 986 kcal/day at the time of referral to the department of rehabilitation medicine and was increased to 2200 kcal/day. The oral intake level in this case improved from "nothing by mouth" level to "total oral diet with no restriction" level. In both the cases, physical function and nutritional status also improved with improvement in oral intake level. These cases indicate that nutritional management and physical rehabilitation in addition to dysphagia rehabilitation can be effective in the treatment of sarcopenic dysphagia. Our study [11] investigated the association between tongue strength, grip strength, and nutritional status, suggesting the effectiveness of physical rehabilitation and nutritional therapy in improving tongue strength. Yoshimura et al. [93] demonstrated that nutritional intervention added to resistance training improved muscle mass and activities of daily living more than resistance training alone in older inpatients in a rehabilitation hospital. Therefore, the combination of nutritional intervention and resistance training can also be effective in the treatment of sarcopenic dysphagia. Wakabayashi and Sakuma [94] have proposed that nutritional rehabilitation is useful for the treatment of sarcopenic dysphagia. In this concept, nutrition management, to increase muscle mass and strength, is proposed to be indispensable for rehabilitation. On the other hand, the effectiveness of nutritional intervention in sarcopenic dysphagia is unclear because of the lack of intervention studies and hence, such studies are warranted in future.

In adults aged 60 years or older, with atrophy of the vocal cords or sulcus vocalis with aging, self-controlled vocal exercise in the sitting position that consists of counting out loud from 1 to 10 while pulling up firmly on both sides of the seat reduced the frequency of hospitalization for aspiration pneumonia (2/199 in the intervention group and 18/216 in the control group) [95]. Subjects in the intervention group exercised for a total of two sets, both in the morning and in the evening for 6 months. The intrinsic laryngeal muscles commonly cause glottal closure insufficiency with aging [96–98]; therefore, sarcopenia can cause atrophy of the vocal cords. Because insufficient glottal closure increases the risk of aspiration [99], atrophy of the vocal cords can lead to aspiration pneumonia in older adults. The vocal exercise mentioned above can be an effective treatment for sarcopenic dysphagia.

As decrease in pharyngeal and supraglottic sensitivity was indicated in older adults with sarcopenic dysphagia, sensory stimulation may be an effective treatment. Ortega et al. [100] demonstrated the effectiveness of two sensory stimulation techniques. One was the chemical sensory stimulation with a natural TRPV1 agonist solution (natural capsaicinoids 1×10^{-5} M). In this study, capsaicin solution was obtained from an alimentary sauce containing 185.5 μg/g of capsaicinoid. Subjects consumed 10 mL of tomato juice mixed with the capsaicinoid sauce three times per day before each meal, 5 days per week for 2 weeks. The other technique was electrical stimulation in the thyrohyoid position using the Intelect VitalStim device (Chattanooga Group, Hixson, TN, USA), consisting of the application, at rest, of 80 Hz of transcutaneous electrical stimulus (biphasic, 700μs). Subjects received this therapy for 1 h per day, 5 days a week for 2 weeks. Aspiration was significantly reduced in the group that received a natural TRPV1 agonist solution (TRPV1 group; 38.46% vs. TSES group; 0%) and the prevalence of penetration decreased significantly in the group receiving electrical stimulation (TSES group; 87.5 vs. TRPV1 group; 25%). In addition, the time for laryngeal vestibule closure was significantly shortened in responder patients in the group receiving electrical stimulation (TSES group; 480 ± 167 ms vs. TRPV1 group; 295 ± 189.9 ms). Because the cause of dysphagia in the subjects in this study was aging (39.5%), or a combination of aging with previous stroke or neurodegenerative diseases, the effectiveness of these techniques for older adults with sarcopenic dysphagia should be examined.

In rehabilitation for sarcopenic dysphagia, risk management for aspiration pneumonia is also important. Frail older patients with oropharyngeal dysphagia have poorer oral health, higher oral bacterial load, and a higher prevalence of oral colonization by respiratory pathogens than healthy older adults [101]. Since these can be potential risk factors of aspiration pneumonia, oral care is important as a risk management strategy in the treatment of sarcopenic dysphagia.

The Dysphagia Working Group from the European Society for Swallowing Disorders and the European Union Geriatric Medicine Society has proposed that oropharyngeal dysphagia is a multifactorial geriatric syndrome [7] and is treatable only with a multidimensional approach. Further research is required to identify the components of this multidimensional approach.

5. Conclusions

Sarcopenic dysphagia is a swallowing disorder caused by sarcopenia of the swallowing muscles, including the general skeletal muscle. Its prevalence seems to be high, particularly in older adults after acute disease. Because sarcopenic dysphagia is caused mainly by inactivity and malnutrition, it is preventable and treatable in most cases. Among published articles on dysphagia, there have been few studies on sarcopenic dysphagia. With an increasing aging population, sarcopenic dysphagia has become an important public health issue. For adequate prevention, diagnosis, and treatment, further studies on the pathophysiology of and intervention for sarcopenic dysphagia are warranted in future.

Author details

Kotomi Sakai[1,2]* and Kunihiro Sakuma[3]

*Address all correspondence to: sakai.kotomi@hmw.gr.jp

1 Department of Rehabilitation, Setagaya Memorial Hospital, Tokyo, Japan

2 Department of Dysphagia Rehabilitation, Nihon University School of Dentistry, Tokyo, Japan

3 Institute for Liberal Arts, Environment and Society, Tokyo Institute of Technology, Tokyo, Japan

References

[1] Rosenberg IH. Sarcopenia: Origins and clinical relevance. The Journal of Nutrition. 1997;**127**:990-991

[2] Cruz-Jentoft AJ, Baeyens JP, Bauer JM, Boirie Y, Cederholm T, Landi F, Martin FC, Michel JP, Rolland Y, Schneider SM, Topinkova E, Vandewoude M, Zamboni M. Sarcopenia:

European consensus on definition and diagnosis: Report of the European Working Group on Sarcopenia in Older People. Age and Ageing. 2010;**39**:412-423

[3] Fielding RA, Vellas B, Evans WJ, Bhasin S, Morley JE, Newman AB, Abellan van Kan G, Andrieu S, Bauer J, Breuille D, Cederholm T, Chandler J, De Meynard C, Donini L, Harris T, Kannt A, Keime Guibert F, Onder G, Papanicolaou D, Rolland Y, Rooks D, Sieber C, Souhami E, Verlaan S, Zamboni M. Sarcopenia: An undiagnosed condition in older adults. Current consensus definition: Prevalence, etiology, and consequences. International Working Group on Sarcopenia. Journal of the American Medical Directors Association. 2011;**12**:249-256

[4] Chen LK, Liu LK, Woo J, Assantachai P, Auyeung TW, Bahyah KS, Chou MY, Chen LY, Hsu PS, Krairit O, Lee JS, Lee WJ, Lee Y, Liang CK, Limpawattana P, Lin CS, Peng LN, Satake S, Suzuki T, Won CW, Wu CH, Wu SN, Zhang T, Zeng P, Akishita M, Arai H. Sarcopenia in Asia: Consensus report of the Asian Working Group for Sarcopenia. Journal of the American Medical Directors Association. 2014;**15**:95-101

[5] Anker SD, Morley JE, Haehling SV. Welcome to the ICD-10 code for sarcopenia. Journal of Cachexia, Sarcopenia and Muscle. 2016;**7**:512-514

[6] WHO. International classification of functioning, disability and health [online]. 2016; **20**:22-27 http://www.who.int/classifications/icf/en/

[7] Baijens LWJ, Clavé P, Cras P, Ekberg O, Forster A, Kolb G, Leners JC, Masiero S, Mateos del Nozal J, Ortega O, Smithard DG, Speyer R, Walshe M. European Society for swallowing disorders—European Union geriatric medicine society white paper: Oropharyngeal dysphagia as a geriatric syndrome. Clinical Interventions in Aging. 2016;**11**:1403-1428

[8] Veldee MS, Peth LD. Can protein-calorie malnutrition cause dysphagia? Dysphagia. 1992;**7**:86-101

[9] Robbins J, Gangnon RE, Theis SM, Kays SA, Hewitt AL, Hind JA. The effects of lingual exercise on swallowing in older adults. Journal of the American Geriatrics Society. 2005;**53**:1483-1489

[10] Kuroda Y, Kuroda R. Relationship between thinness and swallowing function in Japanese older adults: Implications for sarcopenic dysphagia. Journal of the American Geriatrics Society. 2012;**60**:1785-1786

[11] Sakai K, Nakayama E, Tohara H, Maeda T, Sugimoto M, Takehisa T, Takehisa Y, Ueda K. Tongue strength is associated with grip strength and nutritional status in older adult inpatients of a rehabilitation hospital. Dysphagia. 2016. [Epub ahead of print]

[12] Clave P, Shaker R. Dysphagia: Current reality and scope of the problem. Nature Reviews of Gastroenterology and Hepatology. 2015;**12**:259-270

[13] van der Maarel-Wierink CD, Vanobbergen JN, Bronkhorst EM, Schols JM, de Baat C. Meta-analysis of dysphagia and aspiration pneumonia in frail elders. Journal of Dental Research. 2011;**90**:1398-1404

[14] Bonilha HS, Simpson AN, Ellis C, Mauldin P, Martin-Harris B, Simpson K. The one-year attributable cost of post-stroke dysphagia. Dysphagia. 2014;**29**:545-552

[15] Altman KW, Yu GP, Schaefer SD. Consequence of dysphagia in the hospitalized patient: Impact on prognosis and hospital resources. Archives of Otolaryngology—-Head & Neck Surgery. 2010;**136**:784-789

[16] Chen LK, Lee WJ, Peng LN, Liu LK, Arai H, Akishita M. Recent advances in sarcopenia research in Asia: 2016 update from the Asian Working Group for Sarcopenia. Journal of the American Medical Directors Association. 2016;**17**:767.e1-767.e7

[17] Maeda K, Akagi J. Decreased tongue pressure is associated with sarcopenia and sarcopenic dysphagia in the elderly. Dysphagia. 2015;**30**:80-87

[18] Maeda K, Akagi J. Sarcopenia is an independent risk factor of dysphagia in hospitalized older people. Geriatrics & Gerontology International. 2015;**4**:515-21

[19] Maeda K, Takaki M, Akagi J. Decreased skeletal muscle mass and risk factors of sarcopenic dysphagia: A prospective observational cohort study. The Journals of Gerontology Series A, Biological Sciences and Medical Sciences. 2016. [Epub ahead of print]

[20] Madhavan A, LaGorio LA, Crary MA, Dahl WJ, Carnaby GD. Prevalence of and risk factors for dysphagia in the community dwelling elderly: A systematic review. The Journal of Nutrition, Health & Aging. 2016;**20**:806-815

[21] Wakabayashi H, Matsushima M. Dysphagia assessed by the 10-item eating assessment tool is associated with nutritional status and activities of daily living in elderly individuals requiring long-term care. The Journal of Nutrition, Health & Aging. 2016; 20:22-27

[22] Aslam M, Vaezi MF. Dysphagia in the elderly. Gastroenterology & Hepatology. 2013; **9**:784-795

[23] Wakabayashi H, Matsushima M, Uwano R, Watanabe N, Oritsu H, Shimizu Y. Skeletal muscle mass is associated with severe dysphagia in cancer patients. Journal of Cachexia, Sarcopenia and Muscle. 2015;**6**:351-357

[24] Robbins J, Hamilton JW, Lof GL, Kempster GB. Oropharyngeal swallowing in normal adults of different ages. Gastroenterology. 1992;**103**:823-829

[25] Humbert IA, Robbins J. Dysphagia in the elderly. Physical Medicine and Rehabilitation Clinics of North America. 2008;**19**:853-866

[26] Ney DM, Weiss JM, Kind AJ, Robbins J. Senescent swallowing: Impact, strategies, and interventions. Nutrition in Clinical Practice: Official Publication of the American Society for Parenteral and Enteral Nutrition. 2009;**24**:395-413

[27] Maeda K, Koga T, Akagi J. Tentative nil per os leads to poor outcomes in older adults with aspiration pneumonia. Clinical Nutrition (Edinburgh, Scotland). 2016;**35**:1147-1152

[28] Hudson HM, Daubert CR, Mills RH. The interdependency of protein-energy malnutrition, aging, and dysphagia. Dysphagia. 2000;**15**:31-38

[29] Lewis MI, Sieck GC. Effect of acute nutritional deprivation on diaphragm structure and function. Journal of Applied Physiology. 1990;**68**:1938-1944

[30] Sieck GC, Lewis MI, Blanco CE. Effects of undernutrition on diaphragm fiber size, SDH activity, and fatigue resistance. Journal of Applied Physiology. 1989;**66**:2196-2205

[31] Drew JS, Farkas GA, Pearson RD, Rochester DF. Effects of a chronic wasting infection on skeletal muscle size and contractile properties. Journal of Applied Physiology. 1988;**64**:460-465

[32] Lewis MI, Li H, Huang Z-S, Biring MS, Cercek B, Fournier M. Influence of varying degrees of malnutrition on IGF-I expression in the rat diaphragm. Journal of Applied Physiology. 2003;**95**:555-562

[33] Peterson SJ, Braunschweig CA. Prevalence of sarcopenia and associated outcomes in the clinical setting. Nutrition in Clinical Practice: Official Publication of the American Society for Parenteral and Enteral Nutrition. 2016;**31**:40-48

[34] von Haehling S, Anker SD. Prevalence, incidence and clinical impact of cachexia: Facts and numbers-update 2014. Journal of Cachexia, Sarcopenia and Muscle. 2014;**5**:261-263

[35] Takagi D, Hirano H, Watanabe Y, Edahiro A, Ohara Y, Yoshida H, Kim H, Murakami K, Hironaka S. Relationship between skeletal muscle mass and swallowing function in patients with Alzheimer's disease. Geriatrics & Gerontology International. 2016. [Epub ahead of print]

[36] Matsuo K, Palmer JB. Anatomy and physiology of feeding and swallowing: Normal and abnormal. Physical medicine and Rehabilitation Clinics of North America. 2008; **19**:691-707

[37] Leopold NA, Kagel MC. Dysphagia – ingestion or deglutition? A proposed paradigm. Dysphagia. 1997;**12**:202-206

[38] Matsuo K, Palmer JB. Coordination of mastication, swallowing and breathing. The Japanese Dental Science Review. 2009;**45**:31-40

[39] Yokota J, Ogawa Y, Yamanaka S, Takahashi Y, Fujita H, Yamaguchi N, Onoue N, Ishizuka T, Shinozaki T, Kohzuki M. Cognitive dysfunction and malnutrition are independent predictors of dysphagia in patients with acute exacerbation of congestive heart failure. PloS One. 2016;**11**:e0167326

[40] Chang K-V, Hsu T-H, Wu W-T, Huang K-C, Han D-S. Association between sarcopenia and cognitive impairment: A systematic review and meta-analysis. Journal of the American Medical Directors Association. 2016;**12**:1164.e7-1164.e15

[41] Robbins J, Kays SA, Gangnon RE, Hind JA, Hewitt AL, Gentry LR, Taylor AJ. The effects of lingual exercise in stroke patients with dysphagia. Archives of Physical Medicine and Rehabilitation. 2007;**88**:150-158

[42] Robbins J, Levine R, Wood J, Roecker EB, Luschei E. Age effects on lingual pressure generation as a risk factor for dysphagia. The Journals of Gerontology Series A, Biological Sciences and Medical Sciences. 1995;**50**:M257-M262

[43] Nicosia MA, Hind JA, Roecker EB, Carnes M, Doyle J, Dengel GA, Robbins J. Age effects on the temporal evolution of isometric and swallowing pressure. The Journals of Gerontology Series A, Biological Sciences and Medical Sciences. 2000;**55**:M634-M640

[44] Robbins J, Humpal NS, Banaszynski K, Hind J, Rogus-Pulia N. Age-related differences in pressures generated during isometric presses and swallows by healthy adults. Dysphagia. 2016;**31**:90-96

[45] Buehring B, Hind J, Fidler E, Krueger D, Binkley N, Robbins J. Tongue strength is associated with jumping mechanography performance and handgrip strength but not with classic functional tests in older adults. Journal of the American Geriatrics Society. 2013;**61**:418-422

[46] Utanohara Y, Hayashi R, Yoshikawa M, Yoshida M, Tsuga K, Akagawa Y. Standard values of maximum tongue pressure taken using newly developed disposable tongue pressure measurement device. Dysphagia. 2008;**23**:286-290

[47] Mendes AE, Nascimento L, Mansur LL, Callegaro D, Jacob Filho W. Tongue forces and handgrip strength in normal individuals: Association with swallowing. Clinics (Sao Paulo, Brazil). 2015;**70**:41-45

[48] Crow HC, Ship JA. Tongue strength and endurance in different aged individuals. The Journals of Gerontology Series A, Biological Sciences and Medical Sciences. 1996; **51**:M247-M250

[49] Butler SG, Stuart A, Leng X, Wilhelm E, Rees C, Williamson J, Kritchevsky SB. The relationship of aspiration status with tongue and handgrip strength in healthy older adults. The Journals of Gerontology Series A, Biological Sciences and Medical sciences. 2011;**66**:452-458

[50] Miller JL, Watkin KL, Chen MF. Muscle, adipose, and connective tissue variations in intrinsic musculature of the adult human tongue. Journal of Speech, Language, and Hearing Research. 2002;**45**:51-65

[51] Nashi N, Kang S, Barkdull GC, Lucas J, Davidson TM. Lingual fat at autopsy. The Laryngoscope. 2007;**117**:1467-1473

[52] Yamaguchi A, Nasu M, Esaki Y, Shimada H, Yoshiki S. Amyloid deposits in the aged tongue: A postmortem study of 107 individuals over 60 years of age. Journal of Oral Pathology. 1982;**11**:237-244

[53] Tamura F, Kikutani T, Tohara T, Yoshida M, Yaegaki K. Tongue thickness relates to nutritional status in the elderly. Dysphagia. 2012;**27**:556-561

[54] Butler SG, Stuart A, Wilhelm E, Rees C, Williamson J, Kritchevsky S. The effects of aspiration status, liquid type, and bolus volume on pharyngeal peak pressure in healthy older adults. Dysphagia. 2011;**26**:225-231

[55] Feng X, Todd T, Lintzenich CR, Ding J, Carr JJ, Ge Y, Browne JD, Kritchevsky SB, Butler SG. Aging-related geniohyoid muscle atrophy is related to aspiration status in healthy

older adults. The Journals of Gerontology Series A, Biological Sciences and Medical Sciences. 2013;**68**:853-860

[56] Logemann JA, Pauloski BR, Rademaker AW, Colangelo LA, Kahrilas PJ, Smith CH. Temporal and biomechanical characteristics of oropharyngeal swallow in younger and older men. Journal of Speech, Language, and Hearing Research. 2000;**43**:1264-1274

[57] Kang BS, Oh BM, Kim IS, Chung SG, Kim SJ, Han TR. Influence of aging on movement of the hyoid bone and epiglottis during normal swallowing: A motion analysis. Gerontology. 2010;**56**:474-482

[58] Kendall KA, Leonard RJ. Hyoid movement during swallowing in older patients with dysphagia. Archives of Otolaryngology—Head & Neck Surgery. 2001;**127**:1224-1229

[59] Leonard R, Kendall KA, McKenzie S. Structural displacements affecting pharyngeal constriction in nondysphagic elderly and nonelderly adults. Dysphagia. 2004;**19**:133-141

[60] Rofes L, Arreola V, Romea M, Palomera E, Almirall J, Cabre M, Serra-Prat M, Clave P. Pathophysiology of oropharyngeal dysphagia in the frail elderly. Neurogastroenterology and Motility: The Official Journal of the European Gastrointestinal Motility Society. 2010;**22**:851-858, e230

[61] Hara K, Tohara H, Wada S, Iida T, Ueda K, Ansai T. Jaw-opening force test to screen for dysphagia: Preliminary results. Archives of Physical Medicine and Rehabilitation. 2014;**95**:867-874

[62] Iida T, Tohara H, Wada S, Nakane A, Sanpei R, Ueda K. Aging decreases the strength of suprahyoid muscles involved in swallowing movements. The Tohoku Journal of Experimental Medicine. 2013;**231**:223-228

[63] Machida N, Tohara H, Hara K, Kumakura A, Wakasugi Y, Nakane A, Minakuchi S. Effects of aging and sarcopenia on tongue pressure and jaw-opening force. Geriatrics & Gerontology International. 2017;**17**:295-301

[64] Hiramatsu T, Kataoka H, Osaki M, Hagino H. Effect of aging on oral and swallowing function after meal consumption. Clinical Interventions in Aging. 2015;**10**:229-235

[65] Kendall KA, Leonard RJ. Pharyngeal constriction in elderly dysphagic patients compared with young and elderly nondysphagic controls. Dysphagia. 2001;**16**:272-278

[66] Molfenter SM, Amin MR, Branski RC, Brumm JD, Hagiwara M, Roof SA, Lazarus CL. Age-related changes in pharyngeal lumen size: A retrospective MRI analysis. Dysphagia. 2015;**30**:321-327

[67] Butler SG, Stuart A, Leng X, Rees C, Williamson J, Kritchevsky SB. Factors influencing aspiration during swallowing in healthy older adults. The Laryngoscope. 2010;**120**:2147-2152

[68] Aviv JE, Martin JH, Jones ME, Wee TA, Diamond B, Keen MS, Blitzer A. Age-related changes in pharyngeal and supraglottic sensation. The Annals of Otology, Rhinology, and Laryngology. 1994;**103**:749-752

[69] Gumucio J, Flood M, Harning J, Phan A, Roche S, Lynch E, Bedi A, Mendias C. T lymphocytes are not required for the development of fatty degeneration after rotator cuff tear. Bone & Joint Research. 2014;**3**:262-272

[70] Siriett V, Salerno MS, Berry C, Nicholas G, Bower R, Kambadur R, Sharma M. Antagonism of myostatin enhances muscle regeneration during sarcopenia. Molecular Therapy: The Journal of the American Society of Gene Therapy. 2007;**15**:1463-1470

[71] Rhee S, Yamamoto M, Kitamura K, Masaaki K, Katori Y, Murakami G, Abe SI. Macrophage density in pharyngeal and laryngeal muscles greatly exceeds that in other striated muscles: An immunohistochemical study using elderly human cadavers. Anatomy & Cell Biology. 2016;**49**:177-183

[72] Greenslade J, Wyman A. Investigation of dysphagia. Surgery (Oxford). 2006;**24**:89-92

[73] DeVault KR. Presbyesophagus: A reappraisal. Current Gastroenterology Reports. 2002; **4**:193-199

[74] Fulp SR, Dalton CB, Castell JA, Castell DO. Aging-related alterations in human upper esophageal sphincter function. The American Journal of Gastroenterology. 1990;**85**: 1569-1572

[75] van Herwaarden MA, Katz PO, Matthew Gideon R, Barrett J, Castell JA, Achem S, Castell DO. Are manometric parameters of the upper esophageal sphincter and pharynx affected by age and gender? Dysphagia. 2003;**18**:211-217

[76] Nilsson H, Ekberg O, Bulow M, Hindfelt B. Assessment of respiration during video fluoroscopy of dysphagic patients. Academic Radiology. 1997;**4**:503-507

[77] Preiksaitis HG, Mills CA. Coordination of breathing and swallowing: Effects of bolus consistency and presentation in normal adults. Journal of Applied Physiology. 1996; **81**:1707-1714

[78] Wang CM, Chen JY, Chuang CC, Tseng WC, Wong AM, Pei YC. Aging-related changes in swallowing, and in the coordination of swallowing and respiration determined by novel non-invasive measurement techniques. Geriatrics & Gerontology International. 2015;**6**:736-744

[79] Shaker R, Li Q, Ren J, Townsend WF, Dodds WJ, Martin BJ, Kern MK, Rynders A. Coordination of deglutition and phases of respiration: Effect of aging, tachypnea, bolus volume, and chronic obstructive pulmonary disease. The American Journal of Physiology. 1992;**263**:G750-G755

[80] Izawa KP, Watanabe S, Oka K, Kasahara Y, Morio Y, Hiraki K, Hirano Y, Omori Y, Suzuki N, Kida K, Suzuki K, Akashi YJ. Respiratory muscle strength in relation to sarcopenia in elderly cardiac patients. Aging Clinical and Experimental Research. 2016; 28:1143-1148

[81] Elliott JE, Greising SM, Mantilla CB, Sieck GC. Functional impact of sarcopenia in respiratory muscles. Respiratory Physiology & Neurobiology. 2016;**226**:137-146

[82] Cruz-Jentoft AJ, Landi F, Schneider SM, Zuniga C, Arai H, Boirie Y, Chen LK, Fielding RA, Martin FC, Michel JP, Sieber C, Stout JR, Studenski SA, Vellas B, Woo J, Zamboni M, Cederholm T. Prevalence of and interventions for sarcopenia in ageing adults: A systematic review. Report of the International Sarcopenia Initiative (EWGSOP and IWGS). Age and Ageing. 2014;**6**:748-759

[83] Morley JE. Pharmacologic options for the treatment of sarcopenia. Calcified Tissue International. 2016;**98**:319-333

[84] Shaker R, Kern M, Bardan E, Taylor A, Stewart ET, Hoffmann RG, Arndorfer RC, Hofmann C, Bonnevier J. Augmentation of deglutitive upper esophageal sphincter opening in the elderly by exercise. The American Journal of Physiology. 1997;**272**:G1518-G1522

[85] Easterling C. Does an exercise aimed at improving swallow function have an effect on vocal function in the healthy elderly? Dysphagia. 2008;**23**:317-326

[86] Wakabayashi H, Sashika H, Matsushima M. Head lifting strength is associated with dysphagia and malnutrition in frail older adults. Geriatrics & Gerontology International. 2015;**4**:410-416

[87] Yoon WL, Khoo JKP, Rickard Liow SJ. Chin Tuck Against Resistance (CTAR): New Method for enhancing suprahyoid muscle activity using a Shaker-type exercise. Dysphagia. 2014;**29**:243-248

[88] Sze WP, Yoon WL, Escoffier N, Rickard Liow SJ. Evaluating the training effects of two swallowing rehabilitation therapies using surface electromyography – Chin Tuck Against Resistance (CTAR) Exercise and the Shaker exercise. Dysphagia. 2016;**31**:195-205

[89] Wada S, Tohara H, Iida T, Inoue M, Sato M, Ueda K. Jaw-opening exercise for insufficient opening of upper esophageal sphincter. Archives of Physical Medicine and Rehabilitation. 2012;**93**:1995-1999

[90] Maeda K, Akagi J. Treatment of sarcopenic dysphagia with rehabilitation and nutritional support: A comprehensive approach. Journal of the Academy of Nutrition and Diebetics. 2016;**116**:573-577

[91] Crary MA, Mann GD, Groher ME. Initial psychometric assessment of a functional oral intake scale for dysphagia in stroke patients. Archives of Physical Medicine and Rehabilitation. 2005;**86**:1516-1520

[92] Wakabayashi H, Uwano R. Rehabilitation nutrition for possible sarcopenic dysphagia after lung cancer surgery: A case report. American Journal of Physical Medicine & Rehabilitation/Association of Academic Physiatrists. 2016;**95**:e84-e89

[93] Yoshimura Y, Uchida K, Jeong S, Yamaga M. Effects of nutritional supplements on muscle mass and activities of daily living in elderly rehabilitation patients with decreased muscle mass: A randomized controlled trial. The Journal of Nutrition, Health & Aging. 2016; 20:185-191

[94] Wakabayashi H, Sakuma K. Rehabilitation nutrition for sarcopenia with disability: A combination of both rehabilitation and nutrition care management. Journal of Cachexia, Sarcopenia and Muscle. 2014;**5**:269-277

[95] Fujimaki Y, Tsunoda K, Kobayashi R, Tonghyo C, Tanaka F, Kuroda H, Numata T, Ishii T, Kuroda R, Masuda S, Hashimoto S, Misawa H, Shindo N, Mori T, Mori H, Uchiyama N, Kamei Y, Tanaka M, Hamaya H, Funatsuki S, Usui S, Ito I, Hamada K, Shindo A, Tokumaru Y, Morita Y, Ueha R, Nito T, Kikuta S, Sekimoto S, Kondo K, Sakamoto T, Itoh K, Yamasoba T, Matsumoto S. Independent exercise for glottal incompetence to improve vocal problems and prevent aspiration pneumonia in the elderly: A randomized controlled trial. Clinical Rehabilitation. 2016. [Epub ahead of print]

[96] Malmgren LT, Fisher PJ, Bookman LM, Uno T. Age-related changes in muscle fiber types in the human thyroarytenoid muscle: An immunohistochemical and stereological study using confocal laser scanning microscopy. Otolaryngology – head and neck surgery. Official Journal of American Academy of Otolaryngology-Head and Neck Surgery. 1999;**121**:441-451

[97] Malmgren LT, Jones CE, Bookman LM. Muscle fiber and satellite cell apoptosis in the aging human thyroarytenoid muscle: A stereological study with confocal laser scanning microscopy. Otolaryngology – head and neck surgery. Official Journal of American Academy of Otolaryngology-Head and Neck Surgery. 2001;**125**:34-39

[98] Martins RH, Benito Pessin AB, Nassib DJ, Branco A, Rodrigues SA, Matheus SM. Aging voice and the laryngeal muscle atrophy. The Laryngoscope. 2015;**125**:2518-2521

[99] Giraldez-Rodriguez LA, Johns M, 3rd. Glottal insufficiency with aspiration risk in dysphagia. Otolaryngologic Clinics of North America. 2013;**46**:1113-1121

[100] Ortega O, Rofes L, Martin A, Arreola V, Lopez I, Clave P. A Comparative study between two sensory stimulation strategies after two weeks treatment on older patients with oropharyngeal dysphagia. Dysphagia. 2016;**31**:706-716

[101] Ortega O, Sakwinska O, Combremont S, Berger B, Sauser J, Parra C, Zarcero S, Nart J, Carrion S, Clave P. High prevalence of colonization of oral cavity by respiratory pathogens in frail older patients with oropharyngeal dysphagia. Neurogastroenterology and Motility: The Official Journal of the European Gastrointestinal Motility Society. 2015;**27**:1804-1816

6

Rehabilitation in Sarcopenic Elderly

Raoul Saggini, Simona Maria Carmignano,
Lucia Cosenza, Tommaso Palermo and
Rosa Grazia Bellomo

Abstract

Sarcopenia is a complex problem and an important emerging field in rehabilitation of the elderly. In 2010, the European working group on sarcopenia in older people (EWGSOP) described sarcopenia as a syndrome characterised by progressive and generalised loss of skeletal muscle mass and strength, associated with a risk of adverse outcomes such as physical disability, poor quality of life and death. This field of rehabilitation has been defined as 'evaluative, diagnostic and therapeutic interventions whose purpose is to restore functional ability or enhance residual functional capability in elderly people with disabling impairments'. With growing numbers of frail older people, there is an increasing need for appropriate geriatric rehabilitation services. Definitely, sarcopenia needs a specific rehabilitation program to improve muscular mass and strength that must be integrated with a global approach with the aim to recover postural assessment, amplify sensory-motor systems, in order to gain the necessary information for proper motor planning, to reduce risk of falls. Several physical agents in medicine permit to treat sarcopenia, like vibrations or electrical stimulation. The aim of this chapter is to give an overview about rehabilitative medicine for sarcopenia, highlighting the state of the art, presenting the most significative clinical researches and giving some inputs to set a rehabilitation protocol.

Keywords: sarcopenia, physical energies, complex sensory-motor rehabilitation program, vibrations, electrical stimulation

1. Introduction

Sarcopenia (from the Greek sarx 'flesh' and penia 'loss') is a term used for the first time by Rosenberg to describe the age-related decrease in muscle mass. In fact, aging is associated with a progressive decline in muscle mass that can lead to a decrease in muscle quality and strength.

In 2010, the European working group on sarcopenia in older people (EWGSOP) described sarcopenia as a syndrome characterised by progressive and generalised loss of skeletal muscle mass and strength, associated with a risk of adverse outcomes such as physical disability, poor quality of life and death [1]. The reduction in muscle mass is associated with longer hospitalisation, increased need for rehabilitation care after hospital discharge, infective complications, prolonged duration of mechanical ventilation and higher mortality. There are several approaches to treat sarcopenia and it was demonstrated that, regardless of the type of intervention, treatment improves the quality of life preventing falls, disability and loss of independence among elderly patients [2]. Among interventions, resistance training has been shown to be the most effective to reduce the effects of sarcopenia, this because it induces skeletal muscle hypertrophy and enhances muscle strength; unfortunately, resistance training is not always feasible in sarcopenic elderly people [2]. Therefore, in these cases, physical therapies come to the rescue, i.e. vibrations or electrical stimulations. Particularly, it is possible to use focal vibrations, which excite the afferents coming from the neuromuscular spindle, leading to the activation of the proprioceptive sensory system. Electrical stimulation too is an alternative, even more effective than exercise alone, in strengthening muscles in sarcopenic patients [3]. These alternative approaches to exercise offered a safe addition to a traditional, high-intensity volitional strengthening program with the aim to implement muscular mass and strength. It is also a necessary adequate sensory-motor and functional recovery program to reach an acceptable walking ability. The ability to walk is the key to any human movement, despite the fact the human movements are not limited to bipedal locomotion; bipedal locomotion is a fundamental part of daily life and is a prominent target of public health physical activity guidelines [4]. In order to get a better walking performance and a postural global improvement, two integrate procedures may be used: normalisation of the foot-ground reaction to control vertical and shear forces on the foot during the stance phase; second one is the microgravitary environment that determines the sensory-motor and functional recovery of the posture during walking activity in combination to the development of proprioceptive information from periphery to the cortical central system [4]. Definitely, sarcopenia needs a specific rehabilitation program to improve muscular mass and strength that must be integrated with a global approach with the aim to recovery postural assessment, amplify sensory-motor systems, in order to gain the necessary information for proper motor planning, to reduce risk of falls.

2. Background

Aging, as mentioned, is characterised by a progressive loss of skeletal muscle mass and strength, thus leading to the loss of functional capacity. In sarcopenia, the loss of skeletal muscle mass must be due to a chronic disruption in the balance between muscle protein synthesis and degradation.

In active and healthy elderly patients, the mechanism underlying the loss of muscle mass does not seem to be bound to a disorder of protein metabolism in the basal state (fasting). Rather, it was proposed that muscle in the elderly presents a deficiency in the ability to regulate protein synthesis in response to an anabolic stimulus, such as physical activity or food intake [1].

According to epidemiological data in literature, the prevalence of sarcopenia in people ranging in ages from 60 to 70 turns out to be 5–13%, while in patients over 80, it varies between 11 and 50% [2]. In 2000, the number of people worldwide over the age of 60 years was estimated at 600 million, a value that is forecast to rise to 1.2 billion in 2025 and 2 billion in 2050 [5]. Making an approximate estimate about the prevalence, people with sarcopenia nowadays are more than 50 million that should increase to over 200 million in the next 40 years.

The impact of sarcopenia in elderly affects multiple aspects; in fact, its influence can be seen in terms of morbidity [6], disability [7], increasing in costs related to health care [8] and mortality [9].

The underlying causes of sarcopenia and frailty are multifactorial. Although the progressive loss of muscle mass that occurs with aging is well-known for many years, but it is only with the latest techniques and prospective-longitudinal studies that changes related to aging in muscle composition have begun to be described [10].

Several reviews have highlighted cellular and molecular mechanisms underlying the weakness and muscle atrophy related to aging [11]. It has been seen that the loss of muscle strength and mass are the consequence of a progressive atrophy due to a loss of individual muscle fibres associated to a reduction of some motor units; this implies fat and other non-contractile tissue (i.e. fibrous tissue) infiltrations which involves a reduction of 'muscle quality' [1].

Therefore, changes in musculoskeletal age are initially neuromuscular and subsequently others several factors intervene (**Figure 1**) such as neural transmission, protein synthesis and

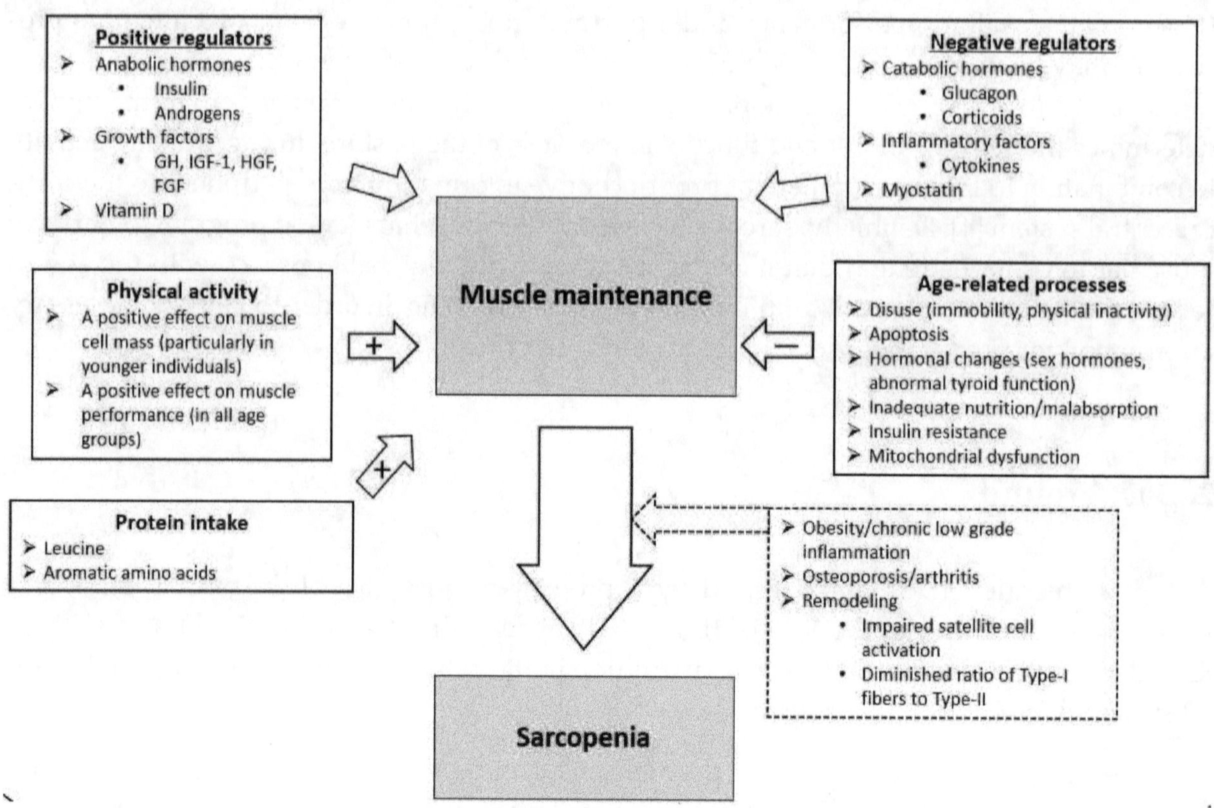

Figure 1. Factors that affect the muscle maintenance and/or the onset of sarcopenia. + positive influence, − negative influence. GH growth hormone, IGF-1 insulin-like growth factor 1, HGF: hepatocyte growth factor, FGF: fibroblast growth factor.

degradation, muscle architecture, composition of muscle fibres, increasing in production of reactive oxygen species, apoptosis of muscle cells, alteration in excitation-contraction coupling and metabolism [11].

In generic terms, sarcopenia is the age-associated loss of skeletal muscle mass and function; this decline is progressive and generalised with the possible risk of adverse outcomes such as physical disability, poor quality of life and even death [12, 13]. The causes are multifactorial and can include disuse, changing endocrine function, chronic diseases, inflammation, insulin resistance and nutritional deficiencies. The pathogenic mechanisms underlying sarcopenia are different from acute muscular atrophy resulting from disuse, cachexia, denervation or other conditions.

In order to make the diagnosis of sarcopenia, the European working group on sarcopenia in older people (EWGSOP) recommends verifying the simultaneous presence of both low muscle mass and reduction in muscle function (understood as strength or performance). Thus, the diagnosis requires the satisfaction of the criterion 1 in combination of criterion 2 or criterion 3 (**Table 1**).

The reason why are necessary at least two criteria for the diagnosis is that the force does not depend only on the muscle mass and also the relationship between strength and mass is not linear [14]. In fact, alterations in muscle quality have a central role in the loss of strength in elderly. Hughes et al. [15] showed that only a variation of 5% in strength depends on muscle mass. Muscle weakness may lead to reduced function, decreased physical activity and immobility, thus leading to secondary muscular 'ex non usu' atrophy. Consequently, diminished muscle mass is the result, but also the cause of age-related loss of strength. This is due to increased levels of pro-inflammatory cytokines and to a damage of type 2 muscle fibres. Furthermore, the growth in muscle mass is not directly related to an increment in strength, which may be increased even in the absence of a visible variation of muscle mass [16]. Neurological changes, hormonal and metabolic milieu, pro-inflammatory cytokines, fat infiltration (lipotoxicity) may conduce to a progressive muscle weakness in elderly [13]. Therefore, defining sarcopenia only in terms of loss of muscle mass is too simplistic and may be of limited clinical value. Precisely for this reason, some authors argue that the term dynapenia would be preferable to describe the loss of strength and function associated with aging [17]. However, 'sarcopenia' is a term so widely spread that replacing it could generate more confusion.

Sarcopenia staging, which reflects the severity degree of the disease, is a concept that can be of assistance in clinical management of the condition; specifically, the EWGSOP suggests a division into 'pre-sarcopenia', 'sarcopenia' and 'severe sarcopenia' (**Table 2**). 'Pre-sarcopenia' stage is characterised by low muscle mass without influencing on muscle strength or physical

Diagnosis is based on documentation of criterion 1 plus criterion 2 or 3
1. Low muscle mass
2. Low muscle strength
3. Low physical performance

Table 1. EWGSOP diagnostic criteria.

Stage	Muscle mass	Muscle strength	Performance
Pre-sarcopenia	↓		
Sarcopenia	↓	↓	Or ↓
Severe sarcopenia	↓	↓	↓

Table 2. EWGSOP stages of sarcopenia.

performance; this phase can only be identified by techniques that measure muscle mass accurately (see later). Concerning to standard populations, 'sarcopenia' stage is characterised by low muscle mass with low muscle strength or low physical performance. The last stage, when the three criteria (low muscle mass, low muscle strength and low physical performance) are present concomitantly, is defined as 'severe sarcopenia'. Recognising different stages of sarcopenia is essential to choose the most appropriate treatment and setting, thus enabling the achievement of therapeutic goals. Staging also allows to program scientific research focused on a particular stage or to evaluate any changes over time [18].

Generally, all the syndromes associated with prominent muscle loss are described as sarcopenia. Only research on the etiopathological mechanisms of age-related sarcopenia can lead to distinction from secondary forms, so the most appropriate therapy for each of them can be chosen such as cachexia, frailty and sarcopenic obesity.

The parameters of sarcopenia are muscle mass and function. The measurable variables are mass, strength and physical performance; for diagnostic and research purposes, it is important to identify the best diagnostic test that is able to measure them accurately. It is also important to recognise changes by repeating the same measures over time in the same individuals [18].

Only a few clinical trials are underway to evaluate the potential for sarcopenia treatments compared to the great impact that reduced mobility and functionality have on the quality of life of older people. The absence of standardised primary outcomes is a major challenge for the design of such studies. For intervention trials, EWGSOP presently recommends three primary outcome variables: muscle mass, muscle strength and physical performance (**Table 3**). Further studies could lead to the finding of outcomes currently considered secondary, but which may play a central role in the diagnostic and prognostic phase of this clinical condition.

Among methods of evaluation computed tomography (CT) and magnetic resonance imaging (MRI) can distinguish fat from other soft tissues of the body, thus representing validate methods for estimating muscle mass for research scope. The high costs and risks related to exposure to radiation (TC), limit their use in clinical practice. Dual energy X-ray absorptiometry (DEXA) distinguishes adipose tissue, bone mineral mass and lean body mass. It can be used both in research and in clinical practice and exposes patients to a smaller quantity of radiations. However, the access to this method is limited for severely obese individuals; furthermore, the equipment is not portable, which limits its use in epidemiological studies on a large scale.

Bioimpedance analysis (BIA) is a test that is not expensive, easy to use, easily reproducible and suitable for both ambulatory patients and bedridden. The bioelectrical impedance measurement

Variable	Exams	Clinical practice
Muscle mass	Computed tomography (CT) Magnetic resonance imaging (MRI) Dual energy X-ray absorptiometry (DXA) Bioimpedance analysis (BIA) Total or partial body potassium per fat-free tissue	BIA DXA Anthropometry
Muscle strength	Handgrip strength Knee flexion/extension Peak expiratory flow	Handgrip strength
Physical performance	Short Physical Performance Battery (SPPB) Usual gait speed Timed up and go test Stair climb power test	SPP Usual gait speed Timed up and go test

Table 3. Measurements of muscle mass, strength and performance in research and clinical practice.

techniques have been studied for many years and the BIA results in standard conditions correlate with the predictions of the MRI [19].

Among measurements to assess muscle strength, it is necessary to emphasise the importance of handgrip test; even if lower limbs are more relevant than the upper limbs in physical function and walking, the evaluation of strength by isometric handgrip has been widely used. Measured under standard conditions, with a well-studied model of dynamometer hand, it is closely correlated with lower limb muscles power and with the area of calf section.

The short physical performance battery (SPPB) is one of the most valid techniques to measure physical performance. It consists of a brief set of tests evaluating the functionality of the lower limbs. This battery is composed of three different sections. The first one is the assessment of balance in three tests: (a) maintenance of balance in stand position with feet together side-by-side for 10 seconds; (b) maintenance of balance in semi-tandem position (heel of one foot against side of big toe of the other) for 10″; (c) maintenance of balance in tandem position (feet aligned heel to toe) for 10″. The second section evaluates gait speed measuring the time required to walk 4 m linear at a normal pace. Finally, the third one measures the time required to perform five rises from a chair to an upright position as fast as possible without the use of the arms.

Other tests can be used in clinical practice, as they require a very simple execution setting. One of these is the sit to stand test, which evaluates the ability to move from sit to stand position without using arms. The timed up-and-go test (TUG), which evaluates the dynamic balance by measuring the time required to complete a series of tasks (getting up from a chair, walking a short distance, turning around an obstacle, walking back and sitting down again) [20, 21].

Specific mode and intensity of physical activity can act synergistically to maintain and even increase muscle mass, strength and power, both in healthy individual and in elderly patients with limited functionality. These interventions also have been found effective for all ages and there is evidence for similar responses in both female and male [22].

During aging, a sedentary lifestyle is associated with a decrease in lean body mass and with an increase in fat mass, which ultimately leads to an increase in mortality and functional limitations. This is demonstrated in studies showing the reduction of cardiovascular-related risk and all causes of mortality in individuals highly physically active than those moderately active or worse sedentary.

Physical activity, in particular resistance exercises, is a powerful stimulus to promote muscle protein anabolism, resulting in specific metabolic and morphological adaptations of the skeletal muscle tissue. Resistance type exercise training can effectively increase muscle strength and muscle mass, thus improving physical performance and functional capacity. To stimulate muscle hypertrophy and to increase strength in elderly patients, it is known [23] that the traditional exercise of resistance at low speed (i.e. performing concentric and eccentric to each muscle in 2–3") is found to be a type of intervention that is safe, feasible and effective. The physiological response to resistance exercises may consist in an increase in protein synthesis, in an activation and proliferation of satellite cells, in a production of anabolic hormones and in a decreased activity of catabolic cytokines. Resistance exercises in elderly subjects appear to lead to an increased number of mitochondria and a reduction in oxidative stress. Recent scientific evidences suggest that muscle performance is a determining factor regarding the functional capabilities. A new and effective approach to increase power in elderly subjects is found to be the fast-contraction-velocity exercise. In addition, the aerobic exercise can generate benefits on elderly muscles through an increment in mitochondrial energy production, increased insulin sensitivity and/or reduction of the oxidative stress [24].

In elderly patients, the clinical relevance of a nutritional and rehabilitative intervention based on exercise, resides with the long-term effects on not only strength and muscle mass but also on the implications concerning functional capacity and risk of developing chronic metabolic diseases. It is well known that the ability to respond to an anabolic stimulus, through the activation of muscle protein synthesis, is kept up even in elderly (though to a lesser extent) [24]. Definitely, it is possible to affirm that resistance-type exercise interventions have been shown effective in increasing skeletal muscle mass, training muscle strength and/or improving functional capacity in elderly [24].

3. Rehabilitation

3.1. Scientific researches

Over the years, we have therefore investigated the effects of exercise and mechanical stimulation in primary prevention and treatment of sarcopenia.

In 2006, the first study [25] evaluated the selective development of muscle strength in 20 female subjects with severe atrophy of the femoral quadriceps muscle, with a mean age of 31 years. Subjects were randomly divided in two groups, named A and B. Group A performed 10 rehabilitation sessions, 5 times per week, lasting 10 minutes each, with mechano-sound vibration (without performing voluntary contraction) with a defined frequency of 300 Hz. Group B performed 10 sessions of strengthening every other day through isokinetic Cybex equipment at 90°/second in concentric-eccentric mode. The evaluation was performed at first visit (T0), after the treatment period (T1) and at a 6 months follow-up (T2) by isokinetic testing (Cybex) with flexion-extension movement of right and left knee at 180 and 60°/second, in both study groups. At T1 evaluation, it was found in both groups a significant increase in muscle strength and working ability as well as an improvement in muscular coordination. The increase in contractile strength in group A was comparable to that obtained with a conventional rehabilitation protocol (group B). Differences between the two groups were the longest duration of treatment effectiveness (about 6 months) and the faster achievement of these results, already during the protocol, in Group A. High speed contractile improvements induced by the local vibrational method appeared more effective; in fact, in group A, contralateral muscle strength improved too, unlike the group B.

In a 2008 study, we compared the efficacy of three methods of training in elderly subjects with postural instability and sarcopenia [26]. Nineteen subjects (11F and 8M, aged between 64 and 80 years) took part in the study. Evaluations at T0 and T1 have been carried out through clinical examination, needle biopsy of the vastus lateralis muscle (measuring specific development of the individual fibres), expression of myosin heavy chains, transcriptional and regenerative capacity profile of satellite cells. Subjects were divided randomly into three groups of six subjects each; group A performed aerobic training (endurance), group B anaerobic training (power), group C mechano-sound vibration at a frequency of 300 Hz. The protocol frequency was three sessions per week for all study groups. The results obtained showed that the development of single fibre strength did not change in any of the training protocols; gene expression profiles showed, for each type of intervention, the stimulation of a specific metabolic pathway, as both resistance and vibration training increased aerobic metabolism, while resistance training stimulated creatine metabolism. All trainings protocols stimulated in a different way the expression of sarcomeric and cytoskeletal proteins; in particular, mechano-sound vibration training has stimulated proteins associated with the Z-line. It was also found that satellite cells contribute to regeneration and trophism of muscle fibre. The results therefore suggested that all training protocols are effective in contrasting the progression of sarcopenia and each one is able to stimulate specific molecular signals. The effects are specific because there is a relationship between the type of exercise and the metabolism stimulated.

In another study, we further evaluated the effect of focused vibration on elderly skeletal muscle [27]. Eleven subjects (5F and 4M, aged between 65 and 82 years), diagnosed with sarcopenia in accordance with the guidelines of the Centers for Disease Control and Prevention (CDC) were evaluated and treated. Inclusion criteria for the study were patients older than 18 years, diagnosis of sarcopenia in absence of joint pathology. Exclusion criteria were cardiovascular and/or metabolic diseases, hereditary or acquired muscular disorders, respiratory and psychiatric disorders, treatment with testosterone or other drugs affecting muscle mass. Mechanical vibrations were applied at local level at a frequency of 300 Hz on thigh muscles for a period of 12 weeks, starting from a 15-minute per session once a week to progressively reach 3 sessions per week. The evaluation consisted of clinical examination, resting ECG and isometric tests. These were carried out the week before the beginning of the study (T0, pre-session), at the end of the therapeutic protocol (T1, post-session) and

16 weeks after the end of treatment (T2, follow-up). Moreover, it was evaluated the body mass index (BMI), the measurement of the circumference of proximal and distal thigh and it was performed the vastus lateralis muscle biopsy. Maximal isometric strength evaluation of lower limb extensor muscles showed an increase in strength since 4 weeks of treatment in women and after 8 weeks in men; increasing strength reached a plateau phase at week 12. As it regards the circumferences, it was found a significant increase of the distal circumference of 0.5–3 cm and a non-significant increase of the thigh circumference at the proximal zone. Vastus lateralis biopsy results showed the increase of muscle fibre section width (T0: 3667 ± 310.7, T1: 4238 ± 357.4 μm^2); changing in myosin chains, which switched from the isoform slow (MyHC-1) to the isoform fast (MyHC-2X). Other interesting observations were the stimulation of genes involved in energetic metabolism (PIK3R3; GSK-3), in protein synthesis and degradation, in calcium homeostasis (ACTA2; MLCB; ARL5A; LCCP; TTID; POP3; RyR3; CHERP) and in oxidative stress processes (P12; PRDX3; MSRA). It was also found a down-regulation of the gene coding for nitric oxide synthase (NOS-1). The results showed that sarcopenic skeletal muscle reduced metabolic power because of several factors, such as a reduction in blood supply, fibrosis processes and atrophy development. Muscle tissue undergoes continuous oxidative phenomena; this leads to imbalance between oxidant and antioxidant capacity; in fact, in elderly, several genes coding for antioxidant factors are down-regulated. The reduced expression of NOS leads to a reduction of the amount of nitric oxide circulating, compromising vasodilatation. Therefore, focused mechano-sound vibration, increasing the expression of genes coding for antioxidant factors, while enhancing the maximal isometric force, can be considered effective in combating sarcopenia.

In a more recent study of 2013, we compared the effectiveness of three types of training on strength and balance ability on a population of elderly male subjects suffering from sarcopenia [4]. In this study, 40 male subjects (mean age 71 years) diagnosed with sarcopenia, in accordance with the guidelines of the CDC, were evaluated and treated. Inclusion criteria of the study were patients over 18 years, sarcopenia diagnosis in absence of joint disorders. Exclusion criteria were cardiovascular or metabolic diseases, hereditary or acquired muscular disorders, respiratory and psychiatric disorders, treatment with testosterone or other substances affecting muscle mass. Forty participants were included randomly into one of the four study groups. Each group performs a specific protocol. Group A carried out a comprehensive sensorimotor training on I-Moove® with 'Reebost' program (for balance and flexibility) for 20 minutes, after warming-up with cycle-ergometer (5 minutes) and stretching of the lower limbs; frequency of sessions was 2 times per week for 12 weeks. Group B performed aerobic endurance training with leg-press and leg-extension: 2 times a week for 12 weeks. Group C underwent training vibration with a frequency of 300 Hz (average size of the transducer of 23.7 cm^2) lasting 15 minutes per session, 1 session a week for the first 8 weeks and 3 sessions per week in the last four weeks; group D (control group) did not perform any kind of rehabilitation program. The assessment was carried out using clinical examination, maximal isometric tests performed on leg-extension equipped with load cell, BMI measurement, gait analysis, stabilometry. At the end of treatment was highlighted statistically significant increase in bilateral isometric force equal to 45% in group B (which performed resistance training) and 43%

in group C, which was treated with mechano-sound vibrations. In the group, which carried out the sensorimotor training on I-Moove (group A), the improvement was only 15%, while no change was observed in the control group. About balance and stability, it was found a significative improvement of the sway area and path length, measured by stabilometry, in groups A and C; no improvements were found in groups B and D. Another observation was the increase in half-step length in all three trained groups (108% in group A, 65% in group B, 92% in group C); step width increased only in the I-Moove group. Significant reduction of 24% in time of contact to the ground was observed only in the vibration training group. The study showed that an overall sensorimotor stimulation produced by focused acoustic vibration and proprioceptive training, carried out with I-Moove, is an effective approach to increase strength and balance in sarcopenic elderly, which could result in a better quality of life.

As a part of primary prevention, we also evaluated the influence of exercise and focused acoustic vibration on blood concentration of some hormones [28]. Aim of the study was to evaluate the effects of focused acoustic vibrations, set to a frequency of 300 Hz, on muscle performance and blood hormone concentrations in healthy young adult males in acute and long-term observations. In this study, 36 male patients (average age 21.5 years) were evaluated and treated; they usually performed moderate intensity level of physical activity (1–2 times per week). The participants were divided into 2 groups: group A performed focused mechano-acoustic vibrations every 3 days for 4 weeks (10 sessions overall); instead, group B performed resistance training every 3 days for 4 weeks (10 sessions). The assessment was carried out every 3 days, during therapeutic session, through haematochemical parameters (to quantify hormone levels), counter-movement jump (CMJ) and maximal voluntary isometric contraction (MVC); assessments were performed before each session, immediately after it and 1 hour after the end of treatment. All subjects also performed isokinetic and MVC tests after 4 weeks of training and at 2 months follow-up. Group A showed a significant increase in growth hormone (GH) and creatine-phosphokinase levels and a reduction of cortisol levels ($P < 0.05$); no change was highlighted in group B. In both groups, it was observed a significant improvement in MVC test ($P < 0.05$). After 4 weeks, the results showed evidence of an increase in isokinetic tests and in maximal strength test in both groups; the improvement persisted in the next 2 months. These results indicate that focused mechano-acoustic vibrations can influence the concentration of particular hormones and can improve neuromuscular performance. The benefit gained is maintained over the medium to long term and it was comparable to what happens after a resistance training treatment.

Other authors have also studied the effectiveness of vibration therapy in improving strength and muscle tone in patients suffering from sarcopenia. Wei et al. [29] try to determine the optimal combination of frequency and exposure time of a whole-body vibration (WBV) training program to improve muscle performance in elderly with age-related muscle loss. A total of 80 community-dwelling older adults with sarcopenia were randomly divided into four groups, 20 patients each: first group treated with WBV set to low-frequency and long duration (20 Hz × 720 seconds), second group treated at medium-frequency and medium duration (40 Hz × 360 seconds), third group set to high-frequency and short duration (60 Hz × 240 seconds) and control group did not perform any training. The treatment period lasted 12 weeks and a follow-up was scheduled at additional 12 weeks. There was a significant time per group interaction effect in isokinetic knee extension at 180°/second. The study found significant time effects in all muscle strength outcome variables. Comparing second group (WBV set at 40 Hz for 360 seconds) with control group, the authors found that the percentage of change from baseline values were significant on isokinetic knee extension tests (at 180 and 60°/second). Therefore, they concluded that the best combination for WBV exercise is to set medium frequency and medium duration (40 Hz × 360 seconds), because of it shows the best outcome among all other combinations tested; moreover, the improvements in knee extension performance can be maintained for 12 weeks after cessation of WBV training.

The effectiveness of electrostimulation in rehabilitation has been long known, especially in muscle strengthening. Kern et al [30] analysed (at functional, structural and molecular level) the effects of electrical stimulation training on healthy seniors with normal lifestyle, without routine sport activity. The study found that electrical stimulation was able to improve muscle torque and functional performances and it increased muscle fibres and most importantly fast fibres, which are related to the power of skeletal muscle. At molecular level, electrical stimulation induced up-regulation of insulin-like growth factor 1 (IGF-1) and modulation of MuRF-1, a muscle-specific atrophy-related gene. Furthermore, it induced up-regulation of relevant markers of differentiating satellite cells and of extracellular matrix remodelling, which might guarantee shape and mechanical forces of trained skeletal muscle as well as maintenance of satellite cell function, reducing fibrosis. This study provide evidence that electrostimulation is a safe method to counteract muscle decline associated with aging.

In 2015, Barberi et al. [31] analysed some downstream pathways activated by IGF-1. They demonstrated that electrical stimulation increases not only anabolic pathways, but it also reduces muscle catabolism. Extracellular matrix during physical exercise shows remodelling processes. The authors demonstrated that this occur also with electrostimulation, due to enhance of collagen expression; in fact, they observed an up-regulation of three different forms of collagen (I, III and VI) in electrical stimulated muscle. The question was if this increase in collagen was due to stimulated fibrosis by electrical stimulation. However, biopsy did not demonstrate any accumulation of fibrotic tissue. Further supporting the morphological evidences, Barberi et al. analysed miR29, one of the most important controllers of fibrosis. Actually, the electrical stimulation regulates miR29, which might down-regulate fibrosis. Then authors verified electrical stimulation in increasing activity of satellite cells, such as physical exercise. In fact, electrostimulation increased the number of these cells, and this is also demonstrated by the increase of their molecular markers (myogenin, miR-206 and miR-1). In conclusion, the electrical stimulation can be applied to elderly sarcopenic patients, which might not carry out normal physical activity, modulating similar factors associated with exercise. In particular, IGF-1 once stimulated through electrostimulation, activates anabolic pathway, increasing protein synthesis and satellite cells. All these modifications lead to an increase in muscle performance.

As part of a bio-progressive rehabilitative approach, treatment of sarcopenic patients may not be limited to muscle strengthening or pain resolution. It appears clear; therefore, the need for a global approach to the patient, which also guarantees postural and gait rehabilitation. To do this, we usually consider the use of SPAD® (dynamic anti-gravitary postural system), the function of which is to provide postural stability and to increase exteroceptive and proprioceptive sensitivity. SPAD® [32] is composed by a conveyor belt, surmounted by a lifting structure, which forces the patient to walk in a straight line on a treadmill, while six proprioceptive blocks (four anterior and two on the back) act on the rotation components.

In a 2008 study [33], the aim was to define the possibility of using SPAD system in elderly rehabilitation. Group A was treated with SPAD system, while group B performed a proprioceptive rehabilitative protocol on Galileo platform (WBV at 28 Hz). Patients were evaluated at the beginning of the treatment (T0), at the end (T1) and at 6 months follow-up (T2) through gait analysis, stabilometry and isokinetic test (Cybex® system). After treatment period, both groups showed a significative improvement in gait alignment, a reduction of sway area and ellipse surface in stabilometry and a significative improvement in isokinetic tests. At follow-up evaluation, better results were found in group A (maintenance of previous results) than in group B, especially in gait and balance. These results show the effectiveness of both treatments suggested, with a better outcome at follow-up in the group that performed a rehabilitative protocol with SPAD system. In conclusion, it can be stated that SPAD treatment allows to comprehensively address the problem of postural disability evident in aging, as it acts on deep spine muscles, improving lower limb muscles tone and associating a motor-vestibular rehabilitation. This means a greater capacity of mobility with a better quality of life for elderly people.

3.2. Rehabilitative protocols

Scientific data illustrated above and those collected by our personal experience allowed us to summarise that each type of physical agents in medicine has a proper applicability in terms of cost/benefit ratio. To modulate muscle activity, enhancing muscle tone, the approach applied is:

Step 1. Focused mechano-acoustic vibrations

Step 2. Focused mechano-acoustic vibrations + SPAD

Step 3. Electrical stimulation + whole-body vibrations + SPAD

With regard to the focused mechano-acoustic vibration, the frequencies related to effects on muscles can be schematically summarised as follows:

- 120 Hz, muscle relaxation
- 200 Hz, strengthening of slow muscle fibres
- 300 Hz, strengthening of fast muscle fibres

Therefore, the treatment protocol we recommend, using Vibration Sound System®, in elderly patients suffering from sarcopenia, consists of 200 Hz for 10 minutes, 300 Hz for 10 minutes and 120 Hz for 5 minutes, applied with segmental strips in standing and/or supine position (**Figure 2**). The aim of this treatment is muscle strengthening and corticalisation.

Integrated protocols involve the use of focal vibrations in combination with active exercises and systems that increase proprioceptive stimulation to determine the synergy between stimuli.

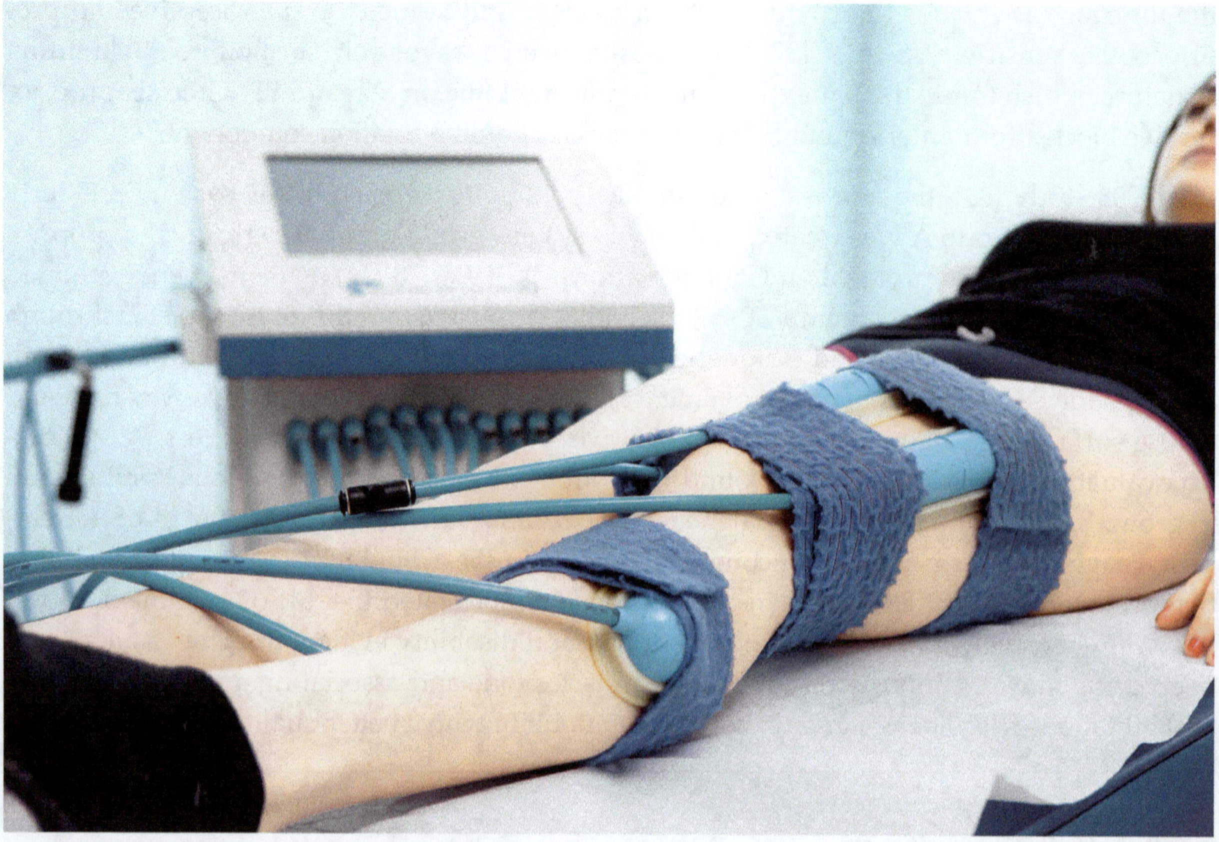

Figure 2. Focused mechano-acoustic vibrations, in supine position.

For example, if the clinical conditions of the patient permit it, we work with Vibration Sound System® to carry out eccentric exercises in upright position.

Treatment goals include increased strength through muscle hypertrophy and improved flexibility. This is also achieved through stretching exercises that improve the absorption of energy and the muscular movement range, and thus the power. Therefore, the reduction of the risk of falling, as well as the improvement of coordination, is achieved.

Another type of integrated protocol, to recover kinetic and kinematic characteristics of gait, includes the use of Vibration Sound System® with a proprioceptive system called Synergy Mat (Human Tecar® Unibell srl, Calco, Italy). It is composed by mats and pillows and it allows training, rehabilitation and natural and harmonious re-education of the body. Different surfaces give the possibility to work barefoot on different levels of instability, responding to the needs of personalised training and rehabilitation (**Figure 3**). Different densities correspond to different level of movement absorption, providing protection of the joints and increasing energy expenditure time. The variety of interchangeable elements that composed the Synergy Mat set (mats and pillows) provides many combinations of routes adapted to the user-specific needs.

To better understand the potential of vibrations and even the feasibility to integrate them with other rehabilitative systems (such as synergy mat), **Table 4** provides a list of protocols related to specific objectives and a brief description of exercises.

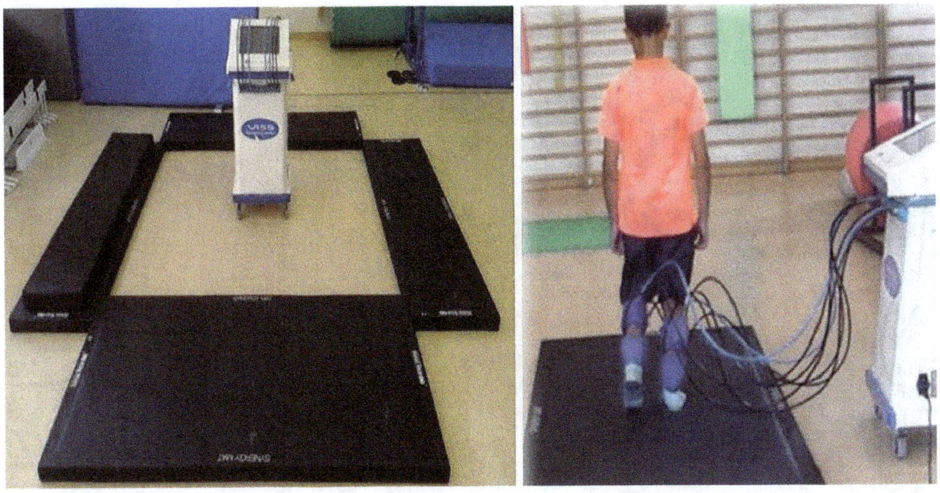

Figure 3. Another possible way to use focused mechano-acoustic vibrations in association with synergy mat.

Aim	Frequencies	Description
Muscle relaxation	50–120 Hz for 10 minutes (applied with an hand piece)	Treatment of tender points and fatigue
	120–200 Hz for 10 minutes (applied with an hand piece)	Treatment of trigger points and taut bands
Muscle strengthening, upright position	200 Hz for 10 minutes 300 Hz for 10 minutes 120 Hz for 5 minutes (applied with segmental strips)	Strengthening of slow muscle fibres Strengthening of fast muscle fibres Deconditioning
Muscle strengthening and corticalisation	200 Hz for 10 minutes 300 Hz for 10 minutes 120 Hz for 5 minutes (applied with segmental strips)	Working with squats through active work or isometric muscle contraction
Proprioceptive exercise in combination with *Synergy Mat* (Human Tecar® Unibell srl, Calco, Italy)	60–80–100–120–140–160–180–200–220–240–260–280–300 Hz, to increase every 2 minutes (applied with segmental strips)	Mono- and bipedal walking on unstable proprioceptive platforms

Table 4. Treatment protocols proposed using mechano-acoustic vibrations.

As mentioned, the second-line treatment we suggest for sarcopenia is the association of focused mechano-acoustic vibrations with SPAD® (**Figure 4**). This system has two alternative and complementary support systems: pneumatic and mechanical, which allow using consistently rates of body weight support even higher than 50%. The aim of this therapy is the recruitment of specific muscle chains, postural reprogramming and optimisation of motor coordination with restoration of the proprioceptive stimuli and physiological recovery of gait motor patterns. Therefore, the goals are both mechanical (partial decompression of lumbar spinal structures during the walk due to the microgravitary environment created) and proprioceptive (automatic-induced adaptations related to walking, once the mechanical action of relieves has achieved the percentage of body weight support established).

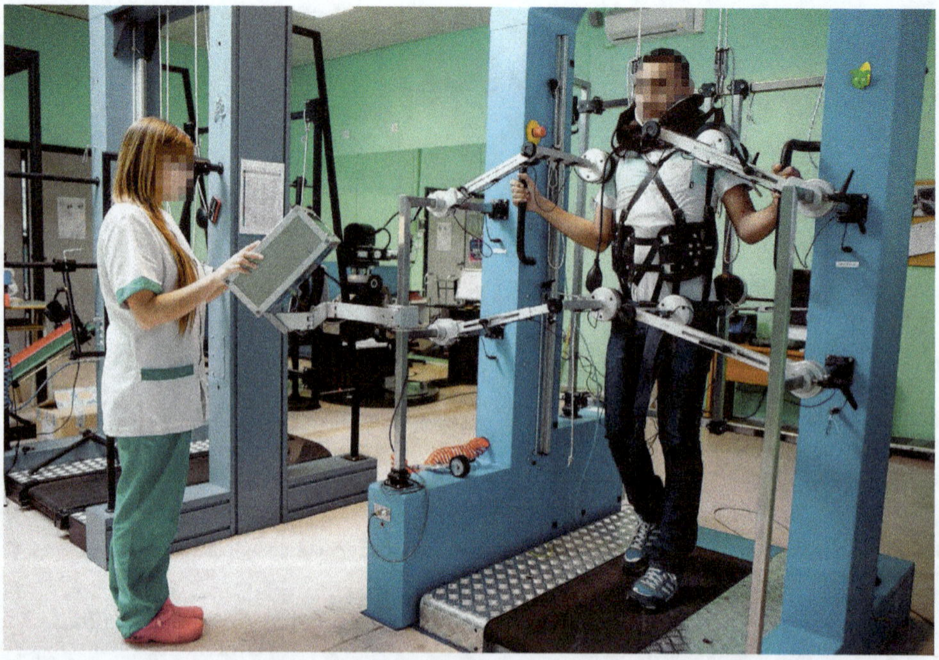

Figure 4. SPAD® system.

Third-line treatment consists of whole-body vibrations, electrical stimulation and SPAD.

Currently available WBV devices (**Figure 5**) deliver vibrations at a range of frequencies from 15 to 60 Hz and displacements from <1 to 10 mm. Considering several combinations of amplitudes and frequencies with current technology, it is clear that there are a wide variety of WBV protocols that could be used in elderly patients suffering from sarcopenia. The duration of treatment varies between individuals as well as frequencies (range 15–45 Hz); moreover, sessions of short duration (2–20 minutes), interspersed in variable-duration periods of rest, are recommended. The exercise on WBV platform would have to be performed in standing with hips and knees in slight flexion, to ensure better transmissibility of the forces to hips and spine. **Table 5** shows our WBV protocols to treat sarcopenia.

Neuromuscular electrical stimulation is defined as the use of electrical stimulation to activate muscles through intact peripheral nerve. Conventional exercise programs to increase strength are based on the overload principle of eliciting a small number of contractions of high-intensity (at least 70% of a maximal contraction 3–10 repetitions or fewer) in a treatment session performed 3–5 times per week. The same frequency of sessions can be applied when using electrical stimulation to increase strength in healthy and healthy-but-injured patients.

Our therapeutical approach involves the use of alternating currents of medium frequency produced by Horizontal Therapy (Hakomed®, **Figure 6**). The rationale is that each induced frequency generates a specific effect; for strengthening, in example, the frequencies at which muscles have to work are 20 or 100 Hz. In particular, our protocol for sarcopenia consists of a stimulation at 20 Hz for 30 minutes per session; this program includes a stimulation phase and a rest phase of 30 seconds each.

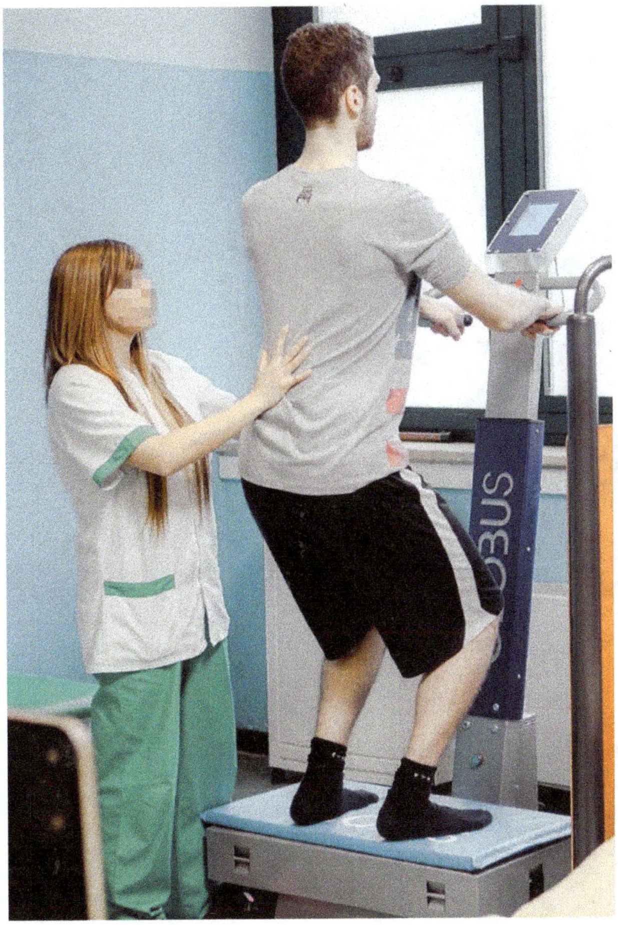

Figure 5. Whole-body vibrations (WBV).

Aim	Parameters	Protocol
Strength training	*Frequency*: 15–12 Hz. *Duration*: 3–5 minutes. *Amplitude*: medium to high, depending on comfort.	Starting position: exercises out of force and power series alternately. Sets of 10, three sets per exercise. 10-to-20-second rest between sets. 1–3-minute rest between the sets. Additional weights 70% of individual's maximal strength.
Stretching/balance exercises	*Frequency*: 15–30 Hz. *Duration*: 3–5 minutes for each exercise. *Amplitude*: low to medium.	Starting position: in standing, carry out exercises from balance and stretching series. The number of repetitions is individually tailored. Importantly, the whole body is gradually brought to an end-of-range stretching position. Balance: placing one foot alternately on the lowest position, slightly lift the other foot and hold at 5 Hz without support for 5–30 seconds.
Power training	*Frequency*: 18–30 Hz. *Duration*: 5–6 minutes. *Amplitude*: medium to high.	Carry out exercises without weights, concentrating on speed and changes in direction.

Table 5. Treatment sequence for the use of whole-body vibration in sarcopenia.

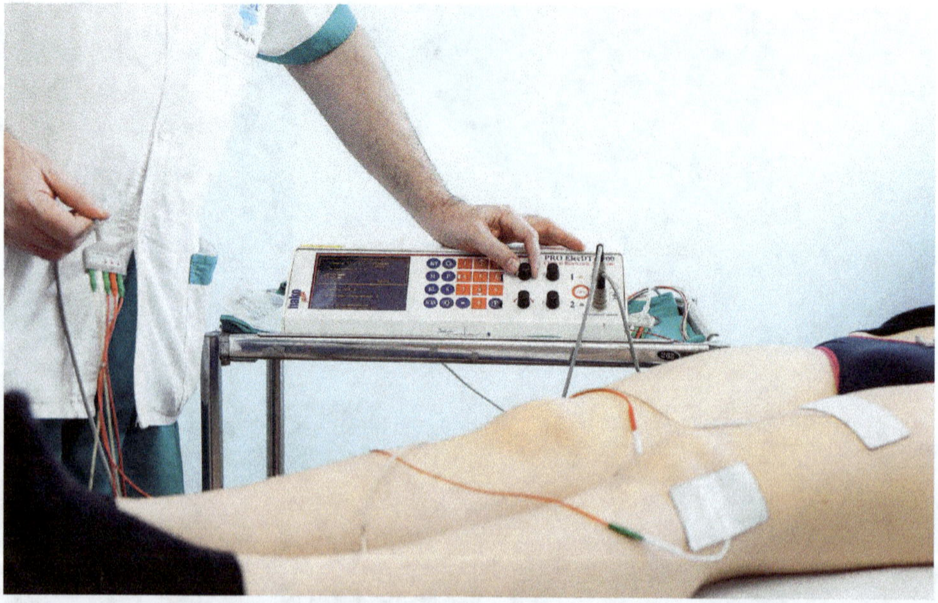

Figure 6. Horizontal therapy.

4. Conclusions

Sarcopenia is a complex problem and an important emerging field in rehabilitation of elderly. The progressive and generalised loss of skeletal muscle mass and strength is associated with the risk of physical disability, poor quality of life and death.

For these reasons, adopting the correct therapeutic solutions results of fundamental importance; to do this is necessary to know, not only the possible pharmacological interventions, but also the therapeutic possibilities that can be used thanks to the increased knowledge in the field of physical therapy. The role of rehabilitation specialist must be to integrate various therapeutic options in order to set a more suitable rehabilitative approach with the purpose of recovery postural assessment and amplify sensory-motor systems.

Author details

Raoul Saggini[1*], Simona Maria Carmignano[2], Lucia Cosenza[2], Tommaso Palermo[2] and Rosa Grazia Bellomo[3]

*Address all correspondence to: saggini@unich.it

1 Department of Medical Sciences, Oral and Biotechnology, "G. d'Annunzio" University, Chieti, Italy

2 School of Specialties in Physical and Rehabilitation Medicine, "G. d'Annunzio" University, Chieti, Italy

3 Department of Medical Sciences, Oral and Biotechnology, "G. d'Annunzio" University, Chieti, Italy

References

[1] Lynch GS, editor. Sarcopenia – Age-Related Muscle Wasting and Weakness. New York: Springer; 2011

[2] Morley JE. Sarcopenia: Diagnosis and treatment. The Journal of Nutrition Health and Aging. 2008;**12**:452-456

[3] Canning A, Grenier S. Does neuromuscular electrical stimulation improve muscular strength gains of the vastus medialis muscle. International Journal of Physical Medicine and Rehabilitation. 2014;**2**:4

[4] Bellomo RG, Iodice P, Maffulli N, Maghradze T, Coco V, Saggini R. Muscle strength and balance training in sarcopenic elderly: A pilot study with randomized controlled trial. European Journal of Inflammation. 2013;**11(1)**:193-201

[5] World Health Organization. Ageing and Life Course [Internet]. 2009. Available from: http://www.who.int/ageing/en/

[6] Sayer AA, Dennison EM, Syddall HE, et al. Type 2 diabetes, muscle strength, and impaired physical function: The tip of the iceberg? Diabetes Care. 2005;**28**:2541-2542

[7] Janssen I, Heymsfield SB, Ross R. Low relative skeletal muscle mass (sarcopenia) in older persons is associated with functional impairment and physical disability. Journal of the American Geriatrics Society. 2002;**50**:889-896

[8] Janssen I, Shepard DS, Katzmarzyk PT, et al. The healthcare costs of sarcopenia in the United States. Journal of the American Geriatrics Society. 2004;**52**:80-85

[9] Gale CR, Martyn CN, Cooper C, et al. Grip strength, body composition, and mortality. International Journal of Epidemiology. 2007;**36**:228-235

[10] Rizzoli R, Reginster JY, Arnal JF, Bautmans I, Beaudart C, Bischoff-Ferrari H, et al. Quality of life in sarcopenia and frailty. Calcified Tissue International. 2013 Aug;**93**(2):101-120

[11] Ryall JG, Schertzer JD, Lynch GS. Cellular and molecular mechanisms underlying age-related skeletal muscle wasting and weakness. Biogerontology. 2008;**9**:213-228

[12] Delmonico MJ, Harris TB, Lee JS, et al. Alternative definitions of sarcopenia, lower extremity performance, and functional impairment with aging in older men and women. Journal of the American Geriatrics Society. 2007;**55**:769-774

[13] Goodpaster BH, Park SW, Harris TB, et al. The loss of skeletal muscle strength, mass, and quality in older adults: The health, aging and body composition study. The Journals of Gerontology Series A Biological Sciences and Medical Sciences. 2006;**61**:1059-1064

[14] Janssen I, Baumgartner R, Ross R, et al. Skeletal muscle cutpoints associated with elevated physical disability risk in older men and women. American Journal of Epidemiology. 2004:**159**:413-421

[15] Hughes VA, Frontera WR, Roubenoff R, Evans WJ, Singh MA. Longitudinal changes in body composition in older men and women: Role of body weight change and physical activity. The American Journal of Clinical Nutrition. 2002;**76**:473-481

[16] Trappe S, Godard M, Gallagher P, Carroll C, Rowden G, Porter D. Resistance training improves single muscle fiber contractile function in older women. American Journal of Physiology Cell Physiology. 2001;**281**:C398-C406

[17] Clark BC, Manini TM. Sarcopenia ≠ dynapenia. The Journals of Gerontology Series A Biological Sciences and Medical Sciences. 2008;**63**:829-834

[18] Cruz-Jentoft AJ, Baeyens JP, Bauer JM, et al. Sarcopenia: European consensus on definition and diagnosis: Report of the European Working Group on Sarcopenia in Older People. Age and Ageing. 2010;**39**(4):412-423

[19] Janssen I, Heymsfield SB, Wang ZM, Ross R. Estimation of skeletal muscle mass by bioelectrical impedance analysis. Journal of Applied Physiology. 2000;**89**:465-471

[20] Guralnik JM, Simonsick EM, Ferrucci L, Robert J, Glynn LF, et al. A short physical performance battery assessing lower extremity function: Association with self-reported disability and prediction of mortality and nursing home admission. The Journals of Gerontology. 1994:**49**:M85-94

[21] Mathias S, Nayak US, Isaacs B. Balance in elderly patients: The "get-up and go" test. Archives of Physical Medicine and Rehabilitation. 1986;**67**:387-389

[22] Chodzko-Zajko WJ, Proctor DN, Fiatarone Singh MA, Minson CT, Nigg CR, Salem GJ, Skinner JS. American College of Sports Medicine position stand. Exercise and physical activity for older adults. Medicine and Science in Sports and Exercise. 2009;**41**:1510-1530

[23] Forbes SC, Little JP, Candow DG. Exercise and nutritional interventions for improving aging muscle health. Endocrine. 2012 Aug;**42**(1):29-38

[24] Snijders T, Verdijk LB, van Loon LJ. The impact of sarcopenia and exercise training on skeletal muscle satellite cells. Ageing Research Reviews. 2009 Oct;**8**(4):328-338

[25] Saggini R, Iodice P, Cancelli F, Di Baldassarre V, Bellomo RG. Lo sviluppo selettivo di forza muscolare nel contesto riabilitativo: metodologie a confronto. Europa Medicophysica. Giugno. 2006;**42**(Suppl. 1):357-358

[26] Saggini R, Bellomo RG, Coco V, Savoia V, Iodice P, Fanò G. Instabilità posturale, sarcopenia e cadute. Geriatric Medicine. Gennaio/Aprile. 2008;**1**(Suppl.):21-25

[27] Pietrangelo T, Mancinelli R, Toniolo L, Cancellara L, Paoli A, Puglielli C, et al. Effects of local vibrations on skeletal muscle trophism in elderly people: Mechanical, cellular, and molecular events. International Journal of Molecular Medicine. 2009 Oct;**24**(4):503-512

[28] Iodice P, Bellomo RG, Gialluca G, Fanò G, Saggini R. Acute and cumulative effects of focused high-frequency vibrations on the endocrine system and muscle strength. European Journal of Applied Physiology. 2011;**111**:897-904

[29] Wei N, Pang MY, Ng SS, Ng GY. Optimal frequency/time combination of whole-body vibration training for improving muscle size and strength of people with age-related muscle loss (sarcopenia): A randomized controlled trial. Geriatrics & Gerontology International; 2016 [Epub ahead of print]. DOI: 10.1111/ggi.12878

[30] Kern H, Barberi L, Löfler S, et al. Electrical stimulation counteracts muscle decline in seniors. Frontiers in Aging Neuroscience. 2014;**6**:189

[31] Barberi L, Scicchitano BM, Musaro A. Molecular and cellular mechanisms of muscle aging and sarcopenia and effects of electrical stimulation in seniors. European Journal of Translational Myology. 2015;**25**(4):5227

[32] Di Pancrazio L, Bellomo RG, Franciotti R, Iodice P, Galati V, et al. Combined rehabilitation program for postural instability in progressive supranuclear palsy. NeuroRehabilitation. 2013;**32**:855-860

[33] Saggini R, Bellomo RG, Savoia V, Iodice P, Di Pancrazio L, et al. Instabilità posturale, sarcopenia e cadute. European Journal of Medical Physics. 2008;**44**(Suppl. 1):21-25

7

Understanding Cachexia, Sarcopenia and Physical Exercise in Patients with Cancer

Shinichiro Morishita, Atsuhiro Tsubaki and Jack B. Fu

Abstract

Many patients with cancer experience muscle wasting and weakness. Muscle wasting in patients with cancer can be caused by cachexia and sarcopenia. Both cachexia and sarcopenia involve inflammation and oxidative stress. However, they differ in the underlying mechanisms that lead to muscle wasting. Cachexia involves the release of inflammatory cytokines due to cancer, while sarcopenia involves inflammation due to aging. Physical exercise has shown effectiveness for improving physical function, ability, and quality of life (QOL) in patients with cancer cachexia. On the other hand, no studies have investigated the relationship between physical exercise and sarcopenia in elderly patients with cancer. Previous studies showed effectiveness for improving physical function in elderly patients with cancer. In the future, more studies are required on physical exercise in sarcopenic elderly patients with cancer.

Keywords: cachexia, sarcopenia, physical exercise, quality of life, patients with cancer

1. Introduction

Muscle wasting and weakness are common in many disease states and conditions including aging and cancer [1]. Muscle wasting in advanced cancer is related to age, sex, tumor type, and inflammation [2]. It can be caused by inflammation and malnutrition in patients with cancer [3]. Patients with cancer have problems including anorexia, weight loss, negative nitrogen balance, and skeletal muscle wasting [4]. The loss of muscle and fat tissue due to chronic illness is referred to as cachexia, and the general loss of muscle mass with advancing age is referred to as sarcopenia [5]. Sarcopenia diagnosis requires documentation of low muscle mass along with either low muscle strength or low physical performance [6]. Cachexia and sarcopenia share some pathological muscle wasting mechanisms characterized by inflammation and oxidative stress [7, 8]. In both cachexia and sarcopenia, muscle loss can lead to frailty and adversely affect various clinical outcomes [9]. Many oncologists and rehabilitation staffs confuse cancer cachexia with simple starvation or physiological processes such as sarcopenia. Since cancer cachexia and sarcopenia can both involve muscle wasting, we speculate that the two conditions can be confused in patients with cancer. However, sarcopenia and cachexia should not be confused in patients with cancer (**Figure 1**). Instead, it should be understood that the loss of skeletal muscle mass occurs in patients with cancer (cachexia) as well as during aging (sarcopenia). Cachexia involves muscle wasting and weakness as a result of cancer-related inflammation, while sarcopenia involves muscle wasting and weakness as a result of age-related inflammation. Thus, the underlying pathological processes leading to muscle wasting and weakness differ between the two conditions.

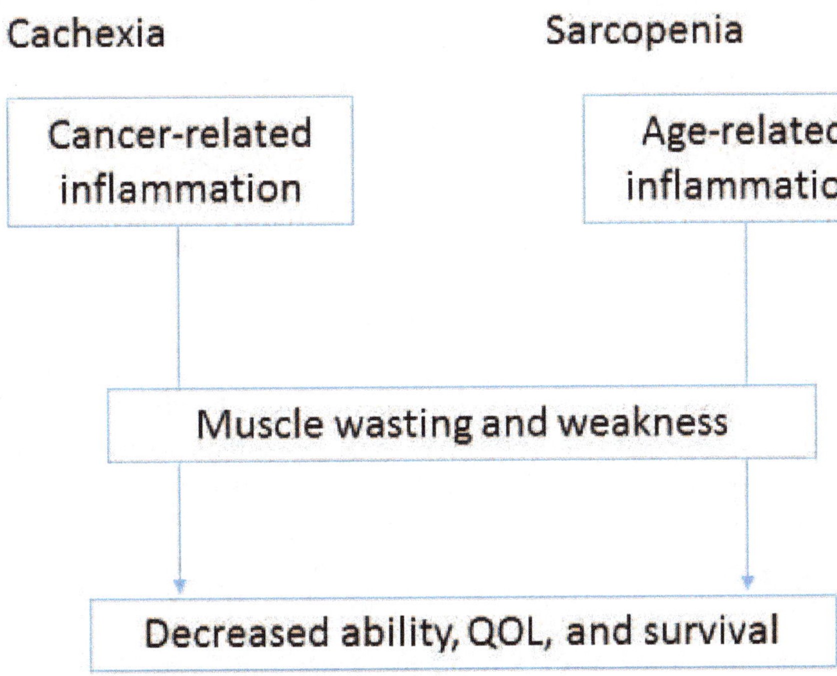

Figure 1. Muscle wasting due to cancer cachexia and sarcopenia.

2. Cachexia

Cachexia is associated with cancer and other chronic diseases, and cachexia patients lose weight and experience a decline in their overall health. The mechanism of cancer cachexia is known to involve inflammatory cytokines such as tumor necrosis factor-alpha and interleukin-6 [10]. Cancer cachexia is a complex syndrome that describes the progressive muscle wasting and weakness observed in many patients with cancer and accounts for at least 20% of cancer deaths [11, 12]. It is caused by numerous complex interactions of tumor and host factors [13, 14], and results in anorexia, wasting syndrome, and subsequent related issues [15].

It is a multifactorial syndrome defined by an ongoing loss of skeletal muscle mass (with or without loss of fat mass) that cannot be fully reversed by conventional nutritional support [16]. A panel of experts has also defined consensus criteria for diagnosing cachexia in patients with cancer [16]: (1) weight loss > 5% over the past 6 months (in the absence of simple starvation); (2) BMI < 20 kg/m^2 and any degree of weight loss > 2%; or (3) appendicular skeletal muscle index consistent with sarcopenia (males < 7.26 kg/m^2; females < 5.45 kg/m^2), and any degree of weight loss > 2%. A defining feature of cancer cachexia is the loss of muscle, but fat may also be lost [17]. Weight loss is involuntary, meaning that there is no desire or attempt to lose weight. Cancer cachexia usually worsens over time, and as weight loss increases, cancer cachexia patients also experience difficulties in daily activities.

Cancer cachexia has three clinical stages: precachexia, cachexia, and refractory cachexia [16]. The condition may occur in stages that are defined by differences in food intake, weight loss, and ability to function. In addition to muscle wasting and appetite loss, patients who have cancer anorexia–cachexia have a poor overall quality of life (QOL) and experience fatigue. They find it difficult to perform regular daily activities [18], and experience a significant symptom burden [19, 20]. Patients with cancer cachexia have significant decrease in physical function [21, 22], with low grip strength, and shorter walking distance even when controlling for muscle wasting [23, 24]. Also, cancer cachexia patients demonstrate lower physical activity [25–27]. In the early or mild stage, patients with cancer may only notice a slight loss of appetite. At the moderate stage, patients will notice more weight loss and often eat less than at the early and mild stages. In the severe stage, muscle wasting becomes markedly increased compared to the moderate stage, and the condition may be resistant to normal treatments such as dietary supplementation and nutritional support. Patients with cancer do not experience weight gain. Furthermore, patients may also have great difficulties in performing routine activities [16, 28]. Cachexia can reduce the physical activities of daily living (ADL) in patients with cancer [29]. Many patients with cancer cachexia experience decrease in physical function and ADL after muscle wasting. Thus, in addition to nutritional support, physical exercise may also contribute to improve the physical function in patients with cancer cachexia.

3. Sarcopenia

Sarcopenia, derived from a Greek word meaning "poverty of flesh," is characterized by the triad of progressive loss of skeletal muscle mass, muscle strength, and physical performance [30]. It is defined as age-related muscle wasting; thus, sarcopenia frequently occurs in elderly people. European Working Group on Sarcopenia in Older People (EWGSOP) recommends that the diagnosis of sarcopenia in elderly patients should be based on the presence of both low muscle mass and low muscle function (strength or performance) [6]. EWGSOP uses these characteristics to further classify the condition into the stages of presarcopenia, sarcopenia, and severe sarcopenia [6]. Sarcopenia has emerged as an important prognostic factor in elderly advanced patients with cancer [6]. Modalities used to assess sarcopenia include magnetic resonance imaging, computed tomography, dual-energy X-ray absorptiometry, and bioelectrical impedance analysis [31]. Sarcopenia is associated with poor performance status, toxicity from chemotherapy, and short time of tumor control [32, 33].

Sarcopenia is now recognized as a multifactorial geriatric syndrome [34, 35], and is a common clinical symptom of elderly patients with cancer [36]. It has been reported to serve as an independent risk factor for poor prognosis indicative of disease and death [37]. It typically co-occurs with cachexia in patients with cancer [38]. However, changes in muscle mass and physical performance may occur before clinically overt cachexia in patients with cancer [35]. In recent years, clinical research on the application of exercise, nutritional support, and drugs, as well as other comprehensive interventions in sarcopenia patients have demonstrated good results [39]. A significant proportion of elderly patients with cancer are at risk of sarcopenia development. However, despite its potential impact on their quality of life [2, 40], limited data are available regarding the factors associated with sarcopenia in elderly patients with cancer, who might have more problems such as malnutrition than non sarcopenic patients.

4. Physical exercise

Physical exercise has the potential to help maintain or slow the loss of physical function [41] as well as sustain and build muscle mass [42]. Aerobic and resistance exercise have been found to better improve upper and lower body strength than usual care in patients with cancer [42]. Aerobic exercise training for skeletal muscles improves wasting in cardiac and cancer cachexia patients [43]. Resistance exercise attenuates muscle wasting associated with a variety of catabolic conditions [44]. Physical exercise has been shown to be effective in improving physical activity levels in cancer survivors [45]. Physical activity intervention significantly improved quality of life for cancer cachexia patients [46, 47]. A systematic review found that physical activity has benefits including improvement in physical activity levels, aerobic fitness, muscle strength, functional quality of life, anxiety, and self-esteem [48] (**Figure 2**).

Physical activity correlated with maximum exercise capacity, weight loss, blood hemoglobin concentration, C-reactive protein, and QOL-related factors of physical functioning and bodily pain in patients with cancer with progressive cachexia [49]. Physical exercise may promote a disruption in the cycle of events leading to cachexia advancement (i.e. muscle tissue loss via anorexigenic proinflammatory cytokines) and, in turn, enhanced functionality and thus, improved QOL in patients with cancer [50]. It has been suggested to counteract sustained disease-related inflammation and the effect of exercise training in cancer cachexia [51]. Furthermore, it has been shown an association with the reduced levels of C-reactive protein in patients with cancer [52].

In patients with cancer, physical exercise represents a function-preserving, anti-inflammatory, and metabolism-modulating strategy with a low cost [53]. It may reverse protein degradation while increasing protein synthesis and lean body mass, thus counteracting the wasting seen in cachexia [54]. It is necessary to develop a better understanding of how to support patients with cancer in starting and maintaining physical activity and exercise programs. It is uncertain whether physical activity during and following cancer treatment has the same benefits

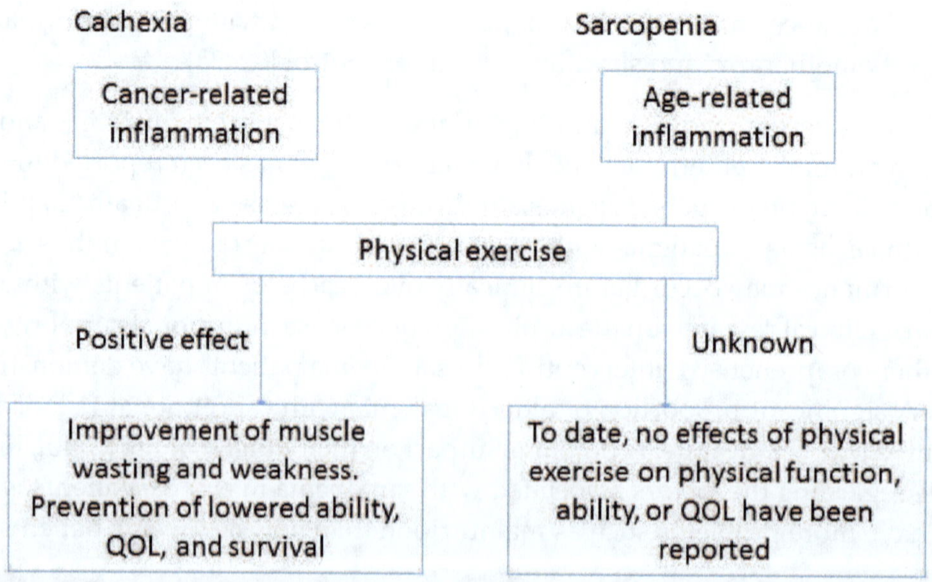

Figure 2. The effectiveness of physical exercise for patients with cancer with cachexia and sarcopenia.

in the weight-stable and weight-losing patients. The question also remains as to whether physical exercise has any health benefit in people with cancer cachexia or those at risk of cancer cachexia. Research investigating physical exercise in patients with cancer undergoing treatment has demonstrated improvements in physical performance, fatigue, and functional quality of life. It is unclear whether these benefits are experienced by patients with cancer cachexia. There is insufficient evidence to establish the safety and effectiveness of physical exercise in cancer cachexia patients, and future trials on exercise and supportive care interventions are required in this population. Aerobic and resistance exercise regimens may have positive effects on decreasing cancer-related fatigue and muscle wasting in patients with cancer cachexia.

To date, no studies have shown a relationship between physical exercise and cancer sarcopenia. In elderly patients with cancer, physical exercise has several benefits including improving immune function [55], hemoglobin and red blood cell count [56], and physical activity [57], not but VO2peak, 1 repetition maximum, functional capacity, anxiety level, or emotional well-being [58]. Physical exercise seems to improve physical function and immune function in elderly patients with cancer [59]. However, it has not shown effectiveness for sarcopenic patients with cancer.

5. Summary and conclusion

Muscle wasting is often encountered in patients with cancer. Both cachexia and sarcopenia lead to muscle wasting in patients with cancer. However, the different mechanisms of muscle wasting in patients with cancer should be recognized. Physical exercise might be effective for improving physical function, physical activity, ADL, and QOL in patients with cancer cachexia. In the future, more studies are required on physical exercise in sarcopenic elderly patients with cancer. Studies investigating the combined effect of physical exercise and nutritional therapies such as branched chain amino acids in cancer rehabilitation are required to improve patient outcomes in the future.

Author details

Shinichiro Morishita[1]*, Atsuhiro Tsubaki[1] and Jack B. Fu[2]

*Address all correspondence to: ptmorishin@yahoo.co.jp

1 Institute for Human Movement and Medical Sciences, Niigata University of Health and Welfare, Niigata, Japan

2 Department of Palliative, Rehabilitation & Integrative Medicine, University of Texas MD Anderson Cancer Center, Houston, TX, USA

References

[1] Lynch GS, Schertzer JD, Ryall JG: Therapeutic approaches for muscle wasting disorders. Pharmacol Ther 2007, **113**(3):461-487.

[2] Wallengren O, Iresjö BM, Lundholm K, Bosaeus I: Loss of muscle mass in the end of life in patients with advanced cancer. Support Care Cancer 2015, **23**(1):79-86.

[3] Argilés JM, López-Soriano FJ, Busquets S: Muscle wasting in cancer: The role of mitochondria. Curr Opin Clin Nutr Metab Care 2015, **18**(3):221-225.

[4] Fearon KC, Baracos VE: Cachexia in pancreatic cancer: New treatment options and measures of success. HPB (Oxford) 2010, **12**(5):323-324.

[5] Muscaritoli M, Anker SD, Argilés J, Aversa Z, Bauer JM, Biolo G, Boirie Y, Bosaeus I, Cederholm T, Costelli P et al: Consensus definition of sarcopenia, cachexia and pre-cachexia: Joint document elaborated by Special Interest Groups (SIG) "cachexia-anorexia in chronic wasting diseases" and "nutrition in geriatrics". Clin Nutr 2010, **29**(2):154-159.

[6] Cruz-Jentoft AJ, Baeyens JP, Bauer JM, Boirie Y, Cederholm T, Landi F, Martin FC, Michel JP, Rolland Y, Schneider SM et al: Sarcopenia: European consensus on definition and diagnosis: Report of the European Working Group on Sarcopenia in Older People. Age Ageing 2010, **39**(4):412-423.

[7] Bowen TS, Schuler G, Adams V: Skeletal muscle wasting in cachexia and sarcopenia: Molecular pathophysiology and impact of exercise training. J Cachexia Sarcopenia Muscle 2015, **6**(3):197-207.

[8] Argilés JM, Busquets S, Stemmler B, López-Soriano FJ: Cachexia and sarcopenia: Mechanisms and potential targets for intervention. Curr Opin Pharmacol 2015, **22**:100-106.

[9] Rolland Y, Abellan van Kan G, Gillette-Guyonnet S, Vellas B: Cachexia versus sarcopenia. Curr Opin Clin Nutr Metab Care 2011, **14**(1):15-21.

[10] Argilés JM, Busquets S, López-Soriano FJ: Cytokines as mediators and targets for cancer cachexia. Cancer Treat Res 2006, **130**:199-217.

[11] Shum AM, Polly P: Cancer cachexia: Molecular targets and pathways for diagnosis and drug intervention. Endocr Metab Immune Disord Drug Targets 2012, **12**(3):247-259.

[12] Murphy KT, Lynch GS: Update on emerging drugs for cancer cachexia. Expert Opin Emerg Drugs 2009, **14**(4):619-632.

[13] Tisdale M: Cancer cachexia. Curr Opin Gastroenterol 2010, **26**(2):146-151.

[14] Tisdale M: Mechanisms of cancer cachexia. Physiol Rev 2009, **89**(2):381-410.

[15] Fearon K, Arends J, Baracos V: Understanding the mechanisms and treatment options in cancer cachexia. Nat Rev Clin Oncol 2013, **10**(2):90-99.

[16] Fearon K, Strasser F, Anker SD, Bosaeus I, Bruera E, Fainsinger RL, Jatoi A, Loprinzi C, MacDonald N, Mantovani G et al: Definition and classification of cancer cachexia: An international consensus. Lancet Oncol 2011, **12**(5):489-495.

[17] Evans WJ, Morley JE, Argilés J, Bales C, Baracos V, Guttridge D, Jatoi A, Kalantar-Zadeh K, Lochs H, Mantovani G et al: Cachexia: A new definition. Clin Nutr 2008, **27**(6):793-799.

[18] Vaughan VC, Martin P, Lewandowski PA: Cancer cachexia: Impact, mechanisms and emerging treatments. J Cachexia Sarcopenia Muscle 2013, **4**(2):95-109.

[19] LeBlanc TW, Nipp RD, Rushing CN, Samsa GP, Locke SC, Kamal AH, Cella DF, Abernethy AP: Correlation between the international consensus definition of the Cancer Anorexia-Cachexia Syndrome (CACS) and patient-centered outcomes in advanced non-small cell lung cancer. J Pain Symptom Manage 2015, **49**(4):680-689.

[20] Tarricone R, Ricca G, Nyanzi-Wakholi B, Medina-Lara A: Impact of cancer anorexia-cachexia syndrome on health-related quality of life and resource utilisation: A systematic review. Crit Rev Oncol Hematol 2016, **99**:49-62.

[21] Dalton JT, Barnette KG, Bohl CE, Hancock ML, Rodriguez D, Dodson ST, Morton RA, Steiner MS: The selective androgen receptor modulator GTx-024 (enobosarm) improves lean body mass and physical function in healthy elderly men and postmenopausal women: Results of a double-blind, placebo-controlled phase II trial. J Cachexia Sarcopenia Muscle 2011, **2**(3):153-161.

[22] Dobs AS, Boccia RV, Croot CC, Gabrail NY, Dalton JT, Hancock ML, Johnston MA, Steiner MS: Effects of enobosarm on muscle wasting and physical function in patients with cancer: A double-blind, randomised controlled phase 2 trial. Lancet Oncol 2013, **14**(4):335-345.

[23] Wallengren O, Lundholm K, Bosaeus I: Diagnostic criteria of cancer cachexia: Relation to quality of life, exercise capacity and survival in unselected palliative care patients. Support Care Cancer 2013, **21**(6):1569-1577.

[24] Mantovani G: Randomised phase III clinical trial of 5 different arms of treatment on 332 patients with cancer cachexia. Eur Rev Med Pharmacol Sci 2010, **14**(4):292-301.

[25] Maddocks M, Byrne A, Johnson CD, Wilson RH, Fearon KC, Wilcock A: Physical activity level as an outcome measure for use in cancer cachexia trials: A feasibility study. Support Care Cancer 2010, **18**(12):1539-1544.

[26] Johns N, Greig C, Fearon KC: Is tissue cross-talk important in cancer cachexia? Crit Rev Oncog 2012, **17**(3):263-276.

[27] Fearon KC: The 2011 ESPEN Arvid Wretlind lecture: Cancer cachexia: The potential impact of translational research on patient-focused outcomes. Clin Nutr 2012, **31**(5):577-582.

[28] Tan BH, Fearon KC: Cachexia: Prevalence and impact in medicine. Curr Opin Clin Nutr Metab Care 2008, **11**(4):400-407.

[29] Massa E, Madeddu C, Lusso MR, Gramignano G, Mantovani G: Evaluation of the effectiveness of treatment with erythropoietin on anemia, cognitive functioning and functions studied by comprehensive geriatric assessment in elderly cancer patients with anemia related to cancer chemotherapy. Crit Rev Oncol Hematol 2006, **57**(2):175-182.

[30] Iannuzzi-Sucich M, Prestwood KM, Kenny AM: Prevalence of sarcopenia and predictors of skeletal muscle mass in healthy, older men and women. J Gerontol A Biol Sci Med Sci 2002, **57**(12):M772–M777.

[31] Cruz-Jentoft AJ, Landi F, Schneider SM, Zúñiga C, Arai H, Boirie Y, Chen LK, Fielding RA, Martin FC, Michel JP et al: Prevalence of and interventions for sarcopenia in ageing adults: A systematic review. Report of the International Sarcopenia Initiative (EWGSOP and IWGS). Age Ageing 2014, **43**(6):748-759.

[32] Peng PD, van Vledder MG, Tsai S, de Jong MC, Makary M, Ng J, Edil BH, Wolfgang CL, Schulick RD, Choti MA et al: Sarcopenia negatively impacts short-term outcomes in patients undergoing hepatic resection for colorectal liver metastasis. HPB (Oxford) 2011, **13**(7):439-446.

[33] Miyamoto Y, Baba Y, Sakamoto Y, Ohuchi M, Tokunaga R, Kurashige J, Hiyoshi Y, Iwagami S, Yoshida N, Watanabe M et al: Negative impact of skeletal muscle loss after systemic chemotherapy in patients with unresectable colorectal cancer. PLoS One 2015, **10**(6):e0129742.

[34] Cruz-Jentoft AJ, Landi F, Topinková E, Michel JP: Understanding sarcopenia as a geriatric syndrome. Curr Opin Clin Nutr Metab Care 2010, **13**(1):1-7.

[35] Collins JT, Noble S, Chester J, Davies HE, Evans WD, Lester J, Parry D, Pettit RJ, Byrne A: Association of sarcopenia and observed physical performance with attainment of multidisciplinary team planned treatment in non-small cell lung cancer: An observational study protocol. BMC Cancer 2015, **15**:544.

[36] Gibson DJ, Burden ST, Strauss BJ, Todd C, Lal S: The role of computed tomography in evaluating body composition and the influence of reduced muscle mass on clinical

outcome in abdominal malignancy: A systematic review. Eur J Clin Nutr 2015, **69**(10):1079-1086.

[37] Zhuang CL, Huang DD, Pang WY, Zhou CJ, Wang SL, Lou N, Ma LL, Yu Z, Shen X: Sarcopenia is an independent predictor of severe postoperative complications and long-term survival after radical gastrectomy for gastric cancer: Analysis from a large-scale cohort. Medicine (Baltimore) 2016, **95**(13):e3164.

[38] Evans WJ: Skeletal muscle loss: Cachexia, sarcopenia, and inactivity. Am J Clin Nutr 2010, **91**(4):1123S–1127S.

[39] Burton LA, Sumukadas D: Optimal management of sarcopenia. Clin Interv Aging 2010, **5**:217-228.

[40] Ugolini G, Pasini F, Ghignone F, Zattoni D, Bacchi Reggiani ML, Parlanti D, Montroni I: How to select elderly colorectal cancer patients for surgery: A pilot study in an Italian academic medical center. Cancer Biol Med 2015, **12**(4):302-307.

[41] Maddocks M, Murton AJ, Wilcock A: Therapeutic exercise in cancer cachexia. Crit Rev Oncog 2012, **17**(3):285-292.

[42] Stene GB, Helbostad JL, Balstad TR, Riphagen II, Kaasa S, Oldervoll LM: Effect of physical exercise on muscle mass and strength in cancer patients during treatment–A systematic review. Crit Rev Oncol Hematol 2013, **88**(3):573-593.

[43] Alves CR, da Cunha TF, da Paixão NA, Brum PC: Aerobic exercise training as therapy for cardiac and cancer cachexia. Life Sci 2015, **125**:9-14.

[44] al-Majid S, McCarthy DO: Cancer-induced fatigue and skeletal muscle wasting: The role of exercise. Biol Res Nurs 2001, **2**(3):186-197.

[45] Bourke L, Homer KE, Thaha MA, Steed L, Rosario DJ, Robb KA, Saxton JM, Taylor SJ: Interventions for promoting habitual exercise in people living with and beyond cancer. Cochrane Database Syst Rev 2013, **9**:CD010192.

[46] Lowe SS: Physical activity and palliative cancer care. Recent Results Cancer Res 2011, **186**:349-365.

[47] Aapro M, Arends J, Bozzetti F, Fearon K, Grunberg SM, Herrstedt J, Hopkinson J, Jaquelin-Ravel N, Jatoi A, Kaasa S et al: Early recognition of malnutrition and cachexia in the cancer patient: A position paper of a European School of Oncology Task Force. Ann Oncol 2014, **25**(8):1492-9.

[48] Speck RM, Courneya KS, Mâsse LC, Duval S, Schmitz KH: An update of controlled physical activity trials in cancer survivors: A systematic review and meta-analysis. J Cancer Surviv 2010, **4**(2):87-100.

[49] Fouladiun M, Körner U, Gunnebo L, Sixt-Ammilon P, Bosaeus I, Lundholm K: Daily physical-rest activities in relation to nutritional state, metabolism, and quality of life in cancer patients with progressive cachexia. Clin Cancer Res 2007, **13**(21):6379-6385.

[50] Battaglini CL, Hackney AC, Goodwin ML: Cancer cachexia: Muscle physiology and exercise training. Cancers (Basel) 2012, **4**(4):1247-1251.

[51] Lira FS, Neto JC, Seelaender M: Exercise training as treatment in cancer cachexia. Appl Physiol Nutr Metab 2014, **39**(6):679-686.

[52] Maddocks M, Jones LW, Wilcock A: Immunological and hormonal effects of exercise: Implications for cancer cachexia. Curr Opin Support Palliat Care 2013, **7**(4):376-382.

[53] Lira FS, Antunes BeM, Seelaender M, Rosa Neto JC: The therapeutic potential of exercise to treat cachexia. Curr Opin Support Palliat Care 2015, **9**(4):317-324.

[54] Gould DW, Lahart I, Carmichael AR, Koutedakis Y, Metsios GS: Cancer cachexia prevention via physical exercise: Molecular mechanisms. J Cachexia Sarcopenia Muscle 2013, **4**(2):111-124.

[55] Bigley AB, Spielmann G, LaVoy EC, Simpson RJ: Can exercise-related improvements in immunity influence cancer prevention and prognosis in the elderly? Maturitas 2013, **76**(1):51-56.

[56] Mohamady HM, Elsisi HF, Aneis YM: Impact of moderate intensity aerobic exercise on chemotherapy-induced anemia in elderly women with breast cancer: A randomized controlled clinical trial. J Adv Res 2017, **8**(1):7-12.

[57] Ying H, Wang Y, Ning X, Zhou J, Zhao L, Shao Y, Bai C, Chen S: Changes of exercise and the clinical effects among eldly non-small cell lung cancer survivors. Zhongguo Fei Ai Za Zhi 2010, **13**(1):64-68.

[58] Quist M, Adamsen L, Rørth M, Laursen JH, Christensen KB, Langer SW: The impact of a multidimensional exercise intervention on physical and functional capacity, anxiety, and depression in patients with advanced-stage lung cancer undergoing chemotherapy. Integr Cancer Ther 2015, **14**(4):341-349.

[59] Miki E, Kataoka T, Okamura H: Feasibility and efficacy of speed-feedback therapy with a bicycle ergometer on cognitive function in elderly cancer patients in Japan. Psychooncology 2014, **23**(8):906-913.

8

Pancreatic Cancer Cachexia: Current Concepts and Clinical Management

Michelle Guan, Arvind M. Shinde and
Andrew E. Hendifar

Abstract

There has been great progress over the last decade in understanding the pathophysiology of cachexia associated with pancreatic cancer. However, there is a large need to find better therapeutic options to successfully manage this complex and challenging condition. Patients with pancreatic cancer have some of the highest prevalence and often the most severe degrees of cachexia, which is described as a multifactorial metabolic syndrome that is associated with unintended weight loss of adipose tissue and skeletal muscle in the setting of anorexia. This chapter will review the current concepts surrounding pancreatic cancer cachexia, its clinical diagnosis, pathophysiology, and its known and proposed therapeutics. A multimodal approach utilizing nutritional support and pharmaceutical therapies is proposed to lead to the most successful management of pancreatic cancer cachexia.

Keywords: pancreatic cancer, cachexia, anorexia, metabolic syndrome, catabolism

1. Introduction

In western countries, pancreatic cancer represents the fourth leading cause of cancer-related death [1]. Among the many complications associated with this disease, cachexia marked by progressive weight loss represents one of the most distressing features related to pancreatic cancer. Cachexia is a multidimensional wasting syndrome that is characterized by unintended loss of both adipose tissue and lean body mass (LBM) that cannot be fully reversed through conventional nutritional support. It is a complex metabolic disorder frequently described in pancreatic cancer and represents a significant physical and psychological burden in approximately 80% of pancreatic cancer patients during the disease progression [2]. The complications associated with cachexia, which include immobility, impaired immunity, and severe respiratory muscle impairment leading to cardiopulmonary failure, result in death in up to one-third of pancreatic cancer patients [3]. Cachectic patients are observed to have lower physical function, decreased tolerance to chemotherapy and radiation treatment, and generally worse prognosis than those with stable weight. Poorer outcomes after pancreaticoduodenectomy have also been observed in patients with preoperative signs of cachexia [4].

While research over the past decade has provided new insights regarding the pathogenesis of pancreatic cancer cachexia, the mechanistic pathology of this condition is still not entirely understood. In this chapter, we will provide a review of the current concepts, potential therapeutic targets, and management of this significant clinical condition.

2. Classification and progression of cancer cachexia

Cachexia has been established to be a common adverse effect of cancer. An international consensus in 2011 defined cachexia as a multifactorial condition recognized by ongoing skeletal muscle loss irreversible by standard nutritional support and eventual functional impairment [5]. The diagnostic criterion established for cancer cachexia is weight loss greater than 5% within 6 months or weight loss greater than 2% in patients already showing depletion (body mass index (BMI) < 20 kg/m^2) or evidence of sarcopenia determined by a dual energy X-ray absorptiometry (DEXA). A skeletal muscle index less than 7.26 kg/m^2 in males and 5.45 kg/m^2 in females is classified as cachexia and the majority of pancreatic cancer patients show signs of cachexia at the time of diagnosis [2].

Cachexia typically develops progressively through a continuum by way of three clinically relevant stages: precachexia, cachexia, and refractory cachexia [5]. A combination of degree of ongoing weight loss as well as depletion of energy stores and body protein mass (using BMI) can be used to classify the severity of the condition. At the precachexia stage, patients show metabolic signs such as anorexia and impaired glucose tolerance prior to significant unintended weight loss. Patients who continue to lose weight and meet the diagnostic criterion described above then transition to full-on cachexia. The cachexia is considered clinically refractory when the cancer is characterized as preterminal or when the individual becomes unresponsive to anticancer therapy. With the presence of uncontrollable catabolism and a life expectancy of less than 3 months, therapeutic interventions usually focus on palliating the symptoms and further preventing the complications of cachexia.

3. Assessment of cancer cachexia

A patient should be assessed for the following features to be characterized with cachexia: anorexia or reduced food intake, catabolic drivers, muscle mass and strength, and functional and psychosocial ability [5]. A recent study indicated that patients who exhibit these components have significantly worse prognosis. Weight loss (>10% weight loss), reduced food intake

(<1500 kcal/day), and indication of systematic inflammation (C-reactive protein (CRP) > 10 mg/L) reduced subjective and objective functional ability in patients with at least two of these components [2].

Many underlying factors could contribute to anorexia or reduced food intake. Pancreatic cancer patients suffer from a reduced drive to eat, chemosensory disturbances (e.g., taste and smell), dysphagia, decreased gastrointestinal (GI) motility (e.g., early satiety and nausea), pain, and fatigue [5]. To detect the presence of these factors, food intake should be assessed routinely by the patient or a family member. At the minimum, the patient should estimate their overall food intake in comparison to their normal intake or have a family member perform a percentile calculation of food consumed during each meal [6]. The early detection of secondary causes of reduced food intake, such as stomatitis, constipation, dyspnoea, and poor dietary habits is important since some complications may be readily reversible [5].

A key component of pancreatic cancer cachexia is hypercatabolism due to tumor metabolism, systemic inflammation, or other tumor-mediated effects. Systemic inflammation is often indexed using serum C-reactive protein (CRP) levels [7]. Indirect indices such as responsiveness to chemotherapy and rate of disease progression should also be evaluated.

As cancer cachexia is characterized by ongoing muscle wasting, a routine assessment of muscle mass is performed with the various techniques currently available. The methods to measure muscle mass include cross-sectional imaging with computed tomography (CT) or magnetic resonance imaging (MRI); appendicular skeletal muscle index obtained from DEXA, anthropometry (mid-upper muscle area); and bioimpedance analysis to obtain a whole body fat-free mass index [5, 8–10]. An imaging-based method is typically selected to quantify changes in body composition by factors such as skeletal muscle wasting, altered body fat distribution, and pathological accumulation of lipids in various tissues. An MRI provides a measurement of quadriceps muscle volume with a coefficient of variation <1% while diagnostic CT scans estimate the cross-sectional area of the abdominal muscle at the L3 area, which can be extrapolated to the lean body mass of the entire body. Muscle strength is typically assessed with an upper-limb hand-grip dynamometry [5].

Among pancreatic cancer patients, those who are overweight were found to be more likely to develop a condition termed as sarcopenic obesity or cachexia hidden in the context of obesity. Sarcopenic obesity is the substantial muscle loss and dysfunction associated with pathological accumulation of adipose tissue. While sarcopenia alone is not associated with decreased survival, being both overweight and sarcopenic does have a significant effect on mortality. With approximately 40% of obese pancreatic patients with detectable sarcopenic obesity, this condition needs to be recognized early on as it was also found to be an important prognostic factor for decreased survival [11]. A comprehensive approach including history, physical examination, and various imaging tests to properly identify this phenomenon can potentially increase the survival of pancreatic cancer patients.

Cancer cachexia contributes substantially to a decreased quality of life by adversely effecting physical and psychosocial functioning. As it is associated with symptoms such as fatigue, weakness, and poor physical performance, it leads to altered body images and can significantly impact the patient's relationships and emotional well-being [12]. A recent study that used an advanced ambulatory pedometer technology found that physical activity was reduced by around 40% in cachectic cancer patients [13]. Since increased bed rest is known to reduce protein synthesis and contribute to the decrease in skeletal muscle mass in healthy patients, this decrease in physical function in cachectic patients adversely affects performance status, quality of social interactions, and ability to performance daily living tasks [14]. Currently, the most widely accepted method for assessing the effects of cancer cachexia is the routine use of patient-reported physical functioning, specifically using the European Organization for Research and Treatment of Cancer (EORTC) quality of life questionnaire (QLQ)-C30 or the Eastern Cooperative Oncology Group (ECOG) questionnaire [15–17]. Physical functioning can also be assessed with physician-reported physical activity (the Karnofsky performance score) and objective methodologies including electric activity meters or checklists of specific activities [17].

4. Mechanisms of cancer cachexia

The pathophysiology of cancer cachexia is characterized by a negative protein and energy balance created by a combination of reduced food intake and abnormal metabolism that is mainly driven by a large increase in the rate of skeletal muscle proteolysis [5, 18, 19]. Anorexia and hypercatabolism have been found in cachectic patients to be driven by mechanical factors such as cytokines, circulating hormones, neuropeptides, neurotransmitters, and tumor-derived factors. Recent studies have also identified other processes that potentially contributed to the pathophysiology of pancreatic cancer cachexia, including neural invasion and abnormalities in muscle microenvironment [20–25]. The following section will review these currently proposed mechanisms that interact and contribute to the development of this disease.

4.1. Mechanical factors

Cancer-associated weight loss can be promoted and maintained by reduced food intake, which can be a result of loss of appetite driven by abnormal mechanical digestion [26]. Tumorigenesis is the main cause of these digestive abnormalities and frequently results in the obstruction of the pancreatic duct and/or GI tract, especially the second portion of the duodenum. This can directly lead to symptoms of pain, fatigue, nausea, dysphagia, gastroparesis, duodenal stenosis, pancreatic insufficiency and malabsorption, and constipation [27]. A pancreaticoduodenectomy to resect a pancreatic head mass is often performed following an obstruction and unfortunately can exacerbate pancreatic insufficiency and reduce oral intake [28, 29].

4.2. Cytokines and systemic inflammation

The hypercatabolic component of cachexia is largely caused by the systemic inflammation response, which in turn promotes fat and protein degradation. Serum C-reactive protein is utilized to indirectly index systemic inflammation, and elevated CRP levels (CRP > 10 mg/L) have been related to cachexia and poor performance in pancreatic cancer patients [2]. Elevated levels of the cytokines IL-6 and IL-10 have also been associated with weight loss, poor prognosis, and decreased survival in patients [7, 30]. The cytokines that are generated by tumor cells or released by the host in response to cancer have been found to contribute to pathways that result in anorexia and hypercatabolism. These pathways can be separated into the hypothalamus-mediated central pathways and the peripheral pathways, which control lipolysis and proteolysis.

4.2.1. Centrally mediated pathways

The hypothalamus typically plays a role in energy intake by responding to peripheral signals regarding energy and adiposity status. A mechanical response is produced via these signaling pathways and abnormalities in these pathways can lead to anorexia. Current findings indicate that systemic inflammation plays a role in inducing cancer anorexia through the activation of a complex neurochemical cascade [24, 25, 31, 32]. Interference with the hypothalamus' normal response to peripheral signals is suggested to be a direct consequence of elevated tumor-mediated cytokine expression, which actively promotes anorexigenic pathways and inhibits orexigenic pathways [24, 25].

Derangements in the ability of the hypothalamus to transduce peripheral signals into neuronal responses may also be associated with cancer anorexia. There are two pathways that are responsible for energy expenditure and food intake within the hypothalamus: neuropeptide Y (NPY)/agouti-related peptide (AgRP) neurons that stimulate energy intake and proopiomelanocortin (POMC)/cocaine and amphetamine-regulated transcript (CART) neurons that inhibit intake. Research suggests that the hyperactivation of the POMC/CART pathways through the IL-1 and other pro-inflammatory cytokines could contribute to developing cancer cachexia [20–23].

Energy homeostasis is also regulated by a protein called leptin through feedback signaling via the central nervous system (CNS). By controlling the synthesis and activation of hypothalamic neuropeptides, such as NPY and corticotropin-releasing factor (CRF), leptin reduces appetite and increases energy expenditure. Since leptin is primarily released by adipose tissue, a lower body fat mass due to starvation leads to lower leptin levels, which allows for the production, release, and action of a potent orexigenic peptide called NPY. NPY then promotes the activation of the NPY/AgRP pathway that stimulates energy intake. Low levels of leptin also decrease the activity of anorexigenic neuropeptides that decrease appetite, which include CRF and melanocortin. Studies have found that cytokines, including tumor necrosis factor-alpha (TNF-α) and interleukin1 (IL-1), increase leptin mRNA expression in adipocytes and in plasma despite decreased adiposity [33–36]. Cancer anorexia might therefore be a consequence of increased leptin levels since compensatory mechanisms that typically occur with reduced food intake are inhibited. However, there is also evidence showing that cytokines can induce anorexia without leptin [37]. In some animal and clinical studies, leptin levels were found to not be elevated in tumor-bearing rats and patients with cancer cachexia [38–41]. Recent research demonstrated that in cancer cachexia, IL-1 and TNF-α mimic leptin signaling and result in the interference of the orexigenic pathway, which is normally a response to reduced leptin levels [24, 42]. This suggests that even during starvation, the inhibition of the orexigenic response and activation of the anorexigenic pathway can occur and lead to unopposed anorexia and elevated energy expenditure.

Serotonin may also contribute to the pathogenesis of cancer anorexia, specifically through the melanocortin system. Research has shown that IL-1 releases hypothalamic serotonin and indirectly alters food intake [43]. High levels of serotonin create a continuous activation of POMC/CART neurons, which causes decreased appetite and anorexia [44]. Additionally, higher levels of tryptophan, which is a precursor of serotonin, were also found in plasma and cerebrospinal fluids of cancer patients with cachexia compared to those without cachexia or healthy controls [45]. After tumor removal, tryptophan concentrations were normalized and subsequently improved appetite [46]. These facts concurrently suggest that serotonin plays a pivotal role in the development of cancer cachexia and is also a potential therapeutic target.

These hypothalamic pathways and neuropeptides were also found to have catabolic effects. The POMC/CART anorexigenic pathway activates the sympathetic nervous system and leads to the induction of mitochondrial uncoupling proteins, including UCP-1 and UCP-2 [47, 48]. By dissipating the proton gradient generated during respiration across the inner mitochondrial membrane and uncoupling respiration from ATP synthesis, UCP-1 and UCP-2 result in thermogenesis and energy expenditure in brown adipose tissue (BAT) [47, 48]. Increases in BAT thermogenesis have been associated with a cachectic state in both humans and experimental animals [49, 50].

4.2.2. Peripheral pathways

Not only have cytokines been proven to corroborate and sustain the neurochemical changes associated with cancer cachexia, but they have also been found to induce lipolysis, muscle catabolism, and the hepatic acute phase protein response (APPR) through multiple pathways [51–57]. The combined action of these cellular activities results in the development of progressive muscle and adipose tissue loss.

4.2.2.1. TNF-α

The cytokine TNF-α has been shown to result in profound metabolic changes, even when administered in low doses. Characterized as a potent anorexigenic agent, it promotes lipolysis, impairs lipogenesis, and increases mobilization of lean tissue reserves from skeletal muscle. TNF-α has been shown to induce lipolysis *in vitro* with increases in glycerol production in mouse and human adipocytes, likely through downregulation of perilipin [51]. Since perilipin typically coats intracellular lipid droplets, the decreased expression of perilipin thus enables the lipolysis regulator hormone-sensitive lipase (HSL) to access the surface of lipid droplets for breakdown [51, 52]. By acting as an inhibitory agent on adipocyte differentiation, TNF-α also results in impaired lipogenesis [53, 54].

Research has also indicated that TNF-α contributes to the muscle wasting that characterizes cancer cachexia. Mouse models demonstrated that TNF-α may promote muscle protein degradation by producing reactive oxygen species (ROS). Nuclear factor κB (NFκB) is activated as a result of this oxidative stress and then subsequently upregulates the ubiquitin-mediated proteasome pathway [55, 56]. Moreover, TNF-α has been shown to upregulate the expression of the 1/2- and 2.4-kb transcripts of ubiquitin and the ubiquitin ligase atrogin 1/MAFbx in skeletal muscle [55, 56]. *In vitro* experiments that involved NFκB-mediated downregulation of MyoD transcripts have also shown the ability of TNF-α to interfere with myogenesis [57].

While these studies indicate that TNF-α is involved in lipolysis and proteolysis, its relevance in cancer cachexia is still not well established. While some studies measuring TNF-α serum levels in pancreatic cancer patients with cachexia found the predicted inverse relationship between TNF-α levels and body weight as well as BMI; other studies involving advance-staged cancer patients demonstrate no such correlation between circulating TNF-α levels, weight loss, and anorexia. Because of the conflicted results produced from these studies, the significance of TNF-α in cancer cachexia still remains an active area of debate.

4.2.2.2. IL-6

Another important pro-inflammatory cytokine implicated in facilitating cachexia is IL-6, which has been associated with weight loss and reduced survival in pancreatic cancer patients [7, 30, 58]. The secretion of IL-6 is known to be induced by TNF-α and works synergistically with TNF-α in many of its cellular functions, including the triggering of other cytokines. Although the role of IL-6 in lipolysis is still unclear, a recent study using cachectic tumor-bearing mice demonstrated enhanced IL-6 signaling in brown adipose tissue, which suggests that IL-6 may be directly involved in activating thermogenesis [59]. More importantly, IL-6 is known to activate the hepatic APPR and stimulate tissue catabolism. The C-26 tumor-bearing mouse model of cancer cachexia established an IL-6 dependent loss of skeletal muscle during cancer cachexia and treatment with an IL-6 targeting antibody attenuated the development of weight loss [60]. Another study confirmed increased CRP levels and IL-6 production in pancreatic cancer patients with cachexia [7]. There is a strong correlation between heightened peripheral blood mononuclear cells (PBMCs) production of IL-6 and the presence of increased APPR [7, 58, 61]. The stimulation of APPR thus promotes the production of acute phase proteins like CRP and gives rise to hypercatabolism at the expense of skeletal muscle [62]. A twofold to threefold increase in fibrinogen production and elevated serum CRP is observed as a consequence of APPR activation [63]. The hepatic synthesis of acute phase proteins occurs due to the mobilization of peripheral amino acid reserves from lean muscle and contributes greatly to the observed weight loss. Both the overproduction of IL-6 and APPR thus have been shown to result in poor responses to chemotherapy in those surviving with pancreatic cancer cachexia [7].

4.3. Tumor-derived factors

In addition to cytokines and systemic inflammation, tumor-derived factors also contribute to the metabolic abnormalities leading to pancreatic cancer cachexia. Two of the most studied factors are lipid mobilizing factor (LMF) and proteolysis-inducing factor (PIF). Other factors that potentially lead to pancreatic cancer cachexia are still being established.

4.3.1. Lipid mobilizing factor

Another molecule associate with cancer is LMF, which was isolated from both a mouse model of cancer cachexia (MAC16 adenocarcinoma) and the urine of patients with unresectable pancreatic cancer and weight loss [64]. Given that LMF was found only in pancreatic patients with weight loss and not in those without weight loss or even normal individuals, LMF/ZAG was identified as a serum protein that is a potential marker of pancreatic cancer cachexia [64, 65]. Additional immunohistochemical findings identified LMF/ZAG expression in pancreatic cancer cells and in the peritumoral stroma, with cachectic pancreatic cancer patients demonstrating stronger immunostaining results than those without cachexia or normal subjects [65].

LMF/ZAG has also been demonstrated through *in vivo* findings to cause selective reduction of carcass fat without altering levels of body water and nonfat mass [66]. This lipolysis is activated by the stimulation of adenylate cyclase in a GTP-dependent fashion and is proposed to be mediated by β3 adrenergic receptors [66–68]. When mice are treated with LMF/ZAG, elevated serum levels of glycerol and 3-hydroxybutyrate are observed as well as an increase of oxygen usage by BAT is observed, demonstrating the role of LMF/ZAG in stimulating lipid utilization [66]. This increase in lipid oxidation and utilization has been shown to be mediated by the $^{14}CO_2$ from [14C-carboxy]triolein and also potentially by β3 adrenergic receptors [69]. This function occurs with the increased expression of mitochondrial UCPs, particularly UCP-1, UCP-2, and UCP-3 in BAT, and UCP-2 in the skeletal muscle and liver [70]. LMF/ZAG also enhances the response of adipose tissues to the lipolytic effects of other stimuli such as catecholamines [66]. The plasma membranes of adipocytes contain Gs α-subunits (Gαs) that stimulate adenylate cyclase and Gi α-subunits (Gαi) that inhibit adenylate cyclase. LMF/ZAG favors mobilization of lipid stores from adipocytes and promotes hypercatabolism by increasing Gαs and decreasing Gαi expression [71]. By promoting both the lipid and substrate utilization as well as mitochondrial oxidative pathways in BAT, LMF/ZAG results in lipolysis, elevated energy expenditure, and a hypercatabolic state.

4.4. Proteolysis-inducing factor

In 1996, PIF was isolated from a murine tumor (MAC16) originating in an adenocarcinoma murine model of cachexia and was discovered to induce skeletal muscle catabolism in MAC16 [72]. In humans, PIF was also discovered in cachectic cancer patients, but not from patients with weight loss due to trauma, cancer patients with little or no weight loss or normal individuals [73]. Moreover, this compound was detected in the urine of 80% of pancreatic cancer patients with significantly higher total weight loss and rate of weight loss than those whose urine did not contain PIF [74]. Immunochemistry analysis also revealed the presence of PIF in the cytoplasm of GI tumors such as pancreatic adenocarcinoma [75].

PIF has been found to induce cachectic symptoms when injected intravenously in normal mice; body composition analysis revealed that PIF extracted from the urine of cachectic cancer patients induced reductions in lean body mass without reduction in food and water intake in murine models [76]. This decrease in muscle mass involved two components: an increase in protein degradation by 50% and a reduction in protein synthesis by 50% observed in gastrocnemius muscle [77]. Additional studies regarding the PIF-mediated reduction in protein mass implicate the ubiquitin-proteasome proteolytic pathway. Upon the administration of PIF in normal mice, mRNA levels for ubiquitin, $E2_{14k}$, and the C9 proteasome subunit are increased. An increase in the expression of the ubiquitin-proteasome pathway in skeletal muscle may contribute to this protein degradation; some studies suggest that this process is found to be mediated by the activation of NFκB [78–80]. While a reduction in protein mass as well as the depletion of myosin is observed, actin levels continue to remain unchanged with the administration of PIF [80].

The role of NFκB in protein degradation following administration of PIF is still not entirely elucidated. However, it is known that arachidonic acid originating from membrane phospholipids is released and then rapidly metabolizes into eicosanoids such as hydroxyeicosatetraenoic acid (15 -HETE) with phospholipase A_2 (PLA_2), which has also been shown to increase in the presence of PIF [81]. 15-HETE was also shown to cause the nuclear accumulation of NFκB and thus protein degradation [82]. The muscle degradation due to the PIF-induced expression of the ubiquitin-proteasome pathway is also largely reliant on NADPH oxidase and production of ROS [81, 83]. Protein kinase C (PKC) is necessary for the activation of NADPH oxidase and may also be dependent on 15-HETE. The generation of ROS stimulates IκB kinase (IKK) and phosphorylates and degrades IκB; this process then releases NFκB from its inactive cytosolic complex [84].

PIF results in the reduction of protein mass not only by causing degradation, but also by inhibiting protein synthesis. PIF activates double-stranded RNA-dependent protein kinase (PKR) through phosphorylation, which leads to the phosphorylation of eIF2; this in turn inhibits translation and subsequently protein synthesis [85]. PKR is also able to elevate the expression and activity of the ubiquitin-proteasome pathway by activating IKK, which then generates excessive NFκB [86].

APPR that is associated with cachectic pancreatic cancer patients may also be driven by PIF, which was found to play a role in excessively generating hepatic cytokines. Human hepatocyte cultures that were treated with PIF had increased NFκB, signal transducers, and activators of transcription (STAT3), which resulted in an increased production of IL-6, IL-8, and CRP, as well as decreased production of transferrin [87]. The same treatment given to human Kupffer cells and monocytes similarly resulted in an increased production of TNF-α, IL-6, and IL-8 [88].

4.5. Other proposed mechanisms

4.5.1. Pax7 dysregulation

Other contributory factors to muscle loss within a cachectic setting have also been investigated in recent studies and further characterize the muscle microenvironment. In pancreatic cancer patients with cachexia, activation of NFκB in satellite muscle progenitor cells resulted in muscle wasting caused by the dysregulation of the self-renewing transcription factor Pax7, which suppressed expression of MyoD and myogenin [89, 90]. These processes subsequently prevented the muscle progenitor cells that typically commit to a myogenic program from completing differentiation and inhibited myoblast fusion, which ultimately impaired muscle regeneration [90]. Furthermore, Pax7 was shown to be induced by serum factors from both cachectic mice and patients in an NFκB-dependent manner [90]. However, the exact circulating factors contributing to NFκB activation and Pax7 dysregulation still require further research.

4.5.2. Neural invasion

Pancreatic cancer patients often develop signs of neural invasion that can result in nerve damage from intraneural tumors of pancreatic cancer. Recent studies suggest that this process involving nerve damage is associated with cachexia as well as astrocyte activation and microglia stimulation in the spinal cord. These activated astrocytes may then stimulate the sympathetic nervous system, which has previously been shown to induce lipolysis and muscle atrophy [47, 91]. However, the mechanisms that potentially lead to cachexia still require further investigation.

4.6. Management of cancer cachexia

Since cachexia is a multifactorial condition, treatments involving combinations of therapies are more likely to be successful. Current therapeutic strategies involve an integrated and multimodal approach including oncological therapy for control of the tumor, nutritional support, and pharmacological treatment. The best supportive care practices also involve the management of the secondary causes of anorexia, such as pain, nausea, pancreatic insufficiency, and constipation.

4.6.1. Nutritional support

Nutritional deficit is one of the highest concerns among pancreatic cancer patients [92]. Involving dieticians and nutrition assessment programs early on in the disease progression is essential for the successful management of pancreatic cancer cachexia. These programs can provide essential dietary suggestions as well as recommendations for oral nutritional supplementation, enteral nutrition, and parenteral nutrition [93–96].

When concerned with appetite and weight management, professional dietary guidance can significantly increase oral caloric and protein intake [97]. Pancreatic cancer patients who were enrolled in studies requiring them to take oral nutritional supplementation found improvements in weight and appetite [98, 99]. Specifically, including L-Carnitine and omega-3 fatty acids as an addition to patients' diets may provide benefits [100, 101]. In a multicenter, randomized, double-blind trial that enrolled patients with advanced pancreatic cancer, L-Carnitine supplementation was found to significantly improve weight and body mass composition, which ultimately resulted in an increased global quality of life [101].

For patients with swallowing difficulties or severe dysphagia, a nasogastric tube or gastrostomy tube can be utilized to administer nutritional support. However, enteral feeding can be linked to morbidity resulting from aspiration, pneumonia, and diarrhea. For patients with bowel dysfunction and progressive weight loss despite enteral support, parenteral nutrition may be used to limit nutritional deterioration and provide temporary benefits [102].

While nutritional interventions can provide temporary stabilization in nutritional status and certain metabolic indices for cachectic cancer patients, response is often limited in these patients and is frequently lower than responses observed in noncancer patients receiving equivalent nutritional support [103]. A unimodal approach is still not sufficient and patients with pancreatic cancer cachexia will therefore require a combination of therapies to successfully manage the cachexia.

4.6.2. Pharmacological approach

Since nutritional interventions produce only limited responses, many studies attempted to manipulate the process of cachexia using a variety of pharmacological agents. The mechanisms of these drugs are all based on modulation of cytokines, hormones, or other pathways involved in the pathophysiology of cancer cachexia.

4.6.2.1. Progestogens

Megestrol acetate (MEGACE) is a synthetic and orally active derivative of the naturally occurring hormone progesterone. It was first developed for the treatment of breast cancer and later for endometrial cancer, MEGACE is now used to stimulate appetite and increase weight in cancer-associated anorexia, as well as for other chronic conditions such as the human acquired immunodeficiency syndrome (AIDS) after being approved by the Food and Drug Administration (FDA) in 1993. Multiple trials have demonstrated that MEGACE (480–800 mg/day) resulted in significant improvements in appetite, food intake, nausea, and weight gain among pancreatic patients with cancer cachexia [27, 104–107]. This efficacy of MEGACE appears to be dose-dependent [106]. MEGACE is generally well-tolerated with low incidence of side effects, including rash, adrenal insufficiency, hyperglycemia, and thromboembolic events, which only have an incidence of less than 5% [105]. Since its approval, many studies have confirmed the effectiveness of MEGACE at increasing weight and thus quality of life when compared to other drugs potentially used for the management of cancer cachexia (cisapride, dronabinol, corticosteroids, and nandrolone) [108, 109]. Body composition analysis has also confirmed that the weight gain observed following MEGACE intake is predominately due to increases in adipose tissue and less from increases in body fluid [110]. However, there were no improvements in survival found in those who were treated with MEGACE [107, 109].

Some studies suggest that the mechanisms by which MEGACE stimulates appetite and weight gain is related to decreased production and release of pro-inflammatory cytokines (IL-1, IL-6, and TNF-α) as well as the stimulation of NPY in the hypothalamus [111–113]. Another progestogen, medroxyprogesterone acetate, was demonstrated through *in vitro* experiments to decrease the production of cytokines and serotonin by PBMC of cancer patients [112, 113].

4.6.2.2. Corticosteroids

Corticosteroids are one of the most widely used appetite stimulants and are effective in inducing food intake and weight gain [114–116]. However, these do not result in lasting changes (less than 4 weeks) and may cause long-term side effects, such as insulin resistance, fluid retention, steroid-induced myopathy, skin fragility, adrenal insufficiency, and sleep and cognitive disorder [116]. The exact mechanisms of action of corticosteroids in a cancer cachexia context still remains unclear, but is likely to be related to the inhibition of IL-1, TNF-α, and leptin as well as the stimulation of NPY [117]. Because of their short duration of effectiveness, corticosteroids may be useful for patient with short expected survival.

4.6.2.3. *Cannabinoids*

Cannabinoids, which are also called dronabinols, are a class of diverse chemical compounds that have a known effect on reducing nausea as well as weight gain and stabilization. A phase II trial found that dronabinol improved anorexia in 68% of patients, but also resulted in dangerous toxicity levels in 16% of patients who eventually suspended treatment [118]. In addition, dronabinol is associated with many adverse side effects, including euphoria, hallucination, psychosis, vertigo, and cardiovascular disorders. The mechanism of action appears to be mediated by interaction with endorphin receptors, interference with IL-1 production, activation of cannabinoid receptors associated with the neurochemical circuit of leptin, and inhibition of prostaglandin synthesis.

In a controlled clinical trial, dronabinol was compared to megestrol acetate in cachectic cancer patients [119]. A total of 469 patients were enrolled in the study and were instructed to take megestrol acetate 800 mg/day or dronabinol 2.5 mg/12 h or both. The findings indicate that megestrol is superior to dronabinol in terms of increasing appetite and weight: 75 vs. 49% ($P = 0.0001$) increase in appetite, respectively and 11 vs. 3% ($P = 0.02$) increase in weight gain of at least 10% from baseline, respectively [114]. There were no differences in appetite and weight between the combination treatment group compared to the megestrol acetate only group (66 vs. 75%, $P = 0.17$, for appetite and 8 vs. 11%, $P = 0.43$, for =10% weight gain, respectively). While megestrol acetate seems to be more effective than dronabinol, cannabinoid is still able to stimulate in appetite and reduce nausea. It is available as an alternative option as an appetite stimulant and antiemetic.

4.6.2.4. *Anti-inflammatory agents*

Systemic inflammation plays an important role in the pathophysiology of pancreatic cancer cachexia. Pro-inflammatory cytokines, including TNF-α, IL-1, and IL-6, have been implicated in the progression of cancer cachexia in a potentially synergistic way. These findings have prompted the development of treatments to curtail the inflammatory response by inhibiting the synthesis or action of cytokines.

Research has indicated that nonsteroidal anti-inflammatory drugs (NSAIDs), including cyclooxygenase-2 (COX-2) inhibitors, indomethacin, and ibuprofen, have the ability to reduce acute phase proteins and cytokines [120–122]. The inhibition of prostaglandin synthesis has been shown *in vivo* to attenuate tumor progression and decrease incidence of cancer cachexia [123, 124]. NSAIDs inhibition of prostaglandin synthesis blocks downstream effects of systemic inflammation; thereby interfering with the cytokines that depend on signal transduction mediated by eicosanoids. In cachectic patients with metastatic solid tumors, indomethacin use may prolong survival and offer palliative support to those with advanced cancer, including pancreatic cancer patients [125]. Other controlled clinical trials have shown that ibuprofen can reduce CRP levels, increase body weight and muscle mass, and improve global quality of life, especially when combined with progestogens [122, 126, 127]. McMillan et al. conducted a multicenter, randomized, control trial that involved 73 cachectic patients with advanced GI cancers, predominately pancreatic cancer (67% of patients) [126]. This study reported that taking a combination of ibuprofen (1200 mg/day) and megestrol acetate (480 mg/day) resulted in more significant improvements in weight and increased quality of life compared to those only consuming megestrol acetate [128]. Similar side effects were present in both groups, including venous thrombosis, upper GI bleeding, and ascites. However, due to disease progression, there was a high attrition rate with 63% failing to complete the 12-week assessment. These provide promising results that would benefit greatly from larger studies that can better evaluate the clinical role of NSAIDs in the management of pancreatic cancer cachexia.

Research has also shown that thalidomide has anti-inflammatory and complex immunomodulatory properties. Thalidomide results in the downregulation of the production of TNF-α as well as other pro-inflammatory cytokines in monocytes, inhibits NFκB, downregulates cyclooxygenase 2, and inhibits angiogenesis [129]. Many controlled trials showed that thalidomide is well-tolerated and successful in improving appetite, weight gain, and sensation of well-being [130, 131]. One specific double-blind, placebo-controlled, randomized clinical trial of thalidomide recruited 50 pancreatic cancer patients with cachexia to take either 200 mg/day of thalidomide or a placebo [131]. The study found that after 4 weeks, patients in the thalidomide group had significant increases in weight compared to the placebo group (0.37 vs. −2.21 kg, $P = 0.005$) and significant improvements in lean body mass (1.0 cm^3 in arm muscle mass vs. −4.46 cm^3, $P = 0.002$) [131]. There were some adverse reactions to thalidomide, including peripheral neuropathy, dizziness, somnolence, constipation, rash, and possible increased risk of venous thromboembolism in the setting of malignancy. These preliminary results are encouraging, but merits further investigation to confirm the efficacy of thalidomide in treating pancreatic cancer cachexia.

Some therapeutic approaches also involve pharmaconutrients with anti-inflammatory activity, such as the omega-3 fatty acids eicosapentaenoic acid (EPA) and docosahexaenoic acid (DHA). Both found abundantly in fish oil, EPA and DHA both have immunomodulatory properties that allow for the suppression of pro-inflammatory cytokines, including IL-1, TNF-α, and IL-6 by PBMC [132, 133]. Research on EPA has also suggested its ability to inhibit the downstream effects of LMF and PIF [134–136]. In past studies involving patients with unresectable pancreatic cancer, fish oil supplementation containing both EPA and DHA as well as high-purity EPA administration have both been associated with weight stabilization [137, 138]. A study conducted by Barber et al. further demonstrated the efficacy of EPA, which were taken through oral supplementation, at producing significant increases in weight, dietary intake, and performance status in cachectic patients with advanced pancreatic cancer [100]. However, recent data from a multicenter, double-blind, placebo-controlled, randomized clinical trial provided conflicting results suggested that single agent EPA administration is not effective in treating cancer cachexia [139]. Another multicenter clinical trial that compared EPA, megestrol acetate, and a combination treatment determined that megestrol acetate alone resulted in more weight gain than EPA administration or a combination therapy [140]. While the role of EPA in the management cancer cachexia still remains unclear, recent data demonstrates EPA's lack of effectiveness as a single agent or even in combination regimens for the management of pancreatic cancer cachexia.

As the mechanisms involved in the development and progression of cancer cachexia continues to be elucidated, the management of this multifactorial syndrome has made improvements towards developing a multimodal approach. Recent data from a large multicenter trial suggests that a combination therapy with megestrol acetate (320 mg/day), EPA supplementation, L-carnitine (4 g/day), and thalidomide (200 mg/day) provides more effective results in improving lean body mass and appetite than single agents [141]. Future progress in the field of cancer cachexia will be realized through the development of combined pharmacological therapies given along with nutritional supplementation in the context of supportive care.

5. Future directions

Despite a significant increase in research on cancer cachexia, there are currently no therapies available for pancreatic cancer cachexia that results in lasting effects on weight management and improvements in prognosis. Developing an effective and powerful treatment for this disease still remains an ongoing challenge.

Recent studies have focused on targeted therapies with anti-inflammatory activity. IL-6 has been identified as a promising target, but most of the studies investigating IL-6 antibodies have involved nonsmall cell lung cancer (NSCLC) patients with cachexia [142–145]. In a phase II randomized, double-blind, placebo-controlled trial with NSCLC patients, the humanized monoclonal IL-6 antibody called ALD518 (also known as BMS-945429) was evaluated for its safety and efficacy in treating cancer cachexia. This safe and well-tolerated antibody effectively increased hemoglobin levels and prevented loss of lean body mass [142, 143]. Rigas et al. also reported statistically significant improvements in fatigue score in the ALD518 group vs. placebo group that persisted over a 12-week period [142].

Another agent that was found to have anti-inflammatory properties is OHR/AVR118, which is an immune modulator that targets both TNF-α and IL-6. In a phase II study by Chasen et al. administering OHR/AVR118 in cachectic patients with advanced cancer resulted in improvements in anorexia, dyspepsia, strength, and depression [146]. A current phase IIb study is advancing the understanding of the role and efficacy of OHR/AVR118 in enhancing appetite as well as improving weight, lean body mass, strength, and quality of life [147]. Additional research is still needed to evaluate the safety and efficacy of these agents in pancreatic cancer patients with cachexia.

Studies have discovered the therapeutic potential of inhibiting myostatin and activin type IIB (ActRIIB) in treating cancer cachexia. ActRIIB is a high affinity activin receptor that mediates signaling through a subset of TGF-β ligands including myostatin and activin and both play a critical role in regulating muscle mass [148]. These ligands inhibit myogenesis and the Akt/mTOR pathway involved in muscle protein synthesis and upregulate the expression of ubiquitin ligases that degrade muscle. In several models of cancer cachexia, Zhou et al. reported the prevention of muscle wasting as well as prolonged survival through the pharmacological inhibition of the ActRIIB pathway [148]. One myostatin inhibitor BYM338 has been developed by Novartis (Hanover, NJ, USA) and is currently being investigated for the efficacy of myostatin inhibitors in attenuating loss of body mass. This compound is currently being evaluated in a multicenter, randomized, double-blind, placebo-controlled phase II trial that involves cachectic patients with either stage IV NSCLC or stage III/IV pancreatic cancer [149]. LY2495655 is another humanized antimyostatin antibody currently investigated in a multicenter, randomized, double-blind, placebo-controlled phase II trial that recruited patients with locally advanced or metastatic pancreatic cancer. Patients were administered with one of two different doses of LY2495655 in combination with gemcitabine to evaluate potential dose-dependent effects on survival, lean body mass, and physical performance [150].

6. Conclusion

Cancer cachexia is still regarded as noncurable and is diagnosed in approximately 80% of pancreatic cancer patients. Among these patients, 30% eventually die from cachexia-related complications [2, 151]. As a multifactorial condition, pancreatic cancer cachexia is complex disease that is associated with anorexia and excessive catabolism mediated by mechanical factors, pro-inflammatory cytokines, neuropeptides, hormones, and tumor-derived factors. The pathophysiology of cachexia in pancreatic cancer is characterized by compromised energy homeostasis driven by decreased food intake and abnormal metabolism. This negative protein and energy balance leads to unintentional skeletal muscle and adipose tissue mass, which greatly decreases the overall prognosis of pancreatic cancer patients.

While the management of cancer cachexia has improved dramatically in the past decade, more research is still needed to further understand the complex mechanisms involved in the pathogenesis and maintenance of pancreatic cancer cachexia. Current research identifies targeted immunotherapy as a promising treatment option for cachexia and successful intervention of this condition will most likely involve a multimodal approach to aid in developing potential therapeutics. Future progress in the management of cancer cachexia will likely be realized through a combined approach that includes nutritional support, multiple agents, and targeted therapies to improve the quality of life and general outlook of patients with pancreatic cancer.

Author details

Michelle Guan[1,2]*, Arvind M. Shinde[1] and Andrew E. Hendifar[1,2]

*Address all correspondence to: michelle8guan@gmail.com

1 Samuel Oschin Comprehensive Cancer Center, Cedars Sinai Medical Center, Los Angeles, CA, USA

2 Department of Medicine, David Geffen School of Medicine, Los Angeles, CA, USA

References

[1] Jemal A, Murray T, Ward E, Samuels A, Tiwari RC, Ghafoor A, et al. Cancer statistics, 2005. CA Cancer J Clin. 2005;**55**(1):10-30. DOI: 10.3322/canjclin.55.1.10.

[2] Fearon KC, Voss AC, Hustead DS, Group CC. Definition of cancer cachexia: effect of weight loss, reduced food intake, and systemic inflammation on functional status and prognosis. Am. J. Clin. Nutr. 2006b;**83**(6):1345-1350.

[3] Bachmann J, Heiligensetzer M, Krakowski-Roosen H, Büchler MW, Friess H, Martignoni ME. Cachexia worsens prognosis in patients with resectable pancreatic cancer. J. Gastrointest. Surg. 2008;**12**(7):1193-1201. DOI: 10.1007/s11605-008-0505-z.

[4] Pausch T, Hartwig W, Hinz U, Swolana T, Bundy BD, Hackert T, et al. Cachexia but not obesity worsens the postoperative outcome after pancreatoduodenectomy in pancreatic cancer. Surgery. 2012;**152**(3):S81–S88. DOI: 10.1016/j.surg.2012.05.028.

[5] Fearon K, Strasser F, Anker SD, Bosaeus I, Bruera E, Fainsinger RL, et al. Definition and classification of cancer cachexia: an international consensus. Lancet Oncol. 2011;**12**(5):489-495. DOI: 10.1016/S1470- 2045(10)70218-7.

[6] Bruera E, Sweeney C. Cachexia and asthenia in cancer patients. Lancet Oncol. 2000;**1**:138-147. DOI: 10.1016/S1470-2045(00)00033-4.

[7] Moses AG, Maingay J, Sangster K, Fearon KC, Ross JA. Pro-inflammatory cytokine release by peripheral blood mononuclear cells from patients with advanced pancreatic cancer: relationship to acute phase response and survival. Oncol. Rep. 2009;**21**(4):1091-1095. DOI: 10.3892/or_00000328.

[8] Simons JP, Schols AM, Westerterp KR, ten Velde GP, Wouters EF. The use of bioelectrical impedance analysis to predict total body water in patients with cancer cachexia. Am. J. Clin. Nutr. 1995;**61**(4):741-745.

[9] Prado CM, Birdsell LA, Baracos VE. The emerging role of computerized tomography in assessing cancer cachexia. Curr. Opin. Support. Palliat. Care. 2009;**3**(4):269-275. DOI: 10.1097/SPC.0b013e328331124a.

[10] Di Sebastiano KM, Mourtzakis M. A critical evaluation of body composition modalities used to assess adipose and skeletal muscle tissue in cancer. Appl. Physiol. Nutr. Metab. 2012;**37**(5):811-821. DOI: 10.1139/h2012-079.

[11] Tan BH, Birdsell LA, Martin L, Baracos VE, Fearon KC. Sarcopenia in an overweight or obese patient is an adverse prognostic factor in pancreatic cancer. Clin. Cancer Res. 2009;**15**(22):6973-6979. DOI: 10.1158/1078- 0432.CCR-09-1525.

[12] Donohoe CL, Ryan AM, Reynolds JV. Cancer cachexia: mechanisms and clinical implications. Gastroenterol. Res. Pract. 2011;**2011**;601434. DOI: 10.1155/2011/601434.

[13] Dahele M, Skipworth RJ, Wall L, Voss A, Preston T, Fearon KC. Objective physical activity and self-reported quality of life in patients receiving palliative chemotherapy. J. Pain Symptom Manage. 2007;**33**(6):676-685. DOI: 10.1016/j.jpainsymman.2006.09.024.

[14] Biolo G, Ciocchi B, Stulle M, Piccoli A, Lorenzon S, Dal MV, et al. Metabolic consequences of physical inactivity. J. Ren. Nutr. 2005;**15**(1):49-53.

[15] Aaronson NK, Ahmedzai S, Bergman B, Bullinger M, Cull A, Duez NJ, Filiberti A, Flechtner H, Fleishman SB, de Haes JC, et al. The European organization for research and treatment of cancer QLQ-C30: a quality-of-life instrument for use in international clinical trials in oncology. J. Natl. Cancer Inst. 1993;**85**(5):365-376.

[16] Luckett T, King MT, Butow PN, Oguchi M, Rankin N, Price MA, Hackl NA, Heading G. Choosing between the EORTC QLQ-C30 and FACT-G for measuring health-related quality of life in cancer clinical research: issues, evidence and recommendations. Ann. Oncol. 2011;**22**(10):2179-2190. DOI: 10.1093/annonc/mdq721.

[17] West H, Jin JO. Performance status in patients with cancer. JAMA Oncol. 2015;**1**(7):998. DOI:10.1001/jamaoncol.2015.3113.

[18] Fearon KC. Cancer cachexia: developing multimodal therapy for a multidimensional problem. Eur. J. Cancer. 2008;44(8):1124-1132. DOI: 10.1016/j.ejca.2008.02.033.

[19] Fearon KC. The 2011 ESPEN Arvid Wretlind lecture: cancer cachexia: the potential impact of translational research on patient-focused outcomes. Clin. Nutr. 2012;33:577– 582. DOI: 10.1016/j.clnu.2012.06.012.

[20] Wisse BE, Frayo RS, Schwartz MW, Cummings DE. Reversal of cancer anorexia by blockade of central melanocortin receptors in rats. Endocrinology. 2001;**142**(8):3292-3301. DOI: 10.1210/endo.142.8.8324.

[21] Marks D, Cone RD. The role of the melanocortin-3 receptor in cachexia. Ann. N.Y. Acad. Sci. 2003;**994**:258-266. DOI: 10.1111/j.1749- 6632.2003.tb03188.x.

[22] Marks DL, Butler AA, Turner R, Brookhart G, Cone RD. Differential role of melanocortin receptor subtypes in cachexia. Endocrinology. 2003;**144**(4):1513-1523. DOI: 10.1210/en.2002-221099.

[23] Scarlett JM, Jobst EE, Enriori PJ, Bowe DD, Batra AK, Grant WF, et al. Regulation of central melanocortin signaling by interleukin-1 beta. Endocrinology. 2007;**148**(9):4217-4225. DOI: 10.1210/en.2007-0017.

[24] Suzuki H, Asakawa A, Amitani H, Fujitsuka N, Nakamura N, Inui A. Cancer cachexia pathophysiology and translational aspect of herbal medicine. Japan J. Clin. Oncol. 2013; 43(7):695-705. DOI: 10.1093/jjco/hyt075.

[25] Tuca A., Jimenez-Fonseca P, Gascón P. Clinical evaluation and optimal management of cancer cachexia. Crit. Rev. Oncol. Hematol. 2013;88(3):625-636. DOI: 10.1016/j. critrevonc. 2013.07.015.

[26] Wigmore SJ, Plester CE, Ross JA, Fearon KC. Contribution of anorexia and hypermetabolism to weight loss in anicteric patients with pancreatic cancer. Br. J. Surg. 1997b;**84**(2):196-197. DOI: 10.1002/bjs.18008 40214.

[27] Deutsch J, Kolhouse JF. Assessment of gastrointestinal function and response to megesterol acetate in subjects with gastrointestinal cancers and weight loss. Support. Care Cancer. 2004;**12**(7):503-510. DOI: 10.1007/s00520-004-0615-4.

[28] Phillips ME. Pancreatic exocrine insufficiency following pancreatic resection. Pancreatology. 2015;**15**(5):449-455. DOI: 10.1016/j.pan.2015.06.003.

[29] Malleo G, Crippa S, Butturini G, Salvia R, Partelli S, Rossini R, Bacchion M, Pederzoli P, Bassi C. Delayed gastric emptying after pylorus-preserving pancreaticoduodenectomy: validation of International Study Group of Pancreatic Surgery classification and analysis of risk factors. HPB (Oxford). 2010;**12**(9):610-618. DOI: 10.1111/j.1477-2574.2010.00203.x.

[30] Ebrahimi B, Tucker SL, Li D, Abbruzzese JL, Kurzrock R. Cytokines in pancreatic carcinoma: correlation with phenotypic characteristics and prognosis. Cancer. 2004;**101**(12): 2727-2736.

[31] Laviano A, Meguid MM, Rossi-Fanelli F. Cancer anorexia: clinical implications, pathogenesis, and therapeutic strategies. Lancet Oncol. 2003;**4**(11):686-694. DOI: 10.1016/S1470-2045 (03)01247-6.

[32] Fearon K, Arends J, Baracos V. Understanding the mechanisms and treatment options in cancer cachexia. Nat. Rev. Clin. Oncol. 2013;**10**(2):90-99. DOI: 10.1038/nrclinonc.2012.209.

[33] Grunfeld C, Zhao C, Fuller J, Pollack A, Moser A, Friedman J, et al. Endotoxin and cytokines induce expression of leptin, the ob gene product, in hamsters. J. Clin. Invest. 1996;**97**(9):2152-2157. DOI: 10.1172/JCI118653.

[34] Janik JE, Curti BD, Considine RV, Rager HC, Powers GC, Alvord WG. Interleukin 1 alpha increases serum leptin concentrations in humans. J. Clin. Endocrinol. Metab. 1997;**82**(9):3084-3086.

[35] Sarraf P, Frederich RC, Turner EM, Ma G, Jaskowiak NT, Rivet DJ 3rd. Multiple cytokines and acute inflammation raise mouse leptin levels: potential role in inflammatory anorexia. J. Exp. Med. 1997;**185**(1):171-175. DOI: 10.1084/jem.185.1.171.

[36] Finck BN, Kelley KW, Dantzer R, Johnson RW. *In vivo* and *in vitro* evidence for the involvement of tumor necrosis factor-alpha in the induction of leptin by lipopolysaccharide. Endocrinology. 1998;**139**(5):2278-2283.

[37] Faggioni R, Fuller J, Moser A, Feingold KR, Grunfeld C. LPS-induced anorexia in leptin-deficient (ob/ob) and leptin receptor-deficient (db/db) mice. Am. J. Physiol. 1997;**273**(1): R181–R186.

[38] Simons JP, Schols AM, Campfield LA, Wouters EF, Saris WH. Plasma concentration of total leptin and human lung-cancer-associated cachexia. Clin. Sci. (Lond.). 1997;**93**(3): 273-277.

[39] Wallace AM, Sattar N, McMillan DC. Effect of weight loss and the inflammatory response on leptin concentrations in gastrointestinal cancer patients. Clin. Cancer Res. 1998;**4**(12):2977-2979.

[40] Mantovani G, Macciò A, Mura L, Massa E, Mudu MC, Mulas C, et al. Serum levels of leptin and proinflammatory cytokines in patients with advanced-stage cancer at different sites. J. Mol. Med. (Berl.). 2000;**78**(10):554-561. DOI: 10.1007/s001090000137.

[41] Bing C, Taylor S, Tisdale MJ, Williams G. Cachexia in MAC16 adenocarcinoma: suppression of hunger despite normal regulation of leptin, insulin and hypothalamic neuropeptide. Y. J. Neurochem. 2001;**79**(5):1004-1012. DOI: 10.1046/j.1471-4159.2001.00639.x.

[42] Inui A. Cancer anorexia-cachexia syndrome: are neuropeptides the key?. Cancer Res. 1999;**59**(18):4493-4501.

[43] Shintani F, Kanba S, Nakaki T, Nibuya M, Kinoshita N, Suzuki E, et al. Interleukin-1 beta augments release of norepinephrine, dopamine, and serotonin in the rat anterior hypothalamus. J. Neurosci. 1993;**13**(8):3574-3581.

[44] Heisler LK, Cowley MA, Tecott LH, Fan W, Low MJ, Smart JL, et al. Activation of central melanocortin pathways by fenfluramine. Science. 2002;**297**(5581):609-611. DOI: 10.1126/science.1072327.

[45] Cangiano C, Cascino A, Ceci F, Laviano A, Mulieri M, Muscaritoli M, et al. Plasma and CSF tryptophan in cancer anorexia. J. Neural Transm. Gen. Sect. 1990;**81**(225):225-233. DOI: 10.1007/BF01245044.

[46] Cangiano C, Testa U, Muscaritoli M, Meguid MM, Mulieri M, Laviano A, et al. Cytokines, tryptophan and anorexia in cancer patients before and after surgical tumor ablation. Anticancer Res. 1994;**14**(3B):1451-1455.

[47] Li G, Klein RL, Matheny M, King MA, Meyer EM, Scarpace PJ. Induction of uncoupling protein 1 by central interleukin-6 gene delivery is dependent on sympathetic innervation of brown adipose tissue and underlies one mechanism of body weight reduction in rats. Neuroscience. 2002;**115**(3):879-889. DOI: 10.1016/S0306-4522(02)00447-5.

[48] Arruda AP, Milanski M, Romanatto T, Solon C, Coope A, Alberici LC, et al. Hypothalamic actions of tumor necrosis factor alpha provide the thermogenic core for the wastage syndrome in cachexia. Endocrinology. 2010;**151**(2):683-694. DOI: 10.1210/en.2009-0865.

[49] Oudart H, Calgari C, Andriamampandry M, Le Maho Y, Malan A. Stimulation of brown adipose tissue activity in tumor-bearing rats. Can. J. Physiol. Pharmacol. 1995;**73**(11):1625-1631.

[50] Roe SY, Cooper AL, Morris ID, Rothwell NJ. Involvement of prostaglandins in cachexia induced by T-cell leukemia in the rat. Metabolism. 1997;**46**(4):359-365.

[51] Rydén M, Arvidsson E, Blomqvist L, Perbeck L, Dicker A, Arner P. Targets for TNF-alpha-induced lipolysis in human adipocytes. Biochem. Biophys. Res. Commun. 2004;**318**(1):168-175. DOI: 10.1016/j.bbrc.2004.04.010.

[52] Zhang HH1, Halbleib M, Ahmad F, Manganiello VC, Greenberg AS. Tumor necrosis factor-alpha stimulates lipolysis in differentiated human adipocytes through activation of extracellular signal-related kinase and elevation of intracellular cAMP. Diabetes. 2002;**51**(10):2929-2935. DOI: 10.2337/diabetes.51.10.2929.

[53] Cawthorn WP, Heyd F, Hegyi K, Sethi JK. Tumour necrosis factor-alpha inhibits adipogenesis via a betacatenin/TCF4(TCF7L2)-dependent pathway. Cell Death Differ. 2007;**14**(7):1361-1373. DOI: 10.1038/sj.cdd.4402127.

[54] Hammarstedt A, Isakson P, Gustafson B, Smith U. Wntsignaling is maintained and adipogenesis inhibited by TNFalpha but not MCP-1 and resistin. Biochem. Biophys. Res. Commun. 2007;**357**(3):700-706. DOI: 10.1016/j.bbrc.2007.03.202.

[55] Llovera M, Carbó N, López-Soriano J, García-Martínez C, Busquets S, Alvarez B, et al. Different cytokines modulate ubiquitin gene expression in rat skeletal muscle. Cancer Lett. 1998;**133**(1):83-87. DOI: 10.1016/S0304- 3835(98)00216-X.

[56] Li YP, Reid MB. NF-kappaB mediates the protein loss induced by TNF-alpha in differentiated skeletal muscle myotubes. Am. J. Physiol. Regul. Integr. Comp. Physiol. 2000;**279**(4): R1165–R1170.

[57] Guttridge DC, Mayo MW, Madrid LV, Wang CY, Baldwin AS Jr. NF-kappaB-induced loss of MyoD messenger RNA: possible role in muscle decay and cachexia . Science. 2000;**289**(5488):2363-2366. DOI: 10.1126/science.289.5488.2363.

[58] Martignoni ME, Kunze P, Hildebrandt W, Künzli B, Berberat P, Giese T, et al. Role of mononuclear cells and inflammatory cytokines in pancreatic cancer-related cachexia. Clin. Cancer Res. 2005;**11**(16):5802-5808. DOI: 10.1158/1078-0432.CCR-05-0185.

[59] Tsoli M, Moore M, Burg D, Painter A, Taylor R, Lockie SH, et al. Activation of thermogenesis in brown adipose tissue and dysregulated lipid metabolism associated with cancer cachexia in mice. Cancer Res. 2012;**72**(17):4372-4382. DOI: 10.1158/0008-5472. CAN-11-3536.

[60] Strassmann G, Fong M, Kenney JS, Jacob CO. Evidence for the involvement of interleukin 6 in experimental cancer cachexia. J. Clin. Invest. 1992;**89**(5):1681-1684. DOI: 10.1172/ JCI115767.

[61] Martignoni ME, Dimitriu C, Bachmann J, Krakowski-Rosen H, Ketterer K, Kinscherf R, et al. Liver macrophages contribute to pancreatic cancerrelated cachexia. Oncol. Rep. 2009;**21**(2):363-369. DOI: 10.3892/or_00000231.

[62] Fearon KC, Barber MD, Falconer JS, McMillan DC, Ross JA, Preston T, et al. Pancreatic cancer as a model: inflammatory mediators, acute-phase response, and cancer cachexia. World J. Surg. 1999;**23**(6):584-588. DOI: 10.1007/PL00012351.

[63] Preston T, Slater C, McMillan DC, Falconer JS, Shenkin A, Fearon KC, et al. Fibrinogen synthesis is elevated in fasting cancer patients with an acute phase response. J. Nutr. 1998;**128**(8):1355-1360.

[64] Todorov PT, McDevitt TM, Meyer DJ, Ueyama H, Ohkubo I, Tisdale MJ, et al. Purification and characterization of a tumor lipid-mobilizing factor. Cancer Res. 1998;**58**(11): 2353-2358.

[65] Felix K, Fakelman F, Hartmann D, Giese NA, Gaida MM, Schnölzer M, et al. Identification of serum proteins involved in pancreatic cancer cachexia. Life Sci. 2011;**88**(5-6):218-225. DOI: 10.1016/j.lfs.2010.11.011.

[66] Hirai K, Hussey HJ, Barber MD, Price SA, Tisdale MJ. Biological evaluation of a lipid-mobilizing factor isolated from the urine of cancer patients. Cancer Res. 1998;**58**(11): 2359-2365.

[67] Khan S, Tisdale MJ. Catabolism of adipose tissue by a tumour-produced lipid-mobilising factor. Int. J. Cancer. 1999;**80**(3):444-447. DOI: 10.1002/(SICI)1097-0215(19990129) 80:3%3C444::AID-IJC18%3E3. 3.CO;2-L.

[68] Russell ST, Hirai K, Tisdale MJ. Role of beta3-adrenergic receptors in the action of a tumour lipid mobilizing factor. Br. J. Cancer. 2002;**86**(3):424-428. DOI: 10.1038/sj.bjc.6600086.

[69] Russell ST, Tisdale MJ. Effect of a tumour-derived lipid-mobilising factor on glucose and lipid metabolism *in vivo*. Br. J. Cancer. 2002;**87**(5):580-584. DOI: 10.1038/sj.bjc.6600493.

[70] Bing C, Russell ST, Beckett EE, Collins P, Taylor S, Barraclough R, et al. Expression of uncoupling proteins-1, -2 and -3 mRNA is induced by an adenocarcinoma-derived lipid-mobilizing factor. Br. J. Cancer. 2002;**86**(4):612-618. DOI: 10.1038/sj.bjc.6600101.

[71] Islam-Ali B, Khan B, Price SA, Tisdale MJ. Modulation of adipocyte G-protein expression in cancer cachexia by a lipid-mobilizing factor (LMF). Br. J. Cancer. 2001;**85**(5):758-763. DOI: 10.1054/bjoc.2001.1992.

[72] Todorov PT, Deacon M, Tisdale MJ. Structural analysis of a tumor-produced sulfated glycoprotein capable of initiating muscle protein degradation. J. Biol. Chem. 1997;**272**(19): 12279-12288. DOI: 10.1074/jbc.272.19.12279.

[73] Todorov P, Cariuk P, McDevitt T, Coles B, Fearon K, Tisdale M. Characterization of a cancer cachectic factor. Nature. 1996;**379**(6567):739-742. DOI: 10.1038/379739a0.

[74] Wigmore SJ, Todorov PT, Barber MD, Ross JA, Tisdale MJ, Fearon KC. Characteristics of patients with pancreatic cancer expressing a novel cancer cachectic factor. Br. J. Surg. 2000b;**87**(1):53-58. DOI: 10.1046/j.1365- 2168.2000.01317.x.

[75] Cabal-Manzano R, Bhargava P, Torres-Duarte A, Marshall J, Bhargava P, Wainer IW. Proteolysis-inducing factor is expressed in tumours of patients with gastrointestinal cancers and correlates with weight loss. Br. J. Cancer. 2001;**84**(12):1599-1601. DOI: 10.1054/ bjoc.2001.1830.

[76] Cariuk P, Lorite MJ, Todorov PT, Field WN, Wigmore SJ, Tisdale MJ. Induction of cachexia in mice by a product isolated from the urine of cachectic cancer patients. Br. J. Cancer. 1997;**76**(5):606-613. DOI: 10.1038/bjc.1997.433.

[77] Lorite MJ, Cariuk P, Tisdale MJ. Induction of muscle protein degradation by a tumour factor. Br. J. Cancer. 1997;**76**(8):1035-1040. DOI: 10.1038/bjc.1997.504.

[78] Lorite MJ, Smith HJ, Arnold JA, Morris A, Thompson MG, Tisdale MJ. Activation of ATP-ubiquitin-dependent proteolysis in skeletal muscle *in vivo* and murine myoblasts *in vitro* by a proteolysis-inducing factor (PIF). Br. J. Cancer. 2001;**85**(2):297-302. DOI: 10.1054/bjoc.2001.1879.

[79] Whitehouse AS, Tisdale MJ. Increased expression of the ubiquitin proteasome pathway in murine myotubes by proteolysis-inducing factor (PIF) is associated with activation of the transcription factor NF-kappaB. Br. J. Cancer. 2003;**89**(6):1116-1122. DOI: 10.1038/sj.bjc.6601132.

[80] Wyke SM, Tisdale MJ. NF-kappaB mediates proteolysis-inducing factor induced protein degradation and expression of the ubiquitin-proteasome system in skeletal muscle. Br. J. Cancer. 2005;**92**(4):711-721. DOI: 10.1038/sj.bjc.66 02402.

[81] Smith HJ, Tisdale MJ. Signal transduction pathways involved in proteolysis-inducing factor induced proteasome expression in murine myotubes. Br. J. Cancer. 2003;**89**(9):1783-1788. DOI: 10.1038/sj.bjc.6601328.

[82] Wyke SM, Khal J, Tisdale MJ. Signalling pathways in the induction of proteasome expression by proteolysis-inducing factor in murine myotubes. Cell Signal. 2005;**17**(1):67-75. DOI: 10.1016/j.cellsig. 2004.05.015.

[83] Russell ST, Eley H, Tisdale MJ. Role of reactive oxygen species in protein degradation in murine myotubes induced by proteolysis-inducing factor and angiotensin II. Cell Signal. 2007;**19**(8):1797-1806. DOI: 10.1016/j.cellsig.2007.04.003.

[84] Smith HJ, Wyke SM, Tisdale MJ. Role of protein kinase C and NF-kappaB in proteolysis-inducing factor-induced proteasome expression in C(2)C(12) myotubes. Br. J. Cancer. 2004;**90**(9):1850-1857. DOI: 10.1038/sj.bjc.6601767.

[85] Eley HL, Tisdale MJ. Skeletal muscle atrophy, a link between depression of protein synthesis and increase in degradation. J. Biol. Chem. 2007;**282**(10):7087-7097. DOI: 10.1074/jbc.M610378200.

[86] Zamanian-Daryoush M, Mogensen TH, DiDonato JA, Williams BR. NF-kappaB activation by double-stranded-RNA-activated protein kinase (PKR) is mediated through NF-kappaB-inducing kinase and IkappaB kinase. Mol. Cell Biol. 2000;**20**(4):1278-1290. DOI: 10.1128/MCB.20.4.1278-1290. 2000.

[87] Watchorn TM, Waddell I, Dowidar N, Ross JA. Proteolysisinducing factor regulates hepatic gene expression via the transcription factors NF-(kappa)B and STAT3. FASEB J. 2001;**15**(3):562-564.

[88] Watchorn TM, Dowidar N, Dejong CH, Waddell ID, Garden OJ, Ross JA. The cachectic mediator proteolysis inducing factor activates NF-kappaB and STAT3 in human Kupffer cells and monocytes. Int. J. Oncol. 2005;**27**(4):1105-1111.

[89] Olguin HC, Olwin BB. Pax-7 up-regulation inhibits myogenesis and cell cycle progression in satellite cells: a potential mechanism for self-renewal. Dev. Biol. 2004;**275**(2):375-388. DOI: 10.1016/j.ydbio.2004.08.015.

[90] He WA, Berardi E, Cardillo VM, Acharyya S, Aulino P, Thomas-Ahner J, et al. NF-κB-mediated Pax7 dysregulation in the muscle microenvironment promotes cancer cachexia. J. Clin. Invest. 2013;**123**(11):4821-4835. DOI: 10.1172/JCI68523.

[91] Imoto A, Mitsunaga S, Inagaki M, Aoyagi K, Sasaki H, Ikeda M, et al. Neural invasion induces cachexia via astrocytic activation of neural route in pancreatic cancer. Int. J. Cancer. 2012;**131**(12):2795-2807. DOI: 10.1002/ijc.27594.

[92] Bozzetti F, Group SW. Screening the nutritional status in oncology: a preliminary report on 1,000 outpatients. Support. Care Cancer. 2009;**17**:279-284. DOI: 10.1007/s00520-008-0476-3.

[93] Ottery F. Supportive nutritional management of the patient with pancreatic cancer. Oncology (Williston Park). 1996;**10**:26-32.

[94] Nitenberg G, Raynard B. Nutritional support of the cancer patient: issues and dilemmas. Crit. Rev. Oncol. Hematol. 2000;**34**:137-168. DOI: 10.1016/S1040-8428(00)00048-2.

[95] Jatoi A, Loprinzi CL. Current management of cancer-associated anorexia and weight loss. Oncology (Williston Park). 2001;**15**(4):497-502.

[96] el-Kamar FG, Grossbard ML, Kozuch PS. Metastatic pancreatic cancer: emerging strategies in chemotherapy and palliative care. Oncologist. 2003;**8**(1):18-34. DOI: 10.1634/theoncologist.8-1-18.

[97] Ovesen L, Allingstrup L, Hannibal J, Mortensen EL, Hansen OP. Effect of dietary counseling on food intake, body weight, response rate, survival, and quality of life in cancer patients undergoing chemotherapy: a prospective, randomized study. J. Clin. Oncol. 1993;**11**(10):2043-2049.

[98] Fearon KC, Von Meyenfeldt MF, Moses AG, Van Geenen R, Roy A, Gouma DJ, et al. Effect of a protein and energy dense N-3 fatty acid enriched oral supplement on loss of weight and lean tissue in cancer cachexia: a randomised double blind trial. Gut. 2003;**52**(10):1479-1486. DOI: 10.1136/gut.52.10.1479.

[99] Bauer JD, Capra S. Nutrition intervention improves outcomes in patients with cancer cachexia receiving chemotherapy–a pilot study. Support. Care Cancer. 2005;**13**:270-274. DOI: 10.1007/s00520-004-0746-7.

[100] Barber MD, Ross JA, Voss AC, Tisdale MJ, Fearon KC. The effect of an oral nutritional supplement enriched with fish oil on weight-loss in patients with pancreatic cancer. Br. J. Cancer. 1999;**81**(1):80-86. DOI: 10.1038/sj.bjc.6690654.

[101] Kraft M, Kraft K, Gärtner S, Mayerle J, Simon P, Weber E, et al. L-Carnitine-supplementation in advanced pancreatic cancer (CARPAN)–a randomized multicentre trial. Nutr. J. 2012;**11**:52. DOI: 10.1186/1475-2891-11-52.

[102] Pelzer U, Arnold D, Gövercin M, Stieler J, Doerken B, Riess H, et al. Parenteral nutrition support for patients with pancreatic cancer. Results of a phase II study. BMC Cancer. 2010;**10**:86. DOI: 10.1186/1471-2407-10-86.

[103] Nixon DW, Lawson DH, Kutner M, Ansley J, Schwarz M, Heymsfield S, et al. Hyperalimentation of the cancer patient with protein-calorie undernutrition. Cancer Res. 1981;**41**(6):2038-2045.

[104] Bruera E, Macmillan K, Kuehn N, Hanson J, MacDonald RN. A controlled trial of megestrol acetate on appetite, caloric intake, nutritional status, and other symptoms in patients with advanced cancer. Cancer. 1990;**66**(6):1279-1282. DOI: 10.1002/1097-0142(19900915)66:6%3C1279::AIDCNCR2820660630%3E3.0.CO;2-R.

[105] Loprinzi CL, Ellison NM, Schaid DJ, Krook JE, Athmann LM, Dose AM, et al. Controlled trial of megestrol acetate for the treatment of cancer anorexia and cachexia. J. Natl. Cancer Inst. 1990;**82**(13):1127-1132. DOI: 10.1093/jnci/82.13.1127.

[106] Loprinzi CL, Michalak JC, Schaid DJ, Mailliard JA, Athmann LM, Goldberg RM, et al. Phase III evaluation of four doses of megestrol acetate as therapy for patients with cancer anorexia and/or cachexia. J. Clin. Oncol. 1993;**11**(4):762-767.

[107] Westman G, Bergman B, Albertsson M, Kadar L, Gustavsson G, Thaning L, et al. Megestrol acetate in advanced, progressive, hormone-insensitive cancer. Effects on the quality of life: a placebo-controlled, randomised, multicentre trial. Eur. J. Cancer. 1999;**35**(4):586-595. DOI: 10.1016/S0959-8049(98)00398-0.

[108] Pascual López A, Roqué i Figuls M, Urrútia Cuchi G, Berenstein EG, Almenar Pasies B, Balcells Alegre M, Herdman M. Systematic review of megestrol acetate in the treatment of anorexia-cachexia syndrome. J Pain Symptom Manage. 2004;**27**(4):360-369. DOI: 10.1016/j.jpainsymman.2003.09.007.

[109] Leśniak W, Bała M, Jaeschke R, Krzakowski M. Effects of megestrol ′ acetate in patients with cancer anorexia-cachexia syndrome–a systematic review and meta-analysis. Pol. Arch. Med. Wewn. 2008;**118**(11):636-644.

[110] Loprinzi CL, Schaid DJ, Dose AM, Burnham NL, Jensen MD. Body-composition changes in patients who gain weight while receiving megestrol acetate. J. Clin. Oncol. 1993b;**11**(1):152-154.

[111] McCarthy HD, Crowder RE, Dryden S, Williams G. Megestrol acetate stimulates food and water intake in the rat: effects on regional hypothalamic neuropeptide Y concentrations. Eur. J. Pharmacol. 1994;**265**:99-102. DOI: 10.1016/0014-2999(94)90229-1.

[112] Mantovani G, Macciò A, Lai P, Massa E, Ghiani M, Santona MC. Cytokine activity in cancer-related anorexia/cachexia: role of megestrol acetate and medroxyprogesterone acetate. Semin Oncol. 1998a;**25**:45-52.

[113] Mantovani G, Macciò A, Lai P, Massa E, Ghiani M, and Santona MC. Cytokine involvement in cancer anorexia/cachexia: role of megestrol acetate and medroxyprogesterone

acetate on cytokine downregulation and improvement of clinical symptoms. Crit. Rev. Oncog. 1998b;**9**:99-106. DOI: 10.1615/CritRevOncog.v9.i2.10.

[114] Willox JC, Corr J, Shaw J, Richardson M, Calman KC, Drennan M. Prednisolone as an appetite stimulant in patients with cancer. Br. Med. J. (Clin. Res. Ed.). 1984;**288**(6410):27. DOI: 10.1136/bmj.288.6410.27.

[115] Bruera E, Roca E, Cedaro L, Carraro S, Chacon R. Action of oral methylprednisolone in terminal cancer patients: a prospective randomized double-blind study. Cancer Treat. Rep. 1985;**69**:751-754.

[116] Loprinzi CL, Kugler JW, Sloan JA, Mailliard JA, Krook JE, Wilwerding MB, et al. Randomized comparison of megestrol acetate versus dexamethasone versus fluoxymesterone for the treatment of cancer anorexia/cachexia. J. Clin. Oncol. 1999;**17**(10):3299-3306.

[117] Plata-Salamán CR. Dexamethasone inhibits food intake suppression induced by low doses of interleukin-1 beta administered intracerebroventricularly. Brain Res. Bull. 1991;**27**:737-738. DOI: 10.1016/0361-9230(91)90055-O.

[118] Nelson K, Walsh D, Deeter P, Sheehan F. A phase II study of delta- 9-tetrahydrocannabinol for appetite stimulation in cancer-associated anorexia. J. Palliat. Care. 1994;**10**:14-18.

[119] Jatoi A, Windschitl HE, Loprinzi CL, Sloan JA, Dakhil SR, Mailliard JA, et al. Dronabinol versus megestrol acetate versus combination therapy for cancer-associated anorexia: a North Central Cancer Treatment Group study. J. Clin. Oncol. 2002;**20**(2):567-573. DOI: 10.1200/JCO.20.2.567.

[120] McMillan DC, Leen E, Smith J, Sturgeon C, Preston T, Cooke TG. Effect of extended ibuprofen administration on the acute phase protein response in colorectal cancer patients. Eur. J. Surg. Oncol. 1995;**21**(5):531-534. DOI: 10.1016/S0748-7983(95)97157-2.

[121] Preston T, Fearon KC, McMillan DC, Winstanley FP, Slater C, Shenkin A, et al. Effect of ibuprofen on the acute-phase response and protein metabolism in patients with cancer and weight loss. Br. J. Surg. 1995;**82**(2):229-234. DOI: 10.1002/bjs.1800820233.

[122] Wigmore SJ, Falconer JS, Plester CE, Ross JA, Maingay JP, Carter DC, et al. Ibuprofen reduces energy expenditure and acute-phase protein production compared with placebo in pancreatic cancer patients. Br. J. Cancer. 1995;**72**(1):185-188. DOI: 10.1038/bjc.1995.300.

[123] Gelin J, Andersson C, Lundholm K. Effects of indomethacin, cytokines, and cyclosporin A on tumor growth and the subsequent development of cancer cachexia. Cancer Res. 1991;**51**(3):880-885.

[124] Gelin J, Moldawer LL, Lönnroth C, Sherry B, Chizzonite R, Lundholm K. Role of endogenous tumor necrosis factor alpha and interleukin 1 for experimental tumor growth and the development of cancer cachexia. Cancer Res. 1991;**51**(1):415-421.

[125] Lundholm K, Gelin J, Hyltander A, Lönnroth C, Sandström R, Svaninger G, et al. Anti-inflammatory treatment may prolong survival in undernourished patients with metastatic solid tumors. Cancer Res. 1994;**54**(21):5602-5606.

[126] McMillan DC, O'Gorman P, Fearon KC, McArdle CS. A pilot study of megestrol acetate and ibuprofen in the treatment of cachexia in gastrointestinal cancer patients. Br. J. Cancer. 1997;**76**(6):788-790. DOI: 10.1038/bjc.1997.463.

[127] Lai V, George J, Richey L, Kim HJ, Cannon T, Shores C, et al. Results of a pilot study of the effects of celecoxib on cancer cachexia in patients with cancer of the head, neck, and gastrointestinal tract. Head Neck. 2008;**30**(1):67-74. DOI: 10.1002/hed.20662.

[128] McMillan DC, Wigmore SJ, Fearon KC, O'Gorman P, Wright CE, McArdle CS. A prospective randomized study of megestrol acetate and ibuprofen in gastrointestinal cancer patients with weight loss. Br. J. Cancer. 1999;**79**:495-500. DOI: 10.1038/sj.bjc.6690077.

[129] Sampaio EP, Sarno EN, Galilly R, Cohn ZA, Kaplan G. Thalidomide selectively inhibits tumor necrosis factor alpha production by stimulated human monocytes. J. Exp. Med. 1991;**173**(3):699-703. DOI: 10.1084/jem.173.3.699.

[130] Bruera E, Neumann CM, Pituskin E, Calder K, Ball G, Hanson J. Thalidomide in patients with cachexia due to terminal cancer: preliminary report. Ann. Oncol. 1999;**10**(7):857-859. DOI: 10.1023/A:1008329821941.

[131] Gordon JN, Trebble TM, Ellis RD, Duncan HD, Johns T, Goggin PM. Thalidomide in the treatment of cancer cachexia: a randomised placebo controlled trial. Gut. 2005;**54**(4):540-545. DOI: 10.1136/gut.2004.047563.

[132] Meydani SN, Lichtenstein AH, Cornwall S, Meydani M, Goldin BR, Rasmussen H, et al. Immunologic effects of national cholesterol education panel step-2 diets with and without fish-derived N-3 fatty acid enrichment. J. Clin. Invest. 1993;**92**:105-113. DOI: 10.1172/JCI116537.

[133] Wigmore SJ, Fearon KC, Maingay JP, Ross JA. Downregulation of the acute-phase response in patients with pancreatic cancer cachexia receiving oral eicosapentaenoic acid is mediated via suppression of interleukin-6. Clin. Sci. (Lond.). 1997;**92**:215-221.

[134] Tisdale MJ, Beck SA. Inhibition of tumour-induced lipolysis *in vitro* and cachexia and tumour growth *in vivo* by eicosapentaenoic acid. Biochem. Pharmacol. 1991;**41**:103-107. DOI: 10.1016/0006-2952(91)90016-X.

[135] Tisdale MJ. Inhibition of lipolysis and muscle protein degradation by EPA in cancer cachexia. Nutrition. 1996;**12**:S31–S33. DOI: 10.1016/0899-9007(95)00066-6.

[136] Hussey HJ, Tisdale MJ. Effect of a cachectic factor on carbohydrate metabolism and attenuation by eicosapentaenoic acid. Br. J. Cancer. 1999;**80**:1231-1235. DOI: 10.1038/sj.bjc.6690490.

[137] Wigmore SJ, Ross JA, Falconer JS, Plester CE, Tisdale MJ, Carter DC. The effect of polyunsaturated fatty acids on the progress of cachexia in patients with pancreatic cancer. Nutrition. 1996;**12**:S27–S30. DOI: 10.1016/0899-9007(95)00078-X.

[138] Wigmore SJ, Barber MD, Ross JA, Tisdale MJ, Fearon KC. Effect of oral eicosapentaenoic acid on weight loss in patients with pancreatic cancer. Nutr. Cancer. 2000b;**36**(2):177-184. DOI: 10.1207/S1532791 4NC3602_6.

[139] Fearon KC, Barber MD, Moses AG, Ahmedzai SH, Taylor GS, Tisdale MJ, et al. Double-blind, placebo-controlled, randomized study of eicosapentaenoic acid diester in patients with cancer cachexia. J. Clin. Oncol. 2006a;**24**(21):3401-3407. DOI: 10.1200/JCO.2005.04.5724.

[140] Jatoi A, Rowland K, Loprinzi CL, Sloan JA, Dakhil SR, MacDonald N, et al. An eicosapentaenoic acid supplement versus megestrol acetate versus both for patients with cancer-associated wasting: a North Central Cancer Treatment Group and National Cancer Institute of Canada collaborative effort. J. Clin. Oncol. 2004;**22**(12):2469-2476. DOI: 10.1200/JCO.2004.06.024.

[141] Mantovani G, Macciò A, Madeddu C, Serpe R, Massa E, Dessì M, et al. Randomized phase III clinical trial of five different arms of treatment in 332 patients with cancer cachexia. Oncologist. 2010;**15**(2):200-211. DOI: 10.1634/theoncologist.2009-0153.

[142] Rigas JR, Schuster M, Orlov SV, Milovanovic B, Prabhash K, Smith JT, et al. Effect of ALD518, a humanized anti-IL-6 antibody, on lean body mass loss and symptoms in patients with advanced non-small cell lung cancer (NSCLC): results of a phase II randomized, double-blind safety and efficacy trial. J. Clin. Oncol. 2010;**28** (abstract 7622).

[143] Schuster M, Rigas JR, Orlov SV, Milovanovic B, Prabhash K, Smith JT. ALD518, a humanized anti-IL-6 antibody, treats anemia in patients with advanced non-small cell lung cancer (NSCLC): results of a phase II, randomized, double-blind, placebo-controlled trial. J. Clin. Oncol. 2010;**28** (abstract 7631.).

[144] Bayliss TJ, Smith JT, Schuster M, Dragnev KH, Rigas JR. A humanized anti-IL-6 antibody (ALD518) in non-small cell lung cancer. Expert Opin. Biol. Ther. 2011;**11**:1663-1668. DOI: 10.1517/14712598.2011.627850.

[145] Ando K, Takahashi F, Motojima S, Nakashima K, Kaneko N, Hoshi K, et al. Possible role for tocilizumab, an anti-interleukin-6 receptor antibody, in treating cancer cachexia. J. Clin. Oncol. 2013;**31**(6):e69–e72. DOI: 10.1200/JCO.2012.44.2020.

[146] Chasen M, Hirschman SZ, Bhargava R. Phase II study of the novel peptide-nucleic acid OHR118 in the management of cancer-related anorexia/cachexia. J. Am. Med. Dir. Assoc. 2011;**12**:62-67. DOI: 10.1016/j.jamda.2010.02.012.

[147] ClinicalTrials.gov. Open label study with OHR/AVR118 in advanced cancer patients with anorexia-cachexia [Internet]. Available from: http://clinicaltrials.gov/ct2/show/NCT01206335 [Accessed: December 2013].

[148] Zhou X, Wang JL, Lu J, Song Y, Kwak KS, Jiao Q, et al. Reversal of cancer cachexia and muscle wasting by ActRIIB antagonism leads to prolonged survival. Cell. 2010;**142**:531-543. DOI: 10.1016/j.cell.2010.07.011.

[149] ClinicalTrials.gov. Clinical study of BYM338 for the treatment of unintentional weight loss in patients with cancer of the lung or the pancreas [Internet]. Available from: http://clinicaltrials.gov/ct2/show/NCT01433263 [Accessed: December 2013].

[150] ClinicalTrials.gov. A Phase 2 study of LY2495655 in participants with pancreatic cancer [Internet]. Available from: http://clinicaltrials.gov/ct2/show/NCT01505530 [Accessed: December 2013].

[151] Bachmann J, Ketterer K, Marsch C, Fechtner K, Krakowski-Roosen H, Büchler MW, et al. Pancreatic cancer related cachexia: influence on metabolism and correlation to weight loss and pulmonary function. BMC Cancer. 2009;**9**:255. DOI: 10.1186/1471-2407-9-255.

9

Sarcopenia in Chronic Illness and Rehabilitative Approaches

Raoul Saggini, Simona Maria Carmignano, Lucia Cosenza, Tommaso Palermo and Rosa Grazia Bellomo

Abstract

Primary sarcopenia is considered to be age-related when no other cause is evident, other than aging itself. Secondary sarcopenia should be considered when one or more other causes are evident, such as multiple chronic conditions. Previous studies have reported that low muscle strength and impaired physical performance can be found in chronic diseases, including metabolic disease (diabetes, hypertension, and obesity), arthritis, osteoporosis, cancer, chronic kidney disease, chronic obstructive pulmonary disease, neuromuscular disease, and chronic infection. The development of preventive and therapeutic strategies against secondary sarcopenia and wasting disorders in general is an epidemiological need. The planning of a complex rehabilitation program in sarcopenia associated to chronic conditions, in the context of a comprehensive treatment, is made up of a nutritional support, exercise, correction of lifestyles, and the use of advanced physical energies. Therefore, for the purposes of the optimal management, it is essential to identify the pathogenesis and clinical characteristics that can affect the different rehabilitative treatment.

Keywords: secondary sarcopenia, chronic illness, rehabilitative approaches

1. Introduction

Many definitions available on sarcopenia agree on to define it as paraphysiological phenomenon, characterized by loss of muscle mass that occurs with aging.

Some authors emphasize the histopathology defining sarcopenia as an increase of the adipose and connective component within the muscle itself, whereas others focus on the reduction of muscle strength and physical function [1, 2].

Cachexia is a composite word from the Greek words "kakos" (bad) and "hexis" (condition) and refers to the prognosis and functionality of patients suffering from cachexia. The characteristic of this complex metabolic disturbance is weight loss due to an underlying cause disease, such as heart failure, chronic pulmonary diseases, or cancer. According to the definition given by Cruz-Jentoft et al. in 2010, cachexia is found in patients with unintentional weight loss of 5% in the past year, a body mass index (BMI) lower than 20, decreased muscle mass as shown with bioimpedance analysis (BIA) or dual-energy X-ray absorptiometry (DEXA), low muscle strength, low serum albumin levels, anemia, and elevated biomarkers of inflammation [2].

Weight loss becomes a clinical sign of any progressive acute or chronic disease state. In its extreme form, it involves a significant lean body mass (including skeletal muscle) and fat loss. Skeletal muscle provides a fundamental basis for human function, enabling locomotion, and respiration. Muscle wasting is related to a poor quality of life and increased morbidity/mortality [3].

2. Sarcopenia in chronic illness

Sarcopenia can be defined as primary sarcopenia when due to the aging process and secondary when due to comorbidities, malnutrition, or immobility (**Figure 1**).

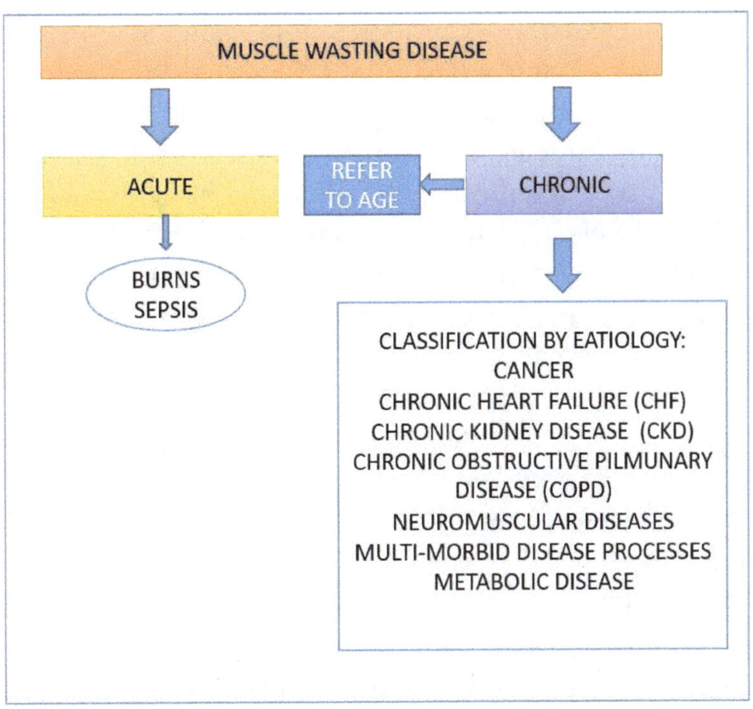

Figure 1. Classification of sarcopenia.

- Comorbidities that induce sarcopenia are organ failure (e.g. heart, kidneys, lungs, brain and liver), inflammatory diseases, cancer, and endocrine diseases.
- Malnutrition due to gastrointestinal disorders, anorexia in cases of polypharmacy, and inadequate intake due to psychosocial disorders lead to secondary sarcopenia.
- Inactivity as a result postoperative deconditioning or prolonged rehabilitation is the reason for activity-related secondary sarcopenia [4].

It has been known for millennia that muscle and fat wasting leads to poor outcomes, including deaths in chronic disease states. It is usually accompanied by physical inactivity, decreased mobility, slow gait, and poor physical endurance, which are also common features of the frailty syndrome. Although the specific contribution of each of these factors is unknown, there are more and more convincing evidence of chronic low-grade inflammation prominent role in the development of sarcopenia. According to recent studies, chronic inflammation is associated with many degenerative diseases [5]. Systemic inflammation is thus dependent on many factors that include diseases such as obesity, type 2 diabetes, dementia [5, 6], heart failure, and rheumatic diseases [7, 8], which can then be the result of this inflammatory condition and/or themselves can be the cause of the increase of inflammation. The impact of inflammation on the development of sarcopenia is supported by many studies. Animal studies show that low-grade inflammation reduction following the administration of ibuprofen in rats have determined a significant decrease in the loss of muscle mass [9]. Other studies, always conducted on animals, have shown that administration of interleukin-6 (IL-6) or tumor necrosis factor alpha (TNF-α) increases the skeletal muscle degradation, decreases protein synthesis, and reduces plasma concentrations of insulin-like growth factor (IGF) [10]. However, considering the studies of healthy elderly people living in the community, it was confirmed that one pro-inflammatory state produces, in the long-term, negative effects on sarcopenia. In the study "Longitudinal Aging Study Amsterdam," high levels of IL-6 and C-reactive protein (CRP) were associated with a double or triple risk of losing more than 40% to the hand grip (strength of the handshake) over 3 years. TNF-α, IL-1a, IL-6, IL-18, C-reactive protein (CRP) and fibrinogen are among the cytokines and acute phase proteins, that result to be more elevated in pro-inflammatory state [11]. Moreover, high levels of muscle catabolic biomarkers, which include IL-6, are important predictors of the decline in muscle strength [12]. Other authors report that IL-6 is a multifunctional cytokine because it has both pro and anti-inflammatory effects by determining muscular growth or atrophy, and according to different conditions, its effect is anabolic or catabolic. Several different pathophysiological processes induce sarcopenia following distinct pathways: neurological diseases produce sarcopenia by loss of motor neurons. Malabsorption leads to protein deficits and muscle catabolism. Disuse of muscles due to physical inactivity is followed by muscle degeneration. Hormonal disturbances of the thyroid, hypercortisolism, and insulin resistance lead to sarcopenia resulting from protein deficiency [13, 14]. These processes are found in combination or alone in many acute and chronic diseases above all in elderly patients, for example heart failure, chronic obstructive pulmonary disease (COPD), diabetes, neurological diseases, musculoskeletal diseases, as well as post-traumatic or postoperative conditions [15].

2.1. Sarcopenia: obesity and diabetes

Although the mechanism by which the potential TNF-α and IL-6 increase and the relationship with sarcopenia is not yet well defined, they may be related to the increase of the intramuscular adipose tissue. Under the pro-inflammatory stimulus, the intramuscular contents and intra-myocellular fat deposits increase creating a vicious circle where adipocytes, which secrete IL-6 and TNF-α as well as adipocines such as leptin and adiponectin, further promote inflammation [16].

More recently, Newman et al. have shown that it is important to consider in sarcopenia the percentage of fat mass. These authors have shown that people with higher body weight is not classified as suffering from sarcopenia, though their lean mass is sufficient compared to the total body weight [17]. Both sarcopenia and obesity represent, as the individual factors, a risk for adverse events, it has been shown that if present in combination, act synergistically increasing the earlier onset of disability [18]. For example, Rolland et al. found in a cohort study of women with sarcopenia, decreased physical performance (climbing stairs) compared to a group of healthy same aged, the worse performance was related to sarcopenia associated with obesity [19].

2.2. Chronic obstructive pulmonary disease

Chronic obstructive pulmonary disease (COPD) is a common cause of morbidity and mortality worldwide. The burden of disease is induced to a great extent by extrapulmonary symptoms, such as osteoporosis, heart failure, and sarcopenia. Using only BMI as a predictor of muscle mass or sarcopenia is misleading in these patients because the combination of abdominal obesity and sarcopenia is often present [20]. Sarcopenia affects 15% of patients with chronic obstructive pulmonary disease (COPD) stable and compromises the independence and the functional state of the musculoskeletal system. This loss of muscle mass does not seem to affect the outcome of pulmonary rehabilitation, which can lead to remission of the syndrome in selected patients. Pulmonary rehabilitation can improve symptoms and quality of life of patients with respiratory disease. It releases dyspnea and fatigue, as well as increasing exercise tolerance, emotional function so in indirect way it decreases frailty such as weakness, inactivity and fatigue, and then sarcopenia [21, 22].

It has been reported that patients with COPD and sarcopenia have nearly overlapping results after pulmonary rehabilitation compared to patients with COPD without sarcopenia, in terms of upper and lower limb strength, exercise capacity and health status [23].

Another important data are the absence of statistical differences about the body composition, functional performance, or health status between patients with and patients without sarcopenia undergone to pulmonary rehabilitation [24].

Musculoskeletal dysfunction is a recognized manifestation of COPD whose characteristics include the weakness of the quadriceps, the atrophy, and the change of type II fibers, all associated with a poor prognosis independent from lung function [25]. COPD determines an imbalance favoring protein breakdown over synthesis, apoptosis, sarcomere and sarcolemma damage, reduced myosin heavy chain-I isoform type I [slow twitch/endurance] muscle fibers, and a decreased density of capillaries and mitochondria [26–28]. This chronic disease is related to abnormalities of oxidative enzymes, mitochondrial activity, and expression of myogenin and m-cadherin—key molecules required for muscle growth and repair [29]. In chronic conditions, the poor peripheral oxygenation linked to abnormalities of gas exchange typical of COPD and anemia, as well as increased oxidation processes [30–32] associated with hypercapnia, create an acidosis condition that alters muscle proteases [33, 34], increasing catabolic activity in the muscle [35]. In addition, the effect of tobacco is associated with the [36] myopathy induced by corticosteroid use (especially systemic steroids) [37, 38], malnutrition that has a negative balance of energy [39], and reduction of physical activity leading sarcopenia [40]. The other mechanism involved in the genesis of sarcopenia is a sedentary lifestyle due not only to previous habits but also to reduced exercise tolerance. This was highlighted by disproportionate impairment of lower limb musculature in comparison to the upper limbs (that are subjected to a lesser degree of physical inactivity than the legs) [41] and by similarity in the structural changes seen in the sarcopenia of COPD and atrophy due to muscle disuse [42]. Furthermore, recovery of strength is possible with muscle training and conditioning [43, 44], and the apparent lack of correlation between the severity of airflow limitation and extent of muscle dysfunction [45]. Rehabilitation would therefore be expected to improve frailty and sarcopenia, but there are little published data on this as an intervention.

2.3. Sarcopenia: chronic renal failure

Patients with end-stage renal disease (ESRD) and chronic renal failure (CRF) receiving dialysis can have altered nutritional status and body composition due to dietary restrictions, level of physical activity, co-morbidities, metabolic alterations, and inflammation. Fatigue and immobility due to low muscle function are frequent symptoms reported by patients with chronic kidney disease. Sarcopenia is found in all stages of the disease and more distinctly in patients with high grades of renal function impairment. Pereira et al. found a significantly higher association of sarcopenia, diagnosed by BPA and hand grip strength measurements and mortality [46]. The degradation of proteins is an important energy production mechanism since the amino acids are rapidly converted to glucose. In conditions of catabolism generates an imbalance in favor of the degradation compared to the synthesis of proteins and, not existing a storage of the same, the muscle proteins are degraded and, if not additional sufficiently, develop muscle atrophy that determines a condition of sarcopenia [47, 48].

Many diseases promote protein catabolism, including the IRC; in particular, it was noted that during and after the hemodialysis session protein degradation is significantly accelerated. Several studies have shown that the ubiquitin-proteasome system (UPS) is the major proteolytic system in renal patients (**Figure 2**); despite prove even other hyperactive pathways (lysosomal cathepsin and calpain-gated calcium), caspase is a protease involved in cell apoptosis process that accelerates the degradation of the muscle through the reduction of complex protein structures in simple proteins, useful substrates for the UPS [49].

Several evidences have shown that patients with CRF, insulin resistance, inflammation, metabolic acidosis, and excess of angiotensin II determine high levels of caspase 3 and

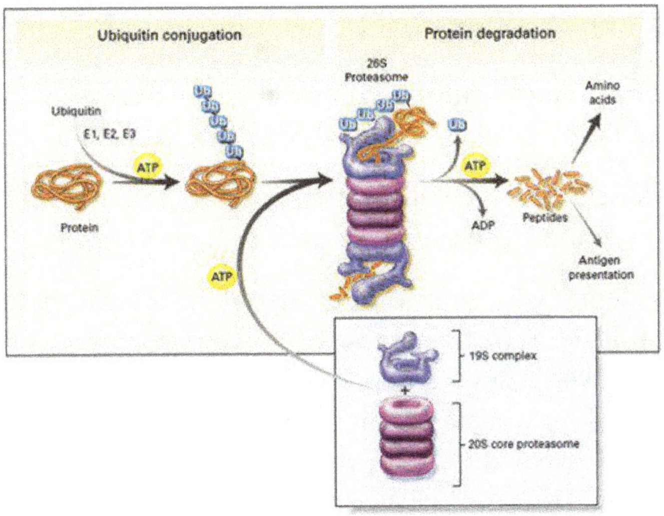

Figure 2. The proteins responsible for muscle degradation are first of all ubiquitin: the enzyme activates the ubiquitin E1, activating a cascade of ATP-dependent events. The ubiquitin chain is recognized by the proteasome 19S, which catalyzes entrance of the protein substrate in the proteasome core 20S, which is cleaved to peptides of the 26S proteasome. The peptides are degraded into amino acids to build cellular proteins or are released from the cells. From: Workeneh BT, Mitch WE. Review of muscle wasting associated with chronic kidney disease. The American Journal of Clinical Nutrition 2010;**91(suppl)**:1128S-1132S.

a significant increase of catabolic processes. These conditions promote the degradation of muscle protein, itself CRF can induce and enhance insulin resistance, encouraging the development of sarcopenia [50–52]. Another consequence of CRF, even more, of the hemodialysis treatment, is the presence of a chronic inflammatory state that, through different modulators, including TNF-alpha, suppresses the action of insulin, increases blood cortisol levels, and activates caspase-3. Glucocorticoids enhance degradation of muscle proteins by upregulation of UPS system. Metabolic acidosis, that is very common, especially in the case of dialysis treatment, determines sarcopenia through multiple mechanisms: induces a negative nitrogen balance and protein synthesis, promotes protein degradation by the UPS system and caspase 3 and alteration of pathway PI3K/Akt, which is a critical transduction signal in cell proliferation and cell cycle progression, apoptosis, and cellular metabolism. It reduces blood levels of IGF-1 and increases those of glucocorticoids. It is probably the main cause of the high prevalence of sarcopenia CFR [53]. The dialysis treatment, by itself, may determine, during each session, a damage to the protein metabolism, with the loss of amino acids and proteins in the dialysate, which reduces the availability of nutrients for muscle synthesis [54]. Many studies, in fact, show that the dialysis catabolic effects induce negative impact on the homeostasis of skeletal muscle protein with reduction of their synthesis and increase of their degradation [55]. Other authors noted that the increased protein lysis persists up to 2 hours after the end of hemodialysis session [56].

The mechanisms underlying this alteration of protein turnover were due not only to the reduction of circulating levels of amino acids and proteins but also to alterations of the factor and EIF2B (eukaryotic translation initiation factor 2 subunit B), which acts in the early steps of protein synthesis and activation of the inflammatory cascade [57].

2.4. Sarcopenia: chronic heart failure (CHF)

Heart dysfunction is a major factor limiting physical performance and skeletal muscle abnormalities, which often accompany CHF, may also contribute to fatigue and dyspnea (**Figure 3**).

Heart dysfunction is associated by metabolic changes that implicate inflammatory and endocrine disorders that determine muscle atrophy and weakness [58].

Cardiac myopathy is defined as muscle fiber atrophy, decreased capillary density, and a low number of type I fibers (fast) compared to type 2, with alteration of the normal ratio between type 1 fibers and type 2 fibers, changes that are responsible for intolerance to physical exercise [59]. Mechanism involved is the ubiquitin-mediated proteolysis and anorexia that exacerbate the weight loss process.

The UPS involves a multi-subunit protease that specifically degrades ubiquitin-conjugated proteins through the action of three enzymes, the ubiquitin-activating enzyme, the ubiquitin-conjugating enzyme, and ubiquitin ligases (atrogin-1 and MuRF-1). A higher frequency of myonuclear apoptosis has also been found in the muscle of patients with CHF relative to age-matched healthy controls [60].

In fact, patients develop anorexia that is secondary to intestinal edema with symptoms like dysgeusia, nausea, and gastroenteropathy and it is also mediated by several drugs such as digoxin, angiotensin-converting enzyme (ACE) inhibitors, β-blockers, and diuretics that favor a loss of nutrients. So, an insufficient intake or absorption of primary nutritional elements, or their loss, determines a malnutrition condition and muscle depletion.

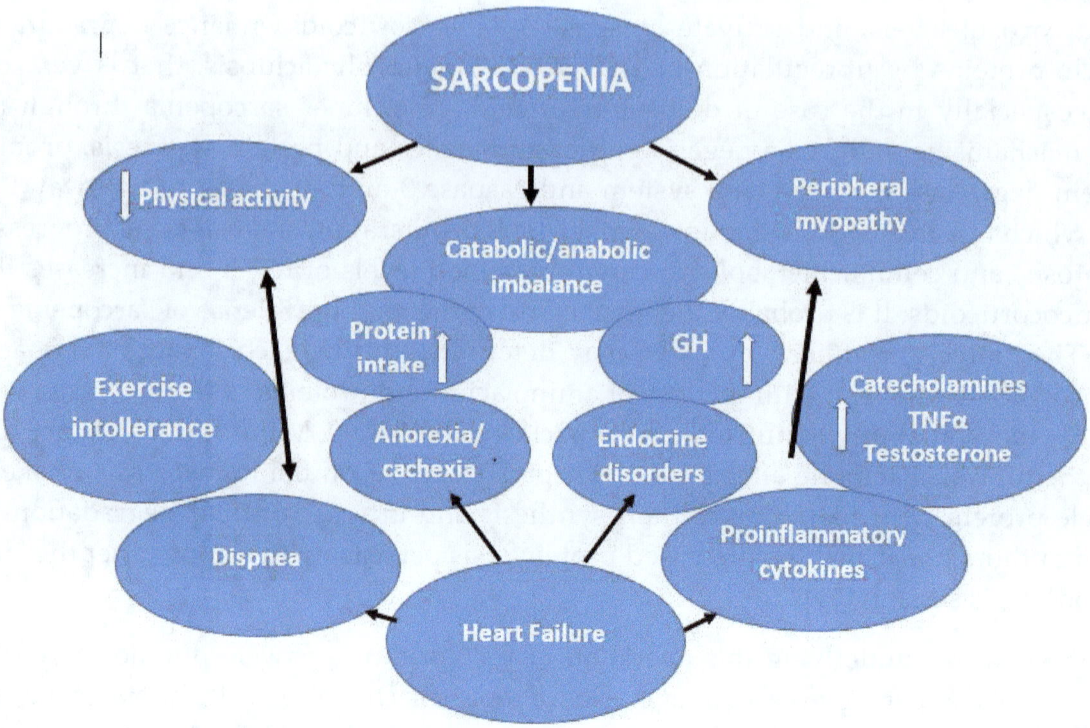

Figure 3. Pathophysiology of secondary sarcopenia.

Furthermore, elevation of angiotensin II levels aggravates these mechanisms. High levels of angiotensin II increase cytokines, such as TNF-alpha, interleukin 6, and glucocorticoids, which induce muscle protein degradation. TNF-α and its soluble receptors have been associated with declines in muscle mass and strength [61]. Another pathophysiological process is related to the decrease of expression of growth hormone (GH) and IGF-1 (anabolic hormones) in muscle, possibly contributing to muscle mass loss [62].

2.5. Sarcopenia: cancer

Within neoplastic sarcopenia definition (often described as cachexia), are included both the real cases of primary cachexia and the cases of nutritional deterioration secondary to obstruction of the digestive tract, chemo-radiotherapy toxicity, and post-surgical intestinal malabsorption syndromes (secondary cachexia). Cachexia is, regardless of the histology and location of the primary tumor, the most common paraneoplastic syndrome in patients with advanced cancer. Over 70% of cancer patients, especially in advanced stages, develop signs and symptoms of cachexia, and about 20% die because of its consequences [63].

Cachexia is characterized by alterations of all metabolic systems, production of circulating factors in part produced by the tumor, in part by the host cells, mainly macrophages, in response to the tumor, and reduced caloric intake.

Some of these alterations appear early in the natural history of neoplastic disease:

a. **Glucose metabolism**: Increased gluconeogenesis from lactate, amino acids, and free fatty acids with loss of protein and lipid reserves.

b. **Protein metabolism**: Increased turnover with decreased muscle and hepatic protein synthesis, increased hepatic synthesis of acute phase proteins, increased serum levels of proteolysis-inducing factor (PIF), and increased protein degradation from muscle tissue. The activation of muscle proteolytic systems, such as that of the ubiquitin-proteasome, is present even before there has been weight loss, suggesting that biomolecular alterations responsible for muscular loss are highlighted early in the natural history of neoplastic disease. Other proteolytic mechanisms provide the activation of calcium-dependent systems, such as that of calpain (regulated by a kinase ATP-dependent and an inhibitor, calpastatin).

c. **Lipid metabolism**: Increased beta-oxidation of fatty acids and the turnover of free fatty acids, increased serum lipoprotein, triglycerides, and production of lipid mobilizing factor (LMF), which induces lipolysis [64].

Some systemic effects of cancer cachexia, such as anorexia, "fatigue," and increased resting energy expenditure, are the result of circulating factors' action in part produced by the tumor and in part by the host cells, mainly macrophages, in response to the tumor. Among them, a central role is given by the pro-inflammatory cytokines (IL-1, IL-6, TNF-α, IFN-γ), which trigger the acute phase response with reduced synthesis of proteins (albumin, prealbumin, and transferrin) [65]. Cytokines such as interleukin-1 (IL-1) and tumor necrosis factor-α (TNF-α) have been suggested as involved in cancer-related anorexia, possibly by increasing the levels of corticotropin-releasing hormone (CRH), a central nervous system neurotransmitter that suppresses food intake, and the firing of glucose-sensitive neurons, which would also decrease food intake [66].

2.6. Secondary sarcopenia: assessment

The variability of weight, even when expressed as body mass index (BMI), is very wide in patients with chronic conditions. There is a correlation between the amount of weight loss and survival. The weight loss cannot be explained only by the decreased supply of food. In fact, it may be related to the size of the increase in basal metabolic rate (resting energy consumption). It is important at the same time in particular for patients suffering from metabolic syndrome and respiratory problems to assess the degree of overweight and obesity.

Therefore, it is necessary to investigate:

- Weight and height (BMI body mass index), and weight loss percentage in the previous period (2 weeks, 1 month, or 6 months).
- Assessment of the quantity and quality of food intake (presence or not of dysphagia). The term sarcopenic dysphagia means a condition characterized by the presence of dysphagia due to sarcopenia of swallowing muscles associated with secondary sarcopenia. Unlike in the elderly dysphagia in stroke outcome, the sarcopenic dysphagia is rarely acknowledged, probably due to the fact that the definition and diagnostic criteria of this condition have not yet been clearly established. According to Butler et al., muscle strength, measured with handgrip, correlates directly with the isometric strength of posterior tongue. This observation indicates that the muscle strength of tongue can be reduced with the generalized deficit in skeletal muscle force, like in sarcopenia [67].

The 10-item Eating Assessment Tool (EAT-10) and a water test (e.g. Toronto Bedside Swallowing Screening Test) or different viscosities (e.g. Volume-Viscosity Swallowing Test) combined with pulse oximetry are useful for dysphagia screening, and if it is confirmed, it requires further secondary clinical evaluations (speech therapist) and possibly instrumental study (Videofluoroscopic Swallowing Study) [68].

The Mini Nutritional Assessment (MNA) [68] is a multidimensional assessment tool, which is easy to complete and allow an easy and feasible large-scale use. The MNA includes 18 items divided into three main sectors (anthropometry and variations in weight, measuring quantitative and qualitative food intake, and disability status and cognitive status); the maximum score is 30. A score below 17 is indicative of malnutrition, a score between 17 and 23.5 is indicative of risk of malnutrition, and a score greater than 24 indicates a normal nutritional status.

The questionnaire allows to classify the nutritional state in an univoque way and has high interpersonal reliability and clearly defined thresholds. It has been validated in several ethnicities and ethnic-specific anthropometric cut-off has been set up [69].

The MNA is also a nutrition guide. Timely intervention blocks the weight loss in people who are at risk of malnutrition or undernourished. It takes in regard anthropometric, global, dietary, and subjective assessment, and it gives to this tool high sensitivity (96%) and specificity (98%) [70].

The scale allows to global assessment of patient as the prevalence of malnutrition increases significantly among hospitalized and institutionalized patients and those with cognitive impairment. The connection is simple enough to guess, the inability to feed on their own, the choice of foods, and the long-lasting immobility.

Perhaps less intuitive, chronic protein energy malnutrition affects the ongoing development of higher cognitive processes rather than simply showing a generalized cognitive and motor impairment.

Deficits of cognitive, emotional, and behavioral functioning are linked to structural abnormalities of different regions of the brain. Brain structures and brain circuits calculate different components of cognitive processes. Malnutrition has long-lasting effects in the processes of cognition and behavior [71].

According to the consensus conference of EWGSOP of 2009, the main parameters to be evaluated in the course of sarcopenia relate to muscle mass, muscle strength, and physical performance of the subject. Based on these three parameters, sarcopenia can be classified into three stages: pre-sarcopenia, sarcopenia, and its severe form [72].

Muscle mass can be assessed by magnetic resonance imaging (MRI) and computed tomography (CT); their use is limited in primary care settings by difficulties in access, costs, the lack of portable equipment, and the requirement of highly specialized personnel [73].

Dual-energy X-ray absorptiometry (DXA) is used to assess body composition and provides reproducible estimates of appendicular skeletal lean mass but it is known that the accuracy of DXA for assessing muscle mass in people of different ages and different pathological conditions may vary [74]. Bio-electrical impedance analysis (BIA) estimates the volume of fat and lean body mass based on the relationship between the volume of a conductor and its electrical resistance. It is not expensive, it can be used easily in clinical practice, both on ambulatory subjects and on hospitalized patients [75, 76]. A still not widely used method, but of extreme interest for the estimation muscular mass, it is represented by the ultrasounds.

Ultrasound allows to explore parenchymas and soft tissue of the human body, responding to all the ideal requirements of a diagnostic method: the almost absolute harmlessness, practicity, rapidity of implementation, and cost contents. According to Fanelli and Kuczmarski, ultrasound application represents a prediction system of body fat that is valid at least as far as plicometry [77], but there are still many limitations related to the application of the method: there is no conventional choice of best frequency to apply, body position, and probe pressure on the surface to be evaluated (**Table 1**).

This method, by measuring thickness of the muscular layers, visceral and subcutaneous fat, was useful in evaluating the regional body composition and where the plicometry is limited [78]. In 2012, Leahy et al. [79] took ultrasound and DXA measurements with good predictive accuracy. In addition, others have used ultrasound to predict the body density of lean men [77], lean women [80], obese adult, Japanese men and women [81], sumo wrestlers [82], the body fat percentage of physically active British and Chinese men [83], and the fat mass of pre-pubertal Japanese children. A new technology, a small, portable, hand-held 2.5 MHz A-mode ultrasound transducer designed specifically for the purpose of body composition assessment; it is connected to a laptop computer using a USB cable, the software assumes the acoustic reflections of the fat-muscle and muscle bone interfaces (Body View, IntelaMetrix, Inc., Livermore, CA) [84].

Advantages	Limitations
Lower cost than laboratory methods	Higher cost than field methods
High accuracy and precision in the hands of an experienced technician	Requires experienced technician, considerable skill is necessary
Capable of regional and segmental measurements	Measurement procedures and techniques are not yet standardized
Minimal tissue compression	Inherent artifacts (fascia etc.)
Noninvasive and no ionizing radiation	
Applicable for testing in the field	
Can measure other tissue thicknesses (muscle and bone)	
Short testing time, rapid procedure	

Table 1. Advantages and limitations of ultrasound application.

Studies reported qualitative changes in muscle related to sarcopenia (e.g. atrophy of type II muscle fibers, increase of intramuscular fat, increase of extracellular water relative to muscle volume) and that these abnormalities can be linked to differences in echo intensity obtained from ultrasonography images.

Enhanced echo intensity (EI) represents changes caused by increase of intramuscular fat and fibrous tissue: an increase of echogenicity indicates greater fibrous tissue and fat between muscular fibers (**Figure 4**) [85]. The simplicity of execution, the low cost, and wide availability make them ideal in the evaluation also for bedridden patients.

Muscle strength was assessed by functional tests: handgrip strength, the walking speed, flexion/extension of the thigh muscles, and forced expiratory flow. Handgrip strength appears to be the most widely used method for the measurement of muscle strength. Isometric handgrip strength shows a good correlation with leg strength and also with lower extremity power, knee extension torque, and calf cross-sectional muscle area [86, 87]. Standardized conditions for the test [88] include seating the subject in a standard chair with their forearms resting flat on the armchairs. Six measures should be taken, three with each arm. Ideally, the patients should be encouraged to squeeze as hard and as tightly as possible for 3–5 seconds for each of the six trials; usually, the highest reading of the six measurements is reported as the final result [89].

The most widely used tool in clinical practice for the assessment of physical performance is measured by gait speed alone or as part of a test battery such as short physical performance battery (SPPB). The SPPB is a test scored to a maximum of 12 points comprising an assessment of gait speed (over 3–4 m), a balance test, and a repeated chair stand test. These tests focus on lower extremity function, as the latter has been shown to correlate with mobility, disability, and patient outcomes, including hospitalization, institutionalization, and mortality. The SPPB takes about 10 min to complete. Participants presenting a score ≤8 points have been described as having a poor physical performance [90]. Other standalone tests can be performed to assess

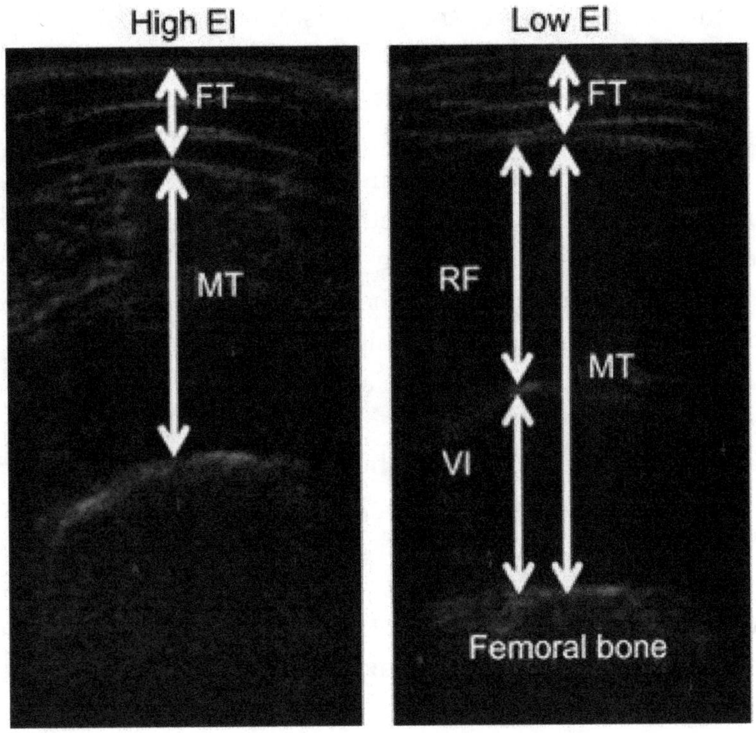

Figure 4. Echo intensity of the rectus femoris muscle. Left: High echo intensity; Right: low echo intensity. EI, echo intensity; FT, subcutaneous fat thickness; MT, muscle thickness; RF, rectus femoris muscle; VI, vastus intermedius muscle. From Watanabe et al. [85].

physical performance. In the Timed Up and Go (TUG) test, individuals are asked to rise from a standard armchair, walk to a marker 3 m away, turn, walk back, and sit down again. The 6-min walk distance or 400 m walk time can be used to measure aerobic capacity. The stair climb power test also shows good correlation with other measures of leg power and physical performance but is mostly restricted to use in research settings [91].

They have been proposed numerous biomarkers to evaluate the catabolic/anabolic balance of skeletal muscle: inflammation biomarkers, such as C-reactive protein, interleukin-6, and tumor necrosis factor-α, and other clinical parameters that express the general state of health like hemoglobin, serum albumin, and urinary creatinine. In the overall evaluation, it is important to measure, also, hormones: dehydroepiandrosterone sulfate, testosterone, insulin-like growth factor-1, and vitamin D, products of oxidative damage like advanced glycation end-products, protein carbonyls, and oxidized low-density lipoproteins, or antioxidants and finally α-tocopherol [92].

3. Rehabilitative approach

3.1. Nutritional-supplementary-integrative—intervention

Malnutrition and peripheral insulin resistance, which increases glucose levels in peripheral blood, are frequent alterations in pathologies that may cause sarcopenia.

The feeding of patient suffering from sarcopenia is essential, mostly the intake of essential amino acids. It should be reminded the importance of 3 protein meals intake and/or supplementation, better if it is given immediately after exercise. The reduced response to the protein synthesis after ingestion of small amounts of essential amino acids can be increased by the ingestion of a mixture with a greater amount of leucine (essential branched-chain amino acid) or a supplementation with hydroxy-methyl butyrate (HMB), a metabolite of leucine; it promotes protein synthesis by preventing protein breakdown. Hormone replacement therapy, if there are no contraindications can be used. According to the recommendations of the European Society for Clinical and Economic Aspects of Osteoporosis, Osteoarthritis and Musculoskeletal Diseases (ESCEO), it must be associated to physical exercise, a high protein diet (1–1.2 g/kg per day with at least 20–25 g of high quality protein, such as those derived from milk) [93]. Rizzoli et al. reported that the recommendations for optimal dietary protein intake are daily 1.0–1.2 g/kg (body weight) with an optimal repartition over each daily meal to prevent sarcopenia [94]. Paddon-Jones et al. proposed a dietary plan that includes 25–30 g of high quality protein per meal as dietary protein recommendations for the prevention of sarcopenia [95]. A protein-enriched diet equivalent to 1.3 g/kg/day achieved through lean red meat is safe and effective for enhancing the effects of progressive resistance training. Carnitine plays a decisive role in the metabolism of long-chain free fatty acids, thus affecting lipid metabolism and energy reserves within the cells. Carnitine is a necessary cofactor for the transport of long-chain fatty acids within the mitochondrial matrix, where they are subjected to oxidation for the production of cellular energy. A clinical study has shown that administration of 6 g/day of L-carnitine for the duration of 30 days was able to significantly improve the symptom "fatigue," appetite, and lean body mass of patients. Therefore, the administration of L-carnitine should be recommended in cachectic patients at a dose of 4–6 g/day orally for a period of time of 3-4 months being usually well tolerated by the patient. Occasional side effects of L-carnitine include epigastralgia and, more rarely, diarrhea [96].

In addition to the now well-known beneficial effects on bone, the vitamin D has positive extraskeletal effects; it acts on the muscle directly (receptor have been identified in skeletal muscle) and indirectly, through increasing of calcium that is essential for muscle contraction; and finally, it promotes the synthesis of contractile proteins [94]. Even supplements, such as omega-3 and carnitine, are widely recommended in this area [96, 97].

Creatine is a molecule produced in the body, and it is a natural amine endogenously synthesized by the liver, kidney, and pancreas from the amino acids arginine, glycine, and methionine. It stores high-energy phosphate groups in the form of phosphocreatine that releases energy to aid cellular function in brain, bones, muscles, and liver. It can be found in some foods, mostly meat, eggs, and fish [98]. Creatine supplementation became popular in the 1990s for enhancing athletic performance and building lean body mass [99]. It has also been used in the treatment of chronic heart failure and mitochondrial disorders. Recent findings have confirmed the potential therapeutic effects of creatine supplementation and have demonstrated that in the elderly, it improves the quality of life by increasing muscle strength and resistance to fatigue, improving performance in daily activities, and preventing bone loss [100, 101]. As a supplement, it is most commonly available as a monohydrate in powder, candy, gum, and liquid. Many synthetic derivatives are available, including creatine malate, creatine pyruvate, creatine citrate, creatine-magnesium chelate, and creatine ethyl ester. Studies with older people have used this regimen 2–5 g per day to ensure the saturation of muscle compound [102], and when it is associated with resistance training, training volume is increased, thereby enhancing strength and muscle mass [103].

The quality of proteins is paramount. A major stimulus in muscle anabolism has been reported as a result of an increase in circulating leucine levels. This was inferred from the observation that the ingestion of whey protein causes even more postprandial muscle protein synthesis rates relative to the ingestion of the intact or hydrolyzed casein and the difference is in the leucine content that has a key role in increasing muscle protein synthesis [104].

Whey protein can be considered a high quality protein, due to the anabolic properties attributed to the faster digestion and absorption of essential amino acids, such as leucine [105].

The mechanism of action of whey proteins is linked to the phosphorylation of p70S6K, which targets the ribosomal subunit S6 and thus promotes protein synthesis. It has been seen that its levels remain elevated even 2 hours after ingestion of whey proteins [106]. In association with amino acid supplementation, it is helpful to administer omega-3 fatty acid because these affect the membrane fluidity, endocytosis, exocytosis, absorption, and release of neurotransmitters such as acetylcholine involved in muscle contraction. They also stimulate the pathway of protein kinase C, enhancing muscle protein synthesis [107].

A recent integrative approach is the use of melatonin. Melatonin, also known as N-acetyl-5-methoxytryptamine, is a derivative of tryptophan, an essential amino acid [108]. It is well known for its role in synchronization of circadian rhythms such as sleep timing, blood pressure, and seasonal reproduction [109, 110], but it is also an antioxidant molecule since it seems to be essential regulator of homeostasis.

Lee et al. found an inverse association between urine melatonin and sarcopenia, suggesting that melatonin may have a protective role in the pathophysiology of sarcopenia. Aging and age-related conditions show an association with low melatonin level. Considering that melatonin has anti-apoptotic effects and attenuates autophagic pathways, its decrease may have a role in the pathogenesis of sarcopenia. Muscle is one of the systems that requires more oxygen and consequently generates more reactive species. Melatonin is a protective factor against this damage, scavenging free radicals, enhancement of antioxidant enzymes, and inhibition of pro-oxidant enzymes [111, 112].

Its antioxidant function is expressed by protection of the electron transport chain and mitochondrial DNA from oxidative damage more efficiently than other conventional antioxidants. So, it increases ATP production in mitochondria [113]. For example, melatonin induces autophagy in myoblast cells collaborating in myogenic differentiation degradation [88], but it inhibits autophagy in muscles from carbon tetrachloride-treated mice by reducing oxidative stress-induced damage. Melatonin reduces endoplasmic reticulum stress in skeletal muscle by increasing the expression of several proteins as well as mRNA levels [114]; this improves protein synthesis. It reduces inflammation in muscle cells, acting specifically against these cytokines in rats [115] and also in humans [116].

Melatonin is more than a regulator of circadian rhythm, it is an antioxidant molecule, and it seems to be essential as a physiological regulator of homeostasis. So, its supplementation may be useful to prevent or treat sarcopenia-associated diseases, including osteoporosis and neuromuscular dysfunction [117].

The management of weight loss in secondary sarcopenia must be evaluated with extreme care since it is known that any treatment of obesity is diet therapy which affects the loss of fat mass and lean mass. This loss of muscle mass is greater when they are prescribed diets with a very low calorie intake or less than 1000 kcal/day, which should be strongly discouraged in chronic diseases. In the management, it is necessary to ensure a moderate caloric restriction ensuring a gradual weight loss, from 0.5 to 1 kg per week, or a decline of 8–10% compared to the initial weight in 6 months. It is also necessary to ensure proper protein intake. Metabolic and epidemiological studies suggest that the current intake recommendations for protein in elderly may not be sufficient.

3.2. Reduction of chronic inflammation

Despite the different chronic conditions can lead to secondary sarcopenia, one of the factors underlying the development and progression is the state of chronic inflammation. The pronounced anti-inflammatory effects of extremely low frequency (ELF) magnetic fields may improve the well-being of patients suffering from illnesses of different etiology. Human studies regarding ultralow frequency magnetic field effects have been carried out in several clinical settings over the past 20 years for treating bone and joint diseases, neuropathies, spinal cord injury, diabetic neuropathy, immune disorders, and cardiomyopathy. Properly configured signals have been demonstrated to regulate major cellular functions, including cell proliferation, differentiation, apoptosis, cell cycle, DNA replication, and cytokine/chemokine expression [118, 119].

The anti-inflammatory effects have demonstrated a decrease in pro-inflammatory cytokines and increase in anti-inflammatory cytokines after traumatic brain injury. Several metabolic parameters change in consequence of exposure to electromagnetic field, as observed in injured rats [120], stroke, decreased pain in osteoarthritis [121], wound healing [122] and postsurgical recovery [123].

Saggini et al. show inflammatory effects of external pulsed electromagnetic fields in the treatment of low back pain with a decrease of pro-inflammatory cytokines (IL-6) after 40 minutes to a sequence of electromagnetic fields of low intensity with inferior frequencies at 100 KHz for a number of 10 sessions in 3 weeks [124]. Furthermore, they allow, as a consequence, a ionic flow capable of optimizing the intrinsic capacity of maintaining the intra and extracellular potential difference essential for the cellular metabolism and homeostasis [125].

The frequency of the field was such to "stimulate" several ions in the sense of the cyclotron frequency. These ions may be involved in the enzymatic chains experimentally affected. This issue needs to be analyzed in detail in the future through well-designed experiments [125].

The term cyclotron frequency points to the form of resonance, which is established at the level of cell membranes, using electromagnetic fields at a very low intensity and at a specific frequency (cyclotron), able to influence and stimulate the metabolism of human cells. It acts to adjust the ordered traffic of selected ions between the internal and external environments of the cell; it stimulates the activity of those ion-dependent enzymes allowing the occurrence of several biological reactions [126].

The bioresonance cyclotron technology (**Figure 5**) (Quantum Electrodynamic Catalysis) is able to provide magnetic fields that respond to the laws of quantum electrodynamics consistency (QUEC), i.e. fields that interact with the "Domains of Consistency" of water, contained in every living being, animal, and plant. The advantage of quanto-elettrodinamica (QUEC) technology is to be able to influence the movement of different ion species to the cell membranes and stimulate the formation of coherent structures by strengthening the metabolism and cell cooperation (homeostasis) [125, 126].

Exposure to bio-cyclotron resonance technology determines: a change of configuration of the water; the normalization of the ion concentration in intracellular and extracellular fluid; the biocatalytic stimulation of intracellular enzymatic functions [127, 128].

With ion cyclotron resonance, we have the possibility to intervene in noninvasive, natural and precise way, on body's homeostasis adjustment mechanisms, where the only pharmacological support can be incomplete.

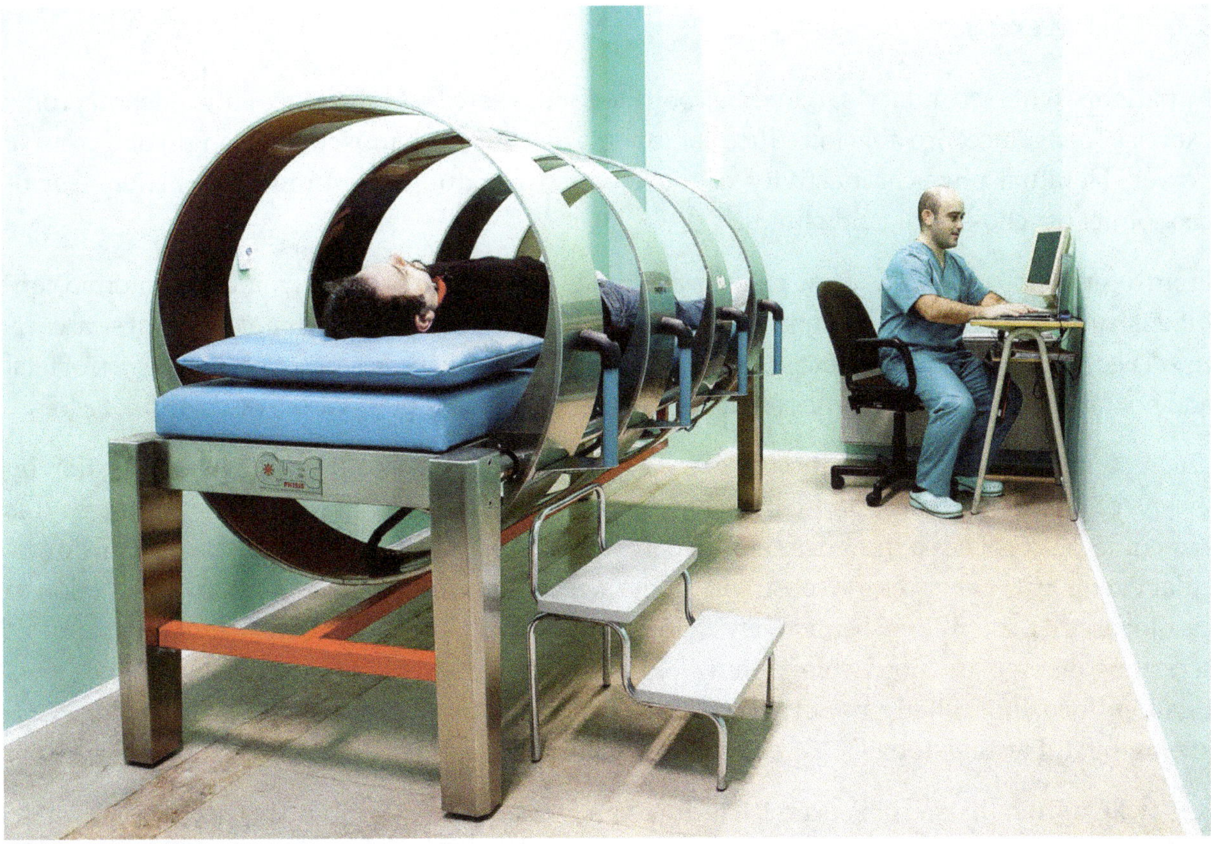

Figure 5. Ion cyclotron resonance with QUEC PHISIS QPS1.

Therefore, it is possible to:

1. Rebalance subjective metabolism
2. Adjust the enzyme functions, the ion channels, and the body pH3.
3. Strengthen the immune system
4. Encourage the bioavailability and absorption of nutrients for cell metabolism
5. Treat neuralgia, headaches, and migraines
6. Stimulate healing in all kinds of wounds, even after surgery
7. Balance the water retention
8. Enhance the effect of drugs and supplements
9. Detoxify and to allow antioxidant function against free radicals, metabolites, and toxins 10.
10. Stimulate a painkiller function (acute and chronic)
11. Get muscle relaxation, from anxiety and stress
12. Improve the homeostasis recovery under stress (physiological microtrauma and muscle protein catabolism).

3.3. Physical exercise

In patients with secondary sarcopenia, both aerobic exercise (endurance) and the anaerobic exercise (resistance) are able to reduce sarcopenia and increase muscular strength and muscle power. Habitual physical inactivity of these patients is due to a number of barriers: socio-economic, psychological, and clinics.

From a clinical point of view, these patients are fragile and sedentary with significant comorbid conditions, such as osteoporosis, anemia, and heart failure, which often limit their access to physical exercise. Theoretically, a physical exercise could be harmful as it may increase temporarily the risk of fatal and nonfatal cardiovascular events, especially if in the presence of other cardiovascular risk factors.

The recommends pre-participation of exercise protocols, provide cardiovascular evaluation by means of history (personal and family history) and physical examination alone, although this screening protocol has a recognized limited power (<10%) to detect potentially lethal cardiovascular event. ECG enhances the sensitivity of the screening process by allowing early detection of cardiovascular conditions distinctively manifesting with ECG abnormalities. If in the course of screening emerge, cardiovascular abnormalities should be assessed the need for further investigation, focusing initially noninvasive, such as echocardiography, Holter monitoring, ECG-averaging, tilt testing, the ECO-stress, myocardial scintigraphy, MRI, and cardiac CT (**Table 2**).

It is well known that aerobic exercise induces an increase in skeletal muscle mitochondria. In fact, adaptations to aerobic training appear to be the result of exercise-induced increases in the transcription of mitochondrial genes.

Absolute	Relative
Unstable coronary heart disease	Major risk factors for coronary heart disease
Decompensated heart failure	Decompensated diabetes
Severe pulmonary arterial hypertension (mean arterial pressure >55 mmHg)	Hypertension above 160/100 mmHg
Uncontrolled arrhythmias	Patients with pacemakers or defibrillators
Uncontrolled high blood pressure (>180/110 mmHg)	
Marfan's syndrome	
Severe symptomatic aortic stenosis, aortic dissection	

Table 2. Contraindications to exercise training.

Many studies have shown an improvement of muscle function even with aerobic or combined aerobic and anaerobic exercises. Aerobic training can include multiple sporting activities, such as stretching, walking, jogging, bicycle ergometer, and aerobic exercises. The latter often based on different tools: weights, elastic bands, rubber balls, rollers, and treadmill. A typical aerobic workout session could last about 90 minutes and be divided as follows: 15–20 minutes of stretching exercises, 20–50 minutes pedaling bicycle ergometer, and 20 minutes of recovery phase [129]. It should start with a lower intensity of training, with the shortest duration and for a few days a week [130]. Several authors showed a significant improvement in aerobic exercise capacity and muscle strength; an improvement in insulin resistance and anorexia; and an increase in ejection fraction, cardiac output, and stroke volume after 6 months of training. Aerobic exercise is related to significant reduction of systolic and diastolic pressure values [108] and an improvement in strength and muscle power [131]. It is well established that traditional, slow-velocity resistance exercise (RE) performing the concentric and eccentric phase of each muscle contraction in 2–3 s is a safe, feasible, and effective intervention to induce muscle hypertrophy and increase strength. It seems to increase muscle protein synthesis [132], satellite cell activation and proliferation [133], anabolic hormone production, and decrease in catabolic cytokine activity [134]. RE has been shown to increase both type I and II muscle fiber cross-sectional areas and whole body leading to an increase in muscle strength. Resistance training needs to use a progressively increasing load to maintain the desired range of repetitions per set of exercise (**Table 3**).

Fast-velocity RE (performing the concentric phase as quickly as possible and taking 2 sec to perform the eccentric phase of each muscle contraction) appears to be a novel intervention for older adults to enhance muscle power. With the subsequent atrophy of type II fibers with aging, fast-velocity movements are important for preserving aging muscle health. Several studies have shown a significant increase in muscle power with fast velocity RE in older adults, because of greater motor unit recruitment of type II fibers [135].

Physical training can improve balance and stability and thus has been recommended as part of rehabilitative exercise protocols. Studies demonstrate significant flexibility improvements (some joints show range of motion improvements of greater than 40%) with supervised exercise programs, including static stretching or a combination of stretching and movements

Type of training	Frequency	Intensity	Duration/set
Aerobic exercise	A minimum of 5 days/week for moderate intensity or 3 days/week for vigorous intensity	Moderate intensity 40–60% VO_2 max 40–60% VO_2 max 40–60% VO_2 max 3–6 METS	Accumulate at least 30 min/day of moderate-intensity activity, in bouts of at least 10 min each; continuous vigorous activity for at least 20 min/day
Resistance exercise involving the major muscle groups (free weights and machines)	At least 2 days/week	Slow-to-moderate lifting velocity 60–80% of 1 RM	8–10 exercises 1–3 sets per exercise 8–12 repetitions (1–3 min of rest among set)
Power training to practice only after the resistance training	2 days/week	Light-to-moderate loading (30–60% of 1 RM) High repetition velocity	1–3 sets per exercise, 6–10 repetitions

HR, heart rate; RM, repetition maximum; and METS, metabolic equivalents.

Table 3. Physical exercise indications.

through a full range of motion [136]. The recovery of proprioception is an essential part of the recovery of sarcopenia for the recovery the motor task is to be made through advanced systems for muscle strength and balance. I-Moove (**Figure 6**) has a balancing platform with helispheric movement and continuous realignment of spatial plans and subsystems of the body in order to maintain an optimal posture in open chain or to exert a tensile force. It also provides a real-time visual feedback that allows to monitor corrections [137].

It is possible to use whole body vibration and focal vibration system that is an effective method to activate the proprioceptive sensory system. It consists of the excitation of the afferents coming from the neuromuscular spindle. This causes the activation of a large number

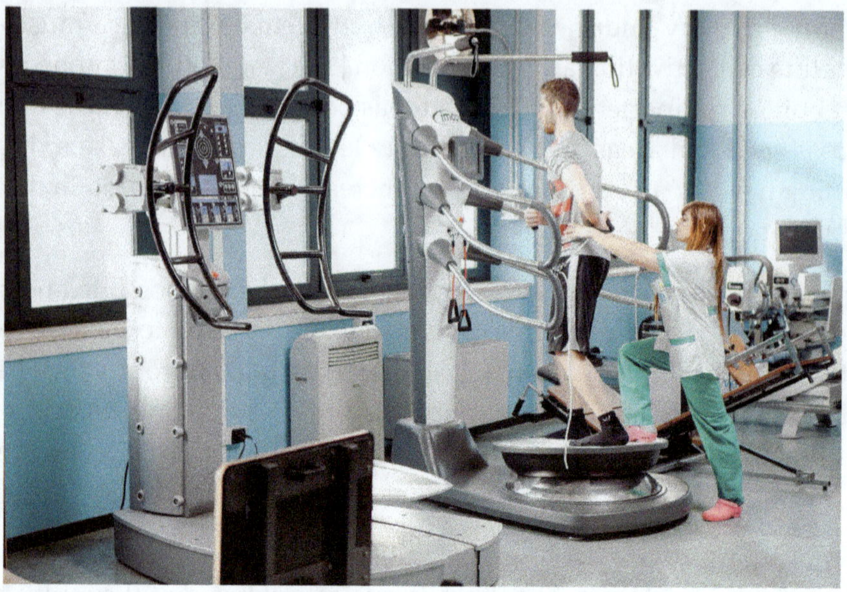

Figure 6. I-Moove and rehabilitative gym at University Centre of Physical Medicine and Rehabilitation University G. d' Annunzio- Chief R. Saggini.

of alpha-motor neurons, leading to the recruitment of muscle fibers, previously inactive, to contribute to muscle contraction. It has been demonstrated that mechanical vibration on a single muscle is able to activate Ia and II afferent nerve fibers of the muscle spindle, and hence the alpha motor neurons: this elicits the so-called Tonic Vibration Reflex (TVR), consisting in sustained contraction of the muscle vibrated and simultaneous relaxation of its prime antagonists. Neuromuscular electrical stimulation (NMES) is an alternative and potentially more effective mean than exercise alone of increasing the force of muscles. These alternative approaches to exercise offered a safe addition to a traditional, high-intensity volitional strengthening program with the aim to implement muscular mass and strength (as described in chapter *Rehabilitation in sarcopenic elderly*)

4. Dynamic antigravity postural system (SPAD)

SPAD®, a device for body weight relief, consisting of a machinery designed to reduce, modify, and condition the force of gravity acting on the body structures of movement during the act of rectilinear motion (**Figure 7**). The system is based on the rational that gait training can be made combining the motor task to sensory feedback, in line with the multisensory approach to postural balance. The system consists of a treadmill on which the patient carries out training in body weight support and of a structure to which the patient is harnessed by means of a pneumatic belt placed between the iliac crests and the costal arches, connected to lifting system with four tie rods attached to the body and to the pelvic girdle. Equipment is completed by four front pads (two on the humeral heads for the shoulder girdle and two on the anterior superior iliac spine for the pelvis), which act as stabilizers (as they prevent possible twisting of the pelvis or shoulder during movement on the treadmill), and at the same time as informants proprioceptive. Two rear pads can be placed on the interscapular region and on the sacral area; according to the characteristics of

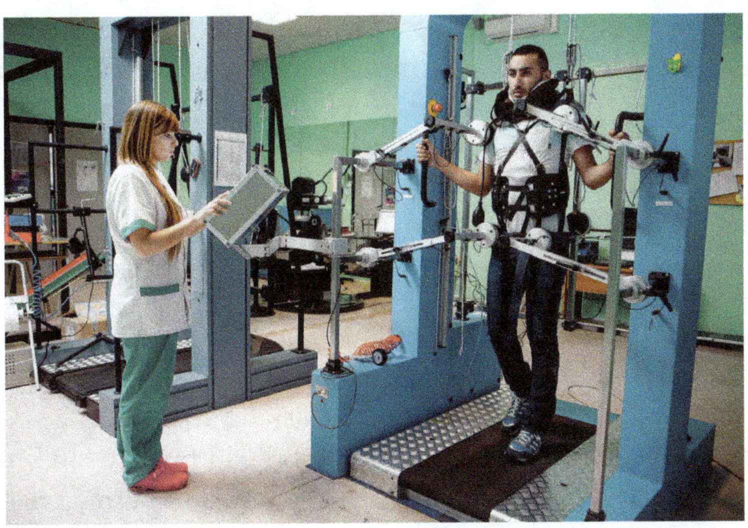

Figure 7. Dynamic antigravity postural system (SPAD).

the patient, an inflatable collar can also be used. Each session of SPAD® provides a 30–50% mean body weight relief and a training on the treadmill with adjustable speed (down to 0.01 km/h during the first session, allowing to become familiar with the machine and thus obtaining a higher compliance). The harnessing in body weight support allows the vertical excursion of the center of gravity of the subject, facilitating the execution of longer steps, according to the possibilities of the individual patient; the step performing is corrected continuously by the operator, inviting the patient to get an ordered cadence with sequential placement of heel-plant-toe. In this way, session after session, SPAD® allows to change asymmetrical gait adaptations, working with a dual action: a mechanical one, which allows a neuromotor retraining with cortical-subcortical learning aimed to the reacquisition of a balanced body schema that minimizes the energy consumption needed to maintain the posture, and a proprioceptive one, which acts on the maintenance of automatic and induced over time walking adaptations. The last part of the session provides for the reduction of body weight relief gradually to 0% and the reduction of the speed of the treadmill until the stop; in this way, in the last part of the session, the patient continuing to maintain the proprioceptive stimulus [138–140].

5. Exercises in virtual reality

Virtual reality exercises in the proposed protocol are based on the most recent findings about the neurophysiology of learning processes and movement memorization. The virtual reality system Riablo® is based on the use of sensors connected to a screen, which in real time sent the exact awareness of the carried out motor task to the patient, with the possibility to focus attention only on the fundamental elements of the movement reducing distracting stimuli from the surrounding real environment. It is possible to set a series of exercises: stand up from the chair; displacement of the load with bending knees; displacement of the load on the sagittal plane; displacement of the load on the sagittal and frontal planes; and bilateral squats with back support. The resulting motor performances and the collected kinematic data are entirely analyzed and recorded in the system, which calculate a score. This motivational input rewards the patient's efforts, ensuring faster progress [141].

6. Microgravity aquatic therapy

Aquatic therapy is based upon several important bioengineering properties. The basic forces acting upon the patient while in the water consist of buoyancy, drag, and inertial forces. Additional factors affecting the patient include hydrostatic pressure and specific heat. Various properties of water contribute to therapeutic effects, including the ability to use water for resistance in place of gravity or weights. Thermal stability that permits maintenance of near-constant temperature; hydrostatic pressure that supports, stabilizes and influences heart and lung function; buoyancy that permits floatation and reduces the effects of gravity; and turbulence and wave propagation that allow gentle manipulation and movement. In our clinical experience, microgravity aquatic therapy can restore active range of motion. In the water, where resistance of water changes depending on walking speed, it is possible to adjust the exercise intensity. Compared to slow movements, such as walking, the body is subjected to greater levels of water resistance with movements that require use of great muscle strength in a short period of time. Previous studies have found that by exercising in the water, where buoyancy makes it difficult to support the body, people can experience postural instability and improve dynamic balance and muscle strength [142]. As far as exercise safety was concerned, in the water buoyancy and viscosity, lower forces applied to body mass-bearing joints, such as the knee, and as a result, the aquatic exercise did not damage muscles and joints. Moreover, in the present aquatic exercise training, the level of intensity can be defined as "moderately strong."

7. Resistance exercise with Kineo system

Changes related to sarcopenia have negative implications on metabolism, cardiovascular, and muscular function. Physical exercise is the most effective intervention to improve quality of life, physical, and psychological health [143].

Physical exercise acts on all the physiopathological mechanisms of sarcopenia: increases mTOR expression that controls protein synthesis in the muscle in response to exercise and nutrition; decreases fat infiltration and prevents lipotoxicity; and regulates oxidative stress through activation of mitochondrial genes and optimization of energy production, increase of capillary density, and muscle perfusion.

A training program that includes endurance and resistance exercises has more positive effects on sarcopenic muscle: resistance exercises are more effective in increasing muscle mass and strength, whereas endurance exercises are more effective for improving maximum aerobic power [144].

Increase of muscle strength and mass can be achieved with an innovative system, such as the KINEO system: a multitasking ergonomic robotic platform that will give you the opportunity to differentiate the activities of muscular work in a highly efficient and accurate way. It is the only robotic platform that allows to differentiate the workload in the two movement phases: concentric and eccentric. This allows to optimize the training of strength and also to work with maximum loads in the concentric phase, as it reduces the load in the return movement.

Kineo (**Figure** 8) is the only robotic platform that allows to differentiate the workload in the two movement phases: concentric and eccentric. This allows to optimize the training of strength and also to work with maximum loads in the concentric phase, as it reduces the load in the return movement.

The Kineo system makes it possible to perform the movement with or without inertia: in the latter case, the displacement of the load requires an application of muscle strength

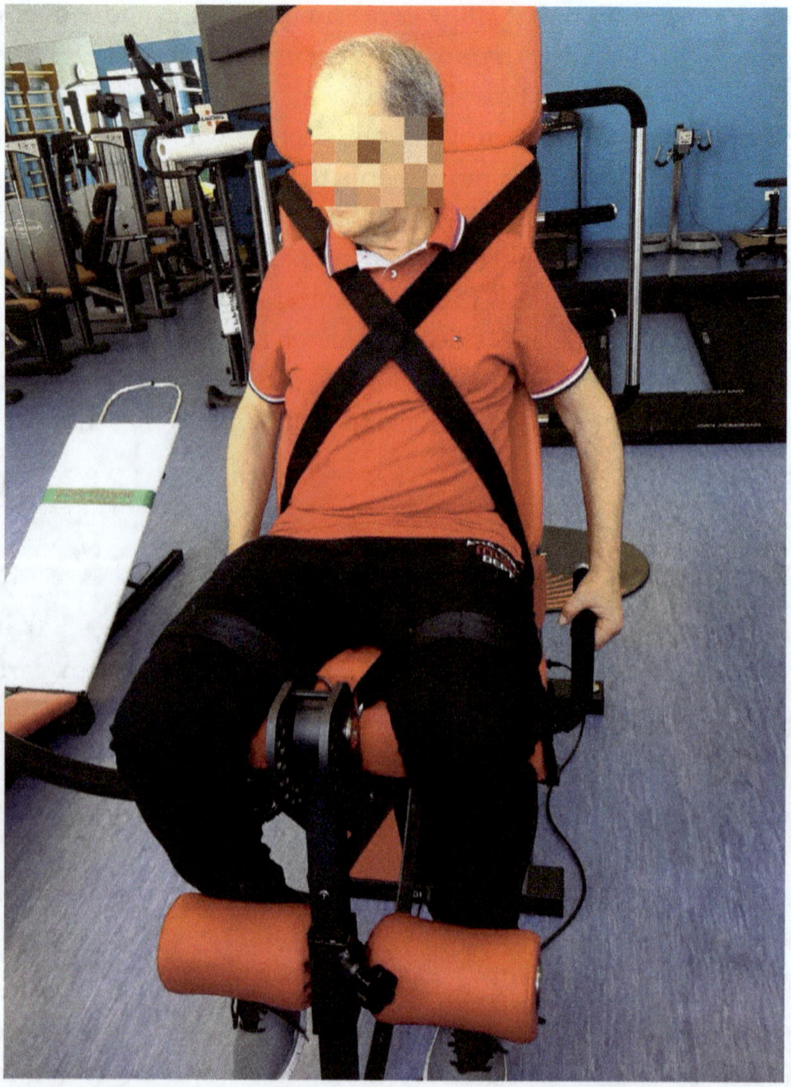

Figure 8. Kineo system.

throughout the movement, even in gestures characterized by great explosiveness. The set load remains constant in all angles and is not modified by inertia, as is the case with a traditional isotonic work. It is possible to differentiate the load between the concentric phase and the eccentric phase. It is possible to work in different conditions, such as elastic and "water viscous method." The elastic method uses resistance bands or springs as external resistance. The elongation of an elastic element depends on the strength applied to it by the subject and the nature of the elastic material (elastic constant). The advantage of the traditional elastic method is constituted by the gradual increase in the muscular effort while varying the workload is laborious.

Kineo elastic method is its ability to use differentiated loads between the concentric and eccentric phase to generate specific muscle adaptations and to use different methods in the concentric and eccentric phase.

Water workout is, universally, recognized as the most appropriate method for prevention and functional rehabilitation, because the load adapts exactly to the real strength of the subject. The "water viscous method," which can be considered as the most innovative, uses the principle of water workout and makes it available in a classic workout station. Kineo offers the possibility to use six levels (**Figure 9**) of viscosity simulating a workout in various fluids, such as water, oil, honey, and so on, which correspond to different levels of muscular effort. One of the most important applications of the water viscous method is the work for the stabilization of the joints, especially the knee joint, because the progressive increase in the viscous load involves the individual muscle groups according to physiologically correct models.

The water viscous method is characterized by the following features: the load increases or decreases depending on the speed of movement and level of viscosity; the speed is not constant but it depends on the level of applied force; and there is no inertia. When the movement stops, the load is immediately set to zero (maximum safety for the subject). Biphasic load: you can independently configure the level of viscosity in the concentric and eccentric phases (**Figure 10**). Unlike other methods, the progressive increase in the load according to the speed allows the subject to use a load that always respects his/her neuromuscular condition and prevents pain.

The training schedule with Kineo should involve two or three sessions a week in nonconsecutive days. The workload is related to the potentialities of the individual subject, which is analyzed with specific tests that evaluate strength, equilibrium, speed, and power. (see http://www.kineosystem.com/)

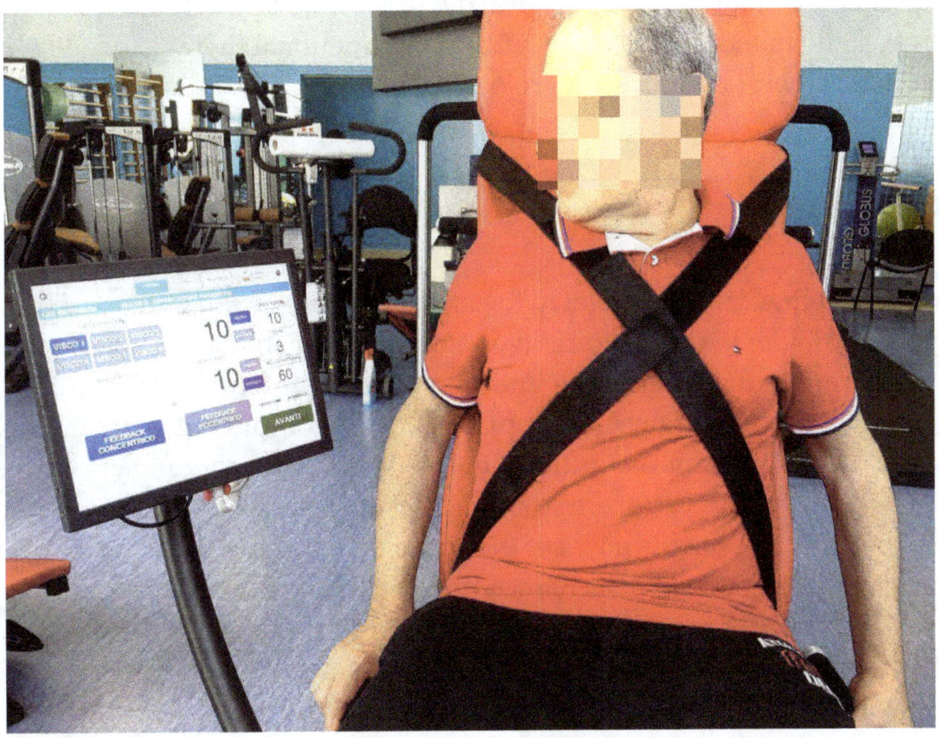

Figure 9. Kineo system, concentric vs. eccentric phase.

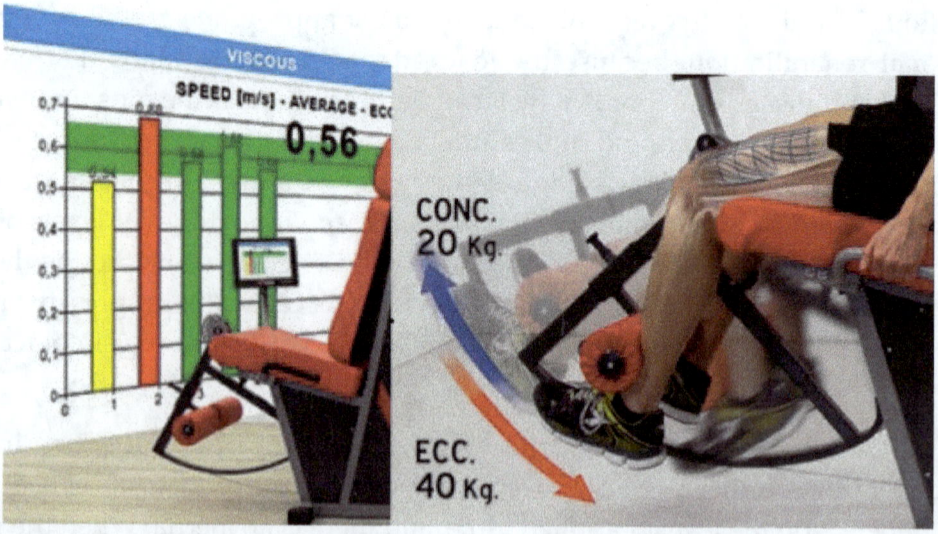

Figure 10. Kineo system, viscous method.

8. Quality of life improvement

The inclusive approach to improve the quality of life includes music therapy relaxation training, diaphragmatic breathing, guided imagery, self-hypnosis, mindfulness meditation, and distracting thoughts and activities outdoor exercises being perceived as energizing and indoor exercises being perceived as relaxing. Using methods deriving from cognitive therapy, patients are taught how to identify and change unhelpful or negative thoughts (cognitive restructuring) that contribute to psychological distress, while facilitating coping thoughts that reduce distress and enhance other coping efforts. Occupational therapists can help patient to maintain or resume their previous social role.

9. Conclusion

Sarcopenia is a disabling condition related to various adverse health outcomes such as mental disorders, poor quality of life, and mortality. Acting with rehabilitation goals is important for promoting positive functional (strength and power) and structural (hypertrophy and phenotypic changes) adaptive responses. The planning of a complex rehabilitation program in sarcopenia associated to chronic conditions, in the context of a comprehensive treatment, is made up of a nutritional support, exercise, correction of lifestyles, and use of advanced physical energies. Therefore, for the purposes of the optimal management, it is essential to identify the pathogenesis aspects and clinical characteristics, which can affect the different treatment choices in rehabilitation. A specialist in the identification, evaluation, and rehabilitation of neuromuscular, musculoskeletal, and functional disorders associated with chronic conditions and its treatment emphasizing the restoration and maintenance of function and quality of life. Future research should focus on better understanding the role of rehabilitation and on defining appropriate interventions for sarcopenia in chronic illness.

Author details

Raoul Saggini[1]*, Simona Maria Carmignano[2], Lucia Cosenza[2], Tommaso Palermo[2] and Rosa Grazia Bellomo[3]

*Address all correspondence to: saggini@unich.it

1 Physical and Rehabilitation Medicine, Department of Medical Oral and Biotechnological Sciences, Director of the School of Specialty in Physical and Rehabilitation Medicine, "Gabriele d'Annunzio" University, National Coordinator of Schools of Specialty in Physical and Rehabilitation Medicine, Chieti-Pescara, Italy

2 School of Specialty in Physical and Rehabilitation Medicine, "Gabriele d'Annunzio" University of Chieti- Pescara, Italy

3 Physical and Rehabilitation Medicine, Department of Medicine and Sciences of Aging, "Gabriele d'Annunzio" University of Chieti-Pescara, Italy

References

[1] Morley JE, Anker SD, von Haehling S. Prevalence, incidence, and clinical impact of sarcopenia: Facts, numbers and epidemiology—update 2014. Journal of Cachexia, Sarcopenia and Muscle 2014;**5**:253-259. DOI: 10.1007/s13539-014-0161-y

[2] Cruz-Jentoft AJ, Baeyens JP, Bauer JM, Boirie Y, Cederholm T et al. European Working Group on Sarcopenia in Older People. Sarcopenia: European consensus on definition and diagnosis—Report of the European Working Group on Sarcopenia in Older People. Age and Ageing; 2010;**39:**412-413

[3] Kalantar-Zadeh K, Rhee C, Sim JJ, Stenvinkel P, Anker SD, Kovesdy CP. Why cachexia kills: Examining the causality of poor outcomes in wasting conditions. Journal of Cachexia, Sarcopenia and Muscle 2013;**4:**89-94

[4] Dovjak P. Sarcopenia in cases of cases of chronic and acute illness. Zeitschrift Fur Gerontologie Und Geriatrie. 2016;**9:**100-106. DOI: 10.1007/s00391-015-0986-9

[5] Berger MJ, Doherty TJ. Sarcopenia: Prevalence, mechanisms, and functional consequences. Interdisciplinary Topics in Gerontology 2010;**37:**94-114

[6] Bruunsgaard H, Andersen-Ranberg K, Jeune B, Pedersen AN, Skinhøj P, Pedersen BK et al. A high plasma concentration of TNF-alpha is associated with dementia in centenarians. The Journals of Gerontology. Series A, Biological Sciences and Medical Sciences. 1999;**54(7)**:M357-M364

[7] Toth MJ, Ades PA, Tischler MD, Tracy RP, LeWinter MM. Immune activation is associated with reduced skeletal muscle mass and physical function in chronic heart failure. International Journal of Cardiology 2006;**109**:179-187

[8] [8] Gratacós J, Collado A, Filella X, Sanmartí R, Cañete J, Llena J et al. Serum cytokines (IL-6, TNF-alpha, IL-1 beta and IFN-gamma) in ankylosing spondylitis: A close

correlation between serum IL-6 and disease activity and severity. British Journal of Rheumatology. 1994;**33(10)**:927-931

[9] Rieu I, Magne H, Savary-Auzeloux I, Averous J, Bos C, Peyron MA et al. Reduction of low grade inflammation restores blunting of postprandial muscle anabolism and limits sarcopenia in old rats. Journal of Physiology. 2009;**587(Pt 22):**5483-5492. DOI: 10.1113/jphysiol.2009.178319.

[10] Degens H. The role of systemic inflammation in age-related muscle weakness and wasting. Scandinavian Journal of Medicine and Science in Sports 2010;**20:**28-38

[11] Ferrucci L, Corsi A, Lauretani F, Bandinelli S, Bartali B, Taub DD et al. The origins of age-related proinflammatory state. Blood. 2005;**105(6)**:2294-2299

[12] Stenholm S, Maggio M, Lauretani F, Bandinelli S, Ceda GP, Di Iorio A et al. Anabolic and catabolic biomarkers as predictors of muscle strength decline: The InCHIANTI study. Rejuvenation Research 2010;**13**:3-11

[13] Ershler WB. Interleukin-6: A cytokine for gerontologists. Journal of the American Geriatrics Society 1993;**41:**176-181

[14] Sieber CC. Malnutrition in the elderly—when too much turns into too few. Zeitschrift für Gerontologie und Geriatrie. 2007;**40(1)**:1-2

[15] Miller MS, Callahan DM, Toth MJ. Skeletal muscle myofilament adaptations to aging, disease, and disuse and their effects on whole muscle performance in older adult humans. Frontiers in Physiology 2014;**5**:369

[16] Degens H. Age-related skeletal muscle dysfunction: Causes and mechanisms. Journal of Musculoskeletal & Neuronal Interactions 2007;**7**:246-252

[17] Mathus-Vliegen EM. Obesity and the elderly. Journal of Clinical Gastroenterology 2012;**46**:533-544

[18] Bouchonville MF, Villareal DT. Sarcopenic obesity: How do we treat it?. Current Opinion in Endocrinology, Diabetes, and Obesity 2013;**20**:412-419

[19] Rolland Y, Lauwers-Cances V, Cristini C, Abellan van Kan G, Janssen I, Morley JE et al. Difficulties with physical function associated with obesity, sarcopenia, and sarcopenic-obesity in community-dwelling elderly women: The EPIDOS (EPIDemiologie de l'OSteoporose) Study. American Journal of Clinical Nutrition. 2009;**89(6)**:1895-1900

[20] Tamene, A et al. Chronic obstructive pulmonary disease (COPD) is a common comorbidity and is independently associated with adverse outcomes in African-American patients with heart failure. Journal of the American College of Cardiology. 2013;**61(10)**:E728

[21] Fragoso CA, Enright PL, McAvay G, Van Ness PH, Gill TM. Frailty and respiratory impairment in older persons. The American Journal of Medicine 2012;125:79-86.

[22] Kon SS, Canavan JL, Nolan CM, Clark AL, Jones SE, Cullinan P et al. The 4-metre gait speed in COPD: Responsiveness and minimal clinically important difference. The European Respiratory Journal 2014;**43**:1298-1305

[23] Liu CK, Leng X, Hsu FC, Kritchevsky SB, Ding J, Earnest CP, et al. The Journal of Nutrition, Health & Aging 2014;**18**:59. DOI: 10.1007/s12603-013-0369-0

[24] Jones SE, Maddocks M, Kon SSC, Canavan JL, Nolan CM, Clark AL et al. Sarcopenia in COPD: Prevalence, clinical correlates and response to pulmonary rehabilitation. Thorax 2015;**70**:213-218

[25] Janssen I, Shepard DS, Katzmarzyk PT, Roubenoff R. The healthcare costs of sarcopenia in the United States. Journal of the American Geriatrics Society. 2004;**52(1)**:80-85

[26] Debigaré R, Marquis K, Côté CH, Tremblay RR, Michaud A, LeBlanc P, et al. Catabolic/anabolic balance and muscle wasting in patients with COPD. CHEST Journal. 2003;**124(1)**:83-89

[27] Gosker H, Van Mameren H, Van Dijk P, Engelen M, Van der Vusse G, Wouters E, et al. Skeletal muscle fibre-type shifting and metabolic profile in patients with chronic obstructive pulmonary disease. European Respiratory Journal. 2002;**19(4)**:617-625

[28] Gosker H, Hesselink M, Duimel H, Ward K, Schols A. Reduced mitochondrial density in the vastus lateralis muscle of patients with COPD. European Respiratory Journal. 2007;**30(1)**:73-79

[29] Gea J, Agustí A, Roca J. Pathophysiology of muscle dysfunction in COPD. Journal of Applied Physiology. 2013;**114(9)**:1222-1234

[30] Pitsiou G, Kyriazis G, Hatzizisi O, Argyropoulou P, Mavrofridis E, Patakas D. Tumor necrosis factor—alpha serum levels, weight loss and tissue oxygenation in chronic obstructive pulmonary disease. Respiratory Medicine. 2002;**96(8)**:594-598

[31] Brunelle J, Chandel N. Oxygen deprivation induced cell death: An update. Apoptosis. 2002;**7(6)**:475-482

[32] Gonzalez NC, Wood JG. Alveolar Hypoxia-Induced Systemic Inflammation: What Low PO2 Does and Does Not Do. Advances in experimental medicine and biology. 2010;662:27-32. doi:10.1007/978-1-4419-1241-1_3

[33] Rafferty GF, Lou Harris M, Polkey MI, Greenough A, Moxham J. Effect of hypercapnia on maximal voluntary ventilation and diaphragm fatigue in normal humans. American Journal of Respiratory and Critical Care Medicine. 1999;**160(5)**:1567-1571

[34] England BK, Chastain JL, Mitch WE. Abnormalities in protein synthesis and degradation induced by extracellular pH in BC3H1 myocytes. American Journal of Physiology. Cell Physiology. 1991;**260(2):**C277-C282

[35] Sanders KJ, Kneppers AE, van de Bool C, Langen RC, Schols AM. Cachexia in chronic obstructive pulmonary disease: New insights and therapeutic perspective. Journal of Cachexia, Sarcopenia and Muscle. 2016;**7(1)**:5-22

[36] Barreiro E, Peinado VI, Galdiz JB, Ferrer E, Marin-Corral J, Sánchez F, et al. Cigarette smoke-induced oxidative stress: A role in chronic obstructive pulmonary disease skeletal muscle dysfunction. American Journal of Respiratory and Critical Care Medicine. 2010;**182(4)**:477-488

[37] Ramsay D, Zochodne D, Robertson D, Nag S, Ludwin S. A syndrome of acute severe muscle necrosis in intensive care unit patients. Journal of Neuropathology and Experimental Neurology. 1993;**52(4)**:387-398

[38] Decramer M, De Bock V, Dom R. Functional and histologic picture of steroid-induced myopathy in chronic obstructive pulmonary disease. American Journal of Respiratory and Critical Care Medicine. 1996;**153(6)**:1958-1964

[39] Calvani R, Miccheli A, Landi F, Bossola M, Cesari M, Leeuwenburgh C, et al. Current nutritional recommendations and novel dietary strategies to manage sarcopenia. The Journal of Frailty & Aging. 2013;**2(1)**:38

[40] Landi F, Marzetti E, Martone AM, Bernabei R, Onder G. Exercise as a remedy for sarcopenia. Current Opinion in Clinical Nutrition and Metabolic Care. 2014;**17(1)**:25-31.

[41] Gea J, Orozco-Levi M, Barreiro E, Ferrer A, Broquetas J. Structural and functional changes in the skeletal muscles of COPD patients: The "compartments" theory. Monaldi Archives for Chest Disease. 2001;**56(3)**:214-224

[42] Chopard A, Hillock S, Jasmin BJ. Molecular events and signalling pathways involved in skeletal muscle disuse-induced atrophy and the impact of countermeasures. Journal of Cellular and Molecular Medicine. 2009;**13(9b):**3032-3050

[43] Maltais F, LeBlanc P, Simard C, Jobin J, Bérubé C, Bruneau J, et al. Skeletal muscle adaptation to endurance training in patients with chronic obstructive pulmonary disease. American Journal of Respiratory and Critical Care Medicine. 1996;**154(2):**442-447

[44] O'Shea SD, Taylor NF, Paratz JD. Progressive resistance exercise improves muscle strength and may improve elements of performance of daily activities for people with COPD: A systematic review. CHEST Journal. 2009;**136(5):**1269-1283

[45] Seymour J, Spruit M, Hopkinson N, Natanek S, Man W-C, Jackson A, et al. The prevalence of quadriceps weakness in COPD and the relationship with disease severity. European Respiratory Journal. 2010;**36(1):**81-88.

[46] Pereira RA, Cordeiro AC, Avesani CM, Carrero JJ, Lindholm B, Amparo FC et al. Sarcopenia in chronic kidney disease on conservative therapy: Prevalence and association with mortality. Nephrol Dial Transplant. 2015;**30(10)**:1718-1725

[47] Zha Y, Qian Q. Protein nutrition and malnutrition in CKD. Nutrients. 2017;**9**:208. DOI: 10.3390/nu9030208

[48] Du J, Wang X, Miereles C, Bailey JL, Debigare R, Zheng B, et al. Activation of caspase-3 is an initial step triggering accelerated muscle proteolysis in catabolic conditions. J Clin Invest. 2004;**113(1)**:115-123

[49] Chauveau P, Combe C, Laville M, Fouque D, Azar R, Cano N et al. Factors influencing survival in hemodialysis patients aged older than 75 years: 2.5-year outcome study. American Journal of Kidney Diseases. 2001;**37(5)**:997-1003

[50] Zhang L, Du J, Hu Z, Han G, Delafontaine P, Garcia G, Mitch WE. IL-6 and serum amyloid A synergy mediates angiotensin II-induced muscle wasting. Journal of the American Society of Nephrology. 2009;**20(3):**604-612

[51] Song YH, Li Y, Du J, Mitch WE, Rosenthal N, Delafontaine P. Muscle-specific expression of IGF-1 blocks angiotensin II-induced skeletal muscle wasting. Journal of Clinical Investigation. 2005;**115(2):**451-458

[52] Kuemmerle N, Krieg RJ Jr, Latta K, Challa A, Hanna JD, Chan JC. Growth hormone and insulin-like growth factor in non-uremic acidosis and uremic acidosis. Kidney International Supplements 1997;**58:**S102-S105

[53] Löfberg E, Essén P, McNurlan M, Wernerman J, Garlick P, Anderstam B et al. Effect of hemodialysis on protein synthesis. Clinical Nephrology. 2000;**54(4)**:284-294

[54] Lim VS, Ikizler TA, Raj DS, Flanigan MJ. Does hemodialysis increase protein breakdown? Dissociation between whole-body amino acid turnover and regional muscle kinetics. Journal of the American Society of Nephrology. 2005;**16(4)**:862-868

[55] Ikizler TA, Flakoll PJ, Parker RA, Hakim RM. Amino acid and albumin losses during hemodialysis. Kidney International. 1994;**46(3)**:830-837

[56] Kobayashi H, Børsheim E, Anthony TG, Traber DL, Badalamenti J, Kimball SR et al. Reduced amino acid availability inhibits muscle protein synthesis and decreases activity of initiation factor eIF2B. American Journal of Physiology. Endocrinology and Metabolism. 2003;**284(3)**:E488-E498

[57] Shyu KG, Lu MJ, Wang BW, Sun HY, Chang H. Myostatin expression in ventricular myocardium in a rat model of volume-overload heart failure. European Journal of Clinical Investigation. 2006;**36(10)**:713-719

[58] Cunha TF, Bacurau AV, Moreira JB, Paixão NA, Campos JC, Ferreira JC et al. Exercise training prevents oxidative stress and ubiquitin-proteasome system overactivity and reverse skeletal muscle atrophy in heart failure. PLoS One. 2012;**7(8)**:e41701

[59] Sakuma K, Yamaguchi A. Sarcopenia and cachexia: The adaptations of negative regulators of skeletal muscle mass. Journal of Cachexia, Sarcopenia and Muscle 2012;**3**:77-94

[60] Forbes SC, Little JP, Candow DG. Exercise and nutritional interventions for improving aging muscle health. Endocrine 2012;**42:**29-38

[61] Hambrecht R, Schulze PC, Gielen S, Linke A, Möbius-Winkler S, Yu J et al. Reduction of insulin-like growth factor-I expression in the skeletal muscle of noncachectic patients with chronic heart failure. Journal of the American College of Cardiology. 2002;**39(7)**:1175-1181

[62] Strasser F, Anker SD, Bosaeus I, Bruera E, Fainsinger RL, et al. Definition and classification of cancer cachexia: An international consensus. The Lancet Oncology 2011;**12**:489-495

[63] Busquets S, Felipe A, Lopez-Soriano, FJ. Molecular mechanisms involved in muscle wasting in cancer and ageing: Cachexia versus sarcopenia. The International Journal of Biochemistry & Cell Biology 2005;**37:**1084-1104

[64] Argiles JM, Busquets S, Lopez-Soriano FJ. The pivotal role of cytokines in muscle wasting during cancer. The International Journal of Biochemistry & Cell Biology. 2005;**37:**1609-1619

[65] Watanobe H, Takebe K. Intravenous administration of tumor necrosis factor-alpha stimulates corticotropin releasing hormone secretion in the push-pull cannulated median eminence of freely moving rats. Neuropeptides. 1992;**22:81-84**

[66] Butler SG, Stuart A, Leng X, Wilhelm E, Rees C, Williamson J. The relationship of aspiration status with tongue and handgrip strength in healthy older adults. The Journals of Gerontology. Series A, Biological Sciences and Medical Sciences. 2011;**66(4)**:452-458

[67] Wakabayashi H. Presbyphagia and sarcopenic dysphagia: Association between aging, sarcopenia, and deglutition disorders. The Journal of Frailty & Aging. 2014;**3(2)**:97-103

[68] Guidoz Y, Wellas BJ, Garry PJ. Mini Nutritional Assessment: A practical assessment tool for grading the nutritional state of elderly patient. In: Wellas BJ, Guidoz Y, Garry PJ, Albarede JL, eds. Nutrition in the Elderly, the Mini Nutritional Assessment (MNA). Facts and Research in Gerontology 1994/1995. 2nd ed. Paris: Serdi Publishing Company; 1995. pp. 15-60

[69] Kaiser MJ, Bauer JM, Ramsch C et al. The Journal of Nutrition, Health & Aging 2009;**13:**782. DOI: 10.1007/s12603-009-0214-7

[70] Kaur S, Miller MD, Halbert J, Giles LC, Crotty M. Nutritional status of adults participating in ambulatory rehabilitation. Asia Pacific Journal of Clinical Nutrition. 2008;**17(2)**:199-207

[71] Strupp BJ, Levitsky DA. Enduring cognitive effects of early malnutrition: A theoretical appraisal. Journal of Nutrition 1995;**125:2221S-2232S.**

[72] Jentoft AJ, Baeyens JP, Bauer JM et al. Sarcopenia: European consensus on definition and diagnosis: Report of the European Working Group on Sarcopenia in Older People. Age and Ageing. 2010;**39(4)**:412-423

[73] Mitsiopoulos N, Baumgartner RN, Heymsfield SB, Lyons W, Gallagher D et al. Cadaver validation of skeletal muscle measurement by magnetic resonance imaging and computerized tomography. Journal of Applied Physiology. 1998;**85(1)**:115-122

[74] Levine JA, Abboud L, Barry M, Reed JE, Sheedy PF, Jensen MD. Measuring leg muscle and fat mass in humans: Comparison of CT and dual-energy X-ray absorptiometry. Journal of Applied Physiology. 2000;**88(2)**:452-456

[75] Vona-Davis, Rose DP. Adipokines as endocrine, paracrine, and autocrine factors in breast cancer risk and progression. Endocrine-Related Cancer. 2007;**14(2)**:189-206

[76] Sullivan DH, Walls RC, Bopp MM. Protein energy undernutrition and the risk of mortality within one years of hospital discharge: A follow-up study. Journal of the American Geriatrics Society 1995b;**43**:507-512

[77] Fanelli MT, Kuczmarski RJ. Ultrasound as an approach to assessing body composition. American Journal of Clinical Nutrition1984;**39(5)**:703-709

[78] Kuczmarski RJ, Fanelli MT, Koch GG. Ultrasonic assessment of body composition in obese adults: Overcoming the limitations of the skinfold caliper. American Journal of Clinical Nutrition. 1987;**45(4)**:717-724

[79] Leahy S, Toomey C, McCreesh K, O'Neill C, Jakeman P. Ultrasound measurement of subcutaneous adipose tissue thickness accurately predicts total and segmental body fat of young adults. Ultrasound in Medicine and Biology. 2012;**38(1)**:28-34

[80] Volz PA, Ostrove SM. Evaluation of a portable ultrasonoscope in assessing the body composition of college-age women. Medicine & Science in Sports & Exercise. 1984;**16(1)**:97-102

[81] Abe T, Kondo M, Kawakami Y, Fukunaga T. Prediction equations for body composition of Japanese adults by B-mode ultrasound. American Journal of Human Biology. 1994;**6(2)**:161-170.

[82] Saito K, Nakaji S, Umeda T, Shimoyama T, Sugawara K, Yamamoto Y. Development of predictive equations for body density of sumo wrestlers using B-mode ultrasound for the determination of subcutaneous fat thickness. British Journal of Sports Medicine. 2003;**37(2)**:144-148.

[83] Eston R, Evans R, Fu F. Estimation of body composition in Chinese and British men by ultrasonographic assessment of segmental adipose tissue volume. British Journal of Sports Medicine. 1994;28(1):9-13.

[84] Silva L. An Introduction to Ultrasound and the BodyMetrixSystem. Livermore, California, USA: IntelaMetrix; 2010.

[85] Watanabe Y, Yamada Y, Fukumoto Y, Ishihara T, Yokoyama K, Yoshida T et al. Echo intensity obtained from ultrasonography images reflecting muscle strength in elderly men. Clinical Interventions in Aging 2013;**8:**993-998

[86] Lauretani F, Russo CR, Bandinelli S, Bartali B, Cavazzini C, Di Iorio A,. Age-associated changes in skeletal muscles and their effect on mobility: An operational diagnosis of sarcopenia. Journal of Applied Physiology. 2003;**95(5)**:1851-1860

[87] Roberts HC, Denison HJ, Martin HJ, Patel HP, Syddall H, Cooper C, Sayer AA. A review of the measurement of grip strength in clinical and epidemiological studies: Towards a standardised approach. Age and Ageing. 2011;**40(4)**:423

[88] Magasi SR, Bubela DJ, Wang Y-C, Gershon RC. Grip and knee extension muscle strength reflect a common construct among adults. Muscle and Nerve 2012; **46**:555-558.

[89] Bean JF, Kiely DK, Herman S, Leveille SG, Mizer K, Frontera WR, Fielding RA. The relationship between leg power and physical performance in mobility-limited older people. Journal of the American Geriatrics Society. 2002;**50(3)**:461-467

[90] National Institute on Aging, Laboratory of Epidemiology, Demography, and Biometry. https://www.nia.nih.gov/

[91] Kiely DK, LaRose S, Alian J, Frontera WR. Is stair climb power a clinically relevant measure of leg power impairments in at-risk older adults? Archives of Physical Medicine and Rehabilitation 2007;**88**:604-609.

[92] Cesari M, Roger A, Pahor M, Goodpaster B, Hellerstein M, Gabor A. Biomarkers of sarcopenia in clinical trials—recommendations from the International Working Group on Sarcopenia. Journal of Cachexia, Sarcopenia and Muscle 2012;**3(3)**:181-190.

[93] Bukhari SS, Phillips BE, Wilkinson DJ, Limb MC, Rankin D, Mitchell WK, et al. Intake of low-dose leucine-rich essential amino acids stimulates muscle anabolism equivalently to bolus whey protein in older women at rest and after exercise. American Journal of Physiology. Endocrinology and Metabolism. 2015;**308(12)**:E1056-E1065.

[94] Rizzoli R. Nutrition and Sarcopenia. Journal of Clinical Densitometry. 2015;**18(4)**:483-487.

[95] Paddon-Jones D, Rasmussen BB. Dietary protein recommendations and the prevention of sarcopenia. Current Opinion in Clinical Nutrition and Metabolic Care. 2009;**12(1)**:86-90

[96] Saggini R, Calvani M. The treatment of cancer: a comprehensive therapeutic model entailing a complex of interaction modalities. DOI: 10.5772/55696

[97] Saggini R, Bellomo RG, Carmignano SM, Saggini A. Cancer pain—The role of an integrated, comprehensive rehabilitation program in its management. In: Rangel LBA, Silva IA, editors. Updates on Cancer Treatment. Rijeka, Croatia, InTech; 2015

[98] Wyss M, Kaddurah-Daouk R. Creatine and creatinine metabolism. Physiological Reviews 2000;**80**:1107-1213.

[99] Candow DG. Sarcopenia: Current theories and the potential beneficial effect of creatine application strategies. Biogerontology. 2011;**12**:273-281.

[100] Gualano B, Artioli GG, Poortmans JR, Lancha Junior AH. Exploring the therapeutic role of creatine supplementation. Amino Acids 2010;**38**:31-44.

[101] Rawson ES, Wehnert ML, Clarkson PM. Effects of 30 days of creatine ingestion in older men. European Journal of Applied Physiology and Occupational Physiology 1999;**80**:139-144.

[102] Hultman E, Söderlund K, Timmons JA, Cederblad G, Greenhaff PL. Muscle creatine loading in men. Journal of Applied Physiology 1996;**81**:232-237.

[103] Gualano B, Roschel H, Lancha-Jr AH, Brightbill CE, Rawson ES. In sickness and in health: The widespread application of creatine supplementation. Amino Acids 2012;**43**:519-529.

[104] Pennings B, Boirie Y, Senden J, Gijsen AP, Kuipers H, van Loon LJ. Whey protein stimulates postprandial muscle protein accretion more effectively than do casein and casein hydrolysate in older men. The American Journal of Clinical Nutrition 2011;**93**:997-1005.

[105] Burd NA, Yang Y, Moore DR, Tang JE, Tarnopolsky MA, Phillips SM. Greater stimulation of myofibrillar protein synthesis with ingestion of whey protein isolate v. micellar casein at rest and after resistance exercise in elderly men. British Journal of Nutrition. 2012;**108**:958-962.

[106] Mitchell CJ, Della Gatta PA, Petersen AC, Cameron-Smith D. Soy protein ingestion results in less prolonged p70S6 kinase phosphorylation compared to whey protein after resistance exercise in older men. Journal of the International Society of Sports Nutrition 2015; **12**:6. DOI: 10.1186/s12970-015-0070-2.

[107] Di Girolamo FG, Situlin R, Mazzucco S. Omega-3 fatty acids and protein metabolism: Enhancement of anabolic interventions for sarcopenia. Nutrition in Clinical Practice. 2013;**28(6)**:684-690. DOI: 10.1177/0884533613507607.

[108] Stehle J, Reuss S, Riemann R, Seidel A, Vollrath L. The role of arginine-vasopressin for pineal melatonin synthesis in the rat: Involvement of vasopressinergic receptors. Neuroscience Letters 1991;**123**:131-134.

[109] Dawson D, Encel N. Melatonin and sleep in humans. Journal of Pineal Research 1993;**15**:1-12.

[110] Pechanova O, Paulis L, Simko F. Peripheral and central effects of melatonin on blood pressure regulation. International Journal of Molecular Sciences 2014, 15, 17920-17937.

[111] Erkanl N K, Kayalar N, Ercan F, Sener G, KNrali K. Melatonin protects against ischemia/reperfusion injury in skeletal muscle. Journal of Pineal Research. 2005;**39**:238-242

[112] Lee JY, Kim JH, Lee DC. Urine melatonin levels are inversely associated with sarcopenia in postmenopausal women. Menopause. 2014; **21(1)**:39-44. DOI: 10.1097/GME.0b013e318291f6c8.

[113] Ramis MR, Esteban S, Miralles A, Tan DX, Reiter R. Protective effects of melatonin and mitochondria-targeted antioxidants against oxidative stress: A review. Current Medicinal Chemistry 2015;**22**:2690-2711

[114] Kim CH, Kim KH, Yoo YM. Melatonin-induced autophagy is associated with degradation of MyoD protein in C2C12 myoblast cells. Journal of Pineal Research 2012;53:289-297

[115] Borges LS, Dermargos A, da Silva J EP, Weimann E, Lambertucci RH, Hatanaka E. Melatonin decreases muscular oxidative stress and inflammation induced by strenuous exercise and stimulates growth factor synthesis. Journal of Pineal Research. 2015;**58**:166-172.

[116] Ochoa JJ, Díaz-Castro J, Kajarabille N, García C, Guisado IM, de Teresa C, Guisado R. Melatonin supplementation ameliorates oxidative stress and inflammatory signaling induced by strenuous exercise in adult human males. Journal of Pineal Research 2011;**51**:373-380.

[117] Coto-Montes A, Boga JA, Reite RJ. Melatonin as a potential agent in the treatment of sarcopenia. International Journal of Molecular Sciences 2016;**17(10)**:177. DOI: 10.3390/ijms17101771

[118] Aaron RK, Ciombor DM, Simon BJ. Treatment of nonunions with electric and electromagnetic fields. Clinical Orthopaedics 2004;**419**:21-29.

[119] Pesce M, Patruno A, Speranza L, and Reale M. Extremely low frequency electromagnetic field and wound healing: Implication of cytokines as biological mediators. European Cytokine Network 2013;**24**:1-10

[120] Rasouli J, Lekhraj R, White NM, Flamm ES, Pilla AA, Strauch B, Casper D. Attenuation of interleukin-1beta by pulsed electromagnetic fields after traumatic brain injury. Neuroscience Letters 2012;**519**:4-8.

[121] Nelson FR, Zvirbulis R, and Pilla AA. Non-invasive electromagnetic field therapy produces rapid and substantial pain reduction in early knee osteoarthritis: A randomized double-blind pilot study. Rheumatology International 2013;**33**:2169-2173.

[122] Pesce M, Patruno A, Speranza L, and Reale M. Extremely low frequency electromagnetic field and wound healing: Implication of cytokines as biological mediators. European Cytokine Network 2013;**24**:1-10.

[123] Heden, P and Pilla AA. Effects of pulsed electromagnetic fields on postoperative pain: A double-blind randomized pilot study in breast augmentation patients. Aesthetic Plastic Surgery 2008; 32, 660-666

[124] Saggini R, Bellomo RG, Saggini A, Iodice P, Toniato E. Rehabilitative treatment for low back pain with external pulsed electromagnetic fields. International Journal of Immunopathology and Pharmacology. 2009;**22(3 suppl)**:25-28

[125] Saggini R, Scarcello L, Carmignano SM, Khodor H, Visciano C, Giuliani L. Complex Rehabilitation Project in Leigh syndrome. Journal of Clinical Trials. 2014;**4**:196

[126] Lappin MS, Lawrie FW, Richards TL, Kramer ED. Effects of a pulsed electromagnetic therapy on multiple sclerosis fatigue and quality of life: A double-blind, placebo controlled trial. Alternative Therapies in Health and Medicine. 2003;**9(4)**:38-48

[127] Di Bonaventura G, Saggini R, Giuliani L, Bellomo RG et al. Exposure to extremely low frequencies electromagnetic field aspects biofilm formation by cystic fibrosis pathogens. Future Microbiology 2014;**10**.

[128] Gerardi G, De Ninno A, Prosdocimi M, Ferrari V, Barbaro F, et al. Effects of electromagnetic fields of low frequency and low intensity on rat metabolism. BioMagnetic Research and Technology 2008;**6**:3.

[129] Hernandez A, Cheng A, Westerblad H. Antioxidants and skeletal muscle performance: "common knowledge" vs. experimental evidence. Frontiers in Physiology. 2012;**3**:46. DOI: 10.3389/fphys.2012.00046

[130] Hurley BF, Hanson ED, Sheaff AK. Strength training as a countermeasure to aging muscle and chronic disease. Sports Medicine 2011;**41**:289.

[131] Binder E, Schechtman K, Ehsani A, Steger-May KMA, Brown M, Sinacore DR, et al. Effects of exercise training on frailty in community-dwelling elderly adults: Results of a randomized, controlled trial. Journal of the American Geriatrics Society. 2002;**50(12)**:1921-1928

[132] Schulte JN, Yarasheski KE. Effects of resistance training on the rate of muscle protein synthesis in frail elderly people. International Journal of Sport Nutrition and Exercise Metabolism 2001;**11**:S111-S118.

[133] Candow DG, Chilibeck PD, Abeysekara S, Zello GA J. Short-term heavy resistance training eliminates age-related deficits in muscle mass and strength in healthy older males. Journal of Strength and Conditioning Research. 2011;**25(2)**:326-333.

[134] Liu CJ, Latham NK. Progressive resistance strength training for improving physical function in older adults. Cochrane Database of Systematic Reviews. 2009;**8(3)**:CD002759.

[135] Reid KF, Callahan DM, Carabello RJ, Phillips EM, Frontera WR, Fielding RA. Lower extremity power training in elderly subjects with mobility limitations: A randomized controlled trial. Aging Clinical and Experimental Research. 2008;**20(4)**:337-343.

[136] American Geriatrics Society, British Geriatrics Society, and American Academy of Orthopaedic Surgeons Panel on Falls Prevention. Guideline for the prevention of falls in older persons. Journal of the American Geriatrics Society. 2001;**49(5)**:664-672

[137] Bellomo RG, Iodice P, Maffulli N, Maghradze T, Coco V, Saggini R. Muscle strength and balance training in sarcopenic elderly: A pilot study with randomized controlled trial. European Journal of Inflammation. 2013;**11**:193-201

[138] Bellomo RG, Khodor H, Barassi G, Carmignano SM, Di Stefano A, Di Pancrazio L, Saggini R. Global bioprogressive rehabilitation program and postural instability in Parkinson's disease. European Scientific Journal. 2014;**2**:310-321

[139] Saggini R, Di Pancrazio L, Pisciella V, Iodice P, Marri A, Bellomo RG. Postural anti-gravitational reprogramming in the elderly with flexed posture. European Journal of Physical and Rehabilitation Medicine. 2010;**46** - suppl.1 - No.2. ISSN: 1973-9087.

[140] Saggini R, Di Stefano A, Capogrosso F, Carmignano SM, D'Ettole S, Iodice P et al.Task-oriented physical exercise using postural re-alignment with body weight support in chronic stroke. European Journal of Inflammation. 2013;**11(3)**:739-749

[141] Bellomo RG, Pisciella V, Di Pancrazio L, Saggini R. The virtual images into physical rehabilitation. In: book abstract SIMFER the Italian Society of Physical and Rehabilitation Medicine 37th National Congress. Campobasso, Italy; 20-23 September 2009; 189.

[142] Devereux K, Robertson D, Briffa NK. Effects of a water-based training on women 65 years and over: A randomised controlled trial. The Australian Journal of Physiotherapy 2005;**51**:102-108

[143] Montero-Fernández N, Serra-Rexach JA. Role of exercise on sarcopenia in the elderly. European Journal of Physical and Rehabilitation Medicine. 2013;**49(1)**:131-143

[144] Phu S, Boersma D, Duque G. Exercise and sarcopenia. Journal of Clinical Densitometry. 2015;**18(4)**:488-492

10

Frailty and Cardiovascular Disease

Vinod Chainani, Russell Riehl, Geeta Chainani,
Abir Abdo, Mauricio G. Cohen, Carlos Alfonso,
Pedro Martinez-Clark, Carl J. Lavie, John P. Reilly and
Nidal Abi-Rafeh

Abstract

Cardiovascular disease (CVD) comprises a vast spectrum of disease states ranging from hypertension (HTN) to valvular heart disease (VHD). CVD is known to be the leading cause of morbidity, mortality, and health-care expenditure throughout the world. According to the World Health Organization, coronary artery disease (CAD) and stroke, both subsets of CVD, are the world's biggest killers, accounting for a combined 15 million deaths in 2015. These diseases have remained the leading causes of death globally in the last 15 years. In 2010, CAD alone was projected to cost the U.S. $108.9 billion including the cost of health-care services, medications, and lost productivity. The presence of frailty significantly worsens outcomes for patients suffering from CAD. With just this one example of how frailty affects CVD, it is clear that understanding the impact of frailty upon patients afflicted with the spectrum of cardiovascular disease is integral for the care of this very significant patient population.

Keywords: frailty, cardiovascular disease, valvular heart disease, outcomes in cardiovascular disease, hypertension, coronary artery disease, peripheral vascular disease, lipid dysregulation

1. Introduction

Cardiovascular disease (CVD) comprises a vast spectrum of disease states ranging from hypertension (HTN) to valvular heart disease (VHD) and is known to be the leading cause of morbidity, mortality, and health-care expenditure throughout the world. According to the World Health Organization, coronary heart disease (CHD) and stroke, both subsets of CVD, are the world's most impactful causes of mortality, accounting for a combined 15 million deaths in

2015. These diseases have remained the leading causes of death globally in the last 15 years. In 2010, CHD alone was projected to cost the United States (US) $108.9 billion including the cost of health-care services, medications, and lost productivity. The presence of frailty significantly worsens outcomes for patients suffering from CHD [1]. With just this one example of how frailty affects CVD, it is clear that understanding the impact of frailty upon patients afflicted with the spectrum of CVD is integral for the care of this very significant patient population.

While frailty as an entity is manifested by the interplay of multiple factors, there are some that are pertinent to the relationship between CVD and frailty. Endocrine dysregulation and higher levels of inflammatory markers have been found in frail compared with non-frail persons, and these derangements have been appreciated in patients with CHD. Elevations in some markers of frailty are also risk factors for the development of progressive vascular and CHD [2]. So while it can be inferred that CVD and frailty share common links, the effect of frailty upon the outcomes of CVD is still an area of interest and continued study [3].

We now know that CVD can worsen sarcopenia and lead to frailty, while frailty worsens morbidity and mortality in CVD [4, 5]. Maximal aerobic power (MAP), a measure of frailty, decreases with age due to a decrease in cardiac output. And though CVD is not the primary cause of decline of MAP, CVD clearly exacerbates the said decline [5]. Recently, in a meta-analysis of 54,250 elderly individuals with a mean follow-up of 6.2 years, the presence of atherosclerotic CVD was associated with the coexistence of frailty syndrome (FS) with an odds ratio (OR) of 2.7–4.1 [6]. Also, in patients who did not begin the study with FS, CVD was associated with the onset of FS during follow-up of these patients. There have been several studies that highlight the relationship between CVD and frailty, as described in **Tables 1** and **2**.

Study	Study type/number of patients	Objective	Outcome
Chin et al. [7]	Population-based cohort study/545 men	Assess association between classic cardiovascular risk factors and subsequent functional disability and mental well-being in elderly men.	Combined classic cardiovascular risk factors are predictive of functional disability.
Newman et al. [8]	Observational cohort/4375 patients	Assess the relationship between subclinical cardiovascular disease and frailty.	Cardiovascular disease was associated with an increased likelihood of frail health.
Chaves et al. [9]	Prospective population based cohort/670 patients	Examined the cross-sectional relationship between hemoglobin (Hb) and a recently-validated measure of frailty in community-dwelling older women, and whether this relationship was modified by cardiovascular disease (CVD) status.	Mildly low and low-normal Hb levels were independently associated with increased frailty risk. This risk was synergistically modified by the presence of CVD.
Woods et al. [10]	Prospective study, the Women's Health Initiative Observational Study/40.657 women	Identified risk factors for frailty as targets for prevention. Investigated the predictive validity of this frailty classification for death, hospitalization, hip fracture, and activity of daily living (ADL) disability.	Community-dwelling older women with CVD and cardiovascular risk factors were at higher risk of developing incident frailty.

Table 1. Effect of cardiovascular disease on frailty.

Study	Study type/ number of patients	Objective	Outcome
Klein et al. [11]	Prospective cohort/2962 patients	Association of measures of frailty to disease outcomes and survival in a population-based study of Midwestern adults.	Greater frailty was significantly associated with cardiovascular disease and hypertension.
Cacciatore et al. [12]	Prospective cohort/1259 patients	This study aimed to examine the predictive role of frailty on long-term mortality in elderly subjects with CHF.	Frailty represents a new independent variable for predicting long-term mortality in elderly subjects with CHF.
Purser et al. [13]	Observational cohort/309 patients	To characterize physiological variation in hospitalized older adults with severe coronary artery disease (CAD) and evaluate the prevalence of frailty in this sample, to determine whether single-item performance measures are good indicators of multidimensional frailty, and to estimate the association between frailty and 6-month mortality.	Gait speed frailty was the strongest predictor of mortality in a population with CAD and may add to traditional risk assessments when predicting outcomes in this population.
Boxer et al. [14]	Prospective cohort/60 patients	To assess the distance on the 6-min walk test (6MWT) as a measure of frailty in 60 older HF patients (ejection fraction <or= 40%) compared with frailty phenotype (FP).	The 6MWT may be useful to identify frailty and those in transition to frailty.
Dumurgier et al. [15]	Prospective cohort study/3208 men and women	Study the relation between low walking speed and the risk of death in older people, both overall and with regard to the main causes of death.	Slow gait speed was associated with a threefold increase in cardiovascular mortality over 5 years but no difference in death due to cancer or death due to other causes, implying a specific effect of frailty on CVD.
Ekerstad et al. [5]	Prospective cohort/307 patients	To analyze how frailty predicts short-term outcomes for elderly non-ST-segment elevation myocardial infarction patients.	Frailty is strongly and independently associated with in-hospital mortality, 1-month mortality, prolonged hospital care, and the study's primary composite outcome which included endpoints like all-cause mortality, reinfarction, revascularization, and even dialysis in older patients after non-ST elevation myocardial infarction (NSTEMI).

Table 2. Effect of frailty on cardiovascular disease.

A scoring system easily used on an inpatient basis highlights the interplay of CVD and frailty [16]. Sanchis et al. described seven independent predictors of frailty: age ≥75 years, female sex, prior CHD, admission for heart failure (HF), hemoglobin ≤12.5 g/dL, vitamin D ≤9 ng/mL, and cystatin-C ≥1.2 mg, which could be measured on an inpatient basis. Defining frailty as positive when there were ≥3 had a good correlation with the Fried score of frailty.

In this chapter, we delve into a basic understanding of the underlying pathophysiology of CVD in relation to frailty and how it is worsened by the latter, inflammatory markers that have proven significant in CVD and frailty, and how frailty affects a vast spectrum of CVD, ranging from lipid dysregulation to outcomes in VHD.

2. Pathophysiology

The pathophysiology of CVD and frailty relates to a baseline chronic inflammatory state [17–20]. This phenomenon is caused by a metabolic imbalance in the body, hereby systemic demand is not met by metabolic supply, and consequently the body becomes primarily catabolic, oxidative stress increases, and ultimately a low-level inflammatory phenotype is established [18, 21–28].

Multiple diseases place systemic stress demands on the body [1] that in turn leads to the inability of the body to keep pace with the demands of daily living, such as thermoregulation, aerobic respiration, glycolysis, and oxidative phosphorylation [17, 22, 29]. As a consequence of this baseline mismatch between the body's demand and its ability to supply, the body enters a pro-catabolic state and begins to metabolize itself for nutrient utilization [17, 25]. During this state, more inefficient systems are used to produce energy, and weakness and weight loss occur [30]. A pro-catabolic state is frequently seen in both CHD and frailty and leads to, as we already know exists in frailty, a pro-inflammatory state [18, 24].

The aforementioned pro-inflammatory state is highlighted by the presence of elevated inflammatory markers. There are markers specific to frailty and others that are common between CVD and frailty. Interleukin (IL)-6 is the most consistently seen inflammatory marker in patients with frailty, and is thought to be central to the pathogenesis of the phenotype [18, 21, 24, 26–28]. Studies have reported seeing elevated plasma uric acid, D-dimer, white blood cells (WBCs), erythrocyte sedimentation rate (ESR), triglycerides, homocysteine, glucose, hemoglobin A1C (HbA1c), creatinine, cystatin C, insulin-like growth factor (IGF)-1, fibrinogen, von Willebrand factor, factors VIII and IX, oxidized proteins, protein carbonylation, as well as decreased vitamin D and testosterone in patients with frailty [31]. In order to highlight the common role inflammation plays in both CVD and frailty, we can appreciate that elevations of C-reactive protein (CRP), factor VIII, and D-dimer are commonly seen even after correction of CVD [32]. Particularly, D-dimer, CRP, IL-6, and tumor necrosis factor (TNF)-alpha will be discussed where pertinent.

3. Frailty and hypertension (HTN)

Though not all frail patients are hypertensive, there is some evidence to suggest that HTN is independently associated with frailty [33]. The mechanism behind this finding is further elucidated by the fact that frail patients have a decreased ability to use adenosine triphosphate (ATP) [23, 29, 34]. This leads to a decreased ability of smooth muscle to use ATP to pump calcium back into the sarcoplasmic reticulum, which is marked by a slower rate of decay of the calcium transit. In practical terms, this means the blood vessels of frail patients have decreased compliance and difficulty relaxing, which leads to HTN.

The renin-angiotensin-aldosterone system (RAAS) is one of the primary systems used by the body to regulate blood pressure (BP) (**Figure 1**) [35, 36]. Chronic inflammation directly stimulates RAAS, which causes HTN [37]. Since frail patients have persistently increased inflammation, stimulating RAAS, they are more likely to develop HTN. Thus, there is a direct link between the chronic inflammation phenotype and HTN in frail patients.

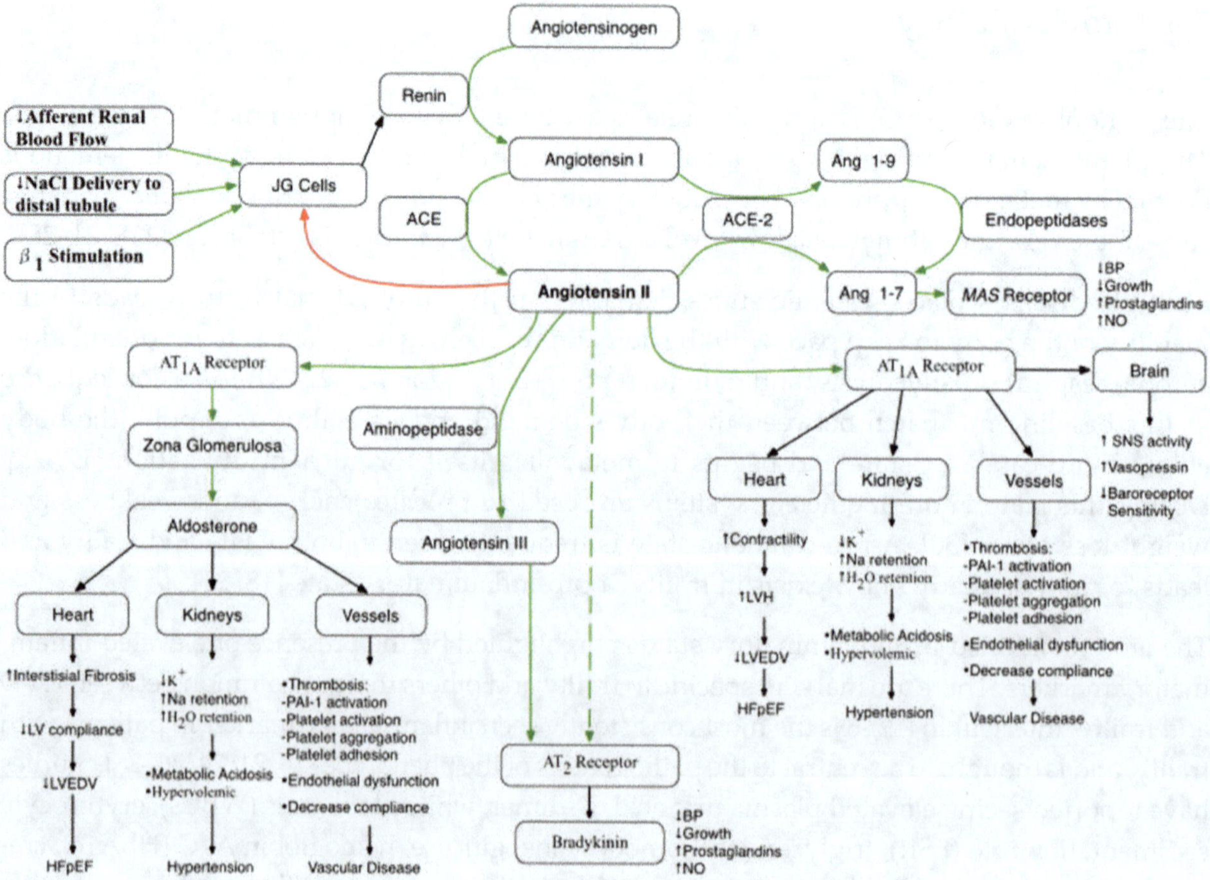

Figure 1. Renin-angiotensin-aldosterone system. ACE I, angiotensin-converting enzyme inhibitor; ACE-2, angiotensin-converting enzyme-2; Ang, angiotensin; BK, bradykinin; BP, blood pressure; HFpEF, heart failure with preserved ejection fraction; JG, juxtaglomerular; LV, left ventricle; LVEDV, left ventricular end diastolic volume; LVH, left ventricular hypertrophy; NO, nitric oxide; PAI-1, plasminogen activator inhibitor-1; SNS, sympathetic nervous system.

Evidence from randomized controlled trials over the past decade indicates there is benefit to treating hypertension in older patients [38, 39]. This is inconsistent with earlier observational and subgroup analyses of previous randomized control trials which were inconclusive [40, 41]. The HYVET trial in 2008 specifically focused the treatment of hypertension in elderly patients and found that antihypertensive treatment in patients older than 80 was beneficial [39]. In 2015, the Systolic Blood Pressure Intervention Trial (SPRINT) was undertaken. This trial should not be confused with the Sarcopenia and Physical Frailty in Older People: Multicomponent Treatment Strategies (SPRINTT) trial, which aims to provide a clear operational definition of physical frailty and assess the impact a multi-component intervention has on its progression [42]. The SPRINT trial showed that among patients >50 years old, lowering BP to <120 mmHg, particularly in the elderly, was associated with a significant decrease in mortality compared to a target of less than 140 mmHg at 5 years (5.2% vs. 6.8%; hazard ratio (HR): 0.75; 95% confidence interval (CI): 0.64–0.89, $p < 0.001$) [38]. Of note, patients who were >75 years old tended to fare better than younger patients. Taken together, this suggests that all elderly patients benefit from antihypertensive treatments, but there is an important caveat to both of these studies: enrolled patients tended to be relatively healthy patients and specifically excluded patients with heart failure, stroke, and end-stage renal disease [35, 38].

The exclusion criteria for HYVET and SPRINT raise concern that their findings may not be generalizable to frail patients [43]. A subgroup analysis of patients enrolled in HYVET addressed this concern [44]. Participants in both the control and treatment groups were given a frailty index according to 60 different variables. The impact of the frailty index on subsequent risk of stroke, mortality, and cardiac events was found to be non-significant, suggesting that benefits associated with BP lowering were conserved in frail patients. A frailty index was calculated for SPRINT participants using a similar set of 36 variables [45]. The frailty index distribution among the participants was comparable to general population cohorts. This suggests the heterogeneity of frailty among participants is similar to the general population.

Another 2015 report as a part of the Zwolle Outpatient Diabetes Project Integrating Available Care-34 (ZODIAC-34) cohort study, this time including all-comers, confirmed what observational studies had shown: for all-cause mortality (especially frail patients), there was an inverse relationship between blood pressure and all-cause mortality with a hazard ratio for systolic blood pressure of 0.92 (95% CI: 0.87–0.98) and 0.83 for diastolic blood pressure (95% CI: 0.73–0.93) [46]. This suggested that among all patients >75 years of age, this time including those with less than 1 year life expectancy and DM, lower BP was associated with an increase in mortality. Contiguously, intensive lowering of BP in patients with low gate speed (a commonly used proxy for frailty) did not reduce mortality and the rate of CVD events ($p = 0.05, 0.28$, respectively) [47].

4. Frailty and lipids

The metabolism of lipids has been shown to affect aging, such that having a high-density lipoprotein (HDL) level above 70 mg/dL is referred to as longevity syndrome. The Invecchiamento e Longevità nel Sirente (ilSERENTE) study showed that the HDL levels of the patients in their study who died during follow-up were significantly lower than the levels of the survivors. This finding contributed to the understanding of the effect of HDL on lifespan, highlighting the role of lipid metabolism in decreasing mortality in the frail, elderly patient [48]. Another study of the same group of patients showed that, among frail patients, those with the highest HDL levels had the best functional states [49]. To further support this idea, another study done in 2015 supported frailty as an independent risk factor for various diseases along the CVD spectrum. A low HDL level was one of the parameters [50]. As a part of the Longitudinal Aging Study Amsterdam, it was described that a lower total cholesterol was related to a higher rate of decline on information-processing speed indicating, ultimately, that lower total cholesterol may be considered to be a marker of frailty and predictive of lower cognitive function in the elderly [51]. As described earlier, there has been significant study regarding the relationship between frailty, HDL status, and its effect on mortality. Conversely, the relation between low-density lipoprotein (LDL) levels and frailty has yet to be established. Also, whereas the effect of lipids in the frail patient has been studied, the effect of frailty on the patient with a lipid disorder has yet to be established.

There has been speculation upon the metabolism of lipids in the frail patient. As there is a pro-inflammatory milieu in the frail patient, this inflammation may affect lipid metabolism and, hence, lipid profiles in those who are frail. There may also be some correlation between dysfunctional lipid metabolism due to endocrine dysregulation evidenced by lower IGF-1 and growth hormone levels in frail patients, lower HDL levels, and resultant poorer outcomes in CHD [52, 53]. A study on metabolic syndrome and disability showed a correlation between high triglycerides and a limitation in mobility and activities of daily living [54]. Overall, the effect of frailty, its pro-inflammatory state, and the collective effect on lipids seems to be contiguous with an elevation in triglycerides (TGs) and a decrease in HDL likely contributing to the elevated CVD risk in the frail population.

5. Frailty and atrial fibrillation (AF)

The up-regulation of the RAAS system in frail patients, as mentioned earlier, mediates an up-regulation of endothelin-1, which in turn mediates an increase in cardiac fibrosis [55]. Cardiac fibrosis, in turn, increases the likelihood of AF by disrupting the cardiac neuroconduction pathways [23]. Additionally, frailty may be an independent risk factor for AF [46] due to a decreased ability to modulate heart rate, resulting in an increased likelihood of a patient developing AF [56, 57]. Additionally, an increased calcium influx, as discussed earlier, causes changes in the trans-cellular membrane potential, which in turn makes a patient more likely to develop AF [23].

Frail patients have a 4.4 times higher chance (95% CI: 2.104–9.080, $p < 0.001$) of having AF compared to the general population [57]. Additionally, Polidoro et al. found that even after adjusting for age, sex, CVD, and CVD risk factors, AF was associated with a fourfold increase in frailtyhighlighting the relation between frailty and AF [58]. Additional evidence supporting the link between frailty and AF is the impairment of autonomic control vis-à-vis decreased heart rate variability which often precedes episodes of paroxysmal AF [57]. Similarly, there is decreased heart rate variability in frail patients.

AF has a significant impact on outcomes, including mortality, in frail patients [59]. Nguyen et al. found that in patients with AF, there was a 2.69 times higher risk of death in frail patients over a 6-month period after hospitalization (HR: 2.69, 95% CI: 1.53–4.74). This relationship held even after correction for potential co-founders (HR: 2.33; 95% CI: 1.31–4.14). It may be plausible to infer that AF also causes significant risk for cognitive decline to these patients seeing as they are already at an increased risk for microbleeds as discussed subsequently in the section on cerebrovascular disease. Furthermore, the strong risk of stroke and TIA outlined in the subsequent text is indubitably linked with AF [60].

Despite the increased risk of death with AF, frail patients have an eightfold less likelihood of being discharged home on an oral anticoagulant after hospitalization [57]. In fact, frailty is the third most cited reason for not prescribing an oral anticoagulant. This makes the report by Granzera et al. more pertinent as the population ages [61]. In this study, he provides an approach to deciding if oral anticoagulation is appropriate in elderly frail patients (**Figure 2**).

Granziera et al. also discussed what factors should go into making the decision of whether to use warfarin or novel oral anticoagulants (NOACs) in frail patients [61]. Severe renal impairment, severe liver impairment, and poor adherence favored the use of warfarin. The exceptions

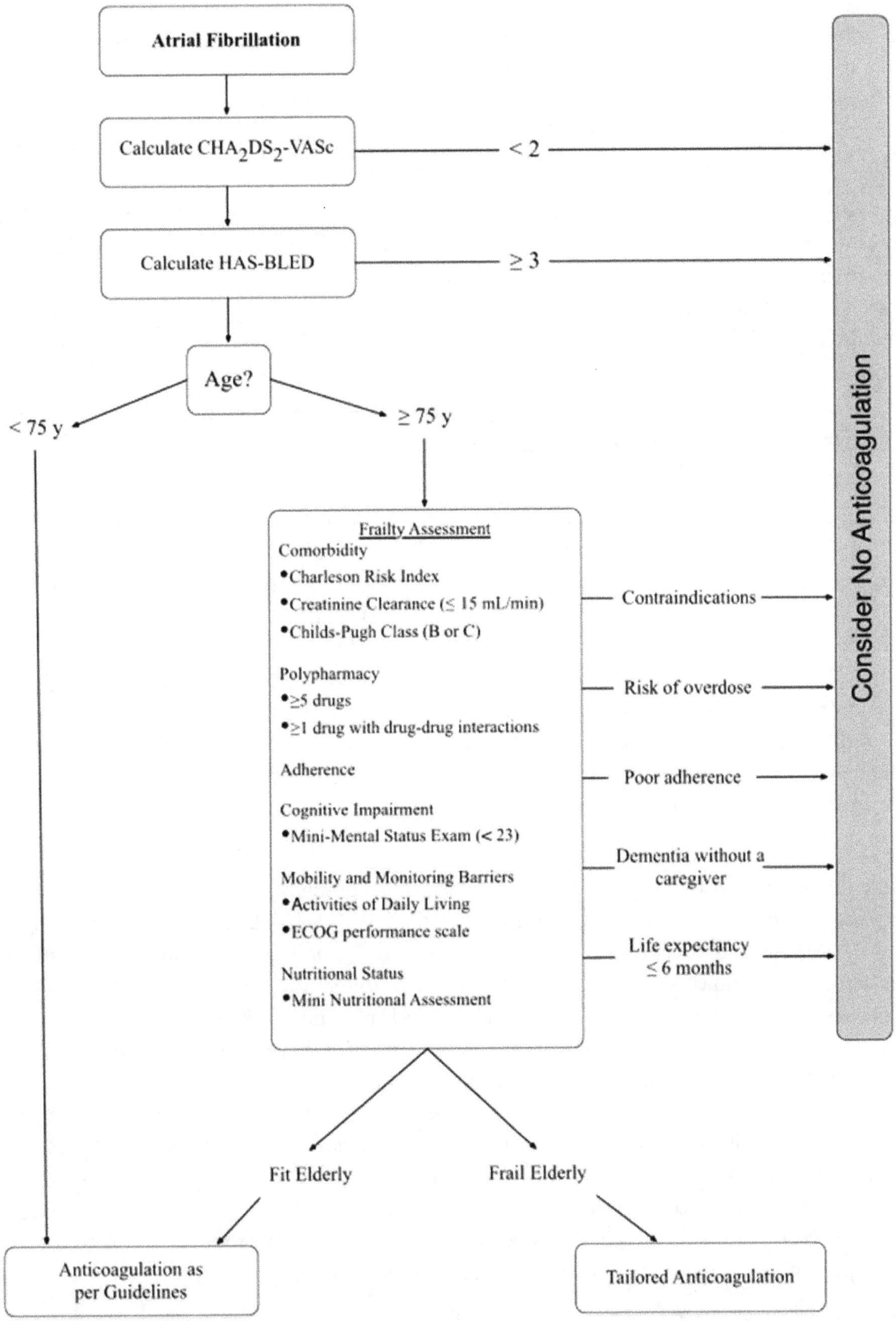

Figure 2. Decision algorithm for use of oral anticoagulants in elderly frail patients (<75 vs. ≥75 years). Adapted from Granziera et al. [61].

to favoring warfarin in renal impairment are apixaban and edoxaban, both of which may be prescribed in patients with compromised renal function. Decreased renal and hepatic clearances have minimal effect on warfarin. In patients at risk for poor compliance, their risk for stroke will not revert to baseline if a dose is missed. For patients with decreased mobility, they are less likely to comply with nutritional changes for warfarin and have polypharmacy; NOACs are the better choice for improved compliance.

Frail patients may have less of a benefit from device therapy than healthy patients [57]. In a combined analysis of four clinical trials, the benefits of implantable cardioverter defibrillators were inversely proportional to the number of comorbidities. This line of thought was further supported by a retrospective study of 83,792 undergoing ICD implantation in which frail patients had a 22% risk of mortality at 1 year compared to 12% overall.

6. Frailty and cerebrovascular disease

Several studies have indicated that frailty is associated with low cognitive performance. This is attributed to multiple causes including increased rates of Alzheimer's disease (AD), mild cognitive impairment, and a distinct subtype of frailty—cognitive frailty [62, 63]. Cognitive frailty is a clinical syndrome found in elderly patients without AD or other dementias, and occurs concurrently with physical frailty [63]. The key feature differentiating this syndrome from AD and other dementias is its potential for reversibility. The proposed mechanism for cognitive frailty is similar to physical frailty—a decrease in physiological reserves for responding to systemic stressors that manifests as an erosion of homeostatic mechanisms. The erosion of homeostatic mechanisms seen in cognitive frailty is manifested as β-amyloid accumulation. These changes are independent other causes of dementia such as vascular and Alzheimer's dementia.

Frail patients were also more likely to have any form of dementia (HR 1.85; 95% CI: 1.01–3.40) and vascular dementia in particular (HF 2.68; 95% CI: 1.16–7.17) [62]. Frail patients are 3.38 times (95% CI: 2.37–4.81, $p < 0.001$) more likely to have a stroke or TIA than non-frail patients [60]. This association with cerebrovascular disease extends to include pre-frail patients, who have a 1.98 times greater risk of having a stroke versus non-frail patients (95% CI: 1.53–2.57, $p < 0.001$). Another manifestation of cerebrovascular disease, cerebromicrobleeds, is one of the primary lesions responsible for vascular dementia. When the number of lesions is low (only one or two), there is usually no clinical evidence of microbleed, but when there is a larger lesion burden, patients present with stroke or dementia [64]. Even when adjusted for age, sex, and presence of vascular risk factors (CHD, chronic kidney disease, and global cognitive impairment), the lesion number was positively correlated with the severity of physical frailty. Chung et al. also found that the severity of physical frailty was positively correlated with proportion of cerebromicrobleeds present in the deep and infratentorial regions of the brain.

Furthermore, a study performed on patients undergoing carotid endarterectomy (CEA) using the American College of Surgeons National Surgical Quality Improvement Program (NSQIP) database from 2005 to 2011 showed that frailty is a predictor of increased stroke, mortality, myocardial infarction, and length of stay after CEA, further supporting the idea that CVD and frailty are strongly interlinked with frail patients suffering poorer outcomes postintervention [65].

6.1. Inflammatory markers in CHD

The relationship between frailty and CHD is one that has been extensively studied as well. Chronic inflammation is a shared mechanism between atherosclerosis and frailty [18, 66, 67]. In Libby et al.'s strong and well-cited review article, they show that, in addition to plaque characteristics, acute coronary syndromes are also caused by a chronic inflammatory state [59]. This link is most strongly seen by four markers of inflammation shared by both frailty and coronary vascular disease: IL-6, CRP, fibrinogen, and D-dimer [26, 27].

Hunter et al. made the strong case that IL-6 is a keystone mediator of systemic inflammation in multiple disease processes, especially CVD [28]. There have been numerous other studies linking IL-6 and CHD [18, 66, 67]. This suggests that IL-6 is central to the immunogenic dysregulation that accounts for the disease burden suffered by patients with both CVD and frailty [28]. Another significant marker of chronic inflammation shared between both CHD and frailty is CRP [26, 27]. Like IL-6, this marker is elevated in frailty even when CHD is accounted for [32].

Fibrinogen is an acute-phase reactant shown to be elevated with chronic inflammation and is strongly correlated with both frailty and atherosclerosis [26, 66]. Elevated fibrinogen is an independent risk factor for CVD events [66]. The mechanism is thought to be caused by fibrinogen affecting the plaque phenotype, causing it to be more permeable, able to accumulate oxidized LDL, increase platelet reactivity, and aggregation. A direct association between frailty and fibrinogen has been observed independent of chronic disease states [26].

Similar to fibrinogen, D-dimer fragments are an independent risk factor for CHD to the point where they are considered a biomarker for atherothrombosis [66]. Moreover, elevated D-dimers are also independently associated with frailty [32].

7. Frailty and CHD

A meta-analysis of 54,250 elderly individuals with a mean follow-up of 6.2 years showed that the presence of atherosclerotic CVD was associated with the coexistence of frailty syndrome with an odds ratio of 2.7–4.1 [6]. The relationship between CVD and frailty is significantly bidirectional [6, 60]. This is highlighted by the twofold increase in mortality among frail CHD patients compared to non-frail patients even when adjusted for age and comorbidities [68]. In the Women's Health Initiative Study, women with CHD were more likely to become frail over the subsequent 6 years; likewise, the Health, Aging, and Body Composition Study showed that older adults with frailty were more likely to develop CHD. This same study showed that the presence of frailty, assessed by gait speed, was associated with an increased risk of incident CVD. After adjustment for potential confounding factors, a slower gait was associated with an increased incidence of CVD events and all-cause mortality compared with individuals having higher walking speed [69]. Furthering the complexity of this disease interplay is the fact that patients with both frailty and CHD have a higher frequency of multivessel disease and left main disease (74%) than non-frail patients (60%) and moderately frail (68%) patients ($p = 0.019$) [70]. These differences persisted even after correcting for age and gender ($p = 0.005$). The wealth of evidence clearly defines the effect of frailty upon CHD.

Interestingly, atherogenesis is also affected by sarcopenia. This effect is partially due to the replacement of muscle with adipose tissue, and partially to the neurohumoral dysregulation and decreased mobility brought on by sarcopenia [71–73]. Atherogenesis is worsened by the presence of sarcopenia and frailty in humans as evidenced by the association between carotid atherosclerosis, arterial stiffness, and sarcopenia [6]. It, therefore, seems natural that frail patients fare worse after an acute CHD event compared to non-frail patients. This notion was validated by Dodson et al., who found that at 1 year after an acute CHD event, older adults with slow gait speed (<0.8 m/s measured 1 month after the event) were more likely to die or be re-admitted to the hospital than those with faster speeds (35.4% vs. 18.5%; $p = 0.006$) [74]. However, it is important to note that the majority of these events were re-admissions—not death.

Regarding interventions, there has been an extensive amount of investigation into whether coronary artery bypass grafting (CABG) is better than percutaneous coronary intervention (PCI) in frail patients. Fifty-six percent of frail patients who underwent CABG had postoperative complications compared to seventeen percent of those who were non-frail ($p < 0.001$) [75]. Frailty was also an independent predictor of in-hospital mortality after CABG (OR 1.8; 92% CI: 1.1–3.0). Similarly, PCI also carried significant risks. Frailty was associated with a longer hospital stay (HR 4.8, 95% CI: 1.4–16.3; $p = 0.013$), higher 30-day mortality (HR 4.8, 95% CI: 1.4–16.3; $p = 0.01$), and higher 1-year mortality (HR 5.9, 95% CI: 2.5–13.8; $p < 0.001$) [76, 77]. Importantly, there is evidence that there is no significant difference in change in frailty at 30 months between CABG and PCI ($p = 0.090$) [78]. In patients ≥75 years old treated with either PCI or CABG, there was a significantly different trajectory in their frailty score at 30 months (0.188 vs. 247, respectively) and at baseline (0.164 vs. 0.189, respectively; $p = 0.041$). Including frailty as part of the three-tiered criterion in the assessment of a patient undergoing PCI improved the discriminatory ability of the Mayo Clinic risk score [79]. Of great importance is the decision as to which modality of intervention is most effective in the frail population with obstructive coronary artery disease (CAD). Although we suspect that being less invasive in frail patients may be preferable, a prospective, randomized trial in the frail population addressing this quandary, as well as whether revascularization impacts frailty, would be beneficial.

8. Frailty and peripheral arterial disease (PAD)

Clearly, PAD is a pandemic condition that could potentially lead to the literal loss of life and limb. It manifests as tissue hypoperfusion caused by acute insult upon a limb with preexisting underlying atherosclerosis. This disease process is a significant cause of morbidity and mortality in both the frail and non-frail populations [80, 81].

Frailty has been shown to be associated with and worsen outcomes in patients with PAD. A study of the participants >50 years of age in the National Health and Nutritional Examination Survey (NHANES) showed that, in multivariable multinomial logistic regression models, ankle brachial index (ABI) <0.9 predicted frailty and pre-frailty. A higher prevalence of frailty was seen in participants with ABI ≥1.4. Frailty predicted general and CVD mortality in participants with ABI <0.9. Hence, this study suggested that frailty mediates increased morbidity and mortality in PAD [82]. A cross-sectional study was carried out in a geriatric population of ≥65-year-old residents of Taichung, Taiwan, in June 2009 to assess the association between frailty and subclinical PAD. It reported findings suggesting that frail individuals had a significantly increased risk for subclinical PAD with an odds ratio of 3.168 [83]. In a study assessing gait in patients with PAD versus non-PAD both with and without frailty, the pre-frail group defined by the Fried Frailty Index had a diminished difference between study groups. This indicated that pre-frail patients have a poor functional status overall, which may overshadow the level of dysfunction imposed upon them by PAD alone [84].

Another study assessing the effect of frailty on outcomes after vascular surgery showed that frailty, assessed by the modified Frailty Index (mFI), predicted mortality in patients undergoing open procedures and Clavien-Dindo class IV (life-threatening) complications for both open and endovascular abdominal aortic aneurysm repairs [85]. Affecting disposition and, hence, patient wellness and health-care expenditure, frailty also increases the propensity of home-dwelling patients classified as frail to be discharged to a facility other than their home after elective vascular interventions [86]. There is also evidence to support the idea that frail females are potentially at the highest risk of death after vascular surgery, suggesting that female gender may be an additive risk factor [87].

9. Frailty and heart failure

The pathogenesis of HF has significant overlap with the processes leading to the frailty phenotype [17, 88]. With HF, much like frailty, the metabolic demands of the body outstrip physiologic reserves. The findings of Lavie et al. likewise show that a loss of fat (reserves) signals a worsening prognosis in HF [30].

Frail patients and patients with HF consistently have a similar biochemical profile of elevated CRP and interleukin-6, which in turn promote mitochondrial dysfunction [18, 22, 31]. Mitochondrial dysfunction produces excessive reactive oxygen species producing a pro-apoptotic intracellular environment. In the case of HF, apoptosis of cardiomyocytes fosters a local pro-inflammatory atmosphere, leading to cardiac fibrosis and ultimately decreased contractility. Likewise, when applied to skeletal muscle, this process causes sarcopenia, one of the hallmarks and precursors of frailty.

The likelihood of a frail patient to manifest HF is 8.76 times higher than that of a non-frail patient and, compared to any other element of CVD, HF is the most strongly linked with frailty [60, 89]. However, it should be noted that frailty is not limited to geriatric heart failure patient, and been observed in up to one-third of younger patients with HF [68]. The prevalence of frailty among heart failure patients is important because frailty is an even stronger predictor of mortality than is HF per se [88]. Cacciatore et al. assessed the role frailty had on mortality in HF patients (n = 1139) over a 12-year period compared to patients without CHF (n = 120) and found that frailty was independently associated with mortality in HF (HR 1.48, 95% CI: 1.04–2.11; p = 0.0032) and control group patients (HR 1.36, 95% CI: 1.17–1.57; p < 0.001), proving that it indeed was a more important predictor of mortality than HF itself [12]. Lupon et al. found that among 622 outpatient HF patients, frailty was an independent predictor of mortality even after adjustment for HF (HR 2.09, 95% CI: 1.11–3.92; p = 0.022) [90].

Discerning which patients are frail versus non-frail also has an impact on clinic resources. Frail patients versus non-frail patients in one study had a 92% increase in Emergency Department (ED) visits (HR 1.92, 1.60; 95% CI: 1.30–2.83) and 65% increased risk for hospitalizations (HR 1.65; 95% CI: 1.17–2.35) [91]. Of note, there was no significant association between outpatient visits in HF patients and frailty. This raises the question as to whether or not more intensive outpatient management of frail HF patients would decrease ED and hospital utilization.

One possible intervention to decrease the amount of hospital utilization in frail patients and, moreover, improve their morbidity and mortality is specifically resistance exercise [92]. As noted by Lavie et al., there is compelling evidence that muscle mass and muscle strength are protective in HF patients [93]. Moreover, a lack of muscular fitness overall is a strong determinant of cardiac cachexia which, as mentioned earlier, may be seen as a classification of frailty. There is evidence to suggest that maximal aerobic power, a measure of frailty, decreases with age, due to a decrease in cardiac output, and is exacerbated by CVD. Importantly, this is a measure of frailty which could be addressed with an increase in muscle mass and anaerobic exercise [94]. It is important to note that resistance training is the most well-validated countermeasure to slow the decline of muscle mass and muscle strength, even in frail patients [92]. By slowing the decline in muscle strength, the decline into frailty is consequently retarded. Taken together, this evidence points to muscle bulk, or the lack thereof, as being a significant marker of disease progression in HF and element of CVD.

The choice of pursuing advanced therapeutic options in the frail population with HF is a difficult one. As Joyce points out, HF itself and its ensuing sequelae can simulate the frailty phenotype [95]. Discerning between frailty caused specifically by HF and frailty attributable to non-CVD causes has significant implications in this selection of patients for destination therapy with left ventricular assist devices (LVADs). In patients with HF as the primary driver of his or her frailty, implantation of an LVAD led to restoration of aberrant cardiac output and metabolism. Flint et al. sorted out frail patients receiving an LVAD into three groups: LVAD-responsive, LVAD-independent, and LVAD-intermediate. In the LVAD-responsive group, whose frailty was primarily due to HF, implantation of LVAD caused a significant decrease in post-LVAD frailty as measured by hand-grip strength compared to both the LVAD-intermediate and LVAD-independent patients. These LVAD-responsive patients may be more accurate representatives of cardiac cachexia versus frailty.

Frailty in the heart-transplant (HT) population has more significant and far-reaching importance. Frail patients who underwent HT in one study had a 1-year survival rate of 52 ± 23% versus 100% in the non-frail control arm. This has significant implications in the way HT therapy is allocated. This is a realm that requires more study, though studies will be sparse given the requirements for HT approval, including appropriate performance on pre-HT cardiopulmonary testing, in which frail and pre-frail patient would likely have suboptimal results.

10. Frailty and valvular heart disease (VHD)

In industrialized countries, the prevalence of VHD is estimated at 2.5%. Degenerative calcification seems to augment the prevalence of VHD markedly after the age of 65 years, particularly regarding aortic stenosis (AS) and mitral regurgitation (MR). These two disease entities account for three in four cases of VHD. Also contributing to the incidence of VHD is infective endocarditis, the incidence of which is approximately 30 cases per million individuals per year worldwide. Finally, rheumatic heart disease (RHD) is another very significant contributor to the incidence of VHD and still represents a significant health burden with over 15 million cases of RHD worldwide, 282,000 new cases, and 233,000 deaths annually [96]. Health-care expenditure for these disease entities is substantial. In fact, US expenditure estimates close to $2 billion annually for symptomatic and asymptomatic aortic VHD, and $2.6 billion for symptomatic and asymptomatic mitral VHD [97, 98].

Patients who meet indications for VHD surgery are frequently not offered surgery due to prohibitive risk features. As an example in the mitral VHD population, among patients who meet the current indications for surgical treatment of MR, almost 50% are not offered therapy due to several factors, including high surgical risk from comorbidities and frailty associated with advanced age [99, 100]. Importantly, though some patients may tolerate a surgical procedure, meaningful functional recovery is not achieved if they demonstrate marked frailty prior to the intervention [101]. Unfortunately, such patients are left with few clinical options, resulting in frequent referrals to palliative care and hospice programs. Fortunately, as we now know, patients earlier deemed inoperable or high risk for conventional VHD surgery have minimally invasive options to address their comorbid state. These include transcatheter aortic valve replacement (TAVR), transcatheter mitral valve replacement (TMVR), and Mitraclip. These procedures may be the ones most suitable for the frail population as they are part of the aforementioned patient populations that would otherwise be left without options. Currently, of the interventions for VHD that are performed, the three mentioned earlier are the ones that have the most impact on the frail population.

In a study aimed at studying inflammatory markers in patients undergoing TAVR in an attempt to estimate preoperative risk, two inflammatory markers were studied. Neopterin, a pteridine synthesized by activated macrophages, and immune activation-mediated tryptophan and its subsequent degradation had both been shown prior to be associated with frailty and chronic disease. Ultimately, increased immune activation and associated tryptophan degradation underscored the prognostic role of baseline inflammation for outcome in patients with severe AS undergoing TAVR [102]. The aforementioned inflammatory markers like IL-6, TNF-alpha, D-dimer, and CRP have not yet been studied in the frail population in regard to outcomes in VHD but may prove to be valuable area of further research.

Frailty is well known in the VHD population to be associated with poorer outcomes when compared to non-frail patients. Patients with a moderate to severe degree of frailty (defined as requiring assistance to ambulate or attend to their own bodily needs, or a modified Rankin score 4) are generally considered high risk for valvular surgery [103]. In a study conducted by Sepeheri et al., frailty had a strong positive relationship with the risk of major adverse cardiovascular and cerebrovascular events (MACCE) (odds ratio, 4.89; 95% confidence interval, 1.64–14.60) [104]. Relationships were stronger in older patients undergoing TAVR than younger patients undergoing CABG and VHD surgery (hazard ratio for frailty in TAVR, 3.31–4.89 vs. hazard ratio for non-TAVR, 1.10–3.16). One single-center experience of all cardiac operations demonstrated frailty to be an independent predictor of in-hospital mortality, institutional discharge, and reduced midterm survival [105]. In a study assessing the effect of frailty on mortality, length of stay (LOS), and discharge destination in patients post-TAVR, Chauhan et al. showed that frailty portended an increase in LOS and mortality [106]. Additionally, a study assessing preoperative computed tomography (CT) scans that are done as part of the workup for transcatheter therapeutic interventions for VHD shows that these CTs have proven useful in measuring the patient's skeletal mass index (SMI) and, thus, preoperative sarcopenia. This correlated directly to length of stay more strongly than the frailty index [107].

Many of the frail patients afflicted with MR, however, tolerate MitraClip and are able to recover from the femoral venotomy and general anesthesia required for this procedure. In one study assessing effectiveness of transcutaneous mitral valve repair with Mitraclip in 564 patients, frailty was noted in 57% of patients. The procedural success rate, nonetheless, was 91% defined as MR less than or equal to grade 2 and surviving the hospital stay. A majority of patients were discharged home with moderate or less MR than prior [108]. Patients with severe frailty who are bedridden and/or require constant nursing care may be too disabled to achieve meaningful benefit from MitraClip and may also be considered prohibitive for TAVR [101]. This, though, has yet to be assessed prospectively.

The interesting aspect of frailty in VHD is that the novel interventions in this field are generally aimed to treat non-operable or high, prohibitive risk individuals. Frail patients comprise a significant portion of this population indicating that understanding how best to treat these patients is of significant import for the field in its gestalt. As this field continues to develop more prolifically, addressing the frail patient will prove to be an area of in-depth study. Many practitioners share the belief that current interventions prove to reverse certain aspects of frailty but this has yet to be studied in a prospective trial.

11. Conclusions

Frailty is a significant disease entity affecting a myriad of clinical situations. How it affects the spectrum of CVD has been an area of interest and study for a number of years. With the advent of novel procedures in the realm of VHD and the expansion of patient populations now being considered as candidates for interventions, the topic of frailty, its interplay with CVD, and how it affects outcomes in patients with CVD are of the utmost import. As discussed earlier, current risk scores for patients undergoing cardiovascular surgery (STS and euroSCORE) have yet to include frailty as official criteria in their scoring systems, yet many practitioners still note frailty to be a condition predisposing patients to unfavorable outcomes and, thus, precluding them from interventions.

That frail patient suffers poorer outcomes is significant. From postintervention mortality to disposition postdischarge, frail patients perform suboptimally when compared to their non-frail counterparts. The generalized debility to which frail patients are predisposed may make them less tolerant of therapeutic postintervention treatments that would otherwise improve their outcomes, such as physical therapy and progressive exercise training. Their subclinical inflammatory state may further prevent wound healing and resolution. Also, their comorbid conditions may prevent complete healing and recovery as well. These hypotheses have not yet been studied and warrant further investigation for the purpose of elucidating ways to counteract the aforementioned poorer outcomes experienced by frail patients.

Frailty can be treated, potentially, with specific modalities, such as exercise, protein-calorie supplementation, vitamin D, and reduction of polypharmacy [109]. This shows that, although frailty is incredibly significant and has undeniable impacts on morbidity and mortality, it is something that is potentially reversible. With further study and therapeutic interventions tailored specifically to the frail patient, we may be able to expand our indications and improve the quality of life for a patient population known to suffer with a disease process different from any other.

Author details

Vinod Chainani[1]*, Russell Riehl[1], Geeta Chainani[5], Abir Abdo[2], Mauricio G. Cohen[3], Carlos Alfonso[3], Pedro Martinez-Clark[3], Carl J. Lavie[1], John P. Reilly[1] and Nidal Abi-Rafeh[4]

*Address all correspondence to: vinod.chainani@gmail.com

1 Ochsner Health System, John Ochsner Heart and Vascular Institute, Jefferson, Louisiana, USA

2 Louisiana State University Health Sciences Center, New Orleans, Louisiana, USA

3 University of Miami Miller School of Medicine, Miami, Florida, USA

4 Tulane University School of Medicine, New Orleans, Louisiana, USA

5 Windsor University School of Medicine, Saint kitts, Carribean

References

[1] Go AS, Mozaffarian D, Roger VL, et al. Heart disease and stroke statistics—2013 update: A report from the American Heart Association. Circulation. 2013;**127**(1):e6-e245

[2] Tracy RP. Emerging relationships of inflammation, cardiovascular disease and chronic diseases of aging. International Journal of Obesity and Related Metabolic Disorders. 2003;**27**(Suppl 3):S29-S34

[3] Singh M, Alexander K, Roger VL, et al. Frailty and its potential relevance to cardiovascular care. Mayo Clinic Proceedings. 2008;**83**(10):1146-1153

[4] Bouillon K, Batty GD, Hamer M, et al. Cardiovascular disease risk scores in identifying future frailty: The Whitehall II prospective cohort study. Heart. 2013;**99**(10):737-742

[5] Ekerstad N, Swahn E, Janzon M, et al. Frailty is independently associated with short-term outcomes for elderly patients with non-ST-segment elevation myocardial infarction. Circulation. 2011;**124**(22):2397-2404

[6] Afilalo J, Karunananthan S, Eisenberg MJ, Alexander KP, Bergman H. Role of frailty in patients with cardiovascular disease. American Journal of Cardiology. 2009;**103**(11): 1616-1621

[7] Chin A Paw MJ, Dekker JM, Feskens EJ, Schouten EG, Kromhout D. How to select a frail elderly population? A comparison of three working definitions. Journal of Clinical Epidemiology. 1999;**52**(11):1015-1021

[8] Newman AB, Gottdiener JS, Mcburnie MA, et al. Associations of subclinical cardiovascular disease with frailty. Journal of Gerontology: Series A Biological Sciences and Medical Sciences. 2001;**56**(3):M158-M166

[9] Chaves PH, Semba RD, Leng SX, et al. Impact of anemia and cardiovascular disease on frailty status of community-dwelling older women: The Women's Health and Aging Studies I and II. Journal of Gerontology: Series A Biological Sciences and Medical Sciences. 2005;**60**(6):729-735

[10] Woods NF, LaCroix AZ, Gray SL, et al. Frailty: Emergence and consequences in women aged 65 and older in the Women's Health Initiative Observational Study. Journal of American Geriatrics Society. 2005;**53**(8):1321-1330

[11] Klein BE, Klein R, Knudtson MD, Lee KE. Frailty, morbidity and survival. Archives of Gerontology and Geriatrics. 2005;**41**(2):141-149

[12] Cacciatore F, Abete P, Mazzella F, et al. Frailty predicts long-term mortality in elderly subjects with chronic heart failure. European Journal of Clinical Investigation. 2005;**35**(12):723-730

[13] Purser JL, Kuchibhatla MN, Fillenbaum GG, Harding T, Peterson ED, Alexander KP. Identifying frailty in hospitalized older adults with significant coronary artery disease. Journal of American Geriatrics Society. 2006;**54**(11):1674-1681

[14] Boxer RS, Wang Z, Walsh SJ, Hager D, Kenny AM. The utility of the 6-minute walk test as a measure of frailty in older adults with heart failure. The American Journal of Geriatric Cardiology. 2008;**17**(1):7-12

[15] Dumurgier J, Elbaz A, Ducimetière P, Tavernier B, Alpérovitch A, Tzourio C. Slow walking speed and cardiovascular death in well functioning older adults: Prospective cohort study. British Medical Journal. 2009;**339**:b4460

[16] Sanchis J, Núñez E, Ruiz V, et al. Usefulness of clinical data and biomarkers for the identification of frailty after acute coronary syndromes. Canadian Journal of Cardiology. 2015;**31**(12):1462-1468

[17] Fried LP, Tangen CM, Walston J, et al. Frailty in older adults: Evidence for a phenotype. The Journal of Gerontology: Series A Biological Sciences and Medical Sciences. 2001;**56**(3):M146-M156

[18] Fedarko NS. The biology of aging and frailty. Clinics in Geriatric Medicine. 2011;**27**(1):27-37

[19] Wang Z, Nakayama T. Inflammation, a link between obesity and cardiovascular disease. Mediators of Inflammation. 2010;**2010**:535918

[20] Zakynthinos E, Pappa N. Inflammatory biomarkers in coronary artery disease. Journal of Cardiology. 2009;**53**(3):317-333

[21] Yao X, Li H, Leng SX. Inflammation and immune system alterations in frailty. Clinics in Geriatric Medicine. 2011;**27**(1):79-87

[22] Biala AK, Dhingra R, Kirshenbaum LA. Mitochondrial dynamics: Orchestrating the journey to advanced age. Journal of Molecular and Cellular Cardiology. 2015;**83**:37-43

[23] Keller KM, Howlett SE. Sex differences in the biology and pathology of the aging heart. Canadian Journal of Cardiology. 2016;**32**(9):1065-1073

[24] Liu CK, Lyass A, Larson MG, et al. Biomarkers of oxidative stress are associated with frailty: The Framingham Offspring Study. Age (Dordr). 2016;**38**(1):1

[25] Morley JE, Malmstrom TK. Frailty, sarcopenia, and hormones. Endocrinology & Metabolism Clinics of North America. 2013;**42**(2):391-405

[26] Soysal P, Stubbs B, Lucato P, et al. Inflammation and frailty in the elderly: A systematic review and meta-analysis. Ageing Research Reviews. 2016;**31**:1-8

[27] Michaud M, Balardy L, Moulis G, et al. Proinflammatory cytokines, aging, and age-related diseases. Journal of the American Medical Directors Association. 2013;**14**(12):877-882

[28] Hunter CA, Jones SA. IL-6 as a keystone cytokine in health and disease. Nature Immunology. 2015;**16**(5):448-457

[29] Akki A, Yang H, Gupta A, et al. Skeletal muscle ATP kinetics are impaired in frail mice. Age (Dordr). 2014;**36**(1):21-30

[30] Lavie CJ, De Schutter A, Alpert MA, Mehra MR, Milani RV, Ventura HO. Obesity paradox, cachexia, frailty, and heart failure. Heart Failure Clinics. 2014;**10**(2):319-326

[31] Niedernhofer LJ, Kirkland JL, Ladiges W. Molecular pathology endpoints useful for aging studies. Ageing Research Reviews. 2016;**35**:241-249

[32] Lang PO, Mitchell WA, Lapenna A, Pitts D, Aspinall R. Immunological pathogenesis of main age-related diseases and frailty: Role of Immunosenescence. European Geriatric Medicine. 2010;**1**:112-121

[33] Khan H, Kalogeropoulos AP, Georgiopoulou VV, et al. Frailty and risk for heart failure in older adults: The health, aging, and body composition study. American Heart Journal. 2013;**166**(5):887-894

[34] Feridooni HA, Dibb KM, Howlett SE. How cardiomyocyte excitation, calcium release and contraction become altered with age. Journal of Molecular and Cellular Cardiology. 2015;**83**:62-72

[35] Kalidindi SR, Tang WH, Francis GS. Drug insight: Aldosterone-receptor antagonists in heart failure--the journey continues. Nature Clinical Practice Cardiovascular Medicine. 2007;**4**(7):368-378

[36] Singh A, Williams GH. Textbook of Nephro-Endocrinology. 1st ed. Amsterdam, Boston: Elsevier/Academic Press; 2009

[37] Muñoz-Durango N, Fuentes CA, Castillo AE, et al. Role of the renin-angiotensin-aldosterone system beyond blood pressure regulation: Molecular and cellular mechanisms involved in end-organ damage during arterial hypertension. International Journal of Molecular Science. 2016;**17**(7):797

[38] Wright JT, Williamson JD, Whelton PK, et al. A randomized trial of intensive versus standard blood-pressure control. New England Journal of Medicine. 2015;**373**(22):2103-2116

[39] Beckett NS, Peters R, Fletcher AE, et al. Treatment of hypertension in patients 80 years of age or older. New England Journal of Medicine. 2008;**358**(18):1887-1898

[40] Langer RD, Criqui MH, Barrett-Connor EL, Klauber MR, Ganiats TG. Blood pressure change and survival after age 75. Hypertension. 1993;**22**(4):551-559

[41] Gueyffier F, Bulpitt C, Boissel JP, et al. Antihypertensive drugs in very old people: A subgroup meta-analysis of randomised controlled trials. INDANA Group. Lancet. 1999;**353**(9155):793-796

[42] Landi F, Cesari M, Calvani R, et al. The "Sarcopenia and Physical fRailty IN older people: Multi-componenT Treatment strategies" (SPRINTT) randomized controlled trial: Design and methods. Aging Clinical and Experimental Research. 2017;**29**(1):89-100

[43] Materson BJ, Garcia-Estrada M, Preston RA. Hypertension in the frail elderly. Journal of the American Society of Hypertension. 2016;**10**(6):536-541

[44] Warwick J, Falaschetti E, Rockwood K, et al. No evidence that frailty modifies the positive impact of antihypertensive treatment in very elderly people: An investigation of the impact of frailty upon treatment effect in the HYpertension in the Very Elderly Trial (HYVET) study, a double-blind, placebo-controlled study of antihypertensives in people with hypertension aged 80 and over. Boston Medical Center Medicine. 2015;**13**:78

[45] Pajewski NM, Williamson JD, Applegate WB, et al. Characterizing Frailty Status in the Systolic Blood Pressure Intervention Trial. The Journal of Gerontology Series A Biological Sciences and Medical Sciences. 2016;**71**(5):649-655

[46] van Hateren KJ, Hendriks SH, Groenier KH, et al. Frailty and the relationship between blood pressure and mortality in elderly patients with type 2 diabetes (Zwolle Outpatient Diabetes project Integrating Available Care-34). Journal of Hypertension. 2015;**33**(6):1162-1166

[47] Won CW, Kim S. Use of frailty in deciding clinical treatment goals for chronic disease in elderly patients in the community. Journal of the American Medical Directors Association. 2016;**17**(11):967-969

[48] Landi F, Russo A, Pahor M, et al. Serum high-density lipoprotein cholesterol levels and mortality in frail, community-living elderly. Gerontology. 2008;**54**(2):71-78

[49] Landi F, Russo A, Cesari M, Pahor M, Bernabei R, Onder G. HDL-cholesterol and physical performance: Results from the ageing and longevity study in the sirente geographic area (ilSIRENTE Study). Age Ageing. 2007;**36**(5):514-520

[50] Ramsay SE, Arianayagam DS, Whincup PH, et al. Cardiovascular risk profile and frailty in a population-based study of older British men. Heart. 2015;**101**(8):616-622

[51] van den Kommer TN, Dik MG, Comijs HC, Fassbender K, Lütjohann D, Jonker C. Total cholesterol and oxysterols: Early markers for cognitive decline in elderly? Neurobiology of Aging. 2009;**30**(4):534-545

[52] Roubenoff R, Parise H, Payette HA, et al. Cytokines, insulin-like growth factor 1, sarcopenia, and mortality in very old community-dwelling men and women: The Framingham Heart Study. American Journal of Medicine. 2003;**115**(6):429-435

[53] Hwang AC, Liu LK, Lee WJ, et al. Association of frailty and cardiometabolic risk among community-dwelling middle-aged and older people: Results from the I-Lan Longitudinal Aging Study. Rejuvenation Research. 2015;**18**(6):564-572

[54] Carriere I, Pérès K, Ancelin ML, et al. Metabolic syndrome and disability: Findings from the prospective three-city study. The Journal of Gerontology Series A Biological Sciences and Medical Sciences. 2014;**69**(1):79-86

[55] Wang X, Guo Z, Ding Z, et al. Endothelin-1 upregulation mediates aging-related cardiac fibrosis. Journal of Molecular and Cellular Cardiology. 2015;**80**:101-109

[56] Pulignano G, Del Sindaco D, Tinti MD, et al. Atrial fibrillation, cognitive impairment, frailty and disability in older heart failure patients. Journal of Cardiovascular Medicine (Hagerstown). 2016;**17**(8):616-623

[57] Bibas L, Levi M, Touchette J, et al. Implications of frailty in elderly patients with electrophysiological conditions. JACC: Clinical Electrophysiology. 2016;**2**(3):288-294

[58] Polidoro A, Stefanelli F, Ciacciarelli M, Pacelli A, Di Sanzo D, Alessandri C. Frailty in patients affected by atrial fibrillation. Archives of Gerontology and Geriatrics. 2013;**57**(3):325-327

[59] Nguyen TN, Cumming RG, Hilmer SN. The impact of frailty on mortality, length of stay and re-hospitalisation in older patients with atrial fibrillation. Heart, Lung and Circulation. 2016;**25**(6):551-557

[60] Veronese N, Cereda E, Stubbs B, et al. Risk of cardiovascular disease morbidity and mortality in frail and pre-frail older adults: Results from a meta-analysis and exploratory meta-regression analysis. Ageing Research Reviews. 2017;**35**:63-73

[61] Granziera S, Cohen AT, Nante G, Manzato E, Sergi G. Thromboembolic prevention in frail elderly patients with atrial fibrillation: A practical algorithm. Journal of the American Medical Directors Association. 2015;**16**(5):358-364

[62] Solfrizzi V, Scafato E, Frisardi V, et al. Frailty syndrome and the risk of vascular dementia: The Italian Longitudinal Study on Aging. Alzheimer's & Dementia. 2013;**9**(2):113-122

[63] Ruan Q, Yu Z, Chen M, Bao Z, Li J, He W. Cognitive frailty, a novel target for the prevention of elderly dependency. Ageing Research Review. 2015;**20**:1-10

[64] Chung CP, Chou KH, Chen WT, et al. Cerebral microbleeds are associated with physical frailty: A community-based study. Neurobiology of Aging. 2016;**44**:143-150

[65] Melin AA, Schmid KK, Lynch TG, et al. Preoperative frailty Risk Analysis Index to stratify patients undergoing carotid endarterectomy. Journal of Vascular Surgery. 2015;**61**(3):683-689

[66] Borissoff JI, Spronk HM, ten Cate H. The hemostatic system as a modulator of atherosclerosis. New England Journal of Medicine. 2011;**364**(18):1746-1760

[67] Libby P. Mechanisms of acute coronary syndromes and their implications for therapy. New England Journal of Medicine. 2013;**368**(21):2004-2013

[68] Afilalo J, Alexander KP, Mack MJ, et al. Frailty assessment in the cardiovascular care of older adults. Journal of American College of Cardiology. 2014;**63**(8):747-762

[69] Newman AB, Simonsick EM, Naydeck BL, et al. Association of long-distance corridor walk performance with mortality, cardiovascular disease, mobility limitation, and disability. Journal of American Medical Association. 2006;**295**(17):2018-2026

[70] Gharacholou SM, Roger VL, Lennon RJ, et al. Comparison of frail patients versus nonfrail patients ≥65 years of age undergoing percutaneous coronary intervention. American Journal of Cardiology. 2012;**109**(11):1569-1575

[71] Goodpaster BH, Carlson CL, Visser M, et al. Attenuation of skeletal muscle and strength in the elderly: The Health ABC Study. Journal of Applied Physiology (1985). 2001;**90**(6):2157-2165

[72] Srinivas-Shankar U, Roberts SA, Connolly MJ, et al. Effects of testosterone on muscle strength, physical function, body composition, and quality of life in intermediate-frail and frail elderly men: A randomized, double-blind, placebo-controlled study. Journal of Clinical Endocrinology and Metabolism. 2010;**95**(2):639-650

[73] Waters DL, Qualls CR, Dorin RI, Veldhuis JD, Baumgartner RN. Altered growth hormone, cortisol, and leptin secretion in healthy elderly persons with sarcopenia and mixed body composition phenotypes. The Journal of Gerontology Series A Biological Sciences and Medical Sciences. 2008;**63**(5):536-541

[74] Dodson JA, Arnold SV, Gosch KL, et al. Slow gait speed and risk of mortality or hospital readmission after myocardial infarction in the translational research investigating underlying disparities in recovery from acute myocardial infarction: Patients' Health Status Registry. Journal of American Geriatric Society. 2016;**64**(3):596-601

[75] O'Neill DE, Knudtson ML, Kieser TM, Graham MM. Considerations in cardiac revascularization for the elderly patient: age isn't everything. Canadian Journal of Cardiology. 2016;**32**(9):1132-1139

[76] Kang L, Zhang SY, Zhu WL, et al. Is frailty associated with short-term outcomes for elderly patients with acute coronary syndrome? Journal of Geriatric Cardiology. 2015;**12**(6):662-667

[77] Murali-Krishnan R, Iqbal J, Rowe R, et al. Impact of frailty on outcomes after percutaneous coronary intervention: A prospective cohort study. Open Heart. 2015;**2**(1):e000294

[78] Freiheit EA, Hogan DB, Patten SB, et al. Frailty trajectories after treatment for coronary artery disease in older patients. Circulation: Cardiovascular Quality and Outcomes. 2016;**9**(3):230-238

[79] Singh M, Rihal CS, Lennon RJ, Spertus JA, Nair KS, Roger VL. Influence of frailty and health status on outcomes in patients with coronary disease undergoing percutaneous revascularization. Circulation: Cardiovascular Quality and Outcomes. 2011;**4**(5):496-502

[80] Thukkani AK, Kinlay S. Endovascular intervention for peripheral artery disease. Circulation Research. 2015;**116**(9):1599-1613

[81] Suzuki J, Shimamura M, Suda H, et al. Current therapies and investigational drugs for peripheral arterial disease. Hypertension Research. 2016;**39**(4):183-191

[82] Ochi M, Kohara K, Tabara Y, et al. Arterial stiffness is associated with low thigh muscle mass in middle-aged to elderly men. Atherosclerosis. 2010;**212**(1):327-332

[83] Lin CH, Chou CY, Liu CS, Huang CY, Li TC, Lin CC. Association between frailty and subclinical peripheral vascular disease in a community-dwelling geriatric population: Taichung Community Health Study for Elders. Geriatrics & Gerontology International. 2015;**15**(3):261-267

[84] Toosizadeh N, Stocker H, Thiede R, Mohler J, Mills JL, Najafi B. Alterations in gait parameters with peripheral artery disease: The importance of pre-frailty as a confounding variable. Vascular Medicine. 2016;**21**(6):520-527

[85] Ehlert BA, Najafian A, Orion KC, Malas MB, Black JH, Abularrage CJ. Validation of a modified Frailty Index to predict mortality in vascular surgery patients. Journal of Vascular Surgery. 2016;**63**(6):1595-1601.e1592

[86] Arya S, Long CA, Brahmbhatt R, et al. Preoperative frailty increases risk of nonhome discharge after elective vascular surgery in home-dwelling patients. Annals in Vascular Surgery. 2016;**35**:19-29

[87] Brahmbhatt R, Brewster LP, Shafii S, et al. Gender and frailty predict poor outcomes in infrainguinal vascular surgery. Journal of Surgical Research. 2016;**201**(1):156-165

[88] Jha SR, Ha HS, Hickman LD, et al. Frailty in advanced heart failure: A systematic review. Heart Failure Reviews. 2015;**20**(5):553-560

[89] Nadruz W, Kitzman D, Windham BG, et al. Cardiovascular dysfunction and frailty among older adults in the community: The ARIC study. The Journal of Gerontology Series A Biological Sciences and Medical Sciences. 2016;**72**:958-964

[90] Lupón J, González B, Santaeugenia S, et al. Prognostic implication of frailty and depressive symptoms in an outpatient population with heart failure. Revista Española de Cardiología. 2008;**61**(8):835-842

[91] McNallan SM, Singh M, Chamberlain AM, et al. Frailty and healthcare utilization among patients with heart failure in the community. JACC Heart Failure. 2013;**1**(2):135-141

[92] Rolland Y, Dupuy C, Abellan van Kan G, Gillette S, Vellas B. Treatment strategies for sarcopenia and frailty. Medical Clinics of North America. 2011;**95**(3):427-438, ix

[93] Lavie CJ, Forman DE, Arena R. Bulking up skeletal muscle to improve heart failure prognosis. JACC Heart Failure. 2016;**4**(4):274-276

[94] Pendergast DR, Fisher NM, Calkins E. Cardiovascular, neuromuscular, and metabolic alterations with age leading to frailty. Journal of Gerontology. 1993;**48** Spec No:61-67

[95] Joyce E. Frailty in advanced heart failure. Heart Failure Clinics. 2016;**12**(3):363-374

[96] Carapetis JR, Steer AC, Mulholland EK, Weber M. The global burden of group A streptococcal diseases. The Lancet Infectious Diseases. 2005;**5**(11):685-694

[97] Kern DM, DeVore S, Kim J, et al. Abstract 53: Health care utilization and cost among type 2 diabetes mellitus (T2DM) patients with cardiovascular disease (CVD) or cardiovascular disease risk factors. Circulation: Cardiovascular Quality and Outcomes. 2015;**6**(Suppl 1):A53

[98] Chen J, Mallow PJ, Moore M, Rizzo JA. Abstract 257: The direct healthcare expenditures of aortic valve disease: Evidence from US National Survey Data. Circulation: Cardiovascular Quality and Outcomes. 2016;**9**(Suppl 2):A257

[99] Mirabel M, Iung B, Baron G, et al. What are the characteristics of patients with severe, symptomatic, mitral regurgitation who are denied surgery? European Heart Journal. 2007;**28**(11):1358-1365

[100] Bach DS, Awais M, Gurm HS, Kohnstamm S. Failure of guideline adherence for intervention in patients with severe mitral regurgitation. Journal of American College of Cardiology. 2009;**54**(9):860-865

[101] Vesely MR, Benitez RM, Robinson SW, Collins JA, Dawood MY, Gammie JS. Surgical and transcatheter mitral valve repair for severe chronic mitral regurgitation: A review of clinical indications and patient assessment. Journal of the American Heart Association. 2015;**4**(12):e002424

[102] Csordas A, Fuchs D, Frangieh AH, et al. Immunological markers of frailty predict outcomes beyond current risk scores in aortic stenosis following transcatheter aortic valve replacement: Role of neopterin and tryptophan. IJC Metabolic & Endocrine. 2016;**10**:7-15

[103] Nishimura RA, Otto CM, Bonow RO, et al. 2014 AHA/ACC guideline for the management of patients with valvular heart disease: a report of the American College of Cardiology/American Heart Association Task Force on Practice Guidelines. Journal of Thoracic and Cardiovascular Surgery. 2014;**148**(1):e1-e132

[104] Sepehri A, Beggs T, Hassan A, et al. The impact of frailty on outcomes after cardiac surgery: A systematic review. Journal of Thoracic and Cardiovascular Surgery. 2014;**148**(6):3110-3117

[105] Lee DH, Buth KJ, Martin BJ, Yip AM, Hirsch GM. Frail patients are at increased risk for mortality and prolonged institutional care after cardiac surgery. Circulation. 2010;**121**(8):973-978

[106] Chauhan D, Haik N, Merlo A, et al. Quantitative increase in frailty is associated with diminished survival after transcatheter aortic valve replacement. American Heart Journal. 2016;**182**:146-154

[107] Dahya V, Xiao J, Prado CM, et al. Computed tomography-derived skeletal muscle index: A novel predictor of frailty and hospital length of stay after transcatheter aortic valve replacement. American Heart Journal. 2016;**182**:21-27

[108] Sorajja P, Mack M, Vemulapalli S, et al. Initial experience with commercial transcatheter mitral valve repair in the United States. Journal of American College of Cardiology. 2016;**67**(10):1129-1140

[109] Morley JE, Vellas B, van Kan GA, et al. Frailty consensus: A call to action. Journal of American Medical Directors Association. 2013;**14**(6):392-397

11

Allogeneic Mesenchymal Stem Cells as a Treatment for Aging Frailty

Bryon A. Tompkins, Ana Marie Landin,
Victoria Florea, Makoto Natsumeda,
Angela C. Rieger, Wayne Balkan,
Ivonne Hernandez Schulman and Joshua M. Hare

Abstract

As life expectancy is projected to increase in the ensuing decades, individuals of older age continue to exceed the previous generation's lifespan. Advancing age is associated with a reduction in physical and mental functional capacity, and chronic inflammation is a major factor contributing to this decline. A heightened inflammatory state can lead to exhaustion, weakness, weight loss, slow gate speed, and an overall decrease in activity level. These phenotypes define the onset of the disease process known as frailty. Frailty is a growing epidemic, which severely undermines a person's ability to deal with outside stressors, and increases their rate of hospitalization, institutionalization, and mortality. Current interventions focus on preventative care by improving exercise capacity, strength, nutritional supplementation, diet, and mobility. However, a biological cure has heretofore remained elusive. Here, we introduce the novel therapeutic principle that mesenchymal stem cell (MSC) therapy may represent a safe, practical, and efficacious both the treatment and prevention of frailty in individuals of advancing age. To date, a phase I safety trial reveals an excellent safety profile and suggests that mesenchymal stem cells can ameliorate signs and symptoms of frailty. These early studies lay the groundwork for future large-scale clinical trials of this exciting and novel therapeutic concept that has the potential to expand health span in the aging population.

Keywords: mesenchymal stem cells, immunomodulation, frailty, tumor necrosis factor-alpha, regenerative medicine

1. Introduction

Projected life expectancy continues to grow worldwide owing to the advancement of new treatments and technologies for leading causes of death such as cardiovascular disease and cancer [1]. Meanwhile, frailty is gaining relevance as a significant clinical syndrome that is associated with increased risk of falls, depression, and disability, leading to higher mortality [2]. Frailty is defined by an age-related decline in reserve and function leading to a reduced ability to cope with acute or external stressors [3] and is characterized by easy tiring, decreased libido, mood disturbance, accelerated osteoporosis, diminished muscle strength, and susceptibility to disease. However, the pathophysiology underlying this syndrome is complex and not clearly understood [4].

Inflammation is a pathophysiologic change that is closely linked with frailty [5]. Aging is associated with immunosenescence or the dysregulation of the innate immune system, resulting in an increase of pro-inflammatory cytokines such as tumor necrosis factor (TNF)-α, interleukin (IL)-6, and IL-1β, further leading to a chronic low-grade inflammatory state [6]. Chronic inflammatory response inhibits the repair, turnover, and adaptation of many tissues, including skeletal muscle [6]. Regeneration of skeletal muscle involves the cross-talk of muscle cells with immune cells, where the pro-inflammatory phenotype of immune cells promotes migration of satellite cells to the injured area, activates satellite cells, and matures newly formed muscle fibers [7]. Muscular degeneration caused by the altered pro-inflammatory state in frail patients is referred to as sarcopenia, another critical physiologic component of frailty.

Aging also produces physiologic changes in the brain, contributing to the development of frailty. Neurons with high metabolic demands, such as the hippocampal pyramidal neurons, are an important mediator in the pathophysiology of cognitive decline and are a key component of the stress response [3]. Concomitant with changes in the immune system, microglial cells, which are the resident immune cells of the central nervous system, are also structurally and functionally altered with aging and undergo senescence, likely causing damage and neuronal death [8]. Accumulating evidence supports an association between frailty, cognitive impairment, and dementia [9, 10].

The brain and endocrine system are intrinsically linked through the hypothalamo-pituitary axis, controlling metabolism via a series of homeostatic hormones. Four major circulating hormones are affected by aging: first, the decrease of insulin-like growth factor 1 (IGF-1) is associated with lower strength and decreased mobility [11]. Second, decreased sex hormone (estradiol and testosterone) increases the release of luteinizing hormone and follicle-stimulating hormone [12]. Third, decreased activity of the adrenocortical cells produces the major sex steroid precursor dehydroepiandrosterone sulfate (DHEA-S), which is associated with a gradual rise in cortisol. DHEA-S directly maintains muscle mass and indirectly prevents the inflammatory pathways that contribute to muscle decline [13, 14]. Finally, the reduced level of 25(OH) vitamin D is associated with the development of osteoporosis [15].

Due to the complexity of multiple inter-related physiological systems that contribute to frailty, there is no gold standard for diagnosing the syndrome. There are currently two models for evaluating frailty: the phenotype model and the cumulative deficit model that forms the basis

Frailty phenotypes	MSC response	Postulated mechanism of action
Weight loss	Maintains total caloric expenditure	↓ Inflammation which suppresses the onset of sarcopenia
Exhaustion	↑ Pulmonary function, ↓ chronic inflammation	↑ Endothelial function, ↓ markers of inflammation
Weakness	↑ Physical performance	↑ Mitochondrial transfer, ↑endogenous stem cell function
Slow gate speed	↑ 6-minute walk distance	↑ Endothelial function, ↑ cardiac performance, ↑skeletal muscle performance
Decreased activity level	↓ Chronic inflammation, ↑ quality of life	↓ TNF-α, ↓ IL-1β, ↑ IL-10

Notes: MSCs home to sites of injury and to enhance repair of damaged tissue (heart, joints, muscle, and blood vessels) and exert their regenerative effects via paracrine signaling, mitochondrial transfer, direct cellular contact, and exosome excretion.

Table 1. The effect of MSCs on the phenotypes of frailty.

of the Canadian Study of Health and Aging (CSHA) frailty index [16]. The phenotype model defines frailty as meeting three or more of five criteria: weight loss (>5% of body weight in the previous year), exhaustion (positive response to questions regarding effort required for activity), weakness (decreased grip strength), slow gait speed (>6–7 seconds for walking 15 feet), decreased physical activity, or low energy expenditure (kcal spent per week: males expending <383 kcal, females expending <270 kcal) (**Table 1**) [17]. This model is simple and easy to use; however, it fails to include factors such as cognitive impairment and highly prevalent conditions associated with functional decline and disability [3].

The cumulative deficit model is based on the accumulation of illnesses, functional and cognitive declines, and social situations that are added together to calculate frailty [16]. This model utilizes 20 or more medically and functionally related questions and 92 baseline variables. The deficit model fashioned the origin of the CSHA frailty index [3]. The frailty index measures a number of age-associated health deficits (signs, symptoms, and laboratory values) [18], which is calculated by dividing each 'deficit' by the total number tested [3]. The higher the number of deficits, the higher the score, with '1' being the maximum index, which indicates a poorer prognosis. Specifically, Rockwood and Mitnitski noted that an index >0.7 indicates a high risk of mortality [19]. In an effort to simplify this index, the same authors proposed the CSHA clinical frailty score, a 7-point rapid screening tool that was highly correlated with the frailty index; with 7 being the maximum score, indicating "severe frailty" [20]. The clinical frailty score is currently widely used in clinical practice [21].

2. Epidemiology

Universal characteristics that are associated with an increased prevalence of frailty include: chronological age, female sex, racial, and ethnic minority, those in supportive residential settings, and lower income [22]. The prevalence among community-dwelling people over 65 years of age ranges from 4 to 17% in studies with varying geographic features [23, 24]. There are similar trends in Japan, the country with the highest life expectancy in the world. The reason for longevity in Japan is multifactorial. The universal health insurance system, the high population density with close access to hospitals, fish-based diets, awareness of healthy aging in the general public, and lower prevalence of lung cancer despite a higher population of smokers are some contributors [25]. Interestingly, a meta-analyses of frail Japanese patients using the phenotype model demonstrated that the age-stratified-weighted prevalence of frailty was lower in younger age groups (1.9% in 65–69 years, 3.8% in 70–74 years), the same in the 75–79-year age groups (10.0%), but higher in older age groups (20.4% in 80–84 years, 35.1% in ≥85 years) when compared to Western countries [25]. One explanation is that non-Japanese frail older individuals die younger, while Japanese frail older individuals survive longer, leading to a higher prevalence of frailty in their 80s.

3. Intervention and preventive care

While there is no cure for frailty, exercise is considered the most effective intervention to improve quality of life and functionality in frail adults. Improvements in muscle strength and mobility [26, 27] are among the most successful changes reported. Several studies have demonstrated an improvement in muscle strength in older persons with resistance exercise [28–30]. A longitudinal study of aging showed that physical activity is associated with a slower progression in functional limitations in older adults over a follow-up period of 6 months [31]. A randomized, placebo-controlled trial compared resistance exercise training, multinutrient supplementation, both interventions, and neither intervention (control group) in frail adults over a period of 10 weeks. The study suggested that high-intensity resistance exercise training improved muscle strength, gait velocity, and stair-climbing power. However, nutritional supplementation did not reduce muscle weakness or physical frailty [28]. Similarly, the LIFE-P (lifestyle interventions and independence for Elders pilot) exploratory study demonstrated that regular physical activity reduces frailty prevalence at a 12-month follow-up time point [32].

Another approach to delay frailty is the use of nutritional supplements, which increase protein and caloric daily intake. Administration of leucine-enriched essential amino acids can increase muscle synthesis through stimulation of the mechanistic target of rapamycin (mTOR) signaling pathway [33]. The PROT-AGE study [34] reviewed the dietary protein intake in older healthy people (>65 years). They found that the optimal protein intake in older persons with sarcopenia is 1.0–1.2 g/kg body weight per day, and higher protein intake >1.2 g/kg body weight per day for those who are exercising. The PROVIDE trial [35] assessed protein supplements enriched in leucine and vitamin D in sarcopenic older adults at high risk for disability. The study demonstrated that the group receiving high quantity protein supplements gained significantly more muscle mass and improved their chair stand ability relative to the control group.

The randomized Controlled Trial of Community-based Nutritional, Physical and Cognitive Training Intervention Programmes for At Risk Frail Elderly (FIT) compared the effects of 6-month interventions with either nutritional supplementation, cognitive training, physical activity, the combination treatments, or no intervention (control) in prefrail and frail adults [36]. Frailty score and status were measured at 3, 6 and 12 months. While these parameters were reduced in all groups, including the controls, the other four groups were significantly improved compared to the controls, at all three time points. However, none of the interventions improved the secondary endpoints, which included: hospitalizations, falls, and performance of activities of daily living [36]. Recent studies suggest that vitamin D plays a role in the pathogenesis and management of frailty [37, 38]. One such study demonstrated that daily doses of ≥800 IU of vitamin D has beneficial effects on balance and muscle strength [39]; while another reported an improvement in balance with a single large dose of vitamin D [40]. While an analysis of 53 trials showed that vitamin D supplementation alone does not prevent fractures in older adults [41], supplementation of vitamin D in combination with calcium can prevent disabling hip fractures among others [41].

While diet and exercise have been thoroughly evaluated, hormone therapy has also been tested. Testosterone undecanoate plus a high-calorie supplement (2108–2416 kJ/day) was compared with a control group (placebo plus a low-calorie supplement (142–191 kJ/day)) in a randomized controlled trial. The results showed that there were no significant differences in frailty scores at either 6- or 12-month follow-up between the groups [42]. While testosterone treatment improves muscle strength, it also increases incidence of adverse cardiovascular events [43]. Estrogen in combination with progestin therapy in postmenopausal women increases the risk of incident breast cancer after 5.6- or 7.1-years of follow-up [44, 45]. Likewise, the benefits of dehydroepiandrosterone sulfate (DHEA-S) supplementation in frail patients have not been demonstrated. Older subjects who received DHEA for 2 years exhibited no beneficial effects on body composition, physical performance, or quality of life [46]. Similarly, 1 year of treatment with insulin-like growth factor 1 (IGF-1) did not alter bone mineral density, fat mass, muscle strength, blood lipid parameters, and measures of postprandial glucose disposal in postmenopausal women [47].

Frailty is increasingly recognized as a clinical state of vulnerability with increased risk of adverse health outcomes. The pathogenesis that underlies this syndrome is multifactorial and elusive, and there is not yet a gold standard for diagnosis or treatment. Exercise and nutritional supplementations are currently the key interventions for frailty. Although helpful, none of them have been proven to treat the disease process. Therefore, an alternative approach to treating frail adults needs to be investigated. Here, we focus on a novel intervention, allogeneic mesenchymal stem cells (allo-MSCs) as a potential therapy for the treatment of frailty. While the mechanism is as yet unclear, we propose that the beneficial effects of MSCs for frailty are due, in large part, to a combination of their immunomodulatory, antifibrotic, and pro-regenerative effects.

4. Regenerative medicine

Frailty is a multifactorial condition triggered by genetic and environmental factors. As previously described, there is a direct association between frailty and the loss of proliferative homeostasis, neurodegeneration, DNA/mitochondrial mutations, free radical accumulation, a rise in pro-inflammatory markers, and increased immunosenescence. Stem cell depletion is a key mechanism postulated to contribute to frailty and its epigenetic dysregulation [48–50]. Thus, the repletion of stem cells is an appealing approach to treat this multifactorial dysregulation and MSCs are a particularly attractive candidate. MSCs are a multipotent, self-renewing somatic progenitor cell type that exhibits immunoprivileged properties [51–53] and are relatively easy to collect (bone marrow harvest), isolate, and expand [54, 55].

MSCs home to sites of injury, upregulate endogenous stem cells, and reduce inflammation and organ dysfunction [56–61]. With respect to age-related diseases, MSCs have demonstrated improvements in ischemic and nonischemic cardiomyopathies [62–64], stroke [65], systemic inflammation [66], and Parkinson's, among others [67]. Although not completely understood, the beneficial effects of stem cells are likely due primarily to paracrine signaling [68, 69] including microvesicle/exosome release [70, 71] and secondarily to direct cellular contact including gap junction formation [72] and mitochondrial exchange via tunneling nanotubes [73, 60].

MSC effects at the molecular level are secondary to the secretion of growth factors, chemokines, and metalloproteinases, including vascular endothelial growth factor (VEGF), angiopoetin-1, fibroblast growth factor, placental growth factor, stem cell-derived factor (SDF), plasminogen activator [74], hepatocyte growth factor/scatter factor (HGF/SF) [75], secreted frizzled-related protein 2 (Sfrp2), hypoxic-induced Akt-regulated stem cell factor (HASF) and IGF-1 and -2 [76]. These molecules stimulate the Akt pathway [77], promote vasculogenesis [56], and protect native cells under hypoxic conditions [68]. In the heart, injection of MSCs produces antifibrotic, anti-inflammatory, and proangiogenic [57–59] effects and upregulates the proliferation of endogenous cardiac stem cells [60, 61], while improving the preservation of function of the cells surrounding the sites of injection.

MSCs mediate metabolic changes and stimulate resident cell activation after injury. *In vitro* studies have shown that MSC-conditioned culture media stimulates resident cardiac stem cells to proliferate, differentiate, and migrate [53, 78] via IGF-1. HASF and Sfrp2 prevent cardiomyocyte apoptosis, promote cardiac stem cell differentiation, and reduce fibrosis after myocardial infarction (MI) [79–81].

The absence of major histocompatibility complex (MHC) class II antigens underlies the lack of allo-MSCs to stimulate a major immune response [82] and has generated an interest in their systemic and local application without the need for immunosuppression [62]. In the clinical setting, multiple trials have evaluated and proven the safety and efficacy of MSC therapy [63, 64, 83–85]. Several disease processes have been studied in humans: autoimmune diseases, organ transplantation, and as a therapeutic agent after solid organ injury.

5. Immune biomarkers in aging and frailty

Aging and frailty are associated with a dramatic impairment of the ability of the immune system to provide protection from new pathogens. Older frail individual has serious complications that cause adverse health outcomes including acute illness, heightened inflammatory state, and immune dysregulation, which cause a severe impairment in both innate and adaptive immunity and greater susceptibility to infectious diseases, comorbidities, and increased mortality [86, 87]. The accumulation of reactive oxygen species (ROS) in the aging process leads, in part, to chronic activation of Toll-like receptors (TLRs), which in turn leads to an increase in the inflammatory process [88–90]. In frailty, the immune phenotype is dysregulated due to incrementing chronic inflammation known as inflammaging and includes increased IL-6, C-reactive peptide (CRP), and TNF-α [87]. Inflammaging plays an important role in the suppression of the immune system and the remodeling of the immune phenotype (**Figure 1**). The remodeling of the immune phenotype in aging is known as immunosenescence and is marked by several immune biomarkers described below.

The immune risk phenotype (IRP), which is the ratio of CD4+ to CD8+ T cells, decreases to <1 in aging and frailty, has been linked to increased risk of mortality [91, 92]. The decreased IRP associated with aging and frailty is due to an expansion of the CD8+ compartment in comparison to the CD4+ compartment. In spite of the expansion of the CD8+ T-cell compartment, the effector T cells in frail individuals have diminished function mostly due to antigen experienced CD8+ T cells re-expressing the naïve marker CD45RA, also known as TEMRA T cells [87]. This expansion of the TEMRA T cell population is exacerbated by factors such as chronic activation due to Cytomegalovirus (CMV) exposure known to be present in >60% of the US population [93]. Finally, the ability to produce protective antibodies upon new antigenic exposure is also severely impaired in aging and frailty due to a remodeling of the B cell compartment. In addition, there is an intrinsic defect in B cells in aging, which causes a decrease in the enzyme, activation-induced cytidine deaminase (AID) leading to diminished ability to switch antibody isotype, which has been correlated to increased TNF-α [94]. The inflammaging process depletes the B cell compartment of switched memory B cells, which are a predictive biomarker for protective vaccine response. In addition, the refractory/exhausted B cell compartment is expanded filling up the B cell niche with unresponsive cells [86, 94, 95].

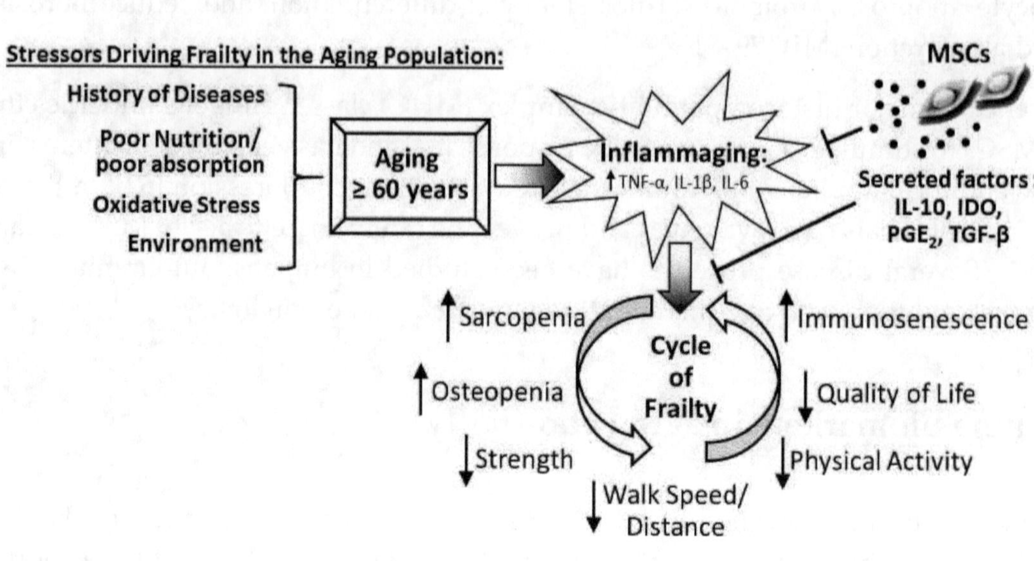

Figure 1. The role of stressors, aging, and inflammation in frailty and the effects of mesenchymal stem cells. As individuals grow older, several stressors (poor nutrition, diseases, oxidative stress, and environmental factors) increase the inflammaging process leading to frailty. Mesenchymal stem cells (MSCs) secrete several factors that block or reverse the inflammaging process and ultimately reverses the effects of frailty.

6. The role of MSCs in inflammaging and immune modulation

Human bone marrow-derived MSCs downregulate the expression of pro-inflammatory cytokines TNF-α, IL-1β, IL-6, and monocyte chemoattractant protein-1 (**Figure 2**) [96, 32]. Other immunomodulatory properties include the inhibition of dendritic cells, natural killer cells [97–99], and T/B cell proliferation via the downregulation of the molecules programmed death-1 (PD-1) transforming growth factor-β, HGF, nitric oxide, indoleamine 2,3-dioxygenase, and prostaglandin-E2 release [52, 68]. Interestingly, MSCs are able to transform pro-inflammatory macrophages (M1) into anti-inflammatory macrophages (M2) by upregulating IGF-1 and IL-10 [100], thereby promoting angiogenesis and cardiomyocyte recovery [101, 102]. Most importantly, MSCs suppress T cell activation, which is crucial due to the high incidence of CMV virus among the US population, causing chronic activation of T cells leading to an exhausted immune phenotype [103].

Ground-breaking immune-modulatory results in the Randomized Comparison of Allogeneic Versus Autologous Mesenchymal Stem Cells for Nonischemic Dilated Cardiomyopathy: POSEIDON-DCM study demonstrated that 6 months post-TESI, allogeneic human mesenchymal stem cells (hMSCs) were more efficient than auto-hMSCs in reducing serum levels of TNF-α, increased switched memory B cells, decreased exhausted B cells concomitant with a decrease in the percentage of B cells expressing TNF-α, decreased T cell activation and decreased TEMRA T cells [62]. This reversal on the effects of chronic inflammation on these immune biomarkers opens up the feasibility of using allo-hMSC as a treatment to reverse the process of inflammaging and immunosenescence.

Together, these findings are indicative of the safety of MSC therapy in a variety of disease processes. Furthermore, given that MSCs are known to elicit immunomodulatory, neoangiogenic,

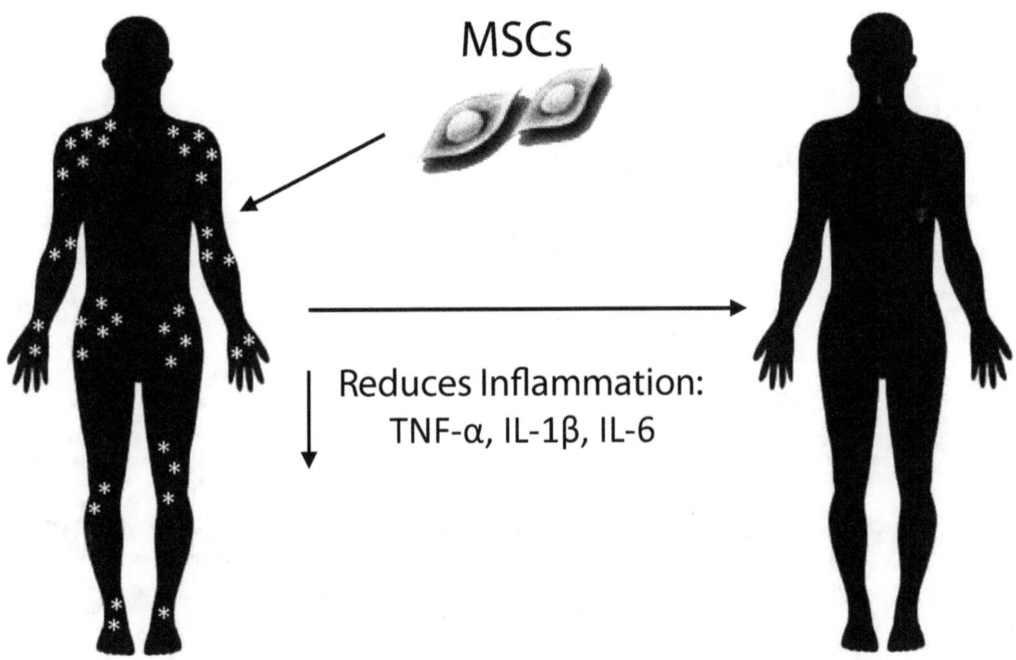

Figure 2. MSCs serve as an anti-inflammatory treatment. (A) Depiction of systemic inflammation (white asterisks'). (B). The anti-inflammatory effects of MSCs. Reproduced from Golpanian et al., with permission from the publisher.

endogenous cellular proliferative, and antifibrotic effects post-MI in both animal models and clinical trials alike, we anticipate that MSC therapy will act in a similar manner and prove beneficial in older individuals with frailty.

7. CRATUS phase I and II

The therapeutic interventions available to frail older individuals focus on improving the functionality of a precipitously declining quality of life. With the understanding that deteriorating endogenous stem cell function is a key mechanism behind this disease process, the allogeneic human mesenchymal stem cells (allo-hMSC) in patients with aging FRAilTy via intravenous delivery (CRATUS) trial (**Figure 3**) was established to reverse the untoward effects of frailty. Conducted at the University of Miami Miller School of Medicine, the pilot phase was designed to establish an optimal dose, and tested the hypothesis that allo-hMSCs were safe, well tolerated, and reduced the signs and symptoms of the disease [104]. The study was conducted in a nonrandomized, nonblinded, escalating dosage via peripheral intravenous infusion in 15 frail subjects [104]. Donors were healthy males and females between the ages of 20 and 45 [104]. Three groups of five patients each received either 20 million (M)-, 100M-, or 200M-cells [104]. Patients were followed out to 1-year postinfusion. The pilot phase revealed the two most salient doses (100M- and 200M-cells) [55] and was followed by

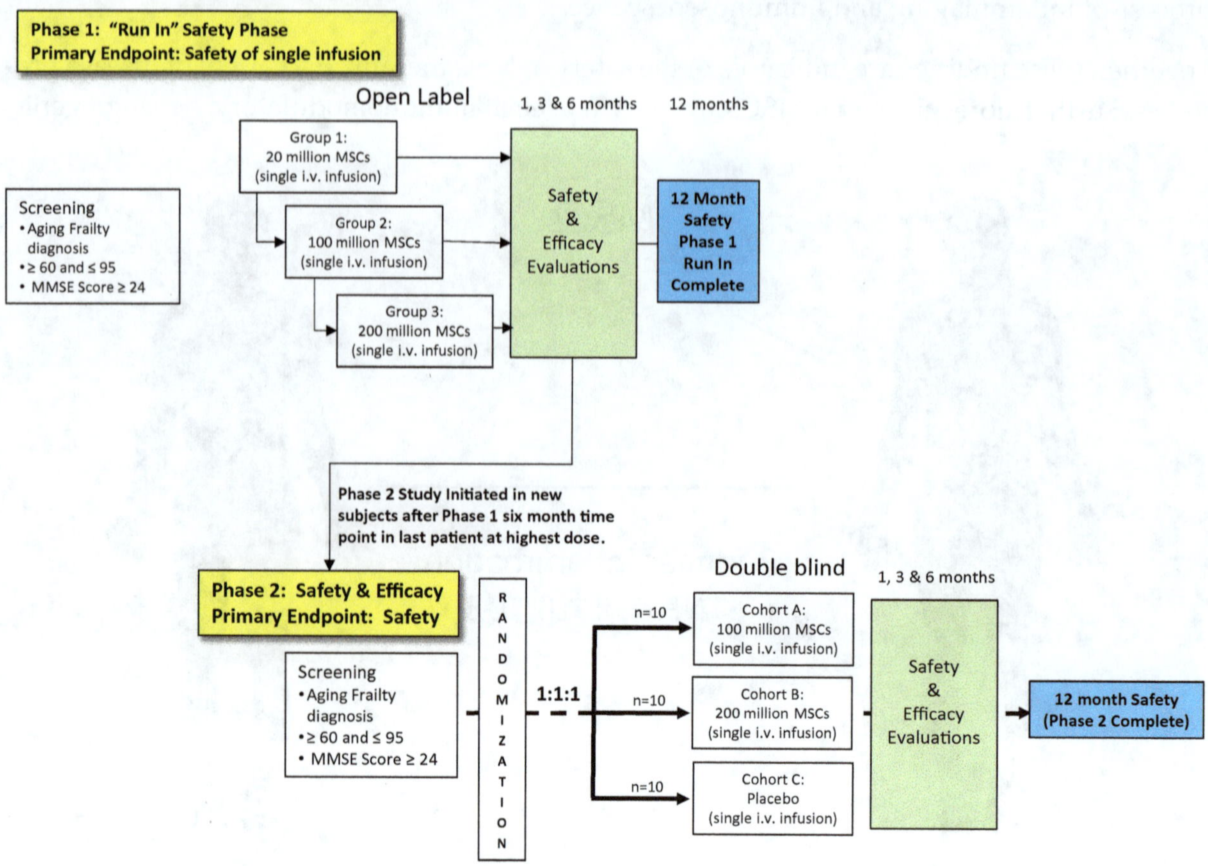

Figure 3. Schematic of the CRATUS pilot and randomized phases.

phase II, a randomized, double-blinded, placebo-controlled trial that further tested the safety and efficacy of allo-hMSCs in frail older individuals.

7.1. Results of the phase I study

The 15 subjects in the pilot phase had an average age of 78.4 ± 4.7 years [55]. Eight patients were categorized as vulnerable to frailty with a CSHA score of 4 and the others were mild, with a score of 6 (n = 6) and moderate with a score of 7 (n = 1) [55]. Most importantly, the primary endpoint, treatment-emergent serious adverse events (TE-SAE) at 1-month postinfusion, was met with no adverse reactions in any group [55].

Efficacy outcomes were measured out to 6 months postinfusion as a secondary endpoint. The 6-minute walk distance (6-MWD) test is a measure of functional exercise capacity [105], which can reflect a frail subject's ability to perform basic activities of daily living. The test has been specifically used to assess subjects with diseases of the musculoskeletal, pulmonary, and cardiovascular systems [106–108]; and as such, the subjects experienced a significant improvement in all treatment groups at 3 and 6 months postinfusion with the greatest improvement in the 100M cell-dose group in the phase I [55]. Pulmonary function was measured via FEV1, and improved in the 200M cell-dose group [55]. In regard to physical and quality of life improvement, the SF-36 questionnaire, which has a physical and mental component, yielded an improvement in the 100M-group in the pilot phase. Immunomodulation was also reported with a significant reduction in the pro-inflammatory biomarker serum TNF-α in the 100M and 200M cell-dose groups at 6 months postinfusion [55].

7.2. Update on the phase II study

The 30 subjects in phase II had a mean age of 75.5 ± 7.3 and a mean frailty score of 4 based on the CSHA Clinical Frailty Scale, and were equally randomized to receive 100M-, 200M-cells, or placebo [109]. Safety was the primary endpoint of the study and was measured via the occurrence of TE-SAE at 1-month postinfusion. The trial has completed enrollment, however, as reported in phase 1, preliminary findings show that the treatment is safe and produces significant improvements in the treated subjects in both quality of life and functional status [109].

8. Conclusion

Frailty has increasingly been recognized as a constellation of waning physical and mental qualities secondary to outside stressors, which relate to aging, and confer a vulnerability to adverse health outcomes [110]. Biologically, inflammation and stem cell depletion are at the forefront of this disease process. Early intervention is warranted at the onset of recognized symptoms to reduce the burden of disease progression, hospitalizations, and associated healthcare costs [111, 112]. To date, several important multimodal interventions are available to manage frailty; however, a disease-specific treatment has yet to emerge [112, 113]. Given the positive results of numerous studies utilizing MSCs in a variety of disease processes common to frailty as defined by the physical phenotype model, we believe stem cell therapy will be a treatment of choice for this disease process.

Future indications applicable to frailty	Response to MSCs	Proposed mechanisms of action
Osteoporosis	Improved bone mineral content and reduced rate of fractures	Reduction in ROS and increased AMPK
Heart disease	Improved function	Increased endothelial function, decreased inflammation, reduced cardiac fibrosis, and increased cardiomyogenesis
Delayed healing in Injury	Increased wound healing	Decrease inflammation (TNF-α and IL-1β), Increased IL-10
Autoimmunity	Delayed onset/prevention	Suppress TH17, induce T regs, and promote TH2 response

Table 2. MSCs and future indications.

Future implications of stem cell administration in frail or prefrail older individuals may be useful in settings where undo stress may cause rapid physical deterioration. There are a number of medical procedures (breast/colorectal cancer treatment, cardiac surgery, non-cardiac elective surgery, etc.) that are taxing to a young healthy individual let alone older individuals [114–116]. A preemptive or perioperative administration of MSCs may dampen the immune response, aid in the healing process, and keep at-risk older individuals from declining in functional status (**Table 2**) [56, 117–120]. Given the results from the CRATUS, pilot dose finding [55] and randomized placebo controlled study [109] and the number of medical procedures older individuals undergo, large, randomized, double-blinded clinical trials are warranted to elucidate the efficacy of stem cell therapy in regard to the disease process in itself and its ability to suppress the progression of frailty after strenuous medical interventions.

In summary, allogeneic MSCs are immunotolerant in frail older individuals providing clinically meaningful improvements in functional capacity, inflammatory biomarkers, and quality of life patient-reported outcomes. Frailty, the multimodal biologically mediated decline in physiologic reserve, may now have an optimistic therapeutic option.

Author details

Bryon A. Tompkins[1,2], Ana Marie Landin[1], Victoria Florea[1], Makoto Natsumeda[1], Angela C. Rieger[1], Wayne Balkan[1,3], Ivonne Hernandez Schulman[1,3] and Joshua M. Hare[1,3]*

*Address all correspondence to: jhare@med.miami.edu

1 The Interdisciplinary Stem Cell Institute, University of Miami Miller School of Medicine, Miami, USA

2 The Department of Surgery, University of Miami Miller School of Medicine, Miami, USA

3 The Department of Medicine, University of Miami Miller School of Medicine, Miami, USA

References

[1] Writing Group M, Mozaffarian D, Benjamin EJ, Go AS, Arnett DK, Blaha MJ, Cushman M, Das SR, de Ferranti S, Despres JP, Fullerton HJ, Howard VJ, Huffman MD, Isasi CR, Jimenez MC, Judd SE, Kissela BM, Lichtman JH, Lisabeth LD, Liu S, Mackey RH, Magid DJ, McGuire DK, Mohler ER, 3rd, Moy CS, Muntner P, Mussolino ME, Nasir K, Neumar RW, Nichol G, Palaniappan L, Pandey DK, Reeves MJ, Rodriguez CJ, Rosamond W, Sorlie PD, Stein J, Towfighi A, Turan TN, Virani SS, Woo D, Yeh RW, Turner MB, American Heart Association Statistics C, Stroke Statistics S. Heart disease and stroke statistics-2016 update: A report from the american heart association. Circulation. 2016;133(4):e38-360. DOI: 10.1161/CIR.0000000000000350

[2] Soysal P, Stubbs B, Lucato P, Luchini C, Solmi M, Peluso R, Sergi G, Isik AT, Manzato E, Maggi S, Maggio M, Prina AM, Cosco TD, Wu YT, Veronese N. Inflammation and frailty in the elderly: A systematic review and meta-analysis. Ageing Research Reviews. 2016;**31**:1-8. DOI: 10.1016/j.arr.2016.08.006

[3] Clegg A, Young J, Iliffe S, Rikkert MO, Rockwood K. Frailty in elderly people. Lancet. 2013;**381**(9868):752-762. DOI: 10.1016/S0140-6736(12)62167-9

[4] Gomes MJ, Martinez PF, Pagan LU, Damatto RL, Cezar MD, Lima AR, Okoshi K, Okoshi MP. Skeletal muscle aging: Influence of oxidative stress and physical exercise. Oncotarget. 2017;**8**(12):20428-20440. DOI: 10.18632/oncotarget.14670

[5] Chen X, Mao G, Leng SX. Frailty syndrome: An overview. Clinical Interventions in Aging. 2014;**9**:433-441. DOI: 10.2147/CIA.S45300

[6] Franceschi C, Campisi J. Chronic inflammation (inflammaging) and its potential contribution to age-associated diseases. The Journals of Gerontology. Series A, Biological Sciences and Medical Sciences. 2014;**69**(Suppl 1):S4-9. DOI: 10.1093/gerona/glu057

[7] Tidball JG, Villalta SA Regulatory interactions between muscle and the immune system during muscle regeneration. The American Journal of Physiology. 2010;**298**(5):R1173-1187. DOI: 10.1152/ajpregu.00735.2009

[8] Luo XG, Ding JQ, Chen SD. Microglia in the aging brain: Relevance to neurodegeneration. Molecular Neurodegeneration. 2010;**5**:12. DOI: 10.1186/1750-1326-5-12

[9] Boyle PA, Buchman AS, Wilson RS, Leurgans SE, Bennett DA. Physical frailty is associated with incident mild cognitive impairment in community-based older persons. Journal of the American Geriatrics Society. 2010;**58**(2):248-255. DOI: 10.1111/j.1532-5415.2009.02671.x

[10] Song X, Mitnitski A, Rockwood K. Nontraditional risk factors combine to predict Alzheimer disease and dementia. Neurology. 2011;**77**(3):227-234. DOI: 10.1212/WNL.0b013e318225c6bc

[11] Cappola AR, Xue QL, Ferrucci L, Guralnik JM, Volpato S, Fried LP. Insulin-like growth factor I and interleukin-6 contribute synergistically to disability and mortality in older women. The Journal of Clinical Endocrinology & Metabolism. 2003;**88**(5):2019-2025. DOI: 10.1210/jc.2002-021694

[12] Travison TG, Nguyen AH, Naganathan V, Stanaway FF, Blyth FM, Cumming RG, Le Couteur DG, Sambrook PN, Handelsman DJ. Changes in reproductive hormone concentrations predict the prevalence and progression of the frailty syndrome in older men: The concord health and ageing in men project. The Journal of Clinical Endocrinology & Metabolism. 2011;**96**(8):2464-2474. DOI: 10.1210/jc.2011-0143

[13] Leng SX, Cappola AR, Andersen RE, Blackman MR, Koenig K, Blair M, Walston JD. Serum levels of insulin-like growth factor-I (IGF-I) and dehydroepiandrosterone sulfate (DHEA-S), and their relationships with serum interleukin-6, in the geriatric syndrome of frailty. Aging Clinical and Experimental Research. 2004;**16**(2):153-157

[14] Lamberts SW. The endocrinology of aging and the brain. Archives of Neurology. 2002; **59**(11):1709-1711

[15] Puts MT, Visser M, Twisk JW, Deeg DJ, Lips P. Endocrine and inflammatory markers as predictors of frailty. Clin Endocrinology (Oxf). 2005;**63**(4):403-411. DOI: 10.1111/j.1365-2265.2005.02355.x

[16] Rockwood K, Mitnitski A. Frailty in relation to the accumulation of deficits. The Journals of Gerontology. Series A, Biological Sciences and Medical Sciences. 2007;**62**(7):722-727

[17] Fried LP, Tangen CM, Walston J, Newman AB, Hirsch C, Gottdiener J, Seeman T, Tracy R, Kop WJ, Burke G, McBurnie MA, Cardiovascular Health Study Collaborative Research G. Frailty in older adults: Evidence for a phenotype. The Journals of Gerontology. Series A, Biological Sciences and Medical Sciences. 2001;**56**(3):M146-156

[18] Rockwood K, Blodgett JM, Theou O, Sun MH, Feridooni HA, Mitnitski A, Rose RA, Godin J, Gregson E, Howlett SE. A frailty index based on deficit accumulation quantifies mortality risk in humans and in mice. Scientific Reports. 2017;7:43068. DOI: 10.1038/srep43068

[19] Rockwood K, Mitnitski A. Limits to deficit accumulation in elderly people. Mechanisms of Ageing and Development. 2006;**127**(5):494-496. DOI: 10.1016/j.mad.2006.01.002

[20] Rockwood K, Song X, MacKnight C, Bergman H, Hogan DB, McDowell I, Mitnitski A. A global clinical measure of fitness and frailty in elderly people. Canadian Medical Association Journal. 2005;**173**(5):489-495. DOI: 10.1503/cmaj.050051

[21] Ritt M, Ritt JI, Sieber CC, Gassmann KG. Comparing the predictive accuracy of frailty, comorbidity, and disability for mortality: A 1-year follow-up in patients hospitalized in geriatric wards. Clinical Interventions in Aging. 2017;**12**:293-304. DOI: 10.2147/CIA.S124342

[22] Bandeen-Roche K, Seplaki CL, Huang J, Buta B, Kalyani RR, Varadhan R, Xue QL, Walston JD, Kasper JD. Frailty in older adults: A nationally representative profile in the United States. The Journals of Gerontology. Series A, Biological Sciences and Medical Sciences. 2015;**70**(11):1427-1434. DOI: 10.1093/gerona/glv133

[23] Collard RM, Boter H, Schoevers RA, Oude Voshaar RC. Prevalence of frailty in community-dwelling older persons: A systematic review. Journal of the American Geriatrics Society. 2012;**60**(8):1487-1492. DOI: 10.1111/j.1532-5415.2012.04054.x

[24] Santos-Eggimann B, Cuenoud P, Spagnoli J, Junod J Prevalence of frailty in middle-aged and older community-dwelling Europeans living in 10 countries. The Journals of Gerontology. Series A, Biological Sciences and Medical Sciences. 2009;**64**(6):675-681. DOI: 10.1093/gerona/glp012

[25] Kojima G, Iliffe S, Taniguchi Y, Shimada H, Rakugi H, Walters K. Prevalence of frailty in Japan: A systematic review and meta-analysis. Journal of Epidemiology. 2016; pii:S0917-5040(16):30083-1. DOI: 10.1016/j.je.2016.09.008

[26] Clegg AP, Barber SE, Young JB, Forster A, Iliffe SJ. Do home-based exercise interventions improve outcomes for frail older people? Findings from a systematic review. Reviews in Clinical Gerontology. 2012;**22**(1):68-78. DOI: 10.1017/S0959259811000165

[27] Theou O, Stathokostas L, Roland KP, Jakobi JM, Patterson C, Vandervoort AA, Jones GR. The effectiveness of exercise interventions for the management of frailty: A systematic review. Journal of Aging Research. 2011;**2011**:569194. DOI: 10.4061/2011/569194

[28] Fiatarone MA, O'Neill EF, Ryan ND, Clements KM, Solares GR, Nelson ME, Roberts SB, Kehayias JJ, Lipsitz LA, Evans WJ. Exercise training and nutritional supplementation for physical frailty in very elderly people. New England Journal of Medicine. 1994;**330**(25):1769-1775. DOI: 10.1056/NEJM199406233302501

[29] Tieland M, Dirks ML, van der Zwaluw N, Verdijk LB, van de Rest O, de Groot LC, van Loon LJ. Protein supplementation increases muscle mass gain during prolonged resistance-type exercise training in frail elderly people: A randomized, double-blind, placebo-controlled trial. Journal of the American Medical Directors Association. 2012;**13**(8):713-719. DOI: 10.1016/j.jamda.2012.05.020

[30] Churchward-Venne TA, Tieland M, Verdijk LB, Leenders M, Dirks ML, de Groot LC, van Loon LJ. There are no nonresponders to resistance-type exercise training in older men and women. Journal of the American Medical Directors Association. 2015;**16**(5):400-411. DOI: 10.1016/j.jamda.2015.01.071

[31] Miller ME, Rejeski WJ, Reboussin BA, Ten Have TR, Ettinger WH. Physical activity, functional limitations, and disability in older adults. Journal of the American Geriatrics Society. 2000;**48**(10):1264-1272

[32] Cesari M, Vellas B, Hsu FC, Newman AB, Doss H, King AC, Manini TM, Church T, Gill TM, Miller ME, Pahor M, Group LS. A physical activity intervention to treat the frailty syndrome in older persons-results from the LIFE-P study. The Journals of Gerontology. Series A, Biological Sciences and Medical Sciences. 2015;**70**(2):216-222. DOI: 10.1093/gerona/glu099

[33] Malafarina V, Uriz-Otano F, Iniesta R, Gil-Guerrero L. Effectiveness of nutritional supplementation on muscle mass in treatment of sarcopenia in old age: A systematic review. Journal of the American Medical Directors Association. 2013;**14**(1):10-17. DOI: 10.1016/j.jamda.2012.08.001

[34] Bauer J, Biolo G, Cederholm T, Cesari M, Cruz-Jentoft AJ, Morley JE, Phillips S, Sieber C, Stehle P, Teta D, Visvanathan R, Volpi E, Boirie Y. Evidence-based recommendations

for optimal dietary protein intake in older people: A position paper from the PROT-AGE Study Group. Journal of the American Medical Directors Association. 2013;**14**(8):542-559. DOI: 10.1016/j.jamda.2013.05.021

[35] Bauer JM, Verlaan S, Bautmans I, Brandt K, Donini LM, Maggio M, McMurdo ME, Mets T, Seal C, Wijers SL, Ceda GP, De Vito G, Donders G, Drey M, Greig C, Holmback U, Narici M, McPhee J, Poggiogalle E, Power D, Scafoglieri A, Schultz R, Sieber CC, Cederholm T. Effects of a vitamin D and leucine-enriched whey protein nutritional supplement on measures of sarcopenia in older adults, the PROVIDE study: A randomized, double-blind, placebo-controlled trial. Journal of the American Medical Directors Association. 2015;**16**(9):740-747. DOI: 10.1016/j.jamda.2015.05.021

[36] Ng TP, Feng L, Nyunt MS, Feng L, Niti M, Tan BY, Chan G, Khoo SA, Chan SM, Yap P, Yap KB. Nutritional, physical, cognitive, and combination interventions and frailty reversal among older adults: A randomized controlled trial. The American Journal of Medicine. 2015;**128**(11):1225-1236 e1221. DOI: 10.1016/j.amjmed.2015.06.017

[37] Wong YY, Flicker L. Hypovitaminosis D and frailty: Epiphenomenon or causal? Maturitas. 2015;**82**(4):328-335. DOI: 10.1016/j.maturitas.2015.07.027

[38] Artaza-Artabe I, Saez-Lopez P, Sanchez-Hernandez N, Fernandez-Gutierrez N, Malafarina V. The relationship between nutrition and frailty: Effects of protein intake, nutritional supplementation, vitamin D and exercise on muscle metabolism in the elderly. A systematic review. Maturitas. 2016;**93**:89-99. DOI: 10.1016/j.maturitas.2016.04.009

[39] Muir SW, Montero-Odasso M. Effect of vitamin D supplementation on muscle strength, gait and balance in older adults: A systematic review and meta-analysis. Journal of the American Geriatrics Society. 2011;**59**(12):2291-2300. DOI: 10.1111/j.1532-5415.2011.03733.x

[40] Dhesi JK, Jackson SH, Bearne LM, Moniz C, Hurley MV, Swift CG, Allain TJ. Vitamin D supplementation improves neuromuscular function in older people who fall. Age and Ageing. 2004;**33**(6):589-595. DOI: 10.1093/ageing/afh209

[41] Avenell A, Mak JC, O'Connell D. Vitamin D and vitamin D analogues for preventing fractures in post-menopausal women and older men. The Cochrane Database of Systematic Reviews. 2014;(4):CD000227. DOI: 10.1002/14651858.CD000227.pub4

[42] Theou O, Chapman I, Wijeyaratne L, Piantadosi C, Lange K, Naganathan V, Hunter P, Cameron ID, Rockwood K, Visvanathan R. Can an intervention with testosterone and nutritional supplement improve the frailty level of under-nourished older people? The Journal of Frailty & Aging. 2016;**5**(4):247-252. DOI: 10.14283/jfa.2016.108

[43] Basaria S, Coviello AD, Travison TG, Storer TW, Farwell WR, Jette AM, Eder R, Tennstedt S, Ulloor J, Zhang A, Choong K, Lakshman KM, Mazer NA, Miciek R, Krasnoff J, Elmi A, Knapp PE, Brooks B, Appleman E, Aggarwal S, Bhasin G, Hede-Brierley L, Bhatia A, Collins L, LeBrasseur N, Fiore LD, Bhasin S. Adverse events associated with testosterone administration. The New England Journal of Medicine. 2010;**363**(2):109-122. DOI: 10.1056/NEJMoa1000485

[44] Rossouw JE, Anderson GL, Prentice RL, LaCroix AZ, Kooperberg C, Stefanick ML, Jackson RD, Beresford SA, Howard BV, Johnson KC, Kotchen JM, Ockene J, Writing Group for the Women's Health Initiative I. Risks and benefits of estrogen plus progestin in healthy postmenopausal women: Principal results from the women's health initiative randomized controlled trial. Journal of the American Medical Association. 2002;**288**(3):321-333

[45] Prentice RL, Manson JE, Langer RD, Anderson GL, Pettinger M, Jackson RD, Johnson KC, Kuller LH, Lane DS, Wactawski-Wende J, Brzyski R, Allison M, Ockene J, Sarto G, Rossouw JE. Benefits and risks of postmenopausal hormone therapy when it is initiated soon after menopause. American Journal of Epidemiology. 2009;**170**(1):12-23. DOI: 10.1093/aje/kwp115

[46] Nair KS, Rizza RA, O'Brien P, Dhatariya K, Short KR, Nehra A, Vittone JL, Klee GG, Basu A, Basu R, Cobelli C, Toffolo G, Dalla Man C, Tindall DJ, Melton 3rd LJ, Smith GE, Khosla S, Jensen MD. DHEA in elderly women and DHEA or testosterone in elderly men. The New England Journal of Medicine. 2006;**355**(16):1647-1659. DOI: 10.1056/NEJMoa054629

[47] Friedlander AL, Butterfield GE, Moynihan S, Grillo J, Pollack M, Holloway L, Friedman L, Yesavage J, Matthias D, Lee S, Marcus R, Hoffman AR. One year of insulin-like growth factor I treatment does not affect bone density, body composition, or psychological measures in postmenopausal women. The Journal of Clinical Endocrinology and Metabolism. 2001;**86**(4):1496-1503. DOI: 10.1210/jcem.86.4.7377

[48] Peffers MJ, Collins J, Loughlin J, Proctor C, Clegg PD.. A proteomic analysis of chondrogenic, osteogenic and tenogenic constructs from ageing mesenchymal stem cells. Stem Cell Research & Therapy. 2016;**7**(1):133. DOI: 10.1186/s13287-016-0384-2

[49] Sethe S, Scutt A, Stolzing A2006. Aging of mesenchymal stem cells. Ageing Research Reviews. 2006;**5**(1):91-116. DOI: 10.1016/j.arr.2005.10.001

[50] Stolzing A, Jones E, McGonagle D, Scutt A. Age-related changes in human bone marrow-derived mesenchymal stem cells: Consequences for cell therapies. Mechanisms of Ageing and Development. 2008;129(3):163-173. DOI: 10.1016/j.mad.2007.12.002

[51] Chapel A, Bertho JM, Bensidhoum M, Fouillard L, Young RG, Frick J, Demarquay C, Cuvelier F, Mathieu E, Trompier F, Dudoignon N, Germain C, Mazurier C, Aigueperse J, Borneman J, Gorin NC, Gourmelon P, Thierry D. Mesenchymal stem cells home to injured tissues when co-infused with hematopoietic cells to treat a radiation-induced multi-organ failure syndrome. The Journal of Gene Medicine 2003;**5**(12):1028-1038. DOI: 10.1002/jgm.452

[52] Augello A, Tasso R, Negrini SM, Amateis A, Indiveri F, Cancedda R, Pennesi G. Bone marrow mesenchymal progenitor cells inhibit lymphocyte proliferation by activation of the programmed death 1 pathway. European Journal of Immunology. 2005;35(5):1482-1490. DOI: 10.1002/eji.200425405

[53] Mourkioti F, Rosenthal N. IGF-1, inflammation and stem cells: Interactions during muscle regeneration. Trends in Immunology. 2005;**26**(10):535-542. DOI: 10.1016/j.it.2005.08.002

[54] Sanina C, Hare JM. Mesenchymal stem cells as a biological drug for heart disease: Where are we with cardiac cell-Based Therapy? Circulation Research. 2005;**117**(3):229-233. DOI: 10.1161/CIRCRESAHA.117.306306

[55] Golpanian S, DiFede DL, Khan A, et al. Allogeneic Human Mesenchymal Stem Cell Infusions for Aging Frailty. J Gerontol A Biol Sci Med Sci. DOI: 10.1093/gerona/glx056.

[56] Golpanian S, Wolf A, Hatzistergos KE, Hare JM. Rebuilding the damaged heart: Mesenchymal stem cells, cell-based therapy, and engineered heart tissue. Physiological Reviews. 2016;**96**(3):1127-1168. DOI: 10.1152/physrev.00019.2015

[57] Cao Y, Gomes S, Rangel EB, Paulino EC, Fonseca TL, Li J, Telxelra MB, Gouvela CH, Bianco AC, Kapiloff MS, Balkan W, Hare JM. S-nitrosoglutathione reductase–dependent PPARγ denitrosylation participates in adipogenesis and osteogenesis. The Journal of Clinical Investigation. 2015;**125**(4):1679-91. DOI: 10.1172/JCI73780

[58] Karantalis V, Hare JM. Use of mesenchymal stem cells for therapy of cardiac disease. Circulation Research. 2015;**116**(8):1413-1430. DOI: 10.1161/CIRCRESAHA.116.303614

[59] Karantalis V, DiFede DL, Gerstenblith G, Pham S, Symes J, Zambrano JP, Fishman J, Pattany P, McNiece I, Conte J, Schulman S, Wu K, Shah A, Breton E, Davis-Sproul J, Schwarz R, Feigenbaum G, Mushtaq M, Suncion VY, Lardo AC, Borrello I, Mendizabal A, Karas TZ, Byrnes J, Lowery M, Heldman AW, Hare JM. Autologous mesenchymal stem cells produce concordant improvements in regional function, tissue perfusion, and fibrotic burden when administered to patients undergoing coronary artery bypass grafting: The prospective randomized study of mesenchymal stem cell therapy in patients undergoing Cardiac Surgery (PROMETHEUS) trial. Circulation Research. 2014;**114**(8):1302-1310. DOI: 10.1161/CIRCRESAHA.114.303180

[60] Hatzistergos KE, Quevedo H, Oskouei BN, Hu Q, Feigenbaum GS, Margitich IS, Mazhari R, Boyle AJ, Zambrano JP, Rodriguez JE, Dulce R, Pattany PM, Valdes D, Revilla C, Heldman AW, McNiece I, Hare JM . Bone marrow mesenchymal stem cells stimulate cardiac stem cell proliferation and differentiation. Circulation Research. 2010;**107**(7):913-922. DOI: 10.1161/CIRCRESAHA.110.222703

[61] Premer C, Blum A, Bellio MA, Schulman IH, Hurwitz BE, Parker M, Dermarkarian CR, DiFede DL, Balkan W, Khan A, Hare JM. Allogeneic mesenchymal stem cells restore endothelial function in heart failure by stimulating endothelial progenitor cells. EBioMedicine. 2015;**2**(5):467-475. DOI: 10.1016/j.ebiom.2015.03.020

[62] Hare JM, DiFede DL, Castellanos AM, Florea V, Landin AM, El-Khorazaty J, Khan A, Mushtaq M, Lowery MH, Byrnes JJ, Hendel RC, Cohen MG, Alfonso CE, Valasaki K, Pujol MV, Golpanian S, Ghersin E, Fishman JE, Pattany P, Gomes SA, Delgado C, Miki R, Abuzeid F, Vidro-Casiano M, Premer C, Medina A, Porras V, Hatzistergos KE, Anderson E, Mendizabal A, Mitrani R, Heldman AW. Randomized comparison of allogeneic

vs. autologous mesenchymal stem cells for non-Ischemic dilated cardiomyopathy: POSEIDON-DCM trial. Journal of the American College of Cardiology. 2016; pii: S0735-1097(16)36906-6. DOI:10.1016/j.jacc.2016.11.009

[63] Hare JM, Traverse JH, Henry TD, Dib N, Strumpf RK, Schulman SP, Gerstenblith G, DeMaria AN, Denktas AE, Gammon RS, Hermiller JB, Jr., Reisman MA, Schaer GL, Sherman W. A randomized, double-blind, placebo-controlled, dose-escalation study of intravenous adult human mesenchymal stem cells (prochymal) after acute myocardial infarction. Journal of the American College of Cardiology. 2009;**54**(24):2277-2286. DOI: 10.1016/j.jacc.2009.06.055

[64] Hare JM, Fishman JE, Gerstenblith G, DiFede Velazquez DL, Zambrano JP, Suncion VY, Tracy M, Ghersin E, Johnston PV, Brinker JA, Breton E, Davis-Sproul J, Schulman IH, Byrnes J, Mendizabal AM, Lowery MH, Rouy D, Altman P, Wong Po Foo C, Ruiz P, Amador A, Da Silva J, McNiece IK, Heldman AW, George R, Lardo A. Comparison of allogeneic vs autologous bone marrow-derived mesenchymal stem cells delivered by transendocardial injection in patients with ischemic cardiomyopathy: The POSEIDON randomized trial. Journal of the American Medical Association. 2012;**308**(22):2369-2379. DOI: 10.1001/jama.2012.25321

[65] Gutierrez-Fernandez M, Rodriguez-Frutos B, Otero-Ortega L, Ramos-Cejudo J, Fuentes B, Diez-Tejedor E. Adipose tissue-derived stem cells in stroke treatment: From bench to bedside. Discovery Medicine. 2013;**16**(86):37-43

[66] Weiss DJ, Casaburi R, Flannery R, LeRoux-Williams M, Tashkin DP. A placebo-controlled, randomized trial of mesenchymal stem cells in COPD. Chest. 2013;**143**(6):1590-1598. DOI: 10.1378/chest.12-2094

[67] Trounson A, McDonald C. Stem cell therapies in clinical trials: Progress and challenges. Cell Stem Cell. 2015;**17**(1):11-22. DOI: http://dx. DOI.org/10.1016/j.stem.2015.06.007

[68] Hodgkinson CP, Bareja A, Gomez JA, Dzau VJ. Emerging concepts in paracrine mechanisms in regenerative cardiovascular medicine and biology. Circulation Research. 2016;**118**(1):95-107. DOI: 10.1161/CIRCRESAHA.115.305373

[69] Ranganath SH, Levy O, Inamdar MS, Karp JM. Harnessing the mesenchymal stem cell secretome for the treatment of cardiovascular disease. Cell Stem Cell. 2012;**10**(3):244-258. DOI: 10.1016/j.stem.2012.02.005

[70] Figeac F, Lesault PF, Le Coz O, Damy T, Souktani R, Trebeau C, Schmitt A, Ribot J, Mounier R, Guguin A, Manier C, Surenaud M, Hittinger L, Dubois-Rande JL, Rodriguez AM.. Nanotubular crosstalk with distressed cardiomyocytes stimulates the paracrine repair function of mesenchymal stem cells. Stem Cells. 2014;**32**(1):216-230. DOI: 10.1002/stem.1560

[71] Akyurekli C, Le Y, Richardson RB, Fergusson D, Tay J, Allan DS. A systematic review of preclinical studies on the therapeutic potential of mesenchymal stromal cell-derived microvesicles. Stem Cell Reviews. 2014;**11**(1):150-60. DOI: 0.1007/s12015-014-9545-9

[72] Hahn JY, Cho HJ, Kang HJ, Kim TS, Kim MH, Chung JH, Bae JW, Oh BH, Park YB, Kim HS. Pre-treatment of mesenchymal stem cells with a combination of growth factors enhances gap junction formation, cytoprotective effect on cardiomyocytes, and therapeutic efficacy for myocardial infarction. Journal of the American College of Cardiology. 2008;**51**(9):933-943. DOI: 10.1016/j.jacc.2007.11.040

[73] Mazhari R, Hare JM. Mechanisms of action of mesenchymal stem cells in cardiac repair: Potential influences on the cardiac stem cell niche. Nature Clinical Practice Cardiovascular Medicine. 2007;**4**(Suppl 1):S21-26. DOI: 10.1038/ncpcardio0770

[74] Kinnaird T, Stabile E, Burnett MS, Lee CW, Barr S, Fuchs S, Epstein SE. Marrow-derived stromal cells express genes encoding a broad spectrum of arteriogenic cytokines and promote in vitro and in vivo arteriogenesis through paracrine mechanisms. Circulation Research. 2004;**94**(5):678-685. DOI: 10.1161/01.RES.0000118601.37875.AC 01.RES.0000118601.37875.AC [pii]

[75] Weimar IS, Miranda N, Muller EJ, Hekman A, Kerst JM, de Gast GC, Gerritsen WR. Hepatocyte growth factor/scatter factor (HGF/SF) is produced by human bone marrow stromal cells and promotes proliferation, adhesion and survival of human hematopoietic progenitor cells (CD34+). Experimental Hematology. 1998;**26**(9):885-894

[76] Cheng SL, Zhang SF, Mohan S, Lecanda F, Fausto A, Hunt AH, Canalis E, Avioli LV. Regulation of insulin-like growth factors I and II and their binding proteins in human bone marrow stromal cells by dexamethasone. The Journal of Cellular Biochemistry. 1998;**71**(3):449-458

[77] Gnecchi M, He H, Liang OD, Melo LG, Morello F, Mu H, Noiseux N, Zhang L, Pratt RE, Ingwall JS, Dzau VJ. Paracrine action accounts for marked protection of ischemic heart by Akt-modified mesenchymal stem cells. Nature Medicine. 2005;**11**(4):367-368

[78] Engels MC, Rajarajan K, Feistritzer R, Sharma A, Nielsen UB, Schalij MJ, de Vries AA, Pijnappels DA, Wu SM. Insulin-like growth factor promotes cardiac lineage induction in vitro by selective expansion of early mesoderm. Stem Cells. 2014;**32**(6):1493-1502. DOI: 10.1002/stem.1660

[79] Schmeckpeper J, Verma A, Yin L, Beigi F, Zhang L, Payne A, Zhang Z, Pratt RE, Dzau VJ, Mirotsou M. Inhibition of Wnt6 by Sfrp2 regulates adult cardiac progenitor cell differentiation by differential modulation of Wnt pathways. Journal of Molecular and Cellular Cardiology. 2015;**85**:215-225. DOI: 10.1016/j.yjmcc.2015.06.003

[80] Kobayashi K, Luo M, Zhang Y, Wilkes DC, Ge G, Grieskamp T, Yamada C, Liu TC, Huang G, Basson CT, Kispert A, Greenspan DS, Sato TN. Secreted frizzled-related protein 2 is a procollagen C proteinase enhancer with a role in fibrosis associated with myocardial infarction. Nature Cell Biology. 2009;**11**(1):46-55. DOI: 10.1038/ncb1811

[81] Mastri M, Shah Z, Hsieh K, Wang X, Wooldridge B, Martin S, Suzuki G, Lee T. Secreted frizzled-related protein 2 as a target in antifibrotic therapeutic intervention. American Journal of Physiology Cell physiology. 2014;**306**(6):C531-539. DOI: 10.1152/ajpcell.00238.2013

[82] Karantalis V, Schulman IH, Balkan W, Hare JM. Allogeneic cell therapy: A new paradigm in therapeutics. Circulation Research. 2015;**116**(1):12-15. DOI: 10.1161/CIRCRESAHA. 114.305495

[83] Hare JM, DiFede DL, Rieger AC, Florea V, Landin AM, El-Khorazaty J, Khan A, Mushtaq M, Lowery MH, Byrnes JJ, Hendel RC, Cohen MG, Alfonso CE, Valasaki K, Pujol MV, Golpanian S, Ghersin E, Fishman JE, Pattany P, Gomes SA, Delgado C, Miki R, Abuzeid F, Vidro-Casiano M, Premer C, Medina A, Porras V, Hatzistergos KE, Anderson E, Mendizabal A, Mitrani R, Heldman AW. Randomized comparison of allogeneic versus autologous mesenchymal stem cells for nonischemic dilated cardiomyopathy: POSEIDON-DCM trial. Journal of the American College of Cardiology. 2017;**69**(5):526-537. DOI: 10.1016/j.jacc.2016.11.009

[84] Chen SL, Fang WW, Ye F, Liu YH, Qian J, Shan SJ, Zhang JJ, Chunhua RZ, Liao LM, Lin S, Sun JP. Effect on left ventricular function of intracoronary transplantation of autologous bone marrow mesenchymal stem cell in patients with acute myocardial infarction. The American Journal of Cardiology. 2004;**94**(1):92-95. DOI: 10.1016/j.amjcard.2004.03.034

[85] Chullikana A, Majumdar AS, Gottipamula S, Krishnamurthy S, Kumar AS, Prakash VS, Gupta PK. Randomized, double-blind, phase I/II study of intravenous allogeneic mesenchymal stromal cells in acute myocardial infarction. Cytotherapy. 2015;**17**(3):250-261. DOI: 10.1016/j.jcyt.2014.10.009

[86] Frasca D, Blomberg BB . Inflammaging decreases adaptive and innate immune responses in mice and humans. Biogerontology. 2016;**17**(1):7-19. DOI: 10.1007/s10522-015-9578-8

[87] Mitnitski A, Collerton J, Martin-Ruiz C, Jagger C, von Zglinicki T, Rockwood K, Kirkwood TB. Age-related frailty and its association with biological markers of ageing. BMC Medicine. 2015;**13**:161. DOI: 10.1186/s12916-015-0400-x

[88] Cannizzo ES, Clement CC, Sahu R, Follo C, Santambrogio L. Oxidative stress, inflamm-aging and immunosenescence. Journal of Proteomics. 2011;**74**(11):2313-2323. DOI: 10.1016/j.jprot.2011.06.005

[89] Albert C. Shaw SJ, Hannah Greenwood, Alexander Panda, and Janet M. Lord. Aging of the Innate Immune System. Current Opinion in Immunology. 2010;**22**(4):507-513. DOI: 10.1016/j.coi.2010.05.003

[90] Dewan SK, Zheng SB, Xia SJ, Bill K . Senescent remodeling of the immune system and its contribution to the predisposition of the elderly to infections. Chinese Medical Journal(Engl)). 2012;**125**(18):3325-3331

[91] Wikby A, Ferguson F, Forsey R, Thompson J, Strindhall J, Lofgren S, Nilsson BO, Ernerudh J, Pawelec G, Johansson B. An immune risk phenotype, cognitive impairment, and survival in very late life: Impact of allostatic load in Swedish octogenarian and nonagenarian humans. Journals of Gerontology Series A Biological Sciences and Medical Sciences. 2005;**60**(5):556-565

[92] Pawelec G. Immunity and ageing in man. Experimental Gerontology. 2006;**41**(12):1239-1242. DOI: 10.1016/j.exger.2006.09.005

[93] Zhang LJ, Hanff P, Rutherford C, Churchill WH, Crumpacker CS. Detection of human cytomegalovirus DNA, RNA, and antibody in normal donor blood. Journal of Infectious Diseases. 1995;**171**(4):1002-1006

[94] Frasca D, Diaz A, Romero M, Landin AM, Phillips M, Lechner SC, Ryan JG, Blomberg BB. Intrinsic defects in B cell response to seasonal influenza vaccination in elderly humans. Vaccine. 2010;**28**(51):8077-8084

[95] Frasca D, Diaz A, Romero M, Phillips M, Mendez NV, Landin AM, Blomberg BB. Unique biomarkers for B-cell function predict the serum response to pandemic H1N1 influenza vaccine. International Immunology. 2012;**24**(3):175-182. DOI: 10.1093/intimm/dxr123

[96] Ortiz LA, Dutreil M, Fattman C, Pandey AC, Torres G, Go K, Phinney DG. Interleukin 1 receptor antagonist mediates the antiinflammatory and antifibrotic effect of mesenchymal stem cells during lung injury. Proceedings of the National Academy of Sciences of the United States of America . 2007;**104**(26):11002-11007. DOI: 10.1073/pnas.0704421104

[97] Djouad F, Charbonnier LM, Bouffi C, Louis-Plence P, Bony C, Apparailly F, Cantos C, Jorgensen C, Noel D. Mesenchymal stem cells inhibit the differentiation of dendritic cells through an interleukin-6-dependent mechanism. Stem Cells. 2007;**25**(8):2025-2032. DOI: 10.1634/stemcells.2006-0548

[98] Spaggiari GM, Abdelrazik H, Becchetti F, Moretta L. MSCs inhibit monocyte-derived DC maturation and function by selectively interfering with the generation of immature DCs: Central role of MSC-derived prostaglandin E2. Blood. 2009;**113**(26):6576-6583. DOI: 10.1182/blood-2009-02-203943

[99] Spaggiari GM, Capobianco A, Abdelrazik H, Becchetti F, Mingari MC, Moretta L. Mesenchymal stem cells inhibit natural killer-cell proliferation, cytotoxicity, and cytokine production: Role of indoleamine 2,3-dioxygenase and prostaglandin E2. Blood. 2008;**111**(3):1327-1333. DOI: 10.1182/blood-2007-02-074997

[100] Burchfield JS, Iwasaki M, Koyanagi M, Urbich C, Rosenthal N, Zeiher AM, Dimmeler S. Interleukin-10 from transplanted bone marrow mononuclear cells contributes to cardiac protection after myocardial infarction. Circulation Research. 2008;**103**(2):203-211. DOI: 10.1161/circresaha.108.178475

[101] Yano T, Miura T, Whittaker P, Miki T, Sakamoto J, Nakamura Y, Ichikawa Y, Ikeda Y, Kobayashi H, Ohori K, Shimamoto K. Macrophage colony-stimulating factor treatment after myocardial infarction attenuates left ventricular dysfunction by accelerating infarct repair. Journal of the American College of Cardiology. 2006;**47**(3):626-634. DOI: 10.1016/j.jacc.2005.09.037

[102] Troidl C, Mollmann H, Nef H, Masseli F, Voss S, Szardien S, Willmer M, Rolf A, Rixe J, Troidl K, Kostin S, Hamm C, Elsasser A. Classically and alternatively activated macrophages

contribute to tissue remodelling after myocardial infarction. Journal of Cellular and Molecular Medicine. 2009;**13**(9b):3485-3496. DOI: 10.1111/j.1582-4934.2009.00707.x

[103] van der Heiden M, van Zelm MC, Bartol SJ, de Rond LG, Berbers GA, Boots AM, Buisman A-M. Differential effects of Cytomegalovirus carriage on the immune phenotype of middle-aged males and females. Scientific Reports. 2016;**6**:26892

[104] Golpanian S, DiFede DL, Pujol MV, Lowery MH, Levis-Dusseau S, Goldstein BJ, Schulman IH, Longsomboon B, Wolf A, Khan A, Heldman AW, Goldschmidt-Clermont PJ, Hare JM. Rationale and design of the allogeneiC human mesenchymal stem cells (hMSC) in patients with aging fRAilTy via intravenoUS delivery (CRATUS) study: A phase I/II, randomized, blinded and placebo controlled trial to evaluate the safety and potential efficacy of allogeneic human mesenchymal stem cell infusion in patients with aging frailty. Oncotarget. 2016;**7**(11):11899-11912. DOI: 10.18632/oncotarget.7727

[105] Guyatt GH, Sullivan MJ, Thompson PJ, Fallen EL, Pugsley SO, Taylor DW, Berman LB.. The 6-minute walk: A new measure of exercise capacity in patients with chronic heart failure. Canadian Medical Association Journal. 1985;**132**(8):919-923

[106] Castillo-Moreno JA, Garcia-Escribano IA, Martinez-Pascual-de-Riquelme M, Jaulent-Huertas L, Dau-Villarreal DF, Rubio-Paton R, Giner-Caro JA, Bonaque-Gonzalez JC, Consuegra-Sanchez L. Prognostic usefulness of the 6-minute walk test in patients with severe aortic stenosis. American Journal of Cardiology. 2016;**118**(8):1239-1243. DOI: 10.1016/j.amjcard.2016.07.042

[107] Albarrati AM, Gale NS, Enright S, Munnery MM, Cockcroft JR, Shale DJ. A simple and rapid test of physical performance inchronic obstructive pulmonary disease. International Journal of Chronic Obstructive Pulmonary Disease. 2016;**11**:1785-1791. DOI: 10.2147/COPD.S106151

[108] Bello L, Campadello P, Barp A, Fanin M, Semplicini C, Soraru G, Caumo L, Calore C, Angelini C, Pegoraro E. Functional changes in Becker muscular dystrophy: Implications for clinical trials in dystrophinopathies. Scientific Reports. 2016;**6**:32439. DOI: 10.1038/srep32439

[109] Hare JM, Difede DL, Khan A, Landin AM, Tompkins B, Goldschmidt PJ, Mendizabal A. Allogeneic mesenchymal stem cells to treat aging frailty: A randomized, placebo-controlled intervention study. The Gerontologist. 2016;**56**(Suppl 3):50-51

[110] Walston J, Hadley EC, Ferrucci L, Guralnik JM, Newman AB, Studenski SA, Ershler WB, Harris T, Fried LP. Research agenda for frailty in older adults: Toward a better understanding of physiology and etiology: Summary from the American Geriatrics Society/National Institute on Aging Research Conference on Frailty in Older Adults. Journal of the American Geriatrics Society. 2006;**54**(6):991-1001. DOI: 10.1111/j.1532-5415.2006.00745.x

[111] Cerreta F, Eichler HG, Rasi G. Drug policy for an aging population--the European Medicines Agency's geriatric medicines strategy. The New England Journal of Medicine. 2012;**367**(21):1972-1974. DOI: 10.1056/NEJMp1209034

[112] Morley JE, Vellas B, van Kan GA, Anker SD, Bauer JM, Bernabei R, Cesari M, Chumlea WC, Doehner W, Evans J, Fried LP, Guralnik JM, Katz PR, Malmstrom TK, McCarter RJ, Gutierrez Robledo LM, Rockwood K, von Haehling S, Vandewoude MF, Walston J. Frailty consensus: A call to action. Journal of the American Medical Directors Association 2013;**14**(6):392-397. DOI: 10.1016/j.jamda.2013.03.022

[113] Xue QL. The frailty syndrome: Definition and natural history. Clinics in Geriatric Medicine 2011;**27**(1):1-15. DOI: 10.1016/j.cger.2010.08.009

[114] van Abbema D, van Vuuren A, van den Berkmortel F, van den Akker M, Deckx L, Buntinx F, van Kampen R, Lambooij E, de Boer M, de Vos-Geelen J, Tjan-Heijnen VC. Functional status decline in older patients with breast and colorectal cancer after cancer treatment: A prospective cohort study. Journal of Geriatric Oncology. 2017; pii: S1879-4068(17)30023-1. DOI:10.1016/j.jgo.2017.01.003

[115] Kim DH, Kim CA, Placide S, Lipsitz LA, Marcantonio ER. Preoperative frailty assessment and outcomes at 6 months or later in older adults undergoing cardiac surgical procedures: A systematic review. Annals of Internal Medicine. 2016;**165**(9):650-660. DOI: 10.7326/M16-0652

[116] CA Polanczyk, E Marcantonio, L Goldman, LEP Rohde, J Orav, CM Mangione, TH Lee. Impact of Age on Perioperative Complications and Length of Stay in Patients Undergoing Noncardiac Surgery. **Annals of Internal Medicine** 2001;**134**:637-643

[117] Sharaf-Eldin WE, Abu-Shahba N, Mahmoud M, El-Badri N. The modulatory effects of mesenchymal stem cells on osteoclastogenesis. Stem Cells International. 2016;2016:1908365. DOI: 10.1155/2016/1908365

[118] Takano T, Li YJ, Kukita A, Yamaza T, Ayukawa Y, Moriyama K, Uehara N, Nomiyama H, Koyano K, Kukita T. Mesenchymal stem cells markedly suppress inflammatory bone destruction in rats with adjuvant-induced arthritis. Laboratory Investigation. 2014;**94**(3):286-296. DOI: 10.1038/labinvest.2013.152

[119] Wei X, Yang X, Han ZP, Qu FF, Shao L, Shi YF. Mesenchymal stem cells: A new trend for cell therapy. Acta Pharmacologica Sinica. 2013;**34**(6):747-754. DOI: 10.1038/aps.2013.50

[120] Rastegar F, Shenaq D, Huang J, Zhang W, Zhang BQ, He BC, Chen L, Zuo GW, Luo Q, Shi Q, Wagner ER, Huang E, Gao Y, Gao JL, Kim SH, Zhou JZ, Bi Y, Su Y, Zhu G, Luo J, Luo X, Qin J, Reid RR, Luu HH, Haydon RC, Deng ZL, He TC. Mesenchymal stem cells: Molecular characteristics and clinical applications. World Journal of Stem Cells. 2010;**2**(4):67-80. DOI: 10.4252/wjsc.v2.i4.67

Permissions

All chapters in this book were first published in FSODCC, by InTech Open; hereby published with permission under the Creative Commons Attribution License or equivalent. Every chapter published in this book has been scrutinized by our experts. Their significance has been extensively debated. The topics covered herein carry significant findings which will fuel the growth of the discipline. They may even be implemented as practical applications or may be referred to as a beginning point for another development.

The contributors of this book come from diverse backgrounds, making this book a truly international effort. This book will bring forth new frontiers with its revolutionizing research information and detailed analysis of the nascent developments around the world.

We would like to thank all the contributing authors for lending their expertise to make the book truly unique. They have played a crucial role in the development of this book. Without their invaluable contributions this book wouldn't have been possible. They have made vital efforts to compile up to date information on the varied aspects of this subject to make this book a valuable addition to the collection of many professionals and students.

This book was conceptualized with the vision of imparting up-to-date information and advanced data in this field. To ensure the same, a matchless editorial board was set up. Every individual on the board went through rigorous rounds of assessment to prove their worth. After which they invested a large part of their time researching and compiling the most relevant data for our readers.

The editorial board has been involved in producing this book since its inception. They have spent rigorous hours researching and exploring the diverse topics which have resulted in the successful publishing of this book. They have passed on their knowledge of decades through this book. To expedite this challenging task, the publisher supported the team at every step. A small team of assistant editors was also appointed to further simplify the editing procedure and attain best results for the readers.

Apart from the editorial board, the designing team has also invested a significant amount of their time in understanding the subject and creating the most relevant covers. They scrutinized every image to scout for the most suitable representation of the subject and create an appropriate cover for the book.

The publishing team has been an ardent support to the editorial, designing and production team. Their endless efforts to recruit the best for this project, has resulted in the accomplishment of this book. They are a veteran in the field of academics and their pool of knowledge is as vast as their experience in printing. Their expertise and guidance has proved useful at every step. Their uncompromising quality standards have made this book an exceptional effort. Their encouragement from time to time has been an inspiration for everyone.

The publisher and the editorial board hope that this book will prove to be a valuable piece of knowledge for researchers, students, practitioners and scholars across the globe.

List of Contributors

Harnish P Patel
Academic Geriatric Medicine, University Hospital Southampton, UK
Department of Medicine for Older People, University Hospital Southampton, UK
NIHR Biomedical Research Centre, Southampton, UK
MRC Lifecourse Epidemiology Unit, University of Southampton, Southampton, UK

Esther Clift and Lucy Lewis
Health Education England, Wessex, UK

Cyrus Cooper
MRC Lifecourse Epidemiology Unit, University of Southampton, Southampton, UK
University of Oxford, Oxford, UK

Rosaly Correa-de-Araujo
Division of Geriatrics and Clinical Gerontology, National Institute on Aging, National Institutes of Health, U.S. Department of Health and Human Services, Bethesda, MD, USA

Zhuowei Yu and Qingwei Ruan
Shanghai Institute of Geriatrics and Gerontology, Shanghai Key Laboratory of Clinical Geriatrics, Huadong Hospital, Shanghai, China
Research Center of Aging and Medicine, Shanghai Medical College, Fudan University, Shanghai, China

Grazia D'Onofrio and Antonio Greco
Department of Medical Sciences, Geriatric Unit & Laboratory of Gerontology and Geriatrics, IRCCS "Casa Sollievo della Sofferenza", San Giovanni Rotondo, Foggia, Italy

Beatriz Lardiés-Sánchez and Alejandro Sanz-París
Universitary Hospital Miguel Servet, Zaragoza, Spain

Kotomi Sakai
Department of Rehabilitation, Setagaya Memorial Hospital, Tokyo, Japan
Department of Dysphagia Rehabilitation, Nihon University School of Dentistry, Tokyo, Japan

Kunihiro Sakuma
Institute for Liberal Arts, Environment and Society, Tokyo Institute of Technology, Tokyo, Japan

Raoul Saggini
Department of Medical Sciences, Oral and Biotechnology, "G. d'Annunzio" University, Chieti, Italy

Simona Maria Carmignano, Lucia Cosenza and Tommaso Palermo
School of Specialties in Physical and Rehabilitation Medicine, "G. d'Annunzio" University, Chieti, Italy

Rosa Grazia Bellomo
Department of Medical Sciences, Oral and Biotechnology, "G. d'Annunzio" University, Chieti, Italy

Shinichiro Morishita and Atsuhiro Tsubaki
Institute for Human Movement and Medical Sciences, Niigata University of Health and Welfare, Niigata, Japan

Jack B. Fu
Department of Palliative, Rehabilitation & Integrative Medicine, University of Texas MD Anderson Cancer Center, Houston, TX, USA

Michelle Guan and Andrew E. Hendifar
Samuel Oschin Comprehensive Cancer Center, Cedars Sinai Medical Center, Los Angeles, CA, USA
Department of Medicine, David Geffen School of Medicine, Los Angeles, CA, USA

Arvind M. Shinde
Samuel Oschin Comprehensive Cancer Center, Cedars Sinai Medical Center, Los Angeles, CA, USA

Raoul Saggini
Physical and Rehabilitation Medicine, Department of Medical Oral and Biotechnological Sciences, Director of the School of Specialty in Physical and Rehabilitation Medicine, "Gabriele d'Annunzio" University, National Coordinator of Schools of Specialty in Physical and Rehabilitation Medicine, Chieti-Pescara, Italy

Simona Maria Carmignano, Lucia Cosenza and Tommaso Palermo
School of Specialty in Physical and Rehabilitation Medicine, "Gabriele d'Annunzio" University of Chieti-Pescara, Italy

Rosa Grazia Bellomo
Physical and Rehabilitation Medicine, Department of Medicine and Sciences of Aging, "Gabriele d'Annunzio" University of Chieti-Pescara, Italy

Vinod Chainani, Russell Riehl, Carl J. Lavie and John P. Reilly
Ochsner Health System, John Ochsner Heart and Vascular Institute, Jefferson, Louisiana, USA

Abir Abdo
Louisiana State University Health Sciences Center, New Orleans, Louisiana, USA

Mauricio G. Cohen, Carlos Alfonso and Pedro Martinez-Clark
University of Miami Miller School of Medicine, Miami, Florida, USA

Nidal Abi-Rafeh
Tulane University School of Medicine, New Orleans, Louisiana, USA

Geeta Chainani
Windsor University School of Medicine, Saint kitts, Carribean

Bryon A. Tompkins
The Interdisciplinary Stem Cell Institute, University of Miami Miller School of Medicine, Miami, USA
The Department of Surgery, University of Miami Miller School of Medicine, Miami, USA

Ana Marie Landin, Victoria Florea, Makoto Natsumeda and Angela C.Rieger
The Interdisciplinary Stem Cell Institute, University of Miami Miller School of Medicine, Miami, USA

Wayne Balkan, Ivonne Hernandez Schulman and Joshua M. Hare
Ochsner Health System, John Ochsner Heart and Vascular Institute, Jefferson, Louisiana, USA
University of Miami Miller School of Medicine, Miami, Florida, USA

Nidal Abi-Rafeh
Tulane University School of Medicine, New Orleans, Louisiana, USA

Geeta Chainani
Windsor University School of Medicine, Saint kitts, Carribean

Bryon A. Tompkins
The Interdisciplinary Stem Cell Institute, University of Miami Miller School of Medicine, Miami, USA
The Department of Surgery, University of Miami Miller School of Medicine, Miami, USA

Ana Marie Landin, Victoria Florea, Makoto Natsumeda and Angela C. Rieger
The Interdisciplinary Stem Cell Institute, University of Miami Miller School of Medicine, Miami, USA

Wayne Balkan, Ivonne Hernandez Schulman and Joshua M. Hare
The Interdisciplinary Stem Cell Institute, University of Miami Miller School of Medicine, Miami, USA
The Department of Medicine, University of Miami Miller School of Medicine, Miami, USA

Index

www.ingramcontent.com/pod-product-compliance
Lightning Source LLC
LaVergne TN
LVHW081012210926
848485LV00004B/843